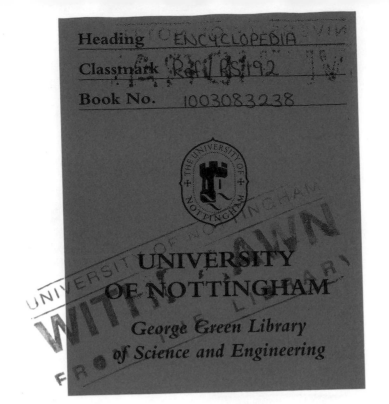

Encyclopedia of Pharmaceutical Technology

Second Edition

Volume 3
Ped–Z
Pages 2045–3032

edited by

James Swarbrick

President
PharmaceuTech, Inc., Pinehurst, North Carolina
and
Vice President for Scientific Affairs, aaiPharma, Inc.
Wilmington, North Carolina, U.S.A.

and

James C. Boylan

Pharmaceutical Consultant
Gurnee, Illinois, U.S.A.

MARCEL DEKKER, INC.   NEW YORK • BASEL

Cover Art: Leigh A. Rondano, Boehringer angelheim Pharmaceuticals, Inc.

ISBN: Volume 1:   0-8247-2822-X
           Volume 2:   0-8247-2823-8
           Volume 3:   0-8247-2824-6
           Prepack: 0-8247-2825-4

ISBN: Online: 0-8247-2820-3

This book is printed on acid-free paper.

Headquarters
Marcel Dekker, Inc.
270 Madison Avenue, New York, NY 10016
tel: 212-696-9000; fax: 212-685-4540

Eastern Hemisphere distribution
Marcel Dekker AG
Hutgasse 4, Postfach 812, CH-4001 Basel, Switzerland
tel: 41-61-261-8482; fax: 41-61-261-8896

World Wide Web
http://www.dekker.com

List of Contributors

Phillip M. Achey/*University of Florida, Gainesville, Florida, U.S.A.*

James P. Agalloco/*Agalloco & Associates, Belle Mead, New Jersey, U.S.A.*

Jean-Marc Aiache/*Faculty of Pharmacy, University of Clermont-Ferrand, Clermont-Ferrand, France*

James E. Akers/*Akers Kennedy & Associates, Kansas City, Missouri, U.S.A.*

Michael J. Akers/*Cook Pharmaceutical Solutions, Bloomington, Indiana, U.S.A.*

Loyd V. Allen, Jr./*International Journal of Pharmaceutical Compounding, Edmond, Oklahoma, U.S.A.*

David G. Allison/*University of Manchester, Manchester, United Kingdom*

Hemant H. Alur/*University of Missouri–Kansas City, Kansas City, Missouri, U.S.A.*

Norman Anthony Armstrong/*Cardiff University, Cardiff, United Kingdom*

Agnès Artiges/*European Directorate for the Quality of Medicines (EDQM), Council of Europe, Strasbourg, France*

Carolyn H. Asbury/*University of Pennsylvania, Philadelphia, Pennsylvania, U.S.A.*

Larry L. Augsburger/*University of Maryland School of Pharmacy, Baltimore, Maryland, U.S.A.*

J. Desmond Baggot/*Monash University, Parkville, Victoria, Australia*

Paul Baldrick/*Regulatory Affairs-Pharmaceuticals, Covance Laboratories Ltd., Harrogate, England*

Debra Barnes/*Hoffmann-LaRoche, Palo Alto, California, U.S.A.*

Onkaram Basavapathruni/*Pharmacia Corporation, Peapack, New Jersey, U.S.A.*

G. J. P. J. Beernink/*University of Florida, Gainesville, Florida, U.S.A.*

Leslie Z. Benet/*University of California San Francisco, San Francisco, California, U.S.A.*

David H. Bergstrom/*Cardinal Health Pharmaceutical Technologies & Services Center, Somerset, New Jersey, U.S.A.*

Ira R. Berry/*International Regulatory Business Consultants, L.L.C., Somerset, New Jersey, U.S.A.*

Guru Betageri/*Western University of Health Sciences, Pomona, California, U.S.A.*

Erick Beyssac/*Faculty of Pharmacy, University of Clermont-Ferrand, Clermont-Ferrand, France*

Haresh Bhagat/*Alcon Research Ltd., Fort Worth, Texas, U.S.A.*

Hridaya Bhargava/*Massachusetts College of Pharmacy and Health Sciences, Boston, Massachusetts, U.S.A.*

M.J. Blanco-Prieto/*Universidad de Navarra, Pamplona, Spain*

Daniel Blankschtein/*Massachusetts Institute of Technology, Cambridge, Massachusetts, U.S.A.*

Roland A. Bodmeier/*Freie Universität Berlin, Berlin, Germany*

Michael J. Bogda/*Barr Laboratories, Inc., Pomona, New York, U.S.A.*

iii

René Bommer/*E. Pfeiffer GmbH, Radolfzell, Germany*

Charles Bon/*AAI International, Wilmington, North Carolina, U.S.A.*

Carol A. Borynec/*University Hospital, Edmonton, Alberta, Canada*

David W.A. Bourne/*University of Oklahoma, Oklahoma City, Oklahoma, U.S.A.*

J. Phillip Bowen/*University of Georgia, Athens, Georgia, U.S.A.*

Gayle A. Brazeau/*University of Florida, Gainesville, Florida, U.S.A.*

Ron J. Brendel/*Mallinckrodt, Inc., St. Louis, Missouri, U.S.A.*

Harry G. Brittain/*Center for Pharmaceutical Physics, Milford, New Jersey, U.S.A.*

Albert W. Brzeczko/*Atlantic Pharmaceutical Services, Owings Mills, Maryland, U.S.A.*

Robert A. Buerki/*The Ohio State University College of Pharmacy, Columbus, Ohio, U.S.A.*

Diane J. Burgess/*University of Connecticut, Storrs, Connecticut, U.S.A.*

John B. Cannon/*Abbott Laboratories, Abbott Park, Illinois, U.S.A.*

Allen Cato III/*Cato Research Ltd., San Diego, California, U.S.A.*

Allen Cato/*Cato Research Ltd., Durham, North Carolina, U.S.A.*

Hak-Kim Chan/*University of Sydney, Sydney, New South Wales, Australia*

L.F. Chasseaud/*Huntingdon Life Sciences, Huntingdon, United Kingdom*

Xiu Xiu Cheng/*Andrx Pharmaceuticals, Inc., Fort Lauderdale, Florida, U.S.A.*

Nora Y.K. Chew/*University of Sydney, Sydney, New South Wales, Australia*

Yie W. Chien/*Kaohsiung Medical University, Kaohsiung, Taiwan*

Masood Chowhan/*Alcon Laboratories, Fort Worth, Texas, U.S.A.*

Sebastian G. Ciancio/*State University of New York at Buffalo, Buffalo, New York, U.S.A.*

Emil W. Ciurczak/*Purdue Pharma LP, Ardsley, New York, U.S.A.*

Bradley A. Clark/*Pharmacia, Skokie, Illinois, U.S.A.*

C. Randall Clark/*Auburn University, Auburn, Alabama, U.S.A.*

Sophie-Dorothée Clas/*Merck Frosst Canada & Co., Pointe Claire-Dorval, Quebec City, Canada*

Sarah M.E. Cockbill/*University of Wales College, Cardiff, United Kingdom*

Douglas L. Cocks/*Indiana University, Bloomington, Indiana, U.S.A.*

James J. Conners/*Dura Pharmaceuticals, San Diego, California, U.S.A.*

Kenneth A. Connors/*University of Wisconsin-Madison, Madison, Wisconsin, U.S.A.*

Chyung S. Cook/*Pharmacia Corporation, Skokie, Illinois, U.S.A.*

James F. Cooper/*Charles River Endosafe, Charleston, South Carolina, U.S.A.*

Geoffrey A. Cordell/*University of Illinois at Chicago, Chicago, Illinois, U.S.A.*

Owen I. Corrigan/*University of Dublin, Trinity College, Dublin, Ireland*

Michael Cory/*GlaxoSmithKline, Research Triangle Park, North Carolina, U.S.A.*

Diane D. Cousins/*United States Pharmacopeia, Rockville, Maryland, U.S.A.*

Alan L. Cripps/*GlaxoSmithKline, Ware, Hertfordshire, United Kingdom*

Patrick J. Crowley/*GlaxoSmithKline, H'arlow, United Kingdom*

Anthony M. Cundell/*Wyeth-Ayerst Pharmaceuticals, Pearl River, New York, U.S.A.*

Chad R. Dalton/*Merck Frosst Canada & Co., Pointe Claire-Dorval, Quebec City, Canada*

James T. Dalton/*The Ohio State University, Columbus, Ohio, U.S.A.*

Ira Das/*St. Louis, Missouri, U.S.A.*

Judith A. Davis/*University of Florida, Gainesville, Florida, U.S.A.*

Jack DeRuiter/*Auburn University, Auburn, Alabama, U.S.A.*

M. Begoña Delgado-Charro/*Centre Interuniversitaire de Recherche et d'Enseignement, Archamps,
France University of Geneva, Switzerland*

Nigel J. Dent/*Country Consultancy Ltd., Northamptonshire, United Kingdom*

Jeffrey Ding/*Battelle Pulmonary Therapeutics, Inc., Columbus, Ohio, U.S.A.*

Marilyn D. Duerst/*University of Wisconsin-River Falls, River Falls, Wisconsin, U.S.A.*

Gillian M. Eccleston/*University of Strathclyde, Glasgow, United Kingdom*

Ronald P. Evens/*Clinical Research, Amgen Inc., Thousand Oaks, California, U.S.A.*

Kevin L. Facchine/*GlaxoSmithKline, Research Triangle Park, North California, U.S.A.*

Gordon J. Farquharson/*Bovis Lend Lease Pharmaceutical, United Kingdom*

Elias Fattal/*University of Paris XI, Châtenay-Malabry, France*

J.C. Ferdinando/*R.P. Scherer Limited, Swindon, United Kingdom*

Charles W. Fetrow/*St. Francis Medical Center, Pittsburgh, Pennsylvania, U.S.A.*

John W.A. Findlay/*Pharmacia, Skokie, Illinois, U.S.A.*

Joseph A. Fix/*Yamanouchi Pharma Technologies, Inc., Palo Alto, California, U.S.A.*

James L. Ford/*Liverpool John Moores University, Liverpool, United Kingdom*

Farrel L. Fort/*TAP Pharmaceutical Products, Inc., Lake Forest, Illinois, U.S.A.*

Cara R. Frosch/*Covance Central Laboratory Services, Inc., Indianapolis, Indiana, U.S.A.*

Kumar G. Gadamasetti/*ChemRx Advanced Technologies, Inc., San Francisco, California, U.S.A.*

Bruno Gander/*Institute of Pharmaceutical Sciences, Zürich, Switzerland*

David Ganderton/*The University of North Carolina at Chapel Hill, Chapel Hill, North Carolina, U.S.A.*

Isaac Ghebre-Sellassie/*Pfizer Global Research and Development, Morris Plains, New Jersey, U.S.A.*

Peter J. Giddings/*SmithKline Beecham plc, Brentford, United Kingdom*

Peter Gilbert/*University of Manchester, Manchester, United Kingdom*

Danièlle Giron/*Novartis Pharma AG, Basel, Switzerland*

Samuel Givens/*Hoffmann-LaRoche, Nutley, New Jersey, U.S.A.*

Igor Gonda/*Aradigm Corporation, Hayward, California, U.S.A.*

Lee T. Grady/*United States Pharmacopoeia, Rockville, Maryland, U.S.A.*

Jerry J. Groen/*Abbott Laboratories, Abbott Park, Illinois, U.S.A.*

Richard A. Guarino/*Oxford Pharmaceutical Resources, Inc., Totowa, New Jersey, U.S.A.*

Pramod K. Gupta/*TAP Pharmaceuticals, Deerfield, Illinois, U.S.A.*

Richard H. Guy/*Centre Interuniversitaire de Recherche et d'Enseignement, Archamps, France University of Geneva, Switzerland*

J. Richard Gyory/*ALZA Corporation, Mountain View, California, U.S.A.*

Huijeong A. Hahm/*University of Maryland School of Pharmacy, Baltimore, Maryland, U.S.A.*

Nigel A. Halls/*GlaxoSmithkline Global Manufacturing and Supply, Uxbridge, United Kingdom*

Jerome A. Halperin/*United States Pharmacopeia, Rockville, Maryland, U.S.A.*

Bruno C. Hancock/*Pfizer Inc., Groton, Connecticut, U.S.A.*

Henri Hansson/*Galenica AB, Meleon, Malmö, Sweden*

D.R. Hawkins/*Huntingdon Life Sciences, Huntingdon, United Kingdom*

Leslie C. Hawley/*Pharmacia Corporation, Kalamazoo, Michigan, U.S.A.*

Anne Marie Healy/*University of Dublin, Trinity College, Dublin, Ireland*

Herbert Michael Heise/*Institute of Spectrochemistry and Applied Spectroscopy, Dortmund, Germany*

Jeffrey M. Herz/*Applied Receptor Sciences, Mill Creek, Washington, U.S.A.*

Anthony J. Hickey/*The University of North Carolina, Chapel Hill, North Carolina, U.S.A.*

Gregory J. Higby/*American Institute of the History of Pharmacy, Madison, Wisconsin, U.S.A.*

Anthony J. Hlinak/*Pharmacia, Skokie, Illinois, U.S.A.*

Harm HogenEsch/*Purdue University, West Lafayette, Indiana, U.S.A.*

R. Gary Hollenbeck/*University of Maryland School of Pharmacy, Baltimore, Maryland, U.S.A.*

Stephen A. Howard/*Purdue Pharma L.P., Ardsley, New York, U.S.A.*

Carmel M. Hughes/*The Queen's University of Belfast, Belfast, United Kingdom*

Jeffrey A. Hughes/*University of Florida, Gainesville, Florida, U.S.A.*

Ho-Wah Hui/*Abbott Laboratories, Abbott Park, Illinois, U.S.A.*

D. Hunkeler/*Laboratoire des Polyélectrolytes et BioMacromolécules, Lausanne, Switzerland*

Anwar A. Hussain/*University of Kentucky, Lexington, Kentucky, U.S.A.*

Daniel A. Hussar/*University of the Sciences in Philadelphia, Philadelphia, Pennsylvania, U.S.A.*

Juhana E. Idänpään-Heikkilä/*Council for International Organizations of Medical Sciences, WHO, Geneva, Switzerland*

Victoria Imber/*CastleRock Technologies, Inc., Sausalito, California, U.S.A.*

David M. Jacobs/*David M. Jacobs Consulting, Basel, Switzerland*

Thomas P. Johnston/*University of Missouri–Kansas City, Kansas City, Missouri, U.S.A.*

Brian E. Jones/*Shionogi Qualicaps, Alcobendas, Spain*

Deborah J. Jones/*Norton Steripak, Cheshire, United Kingdom*

Maik W. Jornitz/*Sartorius Group, Germany*

Jose C. Joseph/*Abbott Laboratories, Abbott Park, Illinois, U.S.A.*

Hans E. Junginger/*Leiden/Amsterdam Center for Drug Research, Leiden University, The Netherlands*

Galina N. Kalinkova/*Medical University, Sofia, Bulgaria*

Isadore Kanfer/*Rhodes University, Grahamstown, South Africa*

Aziz Karim/*Pharmacia Corporation, Skokie, Illinois, U.S.A.*

Brian H. Kaye/*Laurentian University, Sudbury, Ontario, Canada*

David P. Kessler/*Purdue University, West Lafayette, Indiana, U.S.A.*

Ban-An Khaw/*Northeastern University, Boston, Massachusetts, U.S.A.*

Arthur H. Kibbe/*Wilkes University, Wilkes-Barre, Pennsylvania, U.S.A.*

Chris C. Kiesnowski/*Bristol-Myers Squibb Pharmaceutical Research Institute, New Brunswick, New Jersey, U.S.A.*

Kwon H. Kim/*St. John's University, Jamaica, New York, U.S.A.*

Florence K. Kinoshita/*Hercules Incorporated, Arlington, Virginia, U.S.A.*

Cathy M. Klech-Gelotte/*McNeil Consumer Healthcare, Fort Washington, Pennsylvania, U.S.A.*

Axel Knoch/*Pfizer Global Research and Development, Freiburg, Germany*

John J. Koleng, Jr./*The University of Texas at Austin, Austin, Texas, U.S.A.*

Sheldon X. Kong/*Merck & Co. Inc., Whitehouse Station, New Jersey, U.S.A.*

Mark J. Kontny/*Pharmacia, Kalamazoo, Michigan, U.S.A.*

Sylvie Laganière/*Origenix Technologies, Inc., Quebec, Canada*

Duane B. Lakings/*Drug Safety Evaluation Consulting, Inc., Birmingham, Alabama, U.S.A.*

Robert Langer/*Massachusetts Institute of Technology, Cambridge, Massachusetts, U.S.A.*

Destin A. LeBlanc/*Cleaning Validation Technologies, San Antonio, Texas, U.S.A.*

Jason M. LePree/*Boehringer Ingelheim Pharmaceuticals, Ridgefield, Connecticut, U.S.A.*

Chi H. Lee/*The University of Missouri-Kansas City, Kansas City, Missouri, U.S.A.*

Kyung Hee Lee/*University of Illinois at Chicago, Chicago, Illinois, U.S.A.*

Mike S. Lee/*Milestone Development Services, Newtown, Pennsylvania, U.S.A.*

Vincent H.L. Lee/*University of Southern California, Los Angeles, California, U.S.A.*

Yong-Hee Lee/*Trega Biosciences, Inc., San Diego, California, U.S.A.*

Gareth A. Lewis/*Sanofi-Synthelabo, Chilly Mazarin, France*

Luk Chiu Li/*Abbott Laboratories, Abbott Park, Illinois, U.S.A.*

Eric J. Lien/*University of Southern California, Los Angeles, California, U.S.A.*

Senshang Lin/*St. John's University, Jamaica, New York, U.S.A.*

Nils-Olof Lindberg/*Pharamacia AB, Helsingborg, Sweden*

B. Lindsay/*University of Strathclyde, Glasgow, United Kingdom*

John M. Lipari/*Abbott Laboratories, Abbott Park, Illinois, U.S.A.*

Robert L. Maher, Jr./*Duquesne University, Pittsburgh, Pennsylvania, U.S.A.*

Henri R. Manasse, Jr./*American Society of Health-System Pharmacists, Bethesda, Maryland, U.S.A.*

Laviero Mancinelli/*University of California San Francisco, San Francisco, California, U.S.A.*

Peter Markland/*Southern Research Institute, Birmingham, Alabama, U.S.A.*

Diego Marro/*Centre Interuniversitaire de Recherche et d'Enseignement, Archamps, France University of Geneva, Switzerland*

Luigi G. Martini/*GlaxoSmithKline, Harlow, United Kingdom*

Michael B. Maurin/*DuPont Pharmaceuticals Company, Wilmington, Delaware, U.S.A.*

Joachim Mayer/*University of Lausanne, Lausanne, Switzerland*

Orla McCallion/*Vandsons Research, Islington, London, United Kingdom*

James C. McElnay/*The Queen's University of Belfast, Belfast, United Kingdom*

Iain J. McGilveray/*McGilveray Pharmacon, Inc., Ottawa, Ontario, Canada*

Jim W. McGinity/*The University of Texas at Austin, Austin, Texas, U.S.A.*

Michael McKenna/*Pfizer, Inc., New York, New York, U.S.A.*

Marghi R. McKeon/*Lab Safety Corp., Des Plaines, Illinois, U.S.A.*

Eugene J. McNally/*Boehringer Ingelheim Pharmaceuticals, Inc., Ridgefield, Connecticut, U.S.A.*

Duncan E. McVean/*Consultant, Solon, Ohio, U.S.A.*

Robert W. Mendes/*Massachusetts College of Pharmacy and Health Sciences (Retired), Dedham, Massachusetts, U.S.A.*

Marvin C. Meyer/*University of Tennessee, Memphis, Tennessee, U.S.A.*

Ashim K. Mitra/*University of Missouri–Kansas City, Kansas City, Missouri, U.S.A.*

Samir S. Mitragotri/*University of California, Santa Barbara, California, U.S.A.*

Suresh K. Mittal/*Purdue University, West Lafayette, Indiana, U.S.A.*

Lorie Ann Morgan/*GlaxoSmith Kline, Research Triangle Park, North Carolina, U.S.A.*

Karen Morisseau/*University of Rhode Island, Kingston, Rhode Island, U.S.A.*

Gerold Mosher/*CyDex, Inc., Overland Park, Kansas, U.S.A.*

Christel C. Mueller-Goymann/*Universität Braunschweig Mendelssohnstr, Braunschweig, Germany*

Ronald L. Mueller/*GlaxoSmithKline, King of Prussia, Pennsylvania, U.S.A.*

Suman K. Mukherjee/*University of Southern California, Los Angeles, California, U.S.A.*

Sandy J.M. Munro/*GlaxoSmithKline, Ware, Hertfordshire, United Kingdom*

Fernando J. Muzzio/*Rutgers University, Piscataway, New Jersey, U.S.A.*

Paul B. Myrdal/*The University of Arizona, Tucson, Arizona, U.S.A.*

Venkatesh Naini/*Barr Laboratories, Inc., Pomona, New York, U.S.A.*

Jintana M. Napaporn/*University of Florida, Gainesville, Florida, U.S.A.*

Robert A. Nash/*Consultant, Mahwah, New Jersey, U.S.A.*

Deanna J. Nelson/*BioLink Technologies, Inc., Cary, North Carolina, U.S.A.*

Sandeep Nema/*Pharmacia Corporation, Skokie, Illinois, U.S.A.*

Michael T. Newhouse/*Inhale Therapeutic Systems, Inc., San Carlos, California, U.S.A.*

Ann W. Newman/*SSCI, Inc., West Lafayette, Indiana, U.S.A.*

J.M. Newton/*University of London, London, United Kingdom*

Thomas M. Nowak/*Abbott Laboratories, Abbott Park, Illinois, U.S.A.*

Thomas M. O'Connell/*GlaxoSmithKline, Research Triangle Park, North California, U.S.A.*

Christine K. O'Neil/*Duquesne University, Pittsburgh, Pennsylvania, U.S.A.*

B. O'Mahony/*University of Strathclyde, Glasgow, United Kingdom*

John P. Oberdier/*Abbott Laboratories, Abbott Park, Illinois, U.S.A.*

Clyde M. Ofner III/*University of the Sciences in Philadelphia, Philadelphia, Pennsylvania, U.S.A.*

Claudia C. Okeke/*United States Pharmacopeia, Rockville, Maryland, U.S.A.*

Wayne P. Olson/*Consultant, Beecher, Illinois, U.S.A.*

Rama V. Padmanabhan/*ALZA Corporation, Mountain View, California, U.S.A.*

Jagdish Parasrampuria/*Galderma R&D, Cranbury, New Jersey, U.S.A.*

Eun Jung Park/*University of Illinois at Chicago, Chicago, Illinois, U.S.A.*

Jung Y. Park/*Boehringer Ingelheim Pharmaceuticals, Inc., Ridgefield, Connecticut, U.S.A.*

Kinam Park/*Purdue University, West Lafayette, Indiana, U.S.A.*

Barbara Perry/*Hoffmann-LaRoche, Welwyn, United Kingdom*

Adam Persky/*University of Florida, Gainesville, Florida, U.S.A.*

Gregory F. Peters/*Lab Safety Corporation, Des Plaines, Illinois, U.S.A.*

John M. Pezzuto/*University of Illinois at Chicago, Chicago, Illinois, U.S.A.*

J. Bradley Phipps/*ALZA Corporation, Mountain View, California, U.S.A.*

Michael J. Pikal/*University of Connecticut, Storrs, Connecticut, U.S.A.*

Wayne L. Pines/*Pharmaceutical Consultant, Washington, D.C., U.S.A.*

Dario Pistolesi/*Fedegari Autoclavi S.p.A., Albuzzano, PV, Italy*

Michael E. Placke/*Battelle Pulmonary Therapeutics, Inc., Columbus, Ohio, U.S.A.*

Therese I. Poirier/*Duquesne University, Pittsburgh, Pennsylvania, U.S.A.*

Jacques H. Poupaert/*Université Catholique de Louvain, Brussels, Belgium*

Sunil Prabhu/*Western University of Health Sciences, Pomona, California, U.S.A.*

Neil Purdie/*Oklahoma State University, Stillwater, Oklahoma, U.S.A.*

R. Raghavan/*Abbott Laboratories, Abbott Park, Illinois, U.S.A.*

M.S. Rahman/*Cardinal Health Pharmaceutical Technologies & Services Center, Somerset, New Jersey, U.S.A.*

Ali R. Rajabi-Siahboomi/*Colorcon Limited, Kent, United Kingdom*

Suneel Rastogi/*Forest Laboratories, Inc., Inwood, New York, U.S.A.*

William R. Ravis/*Auburn University, Auburn, Alabama, U.S.A.*

Thomas L. Reiland/*Abbott Laboratories, Abbott Park, Illinois, U.S.A.*

Jean Paul Remon/*Ghent University, Ghent, Belgium*

Shijun Ren/*University of Southern California, Los Angeles, California, U.S.A.*

Michael Repka/*The University of Mississippi, University, Mississippi, U.S.A.*

Christopher T. Rhodes/*University of Rhode Island, Kingston, Rhode Island, U.S.A.*

Martin M. Rieger/*M&A Rieger, Morris Plains, New Jersey, U.S.A.*

Jean G. Riess/*University of California at San Diego, San Diego, California, U.S.A.*

Thomas N. Riley/*Auburn University, Auburn, Alabama, U.S.A.*

Ronald J. Roberts/*AstraZeneca, Macclesfield, Cheshire, United Kingdom*

Naír Rodríguez-Hornedo/*University of Michigan, Ann Arbor, Michigan, U.S.A.*

Raymond C. Rowe/*AstraZeneca, Macclesfield, Cheshire, United Kingdom*

Joseph T. Rubino/*Wyeth-Ayerst Research, Pearl River, New York, U.S.A.*

J. Howard Rytting/*The University of Kansas, Lawrence, Kansas, U.S.A.*

Rosalie Sagraves/*University of Illinois at Chicago, Chicago, Illinois, U.S.A.*

Peter C. Schmidt/*University of Tübingen, Tübingen, Germany*

David R. Schoneker/*Colorcon, West Point, Pennsylvania, U.S.A.*

Stephen G. Schulman/*University of Florida, Gainesville, Florida, U.S.A.*

Erik R. Scott/*ALZA Corporation, Mountain View, California, U.S.A.*

Gerald Scucci/*Rutgers University, Piscataway, New Jersey, U.S.A.*

Richard B. Seymour/*Haight Ashbury Free Clinics, San Francisco, California, U.S.A.*

Jaymin C. Shah/*Pfizer Inc., Groton, Connecticut, U.S.A.*

Umang Shah/*Parke-Davis Division, Warner Lambert, Morris Plains, New Jersey, U.S.A.*

Shalaby W. Shalaby/*Poly-Med, Inc., Pendleton, South Carolina, U.S.A.*

Leon Shargel/*Eon Labs Manufacturing, Inc., Laurelton, New York, U.S.A.*

Joseph Sherma/*Lafayette College, Easton, Pennsylvania, U.S.A.*

Troy Shinbrot/*Rutgers University, Piscataway, New Jersey, U.S.A.*

Brent D. Sinclair/*University of Michigan, Ann Arbor, Michigan, U.S.A.*

Ambarish K. Singh/*The Bristol-Myers Squibb Pharmaceutical Research Institute, New Brunswick, New Jersey, U.S.A.*

Brahma N. Singh/*St. John's University, Jamaica, New York, U.S.A.*

Shailesh K. Singh/*Wyeth–Ayerst Research, Pearl River, New York, U.S.A.*

Patrick J. Sinko/*Rutgers University, Piscataway, New Jersey, U.S.A.*

Jerome P. Skelly/*Consultant, Alexandria, Virginia, U.S.A.*

Michael F. Skinner/*Rhodes University, Grahamstown, South Africa*

William H. Slattery III/*House Ear Institute, Los Angeles, California, U.S.A.*

David E. Smith/*Haight Ashbury Free Clinics, San Francisco, California, U.S.A.*

Edward J. Smith/*Packaging Science Resources, King of Prussia, Pennsylvania, U.S.A.*

Marshall Steinberg/*International Pharmaceutical Excipients Council-Americas, Arlington, Virginia, U.S.A.*

Ralph Stone/*Alcon Laboratories, Fort Worth, Texas, U.S.A.*

Raj Suryanarayanan/*University of Minnesota, Minneapolis, Minnesota, U.S.A.*

Stuart R. Suter/*Suter Associates, Glenside, Pennsylvania, U.S.A.*

Lynda Sutton/*Cato Research Ltd., Durham, North Carolina, U.S.A.*

Hanne Hjorth Tønnesen/*University of Oslo, Oslo, Norway*

Hua Tang/*Massachusetts Institute of Technology, Cambridge, Massachusetts, U.S.A.*

Kevin M.G. Taylor/*University of London, London, United Kingdom*

Bernard Testa/*University of Lausanne, Lausanne, Switzerland*

Maya Thanou/*Leiden/Amsterdam Center for Drug Research, Leiden University, The Netherlands*

C. Thomasin/*The R.W. Johnson Pharmaceutical Research Institute, Schaffhausen, Switzerland*

Diane O. Thompson/*CyDex, Inc., Overland Park, Kansas, U.S.A.*

William J. Thomsen/*Arena Pharmaceuticals, San Diego, California, U.S.A.*

Youqin Tian/*Alcon Research, Ltd., Fort Worth, Texas, U.S.A.*

Jeffrey Tidwell/*University of North Carolina, Chapel Hill, North Carolina, U.S.A.*

James E. Tingstad/*Tingstad Associates, Green Valley, Arizona, U.S.A.*

Richard Turton/*West Virginia University, Morgantown, West Virginia, U.S.A.*

Mitsuru Uchiyama/*Japan Pharmacists Education Center, Tokyo, Japan*

Madhu K. Vadnere/*NJ Pharma LLC, Chatham, New Jersey, U.S.A.*

Lynn Van Campen/*Inhale Therapeutic Systems, Inc., San Carlos, California, U.S.A.*

Koen Van Deun/*Janssen Pharmaceutica N.V., Beerse, Belgium*

Mark D. VanArendonk/*Pharmacia Corporation, Kalamazoo, Michigan, U.S.A.*

Christine Vauthier/*University of Paris XI, Châtenay-Malabry, France*

Geraldine Venthoye/*Inhale Therapeutic Systems, Inc., San Carlos, California, U.S.A.*

J. Coos Verhoef/*Leiden/Amsterdam Center for Drug Research, Leiden University, The Netherlands*

Vesa Virtanen/*Orion Pharma, Kuopio, Finland*

Imre M. Vitez/*Bristol-Myers Squibb Pharmaceutical Research Institute, New Brunswick, New Jersey, U.S.A.*

Karel Vytras/*University of Pardubice, Pardubice, Czech Republic*

Roderick B. Walker/*Rhodes University, Grahamstown, South Africa*

Kenneth A. Walters/*An-eX Analytical Services Ltd, Cardiff, United Kingdom*

Ch. Wandrey/*Laboratoire des Polyélectrolytes et BioMacromolécules, Lausanne, Switzerland*

R.P. Waranis/*Cardinal Health Pharmaceutical Technologies & Services Center, Somerset, New Jersey, U.S.A.*

Richard J. Washkuhn/*Lexington, Kentucky, U.S.A.*

Alan L. Weiner/*Alcon Research, Ltd., Fort Worth, Texas, U.S.A.*

Peter G. Welling/*University of Strathclyde, Glasgow, Scotland*

Albert I. Wertheimer/*Temple University, Philadelphia, Pennsylvania, U.S.A.*

Cheryl A. Wiens/*University of Alberta, Edmonton, Alberta, Canada*

Ellen M. Williams/*Pfizer, Inc., New York, New York, U.S.A.*

Roger L. Williams/*U.S. Pharmacopeia, Rockville, Marryland, U.S.A.*

C. G. Wilson/*University of Strathclyde, Glasgow, United Kingdom*

A. David Woolfson/*The Queen's University of Belfast, Belfast, United Kingdom*

Samuel H. Yalkowsky/*The University of Arizona, Tucson, Arizona, U.S.A.*

Victor C. Yang/*The University of Michigan, Ann Arbor, Michigan, U.S.A.*

Andrew B.C. Yu/*U.S. Food and Drug Administration, Rockville, Maryland, U.S.A.*

Mark J. Zellhofer/*University Pharmaceuticals of Maryland, Inc., Baltimore, Maryland, U.S.A.*

Feng Zhang/*The University of Texas at Austin, Austin, Texas, U.S.A.*

William C. Zimlich, Jr./*Battelle Pulmonary Therapeutics, Inc., Columbus, Ohio, U.S.A.*

Preface to the Second Edition

Pharmaceutical science and technology have progressed enormously in recent years. Significant advances in therapeutics and a greater understanding of the need to optimize drug delivery in the body have brought about an increased awareness of the valuable role played by the dosage form in therapy. This, in turn, has resulted in an increased sophistication and level of expertise in the design, development, manufacture, testing, and regulation of drugs and dosage forms.

The *Encyclopedia of Pharmaceutical Technology* is a unique, comprehensive compilation that brings together knowledge from every specialty encompassed by pharmaceutical technology. It is the ideal place for initiation of research projects or for becoming acquainted with or updating oneself in a specific topic.

It has been 17 years since we first began organizing topics and contacting potential authors for the first edition of the *Encyclopedia of Pharmaceutical Technology*. The first volume appeared in 1988. The last volume of the first edition, Volume 20, appeared in 2001. As the usefulness of the encyclopedia became evident, a second edition was launched. The constant progress in the many fields comprising pharmaceutical technology has resulted in a second edition that will be available in print and online, which will allow for quarterly updates and expansions.

The print version of the encyclopedia consists of three volumes totaling over 3,000 pages and over 200 articles arranged alphabetically by subject. Each article is written by an expert in a particular specialty and represents the latest advances in the field.

The online version includes everything in the print version and also offers the convenience of a keyword search engine as well as the inclusion of color illustrations. New articles and revised articles will be digitally posted quarterly and available to all subscribers of the electronic version.

The production and publishing of a work of this nature is not possible without the dedication and talent of numerous individuals. In particular, we gratefully acknowledge the efforts of the authors, several of whom have contributed multiple articles. Clearly, without this talented and responsive cadre of world class scientists, there would be no *Encyclopedia of Pharmaceutical Technology*.

Our publisher, Marcel Dekker, Inc., has always been supportive of our efforts and receptive to our editorial needs. We are especially indebted to Carolyn Hall, Managing Editor of the Encyclopedia Department, for her marvelous assistance in working with us to bring this work to fruition.

Finally, we would be remiss if we did not thank you, our readers, for your numerous comments and continuing support. We hope the second edition meets and exceeds your expectations. As always, we welcome your comments.

James Swarbrick
James C. Boylan
Editors

Aims and Scope

The need for a comprehensive, authoritative, contemporary, and relevant collection of articles detailing that area of the pharmaceutical sciences embraced by the term "pharmaceutical technology" has been amply confirmed by the success of the First Edition of the *Encyclopedia of Pharmaceutical Technology*.

With the first volume published in 1988 and the last in 2000, this 20 volume set contained over 300 articles covering a wide range of topics described in over 9000 pages of text, illustrations, tables, references, and indices.

As with the First Edition, the new, Second Edition focuses on a list of topics relevant to the discovery, development, regulation, manufacture, and commercialization of drugs and dosage forms. Consistent with the phrase "pharmaceutical technology," it emphasizes contributions in such areas as pharmaceutics, pharmacokinetics, analytical chemistry, quality assurance, drug safety, and the manufacturing process—not solely on discussion of the chemical and/or pharmacological profiles of individual drugs or classes of drugs.

The aim of the Second Edition is to essentially match the breadth of coverage found in the First Edition but with a more consistent format and style for the approximately 200 topics. At the same time, the number of volumes is being reduced to three, each of approximately 1000 pages, which will be published simultaneously. This more condensed, but consistent, three-volume presentation will appeal to institutional libraries and organizations, as well as individual pharmaceutical scientists.

All First Edition entries selected for inclusion in the Second Edition have been updated. New topics have been included, and some topics reorganized from multiple headings in the First Edition to single entries in the Second Edition, and vice versa, to reflect the current significance of a particular area. As before, the authors are recognized experts in their respective fields of activity.

The online version of the *Encyclopedia* has a powerful search engine, user-friendly interface, and customer-focused features. The database that is *EPT Online* is dynamic, with a number of articles added each quarter. Users can browse the Table of Contents and search the full text in query-based and menu-driven modes. Search features ensure the return of a limited number of useful search results quickly.

EPT Online will be marketed as a subscription product updated quarterly. Purchase of the print *Encyclopedia* will not be a prerequisite for purchase of *EPT Online*. We plan to track the activities of users and broaden our business plan.

Contents

xvi

Volume 2

xviii

PEDIATRIC DOSING AND DOSAGE FORMS

Rosalie Sagraves
University of Illinois at Chicago, Chicago, Illionis

INTRODUCTION

The administration of medications to pediatric patients is in many ways difficult because health care providers and parents are faced with many challenges not experienced, or experienced to a lesser degree, than when medications are prescribed for and taken by adults. First, less information is available about the use of most medications for pediatric patients. In fact only about 20% of drugs marketed in the United States have labeling for pediatric use (1). Milap Nahata, in a 1999 article on pediatric drug formulations, stated that "only five of the 80 drugs most commonly used in newborns, and infants are approved for pediatric use" (1). Second, many drugs that are used for some pediatric patients are not in appropriate dosage forms for use by children. This includes even some medications approved for use in pediatric patients. These issues have resulted in many questions that need to be answered about drug administration to pediatric patients. For example, is the drug approved for use in pediatric patients and in what age groups? If not approved, is there scientific information that enables us to determine whether the drug is safe and effective for pediatric patients of various ages? If the drug is available commercially for pediatric use, what dose should be administered and how frequently? What route should be used for administration, and what dosage form selected? If the drug is not available in an appropriate dosage form for childhood use, can it be prepared extemporaneously? Is there stability studies, palatability tests, clinical data in children, etc. that pertain to the extemporaneous formulation? How should the drug be monitored for effectiveness as well as for adverse effects? Information determined in adult medication studies may not be applicable to pediatric patients because of pharmacokinetic and pharmacodynamic differences as well as differences in disease states for which a particular drug might be used. Many questions about the use of particular drugs in various age groups of pediatric patients can only be answered through well-designed, randomized controlled studies in pediatric patients who need certain medications for particular health problems.

In 1997, the Food and Drug Administration (FDA) proposed new regulations for how pharmaceutical manufacturers would access safety and efficacy of certain new drugs that could have pediatric indications (1, 2). Thereafter, the FDA and the American Association of Pharmaceutical Scientists (AAPS) held a conference with academicians, pharmaceutical industry representatives, and U.S. Pharmacopeia (USP) representatives to discuss these proposed FDA regulations.

The FDA Modernization Act (FDAMA) of 1997 contains within it financial incentives for the development and marketing of drugs that could be used for pediatric patients (3). Some of these incentives include an extension of 6 months on market exclusivity and waiving fees for supplemental applications needed for receiving the approval of drugs for pediatric use that are already approved for adult use. In addition, the FDA published a list of drugs approved in adults for which additional pediatric data may produce health benefits for pediatric patients (4). For drugs on this list, FDA may ask a pharmaceutical manufacturer why it has not sought approval of a particular drug for pediatric use. So far there has not been much advancement in this area. This may be due to the wait for final approval of FDAMA.

Various medical and pharmacy organizations have worked hard throughout the years in their efforts to better educate children, parents, educators, and health care providers about the medications and their appropriate use. Indeed, individuals who help care for children may not be adequately trained to educate children about medications that they need to use. Therefore in June 2000, the USP started the development of three target initiatives: principles for educating children about their medications, guidelines for developing and evaluating information for children, and developing specific curricular information in a modular format (5). The USP position about educating children about medications may be found on their website (www.usp.org). The following information pieces have been developed by the USP (5):

- *Guide to Developing and Evaluating Medicine Education Programs and Materials for Children and*

Adolescents (joint publication of the American Health Association and USP)

- *A Kid's Guide to Asking Questions about Medicines*
- *Teaching Kids about Medicines*
- *Talking to Children about Their Medicines* (pamphlet developed jointly by Pfizer and USP to be disseminated to pediatricians and children's families)
- An Annotated Bibliography of Research and Programs Relating to Children and Medications

The USP has started working with the National Center for Health Education in New York to develop educational materials that can help school systems nationwide to know more about medications that students may need to take. The USP also adopted the following resolution to address the work that needs to be done in the area of health education (5):

Facilitate and contribute to the development of a rational school medicines policy, including guidelines for student, faculty, and staff medicine education, for acquisition, transport, storage, administration, use, and disposal of medicines; for protection of privacy; and for record-keeping in primary and secondary schools. Initiatives should be undertaken in collaboration with appropriate partners.

The USP has been working with the National Institute of Child Health and Human Development (NICHD) to develop a list of drugs for which more pediatric information is needed to insure proper use in children. The USP is also evaluating similarities and differences among neonates, children, and adults that may affect medication dosing and which might help in the appropriate labeling of medicines for pediatric use. The USP is reviewing the literature and developing tables for drugs, using evidence-based information. USP members can find this information by contacting Joyce Weaver (jpw@usp.org).

This overview of pediatric dosing and dosage forms covers issues that peditric health care providers face daily, such as age-related drug pharmacokinetic and pharmacodynamic changes that occur secondarily to physiologic changes in maturing neonates, infants, children, and adolescents that can affect drug absorption from various routes of administration as well as drug distribution, metabolism, and elimination. To be more knowledgeable about pharmacokinetic changes, therapeutic drug monitoring (TDM) must be undertaken for drugs with narrow therapeutic indexes and for those for which pharmacodynamic data (i.e., pharmacologic response that correlates to the drug concentration at the receptor site) correlates with pharmacokinetic information. Also addressed will be drug administration by various routes including intravenous (i.v.), oral (p.o.), intramuscular (i.m.), subcutaneous (s.c.), percutaneous, rectal, otic, nasal, ophthalmic, and inhalation. Another issue discussed is product selection for pediatric patients.

To better understand changes in drug disposition, the pediatric population needs to be categorized into various groups (Table 1) because children vary markedly in their absorption, distribution, metabolism, and elimination of medications. This occurs because neonates, infants, children, adolescents, and adults have different body compositions (i.e., as to their percentages of body water and fat) and have their body organs in different stages of development.

Table 1 Pediatric age groups terminology

Terms	Definition
Gestational age	Time from the mother's last menstrual period to the time the baby is born; at birth, a Dubowitz score in weeks gestational age is assigned, based on the physical examination of the newborn
Postnatal age	Age since birth
Postconceptional age	Age since conception, i.e., gestational plus postnatal age
Neonate	First 4 weeks or first month of life
Premature neonates	Born at less than 37-weeks gestation
Fullterm neonates	Born between 37- and 42-weeks gestation
Postterm neonates	Born after 42-weeks gestation
Infant	1 month to 1 year of age
Child	1–12 years of age
Adolescent	12–18 years of age

PEDIATRIC PHARMACOKINETICS AND PHARMACODYNAMICS

Effect of Developmental Physiologic Changes on Pharmacokinetics and Pharmacodynamics of Drugs

Rational pediatric pharmacotherapy is primarily based on the knowledge about a particular drug, including its pharmacokinetics and pharmacodynamics, that may be modified by physiologic maturation of the child from birth through adolescence. Physiologic changes that occur can affect drug absorption, distribution, metabolism, and elimination. The most dramatic changes occur during the neonatal period.

Oral Absorption

Drug absorption from the gastrointestinal (GI) tract is dependent on patient factors, physicochemical properties of the orally administered drug, and the drug formulation. Patient factors that affect GI absorption include absorptive surface area, maturation of the mucosal membrane, gastric and duodenal pH, gastric emptying time, GI motility, enzyme activity, bacterial colonization of the GI tract, and dietary intake, including the specific gastric content status at the time when a medication is ingested (6–8). Patient factors are influenced by rapid maturational changes that occur throughout early childhood, but which occur primarily during the first few months of life.

Most drugs are absorbed across the GI tract by passive diffusion, but a variety of drug physiCochemical factors influence the extent of absorption. These factors include molecular weight, lipid solubility, ionization as well as disintegration and dissolution rates (7). In addition, drug absorption may be dependent on the dosage form selected (e.g., a liquid, a tablet that may need to be crushed, or a sustained-release product), and the particular brand selected. For timed-release preparations, the release characteristics must also be taken into consideration.

Gastric pH

When examining patient-specific factors such as gastric pH, which affect oral absorption, it should be noted that infants born vaginally who are at least 32-weeks gestation, usually have gastric pHs between 6 and 8 at birth (7, 8). Gastric pH then falls rapidly within a few hours after delivery to a pH of less than 3 (7, 8). The initial gastric pH is alkaline compared to that of adults and results from the presence of amniotic fluid in the infant's stomach (9, 10). Thereafter, gastric pH remains acidic until approximately day 10, then a nadir in acid production occurs between days 10 and 30 of life. Then gastric acid production begins to increase, but gastric pH and maximal gastric output may not mirror that of adults on a per kilogram basis until after the neonatal period (7).

Gastric emptying and gastrointestinal motility

Gastric emptying time in neonates, especially those less than 24 h of age, may be variable (7). It may not reach adult levels until 6–8 months of age and may be associated with diet (11, 12). Gastrointestinal transit time may be prolonged and peristaltic activity unpredictable in young infants (8, 13); both appear affected by the feeding (13). Lebenthal and colleagues noted that breast-fed infants, older than 45 days of age, had gastric transit times longer than 10 h while formula-fed infants had transit times less than 10 h (14). It should also be noted that young infants have a propensity to reflux their gastric contents because of GI immaturity. All these factors affect the extent to which a drug may be absorbed.

Enzyme activity and microflora in the gastrointestinal tract

Pancreatic enzyme activity may be low at birth, but enzymes such as amylase, lipase, and trypsin develop to adult levels within the first year of life (15). Premature infants appear to have lower amylase levels than do full-term infants. Low concentrations of pancreatic enzymes may be the reason why newborns have a decreased ability to cleave prodrug esters such as chloramphenicol palmitate (7). Lipid-soluble drugs may not be well absorbed by neonates because of low lipase concentrations and bile acid pool (8).

More information is needed about the microflora of the GI tract and its effect on drug absorption. In addition, the effects of various diets and antibiotic use can alter the microflora of the GI tract (7).

Absorptive surface area

The surface area of the small intestine in young infants is proportionately greater than in adults. This physiologic difference may allow for increased drug absorption from the GI tract.

Intramuscular Absorption

When a child is unable to take a medication orally or the drug is unavailable for oral use, there may be a need to administer a drug parenterally by either the i.v. or i.m. route. Of these, the latter may be less desirable because of pain, irritation, and decreased drug delivery as compared to i.v. administration. Drug absorption after i.m. administration depends on various physicochemical and patient factors. Physicochemical factors to be considered include lipid or water solubility, drug concentration, and surface area. When addressing drug solubility, it should be noted that lipophilic drugs readily diffuse through the capillary walls of endothelial cells whereas water-soluble drugs diffuse at fairly rapid rates from interstitial fluid to plasma via pores in capillary membranes (16). A lipid-soluble drug may be more rapidly absorbed i.m., but a water-soluble drug may be more desirable because the drug must be stable in an aqueous solution until administered. After administration, the drug must then be water soluble at physiologic pH until absorption occurs (16).

Drug absorption may be dependent on concentration, but available data do not allow us to determine whether an increased or decreased drug concentration results in better absorption. An increase in the osmolality of a pharmaceutical preparation secondary to the addition of another substance such as an excipient may decrease or slow down i.m. adsorption (16). Absorption occurs more rapidly when diffusion involves a large area of muscle or the drug spreads over a large muscle mass. The massaging of an injection site after i.m. administration increases the rate of absorption (16).

A physiologic determination of i.m. drug absorption is dependent on the adequacy of blood flow to muscle groups used for drug administration. Absorption rates differ at injection sites because blood flow varies among different muscle groups. For example, the absorption of a drug-administered i.m. in the deltoid muscle is faster than from the vastus lateralis that, in turn, is more rapid than from the gluteus (16, 17). This occurs because blood flow to the deltoid muscle is 7% higher than to vastus lateralis and 17% higher than to gluteal muscle groups (18). Physiologic conditions that reduce blood flow to a muscle group may adversely alter the rate and/or extent of a drug-administered i.m. Decreased perfusion or hemostatic decompensation, frequently observed in ill neonates and young infants, may reduce i.m. drug absorption. Drug absorption may be adversely affected in neonates who receive a skeletal muscle-paralyzing agent such as pancuronium (16) because of decreased muscle contraction. A small muscle mass in neonates and young infants may also reduce the ability of a drug to be adequately absorbed.

The injection technique used may alter i.m. absorption. This was noted when needles of different lengths were used. The use of a longer needle (38 vs. 31 mm, 1 1/2 vs. 1 1/4 in.) for i.m. administration in adult patients resulted in higher diazepam serum concentrations (18). This probably occurred because the drug administered with the shorter needle was actually administered s.c. rather than i.m.

Some drugs are absorbed more slowly after i.m. than oral administration; examples include diazepam, digoxin,

and phenytoin. This probably occurs because these drugs require a mixture of alcohol, propylene glycol, and water for solubility, and they are insoluble in the muscle after i.m. administration (18).

Complications associated with i.m. administration include nerve injury, muscle contracture, and abscess formation (19). Less common problems include intramuscular hemorrhage, cellulitis, skin pigmentation, tissue necrosis, muscle atrophy, gangrene, and cyst or scar formation. In addition, injury may occur from broken needles and inadvertent injection into a joint or vein (19).

Subcutaneous Absorption

The s.c. route is used for the administration of drugs such as insulin that require slow absorption. Injection technique and patient factors, such as fluid status and physical build, are important (18). Exercise, elevation or warming of the injection site, or inadvertently administrating a drug i.m. rather than s.c. can increase absorption and be dangerous in some situations, such as hypoglycemia occurring in a diabetic patient from excessive insulin absorption (18). Adverse effects that can occur secondarily to s.c. administration include tissue ischemia, sterile and nonsterile abscesses, lipodystrophy, cysts, and granulomatous formation.

Intraosseous Drug Absorption

If an i.v. line cannot be placed, the intraosseous drug administration route can be used for pediatric patients during, for example, cardiopulmonary resuscitation (CPR) because drug delivery by this route is similar to that for i.v. administration (20). If drug or fluid deliver by this route is sluggish, a saline flush can be used to clear the needle. Intraosseous administration is used to deliver medications such as epinephrine, atropine, sodium bicarbonate, dopamine, diazepam, isoproterenol, phenytoin, phenobarbital, dexamethasone, and various antibiotics (20).

Percutaneous or Transdermal Absorption

The percutaneous (transdermal or topical) route for systemic drug delivery is used infrequently for pediatric patients. Medications are typically applied to the skin for their local effect. In the future, this route may be used more frequently for systemic effects as more transdermal systems are developed for drug delivery.

The percutaneous absorption or the transdermal delivery of a drug occurs in the following manner. Initially a topically applied drug is absorbed into the stratum corneum and diffuses through that layer of skin into the epidermis and then into the dermis where drug molecules reach capillaries and enter the circulatory system. Diffusion through the stratum corneum is the rate-determining step unless skin perfusion is decreased. If the latter case, diffusion is controlled by the transfer of drug molecules into capillaries rather than by the diffusion process previously explained. Percutaneous or transdermal absorption (21, 22) is affected by

- Patient age.
- Application site.
- State of hydration of the stratum corneum.
- Thickness and intactness of the stratum corneum.
- Physical characteristics of the solute, and
- Physical characteristics of the vehicle or solvent.

Drug diffusion may be explained by Eq. 1:

$$J = \frac{K_m \times D_m \times C_s}{\ell} \tag{1}$$

where J is flux, K_m is the partition coefficient, D_m is the diffusion constant under specific conditions such as temperature and hydration, C_s is the concentration gradient, and ℓ is the length or thickness of stratum corneum (21).

Lipid-soluble drugs are better absorbed into the stratum corneum than are water-soluble drugs, but the latter do not easily traverse the stratum corneum. Thus, lipid-soluble drugs are more likely to be stored in the stratum corneum, whereas water-soluble drugs are more likely to diffuse across the stratum corneum to the epidermis and dermis (21).

Patient age

Drug absorption transdermally is not appreciably different in various age groups of patients except for neonates less than 32-week gestation at birth (23). Drug absorption is increased in premature neonates, because the stratum corneum is not completely formed at birth. An example of increased drug absorption occurred in two premature neonates who were repeatedly washed with 3% hexachlorophene and developed encephalopathy secondary to drug absorption (21). The absorption of the corticosteroid betamethasone valerate after topical application in children resulted in hypothalamus–pituitary–adrenal axis suppression. Children may have increased drug absorption from the percutaneous application of drugs not because of higher absorption rate but because of a greater topical application or a larger dose per kilogram. Examples of deaths in children from percutaneous drug absorption include those caused by salicylic acid and phenol absorption (21). Toxicity has also been noted with the topical application of iodine and alcohol-containing products (23).

Application site

The ability of a drug to be absorbed transdermally depends on the thickness of the stratum corneum. For example, absorption occurs more readily through abdominal skin than through skin on the plantar surface of the foot. Topical absorption may be enhanced from a particular site by the application of an occlusive dressing.

Status of the stratum corneum

Percutaneous absorption of a drug is enhanced by the hydration of the stratum corneum. Such hydration affects the absorption of hydrophilic drugs more than lipophilic drugs. Drugs will penetrate damaged skin more than intact skin. Skin damaged because of dryness will allow for increased drug penetration through areas where the skin is cracked or broken.

Solute

The penetration of the solute (or drug) depends on its polarity and on the polarity of the delivery vehicle.

Vehicle or solvent

Drug-delivery vehicles typically used for topical application include lotions, ointments, creams, emulsions, and gels. Substances such as emulsifiers may be added to the drug and vehicle to improve the texture of an emulsion, a stabilizer to preserve drug stability, the vehicle, or both, a thickening agent to increase viscosity, or a humectant to draw moisture into the skin (21). It is particularly important to consider the vehicle and other additives when selecting a topical drug preparation for a neonate, especially when premature, because of the greater possibility of absorption of not only the drug but also other product ingredients. Toxic reactions have occurred in neonates from ingredients considered "inactive."

Transdermal Drug-Delivery Systems

Drugs chosen for delivery via a transdermal drug-delivery system must adequately penetrate the skin in such a way that the system determines the delivery rate that should be fairly constant (21). In addition, the drug must not irritate or sensitize the skin. It is hoped that in the future more drugs will be developed for transdermal delivery. This could become an alternative route for drug delivery to children who have difficulty with oral administration.

Endotracheal Absorption

The endotracheal (ET) route has been used to administer medications during CPR when other routes, such as the i.v. route, are unavailable. It provides rapid access as well as rapid drug absorption and distribution (24). Some studies have shown that the time to reach peak absorption is similar to that for the i.v. route, but serum concentrations achieved were 10–33% of that achieved with i.v. administration, resulting in a weaker response. A depot effect has also been demonstrated for drugs such as epinephrine. Work needs to be done to determine the optimal dose by this route, drug-delivery vehicle, and the most effective delivery technique.

Rectal Absorption

The rectal route is used for local and systemic therapy for the following reasons (25):

- Nausea or vomiting.
- Rejection of oral education because of its taste, texture, etc.
- Upper GI disease that might affect absorption.
- Medication absorption affected by food or gastric emptying.
- Medication is readily decomposed in gastric fluid but may be stable in rectal fluid, and
- First-pass effect of high-clearance drug may be partially avoided.

Absorption from the rectum depends on various physiological factors such as surface area, blood supply, pH, fluid volume, and possible metabolism by microorganisms in the rectum. The rectum is perfused by the inferior and middle rectal arteries, whereas the superior, the middle, and the inferior rectal veins drain the rectum (25). The latter two are directly connected to the systemic circulation; the superior rectal vein drains into the portal system. Drugs absorbed from the lower rectum are carried directly into the systemic circulation, whereas drugs absorbed from the upper rectum are subjected to hepatic first-pass effect (25). Therefore, a high-clearance drug should be more bioavailable after rectal than oral administration. The volume of fluid in the rectum, the pH of that fluid, and the presence of stool in the rectal vault may affect drug absorption. Because the fluid volume is usually low compared to that in other areas of the GI tract, a drug may not be completely soluble. In addition, a variety of organisms colonize the rectum, and it is debated whether these organisms are involved in drug metabolism (25). Absorption is also influenced by the dosage form used. For example, drugs are rapidly absorbed rectally from aqueous or alcoholic solutions, whereas absorption

from a suppository depends on its base, the presence of a surfactant, particle size of the active ingredient(s), and drug concentration (25). The following problems may be associated with the rectal route for drug administration (25):

- Decreased absorption secondary to defecation of the rectally administered pharmaceutical product.
- Less absorption rectally than orally because the absorbing surface area of the rectum is smaller.
- Dissolution problems for rectally administered medications because of lower fluid volume in the rectum than in the stomach, duodenum, etc..
- Microorganisms in rectum may cause degradation of some medications, and
- Patient or parent acceptance.

Distribution

A drug is distributed by moving from a patient's systemic circulation to various compartments, tissues, and cells. Distribution depends on patient factors, drug physiochemical properties, and the route of drug administration. Patient factors that influence drug distribution or the volume of drug distribution (V_d) include body composition, perfusion, protein- and tissue-binding characteristics, and permeability (7, 8). Many of these characteristics are age dependent. Drug physiochemical properties that may influence distribution include molecular weight, pK_a, and partition coefficient.

Differences in body composition

Age-related changes in body composition can alter the V_d of a drug. At birth, 85% of the weight of a premature infant may be water, compared to approximately 75% as total body water (TBW) in a full-term infant (13). Neonates have the highest percentage of extracellular water (65% of TBW in premature infants as compared to 35–44% in full-term neonates and 20% in adults). The intracellular water (ICW) is more stable throughout life (i.e., 25% in premature neonates, 33% in full-term neonates, and 40% in adults) (7). An infant's percentage of TBW approaches that of an adult male by 1 year of age (60% TBW); it reaches the same about the time of puberty or 12 years of age (8). Women have a lower percentage of TBW (50%) than men do because they have a higher concentration of body fat. Thus, neonates, because of their high TBW, have a higher V_d for water-soluble drugs such as aminoglycosides than older children or adults. For example, the V_d for an aminoglycoside such as gentamicin approximates that of extracellular cellular fluid volume, 0.5–1.2 L/kg for a neonate, but only 0.2–0.3 L/kg for an older child or an adult (8).

Adipose tissue increases from as little as 0.5% in a premature infant to approximately 16% of body weight for a full-term infant (26, 27). Boys experiene a spurt in body fat between the ages of 5 and 10 years, and then a gradual decrease in fat content until about 17 years of age; girls usually have a rapid increase in adipose tissue at puberty (9). Thus, one would expect neonates and young infants to have a decreased V_d for lipid-soluble drugs. This has been noted for diazepam in neonates who have exhibited an apparent V_d of 1.4–1.8 L/kg compared to 2.2–2.6 L/kg in adults (28).

Protein binding

Neonates have lower concentrations of various plasma proteins (e.g., albumin concentrations about 80% of those in adults) for drug binding, but the albumin present may also have a lower affinity for binding drugs than noted for adults who are receiving the same medications. This lower affinity for binding drugs may result in a competition for various albumin-binding sites with substances such as bilirubin. Plasma protein binding noted in adults is usually achieved in children by the age of 1 year (13).

In neonates drugs such as various penicillins, phenobarbital, phenytoin, and theophylline have lower protein-binding affinity than in adults. This may increase the concentration of free or pharmacological active drug in neonates, and may also change the apparent volume of distribution. Thus, neonates may require different doses on a mg/kg basis compared to that for adults for these drugs to achieve appropriate therapeutic serum concentrations.

In addition to binding to plasma proteins in the neonate, some drugs such as sulfonamides may displace plasma bilirubin from binding sites. This may increase an infant's risk for developing kernicterus. The significance of drugs displacing bilirubin is controversial because bilirubin may have a greater affinity for albumin than drugs have (29).

Tissue binding

The binding of drugs to various body tissues appears to vary with age; for example, digoxin binding to erythrocytes is higher in neonates than in adults. This may be due to the increased number of binding sties on neonatal erythrocytes (30).

Drug penetration into the central nervous system

A drug is more likely to cross into the central nervous system (CNS) of a neonate rather than an older child or an adult. This most likely occurs because its CNS is less mature and the blood–brain barrier is less formed. This is an important consideration when antimicrobial therapy is needed for the treatment of bacterial meningitis or anticonvulsant for seizures.

Metabolism

Although drug metabolism can occur in various body organs including the lungs, GI tract, liver, and kidneys as well as in the blood, the liver is the primary organ for metabolism. Most drugs are metabolized from lipid-soluble parent compounds to more polar, less lipophilic metabolites that are more readily eliminated renally (9).

Hepatic metabolism

Most drug metabolism occurs in the liver by phase I or phase II metabolic processes. Phase I reactions primarily biotransform an active drug to a more water-soluble compound that typically is inactive or has less activity than the parent compound. Oxidation, reduction, hydralysis, and hydroxylation are examples of phase I reactions (6, 8, 16) Oxidation is primarily catalyzed by the cytochrome (CYP) P450 system that has a multitude of isozymes (at least 13 primary enzymes) with a multitude of isozymes of specific gene families (6). It appears that isozymes CYP450 1A2, 2D6, 2C19, and 3A3/4 are involved in drug metabolism in humans (6). Oxidizing enzyme systems appear to mature after birth so that by the age of 6 months, activity is similar to or even exceeds adult levels. More information about drugs affected by phase I reactions may be found in (6).

Phase II reactions (glucuronidation, sulfation, acetylation, and glutathione conjugation) usually involve the conjugation of active drugs with endogenous molecules to form metabolites that are more water soluble (16); glucuronidation is the most thoroughly studied reaction. It is postulated that maternal glucocorticoids inhibit the development of glucuronyltransferase, the enzyme involved in glucuronidation in utero. After birth this metabolic system matures rapidly and reaches adult levels by the age of 2 years (29).

Sulfate conjugation appears to be fully developed immediately prior to or at the time of birth. Infants and young children readily sulfate acetaminophen; in adults the major metabolic route is glucuronidation (31). Little is known about acetylation in neonates or infants. It is believed that neonates have an extremely low capacity for acetylation at birth, but this pathway matures at approximately 20 days of age (29).

Theophylline is an example of a drug that is readily metabolized in neonates by N-methylation to caffeine (process not relevant clinically in older infants, children, and adults). It is also a compound that has pharmacologic activity versus apnea (like theophylline), but which may have toxicity when it is not readily metabolized by the liver, and its elimination is slowed by immature kidneys (6).

Neonates require close monitoring if their mothers received enzyme inducers such as phenytoin, phenobarbital, carbamazepine, or rifampin during pregnancy or if they need one of these drugs themselves (16). Examples of drugs that inhibit the metabolism of other medications include cimetidine, erythromycin, and ketoconazole (16).

Renal Elimination

The kidneys are the major route for drug elimination, especially for water-soluble compounds or the metabolites of lipid-soluble drugs. Renal drug elimination is dependent on renal blood flow, glomerular filtration, and tubular secretion and reabsorption. These functions appear to mature at different rates in the neonate and infant. Full-term infants achieve renal blood flow similar to that of adults by the age of 5–12 months; glomerular filtration approaches adult values by the age of 3–5 months (6). Premature neonates exhibit lower rates for glomerular filtration at birth than do full-term neonates, and more time is required of them postnatally to develop filtration ability (32). This is probably due to their lack of as many functional nephrons at birth. Tubular function is less mature in the neonate at birth than is glomerular filtration, and it matures at a slower rate. Tubular function begins to approach adult values by 7 months of age. Renal function is equal to that of adults by 1 year of age.

Aminoglycosides (e.g., gentamicin, tobramycin, amikacin) and digoxin are drugs whose eliminations are affected by renal maturation. The renal elimination of aminoglycosides in neonates and young infants parallels the maturation of glomerular function and correlates with creatinine clearance (33). The renal elimination of digoxin parallels kidney maturation. Dosage adjustment for this drug is necessary as renal function matures in neonates and young infants. In addition, older infants and children require higher mg/kg doses of digoxin than do adults to achieve the same serum concentrations. This may be due to decreased digoxin absorption or increased renal elimination (8).

THERAPEUTIC DRUG MONITORING

Therapeutic drug monitoring should encompass the entire drug-use process including drug selection, product selection, administration route, patient age, appropriate dosing on a mg/kg or mg/m^2 basis, and monitoring serum concentrations when appropriate and observing the patient for optimal drug effect(s) and possible adverse drug events.

Important Differences in Pediatric Serum Drug Concentrations

For many drugs, especially for those with narrow therapeutic indexes, serum concentration ranges have been determined that correlate to minimum and maximum therapeutic effects as well as to the development of toxicity. Therapeutic serum concentration ranges for various drugs have been developed for adults, and these data have been applied to pediatric patients including neonates. Such data may be appropriate to monitor drug therapy in children, but possibly not in children of all ages or possibly not in children at all. For example, Painter et al. (34) noted that neonates need higher serum phenobarbital concentrations than do older children and adults to terminate seizures. Gilman et al. (35) observed that higher phenobarbital loading doses were needed to achieve serum concentrations in neonates that would reduce the occurrence of seizures. Thus, there may be a need for different serum concentration ranges for various drugs needed by different age groups of patients for a similar pharmacodynamic or therapeutic outcome.

Free serum concentrations, rather than total concentrations, of some drugs such as phenytoin may need to be monitored in some patients, including neonates, who have low serum albumin. Gilman has advocated the possibility of using individualized dosing and serum concentration range for pediatric patients because children, especially neonates, have rapidly maturing functions of various organs and changes in albumin for drug binding (36).

Serum concentration monitoring of various drugs administered to pediatric patients may appropriately give information about the drug but not its metabolites. This may be a problem when children metabolize specific drugs differently than adults with resulting differences in metabolite concentrations or the presence of different metabolites. This has been noted when premature infants have been administered theophylline for central apnea. A major metabolite of theophylline in neonates is caffeine, although only small concentrations of this metabolite are noted in older children and adults (37, 38). Caffeine is effective in treating apnea, and thus may add to the effectiveness of theophylline. This may help explain why lower theophylline serum concentrations may be needed for apnea rather than asthma. In addition, the presence of the 4-en metabolite of valproic acid noted in the serum of infants and young children, but not adults, receiving this medication for seizures may be responsible for the hepatoxicity of this drug in young pediatric patients (36, 39).

Serum Drug Concentrations

Because of the cost associated with therapeutic drug monitoring, serum drug concentrations must be drawn appropriately to provide useful information. Drugs typically followed pharmacokinetically are those with narrow therapeutic indexes for which there is an association between pharmacokinetic and pharmacodynamic data or toxicity. For many drugs, especially for those administered orally, the determination of trough concentrations (serum concentrations obtained prior to administration) may be most appropriate. This eliminates differences in absorption rates that could influence peak concentrations (e.g., orally administered phenobarbital, phenytoin, carbamazepine, or valproic acid). Trough concentrations may be important for drugs such as digoxin that take time to distribute to tissue receptors in such a way that serum concentrations reflect pharmacodynamic effects. Peak concentrations are best used for determining toxicity and therapeutic effects of drugs with short half-lives.

Table 2 gives therapeutic serum concentrations and pharmacokinetic information for some drugs administered to pediatric patients.

Technical Factors

Sample size and timing of blood drawing for serum concentration determination

Because of the small blood volume and the small size of veins, it is technically difficult to draw blood from neonates, infants, and young children for therapeutic drug monitoring, and it is therefore important to determine the best drawing schedule. For example, when are peak and trough data needed compared to trough data only? For anticonvulsants administered orally or i.v., trough concentrations are needed, whereas for aminoglycosides it may be important to obtain both peaks and troughs.

DOSING REGIMENS

Drugs for pediatric patients should be dosed on a mg/kg or a mg/m^2 basis using information available for the patient's age group. In addition, the patient's renal and hepatic functions must be considered. The route for administration must be determined based on the severity of the illness, the availability of the medication for a particular route of administration, and whether the patient is able to take a medication orally.

The Bibliography succeeding the References at the end of this chapter contains a list of handbooks and other references that are useful sources of dosing information for neonatal and/or pediatric pediatrics. In addition, drug information centers in pediatric hospitals or university settings are another excellent resource for pediatric drug information.

EXCIPIENTS OR ADDITIVES IN MEDICATIONS

Pharmaceutical products may contain, in addition to the active or therapeutic agent(s), a variety of other ingredients that are termed inactive or inert that are categorized as excipients or additives (flavorings, sweeteners, preservatives, stabilizers, diluents, lubricants, etc.). The words inert or inactive are misnomers for some excipients because some have been shown to cause adverse effects. Neonates and young children are at risk for such adverse effects, because they may not be able to metabolize or eliminate an ingredient in a pharmaceutical product in the same manner as an adult. In addition, patients of various ages have experienced allergic reactions to excipients such as tartrazine dyes.

Benzyl alcohol is a preservative that may be present in multidose vials of bacteriostatic sodium chloride and bacteriostatic water for injection and pharmaceuticals available in multidose vials for parenteral use. An association between the presence of benzyl alcohol in solutions used for flushing intravascular catheters and to reconstitute medications and a gasping syndrome and deaths in neonates was first reported in the early 1980s (40, 41). The neonates also displayed clinical findings such as an elevated anion gap, metabolic acidosis, CNS depression, seizures, respiratory failure, renal and hepatic failures, cardiovascular collapse, and death. Those at highest risk were premature infants who weighted less than 1250 g at birth (40–42). In a study by Benda et al., premature neonates who survived benzyl alcohol administration were compared to neonates born after the use of benzyl alcohol-containing flush solutions was discontinued (43). They noted that survivors had a higher incidence of cerebral palsy (50%) compared to infants who did not receive benzyl alcohol flushes (2.4%) ($P < 0.001$). In addition, the incidence of cerebral palsy and developmental delay was 53.9 versus 11.9% in the two populations ($P < 0.001$). The cause is probably associated with benzyl alcohol use and the inability of neonates, especially those who are premature, to adequately metabolize benzyl

Table 2 Pediatric pharmacokinetic data of some medications[a]

Drug	Therapeutic serum concentration (μg/ml)	Bioavailability (for oral drugs) (%)	Plasma protein binding (%)	V_d (L/kg)	$t_{1/2}$ (h)
Carbamazepine	4–12	>70	40–90	1.5 (neonate) 0.8–1.9 (child)	8–25 (child) $t_{1/2}$ varies with multiple dosing
Clonazepam	20–80 ng/mL	>85	47–80	3.2 (child)	20–40 (child)
Ethosuximide	40–100	~100	0	0.6–0.7 (child)	24–36 (child)
Gentamicin	trough $\leqq$ 2 peak 4–10	Not available	<30	0.4–0.6 (neonate) 0.3–0.35 (child)	3–11.5 (<1 wk) 3–6 (1 wk-6 mo) 1.2 (child)
Phenobarbital	15–40	80–100	40–60	0.6–1.2 (neonate) 0.7–1 (child)	45–173 (neonate) 37–72 (child)
Phenytoin	10–20	85–95	>90	1–1.2 (premature neonate) 0.8–0.9 (full-term neonate) 0.7–0.8 (child)	6–140 (<8 days)[b] 5–80 (9–21 days)[b] 2–20 (21–36 days)[b] 5–18 (child)[b]
Theophylline	5–15	up to 100%, depending on the formulation	32–40 (neonate) 55–60 (child)	0.4–1 (premature neonate) 0.3–0.7 (child)	19.9–35 (neonate) 3.4 ± 1.1 (1–4 yrs)
Valproic acid	40–100 (150)[c]	100	>90[d]	0.2 (child)	23–35 (neonate) 4–14 (child)

[a]Age or stage of life in parentheses.
[b]Michaelis–Menton pharmacokinetics; $T_{1/2}$ varies with serum concentration.
[c]Upper end of the serum concentration range is not definitely established.
[d]May vary with serum concentration.

(Adapted from Sagraves, R. Epilepsy and other Convulsive Disorders. In *Pediatric Pharmacotherapy*, 2nd Edn: Kuhn, R.J., Ed.) University of Kentucky: Lexington, 1993; Taketomo, C.K.; Hodding, J.H.; Kraus, D.M. *Pediatric Dosage Handbook*; LEXI-COMP, Inc.: Hudson, OH, 2000; Kauffman, R.E. Drug Therapeutics in the Infant and Child. In *Pediatric Pharmacology: Therapeutic Principles in Practice*; Yaffe, S.J., Aranda, J.V., Eds.; W.B. Saunders Co.: Philadelphia, 1992; 212–219; Rane, A. Drug Disposition and Action in Infants and Children. In *Pediatric Pharmacology: Therapeutic Principles in Practice*; Yaffe, S.J., Aranda, J.V., Eds.; W.B. Saunders Co. Philadelphia, 1992; 10–19.)

alcohol (44). The American Academy of Pediatrics (45), the Centers for Disease Control (46), and the FDA (47) recommend that the administration of products containing benzyl alcohol be avoided in infants. Preservative-free i.v. flush solutions are recommended (45–47).

Initially, it was believed that benzyl alcohol was only toxic in neonates who received doses greater than 99 mg/kg (42), but it has been suggested that lower doses may be toxic, resulting in kernicterus and intraventricular hemorrhages (48, 49). Therefore, pharmaceutical preparations and fluids containing benzyl alcohol should be avoided in premature neonates.

Benzoic acid and sodium benzoate are added in low concentrations to various pharmaceutical preparations as bacteriostatic and fungistatic agents. Hypersensitivity reactions to benzoates have occurred when administered to allergic patients, such as those with asthma, those who do not tolerate aspirin, and those with a history of urticaria (44). Hyperbilirubinemia and systemic effects attributed to benzyl alcohol may occur in premature neonates because benzyl alcohol is metabolized to benzoic acid (44).

Propylene glycol is found as a solvent in some i.v. multiple vitamin preparations and a variety of pharmaceutical preparations for parenteral administration including phenytoin, digoxin, and diazepam. MacDonald et al. (50) noted that neonates who received MVI-12 (propylene glycol dose of approximately 3 g/day) versus those who received MVI concentrate (propylene glycol dose of approximately 300 mg/day) had a significant increase in seizures. In addition, infants in the first group suffered from hyperbilirubinemia and renal failure. (Although MVI concentrate is no longer on the market in the United States, it was used in the early 1980s.)

Serum hyperosmolality has been reported in infants who received vitamin preparations (51), and in burn patients due to the topical absorption of propylene glycol-containing products (52, 53). In addition, burn patients have experienced metabolic acidosis with a high anion gap, decreased ionized calcium concentrations, acute renal failure, and death from topical propylene glycol absorption (44, 54). Problems associated with the oral ingestion of propylene glycol-containing products by children include CNS depression, seizures, and cardiac dysrhythmias (55). Hypotension, cardiac dysrhythmias, respiratory depression, and seizures have occurred after the rapid administration of phenytoin that may be associated with the propylene glycol (56).

The American Academy of Pediatrics Committee on Drugs recommends that medications intended for pediatric use be ethanol free (57). If, because of stability or solubility problems with the active ingredients(s), liquid medications need ethanol as an ingredient, but they should

not contain more than 5% v/v ethanol (57). The Academy also recommends that the ingestion of a single dose of an ethanol-containing product by a pediatric patient should not result in blood ethanol concentrations greater than 25 mg/100 mL, the volume of a packaged liquid medication should be of a minimal amount so that its entire ingestion would not result in a lethal dose and safety closures should be on all medicinals containing greater than 5% v/v ethanol. In addition, the Academy suggests that children under 6 years of age who need an ethanol-containing OTC preparation be under medical supervision and that doses of any ethanol-containing product be spaced at intervals to avoid ethanol accumulation (57).

The Academy of Pediatrics made their recommendations concerning ethanol exposure from medications based on potential acute and chronic ethanol-related problems. Acutely, the coadministration of ethanol may alter drug adsorption or metabolism, and may result in drug interactions (e.g., increased sedation when taken with sedatives). Disulfiram-like reactions have occurred after the ingestion of an alcohol-containing medication or when an ethanol-containing product is used in conjunction with medications such as metronidazole, sulfonamides, chloramphenicol, or cefamandole (57). The CNS effects (muscle incoordination, a longer reaction time, behavioral changes) are the most commonly reported acute adverse reactions associated with ethanol ingestion. Such reactions have occurred with blood ethanol concentrations in the range of 1–100 mg/100 ml (57). Lethal ethanol doses in children occur at approximately 3 gm/kg although deaths due to ethanol-induced hypoglycemia have occurred at lower doses or because of interactions with other medications (57, 58). Chronic ethanol exposure may induce hepatic enzymes, and may thus alter the clearance of drugs such as phenytoin, phenobarbital, and warfarin (59). Examples of other additives that have been problematic in pediatric patients include lactose (55), tartrazine dyes (44, 55) and sulfites (55).

It is therefore important for health care professionals, and especially those who are responsible for selecting and administering medications to premature neonates, to examine pharmaceutical preparations for the presence of inactive ingredients as well as for the active drug. The provision of medications should be based on choosing the safest preparations possible. Various brands of medications should be compared to ensure that products without hazardous excipients. In the hospital setting, pharmacy and therapeutics committees and the pharmacy department play important roles in this process because they compare pharmaceutical preparations for formulary selection. In the outpatient setting, physicians and pharmacists must responsibly select the most appropriate brand of a particular medication. Kumar et al. (60) recommend that labeling for pharmaceutical products should include the names and the amounts of excipients as well as active ingredients to help health care professionals select appropriate drug products for neonates.

INTRAVENOUS ADMINISTRATION

Without being properly instructed about methods used for administering i.v. medications to pediatric patients, health care personnel may give a medication incorrectly, resulting in an inappropriate or unexpected therapeutic response. Therefore, it is important that health care personnel (nurses, physicians, pharmacists) understand how medications are administered by this route.

The i.v. route is most frequently chosen for medication delivery when a patient's clinical condition requires that a medication be administered by the most expeditious and complete method possible. In addition, some drugs are only available for i.v. administration. Although this route is the most reliable for drug delivery to the systemic circulation, problems can occur that reduce and/or delay medication delivery because of the product selected, dosage volume needed, or frequency of administration, but problems can also be associated with the i.v. delivery system used. The latter occur most frequently when a small medication volume is administered at a slow rate as is often needed for a neonate or young infant. A brief discussion of problems associated with i.v. drug delivery to pediatric patients is given here. A thorough overview of i.v. drug administration to pediatric patients is provided in Refs. (61 and 62).

Disposable IV Equipment, Effects on Drug Delivery

Infusion rates and location of injection sites

The first article to explore problems that can occur with i.v. drug delivery to pediatric patients was published in 1979 by Gould and Roberts (63). They demonstrated in their study using an in vitro system for drug administration (Fig. 1) that infusion rates as well as the location of the injection sites in the i.v. infusion system influence the infusion profile of i.v. administered medications. Figure 1 shows the effects of different i.v. fluid rates on the length of time to infuse 95% of a gentamicin dose administered at various sites in the infusion system (63). It was reported that at a slow infusion rate of 3 ml/h, a drug takes longer to be infused and that the time for infusion time depends on the site of administration (i.e., the further the drug

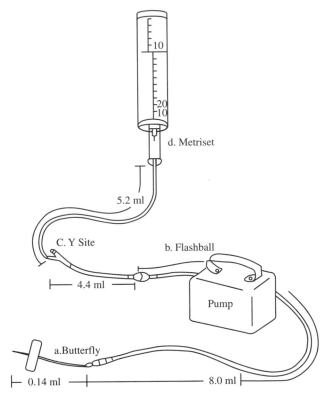

Fig. 1 Intravenous administration system used by Gould and Roberts. (From Ref. 63.)

injection from a patient, the longer to administer 95% of the medication, see Figs. 2,3). Thus, it took approximately 400 min to infuse gentamicin at an infusion rate of 3 ml/h via a Y-site in the administration system. However, the same drug administered at a butterfly injection site at the same fluid flow rate reduced the length of time to administer 95% of the drug to less than 20 min. Gould and Roberts also stated that the time needed for drug administration in their i.v. system was longer than what had been expected (63).

Type of injection site

Leff and Roberts (61) demonstrated that the amount of drug received by a pediatric patient and the drug-delivery rate are influenced by the type of injection site (Y-site, T-type, T-connector, stopcock, etc.) and the volume (dead space) contained in the particular site. For the delivery of small dosage volumes (less than 1 ml) i.v. tubing should have microinjection sites that prevent a drug from being sequestered in the injection site. In addition, the amount of i.v. fluid needed to adequately flush microinjection sites to clear the medication would be less than needed to flush injection sites found on tubing used to administer drugs to adults.

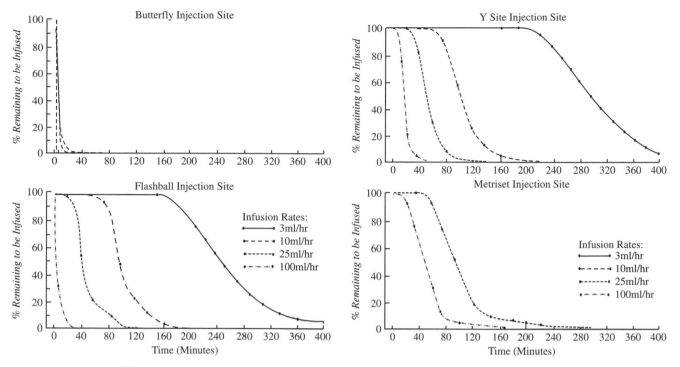

Fig. 2 Influence of i.v. flow rate on the infusion profile of gentamicin. (From Ref. 61.)

Fluid flow dynamics

Another characteristic of i.v. tubing that affects drug delivery is fluid flow dynamics. It appears that flow in i.v. tubing is best characterized by laminar flow, and the radius of the tubing. Poiseuille's law describes flow in i.v. tubing as

$$\frac{q_v = Pr^4}{4nL} \tag{2}$$

where q_v is the volumetric flow rate, P is the pressure change in the i.v. tubing, r is the radius of the i.v. tubing, n is the viscosity of the fluid, and L is the length of the i.v. tubing.

Thus, for i.v. delivery to pediatric patients, microbore tubing with an intraluminal diameter of <0.06 in. should be used rather than macrobore tubing. The use of microbore tubing allows the use of longer tubing lengths without significantly increasing delivery time.

Filters

A filter, especially one with a large reservoir volume, may prolong and/or reduce drug delivery. This occurs if the drug and its diluent are of different densities and there is a layering out of the drug in the filter (64). Therefore, a filter with a smaller reservoir volume should be selected.

Drug and Fluid Considerations for Intravenous Drug Administration

Characteristics of the drug and the fluid such as drug volume, osmolality, pH, and density may affect i.v. drug delivery. The frequency and duration of drug administration is also important as is the need for the infusion system to handle multiple drugs. This may lead to drug incompatibilities and problems in medication scheduling.

Osmolality and pH

Osmolality and pH must be considered when preparing a drug solution for i.v. administration to pediatric patients. Problems such as tissue irritation, pain on injection, phlebitis, electrolyte shifts, and even intraventricular hemorrhages in neonates have been associated with the administration of drug solutions with high osmolalities (65). Drug solutions should have osmolalities similar to serum osmolality, if possible. To control the osmolality, a drug can be diluted with a vehicle selected for i.v. infusion via a syringe infusion system (65) or the i.v. flow rate can be adjusted to achieve a particular drug-vehicle osmolality (61).

Density

If the density of a drug is significantly different from that of the diluent, the drug may layer out on the filter or in the i.v. tubing. The latter occurs more frequently if macrobore tubing, a low flow rate, the i.v. system, or if the tubing is in a particular position. A density problem can be avoided by using microbore tubing which promotes mixing; this is especially important when i.v. flow rates are low, as are needed for neonates or young infants.

Frequency and Duration of Drug Administration; Multiple Drugs

To ensure that frequent doses are administered at appropriate intervals or that multiple drugs are administered to avoid drug incompatibilities, a syringe infusion pump can be used to administer drug volumes over a specific length of time. This helps avoid a situation where part of a drug dose is left in the tubing when the i.v. set is changed, as has been reported for manual administration techniques. More than one syringe pump can be used to simultaneously administer compatible drugs in a parallel system into a micro-Y-site or stopcock.

Types of Intravenous Administration

Drugs may require i.v. administration as continuous infusions or at intervals (q4h, q6h, q12h, etc.). Manual methods require the administration of the drug into the i.v. system at an injection site (Y-site, T-connector, stopcock, etc.), added to the i.v. solution in a mixing chamber, or added to an i.v. bag to be administered via gravity. A syringe pump or another mechanical device may be used for drug administration.

Manual administration

Manual administration is not as accurate as using a syringe pump for drug administration. It has been used for small volumes of medication (< 3 ml), a low flow rate (< 20 ml/h), or if the antegrade (forward toward the patient) injection of a drug bolus is safe (61). If a medication is to be administered antegrade, it should be administered slowly into a microinjection site toward the patient; microbore tubing should be placed between the injection site and the patient to reduce the time to get the drug to the patient. Leff and Roberts (61) recommended that the volume of the drug to be injected by the antegrade technique should be a smaller volume than the tubing fluid volume between the injection site and the patient. If the medication volume is too large to be safely given by antegrade administration, but the i.v. fluid flow rate is low (< 20 ml/h), the drug may be administered by a retrograde technique (Fig. 3).

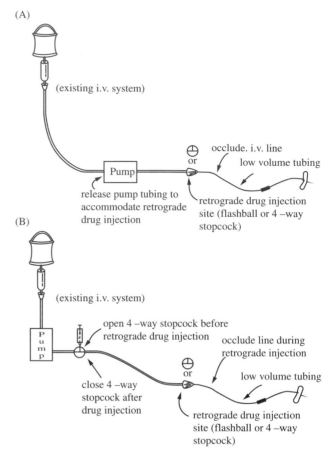

Fig. 3 Examples of retrograde system setups. (From Leff, R.D.; Roberts, R.J. Methods for intravenous drug administration in the pediatric patient. J. Pediatr. 1981, *98*, 631–635.)

Mechanical system for drug administration

If a mechanical system is chosen for drug administration, the appropriate infusion device must be selected based on its operating mechanism, flow accuracy, flow continuity, and ability to detect occlusions. Other important factors include an alarm system, ease of operation, ability to be cleaned easily, and safety from children inadvertently trying to change pump settings. A syringe pump is best for delivering small dosage volumes and when intermittent intervals are needed for medications. It is the mechanical device most often selected for medication administration because it can be used for intermittent administration of small and large doses, or for the continuous infusion of medications at low rates. A drug can be administered separately from the primary i.v. fluid flow rate, with the drug and the fluid mixing for a short distance therefore in microbore tubing (see Fig. 4) before reaching the patient. In addition to being able to more accurately deliver medications than by manual methods,

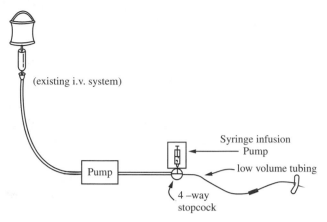

(existing i.v. system)

Syringe infusion
Pump

Pump

low volume tubing

4 –way
stopcock

Fig. 4 Syringe pump setup with drug administered separately of the primary i.v. fluid flow rate. Mixing of the drug and i.v. fluid occurs at a stopcock and for a short distance in microbore tubing. (From Leff, R.D.; Roberts, R.J. Methods for intravenous drug administration in the pediatric patient. J. Pediatr. 1981, *98*, 631–635.)

syringe pump systems have the advantage of being able to separate the administration of incompatible drugs, reduce difficulties associated with the administration of multiple doses, and shorten the time required to administer medications.

Additional Comments about IV Drug Administration

Reed and Gal (6) recommended the following steps to decrease problems associated with i.v. drug administration to pediatric patients:

1. Standardize and document total time for drug administration.
2. Document the volume of any solution used to flush an i.v. dose.
3. Standardize infusion techniques for drugs administration, especially for those with a narrow therapeutic index.
4. Use the largest gauge cannula that can be used.
5. Standardize dilution and infusion volumes for drugs given by intermittent i.v. injection, and avoid attaching lines for drug infusion to a central hub with solutions infused at widely disparate rates, and
6. Use low-volume i.v. tubing and use the most distal sites for drug administration.

In addition, one must remember that for infants the amount of fluid required for drug administration may take away from the amount of fluid available for nutrition. Thus, with medication administration, the fluid volume must be as restrictive as possible so that the bulk of the daily fluid intake can be saved for nutrition. Health care providers must closely monitor daily fluid intake from all sources to prevent fluid overload and must also watch the osmolality of medications with diluents.

ADMINISTRATION OF ORAL MEDICATIONS

The oral route is typically the preferred route for medication administration to pediatric patients. Other routes may be used, if the patient cannot take a medication orally because of vomiting, being unable to swallow, or the medication is unavailable for oral use. In addition, for specific problems it may be better to deliver the medication directly to the area being treated, for example, inhalation, ophthalmic administration, or otic administration.

Dosage Forms

Oral liquids

Liquid medications are the most commonly administered oral medications to pediatric patients because of the ease of swallowing by infants and young children who cannot swallow solid dosage forms. However, availability of some medications as liquid formulations may be limited. If not available in liquid form, a solid dosage form may need to be modified by the pharmacist, other health care provider, or by the parent. If a solid dosage form is modified, for example a suspension is prepared, will the drug be stable and for how long, and will it be absorbed differently than the original dosage form? These are just a few questions that must be answered about the extemporaneous preparation of a drug product for a pediatric patient.

Alcohol-free products should be selected for pediatric patients whenever possible. Furthermore, the inactive ingredients or excipients contained in an oral preparation should be identified. this is especially important if the patient is known to have had an adverse reaction to a particular excipient or there is another reason to avoid a particular additive in a medication. The Committee on Drugs of the American Academy of Pediatrics recommended that pharmaceutical products contain a qualitative listing of inactive ingredients in order that products containing these substance could be avoided in patients who had problems with specific adjuvants (55). Kumar et al. (60) contains lists of inactive ingredients (sweeteners, flavorings, dyes, and preservatives) found in

Table 3 Osmolalities of liquid pharmaceuticals for oral administration

Liquid preparation	Osmolality (Mean ± SEM)
Propylene glycol	8326 ± 1467
Saccharin-containing drugs	
Albuterol	65
Haloperidol	47
Suspensions	2500 ± 246
Sugar-containing[a] drugs	5574 ± 594

[a]Sucrose, mannitol, glucose, and others.
(From Ref. 66.)

many liquid medications such as analgesics, antipyretics, antihistamine decongestants, cough and cold remedies, antidiarrheal agents, and theophylline preparations. The authors of the previous article and Golightly et al. have reviewed adverse effects associated with many inactive ingredients (44, 60).

Liquid medications, taken orally, can cause diarrhea and other GI symptoms, or they may aggravate GI distress that a patient is already experiencing. These GI effects can be associated with the high osmolality of some oral liquids. Osmolalities have been determined for various oral liquids (66). For preparations containing propylene glycol, or various sugars (e.g., sucrose, mannitol, glucose), osmolalities were noted to be high (see Table 3). It is important to compare various brands of liquid medications because they may contain different excipients and may have different osmolalities.

Sustained-Release Preparations

Most medications have shorter half-lives in children than in adults, and therefore children may need sustained-release products to maintain serum concentrations in the therapeutic range. For example, a sustained-release theophylline product may be needed for a child with asthma. It may need to be administered every 8 h to the child as compared to every 12 h for a healthy, nonsmoking adult to maintain therapeutic serum concentrations. When choosing a sustained-release theophylline preparation for a child, it must be remembered that because of differences in release properties, theophylline sustained-release products are not interchangeable. A product selected for the pediatric asthma patient should be reliably absorbed with a minimal serum concentration variation and not a preparation that has exhibited a difference in bioavailability when administered with or without food (67–69).

Extemporaneous liquid preparations

Because many medications are not available as liquid preparations, there are times when powder papers or suspensions must be prepared. An excellent information source about the preparation of liquid dosage forms for pediatric patients has been published by Nahata and Hipple (Nahata, M. C., Hipple, T. F. Pediatric Drug Formulations, 4th Ed. Harvey Whitney Books: Cincinnati, 2000).

Product selection

Products for oral administration should be in a dosage form most readily taken by the child. If the child is old enough to participate in the decision-making process, he or she may state a preference for a liquid, chewable tablet, tablet, or capsule, if the needed drug is available in a variety of dosage forms and appropriate dosage. If a liquid medication is needed, a product should be chosen based on texture, taste, and ease of administration. Other factors that must be considered are the absence of alcohol and dyes, and an osmolality that is close to physiologic (280–290 mOsm/kg). Are there excipients or adjuvants in the product, and if so, what are they and what is their concentration? Is there bioavailability information or pharmacokinetic information for the oral medication in pediatric patients, and if so, in what age groups? Is there information about the extemporaneous product that is to be prepared?

Rebecca Chater, a North Carolina pharmacist, recommends that pediatric patients be involved in medication counseling in order to improve their understanding of why a medication is needed. In the counseling process, the word medication should be used and not drug because of the connotation associated with the latter in today's society (70, 71). Wheeler recommends that, when possible, a product be selected that requires the fewest number of doses administered per day, for example, every 12 h dosing rather than every 8 h, so the medication does not need to be taken to school or day care for administration. If a medication must be given outside of the home, she recommends that two small labeled bottles be dispensed or one large bottle with a small empty bottle labeled to be used for medication administration at day care or school.

Health care providers including nurses, pharmacists, and physicians should demonstrate to parents and older children how medications should be administered and offer appropriate dosing devices (oral syringe, dropper, cylindrical medication spoon, or a small-volume doser with attachable nipple) to enable parents to accurately measure liquid products. A household teaspoon or tablespoon should not be used for medication administration because they are inaccurate. Kraus and Stohlmeyer

(72) explain the use of a new oral liquid medication delivery system that can be used for infants and young children who still use a bottle for feeding.

Administration techniques

The following information is presented to help health care providers counsel parents and older children on how medication should be administered by various routes.

Oral liquids

An oral liquid medication needed for an infant or young child should be shaken well, if required, accurately using an appropriate device. If a dropper or an oral syringe is used, the liquid should be administered toward the inner cheek. Administration in the front of the mouth may allow the child to spit out the medication, whereas administration toward the back of the mouth may result in gagging or choking. The oral syringe should be of an appropriate size to allow for administration into the inner cheek.

Oral solid dosage forms

A medication available only as a solid dosage form, may be prepared as an extemporaneous liquid (e.g., suspension) or it may be modified for oral use, for example, by crushing. As mentioned previously, a sustained-release product should not be crushed or chewed. For a solid, nonsustained-release medication, the product can be crushed and mixed with a small amount of food just prior to administration. Examples of foods that may be used for mixing include applesauce, yogurt, or instant pudding, but the medication should not be added to an entire dish of food or to infant formula, because the infant or child may not eat/drink the entire portion and thus not receive the total amount of medication.

OTHER ROUTES

Intramuscular Administration

Absorption of i.m. administered medications depends on the injection site because perfusion of individual muscle groups differs. For example, drug absorption from the deltoid muscle is faster than that from the vastus lateralis that is more rapid than from the gluteus (16, 17). In addition, lower perfusion or hemostatic decompensation, frequently observed in ill neonates and young infants, may reduce i.m. absorption. It may also be decreased in neonates who receive a skeletal muscle-paralyzing agent such as pancuronium because of decreased muscle contraction.

In addition, the smaller muscle mass of neonates and young infants provides a small absorptive area.

The injection technique and the length of the needle used may affect drug absorption, and thus serum concentrations. For example, using a longer needle ($1^{1}/_{2}$ vs. $1^{1}/_{4}$ in. or 3.8 vs. 3.1 cm.) for i.m. administration resulted in higher diazepam serum concentrations in adults (18). Therefore, it is important to select the appropriate site for drug administration as well as the appropriate length and needle bore. Sites that can be used for i.m. administration include anterior thigh and vastus lateralis, gluteal area and deltoid.

The midanterior thigh (rectus femoris) and the middle third of the vastus lateralis are used for i.m. administration to young infants as well as to older children (19). These sites are better developed and larger than other muscle groups that are used for drug administration to older children or adults. The technique is shown in Fig. 5 (19). With the patient lying supine, the "needle should be inserted in the upper lateral quadrant of the thigh, directed inferiorly at an angle of 45° with the long axis of the leg and posteriorly at a 45° angle" (19) to the surface on which the patient is lying. The person administering the injection should compress the tissues of the injection site to help stabilize the extremity. A 1-in. (2.5-cm) needle has been recommended for pediatric patients by Bergeson et al. (19) while Newton et al. (18) recommend a 23–26 gauge 11/2-in. (3.8-cm) needle. The volume of drug that can be administered in this manner is 0.1–1 ml in infants and 0.1–5 ml in older children and adults (18).

The gluteal musculature develops as the infant or child increases his or her mobility; it becomes a more suitable injection site in children who are walking (18, 19). Damage to the sciatic nerve is the major problem associated with this injection site, and it occurs more commonly in infants because of their lack of gluteal muscle mass (73). Injury to the gluteal nerve, resulting in muscle atrophy, has occurred even when the injection technique was appropriately performed (19). Other nerves including the pudendal, posterior femoral cutaneous, and the inferior cluneal nerves have been damaged because of poor injection technique (19). Additional adverse effects associated with this drug administration route are discussed by Bergeson et al. (19).

A technique for gluteal administration is shown in Fig. 6 although other techniques are also used (19). All techniques involve the determination of the upper outer quadrant (see Fig. 6 for anatomical landmarks). After the location of the upper outer quadrant is determined, the needle should be inserted at a 90° angle to the surface on which the patient is lying, not to the patient's skin (19). This site can be used for older children. A 1-in. (2.5-cm)

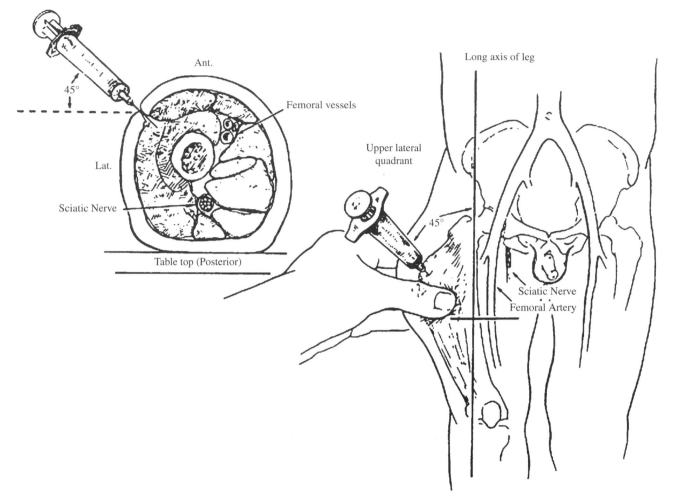

Fig. 5 A technique for anterior lateral-thigh intramuscular injection. (From Ref. 19.)

needle has been recommended (19). The volume of drug that can be administered in this manner is 0.1–5 ml for older children and adults (18).

The ventrogluteal (gluteus medius and minimus) site may be less hazardous for i.m. administration than the dorsogluteal (gluteus maximus) site (19). The technique is shown in Fig. 7 (19). The person administering a drug i.m. ventrogluteally should first note the anatomical landmarks (anterior superior iliac spine, tubercle of the iliac crest, and upper border of the greater trochanter). The needle is inserted into a triangular area bounded by these landmarks while the patient is in the supine position. The location for this injection can be determined "by placing the palm over the greater trochanter, the index finger over the anterior superior iliac spine, and spreading the index and middle fingers as far as possible" (19).

The deltoid muscle can be used for i.m. injections in older children, but it is not an option for young infants and children because of their limited muscle mass. Although

there are few complications associated with this administration route, nerve injury can occur (21). The technique is shown in Fig. 8 (19). The area for deltoid administration should be fully visible so that the anatomical landmarks can be visualized. Then the needle for deltoid injection should enter the muscle halfway between the acromium process and the deltoid tuberosity to avoid hitting the underlying nerves (19). The drug volume that can be administered by this route to older children and adults is 0.1–2 ml (18). The recommended needle length for older children is 1 in. (2.5 cm).

Subcutaneous Administration

The s.c. route is used for drug administration, such as insulin, that requires slow absorption. It is not commonly employed for medication administration for pediatric patients but is used for specific drugs. Typically a 1/2- or 1-in. (1.25- or 2.5-cm) needle is used with the volume of

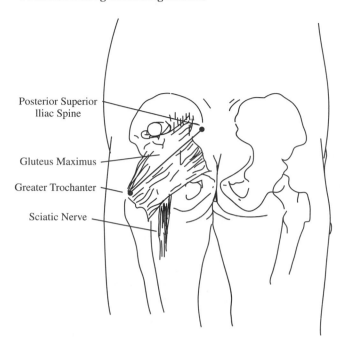

Fig. 6 A technique for gluteal-area intramuscular injection. (From Ref. 19.)

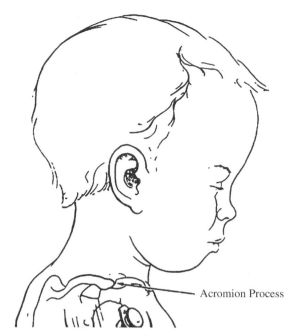

Fig. 8 A technique for deltoid intramuscular injection. (From Ref. 19.)

drug that can be administered by this route ranging from 0.1 to 1 ml (drug volume administered depends on patient size).

Percutaneous Administration

The skin should be thoroughly cleaned prior to applying a topical ointment, cream, etc. A thin layer of ointment or

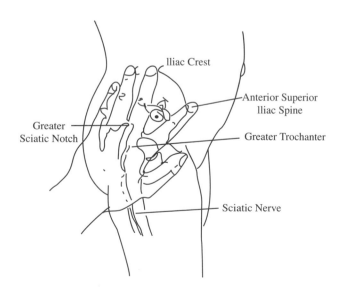

Fig. 7 von Hochstetter technique for ventrogluteal intramuscular injection. (From Ref. 19.)

cream should be applied to the prescribed area to reduce the possibility of a toxic reaction. The area of the skin where the medication is applied should not be covered or occluded unless instructed to do so by the physician because this procedure may increase drug absorption. Specific information should be given on how to cover the area.

Rectal Administration

Before the administration of a rectal suppository, the child's rectal area should be thoroughly cleaned. The infant or child should be placed on his or her side or stomach. The wrapper should be removed from the suppository and its pointed end should be inserted into the rectum above the anal sphincter. (If only half a suppository is prescribed, the suppository should be cut lengthwise before administration.) A finger cot or finger wrapped in plastic can be used for administering the suppository (74). Because an infant or small child cannot adequately retain a suppository in the rectum, the buttocks can be held together firmly for a few minutes after rectal administration to hold the suppository in place (74).

Otic Administration

Otic preparations should be at room temperature prior to administration. If the otic product is a suspension, it should be gently shaken for approximately 10 sec. before administration (74). The child should be lying on his or her side, and the earlobe should be gently pulled down and back to straighten the outer ear canal (for adults the earlobe is pulled up and back). Then the prescribed number of drops should be instilled into the ear without placing the dropper in the ear canal. The patient should be kept in a position with the ear tilted for approximately 2 min to help keep the drops in the ear (75). This procedure may be repeated for the treatment of the other ear, if needed. The tip of the dropper should wiped with a clean tissue after use.

Nasal Administration

For adults, the first step in administering nose drops or a nasal spray is blowing the nose to clear the nasal passages of mucus and other secretions, but infants and young children are unable to do this. Therefore, the nasal passages may need be cleared with a bulb syringe prior to medication administration. A child should lie down on his or her back, or a young infant or child should be placed in a lying position, and the head should be tilted slightly backwards. An appropriate amount of medication should then be placed in each nostril. Thereafter, the infant or child should remain quiet for a few minutes to allow the medication to be absorbed. The dropper should be rinsed with hot water before it is returned to the medication container.

Ophthalmic Administration

An ophthalmic medication should be at room temperature prior to administration. If the eye drops are in a suspension, the container should be gently shaken before administration. A child old enough to follow directions should tilt his or her head slightly backward and to the side so that the eye drops will not drain into the tear ducts near the nose. The eyelids should be separated and the patient should be asked to look up. The appropriate amount of medication is instilled into the lower eyelid, using the medication dropper, which should be accomplished without touching the eyelids. The patient should look downward for a few seconds after drug administration. The eye(s) should then be closed for several minutes in order to spread the medication across the eyeball and be absorbed if the effect is to be systemic (76). In addition, it has been recommended to gently put pressure on the inside corner of the eye for at least a minute to retard drainage of the medication (74). If a squeeze bottle is used, the appropriate amount of medication should be gently squeezed into the eye(s). For each of these methods, the dropper or the tip of the squeeze bottle should be kept away from the eye or skin to avoid contamination of the administration device (76). The

dropper should not rinsed after use because this could lead to contamination of the dropper and the medication. The package insert should be reviewed for specific information.

Another method for administering eyedrops to children recommends that the drops be applied to the inner canthus of the eye while the patient keeps his/her eyes closed until told to open them after medication administration (77). Approximately 66% of the medication administered in this fashion was absorbed. In addition, this method may increase compliance and make children more cooperative.

For the administration of an ophthalmic ointment to a child who can cooperate, the child should tilt his or her head backwards and look up. After the hands have been washed, the person to administer the medication should gently pull down the lower eyelid(s) for drug administration. A thin layer of ointment should then be placed in the lower eyelid(s). Afterwards, the eyelid(s) should be closed for 1 to 2 min to allow for the spreading of the medication and absorption. During this process, the tip of the ophthalmic applicator should not touch the eye. After administration is completed, the tip of the applicator tube should be cleaned with a clean tissue and be tightly capped (76). The package insert should also be reviewed for specific information.

Inhalers

For the use of an inhaled medication (e.g., β2-agonists, corticosteroids, antivirals, cromolyn, etc.), it is crucial for the child and parents to understand the mechanism of the metered dose inhaler (MDI) or nebulizer, if used. The package insert should also be reviewed for information about the specific drug product. A decision may also need to be made as to whether a spacer may be needed for use with the medication canister.

REFERENCES

1. Nahata, M.C. Pediatric Drug Formulations: Challenges and Potential Solutions. Ann. Pharmacother. **1999**, *33*, 247–249.
2. Food and Drug Administration. Regulations Requiring Manufacturers to Assess the Safety and Effectiveness of New Drugs and Biological Products in Pediatric Patients, 21 CFR Parts 201, 312, 314, and 601, Docket No. 97N-0165, U.S. Department of Health and Human Services; Washington, DC, August 17, 1997.
3. FDA Modernization Act of 1997 Public Law 105–115 105th Congress, Washington, DC, 1997.
4. Food and Drug Administration. List of Approved Drugs for Which Additional Pediatric Information May Produce Health Benefits in the Pediatric Population, Docket No. 98N-0056, U.S. Department of Health and Human Services: Washington, DC, May 20, 1998.

5.   USP Member Memorandum, U.S. Pharmacopoeia, Rockville, MD, June 22, 2000.

6.   Reed, M.D.; Gal, P. Principles of Drug Therapy. *Nelson Textbook of Pediatrics*, 16th Ed.; Behrman, R.E., Kliegman, R.M., Jenson, H.B., Eds.; W.B. Saunders Company: Philadelphia, 2000; 2229–2234.

7.   Reed, M.D. The Ontogeny of Drug Disposition: Focus on Drug Absorption, Distribution, and Excretion. Drug Inform. J. **1996**, *30*, 1129–1134.

8.   Milsap, R.L.; Hill, M.R.; Szefler, S.J. Special Pharmacokinetic Considerations in Children. *Applied Pharmacokinetics: Principles of Therapeutic Drug Monitoring*, 3rd Ed.; Evans, W.E., Schentag, J.J., Jusko, W.J., Eds.; Applied Therapeutics: Vancouver, WA, 1992; 10.1–10.32.

9.   Stewart, C.F.; Hampton, E.M. Effect of Maturation on Drug Disposition in Pediatric Patients. Clin. Pharm. **1987**, *6*, 548–564.

10. Christie, D.L. Development of Gastric Function during the First Month of Life. *Infancy*; Lebenthal, E., Ed.; Raven Press: New York, 1981; 109–120.

11. Cavell, B. Gastric Emptying in Preterm Infants. Acta Paediatr. Scand. **1979**, *68*, 725–730.

12. Cavell, B. Gastric Emptying in Infants Fed Human Milk or Infant Formula. Acta Pediatr. Scand. **1981**, *70*, 639–641.

13. Blumer, J.L.; Reed, M.D. Principles of Neonatal Pharmacology. *Pediatric Pharmacology: Therapeutic Principles in Practice*; Yaffe, S.J., Aranda, J.V., Eds.; W.B. Saunders Co.: Philadelphia, 1992; 164–177.

14. Lebenthal, E.; Lee, P.C.; Heitlinger, L.A. Impact of the Development of the GI Tract on Infant Feeding. J. Pediatr. **1983**, *101*, 1–9.

15. Kearns, G.L.; Reed, M.D. Clinical Pharmacokinetics in Infants and Children: A Reappraisal. Clin. Pharmacokinet. **1989**, *17* (Suppl. 1), 29–67.

16. Greenblatt, D.J.; Koch-Weser, J. Intramuscular Injection of Drugs. N. Engl. J. Med. **1976**, *295*, 542–546.

17. Evans, E.F.; Proctor, J.D.; Frantkin, M.J.; Velandia, J.; Wasserman, A.J. Blood Low in Muscle Groups and Drug Absorption. Clin. Pharmacol. Ther. **1975**, *17*, 44–47.

18. Newton, M.; Newton, D.; Fudin, J. Reviewing the Big Three Injection Routes. Nursing **Feb 1992**, *92*, 34–42.

19. Bergeson, P.S.; Singer, S.A.; Kaplan, A.M. Intramuscular Injections in Children. Pediatrics **1982**, *70*, 944–948.

20. Sagraves, R.; Kamper, C. Controversies in Cardiopulmonary Resuscitation: Pediatric Considerations. DICP, Ann. Pharmacother. **1991**, *25*, 760–772.

21. Ghadially, R.; Shear, N.H. Topical Therapy and Percutaneous Absorption. *Pediatric Pharmacology: Therapeutic Principles in Practice*; Yaffe, S.J., Aranda, J.V., Eds.; W.B. Saunders Co.: Philadelphia, 1992; 72–77.

22. American Academy of Pediatrics Committee on Drugs. Alternative Routes of Drug Administration—Advantages and Disadvantages (Subject Review). Pediatrics **1998**, *100*, 143–153.

23. McRorie, T. Quality Drug Therapy in Children: Formulations and Delivery. Drug Inform. J. **1996**, *30*, 1173–1177.

24. Ward, J.T., Jr. Endotracheal Drug Therapy. Am. J. Emerg. Med. **1983**, *1*, 71–82.

25. de Boer, A.G.; Moolenaar, F.; de Leede, L.G.J.; Breimer, D.D. Rectal Drug Administration: Clinical Pharmacokinetic Considerations. Clin. Pharmacokinet. **1982**, *7*, 285–311.

26. Iob, V.; Swanson, W.W. Mineral Growth of the Human Fetus. Am. J. Dis. Child **1934**, *47*, 302–306.

27. Widdowson, E.; Spray, C.M. Chemical Development in Utero. Arch. Dis. Child. **1951**, *26*, 205–214.

28. Morselli, P.L. Clinical Pharmacokinetics in Neonates. Clin. Pharmacokinet. **1976**, *1*, 81–98.

29. Reed, M.D.; Besunder, J.B. Developmental Pharmacology: Ontogenic Basis of Drug Disposition. Pediatr. Clin. North Am. **1989**, *36*, 1053–1074.

30. Kearin, M.; Kelly, J.G.; O'Malley, K. Digoxin "Receptors" In Neonates: An Explanation of Less Sensitivity to Digoxin in Adults. Clin. Pharmacol. Ther. **1980**, *28*, 346–349.

31. Levy, G.; Khanna, N.N.; Soda, D.M.; Tsuzuki, O.; Stern, L. Pharmacokinetics of Acetaminophen in the Human Neonate: Formation of Acetaminophen Glucuronide and Sulfate in Relation to Plasma Bilirubin Concentration and D-Glucaric Acid Excretion. Pediatrics **1975**, *55*, 818–825.

32. Siegel, S.R.; Oh, W. Renal Function as a Marker of Human Fetal Maturation. Acta Paediatr. Scand. **1976**, *65*, 481–485.

33. Siber, G.R.; Smith, A.L.; Levin, M.J. Predictability of Peak Serum Gentamicin Concentration with Dosage Based on Body Surface Area. J. Pediatr. **1978**, *94*, 135–138.

34. Painter, M.J.; Pippenger, C.E.; Wasterlein, C.; Barmada, M.; Pitlick, W.; Carter, G.; Aberin, S. Phenobarbital and Phenytoin in Neonatal Seizures: Metabolism and Tissue Distribution. Neurology **1981**, *31*, 1107–1112.

35. Gilman, J.T.; Gal, P.; Duchowny, M.S.; Weaver, R.L.; Ransom, J.L. Rapid Sequential Phenobarbital Treatment of Neonatal Seizures. Pediatrics **1989**, *83*, 674–678.

36. Gilman, J.T. Therapeutic Drug Monitoring in Neonate and Paediatric Age Group. Problems and Clinical Pharmacokinetic Implications. Clin. Pharmacokinet. **1990**, *19*, 1–10.

37. Tserng, K.Y.; Takieddine, F.N.; King, K.C. Developmental Aspects of Theophylline Metabolism in Premature Infants. Clin. Pharmacol. Ther. **1983**, *33*, 522–528.

38. Lonnerholm, G.; Lindstrom, B.; Paalzow, L.; Sedin, G. Plasma Theophylline and Caffeine and Plasma Clearance of Theophylline During Theophylline Treatment in the First Year of Life. Eur. J. Clin. Pharmacol. **1983**, *24*, 371–374.

39. Dreifuss, F.E.; Santilli, N.; Langer, D.H.; Sweeney, K.P.; Moline, K.A.; Menander, K.B. Valproic Acid Hepatic Fatalities: A Retrospective Review. Neurology **1987**, *37*, 379–385.

40. Gershanik, J.J.; Boecler, B.; George, W.; Sola, A.; Leitner, M.; Kapadia, C. The Gasping Syndrome: Benzyl Alcohol (BA) Poisoning. Clin. Res. **1981**, *29*, 895A, Abstract.

41. Brown, W.J.; Buist, N.R.M.; Gipson, H.T.C.; Huston, R.K.; Kennaway, N.G. Fatal Benzyl Alcohol Poisoning in a Neonatal Intensive Care Unit. Lancet **1982**, *1*, 1250, Letter.

42. Gershanik, J.J.; Boecler, B.; Ensley, H.; McCloskey, S.; George, W. The Gasping Syndrome and Benzyl Alcohol Poisoning. N. Engl. J. Med. **1982**, *307*, 1384–1388.

43. Benda, G.I.; Hiller, J.L.; Reynolds, J.W. Benzyl Alcohol Toxicity: Impact on Neurologic Handicaps Among Surviving Very Low Birth Weight Infants. Pediatrics **1986**, *77*, 507–512.

44. Golightly, L.K.; Smolinske, S.S.; Bennett, M.L.; Sutherland, E.W., III; Rumack, B.H. Pharmaceutical Excipients. Adverse Effects Associated with Inactive Ingredients in Drugs Products (Part I). Med. Toxicol. **1988**, *3*, 128–165.

45. American Academy of Pediatrics Committee on Fetus and Newborn and Committee on Drugs. Benzyl Alcohol: Toxic Agent in Neonatal Units. Pediatrics **1983**, *72*, 356–358.
46. Centers for Disease Control. Neonatal Death Associated with Use of Benzyl Alcohol—United States. MMWR **1982**, *31*, 290–291.
47. Benzyl Alcohol May be Toxic to Newborns. FDA Drug Bull. **1982**, *12*, 10–11.
48. Hiller, J.L.; Benda, G.I.; Rahatzad, M.; Alen, J.R.; Culver, D.H.; Carlson, C.V.; Reynolds, J.W. Benzyl Alcohol Toxicity: Impact on Mortality and Intraventricular Hemorrhage Among Very Low Birth Weight Infants. Pediatrics **1986**, *77*, 500–506.
49. Jadine, D.S.; Rogers, K. Relationship of Benzyl Alcohol to Kernicterus, Intraventricular Hemorrhage, and Mortality in Preterm Infants. Pediatrics **1989**, *83*, 153–160.
50. MacDonald, M.G.; Getson, P.R.; Glasgow, A.M.; Miller, M.K.; Boeckx, R.L.; Johnson, E.L. Propylene Glycol: Increased Incidence of Seizures in Low Birth Weight Infants. Pediatrics **1987**, *79*, 622–625.
51. Glascow, A.M.; Boeckx, R.L.; Miller, M.K.; MacDonald, M.G.; August, G.P. Hyperosmolality in Small Infants Due to Propylene Glycol. Pediatrics **1983**, *72*, 353–355.
52. Berkeris, L.; Baker, C.; Fenton, J.; Propylene Glycol as a Cause of an Elevated Serum Osmolality. Am. J. Clin. Pathol. **1979**, *72*, 633–636.
53. Fligner, C.L.; Jack, R.; Twiggs, G.A.; Raisys, V.A. Hyperosmolality Induced by Propylene Glycol. JAMA **1985**, *253*, 1606–1609.
54. Kulick, M.I.; Lewis, N.S.; Bansal, V.; Warpeha, R. Hyperosmolality in the Burn Patient: Analysis of an Osmolal Discrepancy. J. Trauma **1980**, *20*, 223–228.
55. American Academy of Pediatrics Committee on Drugs. "Inactive" Ingredients in Pharmaceutical Products. Pediatrics **1985**, *76*, 635–643.
56. Louis, S.; Jutt, H.; McDowell, F. The Cardiocirculatory Changes Caused by Intravenous Dilantin and Its Solvent. Am. Heart J. **1967**, *74*, 523–529.
57. American Academy of Pediatrics Committee on Drugs. Ethanol in Liquid Preparations Intended for Children. Pediatrics **1984**, *73*, 405–407.
58. Rumack, B.H.; Spoerke, D.G.; *Poisindex Information System*; Micromedex, Inc.: Denver, 2000.
59. Hoyumpa, A.M.; Schenker, S. Major Drug Interactions. Effect of Liver Disease, Alcohol, and Malnutrition. Ann. Rev. Med. **1982**, *33*, 113–149.
60. Kumar, A.; Rawlings, R.D.; Beaman, D.C. The Mystery Ingredients: Sweeteners, Flavorings, Dyes, and Preservative in Analgesic/Antipyretic, Antihistamine/Decongestant, Cough and Cold, Antidiarrheal, and Liquid Theophylline Preparations. Pediatrics **1993**, *91*, 927–933.
61. Leff, R.D.; Roberts, R.J.; *Practical Aspects of Intravenous Drug Administration*; American Society of Hospital Pharmacists: Bethesda, MD, 1992.
62. Nahata, M.C. Intravenous Infusion Conditions: Implications for Pharmacokinetic Monitoring. Clin. Pharmacokinet. **1993**, *24*, 221–229.
63. Gould, T.; Roberts, R.J. Therapeutic Problems Arising from the Use of the Intravenous Route for Drug Administration. J. Pediatr. **1979**, *95*, 465–471.
64. Rajchgot, P.; Radde, I.C.; MacLeod, S.M. Influence of Specific Gravity on Intravenous Drug Delivery. J. Pediatr. **1981**, *99*, 658–661.
65. Santeiro, M.L.; Sagraves, R.; Allen, L.V. Osmolality of Small-Volume I.V. Admixtures for Pediatric Patients. Am. J. Hosp. Pharm. **1990**, *47*, 1359–1364.
66. Bloss, C.S., Sybert, K. Osmolality of Commercially Available Oral Liquid Drug Preparations. In ASHP Annual Meeting June 1991; *48*, P-35 Abstract.
67. Maish, W.; Sagraves, R. Childhood Asthma. U.S. Pharmacist **1993**, Jan, *36–58, 105*.
68. Hendeles, L.; Weinberger, M.; Szefler, S. Safety and Efficacy of Theophylline in Children with Asthma. J. Pediatr. **1992**, *120*, 177–183.
69. Hendeles, L.; Weinberger, M. Selection of a Slow-Release Theophylline Product. J. Allergy Clin. Immunol. **1986**, *78*, 743–751.
70. Martin, S. Catering to Pediatric Patients. Am. Pharm. **1992**, *32*, 47–50.
71. Chater, R.W. Pediatric Dosing: Tips for Tots. Am. Pharm. **1993**, *33*, 55–56.
72. Kraus, D.M.; Stohlmeyer, L.A.; Hannon, P.R. Infant Acceptance and Effectiveness of a New Oral Liquid Medication Delivery System. Am. J. Health-Syst. Pharm. **1999**, *56*, 1094–1101.
73. Gilles, F.H.; Matson, D.D. Sciatic Nerve Injury Following Misplaced Gluteal Injection. J. Pediatr. **1970**, *76*, 247–254.
74. Administration Guides. Drug Store News **1993**, Dec *13*, 7–14.
75. Otic Preparations Monograph. *Facts and Comparisons*; Olin, B.R., Ed.; J.B. Lippincott Co.: St. Louis, November 1992; 517.
76. Topical Ophthalmic Monograph. *Facts and Comparisons*; Olin, B.R., Ed.; J.B. Lippincott Co.: St. Louis, May 1993; 477b–477c.
77. Smith, S.E. Eyedrop Instillation for Reluctant Children. Br. J. Ophthalmol. **1991**, *75*, 480–481.

BIBLIOGRAPHY

Benitz, W.E., Tatro, D.S., Davis, S., Eds. *The Pediatric Drug Handbook*, 3rd Ed.; Harcourt Health Sciences Group: St. Louis, 1995.

Leff, R.D.; Roberts, R.J. *Practical Aspects of Intravenous Drug Administration*; American Society of Health-System Pharmacists: Bethesda, 1992.

Nahata, M.C.; Hipple, T.F. *Pediatric Drug Formulations*, 4th Ed.; Harvey Whitney Books: Cincinnati, 2000.

Nelson, J.; Bradley, J. *Nelson's 2000–2001 Pocket Book of Pediatric Antimicrobial Therapy*, 14th Ed.; Lippincott Williams & Wilkins: Philadelphia, 2000.

Phelps, S.; Hak, E. *Guidelines for Administration of Intravenous Medications to Pediatric Patients*, 6th Ed.; American Society of Health-System Pharmacists: Bethesda, 1999.

Siberry, G.K., Iannone, Eds.; *Harriett Lane Handbook*, 15th Ed.; Mosby: St. Louis, 2000.

Taketomo, C.K.; Hodding, J.H.; Kraus, D.M.; *Pediatric Dosage Handbook*, 5th Ed.; Lexi-Comp., Inc.: Hudson, OH, 2000.

Young, T.; Mangum, B.; *Neofax 2000*, 13th Ed.; Blackwell Science: Oxford, 2000.

PELLETIZATION TECHNIQUES

Isaac Ghebre-Sellassie
Pfizer Global Research and Development, Morris Plains, New Jersey

Axel Knoch
Pfizer Global Research and Development, Freiburg, Germany

INTRODUCTION

Historically, the term *pellet* has been used by a number of industries to describe a variety of agglomerates produced from diverse raw materials, using different pieces of manufacturing equipment. These agglomerates include fertilizers, animal feeds, iron ores, and pharmaceutical dosage units and thus do not only differ in composition but also encompass different sizes and shapes. As a result, pellets meant different things for different industries. In the pharmaceutical industry, pellets can be defined as small, free-flowing, spherical particulates manufactured by the agglomeration of fine powders or granules of drug substances and excipients using appropriate processing equipment. The term also has been used to describe small rods with aspect ratios of close to unity. Although pellets have been used in the pharmaceutical industry for more than 4 decades, it has only been since the late 1970s, with the advent of controlled-release technology, that the advantages of pellets over single-unit dosage forms have been realized.

Pellets offer a high degree of flexibility in the design and development of oral dosage forms. They can be divided into desired dose strengths without formulation or process changes and also can be blended to deliver incompatible bioactive agents simultaneously and/or to provide different release profiles at the same or different sites in the gastrointestinal (GI) tract. In addition, pellets, taken orally, disperse freely in the GI tract, maximize drug absorption, minimize local irritation of the mucosa by certain irritant drugs, and reduce inter- and intrapatient variability (1).

Given the enormous advantages of multiparticulate systems over single-unit oral dosage forms, extensive research has focused recently on refining and optimizing existing pelletization techniques as well as on the development of novel manufacturing approaches that use innovative formulations and processing equipment. The most commonly used and intensely investigated pelletization processes are powder layering, solution/suspension layering, and extrusion–spheronization and are defined first and then addressed in detail.

Powder layering involves the deposition of successive layers of dry powder of drug or excipients or both on preformed nuclei or cores with the help of a binding liquid. Because powder layering involves the simultaneous application of the binding liquid and dry powder, it generally requires specialized equipment. The primary equipment-related requirement in a powder-layering process is that the product container should have solid walls with no perforations to avoid powder loss beneath the product chamber before the powder is picked up by the wet mass of pellets that is being layered on.

Solution/suspension layering involves the deposition of successive layers of solutions and/or suspensions of drug substances and binders on starter seeds, which may be inert materials or crystals/granules of the same drug. In principle, the factors that control coating processes apply to solution or suspension layering and, as a result, require basically the same processing equipment. Consequently, conventional coating pans, fluid-bed centrifugal granulators, and Wurster coaters have been used successfully to manufacture pellets. The efficiency of the process and the quality of pellets produced are in part related to the type of equipment used.

Extrusion–spheronization is a multistep process involving dry mixing, wet granulation, extrusion, spheronization, drying, and screening. The first step is dry mixing of the drug and excipients in suitable mixers followed by wet granulation, in which the powder is converted into a plastic mass that can be easily extruded. The extruded strands are transferred into a spheronizer, where they are instantaneously broken into short cylindrical rods on contact with the rotating friction plate and are pushed outward and up the stationary wall of the processing chamber by centrifugal force. Finally, owing to gravity, the particles fall back to the friction plate, and the cycle is repeated until the desired sphericity is achieved.

Other pelletization processes that either have limited application or are still at the development stage include

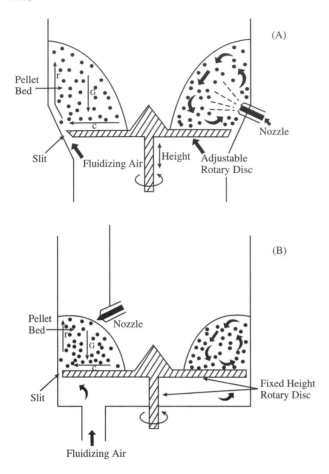

Fig. 1 Schematic representation of centrifugal fluid-bed equipment and process with a single-walled product chamber. (A) Glatt GPCG and GRG Granulators. (B) Freund CF-Granulators. (Adapted from Ref. 5).

spherical agglomeration or balling, spray congealing/drying, and emerging technologies such as cryopelletization and melt spheronization. These processes are addressed briefly.

POWDER LAYERING

The first equipment used to manufacture pellets on a commercial scale was the conventional coating pan, a machine that has been used by pharmaceutical firms, primarily for sugar coating, for a long time. During the 1950s, the industry, in an attempt to prolong the release of drugs from solid oral dosage forms, explored new processes that allowed the manufacture of multiparticulate drug-delivery systems. The turning point came when candy seeds, which had been used for topping decorations

in foodstuffs such as pastries, were used as starter seeds to develop and manufacture sustained-release pellets using conventional coating pans (2). The process was an extension of a procedure that was used to manufacture the candy seeds themselves and involved the successive layering of powder and binder solution on sugar crystals (3). Consequently, the conventional coating pan became the first pharmaceutical equipment used not only to manufacture nonpareils but also to develop sustained-release products of a number of prescription drugs using nonpareils as starter seeds.

Conventional coating pans, however, have had significant limitations as pelletization equipment. The degree of mixing is very poor, and the drying process is not efficient. Mixing is a function of the pan shape, the tilt angle, the baffle arrangement, and the rotational speed of the pan itself. These parameters must be optimized to provide uniform drying and sufficient particle movement to eliminate the potential formation of dead spots during the operation and to maximize yield. For instance, during pelletization, elliptical pans tend to have fewer stagnant spots than do cylindrical pans and, consequently, are the equipment of choice (4). Reducing the tilt angle can also minimize formation of dead spots. If the rotational speed of the pan is too slow, segregation may occur owing to percolation and induce the preferential layering of drug onto larger particles. In addition, prolonged contact time among the particles could favor particle agglomeration if the liquid feed rate leads to surface wetness and stickiness that induce coalescence.

During powder layering, a binding solution and a finely milled powder are added simultaneously to a bed of starter seeds at a controlled rate. In the initial stages, the drug particles are bound to the starter seeds and subsequently to the forming pellets with the help of liquid bridges originated from the sprayed liquid. These liquid bridges are eventually replaced by solid bridges derived either from a binder in the application medium or from any material, including the drug substance, that is soluble in the liquid. Successive layering of the drug and binder solution continues until the desired pellet size is reached. Throughout the process, it is extremely important to deliver the powder accurately at a predetermined rate and in a manner that maintains equilibrium between the binder liquid application rate and the powder delivery rate. If the powder delivery rate is not maintained at predetermined equilibrium levels, overwetting or dust generation may occur, and neither the quality nor the yield of the product can be maximized. Toward the end of the layering process, it is likely that fines may be generated owing to potential interparticle and wall-to-particle friction and appear in the final product, thereby lowering the yield. The problem can be overcome if the application medium is sprayed on the cascading pellets at the end of the layering process to increase the moisture level at the pellet surface and facilitate layering of the fines onto the pellets. Caution must be exercised, however, not to overwet the product bed because the powder–liquid equilibrium that has been established will change and will need to be adjusted accordingly. In an ideal process, no agglomeration occurs, and the particle population at the end of the process remains the same as that of the starter seeds or cores, with the only difference being an increase in the size of the pellets and thus in the total mass in the pan.

Pieces of equipment that overcame the limitations of coating pans and revolutionized powder-layering processing as a pelletization technique are tangential spray or centrifugal fluid-bed granulators. Although tangential spray equipment was originally developed to perform granulation processes, its application was later expanded

to cover other unit operations including the manufacture and coating of pellets.

Although there are variations in the design of centrifugal or rotary granulators, the basic operational principle that determines the degree of mixing and thus the efficiency of the process remains the same and includes centrifugal force, fluidization air velocity, and gravitational force (Fig. 1). During a layering process, these three forces act in concert to generate a spiral, rope-like motion of the particles in the product bed. The rotating disk, which may have fixed or variable speeds, creates a centrifugal force that pushes the particles outward to the vertical wall of the product chamber or stator. The fluidization air, which is directed toward the slit between the periphery of the disk and the stator, generates a force that carries the particles vertically along the wall of the product container into the expansion chamber. The particles lose their momentum and cascade down toward the center of the rotating disk owing to gravitational force. The cycle repeats itself, bringing about a thorough mixing unparalleled by any other powder-layering equipment. The degree of mixing depends on the fluidization air volume and velocity, the slit width, the bed size, and the disk speed. These variables, as well as liquid and powder application rates, atomization air pressure, fluidization air temperature, and degree of moisture saturation determine the yield and quality of pellets.

As mentioned earlier, the key process variable that determines the success of any pelletization process in centrifugal fluid-bed granulators is the degree of mixing, which is partly dictated by the radial velocity of the disk. At low radial velocities, the extent of mixing becomes inadequate, as indicated by the loss in the spiral rope-like motion of the particles. Thus, the rate at which the particles traverse the spray zone is prolonged and could potentially lead to excessive agglomeration. Caking is another serious problem encountered during powder layering at low radial velocities. At high radial velocities, the particle-to-particle and particle-to-wall frictional forces become intense with a very rapid pellet turnover. Generally, this condition leads to an uncontrollable, wobbly bed, resulting in severe particle attrition; that is, the breaking forces overcome the forces that contribute to particle growth through layering, and the pelletization process cannot proceed as intended. In such a situation, not only is a large amount of fines generated, but some of the attrited particles may agglomerate to form nuclei that are subsequently layered upon. Because the drug content of the pellets that contain inert starter seeds and those that use the newly formed nuclei are different, the process may create content uniformity problems. The optimum radial velocities of the disk are generally 3–8 m/s irrespective

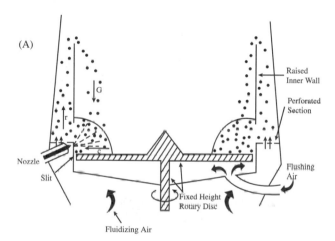

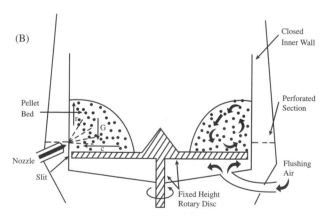

Fig. 2 Schematic representation of centrifugal fluid-bed equipment and process with a double-walled product chamber (Niro-Aeromatic). (A) open position. (B) closed position. (Adapted from Ref. 5.)

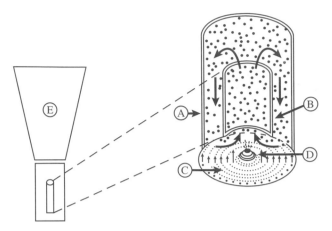

Fig. 3 Schematic representation of the Wurster product chamber and process. (A) product chamber. (B) partition. (C) orifice plate. (D) nozzle. (E) expansion chamber. (Adapted from Ref. 6.)

of the granulator size (6). At the initial stages of the pelletization process, the radial velocity may be kept low and increased as the mass of the batch size increases. After the layering process is completed, the radial disk velocity is usually reduced to avoid particle attrition during the drying step.

Another parameter that plays a key role during layering is the disk clearance or slit width. In some centrifugal granulators, the slit width is fixed, and the fluidization air velocity can be varied only with a change in the fluidization air volume. In others, the slit width is variable and is adjusted to meet the processing requirements. As the disk

clearance is increased, the air velocity decreases, and pellet turnover is reduced. Conversely, as disk clearance decreases, the air velocity increases, resulting in a rapid pellet turnover. Therefore, for maximum process efficiency, the disk clearance is chosen not only to avoid loss of pellets through the gap between the disk and the vertical wall into the plenum and to minimize the loss of powder into the exhaust system but also to generate an air velocity that provides the desired degree of pellet turnover.

Aside from the rotary disk, the other unique feature of the centrifugal equipment is the spray method. During layering, the liquid is sprayed tangentially to and concurrent with particle movement. This feature is primarily responsible for the high yield that is typically obtained from a process involving this type of equipment. The distance the droplets travel before they impinge on the particles is short, and consequently, the droplets are picked up by the particles almost completely with little, if any, loss to the wall of the product chamber or because of spray drying, assuming that the other process variables are optimized.

In addition, powder and binder liquid delivery rates are critical parameters that must be carefully evaluated. Because the surface moisture/solvent determines the extent of binding between the forming pellets and the powder being introduced, the powder delivery and the liquid application rates should be adjusted to establish an equilibrium conducive to layering. It is essential that the powder delivery remains well-controlled during processing, whether airflow is mediated by suction

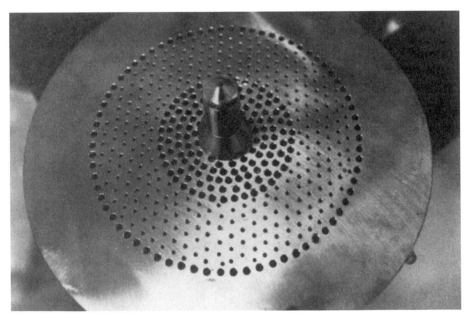

Fig. 4 Air distributer or orifice plate of a Wurster coater. (From Ref. 5.)

(negative pressure), as in the Glatt centrifugal granulators, or by positive air flow, as with the Freund CF granulators.

With a double-walled centrifugal granulator, the process is carried out with the inner wall in the open or closed position (Fig. 2) (7). With powder layering, the inner wall is closed so that simultaneous application of liquid and powder could proceed until the pellets have reached the desired size. The inner wall is then raised, and the spheres enter the drying zone. The pellets are lifted by the fluidization air up and over the inner wall back into the forming zone. The cycle is repeated until the desired residual moisture level in the pellets is achieved.

Scaling up of a layering process from the laboratory to production equipment is straightforward. As with all fluid-bed equipment, the most critical parameters that need to be met, in addition to the spiral rope-like motion of the particles, are the density of the particles and the droplet size within the spray zone. Because more than one spray gun is used in production equipment, it is imperative that the guns are positioned in such a way that optimum drying of the layered drug is attained before the pellets entering the next spray zone. Generally, the rate-limiting step in the process is saturation of the fluidization air by the application medium. Sometimes, it is likely that the spiral rope-like motion of the particles could be lost during scale up, and baffles must be inserted to enhance particle motion) (5).

As for formulation components, they also must meet certain requirements. Binder solutions must have a high binding capacity. Micronizing or finely milling the drug before layering improves the efficiency of the layering process significantly and provides morphologically smooth pellets that are suitable for film coating. However, in the majority of cases, micronization tends to impact flow and thus the delivery rate, a critical process parameter. Therefore, it is likely that during processing, powders may adhere to the sides of the hopper or the feed screw and may even form rat holes within the hopper. To improve the flow properties of the drug substance, glidants are incorporated into the powder before processing. Chemically, glidants could be hydrophobic or hydrophilic and are chosen based on the type of formulation selected.

Finally, the rheological properties of the binding liquid, the liquid application rate, and drying air temperature should be optimized to produce the desired product temperature. In addition, the powder should be delivered at a rate that maintains a balance between the surface wetness of the cores and powder adhesion. If the product bed temperature is high, powder is lost to the exhaust system. If it is too low, it leads to agglomeration and/or the formation of new nuclei that serve as cores for further layering. If that happens, content uniformity of the product

could be severely impacted. Therefore, the product temperature should be optimized to keep the particle population the same throughout the layering and subsequent drying steps.

SOLUTION/SUSPENSION LAYERING

The Wurster coating process, which was invented about 30 years ago, had evolved through elaborate design modifications and refinement into ideal equipment for the manufacture of pellets by solution/suspension layering. The high drying efficiency inherent in fluid-bed equipment, coupled with the innovative and efficient design features of the Wurster process, has allowed the machines to hold center stage in pharmaceutical processing technology. Not only have the manufacture and coating of pellets become routine and efficient, but scaling up of the process, which is key to the viability of any processing technique, has proved to be predictable and economically feasible.

The primary features that distinguish Wurster equipment from other fluid-bed equipment are the cylindrical partition located in the product chamber and the configuration of the air distributor plate, also known as the orifice plate (Figs. 3 and 4). The latter is configured to allow most of the fluidization or drying air to pass at high velocity around the nozzle and through the partition, carrying with it the particles that are being layered on. Once the particles exit the partition, they enter the expansion chamber, where the velocity of the air is reduced below the entrainment velocity, and the particles fall back to the area surrounding the partition (referred to as the down bed). The down bed is kept aerated by the small fraction of air that passes through the small holes on the periphery of the orifice plate. The particles in the down bed are transported horizontally through the gap between the air distributor plate and the partition by suction generated by the high air velocity that prevails around the nozzle and immediately below the partition. The volume of air that passes through the down bed outside the partition is just enough to generate modest particle movement. Because the spray direction is concurrent with particle movement, and particle motion is well-organized under optimum conditions, uniform layering of drug substances is consistently achieved. Because the partition height, that is, the gap between the partition and the orifice plate, controls the rate at which the particles enter the spray zone, it is an important variable that needs to be optimized for every batch size. For instance, at a given load size and fluidization air volume, the partition height can be reduced or increased to provide either a well-controlled particle motion that produces the desired pellet movement or a bubbling down bed that leads to disorganized particle movement and inefficient process.

The disadvantage of the Wurster process is the inaccessibility of the nozzles. If the nozzles are clogged at any time during the layering process, the operation has to be interrupted, and the spray guns must be removed for cleaning. The problem can be alleviated by screening the formulation or by using a spray gun with a bigger nozzle. Another aspect of the process that is challenging when multiple nozzles are used is the potential overlap of adjacent spray zones. Although the position of the nozzle is fixed, the spray zone overlap can be minimized using the air cap at the end of the spray gun.

During scale up, the number of partitions in the product container is increased with an increase in batch size; the diameter of the partitions, however, is kept the same. The intent is to maintain the particle movement and processing dynamics that were established during the development phase when a single partition was used. The fluidization air volume is increased to compensate for the increase in the number of spray zones and consequently to create well-organized particle movement in all partitions. If the fluidization air volume is too high,

it is likely to produce a disorganized bed that in turn adversely affects the layering process. The fluidization air volume is also critical because it, rather than the size of the batch, dictates the liquid application rate.

Another piece of equipment that has been used to manufacture pellets by solution/suspension layering is the tangential spray or centrifugal granulator. An important parameter that needs to be established early in the process is quantity of starter seeds or cores charged into the machine that should, at the minimum, cover the nozzles during start-up; otherwise, the sprayed liquid droplets will either be sprayed onto the wall of the product container or become entrained in the fluidization air. The latter could lead to clogging of the filters, which would then not only increase the pressure differential across the filters and compromise the batch but also may complicate equipment cleanup. In either case, the yield, and probably the quality of the pellets, will be reduced dramatically. As the size of the forming pellets increases, the mass in the bed increases, and the fluidization air volume is continuously increased to provide optimum expansion and mixing of the product bed, as indicated by the spiral rope-like motion of the bed. If such particle movement is not achieved, the bed load may be excessive, and the process may have to be terminated. During layering, the product bed expands both vertically and horizontally, and

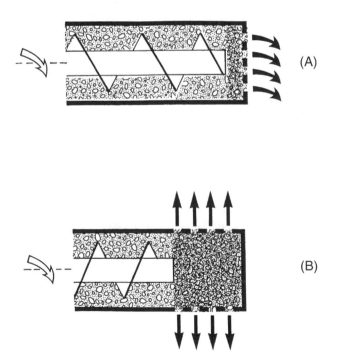

Fig. 5 Schematic representation of screw-fed extruders: (A) axial extruder. (B) radial extruder.

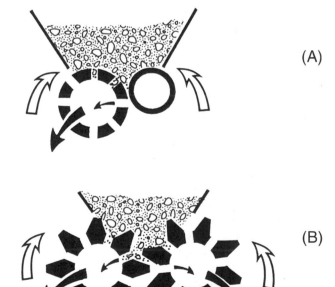

Fig. 6 Schematic representation of gravity-fed extruders: (A) rotary-cylinder extruder. (B) rotary-gear extruder.

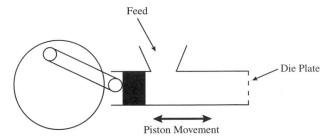

Feed

Die Plate

Piston Movement

Fig. 7 Schematic representation of a ram extruder. (From Ref. 9.)

consequently a several-fold increase in batch weight can be realized in a single step.

During processing, all the components of the formulation are first dissolved or suspended in an appropriate quantity of application medium to provide a formulation with the desired viscosity and is then sprayed onto the product bed. The sprayed droplets immediately impinge on the starter seeds and spread evenly on the surface, provided the drying conditions and fluid dynamics are favorable. This is followed by a drying phase that renders dissolved materials to precipitate and form solid bridges that would hold the formulation components together as successive layers on the starter seeds. The process continues until the desired quantity of drug substance and thus the target potency of the pellets are achieved. The rate of particle growth is rather slow and is limited by the rate of solvent removal. Furthermore, the sprayed droplets must have the necessary rheological properties to spread evenly over the cores, as with coating processes. This must be followed immediately by a very rapid evaporation of the application medium. The evaporation rate should neither impair binder effectiveness nor lead to overwetting and subsequent agglomeration. Ideally, no new nuclei are formed, and the particle population remains the same; however, the sizes of the pellets increase as a function of time, and as a result, the total mass of the system also increases.

Although optimization of process variables is critical for the successful development of a pelletized product, pellets can only be manufactured routinely on a large scale if the formulation is not sensitive to slight variations in processing parameters. Therefore, it is imperative that the formulation characteristics are carefully identified and optimized, both qualitatively and quantitatively, during the development phase. These include drug solubility, type and concentration of binder, and viscosity of the solution/suspension. The working viscosity range usually determines the solid content of the formulation that can be sprayed successfully onto the starter seeds and forming pellets.

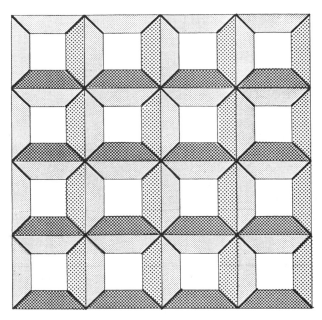

Fig. 8 Schematic representation of a spheronizer friction plate with a cross-hatch pattern.

Solution/suspension layering is usually used when the desired drug loading of the pellets is low because production of high-potency pellets from a low solids content formulation is not economically feasible. An important factor that needs to be considered when suspensions are used as opposed to solutions is the particle size of the drug. Micronized drug particles tend to provide pellets that are smooth in appearance, a property that is extremely desirable during subsequent film coating, particularly for controlled-release applications. If the particle size of the drug in the suspension is large, the amount of binder required to immobilize the particles onto the cores will be high, and, consequently, pellets of low potency are produced. The morphology of the finished pellets also tends to be rough and may adversely affect the coating process and the coated product. Moreover, because particles detach easily from the core they are being layered on owing to frictional forces, yield is usually low.

Although it is possible to manufacture pellets from a formulation that does not contain binders, almost invariably, the layers of drug applied tend to delaminate or break off from the cores in the later stages of the layering process or in the subsequent drying step. Therefore, binders are consistently used during solution/suspension layering to impart strength to the pellets. They are usually low-molecular-weight polymers that are compatible with the drug substance. They should not increase the viscosities of the formulations appreciably and should not, unless intended to do so, modify the release characteristics of the pellets.

EXTRUSION–SPHERONIZATION

Extrusion–spheronization as a pelletization technique was developed in the early 1960s and since then has been researched and discussed extensively. Interest in the technology is still strong, as witnessed by the extent of coverage of the topic in scientific meetings and symposium proceedings, as well as in the scientific literature. The technology is unique in that it is not only suitable for the manufacture of pellets with a high drug loading but it also can be used to produce extended-release pellets in certain situations in a single step and thus can obviate the need for subsequent film coating.

Extrusion–spheronization is a multistep process involving a number of unit operations and equipment. However, the most critical pieces of processing equipment that, in effect, dictate the outcome of the overall process are the extruders and the spheronizers (8).

A variety of extruders, which differ in design features and operational principles, are currently on the market and can be classified as screw-fed extruders, gravity-fed extruders, and ram extruders.

Screw-fed extruders have screws that rotate along the horizontal axis and hence transport the material horizontally; they may be axial or radial screw extruders (Fig. 5). Axial extruders, which have a die plate that is positioned axially, consist of a feeding zone, a compression zone, and an extrusion zone. The product temperature is controlled during extrusion by jacketed barrels. In radial extruders, the transport zone is short, and the material is extruded radially through screens mounted around the horizontal axis of the screws.

Gravity-fed extruders include the rotary cylinder and rotary gear extruders, which differ primarily in the design of the two counter-rotating cylinders (Fig. 6). In the rotary-cylinder extruder, one of the two counter-rotating cylinders is hollow and perforated, whereas the other cylinder is solid and acts as a pressure roller. In the so-called rotary-gear extruder, there are two hollow counter-rotating gear cylinders with counterbored holes.

In ram extruders, a piston displaces and forces the material through a die at the end (Fig. 7). Ram extruders are preferred during formulation development because they are designed to allow for measurement of the rheological properties of formulations (9–11).

Because extruders were initially developed to serve industries other than the pharmaceutical industry, they were

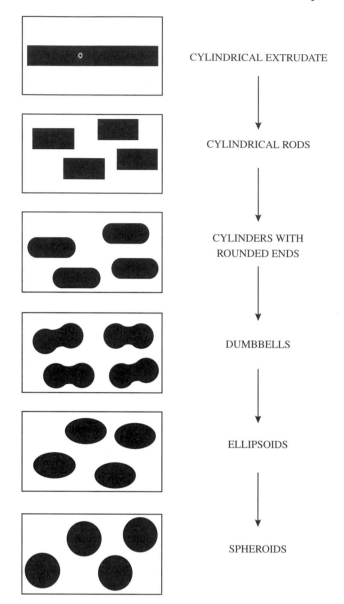

Fig. 9 Shape transitions during a spheronization process.

designed without GMP considerations. Therefore, changes are made to ensure pharmaceutical regulatory compliance, including qualification requirements. At the minimum, all the parts of the extruder that come in contact with the product must be of high-quality stainless steel, and the construction must be such that cleaning requirements are easily met. Whenever possible, the machine should permit easy monitoring and documentation of all critical process parameters such as pressure at the die plate, product temperature, power consumption or torque of the drive unit, and rotational speed of the screw. Some of the GMP requirements surroundings extruders have been highlighted in an article that described a qualification procedure for an extruder that is suitable for the manufacture of clinical samples (12).

The extrusion/spheronization process was first introduced to the pharmaceutical industry in 1964 with the invention of the marumerizer (13). Since then, significant improvements have been made to the machine, and currently well-designed marumerizers of different sizes are commercially available. A marumerizer or spheronizer consists of a static cylinder or stator and a rotating friction plate at the base. The stator can be jacketed for temperature control. The friction plate, which has a grooved surface, is the most critical part of the equipment that initiates the spheronization process. A typical friction plate has a crosshatch pattern, where the grooves intersect at a 90° angle, as shown in Fig. 8. The groove width is selected based on the desired pellet diameter. Usually, groove diameters 1.5–2 times the target pellet diameter are used. The diameter of the friction plate is approximately 20 cm for laboratory-scale equipment or up to 1.0 m for production-scale units. The rotational speed of the friction plate is variable and ranges from 100 to 2000 rpm, depending on the diameter of the unit.

A new variation of spheronizers that was introduced into the market are the so-called air-assisted spheronizers. Basically, they are similar to the standard spheronizers except that they are designed to permit a conditioned air stream to pass from beneath the rotating disk through the gap or slit between the cylindrical wall and the

rotating friction plate into the product bed. The addition of such a feature presumably improves pellet turnover and brings about a spiral rope-like motion that facilitates spheronization.

Axial-type extruders tend to produce extrudates with slightly higher densities. Twin-screw extruders have better material transport characteristics and higher capacity or throughput than do single screw extruders. Radial-type extruders have higher throughput but produce less dense extrudates than those obtained from axial-type extruders. The product temperature in radial extruders increases very little during the extrusion process, probably because of a shorter compression zone and shorter die opening depth. Absence of heat build-up during extrusion leads not only to well-controlled spheronization process but also allows for the processing of thermolabile drug substances.

Although the extrusion step is a continuous process with a very high throughput, the subsequent steps (spheronization, drying, and sizing) are batch processes, and thus are rate limiting. As a result, the overall extrusion–spheronization process is a batch rather than a continuous process. However, a semicontinuous process can be implemented by having an extruder feed, alternatively, into two spheronizers. As one of the spheronizers is spheronizing the extrudates, the other discharges the formed pellets and is recharged with fresh extrudates. The process is then repeated as the roles of the spheronizers are reversed alternately.

In a batch process, a defined quantity of extrudate is fed into the spheronizer from the top, and the spheronized

Table 1 Critical factors in extrusion–spheronization

	Characteristic	Significance[a]	References
Drug substance	Particle size	+++	
	Particle size distribution	++	
	Particle shape	+++	
	Solubility	++	(26)
Formulation	Water content	+++	(23–25, 27, 28)
	Water temperature	+	(25)
	Excipients type	+++	(13, 18, 19, 24, 19, 26)
	Excipients concentration	++	(24, 26)
	Excipients particle size	++	(12, 13, 28)
Extrusion	Extruder type	++	(13)
	Extruder speed	++	(14, 15, 22–23, 25)
	Extrusion screen size	+++	(22, 24)
	Thickness of the die plate	+	(14, 15, 30)
Spheronization	Spheronizer speed (rpm)	+++	(23–25, 27, 25, 29)
	Spheronizer load	+	(23, 24)
	Spheronization time	+++	(23–25)
	Friction plate design	+	

[a]Relative significance: +, low; ++, medium; +++, high.

particles are discharged by centrifugal force via a discharge chute located at the base of the stator or vertical wall of the cylinder. The extrudates are spheronized by interparticle collisions and particle-to-wall frictional forces. The various stages of the spheronization process are shown in Fig. 9. The spheronizing time is usually 2–15 min, depending on the formulation characteristics. Processing time remains constant, provided the composition of the extrudate, including the water content, is kept constant. Because relatively large amounts of water or solvent are incorporated into the formulation, the final pellets contain significant quantities of residual moisture or solvent and are oven-dried or dried in a fluid-bed dryer before further processing. A sizing step might be necessary to separate the fractions if the particle size distribution is wider than intended. In general, the pellets are spherical and have a narrow particle size distribution. The most critical process parameters in the spheronization step that influence the yield and quality are the design of the grooves and rotational speed of the friction plate and the residence time in the spheronizer.

In an extrusion–spheronization process, formulation components such as fillers, lubricants, and pH modifiers play a critical role in producing pellets with the desired attributes. The granulated mass must be plastic and sufficiently cohesive and self-lubricating during extrusion. During the spheronization step, it is essential that the extrudates break at appropriate length and have sufficient surface moisture to enhance formation of uniform spherical pellets.

The degree of liquid saturation of the granulation is another critical factor that needs to be optimized. Granulations containing low moisture content may generate extrudates that produce large quantities of fines during the spheronization step. If the moisture level is too high, the extrudates may adhere to each other and form bundles of strands that cannot be processed further. Therefore, the extrudates must have sufficient mechanical strength to form strands during the extrusion but must also be easily broken into uniform rods during spheronization to provide pellets with a narrow particle size distribution. Generally, the liquid content of the wet powder mixture is approximately 20–30% (w/w). Solvents such as ethanol or mixtures of water and ethanol may be used as granulating liquids when pure water cannot be used for stability or solubility reasons.

Excipients play a more significant role during extrusion–spheronization than during with any other pelletization process (14). They facilitate extrusion and determine the sphericity of the wet pellets; they also impart strength and integrity to the pellets. Microcrystalline cellulose is one of the most widely investigated excipients. It is used as filler and a spheronization aid, regulating the water content and distribution in the granulation. In effect, it modifies the rheological properties of the formulation and imparts plasticity to the pellets. Lactose is another excipient that has been studied extensively and used to evaluate the factors that govern the mechanism of pellet formation by extrusion–spheronization.

In contrast to layering processes, extrusion–spheronization can be used to manufacture pellets with sustained-release characteristics without the application of functional membranes to control release. For instance, matrix-type pellets can be produced with the help of mixture of microcrystalline cellulose and sodium carboxymethylcellulose (15, 16). Organic acids can be incorporated into the pellet matrix to stabilize sensitive drug substances or modify the release characteristics, especially if the solubility of the drug substance being formulated is pH-dependent (17). Although water or other granulation media act as lubricating agents during extrusion, lubricants are sometimes incorporated to improve processing.

Finally, it is not surprising that the drug substance itself plays an important role in the pelletization process, particularly at high drug loading. Physicochemical properties such as particle size, polymorphism, wettability, and solubility determine not only the amount of active ingredient that can be incorporated in the formulation but also the quality and thus the shape and surface smoothness of the final pellets.

Because extrusion–spheronization is a very complex manufacturing process that depends on a number of formulation and processing factors (Table 1), it has been studied extensively. Some of these studies used multifactorial statistical designs to determine the significance of the various factors identified above (12, 18–20). Despite the extensive work that had been done, additional research is still ongoing as demonstrated by the number of publications in various scientific journals (21–28).

SPHERICAL AGGLOMERATION

Spherical agglomeration, or balling, is a pelletization process in which powders, on addition of an appropriate quantity of liquid or when subjected to high temperatures, are converted to spherical particles by a continuous rolling or tumbling action. Spherical agglomeration can be divided into two categories—liquid-induced and melt-induced agglomerations. Over the years, spherical agglomeration has been carried out in horizontal drum pelletizers, inclined dish pelletizers, and tumbling blenders; more recent technologies use rotary fluid-bed granulators and high-shear mixers. Although spherical agglomeration has been practiced routinely in the iron ore and fertilizer industries, its application in the pharmaceutical industry is marginal at best. Nevertheless, the process is one of the most thoroughly investigated pelletization processes, and as a result, a number of mechanisms describing the various phases of pellet formation and growth during spherical agglomeration have been proposed (29).

During liquid-induced agglomeration, liquid is added to the powder before or during the agitation step. As powders come in contact with a liquid phase, they form agglomerates or nuclei, which initially are bound together by liquid bridges. These are subsequently replaced by solid bridges, which are derived from the hardening binder or any other dissolved material within the liquid phase. The nuclei formed collide with other adjacent nuclei and coalesce to form larger nuclei or pellets. The coalescence process continues until a condition arises in which bonding forces are overcome by breaking forces. At this point, coalescence is replaced by layering, whereby small particles adhere on much larger particles and increase the size of the latter until pelletization is completed (30, 31). If the surface moisture is not optimum, some particles may undergo nucleation and coalescence at different rates and form different sizes of nuclei admixed with the larger pellets. As a result, spherical agglomeration tends to produce pellets with a wide particle size distribution.

The rate and extent of agglomerate formation depend, in part, on formulation variables such as particle size and solubility of the powder, the degree of liquid saturation, and the viscosity of the liquid phase. The moisture content is particularly critical because it determines whether nucleation occurs to initiate pelletization or whether the nuclei formed have the necessary plasticity to bring about coalescence after collisions between two nuclei. Further-more, layering of fine particles on the larger nuclei or pellets occurs only if the surface moisture is above the critical level. The rate and extent of agglomerate formation also depend on processing variables, which are specific to a given piece of equipment. In the case of drum pelletizers, drum speed, residence time, load size, and angle of inclination, relative to the horizontal, are critical process variables that need to be optimized. Variables critical to a spherical agglomeration process using centrifugal fluid-bed granulators are disk speed, load size, residence time, fluidization air volume and temperature, and disk clearance (32–43).

Melt-induced agglomeration processes are similar to liquid-induced processes except that the binding material is a melt. Therefore, the pellets are formed with the help of congealed material without having to go through the formation of solvent-based liquid bridges (44–55).

SPRAY DRYING AND SPRAY CONGEALING

Spray drying and spray congealing, known as globulation processes, involve atomization of hot melts, solutions, or suspensions to generate spherical particles or pellets. The droplet size in both processes is kept small to maximize the rate of evaporation or congealing, and consequently the particle size of the pellets produced is usually very small. During spray drying, drug entities in solution or suspension are sprayed, with or without excipients, into a hot air stream to generate dry and highly spherical particles. As the atomized droplets come in contact with hot air, evaporation of the application medium is initiated. This drying process continues through a series of stages whereby the viscosity of the droplets constantly increases until finally almost the entire application medium is driven off and solid particles are formed. Generally, spray-dried pellets tend to be porous. For a thorough discussion on spray drying technology, see Masters (56).

During spray congealing, a drug substance is allowed to melt, disperse, or dissolve in hot melts of waxes, fatty acids, etc., and sprayed into an air chamber, where the temperature is below the melting temperatures of the formulation components, to provide spherical congealed pellets under appropriate processing conditions. A critical requirement in a spray-congealing process is that the formulation components have well-defined, sharp melting points or narrow melting zones. Because the process does not involve evaporation of solvents, the pellets produced are dense and nonporous. See Atilla and Suheylo (57) for a detailed description of the formulation and processing requirements of spray congealing as a pelletization technique.

CRYOPELLETIZATION

Cryopelletization is a process whereby droplets of a liquid formulation are converted into solid spherical particles or pellets by using liquid nitrogen as the fixing medium. The technology, which was initially developed for lyophilization of viscous bacterial suspensions, can be used to produce drug-loaded pellets in liquid nitrogen at $-160°C$. The procedure permits instantaneous and uniform freezing of the processed material owing to the rapid heat transfer that occurs between the droplets and liquid nitrogen. The pellets are dried in conventional freeze dryers. The small size of the droplets and thus the large surface area facilitate the drying process. The amount of liquid nitrogen required for manufacturing a given quantity depends on the solids content and temperature of the solution or suspension being processed. It is usually between 3 and 5 kg per kilogram of finished pellets.

The equipment consists of a container equipped with perforated plates at the bottom. Immediately below the plates at a predetermined distance is a reservoir of liquid nitrogen. in which a conveyor belt with transport baffles is immersed. The conveyor belt has a variable speed and can be adjusted to provide the residence time required for freezing the pellets. The perforated plates generate droplets that fall and freeze instantaneously as they come in contact with the liquid nitrogen below. The frozen pellets are transported out of the nitrogen bath into a storage container at −60°C before drying. Equipment of different size, ranging from laboratory scale to production size, is available commercially. (See Refs. (58, 59) for a detailed description.)

The most critical step in cryopelletization is droplet formation, which is influenced not only by formulations-related variables such as viscosity, surface tension, and solids content but also by equipment design and the corresponding processing variables. The diameter and design of the shearing edge of the holes on the container plates are critical. For instance, the diameter of the holes determines the flow rate, which, in turn, is governed by the viscosity of the formulation. The diameter of the holes also influences the size and shape of the pellets. The smaller the holes, the smaller the pellets produced.

The shape of the droplets depends in part on the distance the droplets travel before contacting the liquid nitrogen. The distance has to allow sufficient time for the formulation of spherical droplets as they contact the liquid nitrogen. When all processing parameters are carefully characterized and optimized, smooth, spherical pellets can be routinely manufactured. In cases, in which the desired pellet diameter is less than 2 mm, the liquid nitrogen is stirred to prevent agglomeration.

Solutions or suspensions suitable for cryopelletization have high solids content and low viscosities. Another important property is the surface tension of the liquid formulation, which partly determines the pellet size. The addition of a surfactant to the formulation reduces the surface tension and results in smaller particle size. Pellet size also depends on the properties of the drug substance.

Immediate-release formulations typically consist of the drug substance, fillers such as mannitol and lactose and binders such as gelatin, gelatin hydrolysates, and polyvinylpyrolidone. Cross-linked biopolymers based on collagen derivatives are used for sustained-release pellets.

See Refs. (59, 60) for a detailed discussion on the formulation and processing variables.

MELT SPHERONIZATION

Melt spheronization is a process whereby a drug substance and excipients are converted into a molten or semimolten state and subsequently shaped using appropriate equipment to provide solid spheres or pellets. The process requires several pieces of equipment such as blenders, extruders, cutters (known as pelletizers in the plastics industry), and spheronizers. The drug substance is first blended with the appropriate pharmaceutical excipients, such as polymers and waxes, and extruded at a predetermined temperature. The extrusion temperature must be high enough to melt at least one or more of the formulation components. The extrudate is cut into uniform cylindrical segments with a cutter. The segments are spheronized in a jacketed spheronizer to generate uniformly sized pellets. The spheronization temperature needs to be high to partially soften the extrudate and facilitate deformation and eventual spheronization (61). Depending on the characteristics of the formulation ingredients, pellets that exhibit immediate- or sustained-release characteristics can be manufactured in a single step. The pellets produced are unique in that they are monosize, a property unmatched by any other pelletization technique. However, the process is still in the development stage, and additional work is needed before the process becomes a viable pelletization technique.

REFERENCES

1. Beachgaard, H.; Nielson, G.H. Controlled Release Multiple Units and Single Unit Doses. Drug Dev. Ind. Pharm. **1978**, 4, 53−67.
2. Special Delivery: Advances in Drug Therapy. *The Research News*; University of Michigan, 1986; 1.
3. Cimicata, L.E. How to Manufacture and Polish Smallest Pan Goods-Nonpareil Seeds. Confectioners J. **1951**, 41−43.
4. Chambliss, W.C. Conventional and Specialized Coating Pans. *Pharmaceutical Pelletization Technology*; Ghebre-Sellassie, I., Ed.; Marcel Dekker, Inc.: New York, 1989; 16−17.
5. Jan, S.; Goodhart, F.W. Dry Powder Layering. *Pharmaceutical Pelletization Technology*; Ghebre-Sellassie, I., Ed.; Marcel Dekker, Inc.: New York, 1989; 182−183.
6. Jones, D.M. Solution and Suspension Layering. *Pharmaceutical Pelletization Technology*; Ghebre-Sellassie, I., Ed.; Marcel Dekker, Inc.: New York, 1989; 158−159.
7. *Niro-Aeromatic Product Manual* Niro-Aeromatic, Inc.: Columbia, MD, 1992.

8. Hicks, D.C.; Freese, H.L. Extrusion Spheronization Equipment. *Pharmaceutical Pelletization Technology*; Ghebre-Sellassie, I., Ed.; Marcel Dekker, Inc.: New York, 1989; 71–100.

9. Fielden, K.E.; Newton, J.M.; Rowe, R.C. A Comparison of the Extrusion and Spheronization Behavior of Wet Powder Masses Processed by a Ram Extruder and a Cylinder Extruder. Int. J. Pharm. **1992**, *81*, 225–233.

10. Fielden, K.E.; Newton, J.M.; Rowe, R.C. The Effect of Lactose Particle Size on the Extrusion Properties of Microcrystalline Cellulose-Lactose Mixtures. J. Pharm. Pharmacol. **1989**, *41*, 217–221.

11. Dietrich, R.; Brausse, R. Erste Erfahrungen Und Validierungsversuche an Einem Neu Entwickelten GMP-Gerechten Und Instrumentierten Pharma-Extruder. Pharm. Ind. **1988**, *50* (10), 1179–1186.

12. Dietrich, R. Food Technology Transfers to Pellet Production. Manuf. Chem. **1989**, *8*, 29–33.

13. Nakahara N. Method and Apparatus for Making Spherical Granules U.S. Patent. 3,277,520, 1964.

14. Harris, M.R.; Ghebre-Sellassie, I. Formulation Variables. *Pharmaceutical Pelletization Technology*; Ghebre-Sellassie, I., Ed.; Marcel Dekker, Inc.: New York, 1989, 217–239.

15. O'Conner, R.E.; Schwartz, J.B. Spheronization II. Drug Release from Drug Diluent Mixtures. Drug Dev. Ind. Pharm. **1985**, *11* (9, 10), 1837–1857.

16. Ghali, E.S.; Klinger, G.H.; Schwartz, J.B. Modified Drug Release from Beads Prepared with Combinations of Two Grades of Microcrystalline Cellulose. Drug Dev. Ind. Pharm. **1989**, *15* (9), 1455–1473.

17. Blanchini, R.; Bruni, R.; Gazzaniga, A.; Vecchio, C. Influence of Extrusion/Spheronization Processing on the Physical Properties of D-Indobufen Pellets Containing pH Adjusters. Drug Dev. Ind. Pharm. **1992**, *18* (14), 1485–1503.

18. Mesiha, M.S.; Valles, J. A Screening Study of Lubricants in Wet Powder Masses Suitable for Extrusion-Spheronization. Drug Dev. Ind. Pharm. **1993**, *19* (8), 943–959.

19. Hasznos, L.; Langer, I.; Gyarmathy, M. Some Factors Influencing Pellet Characteristics Made by an Extrusion/Spheronization Process. I. Effects on Size Characteristics and Moisture Content Decrease of Pellets. Drug Dev. Ind. Pharm. **1992**, *18* (4), 409–439.

20. Hileman, G.A.; Goskonda, S.R.; Spalitto, A.J.; Upadrashta, S.M. A Factorial Approach to High Dose Product Development by an Extrusion/Spheronization Process. Drug Dev. Ind. Pharm. **1993**, *19* (4), 483–491.

21. Ku, C.C.; Joshi, Y.M.; Bergum, J.S.; Jain, N.B. Bead Manufacture by Extrusion/Spheronization. A Statistical Design for Process Optimization. Drug Dev. Ind. Pharm. **1993**, *19* (13), 1505–1519.

22. Baert, L.; Fanara, D.; Remon, J.P.; Massart, D. Correlation of Extrusion Forces, Raw Materials and Sphere Characteristics. J. Pharm. Pharmacol. **1992**, *44*, 676–678.

23. Battaille, B.; Rahman, L.; Jacob, M. Etude Des Parametres de Formulation Sur Les Characteristiques Physico-Techniques de Granules de Theophylline Obtenus Par Extrusion-Spheronisation. Pharma. Acta Helv. **1991**, *66* (8), 223–236.

24. Newton, J.M.; Chow, A.K.; Jeewa, K.B. The Effect of Excipient Source on Spherical Granules Made by Extrusion/Spheronization. Pharm. Tech. **1993**, *3*, 166–174.

25. Bataille, B.; Ligarski, K.; Jacob, M.; Thomas, C.; Duru, C. Study of the Influence of Spheronization and Drying Conditions on the Physico-Mechanical Properties of Neutral Spheroids Containing Avicel pH 101 and Lactose. Drug Dev. Ind. Pharm. **1993**, *19* (6), 653–671.

26. Helen, L.; Yliruusi, J.; Muttonen, E. Process Variables of the Radial Screen Extruder, II, Size and Size Distribution of Pellets. Pharm. Tech. Int. **1993**, *1*, 44–53.

27. Lindner, H.; Kleinebudde, P. Use of Powdered Cellulose for the Production of Pellets by Extrusion/Spheronization. J. Pharm. Pharmacol. **1994**, *46*, 2–7.

28. Kleinebudde, P. Use of a Power-Consumption-Controlled Extruder in the Development of Pellet Formulations. J. Pharm. Sci. **1997**, *84* (10), 1259–1264.

29. Kleinebudde, P. Crystallite-Gel-Model for Microcrystalline Cellulose in Wet-Granulation, Extrusion, and Spheronization. Pharm. Res. **1997**, *14*, 804–809.

30. Ghebre-Sellassie, I. Mechanism of Pellet Formation and Growth. *Pharmaceutical Pelletization Technology*; Ghebre-Sellassie, I., Ed.; Marcel Dekker, Inc.: New York, 1989; 123–143.

31. Wan, L.S.C. Manufacture of Core Pellet Formation and Growth. *Pharmaceutical Pelletization Technology*; Ghebre-Sellassie, I., Ed.; Marcel Dekker, Inc.: New York, 1989; 123–143.

32. Vecchio, C.; Bruni, G.; Gazzaniga, A. Preparation of Indobufen Pellets by Using Centrifugal Rotary Fluidized Bed Equipment Without Starting Seeds. Drug Dev. Ind. Pharm. **1994**, *20* (12), 1943–1956.

33. Holm, P.; Bonde, M.; Wigmore, T. Pelletization by Granulation in a Roto-Processor RP-2. I. Effects of Process and Product Variables on Granule Growth. Pharm. Technol. Eur. **Sep, 1996**, *8*,, 22, 24, 26, 28, 30, 32, 34, 36.

34. Holm, P. Pelletization by Granulation in a Roto-Processor RP-2. Effects of Process and Product Variables on Agglomerates' Shape and Porosity. Pharm. Technol. Eur. **Oct, 1996**, *8*, 38–45.

35. Vertommen, J.; Kinget, R. Influence of Five Selected Processing and Formulation Variables on the Particle Size Distribution, and Friability of Pellets Produced in a Rotary Processor. Drug Dev. Ind. Pharm. **1997**, *23* (1), 39–46.

36. Vertommen, J.; Rombaut, P.; Kinget, R. Shape and Surface Smoothness of Pellets Made in a Rotary Processor. Int. J. Pharm. **Jan 1, 1997**, *146*, 21–29.

37. Vertommen, J.; Rombaut, P.; Kinget, R. Internal and External Structure of Pellets Made in a Rotary Processor. Int. J. Pharm. **Feb 23, 1998**, *161*, 225–236.

38. Vertommen, J.; Rombaut, P.; Michoel, A.; Kinget, R. Estimation of the Amount of Water Removed by Gap and Atomization Air Streams During Pelletization in a Rotary Processor. Pharm. Dev. Technol. **1998**, *3* (1), 63–72.

39. Vojnovic, D.; Rupena, P.; Moneghini, M.; Rubessa, F.; Sergent, M.; Experimental Research Methodology Applied to Wet Granulation in a High-Shear Mixer. I. S. T. P. II Pharma Sci. **1993**, *3* (2), 130–135.

40. Holm, P.; Shaefer, T.; Kristensen, H.G. Pelletization by Controlled Wet Granulation in a High-Shear Mixer. S. T. P. Pharma Sci. **1993**, *3* (2), 130–135.

41. Vertommen, J.; Michoel, A.; Rombaut, P.; Kinget, R. Production of Pseudophedrine HCl Pellets in a High Shear Mixer-Granulator. Eur. J. Pharm. Biopharm. **1994**, *40* (1), 32–35.

42. Vojnovic, D.; Moneghini, M.; Masiello, S. Design and Optimization of Theophylline Pellets Obtained by Wet Speronization in a High-Shear Mixer. Drug Dev. Ind. Pharm. **1995**, *21* (18), 2129–2137.

43. Maggi, L.; Bonfanti, A.; Santi, P.; Massimo, G.; Catellani, P.L.; Belloti, A.; Colombo, P.; Zanchetta, A.; Suitability of a Small Scale High-Shear Mixer for Powder Pelletization. Pharm. Technol. Eur. **Oct, 1996**, *8*, 82, 84, 86, 88–90.

44. Schaefer, T.; Holm, P.; Kristensen, H.G. Melt Granulation in a Laboratory Scale High Shear Mixer. Drug Dev. Ind. Pharm. **1990**, *16* (8), 1249–1277.

45. Shaefer, T.; Holm, P.; Kristensen, H.G. Melt Pelletization in a High Shear Mixer. 1. Effects of Process Variables and Binder. Acta Pharm. Nordica **1992**, *4* (3), 133–140.

46. Shaefer, T.; Holm, P.; Kristensen, H.G. Melt Pelletization in a High Shear Mixer. II. Power Consumption and Granule Growth. Acta Pharm. Nordica **1992**, *4* (3), 141–148.

47. Shaefer, T.; Holm, P.; Kristensen, H.G. Melt Pelletization in a High Shear Mixer. III. Effects of Lactose Quality. Acta Pharm. Nordica **1992**, *4* (4), 245–252.

48. Schaefer, T.; Taagegaard, B.; Thomsen, L.J.; Kristensen, H.G. Melt Pelletization in a High Shear Mixer. IV. Effects of Process Variables in a Laboratory Scale Mixer. Eur. J. Pharm. Sci. **1993**, *1* (3), 125–131.

49. Shaefer, T.; Taageraard, B.; Thomsen, L.J.; Kristensen, H.G. Melt Pelletization in a High Shear Mixer. V. Effects of Apparatus Variables. Eur. J. Pharm. Sci. **1993**, *1* (3), 133–141.

50. Shaefer, T. Melt Pelletization in a High Shear Mixer. X. Agglomeration of Binary Mixtures. Int. J. Pharm. **Aug 9, 1996**, 149–159.

51. Shaefer, T.; Mathiesen, C. Melt Pelletization in a High Shear Mixer. VII. Effects of Product Temperature. Int. J. Pharm. **May 28, 1996**, *134*, 105–117.

52. Schaefer, T.; Mathieson, C. Melt Pelletization in a High Shear Mixer. VIII Effects of Binder Viscosity. Int. J. Pharm. **Aug 9, 1996**, *139*, 125–138.

53. Shaefer, T.; Mathiesen, C. Melt Pelletization in a High Shear Mixer. IX. Effects of Binder Particle Size. Int. J. Pharm. **Aug 9, 1996**, *139*, 139–148.

54. Maejima, T.; Osawa, T.; Nakajima, K.; Kobayashi, M. Preparation of Spherical Beads without Any Use of Solvents by a Novel Tumbling Melt Granulation (TMG) Method. Chem. Pharm. Bull. **1997**, *45*, 518–524.

55. Maejima, T.; Osawa, T.; Nakajima, K.; Kobayashi, M. Effects of Species of Non-Meltable and Meltable Materials and Their Physical Properties on Granulatability in Tumbling Melt Granulation Method. Chem. Pharm. Bull. **1997**, *45*, 1833–1839.

56. Masters, K. *Spray Drying Handbook*, 4th Ed.; John Wiley & Sons: New York, 1985.

57. Atilla, H.A.; Suheyla, K.H. Preparation of Micropellets by Spray Congealing. *Multiparticulate Oral Drug Delivery*; Ghebre-Sellassie, I., Ed.; Marcel Dekker, Inc.: New York, 1994; 17–34.

58. European Patent EP 0, 081, 913, 1985.

59. German Patent DE 37 11 169, 1988.

60. Knoch, A. Cryopelletization. *Multiparticulate Oral Drug Delivery*; Ghebre-Sellassie, I. Ed.; Marcel Dekker, Inc. New York, 1994; 35–50.

61. Ghebre-Sellassie, I.; Nesbitt, R.; Fawzi M. Novel Pharmaceutical Pellets and Process for Their Production PCT Application, WO 93/07859, April 29, 1993.

62. Harrison, P.J.; Newton, J.M.; Rowe, R.C. The Characterization of Wet Powder Masses Suitable for Extrusion/Spheronization. J. Pharm. Pharmacol. **1985**, *37*, 686–691.

PEPTIDES AND PROTEINS—BUCCAL ABSORPTION

Ashim K. Mitra
Hemant H. Alur
Thomas P. Johnston
University of Missouri–Kansas City, Kansas City, Missouri

INTRODUCTION

Background and Rationale

In recent years, proteins and peptides are emerging as a major class of therapeutic agents. Pharmaceutical scientists are faced with the challenges of a) selection of a suitable route of drug delivery and b) formulation of these bioengineered drugs. The most common route of protein and peptide drug delivery has been parenteral. However, this route is associated with pain on administration, resulting in poor patient compliance, and the formulation needs to be sterile. Drugs administered by the gastrointestinal route are subjected to acid hydrolysis and extensive gut and/or hepatic first-pass metabolism. Thus, these protein drugs may exhibit poor oral bioavailability. Noninvasive mucosal and transdermal routes offer effective alternative routes for systemic drug delivery. The transdermal delivery route is limited to potent, lipophilic compounds, does not provide rapid blood levels, and is less permeable than oral mucosa (1). Various absorptive mucosae have been identified and investigated for systemic drug delivery. These include nasal, ocular, pulmonary, rectal, vaginal, buccal, and sublingual. Certain associated drawbacks limit extensive use of the nasal, ocular, pulmonary, rectal, and vaginal mucosae. The buccal and sublingual routes do not have many of these limitations; hence, both routes seem attractive alternative routes for systemic drug delivery. In this article, only buccal drug delivery is addressed.

Advantages

Because of rich buccal vascularity, drugs delivered by the buccal route gain direct access to the systemic circulation and are not subject to first-pass metabolism. Also, therapeutic agents do not come in contact with the acidic digestive fluids secreted by the gastrointestinal tract.

Relative to the nasal and rectal routes, the buccal mucosa has low enzymatic activity, and drug inactivation owing biochemical degradation is not as rapid and extensive (2).

Excellent accessibility to the buccal mucosa makes application of the dosage form painless, precisely located, and easily removable without discomfort at the end of the application period. The oral cavity consists of a pair of buccal mucosae. Thus, a drug-delivery system can be applied at various sites either on the same mucosa or, alternatively, on the left or right buccal mucosa on different applications. This is particularly advantageous if the delivery system contains a drug or excipient that mildly and reversibly damages or irritates the mucosa.

A buccal drug-delivery system is applied to a specific area on the buccal membrane. Moreover, the delivery system can be designed to be unidirectional in drug release so that it can be protected from the local environment of the oral cavity. It also permits the inclusion of a permeation enhancer/protease inhibitor or pH modifier in the formulation to modulate the membrane or the tablet–mucosal environment at or near that particular application site. Although the irritation is limited to a well-defined area, the systemic toxicity of these enhancers/inhibitors and modifiers can be reduced. The buccal mucosa is well-suited for this type of modification because it is less prone to irreversible damage (3). In the event of drug toxicity, the delivery of drugs can be terminated promptly by removal of the dosage form.

In addition, the buccal route may be useful for unconscious patients and in patients who have recently undergone surgery or have experienced upper gastrointestinal tract disease that would affect oral drug absorption.

Disadvantages

The surface area available for absorption in the buccal mucosa is much smaller than the gastrointestinal, nasal, rectal, and vaginal mucosae. The buccal mucosa is continuously bathed by saliva, and the secreted saliva lowers the drug concentration at the absorbing membrane. These two factors, along with the permeability coefficient of the drug, affect the overall absorption rate by this route. In addition, the buccal mucosa is less permeable than any of the mucosae noted above.

Involuntary swallowing of saliva containing dissolved drug or swallowing the delivery system itself would lead to a major loss of drug from the site of absorption. Talking, eating, and drinking affect the retention of the delivery system and therefore may constitute limitations associated with this route of drug administration (1). In addition, there is a risk of choking on the dislodged drug-delivery device.

Taste, irritancy, and allergenicity also may limit the number of drugs that can be delivered by the buccal route.

ANATOMY AND PHYSIOLOGY OF THE ORAL MUCOSA

Structure

The oral mucosa is anatomically divided into three tissue layers (Fig. 1) (4). These three layers are the 1) epithelium, 2) basement membrane, and 3) connective tissues.

Epithelium

The epithelium consists of approximately 40–50 layers of stratified squamous epithelial cells. The epithelial cells originate from a layer of basal cells, which are cuboidal in shape, undergo continuous mitosis, and move to the surface. As the cells migrate to the surface through the intermediate layers, they differentiate and become larger, flattened, and surrounded by an external lipid matrix (membrane-coating granules). This external lipid matrix

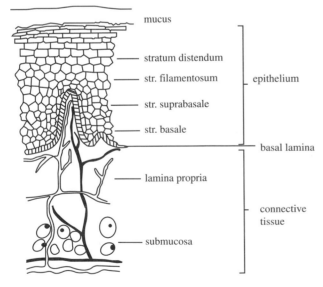

Fig. 1 Schematic diagram showing the principal components of oral mucosa. (From Ref. 4.)

determines the drug permeability of the tissue. Although gingiva (gum) and the hard palate are keratinized, areas such as buccal, sublingual, and the soft palate are nonkeratinized. The thickness of buccal epithelium varies with location and typically ranges from 500 to 800 μm in humans, dogs, and rabbits. The estimated cell turnover time is 5–6 days (5). In addition, the buccal epithelium is also characterized by the presence of intercellular gap junctions.

Basement membrane

The basement membrane (BM) is a continuous layer of extracellular materials and forms a boundary between the basal layer of epithelium and the connective tissues of the lamina propria and the submucosa. The BM can be subdivided into the a) lamina lucida, b) lamina densa, and c) a sublayer of fibrous material. The functions of the BM include providing 1) adherence between epithelium and underlying connective tissues, 2) mechanical support for epithelium, and 3) a barrier to the passage of cells and some large molecules.

Connective tissues

Connective tissues consist of lamina propria and submucosa, if present. The lamina propria is a continuous sheet of connective tissue composed of blood capillaries and nerve fibers serving the oral mucosa.

Vascular drainage from the oral mucosa is principally by way of the lingual, facial, and retromandibular veins. These veins open into the internal jugular vein and thus avoid first-pass metabolism.

The buccal mucosae from monkeys, apes, dogs, pigs, and rabbits possess physiology very similar to that of human buccal mucosa (5).

Permeability

Permeability barriers

The permeability of buccal mucosa lies somewhat between the skin epidermis and intestinal mucosa.

Epithelium: The predominant barrier to drug diffusion resides approximately within the outermost one-third of the epithelium. This is true of both keratinized and nonkeratinized epithelia. Therefore, keratinization is unlikely to offer major resistance to buccal permeation.

Membrane coating granules (MCG): MCGs are spherical or oval organelles (100–300 nm in diameter) found both in keratinized as well as in nonkeratinized epithelia but are different with regard to composition in both epithelia. MCGs discharge their contents into the intercellular space and thus form the permeability barrier.

Permeant factors: The permeation of a drug molecule across the buccal mucosa is dependent on the following.

1. Molecular size—for hydrophilic substances, as molecular weight and molecular size/radius ascends, permeability typically diminishes. Small molecular weight permeants (MW < 100 Da) are rapidly transported through buccal mucosa.
2. Lipid solubility—for non-ionizable compounds, as the lipophilicity rises, the drug permeability typically increases. To maximize the absorption rate, a drug should be available in the salivary film at its solubility limit.
3. Ionization—for ionizable drugs, maximal permeation occurs at the pH at which ionization is least, i.e., where the drug is predominantly in the unionized form (6, 7).

The rate of drug absorption for the transcellular route is pH-dependent. Such dependency results from the fact that the membrane/aqueous partition coefficient for an ionizable drug is pH-dependent.

Basement membrane (BM): The BM has an enormous surface area compared with the epithelium owing to connective tissue papillae, which may affect the effective diffusional pathlength.

Mechanism of Drug Transport

The major pathway of drug transport across buccal mucosa seems to follow simple Fickian diffusion (8, 9). Passive diffusion occurs in accordance with the pH-partition theory. Considerable evidence also exists in the literature regarding the presence of carrier-mediated transport in the buccal mucosa (10, 11). Examination of the equation for drug flux is shown by Eq. 1:

$$J = \frac{DK_P}{h}\Delta C_e \qquad (1)$$

where J = drug flux, D = diffusivity, K_p = partition coefficient, ΔC_e = concentration gradient, and h = diffusional pathlength shows that the flux may be increased by decreasing the diffusional resistance of the membrane by making it more fluid, increasing the solubility of the drug in the saliva immediately adjacent to the epithelium, or enhancing lipophilicity through prodrug modification. Because of the barrier properties of the tight buccal mucosa, the rate-limiting step is the movement of drug molecules across the epithelium.

Two pathways of permeation across buccal mucosa are transcellular, in which the passage of drug occurs through the individual cells of the mucosa, and paracellular, in which the passage of drug occurs through intercellular junctions of the mucosa. Permeability coefficients typically range from 1×10^{-5} to 2×10^{-9} cm/s for oral mucosa (12). The pathway of drug transport across oral mucosa may be studied using: 1) microscopic techniques using fluorescent dyes (12), 2) autoradiography (5), and 3) confocal laser scanning microscopic procedures (13).

FACTORS AFFECTING SYSTEMIC ORAL MUCOSAL DELIVERY

Membrane Factors

Regional differences in both permeability and thickness affect both the rate and extent of drug reaching the systemic circulation (14). Keratinization and composition, although not major factors, of the various oral mucosae affect systemic mucosal drug delivery. Additional factors such as absorptive membrane thickness, blood supply, blood/lymph drainage, cell renewal rate, and enzyme content will also govern the rate and extent of drug absorption into the systemic circulation.

Environmental Factors

Saliva

A major portion of saliva is composed of water (99%) and has a pH of 6.5–7.5 depending on the flow rate and location (15). An increase in the salivary flow rate leads to the secretion of watery saliva. Stimulated salivary secretion affects the film thickness and aids in easy migration of test compounds from one region of the mouth to another. Salivary pH is also important because passive diffusion of unionized drug is the major mechanism of oral absorption (16, 17).

Salivary glands

Drug-delivery systems, therefore, should not be placed either over a duct or adjacent to a salivary duct because this may dislodge the retentive system or may result in excessive washout of the drug or rapid dissolution/erosion of the delivery system, making it difficult to achieve high local drug concentrations. Also, if a retentive system is placed over salivary ducts, the reduced salivary flow rate may produce less/no mucus that is required for proper attachment of a mucoadhesive delivery device.

Movement of the oral tissues

Talking, eating, and swallowing may cause some mouth movement leading to dislodgment of the delivery device (1). The movement of the tongue may also influence the delivery of drugs from a mucoadhesive, retentive system owing to the tongue swiping across the dosage form and adjacent tissues as well as to induction of suction pressures from the tongue compressing against the hard palate.

Dosage Form Design Considerations

Overview

A mucoadhesive buccal drug delivery system should

1. be convenient to apply and unobtrusive when in place,
2. not incorporate a bitter-tasting drug,
3. have a smooth surface rather than a textured surface,
4. preferably achieve unidirectional release of the drug, and
5. use excipients (both diluents and the mucoadhesive polymers) that do not irritate or damage the mucosa, that are nontoxic, and that do not stimulate salivary secretion.

The *size* of the delivery system varies with the type of formulation, i.e., a buccal tablet may be approximately 5–8 mm in diameter, whereas a flexible buccal patch may be as large as 10–15 cm^2 in area. Mucoadhesive buccal patches with a surface area of 1–3 cm^2 are most acceptable (18). It has been estimated that the total amount of drug that can be delivered across the buccal mucosa from a 2-cm^2 system in 1 day is approximately 10–20 mg (12). The *shape* of the delivery system may also vary, although for buccal drug administration, an ellipsoid shape appears to be most acceptable (18). The *thickness* of the delivery device is usually restricted to only a few millimeters. The *location* of the delivery device also needs to be considered. A mucoadhesive retentive system is preferred over a conventional dosage form. A bioadhesive buccal patch would appear to be the most appropriate delivery system because of its flexibility and the area of the buccal mucosa available for its application. The maximal duration of buccal drug retention and absorption is approximately 4–6 h because food and/or liquid intake may require removal of the delivery device.

BIOADHESION

The word *bioadhesion* can be defined as the ability of a material (synthetic or natural) to "stick" (adhere) to a biological tissue for extended periods (18). The phenomenon of bioadhesion can be visualized as a two-step process. The first step involves the initial contact between polymer and the biological tissue. The second step is the formation of secondary bonds owing to noncovalent interactions.

Biomembrane Characteristics

Oral mucosae are covered with mucus that serves as a link between the adhesive and the membrane. Mucin is a polyelectrolyte under neutral or slightly acidic conditions because of the terminal sialic acid residues having a pK_a value of 2.6 (19). At physiological pH (7.4), the mucin molecule is polyanionic, which contributes to bioadhesion.

Adhesive Characteristics

A variety of polymers including water-soluble and water-insoluble and ionic and non-ionic hydrocolloids and water-insoluble hydrogels can be used in bioadhesive systems (20). Factors affecting the bioadhesive properties of the polymer include the following.

Molecular weight and polymer conformation

In general, the adhesive strength of a polymer increases with molecular weights greater than 100,000 (21). The molecule must have adequate length to allow chain interpenetration into the mucus layer. However, the size and conformation of the polymer molecule play an important role as well (22).

Cross-linking density of the polymer

The strength of mucoadhesion decreases with an increase in cross-linking as this leads to a decrease in the polymer's diffusion coefficient (23) and chain segment flexibility and mobility (which in turn reduces interpenetration).

Charge and ionization of the polymer

Anionic polymers provide better efficiency than do cationic or uncharged polymers with respect to both adhesiveness and toxicity (24). Also, polymeric adhesives with carboxyl groups are preferred over those with sulfate groups (25).

Concentration of the polymeric adhesive

In general, the more concentrated the polymeric adhesive becomes, the more the bioadhesive strength diminishes.

The coiled molecules become solvent-poor in a concentrated solution, which, in turn, decreases the available chain length for interpenetration into the mucus layer. Therefore, a critical concentration of the polymeric adhesive is required for optimum bioadhesion (26).

pH of the medium

pH influences the charge on the surface of the mucus and the polymer (27). Charge density on the surface of mucus will vary with pH owing to the differences in dissociation of the functional groups on the carbohydrate and amino acid moieties.

Hydration of the polymer

Swelling affects bioadhesion (28), although an increase in the degree of swelling does not always result in an increase in the bioadhesive strength. However, a high water activity is required to hydrate the mucoadhesive component to expose the bioadhesive site(s) for secondary bond formation, to expand the gel to create pores of sufficient size, and to mobilize all flexible polymer chains for interpenetration. A critical degree of hydration of the mucoadhesive polymer is needed for optimum bioadhesion (20). A greater degree of hydration lowers the adhesive strength owing to the formation of a slippery mucilage.

Theories of Bioadhesion

In general, both physical and weak chemical bonds are responsible for mucoadhesion. Physical/mechanical bond formation can be explained as the entanglement of the adhesive polymer and the extended mucin chains. When this diffusion is mutual, it leads to maximum bioadhesive strength.

Attaching bonds may be either primary owing to covalent bonding or secondary owing to electrostatic, hydrogen, or hydrophobic bonding. Electrostatic or hydrogen bonding results primarily because of hydroxyl (—OH), carboxyl (—COOH), sulfonate (—SO₃H), and amino (—NH₂) groups. Several theories of bioadhesion have been proposed, i.e., wetting, diffusion, electronic, fracture, and adsorption. The mechanism of bioadhesion appears to be best explained by a combination of the wetting, diffusion, and electronic theories.

Measurement of Bioadhesion

Measurement of bioadhesion not only helps in screening the candidate polymer but also assists in studying the mechanism of bioadhesion. However, performance of the final dosage form containing the polymer and the drug is the best test for bioadhesion.

In vitro measurements

Measurement of either tensile or shear stress is the most commonly used in vitro method to measure bioadhesion. All in vitro measurements provide a rank order of bioadhesive strength for a series of candidate polymers. Measurement of tensile strength involves quantitating the force required to break the adhesive bond between the test polymer and a model membrane. This method typically uses a modified balance or tensile tester. A section of freshly excised rabbit stomach tissue with the mucosal side exposed is secured on a weighed glass vial and placed in a beaker containing USP-simulated gastric fluid. Another section of the same tissue is secured onto a rubber stopper with a vial cap with the mucus side exposed (Fig. 2). A small quantity of the test polymer is placed between the two mucosal tissues. The force required to detach the polymer from the tissue is then recorded (29). Measurement of shear strength involves quantitating the force that causes the polymer to slide in a direction parallel to the plane of contact between the polymer and the mucus. This method uses a glass plate suspended from a microbalance on which the test polymer is coated (Fig. 3). This plate is then dipped in a temperature-controlled mucus sample. The force required to pull the plate out of the mucus sample is determined under constant experimental conditions (22).

Additional in vitro methods include adhesion weight (30), fluorescent probe (24), flow channel (31), mechanical spectroscopic (32), falling film (33), colloidal gold staining

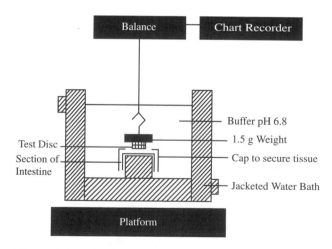

Fig. 2 Schematic diagram showing the apparatus and the setup for assessing the tensile strength. (From Ref. 93.)

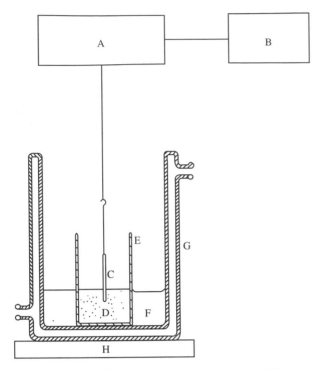

Fig. 3 Schematic diagram showing the apparatus and the set up for assessing the shear strength. Key: (A) Microforce balance; (B) Chart recorder; (C) Glass plate (side on); (D) 1 ml Homogenized mucus; (E) Glass vial; (F) Water; (G) Water jacket at 20°C; (H) Platform moving in vertical direction. (From Ref. 22.)

(34), viscometric method (35), thumb test (36), adhesion number (36), and electrical conductance (36).

In vivo measurements

In vivo methods are relatively few and measure the residence time of bioadhesives at the application site (36). Techniques such as γ-scintigraphy, perfused intestinal loop and radiolabeled transit studies using ^{55}Cr-labeled bioadhesive polymer (37), and ^{99m}Tc-labeled polycarbophil (38) have been used for this purpose.

Bioadhesive Polymers in Buccal Drug Delivery

A variety of water-soluble and water-insoluble polymers of both synthetic and natural origin (20) have been studied as bioadhesives.

Overview

Bioadhesive polymers are used mainly to overcome the short residence time of drug and the dosage form to improve localization of the drug and to achieve controlled or sustained release of the drug. Bioadhesive polymers can be divided into three broad categories: 1) "wet" adhesives,

i.e., polymers that become sticky on hydration, 2) polymers that are electrostatic in nature and adhere primarily owing to nonspecific and noncovalent interactions, and 3) polymers that can bind to a specific site on the cell surface (39).

An ideal bioadhesive should

i.   be nontoxic, nonabsorbable, and nonirritating to the mucus membrane,
ii. form a strong noncovalent bond with the mucin-epithelial cell surfaces,
iii. allow easy incorporation of drug and should not offer hindrance to drug release, and
iv. not decompose on storage or during the shelf life of the dosage form.

Some of the other desirable characteristics of the polymer have been presented previously in *Bioadhesion*.

Drug release from soluble polymers is accompanied by the gradual erosion-type dissolution of the polymer. Therefore, polymer dissolution/drug diffusion may be the overall hybrid mechanism of release. Drug release from nonsoluble hydrogels generally follows Fickian or non-Fickian diffusion kinetics (40). The mechanism of release may be determined by modeling the drug release (first 60%) to the empirical equation (Eq. 2),

$$\frac{M_t}{M_\infty} = kt^n \qquad (2)$$

where M_t/M_∞ = fraction of drug released, k = kinetic constant, t = time, and n = diffusional exponent. The mechanism of drug release may be Fickian diffusion when the value of $n = 0.5$; anomalous (non-Fickian) transport when $n = 0.5 < n < 1.0$, and case-II transport when $n = 1.0$. A value of n greater than 1 signifies super case-II transport as the mechanism of drug release (41).

DOSAGE FORMS

Several bio/mucoadhesive dosage forms have been developed, and mechanism(s) of bioadhesion have been delineated.

Buccal Dosage Forms

Buccal mucosa presents a relatively smooth and immobile surface for the placement of a bioadhesive dosage form. The amount of drug that can be incorporated is limited because of the size limitation of the buccal dosage form. In general, a drug with a daily requirement of 25 mg or less is suitable for buccal delivery. Drugs with a short half-life, requiring sustained/controlled delivery, or exhibiting poor

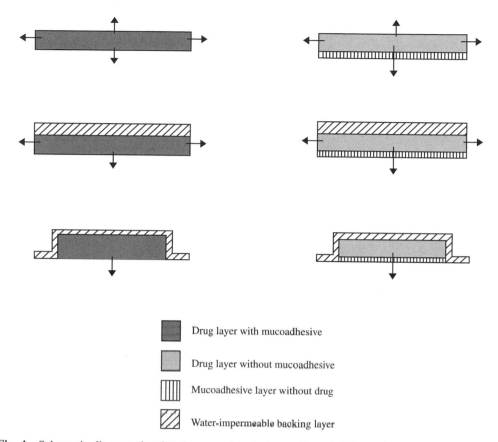

Drug layer with mucoadhesive

Drug layer without mucoadhesive

Mucoadhesive layer without drug

Water-impermeable backing layer

Fig. 4 Schematic diagram showing the geometric designs of buccal delivery devices. (From Ref. 91.)

aqueous solubility and drugs that are sensitive to enzymatic degradation may be delivered successfully across the buccal mucosa. The dosage forms developed for this purpose include tablets, adhesive patches, adhesive gels, and adhesive ointment. Adhesive tablets and patches can be formulated to release the drug either unidirectionally or multidirectionally by varying the extent and permeability of the backing (Fig. 4).

Formulation Development of Buccal Dosage Forms

Novel dosage forms such as adhesive tablets, patches, gels, and ointments have been developed primarily for systemic delivery of therapeutic agents. These dosage forms are also capable of providing sustained drug delivery.

Buccal dosage forms can be of 1) reservoir type and 2) matrix type.

Reservoir type

Drug formulations of the reservoir type are surrounded by a polymeric membrane, which controls the release rate. Reservoir systems present a constant release profile, provided 1) the polymeric membrane is rate limiting and 2) an excess amount of drug is present in the reservoir.

Matrix type

Drug is uniformly dispersed in the polymer in matrix-type systems, and drug release is controlled by the matrix. Drug molecules dispersed in the polymer have to dissolve in the medium and then diffuse through the polymer network. Therefore, a drug dispersion and drug-depletion zone always exists in the matrix. A thin hydrodynamic diffusion layer also exists at the interface of the drug and the matrix. A matrix system may result in a constant release profile only at early times when the drug-depletion zone is rather insignificant.

The parameters that determine the release rate of a drug from a delivery device include polymer solubility, polymer diffusivity, and thickness of the polymer diffusional path, and the drug's aqueous solubility, partition coefficient, and aqueous diffusivity. Finally, the thickness of the hydrodynamic diffusion layer, the amount of drug loaded into the matrix, and the surface area of the device all affect the drug's release rate.

Buccal adhesive tablets

Adhesive tablets may be either monolithic or multilayered devices. Monolithic tablets can be prepared by conventional techniques of either direct compression or wet granulation. These tablets provide the possibility of holding large amounts of drug. Using either compression or spray coating, a partial coating of every face except one that is in contact with the mucosa with a water-impermeable material such as cellophane, hydrogenated castor oil, Teflon, ethyl cellulose, etc., may cause unidirectional drug release. Multilayered tablets may be prepared by adding each formulation ingredient layer by layer into a die and by compressing it on a tablet press (Fig. 4). These tablets can be designed to deliver drugs either systemically or locally. For multilayered tablets, incorporation of the drug into the adhesive layer, which is immediately adjacent to the mucosal surface, may aid in optimizing bioadhesion.

Buccal adhesive patches

Adhesive patches may also be monolithic or multilayered devices of the reservoir or matrix type for either systemic or local drug delivery. Two primary types of manufacturing processes are usually used to prepare adhesive patches. These include solvent casting and direct milling (with or without a solvent). The intermediate product is a sheet from which patches are punched. A backing is then applied to control the direction of drug release and to minimize deformation and disintegration of the device during residence in the mouth. Preparation of adhesive patches by the solvent–casting method involves casting of appropriately prepared aqueous solutions of either polymer (for drug-free patches) or a drug/polymer mixture onto a backing layer sheet mounted on a stainless steel plate by means of a frame. Drying may then be performed by perfusing with a thermostated stream of water or by air drying. The temperature is typically selected based on the exicipients used in the formulation. On complete drying, the laminate may be cut into the desired shape and size

using a suitable punch and a die set. Preparation of adhesive patches by direct milling is done by homogeneously mixing the drug and the bioadhesive, with or without the aid of a solvent, using a two-roll mill. The polymer/drug mixture may then be compressed to its desired thickness, and patches of appropriate size may be cut or punched out. The polymer/drug mixture prepared with a solvent may require an additional drying step afforded by air or oven drying (Fig. 5).

Design of Experiments

A formulation may be evaluated for both in vitro and in vivo release and mucosal permeation by designing appropriate experiments.

In vitro release/permeation studies

In vitro release studies may be designed depending on the shape and application of the dosage form because no standard method is available. A survey of the literature indicates that the apparatus used for the release study varied from a typical USP type I/II apparatus to a rotating basket immersed in a beaker with agitation conditions being rotational (50–250 rpm) to magnetic stirring or mechanical shaking (39). A variety of testing media have been used such as distilled water, chloroform, phosphate buffer, saline, a mixture of methanol, and water, etc. (39). In vitro release studies provide valuable information regarding the behavior of the delivery device and the mechanism of drug release from the delivery device.

In vitro permeation studies can be conducted using a glass diffusion cell with the buccal tissue mounted between the two halves of the cell, which may be filled with constantly stirred buffer solutions. Buccal mucosa may then be excised from the canine or porcine or rabbit cheek immediately after sacrifice. Such permeation studies may provide meaningful results on the simultaneous processes of drug transport and metabolism in the tissue. Attention must be given to the viability of the excised tissue under in vitro conditions. Electrophysiologic characterization appears to be a valuable tool to indicate the viability of the tissue after excision. To retain tissue viability, continuous bubbling with O_2/CO_2 mixtures and the addition of glucose to the buffer media may be useful. Viability can be determined using MTT assay and confocal imaging of vital staining (42). Alternatively, cell culture technique can be used, where by several parameters can be varied to arrive at an optimum delivery device. This technique also helps in understanding the possible mechanism of drug transport and therefore may provide strategies for modification of either the drug molecule or the drug-delivery device (43).

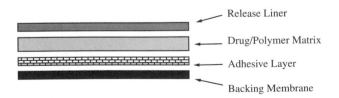

Release Liner

Drug/Polymer Matrix

Adhesive Layer

Backing Membrane

Fig. 5 Schematic diagram showing the design of mucoadhesive buccal patch. (From Ref. 81.)

In vivo absorption studies

Animal studies: Only a small number of absorption studies have been conducted in animals. This may be because buccal administration of drugs to animals is difficult and often produces artifactual results (44). Animals selected as models should be representative of human absorption, tissue, enzymes, degree of keratinization, etc. Conscious or anesthetized animals may be used for absorption studies. Conscious animals should be preconditioned by administering placebos for several consecutive days. The experimental dosage form may then be administered/applied to the buccal mucosa. Absorption may be followed by monitoring plasma and/or urinary drug concentrations as well as the amount of drug remaining in the dosage form after the experiment.

Human studies: Human studies are conducted after the dosage form has been optimized with respect to release of the drug, shape of the dosage form, amount of the drug to be incorporated, and completion of preclinical toxicity studies in animals. Human volunteers may be asked to place the dosage form on the buccal mucosa, and the absorption process may be followed by monitoring the amount of drug remaining in the dosage form after certain time intervals and/or by sampling biological matrices (blood, urine, etc.) with appropriate pharmacokinetic/pharmacodynamic analyses. The amount of drug remaining in the dosage form may reflect absorption only if the absorption step is not rate limiting, and an attempt to prevent swallowing a drug/saliva solution has been made (45).

Evaluation of toxicity and irritation

Irritation is very subjective and may differ widely from treatment to control subjects. Most irritation occurs as a result of penetration enhancers. Evaluation of toxicity and irritation should be concerned with: 1) mucosal tissue irritation, 2) extent of damage to the mucosal cells, and 3) rate of recovery.

Mucosal tissue irritation: Irritation is a complex phenomenon involving interaction among the solution properties of the vehicle, mucosal transport, biological transport, and local drug disposition. To date, no definite relationship has been established between the structure of a penetration enhancer, for example, and the degree of irritation it may cause following buccal application. However, a relationship between the pK_a value of an ionizable compound (benzoic acid derivatives) and irritation as measured by the degree of erythema has been reported (46, 47). Azacycloalkanone enhancers demonstrated more irritancy with alkyl than those with alkenyl chains (48). In general, it would appear that the most effective penetration enhancers induce the greatest degree of irritation to mucosal tissues.

Extent of Damage to Mucosal Cells: Permeation enhancement implies possible alteration of the protective permeability barrier either by: 1) an increase in the fluidity of intercellular lipids (relatively nontoxic) and/or 2) extraction of intercellular lipids or denaturation of cellular proteins (much more damaging/toxic). Therefore, it is imperative that the permeation enhancer: 1) exert a reversible effect, 2) not be systemically absorbed, and 3) not cause cumulative toxicity or permanent changes in the barrier properties. Application of up to 1% sodium lauryl sulfate or cetylpyridinium chloride to the ventral surface of the tongue of dogs resulted in desquamation, widening and separation of keratin (49). The buccal mucosa of rabbits treated with 0.5% sodium deoxycholate or 0.1% sodium lauryl sulfate demonstrated loss of surface epithelial cells (50). Sodium taurocholate and lysophosphatidyl chloride increased buccal insulin absorption in dogs with no mucosal irritation (51).

Methods used to assess membrane damage: Several methods are commonly used to estimate the degree of damage to biological membranes induced by various permeation enhancers. The following methods are a partial listing:

1. morphological examination by scanning or transmission electron microscopy (52),
2. morphological examination using light microscopy and appropriate staining, e.g., hematoxylin and eosin (H&E) (53),
3. determination of the extent of hemolysis caused by a permeation enhancer (54),
4. determination of the release of cellular constituents, e.g., lactate dehydrogenase (LDH) (55),
5. measurements of the changes in the electrical resistance of the membrane,
6. measurements of the changes in the permeability to various markers, e.g., insulin, mannitol, and FITC–dextran, and
7. measurements of changes in cilia movement, e.g., with nasal mucosa.

Rate of recovery of mucosal membranes: The rate of recovery is generally inversely related to the extent of membrane damage, i.e., a greater and more rapid recovery from permeation enhancers that induce minimal damage such as acylcarnitines (56) and sodium glycocholate compared with enhancers such as sodium deoxycholate (57) and polyoxyethylene-9-lauryl ether. The permeability of the tight junction is sensitive to the extracellular calcium concentration. Resealing of tight junctions has been shown to be accelerated if there is a high extracellular calcium concentration rather than an elevated cytoplasmic calcium concentration (58).

Miscellaneous toxicity concerns: Additional toxicity concerns include interference with normal metabolism and function of mucosal cells, e.g., water absorption by these cells (59). The unconjugated bile acids are known to block amino acid metabolism and glucose transport (60). There is a possibility of biotransformation of these enhancers to toxic or carcinogenic substances by hepatic monooxygenases. Absorption of permeation enhancers into the systemic circulation can also cause toxicity, e.g., azone and hexamethylene lauramide (61), which are absorbed across skin. Moreover, changes in membrane fluidity may alter the activity of membrane-bound transport proteins and enzymes.

BUCCAL DRUG DELIVERY OF PEPTIDES AND PROTEINS

Buccal drug delivery avoids acid- and enzyme-mediated degradation and hepatic first-pass metabolism. However, the bioavailability of therapeutic polypeptides and proteins is generally very low (<5%) owing to low lipid solubility and their inherent larger molecular weight compared with conventional small molecules. Degradation of proteins and peptides by enzymes such as aminopeptidases, carboxypeptidases, several endopeptidases, and esterases is also a reason for their low bioavailability. The premise of passive transport as the mechanism of peptide and protein absorption across the buccal mucosa is widely accepted. Endocytotic processes are not apparent in buccal epithelium. No active or carrier-mediated peptide transport systems are present in the buccal epithelium except those responsible for the absorption of a few amino acids such as glutamic acid (anionic) and lysine (cationic) (62). In general, the various aspects addressed thus far can be applied for buccal drug delivery of peptides and proteins (Table 1). It can be noted from the data presented in Table 2 that in general as the molecular weight of the peptide increases, the bioavailability decreases. This suggests that the peptides and proteins, being hydrophilic and globular in nature, are transported by paracellular route.

Biological Activity

Biological activity is the most important concern with the delivery of therapeutic peptides and proteins. Suscepti-

Table 1 Chronological survey of in vivo experiments on buccal delivery of peptides and proteins

Author(s)	Year (REF)	Peptide (in vivo model)
Dillon et al.	1960 (63)	Pitocin (human)
Miller	1973 (64)	Oxytocin (human)
Dawood et al.	1980 (65)	Oxytocin (human)
Ishida et al.	1981 (66)	Insulin (dog)
Anders et al.	1983 (67)	Protirelin (human)
Schurr et al.	1985 (68)	Protirelin (human)
Aungst and Rogers	1988 (69)	Insulin (rat)
Aungst et al.	1988 (70)	Insulin (rat)
Nakada et al.	1988 (71)	Calcitonin (rat)
Oh and Ritschel	1988 (51)	Insulin (rabbit)
Ritschel et al.	1988 (72)	Insulin (dog)
Ho and Barsuhn	1989 (73)	Protirelin, oxytocin (dog)
Wolany et al.	1990 (74)	Octreotide (dog)
al-Achi and Greenwood	1993 (75)	Insulin (rat)
Heiber et al.	1994 (76)	Calcitonin (dog)
Bayley et al.	1995 (77)	Recombinant human interferon-α B/D hybrid (rat, rabbit)
Gutnaik et al.	1996 (78)	Glucagon-like peptide I (human)
Nakane et al.	1996 (79)	Leuteinizing hormone-releasing hormone (dog)
Hoogstraate et al.	1996 (80)	Buserelin (pig)
Li et al.	1997 (81)	Thyrotropin-releasing hormone (rat)
Li et al.	1997 (54)	Oxytocin (rabbit)
Alur et al.	1999 (82)	Calcitonin (rabbit)

Table 2 Data from in vivo experiments on buccal delivery of peptides and proteins

Peptide/protein	MW (Da)	Species				
		Rat	Rabbit	Dog	Pig	Human
TRH	362	—	—	—	—	4%
Oxytocin	1007	—	0.1%	—	—	<10%
LHRH	1182	—	—	0.41% (alone) 0.34–1.62% (with enhancers)	—	—
Buserelin (analog of LHRH)	≈1182	—	—	—	1% (alone) 5% (with enhancers)	—
Calcitonin	3432	—	16 and 37%	550 IU over 6 h	—	—
GLP-I	4169	—	—	—	—	7% (7–36 amide fragment)
Insulin	5808	0% (alone) 25% (with enhancers)	0% (alone) 5% (with enhancers)	0% (alone) 0.5% (with enhancers)	—	0–4%
IFN α-B/D hybrid	19,000	<1%	<1%	—	—	—

bility of these molecules to denaturation by various manufacturing processes may seriously limit the number of methods that can be used in the fabrication of delivery systems. Important process variables such as temperature, pressure, and exposure to organic solvents, etc., during manufacturing need to be considered. The formulation strategies presented above can be applied to the development of peptide and protein formulation in general, or they can be modified according to special needs.

Temperature

High temperatures can break native S—S bonds and form new S—S bonds that can "lock" the protein into a denatured configuration. Low pH, sodium dodecyl sulfate, Tween 80® , chaotropic salts, and exogenous proteins have been used to protect proteins from thermal inactivation (83). Ethylene glycol at 30–50% was used as a protectant of antiviral activity of β-Interferon preparations (84). Human serum albumin was used in recombinant human interferon-β_{ser-17}, which resulted in increased thermal stability (47). Water-soluble polysaccharides such as

dextrans and amylose and point-specific (site-directed) mutagenesis (85) have also been used to increase thermal stability of therapeutic proteins and peptides.

Pressure

Proteins are not very sensitive to pressure changes, and only at large values of pressure do they exhibit conformational changes observed when denatured by heat or changes in solution pH (86). A model enzyme (protein), namely, urease, did not lose much of its activity until the compaction pressure exceeded 474 mPa, above which 50% of the relative activity was lost (87).

Pharmacokinetics and Pharmacodynamic Responses

Pharmacokinetics and pharmacodynamic responses have to be evaluated separately. Initial consideration of a drug candidate for buccal delivery may be its low biological half-life ($t_{\frac{1}{2}}$) possibly owing to high first-pass metabolism and gastrointestinal degradation. It should be noted that both the t_{max} and C_{max} increase (88) with an increase in

$t_{\frac{1}{2}}$. The fraction of the therapeutic peptide absorbed via the oral mucosa should not be calculated from pharmacodynamic response data alone because the efficiency of peptide absorption with respect to its pharmacodynamic response depends not only on the total dose absorbed but also on the rate at which the peptide is taken up by the target organ. Pharmacokinetics after buccal dosing can also be performed using moment analysis (89).

Enzymatic Degradation

The proteolytic activity of the buccal mucosa presents a significant barrier to the delivery of proteins and peptides. Buccal homogenate studies may provide initial data concerning the rate and extent of biochemical degradation of peptides when delivered by the buccal route (90). The disadvantage of homogenate studies includes the inability to distinguish among cytosolic, membrane-bound, and intercellular proteolytic activity. Because protein and peptide transport can be either trans- or paracellular in nature, the exact location of these proteolytic enzymes is important.

A novel concept of using bioadhesive polymers such as derivatives of poly(acrylic acid), polycarbophil, and carbomer to protect therapeutically important proteins and peptides from proteolytic activity of enzymes, endopeptidases (trypsin and α-chymotrypsin), exopeptidases (carboxypeptidases A and B), and microsomal and cytosolic leucine aminopeptidase (91) has been developed. However, cysteine protease (pyroglutamyl aminopeptidase) may not be inhibited by polycarbophil and carbomer (91).

Table 3 Exemplary absorption enhancers under investigation for buccal administration

Class	Exemplary compounds
Chelators	EDTA
Surfactants	Benzalkonium chloride Brij 35 Laureth-9 Sodium dodecylsulfate
Bile salts	Sodium deoxycholate Sodium glycocholate
Fatty acids	Sodium myristate
Peptidase inhibitors	Aprotinin
Miscellaneous	Chondroitinase ABC 1-Dodecylazacycloheptan-2-one Cyclodextrin Quillajasaponine Sodium salicylate

Enzyme Inhibitors

Protease inhibitors are generally used as enzyme inhibitors. These include aprotinin (79), bestatin (92), chondroitinase, and hyaluronidase. According to several published reports, these inhibitors appear to lack adequate effectiveness when administered simultaneously with various peptides in vivo (79).

Permeation Enhancers

Generally, these enhancers fall into six categories: 1) chelators (e.g., EDTA, EGTA); 2) surfactants, which are subdivided into non-ionic, e.g., laureth-9, polysorbate 80, sucrose esters and dodecylmaltoside, cationic; (e.g., cetylmethylammonium bromide), and anionic (e.g., sodium dodecyl glycocholate, sodium lauryl sulfate); 3) Bile salts and other steroidal detergents (e.g., sodium glycocholate, sodium taurocholate, saponins, sodium taurodihydrofusidate, and sodium glycodihydrofusidate); 4) fatty acids (e.g., caprylic acid); 5) nonsurfactants (e.g., 1-dodecylazacycloheptane-2-one (Azone), salicylates, and sulfoxides); and 6) enzymes (e.g., phopholipases, hyaluronidases, neuraminidase, and chondroitinase ABC).

Different mechanisms of absorption enhancement for these permeation enhancers have been proposed. Most permeation enhancers are thought to disrupt the lipid bilayer, which increases membrane fluidity. Some enhancers (nonionic and presumably ionic surfactants) may solubilize and extract lipids (92). Bile salts enhance absorption, stabilize enzyme-labile drugs, and potentially inhibit proteolytic degradation and aggregation of therapeutic proteins by formation of micelles (92). Permeation enhancers, which open tight junctions, are of little benefit in oral mucosal drug delivery because tight junctions are uncommon in these tissues. Structure/-absorption enhancement activity relationships have not been completely characterized for permeation enhancers (Table 3). However, for surfactants, the structure of the polar head groups strongly influences the permeability. For example, it has been reported that for surfactants, absorption enhancement was greatest for ether-based surfactants rather than for esters with similar structure (92).

SUMMARY

In recent years, there has been explosive growth in our understanding of the mechanisms associated with the absorption of drugs, especially of therapeutic peptides and proteins. Scientists from a variety of disciplines continue to elucidate the variables associated with the optimal formulation and delivery of drugs via the oral mucosa. A greater understanding of the para- and transcellular route of drug absorption, proteolytic enzyme activity that may potentially degrade therapeutic peptides, and simultaneous degradation of compounds during the mucosal transport process is essential to the development of buccal delivery systems. Moreover, methods to increase drug flux (e.g., use of permeation enhancers) without associated toxicity, strategies to inactivate proteolytic enzymes, and innovative approaches with regard to controlled drug-delivery and mucoadhesive dosage forms will all improve the delivery of drug substances via the oral cavity.

ACKNOWLEDGMENT

This work was supported in part by NIH grants (AI 36624, EY 09171, and EY 10659; A.K.M.).

REFERENCES

1. Rathbone, M.J.; Drummond, B.K.; Tucker, I.G. The Oral Cavity as Site for Systemic Drug Delivery. Adv. Drug Del. Rev. **1994**, *13*, 1–22.
2. de Varies, M.E.; Bodde, H.E.; Verhoef, J.C.; Junginger, H.E. Developments in Buccal Drug Delivery. Crit. Rev. Ther. Drug. Carr. Syst. **1991**, *8*, 271–303.
3. Merkle, H.P.; Anders, R.; Wermerskirchen, A. Mucoadhesive Buccal Patches for Peptide Delivery. *Bioadhesive Drug Delivery Systems*; Lenaerts, V., Gurney, R., Eds.; CRC Press; Boca Raton, FL, 1990; 105.
4. Chen, S.Y.; Squier, C.A. The Ultrastructure of the Oral Epithelium. *The Structure and Function of Oral Mucosa*; Meyer, J., Squier, C.A., Gerson, S.J., Eds.; Pergamon, NY, 1984; 7.
5. Harris, D.; Robinson, J.R. Drug Delivery Via the Mucous Membranes of the Oral Cavity. J. Pharm. Sci. **1992**, *81*, 1–10.
6. Moffat, A.C. Absorption of Drugs Through the Oral Mucosa. Top Med. Chem. **1972**, *4*, 1.
7. Beckett, A.H.; Hossie, R.D. Buccal Absorption of Drugs. *Handbook of Pharmacology*; Brodie, B.B., Gillette, J.R., Eds.; Springer: NY, 1971; 25.
8. Siegel, I.A.; Hall, S.H.; Stambaugh, R. Permeability of the Oral Mucosa. *Current Concepts of the Histology of Oral Mucosa*; Squier, C.A., Meyer, J., Eds.; Charles C. Thomas: IL, 1971; 274.
9. Dali M.M.; Heran C.L.; Kaeppeli M.; Stetsko P.I.; Smith R.L. Intra-Oral (Buccal/Sublingual) Bioavailablity of Propranolol in Conscious Rabbits as a Function of PH and Dosing Variables Proceedings of the American Association of Pharmaceutical Scientists Annual Meeting New Orleans LA Nov 19–23 1999, 1394, Abstract Number 2559.
10. Evered, D.F.; Sadoogh-Abasian, F.; Patel, P.D. Absorption of Nicotinic Acid and Nicotinamide Across Human Buccal Mucosa In Vivo. Life Sci. **1983**, *27*, 1649–1661.
11. Evered, D.F.; Mallet, C. Thiamine Absorption Across Human Buccal Mucosa In Vivo. Life Sci. **1983**, *32*, 1355–1358.
12. Gandhi, R.B.; Robinson, J.R. Oral Cavity as a Site for Bioadhesive Drug Delivery. Adv. Drug Del. Rev. **1994**, *13*, 43–74.
13. Junginger, H.E.; Hoogstraate, J.A.; Verhoef, J.C. Recent Advances in Buccal Drug Delivery and Absorption— In Vitro and In Vivo Studies. J. Control. Rel. **1999**, *62*, 149–159.
14. Squier, C.A.; Johnson, N.W.; Hopps, R.M. *Human Oral Mucosa Development, Structure and Function*; Blackwell Scientific: Oxford, 1976; 7.
15. Edgar, W.M. Saliva: Its Secretion, Composition and Functions. Br. Dent. J. **1992**, *172*, 305–312.
16. Beckett, A.H.; Triggs, E.J. Buccal Absorption of Basic Drugs and Its Application as an In Vivo Model of Passive Drug Transfer Through Lipid Membranes. J. Pharm. Pharmacol. **1967**, *19*, 31S–41S.
17. Al-Sayed-Omar, O.; Johnston, A.; Turner, P. Influence of PH on the Buccal Absorption of Morphine Sulphate and Its Major Metabolite, Morphine-3-Glucuronide. J. Pharm. Pharmacol. **1987**, *39*, 934–935.
18. Anders, R.; Merkle, H.P. Evaluation of Laminated Muco-Adhesive Patches for Buccal Drug Delivery. Int. J. Pharm. **1989**, *49*, 231–240.
19. Kornfeld, R.; Kornfeld, S. Comparative Aspects of Glycoprotein Structure. Annu. Rev. Biochem. **1976**, *45*, 217.
20. Peppas, N.A.; Buri, P.A. Surface, Interfacial and Molecular Aspects of Polymer Bioadhesion on Soft Tissues. *Advances in Drug Delivery Systems Controlled Release Series*; Anderson, J.M., Kim, S.W., Eds.; Elsevier: Amsterdam, 1986; 1, 257.
21. Chen, J.L.; Cyr, G.N. Compositions Producing Adhesion Through Adhesion. *Adhesive Biological Systems*; Manly, R.S., Ed.; Academic Press: NY, 1970; 163, Chap. 10.
22. Smart, J.D.; Kellaway, I.W.; Worthington, H.E.C. An In Vitro Investigation of Mucosa-Adhesive Materials for Use in Controlled Drug Delivery. J. Pharm. Pharmacol. **1984**, *36*, 295–299.
23. Barrer, R.M.; Barrie, J.A.; Wong, P.S.L. The Diffusion and Solution of Gases in Highly Crosslinked Copolymers. Polymers **1968**, *9*, 609–627.
24. Park, K.; Ch'ng, H.S.; Robinson, J.R. Alternative Approaches to Oral Controlled Drug Delivery Bioadhesives and In Situ Systems. *Recent Advances in Drug Delivery Systems*; Anderson, J.M., Kim, S.W., Eds.; Plenum Press: NY, 1984; 163.
25. Park, K.; Robinson, J.R. Bioadhesive Polymers as Platforms for Oral Controlled Drug Delivery. Int. J. Pharm. **1984**, *19*, 107–127.
26. Gurny, R.; Meyer, J.M.; Peppas, N.A. Bioadhesive Intraoral Release Systems: Design, Testing, and Analysis. Biomaterials **1984**, *5*, 336–340.
27. Ch'ng, H.S.; Park, H.; Kelley, P.; Robinson, J.R. Bioadhesive Polymers as Platforms for Oral Controlled Drug Delivery II: Synthesis and Evaluation of Some

Swelling, Water-Insoluble Bioadhesive Polymers. J. Pharm. Sci. **1985**, *74*, 399–405.

28. Flory, P.J. *Principles of Polymer Chemistry*; Cornell University Press: NY, 1953; 541.

29. Park, H.; Robinson, J.R. Physicochemical Properties of Water Insoluble Polymers Important to Mucin/Epithelial Adhesion. J. Control. Rel. **1985**, *2*, 47–57.

30. Smart, J.D.; Kellaway, I.W. In Vitro Techniques for Measuring Mucoadhesion. J. Pharm. Pharmacol. **1982**, *34*(Suppl.), 70.

31. Mikos, S.A.; Smart, J.D. Scaling Concepts and Molecular Theories of Synthetic Polymers to Glycoproteinic Networks. *Bioadhesive Drug Delivery Systems*; Lenaerts, V., Gurney, R., Eds.; CRC Press: Boca Raton FL, 1990; 25.

32. Mortazavi, S.A.; Smart, J.D. Factors Influencing Gel-Strengthening at the Mucoadhesive-Mucus Interface. J. Pharm. Pharmacol. **1994**, *46*, 86–90.

33. Teng, C.L.C.; Ho, N.F.L. Mechanistic Studies in the Simultaneous Flow and Adsorption of Polymer Coated Latex Particles on Intestinal Mucus. J. Control. Rel. **1987**, *6*, 133–149.

34. Park, K.A. A New Approach to Study Mucoadhesion: Collioidal Gold Staining. Int. J. Pharm. **1989**, *53*, 209–217.

35. Hassan, E.E.; Gallo, J.M. A Simple Rheological Method for the In Vitro Assessment of Mucin-Polymer Bioadhesive Bond Strength. Pharm. Res. **1990**, *7*, 491–495.

36. Kamath, K.R.; Park, K. Mucosal Adhesive Preparations. *Encyclopedia of Pharmaceutical Technology*; Swarbrick, J., Boylan, J.C., Eds.; Marcel Dekker, Inc.: New York, 1994; 10, 133.

37. Ch'ng, H.S.; Park, H.; Kelly, P.; Robinson, J.R. Bioadhesive Polymers as Platforms for Oral Controlled Drug Delivery II: Synthesis and Evaluation of Some Swelling, Water-Insoluble Bioadhesive Polymers. J. Pharm. Sci. **1985**, *74*, 399–405.

38. Khosla, R.; Davis, S.S. The Effect of Polycarbophil on the Gastric Emptying of Pellets. J. Pharm. Pharmacol. **1987**, *39*, 47–49.

39. Ahuja, A.; Khar, R.K.; Ali, J. Mucoadhesive Drug Delivery Systems. Drug Dev. Ind. Phar. **1997**, *23*, 489–515.

40. Lee, P.I. Kinetics of Drug Release from Hydrogel Matrices. *Advances in Drug Delivery Systems*; Anderson, J.M., Kim, S.W., Eds.; (Controlled Release Series) Elsevier: Amsterdam, 1986; 1, 277.

41. Peppas, N.A.; Sahlin, J.J. A Simple Equation for the Description of Solute Release. III. Coupling of Diffusion and Relaxation. Int. J. Pharm. **1989**, *57*, 169–172.

42. Imbert, D.; Cullander, C. Buccal Mucosa In Vitro Experiments. I. Confocal Imaging of Vital Staining and MTT Assays for the Determination of Tissue Viability. J. Control. Rel. **1999**, *58*, 39–50.

43. Audus, K.L.; Bartel, R.L.; Hidalgo, I.J.; Borchardt, R.T. The Use of Cultured Epithelial and Endothelial Cells for Drug Transport and Metabolism Studies. Pharm. Res. **1990**, *7*, 434–451.

44. Pitha, J.; Harman, S.M.; Michel, M.E. Hydrophilic Cyclodextrin Derivatives Enable Effective Oral Administration of Steroidal Hormones. J. Pharm. Sci. **1986**, *75*, 165–167.

45. Merkle, H.P.; Anders, R.; Wermerskirchen, A.; Raechs, S. Buccal Route of Peptide and Protein Drug Delivery. *Peptide and Protein Drug Delivery*; Lee, V.H.L., Ed.; Marcel Dekker, Inc.: New York, 1990; 545.

46. Lee, V.H.L. *Peptide and Protein Drug Delivery*; Lee, V.H.L., Ed.; Marcel Dekker, Inc.: New York, 1990; 1.

47. Berner, B.; Wilson, D.R.; Guy, R.H.; Mazzenfa, G.C.; Clarke, F.H.; Maibach, H.I. The Relationship of pKa and Acute Skin Irritation in Man. Phar. Res. **1988**, *5*, 660–663.

48. Okamoto, H.; Hashida, M.; Sezaki, H. Structure-Activity Relationship of 1-Alkyl- or 1-Alkenylazacycloalkanone Derivatives as Percutaneous Penetration Enhancers. J. Pharm. Sci. **1988**, *77*, 418–424.

49. Siegel, I.A.; Gordon, H.P. Effects of Surfactants on the Permeability of Canine Oral Mucosa In Vitro. Toxicol. Lett. **1985**, *26*, 153–158.

50. Oh, C.K.; Ritschel, W.A. Biopharmaceutic Aspects of Buccal Absorption of Insulin. Methods Find. Exp. Clin. Pharmacol. **1990**, *12*, 205–212.

51. Ritschel, W.A.; Ritschel, G.B.; Forusz, H.; Kraeling, M. Buccal Absorption of Insulin in the Dog. Res. Commun. Chem. Pathol. Pharmacol. **1989**, *63*, 53–67.

52. Sithigornugul, P.; Burton, P.; Nishihata, T.; Caldwell, L. Effects of Sodium Salicylate on Epithelial Cells of the Rectal Mucosa of the Rat: A Light and Electron Microscopic Study. Life Sci. **1983**, *33*, 1025–1032.

53. Li, C.; Bhatt, P.P.; Johnston, T.P. Transmucosal Delivery of Oxytocin to Rabbits Using a Mucoadhesive Buccal Patch. Pharm. Dev. Technol. **1997**, *2*, 265–274.

54. Longenecker, J.P.; Moses, A.C.; Flier, J.S.; Silver, R.D.; Carey, M.; Dubovi, E.J. Effects of Sodium Taurodihydrofusidate on Nasal Absorption of Insulin in Sheep. J. Pharm. Sci. **1987**, *76*, 351–355.

55. Sakai, K.; Kutsuna, T.M.; Nishino, T.; Fujihara, Y.; Yata, N. Contribution of Calcium Ion Sequestration by Polyoxyethylated Nonionic Surfactants to the Enhanced Colonic Absorption of *p*-Aminobenzoic Acid. J. Pharm. Sci. **1986**, *75*, 387–390.

56. Fix, J.A.; Engle, K.; Porter, P.A.; Leppert, P.S.; Selk, S.J.; Gardner, C.R.; Alexander, J. Acylcarnitines: Drug Absorption-Enhancing Agents in the Gastrointestinal Tract. Am. J. Physiol. **1986**, *251*, G332–G340.

57. Hersey, S.J.; Jackson, R.T. Effect of Bile Salts on Nasal Permeability In Vitro. J. Pharm. Sci. **1987**, *76*, 876–879.

58. Pitelka, D.R.; Taggart, B.N.; Hamamoto, S.T. Effects of Extracellular Calcium Depletion on Membrane Topography and Occluding Junctions of Mammary Epithelial Cells in Culture. J. Cell Biol. **1983**, *96*, 613–624.

59. Teem, M.V.; Phillips, S.F. Perfusion of the Hamster Jejunum with Conjugated and Unconjugated Bile Acids: Inhibition of Water Absorption and Effects on Morphology. Gastroenterology **1972**, *62*, 261–267.

60. Clark, M.L.; Lanz, H.C.; Senior, J.R. Bile Salt Regulation of Fatty Acid Absorption and Esterification in Rat Everted Jejunal Sacs In Vitro and into Thoracic Duct Lymph In Vivo. J. Clin. Invest. **1969**, *48*, 1587–1599.

61. Tang-Liu, D.D.S.; Neff, J.; Zolezio, H.; Sandri, R. Percutaneous and Systemic Disposition of Hexamethylene Lauramide and Its Penetration Enhancement Effect on Hydrocortisone in a Rat Sandwich Skin-Flap Model. Pharm. Res. **1988**, *5*, 477–481.

62. Gandhi, R.B. *Some Permselectivity and Permeability Characteristics of Rabbit Buccal Mucosa*; Ph.D. Thesis, University of Wisconsin, Madison, 1990.

63. Dillon, T.F.; Douglas, R.G.; du Vigneaud, V.; Barber, M.L. Transbuccal Administration of Pitocin for Induction of Labor. Obstet. Gynecol. **1960**, *15*, 587–592.

64. Miller, G.W. Induction of Labor by Buccal Administration of Oxytocin: Review of 50 Cases. J. Am. Osteopath. Assoc. **1973**, *72*, 1110–1113.

65. Dawood, M.Y.; Ylikorkala, O.; Fuchs, F. Plasma Oxytocin Levels and Disappearance Rate After Buccal Pitocin. Am. J. Obstet. Gynecol. **1980**, *138*, 20–24.

66. Ishida, M.; Machida, Y.; Nambu, N.; Nagai, T. New Mucosal Dosage Form of Insulin. Chem. Pharm. Bull. **1981**, *29*, 810–816.

67. Anders, R.; Merkle, H.P.; Schurr, W.; Ziegler, R. Buccal Absorption of Protirelin: An Effective Way to Stimulate Thyrotropin and Prolactin. J. Pharm. Sci. **1983**, *72*, 1481–1483.

68. Schurr, W.; Knoll, B.; Ziegler, R.; Anders, R.; Merkle, H.P. Comparative Study of Intravenous, Nasal, Oral, and Buccal TRH Administration Among Healthy Subjects. J. Endocrinol. Invest. **1985**, *8*, 41–44.

69. Aungst, B.J.; Rogers, N.J. Site Dependence of Absorption-Promoting Actions of Laureth-9, Na Salicylate, Na_2EDTA, and Aprotinin on Rectal, Nasal, and Buccal Insulin Delivery. Pharm. Res. **1988**, *5*, 305–308.

70. Aungst, B.J.; Rogers, N.J.; Shefter, E. Comparison of Nasal, Rectal, Buccal, Sublingual, and Intramuscular Insulin Efficacy and the Effects of a Bile Salt Absorption Promoter. J. Pharmacol. Exp. Ther. **1988**, *244*, 23–27.

71. Nakada, Y.; Awata, N.; Nakamichi, C.; Sugimoto, I. The Effect of Additives on the Oral Mucosal Absorption of Human Calcitonin. J. Pharmacobiol. Dyn. **1988**, *11*, 395–401.

72. Ritschel, W.A.; Ritschel, G.B.; Forusz, H.; Kraeling, M. Buccal Absorption of Insulin in the Dog. Res. Commun. Chem. Pathol. Pharmacol. **1989**, *63*, 53–67.

73. Ho N.F.H. Barsuhn C.L. Buccal Delivery of Drugs Proceeding of the International Symposium on Controlled Release Bioactive Materials CH-Basel 1989; *16*, 24.

74. Wolany G.J.M. Munzer J. Rummelt A. Merkle H.P. Buccal Absorption of Sandostatin (Octreotide) in Conscious Beagle Dogs Proceeding of the International Symposium on Controlled Release Bioactive Materials CH-Basel 1990; *17*, Abstract D341.

75. al-Achi, A.; Greenwood, R. *Buccal Administration of Human Insulin in Streptozocin-Diabetic Rats, Res. Commun. Chem. Pathol. Pharmacol*; 1993; 82, 297–306.

76. Heiber, S.J.; Ebert, C.D.; Dave, S.C.; Smith, K.; Kim, S.W.; Mix, D. In Vivo Buccal Delivery of Calcitonin. J. Control. Rel. **1994**, *28*, 269–270.

77. Bayley, D.; Temple, C.; Clay, V.; Steward, A.; Lowther, N. The Transmucosal Absorption of Recombinant Human Interferon-Alpha B/D Hybrid in the Rat and Rabbit. J. Pharm. Pharmacol. **1995**, *47*, 721–724.

78. Gutniak, M.K.; Larsson, H.; Heiber, S.J.; Juneskans, O.T.; Holst, J.J.; Ahren, B. Potential Therapeutic Levels of Glucagon-Like Peptide I Achieved in Humans by a Buccal Tablet. Diabetes Care **1996**, *19*, 843–848.

79. Nakane, S.; Kakumoto, M.; Yukimatsu, K.; Chien, Y.W. Oramucosal Delivery of LHRH: Pharmacokinetic Studies of Controlled and Enhanced Transmucosal Permeation. Pharm. Dev. Technol. **1996**, *1*, 251–259.

80. Hoogstraate, A.J.; Coos Verhoef, J.; Pijpers, A.; van Leengoed, L.A.; Verheijden, J.H.; Junginger, H.E.; Bodde, H.E. In Vivo Buccal Delivery of the Peptide Drug Buserelin with Glycodeoxycholate as an Absorption Enhancer in Pigs. Pharm. Res. **1996**, *13*, 1233–1237.

81. Li, C.; Koch, R.L.; Raul, V.A.; Bhatt, P.P.; Johnston, T.P. Absorption of Thyrotropin Releasing Hormone in Rats Using a Mucoadhesive Buccal Patch. Drug Dev. Ind. Pharm. **1997**, *23*, 239–246.

82. Alur, H.H.; Beal, J.D.; Pather, S.I.; Mitra, A.K.; Johnston, T.P. Evaluation of a Novel, Natural Oligosaccharide Gum as a Sustained-Release and Mucoadhesive Component of Calcitonin Buccal Tablets. J. Pharm. Sci. **1999**, *88*, 1313–1319.

83. Sedmak, J.J.; Grossberg, S.E. Interferon Stabilization and Enhancement by Rare Earth Salts. J. Gen. Virol. **1981**, *52*, 195–197.

84. Knight, E., Jr.; Fathey, D. Human Fibroblast Interferon: An Improved Purification. J. Biol. Chem. **1981**, *256*, 3609–3611.

85. Wells, J.A.; Powers, D.B. In Vivo Formation and Stability of Engineered Disulfide Bonds in Subtilisin. J. Biol. Chem. **1986**, *261*, 6564–6570.

86. Kornblatt, M.J.; Hoa, G.H.B. The Pressure-Induced Inactivation of Mammalian Enolases is Accompanied by Dissociation of the Dimeric Enzyme. Arch. Biochem. Biophys. **1987**, *252*, 277–283.

87. Teng, C.L.D.; Groves, M.J. The Effect of Compactional Pressure on Urease Activity. Pharm. Res. **1988**, *5*, 776–780.

88. Alur, H.H.; Paher, S.I.; Mitra, A.K.; Johnston, T.P. Transmucosal Sustained Delivery of Chlorphenlramine Maleate in Rabbits Using a Novel, Natural Mucoadhesive Gum as an Excipient in Buccal Tablets. Int. J. Pharm. **1999**, *188*, 1–10.

89. Kondo, S.; Sugimoto, I. Moment Analysis of Intravenous, Intraduodenal, Buccal, Rectal, and Percutaneous Nifedipine in Rats. J. Pharmacobio. Dyn. **1987**, *10*, 462–469.

90. Yamamoto, A.; Hayakawa, E.; Lee, V.H. Insulin and Proinsulin Proteolysis in Mucosal Homogenates of the Albino Rabbit: Implications in Peptide Delivery from Nonoral Routes. Life Sci. **1990**, *26*, 2465–2474.

91. Luessen, H.L.; Verhoef, J.C.; de Boer, G.; Junginger, H.E.; de Leeuz, B.J.; Borchard, G.; Lehr, C.M. Multifuntional Polymers for the Peroral Delivery of Peptide Drugs. *Bioadhesive Drug Delivery Systems*; Mathiowitz, E., Chickering, D.E., III, Lehr, C.M., Eds.; Marcel Dekker, Inc.: New York, 1999; 299.

92. Lee, V.H.L. Enzymatic Barriers to Peptide and Protein Absorption. CRC Crit. Rev. Ther. Drug. Carrier Syst. **1988**, *5*, 69–97.

93. Smart, J.D. An In Vitro Assessment of Some Mucosa Adhesive Dosage Forms. Int. J. Pharm. **1991**, *73*, 69–74.

PEPTIDES AND PROTEINS—ORAL ABSORPTION

Eugene J. McNally
Jung Y. Park
Boehringer Ingelheim Pharmaceuticals, Inc., Ridgefield, Connecticut

INTRODUCTION

Rapid developments in biotechnology have posed new challenges for pharmaceutical research scientists to develop peptide (>3 amino acids) and protein drugs. Although these peptide and protein drugs are highly potent and specific in their physiological actions, they are in general difficult to administer orally. The reason is that most peptide and protein drugs are very unstable in the gastrointestinal (GI) tract and show poor oral absorption because of their size and hydrophilic nature (there are specific exceptions, e.g., cyclosporine). Although each nonparenteral delivery route has its own advantages and disadvantages, based on the available published data and the known permeability of mucosal membranes, it may be possible to rank them as the preferred route for the delivery of peptide and protein drugs. It appears that the nasal cavity is the preferred route for the delivery of peptide and protein drugs, followed by the vaginal, pulmonary, oral, and transdermal routes, respectively. It is common knowledge that peptide and protein drugs are easily hydrolyzed and digested by acids and enzymes in the GI tract. In addition, these drugs usually show low bioavailability because of their poor membrane permeability in the GI tract.

To deliver peptide and protein drugs orally, it is necessary to protect them from the hostile GI environment. Many strategies, such as coadministration with nonspecific protease inhibitors as well as the use of chemical modification approaches to improve resistance to enzymatic degradation, have been reported in the scientific and patent literature. In recent years, a number of drug-delivery companies specializing in protein delivery have emerged. A number of these companies are attempting to apply formulation approaches such as liposomes or microspheres to protect protein drugs from enzymatic degradation in the GI tract or using site-specific delivery to the colon or rectum to bypass the harsh GI environment. In addition, to increase the GI absorption of the peptide and protein drugs, absorption enhancers as well as carriers or prodrug approaches are being explored.

The purposes of this article are sixfold: 1) to review the GI tract as it relates to the absorption of drugs; 2) to review briefly the structures of peptides and proteins; 3) to review the enzymatic and physical barriers for intestinal permeability of peptides and proteins; 4) to review the absorption of amino acids, peptides, and proteins across the GI tract; 5) to review the kinds of absorption enhancers and how they work; and 6) to review possible ways to improve the absorption of poorly bioavailable peptide and protein drugs.

GASTROINTESTINAL PHYSIOLOGY RELEVANT TO ABSORPTION

A rational approach to understanding the GI absorption of peptides and proteins requires some knowledge of the GI tract such as morphology, function of different components of the cells, geometry, ultrastructure, biochemical processes, hydrodynamics in the intestinal lumen, and transport mechanisms.

The Digestive System

The digestive system consists of the canal from the mouth to the anus (oropharynx, esophagus, stomach, small intestine, and large intestine) and associated organs (salivary glands, liver, gallbladder, and pancreas) (Fig. 1).The small intestine is divided into three parts, the duodenum, jejunum, and ileum, and is the primary site of absorption for most drugs. The large intestine, which is also called the colon, is divided into the caecum, ascending colon, transverse colon, descending colon, sigmoid colon, rectum, and anus. The salivary glands, liver, gallbladder, and pancreas deliver digestive secretions and help digestion and absorption of peptide and protein drugs.

Stomach

The inner surface of the stomach consists of well-defined tissue layers: the muscle and the submucosal and mucosal layers. The absorption function of stomach is minimal

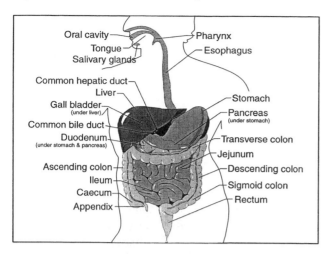

Fig. 1 The human digestive system. (Illustration by Leigh A. Rondano, Boehringer Ingelheim Pharmaceuticals, Inc.)

owing to the limited surface area, lack of villi, thick mucosal layer, and short residence time. The epithelium of the gastric mucosa secretes hydrochloric acid, pepsin, intrinsic factor, and bicarbonate (1). The low pH of gastric juice generated by hydrochloric acid causes protein denaturation (unfolding), which results in increased exposure of peptide bonds to pepsin, which breaks down the proteins into peptides. However, hydrolysis in the stomach is incomplete because pepsin can only break peptide bonds between specific amino acids.

Small intestine

Most enzymatic hydrolysis of the macromolecules in food occurs in the small intestine. The small intestine is approximately 5 m long with a radius of approximately 2 cm, and is divided into three anatomical regions: the duodenum (the first 25 cm), the jejunum (the second 2.0 m), and the ileum (the last 2.75 m) (1). The intestinal membrane wall consists of four basic layers: the mucosa, submucosa, muscularis, and serosa.

The mucosal layer, comprising the lumenal surface of the small intestine, is responsible for the digestive and absorptive functions of the small intestine. The mucosal surface area is much larger than predicted for a simple cylinder. Circular folds account for this amplification. The mucosal surface area is extended further by fingerlike projections called villi and depressions called crypts. The villi are 0.5–1.0 mm in height. Each villus and crypt is lined by epithelial cells that are covered with many closely packed microvilli that project into the intestinal lumen. If the small intestine is viewed as a simple cylinder, its mucosal surface area would be on the order of half of a square meter. However, in reality, the mucosal surface

area of the small intestine is approximately 250 square meters, comparable with size of a tennis court.

Mucous surface: The mucosa of the small intestine consists of three layers (Fig. 2): an absorptive layer, a continuous single sheet of columnar epithelium; the lamina propria, a layer heterogeneous in composition and cell type; and the muscularis mucosa, a muscular layer separating the mucosa and submucosa.

The lamina propria consists primarily of connective tissue and supports the epithelium lining. There is ample evidence that the lymphoid cells and associated structures of the lamina propria play an important role immunologically. Small lymphoid nodules are present in the upper small intestine, whereas large organized aggregates of lymphoid tissue (Peyer's patches) are present in the ileum. The lymphoid cells, nodules, and Peyer's patches of the lamina propria, along with the intraepithelial lymphocytes, establish the so-called gut-associated lymphoid tissue (GALT), which is a major subgroup of the immune system and makes up as much as 25% of the gastrointestinal mucosa.

A one-cell thick sheet of epithelial cells covers the surfaces of the villi and lines of crypts. Some of the cell types identified in the epithelial lining of the small intestine are enterocytes (digestion and absorption), goblet cells (mucus secretion), endocrine cells (hormone secretion), and M cells (absorption of food and antigens).

Absorptive cells: Absorptive cells (commonly called enterocytes or brush border cells) are the most prevalent type of cells on the tips of villi and are the most important for absorption (Fig. 3). In humans, these cells are 20–30 μm in height and 8–10 μm in width. The mucosal surface of this cell is characterized by the presence of microvilli (the brush border, approximately 1.0 μm in height and 0.1–0.2 in width). The microvilli look something like a brush, as shown in Fig. 3. For this reason, the microvillus border of intestinal epithelial absorptive cells is called the brush border. The microvillus plasma membrane has a trilaminar structure (70–90° A thick) composed of proteins, neutral lipids, phospholipids, and glycolipids. An integral and dynamic part of the plasma membrane is the glycocalyx, which is a uniform layer of filamentous glycoproteins (Fig. 4) (2). This glycocalyx layer has a negative charge at physiological pH primarily owing to the presence of sialic acids at the terminal position in the carbohydrate chain. The microvillus and its glycocalyx are viewed as the digestive-absorptive unit of the enterocyte. The plasma membrane of microvilli has an unusually high protein-to-lipid ratio, owing to the presence of specialized proteins possessing enzymatic, receptor, and transport properties. This microvillus plasma membrane contains a number of

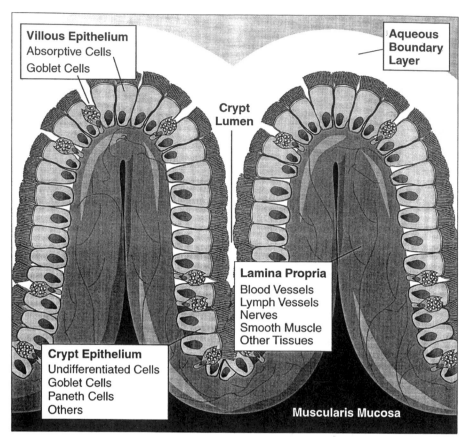

Fig. 2 Schematic depiction of two-section villi and a crypt to illustrate the small intestine mucosa. Also shown is an aqueous boundary layer located at the intestinal lumen and membrane interface. (Illustration by Leigh A. Rondano, Boehringer Ingelheim Pharmaceuticals, Inc.)

enzymes (peptidases) involved in the hydrolysis of peptides. In addition, proteins responsible for the cotransport of sodium and amino acids have been found in the microvillus plasma membrane. Receptor proteins specific for certain substances have been found on the microvilli of enterocytes in different regions of the small intestine. For example, the receptors for the intrinsic factor vitamin B_{12} complex are present in the microvilli of ileal enterocytes but are not found on jejunal cells. This is why vitamin B_{12} is absorbed exclusively from the ileum. Vitamin B_{12} has been explored as a delivery system for peptide and proteins by covalently conjugating vitamin B_{12} to peptides (leuteinizing hormone-releasing hormone, LHRH) or proteins (bovine serum albumin, BSA) (3).

The absorptive cell basolateral membrane rests on the lamina propria. The basolateral membrane is different from the apical membrane. It has a low protein-lipid ratio and is thinner and more permeable than the apical membrane. In addition, different enzymes are present at the basolateral membrane compared with the apical membrane. Adjacent cells are connected by a junctional complex called the tight junction. This tight junction is important because it represents one possible route of intestinal absorption, known as the paracellular route. The other major route of absorption is across the cell, also known as the transcellular route. These routes will be discussed later.

Aqueous boundary (diffusion) layer: The aqueous boundary layer (often referred to as the stagnant, unstirred, or aqueous diffusion layer) is an important hydrodynamic barrier that a drug must traverse before reaching the surface of the mucosal membrane (4). Before a molecule in the intestinal lumen passes through the membrane, it must first cross the aqueous boundary layer located at the intestinal lumen and membrane interface (Fig. 2). The liquid in this layer, in reality, is not static, as the term "unstirred" implies, but represents a film at the surface where diffuse and natural convective mixing occurs. This unstirred layer can be a rate-limiting step for the absorption of hydrophobic molecules. However, hydrophilic molecules such as peptides will diffuse through the

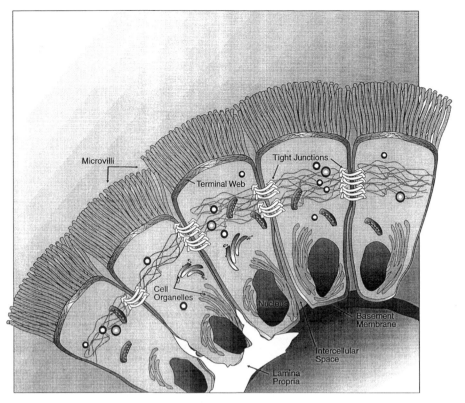

Fig. 3 Schematic depiction of intestinal epithelial absorptive cells. (Illustration by Leigh A. Rondano, Boehringer Ingelheim Pharmaceuticals, Inc.)

aqueous boundary layer with less resistance. The effective thickness of the aqueous boundary layer is thinner around the tips of the villi and thicker and less stirred in the valleys of the villi. The existence of the aqueous boundary layer is physically sound and experimentally demonstrable (5).

Luminal and membrane metabolism of peptides and proteins: In meaningful studies on peptide and protein drug absorption in the small intestine, it is prerequisite to distinguish among cavital, membrane contact, and intracellular drug metabolism (4). Cavital metabolism takes place in the lumen of the small intestine by enzymes such as trypsin, chymotrypsin, carboxypeptidase, and elastase, which are secreted by the pancreas. Membrane contact metabolism is carried out by aminopeptidases localized on the brush border membrane. Intracellular metabolism occurs inside of the cells. The known intracelluar enzymes are cytoplasmic peptidases, prolidase, dipeptidase, and tripeptidase (1). A more detailed discussion of this topic is presented in "Intestinal Absorption Barriers," later.

Intestinal blood flow: The mechanistic relationship among intestinal blood flow and absorption, secretion, and metabolic activity of the intestinal mucosa is unclear. However, there is evidence that impaired intestinal blood flow rate correlates with a decrease in drug absorption rate. It has been postulated that reduced blood flow slows down the absorption rate by: 1) decreasing the effective concentration gradient across the epithelial layer for passively absorbed molecules, by not rapidly carrying the molecule away, and 2) by lowering oxygen supply to the absorption cells needed to maintain the active transport mechanism for absorption.

In general, when molecules transport through the epithelium cell layer directly into the mesenteric blood draining the small intestine, the total mass transfer resistance may be described by the sum of resistance for barriers (aqueous boundary layer in front of the membrane, the membrane itself, and the aqueous boundary layer in blood side) in series (6):

$$\frac{1}{P_{app}} = \frac{1}{P_{aq}} + \frac{1}{P_{membrane}} + \frac{1}{P_{blood}} \tag{1}$$

where P_{app} is apparent permeability coefficient; P_{aq} is permeability coefficient of the aqueous boundary layer; $P_{membrane}$ is permeability coefficient of the membrane; and

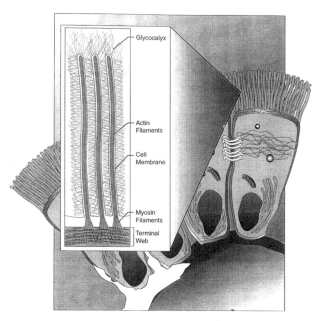

Fig. 4 Schematic depiction of glycocalyx. (Illustration by Leigh A. Rondano, Boehringer Ingelheim Pharmaceuticals, Inc.)

P_{blood} is permeability coefficient of the blood boundary layer.

When the permeabilities of the aqueous boundary layer and membrane are relatively large, reduced blood flow becomes the rate-limiting step. For example, the apparent permeability coefficient is approximately 85% controlled by blood flow when P_{aq} and $P_{membrane}$ are each approximately 10 times greater than P_{blood}.

Large intestine (colon)

The large intestine (or colon) is divided into five parts: 1) the caecum, or opening into the colon; 2) the ascending colon, or second section of the large intestine; 3) the transverse colon; 4) the descending colon; and 5) the sigmoid colon, which is at the end of the colon, ending in the rectum (Fig. 1). The large intestine is approximately 1.5 m long, and its proximal diameter is approximately 2 inches. The wall of the large intestine is divided into four layers, exactly the same as the small intestine: the serosa, muscularis externa, submucosa, and mucosa. However, the mucosa does not contain villi, and the microvilli and the cells are much less dense than those in the small intestine. It also contains a large number of bacteria, which digest food residues into caloric substance that are subsequently absorbed. The total bacteria count in the large intestine is higher than that in the stomach and small intestine. Attempts have been made to deliver peptide and protein drugs to the colon by coating the drug particles with co-polymers that are sensitive to bacterial azo-reductases (7).

In addition, the colon has recently received considerable attention as a possible delivery site for peptide and protein drugs because of low proteolytic activity in this region of the GI tract.

Rectum

The rectum is the terminal 15 to 19 cm of the large intestine. The mucous membrane of the rectum consists of a layer of cylindrical epithelial cells, without villi. The pH in the rectum is between 7.2 and 7.4. The surface area is only 200–400 cm^2. Drug absorption takes place through three veins of the submucous plexus. Superior rectal veins enter into the portal veins and deliver drugs to the liver. However, the inferior and middle rectal veins connect with the inferior vena cava and thus bypass the liver. This may provide an advantage for the delivery of some peptide and protein drugs through the rectal membrane, thus bypassing the liver.

STRUCTURAL AND FUNCTIONAL ASPECTS OF PEPTIDES AND PROTEINS

In addition to understanding the morphology and function of the GI tract, it is also important to have a thorough understanding of the physical/chemical properties of peptides and proteins to rationally formulate them for successful oral delivery. An extensive review is beyond the scope of this article [see other sections in this text and a recent text on formulation and delivery of proteins (8)]. Instead, a brief description of peptides and proteins is provided that focuses on those characteristics that give rise to the unique biological activity of these molecules. Peptides are formed by loss of water from the NH_2 and COOH groups of adjacent amino acids; they are referred to as di-, tri-, tetra- (etc.) peptides depending on the number of amino acids composing them. The term oligopeptides refers to peptides that have fewer than eight amino acids, whereas polypeptide refers to those peptides that contain approximately eight or more amino acids. An amino acid unit in a polypeptide is called a residue. Polypeptides that contain from approximately 50 (molecular weight ≈6000) to more than 8000 amino acid residues (molecular weight ≈1,000,000) are called proteins (9). Each protein molecule is a polymer of α-amino acids linked together in a sequential manner by peptide bonds. Although more than 100 amino acids occur in nature, particularly in plants, only 20 are commonly found in most proteins.

Proteins are one of the major naturally occurring organic compounds, and they constitute much of animal and plant tissue. The word protein comes from the Greek word *proteios*, meaning first place, because proteins are thought to be the most important part of living matter. They are instrumental in almost everything cells do. Proteins are the most abundant components of cells. They account for more than 50% of the dry weight of most cells (9). They serve as antibodies, enzymes, hormones, transport mediators, and structural elements.

Unlike traditional small molecular weight chemical drugs, peptide and especially protein drugs are highly complex molecules that possess primary, secondary, tertiary, and quaternary structures. The primary structure refers to the linear amino acid sequence of a peptide or protein. The secondary structure refers to the way in which segments of the peptide backbone orient into regular patterns such as a α-helix or β-sheet. The tertiary structure refers to the native conformation that is formed by the folding of the secondary structures to a compact, tightly folded structure to reach the most thermodynamically stable state. Quaternary structure occurs when a protein molecule consists of two or more polypeptide chains (10).

A protein's biological function depends on its unique conformation. This conformation is a consequence of the specific linear sequence of the amino acids that makes up the polypeptide chain (primary structure) and the specific three-dimensional structure (conformation) the protein molecule adopts. In general, nonpolar residues tend to fold into the center of the structure to get away from water, whereas the polar residues tend to stay on the surface in contact with water. To maintain the biological activity of the protein drug, this unique higher-order physical structure must be preserved during passage through the GI tract and upon absorption. Subtle changes in the chemical and physical structure can lead to a loss of biological activity.

INTESTINAL ABSORPTION BARRIERS

Enzymatic Barriers

Most dietary proteins are known not to be absorbed in humans as intact forms. Instead, they are usually broken down into amino acids or di- and tripeptides first in the GI tract. The stomach secretes pepsinogen, which is converted to the active protease pepsin by the action of acid. Pepsins, which are most active at pH 2 to 3, hydrolyze partially digested dietary proteins. The partially digested dietary proteins are further broken down by proteolytic enzymes (peptidases) produced by the pancreas and secreted in the duodenum of the small

intestine. The peptidases that break the internal peptide linkages are known as endopeptidases, whereas those that attack the terminal, or end, groups of amino acids are called exopeptidases. The endopeptidases are trypsin, chymotrypsin, and elastase, and the only exopeptidase enzymes are carboxypeptidases (1). All four enzymes (trypsin, chymotrypsin, carcoxypeptidases, and elastase) are secreted by the pancreas as inactive, proenzyme forms of trypsinogen, chemotrypsinogen, procarboxypeptidases, and proelastase. The enzyme enterokinase (also called enteropeptidase) within the lumen of the small intestine converts trypsinogen to trypsin. Then, trypsin converts chymotrypsinogen, procarboxypeptidases, and proelastase to chymotrypsin, carboxypeptidases, and elastase, respectively (1). These enzymes, whose function in vivo is to break down food proteins into amino acids that can be then absorbed and turned into energy, will also degrade a protein drug. It is important to understand the function and sites of secretion of these enzymes so that strategies to protect protein drugs from degradation can be developed.

These four peptidases secreted from the pancreas convert proteins and polypeptides to oligopeptides. The luminal degradation is up to 20% of the total degradation in a given small intestinal segment (11). The rest of the degradation occurs on contact with the brush border membrane or after entry into the cell. Brush border peptidases such as amino oligopeptidase, amino peptidase, and dipeptidyl aminopeptidase then break down the oligopeptides to amino acids (up to 70%) and di- and tripeptides (up to 30%) (1). The di- and tripeptides that cross the brush border membrane are converted to single amino acids by the intracellular enzymes known as cytopasmic peptidases, prolidase, dipeptidase, and tripeptidase (1).

The above-mentioned enzymatic barriers must be overcome to improve oral absorption of peptide and protein drugs from the GI tract. This may be possible to achieve to some extent by the coadministion of proteolytic enzyme inhibitor or by chemical modification of peptides or proteins and by other formulation approaches (see "Intestinal Absorption of Amino Acids, Peptides, and Proteins," later).

Physical Barriers

Absorption barriers are related to the permeability of drug molecules across the gastrointestinal membrane including the colonic membrane. There are two distinct mechanisms for molecules to cross the membrane: via paracellular transport and transcellular transport (Fig. 5) (12). Paracellular transport involves only passive diffusion where the molecules pass through the tight junctions between the epithelial cells. In contrast, transcellular transport can occur

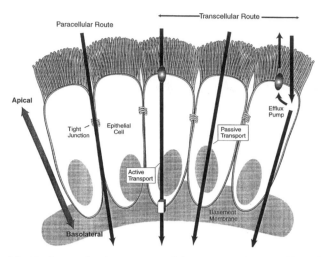

Fig. 5 Routes for the transport of drugs across the GI epithelial cells. (Illustration by Leigh A. Rondano, Boehringer Ingelheim Pharmaceuticals, Inc.)

by passive diffusion as well as by active transport, or endocytosis. In general, the hydrophilic molecules diffuse predominantly through the paracellular route, whereas the lipophilic molecules traverse predominantly through the epithelial cells.

Transcellular transport

Three processes are involved in transcellular transport across the intestinal epithelial cells: simple passive trans-

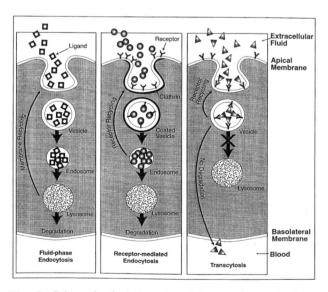

Fig. 6 Schematic depiction of cellular uptake mechanisms: fluid-phase endocytosis, receptor-mediated endocytosis, and transcytosis. (Illustration by Leigh A. Rondano, Boehringer Ingelheim Pharmaceuticals, Inc.)

port, passive diffusion together with an efflux pump, and active transport and endocytosis. Simple passive transport is the diffusion of molecules across the membrane by thermodynamic driving forces and does not require direct expenditure of metabolic energy. In contrast, active transport is the movement of molecules across the membrane resulting directly from the expenditure of metabolic energy and transport against a concentration gradient. Endocytosis processes include three mechanisms: fluid-phase endocytosis (pinocytosis), receptor-mediated endocytosis, and transcytosis (Fig. 6). Endocytosis processes are covered in detail in "Absorption of Polypeptides and Proteins," later.

The mechanism whereby drugs are absorbed from the GI tract is complex. Understanding the intestinal transport mechanism is crucial to the prediction of oral drug absorption. The physical model (13–15) utilizes the basic principles of thermodynamics and mass transport. The physical model for the simultaneous passive and active membrane transport of drugs in the intestinal lumen is depicted in Fig. 7. The bulk aqueous solution with an aqueous boundary layer on the mucosal side is followed by a series of heterogeneous membranes consisting of parallel lipoidal and aqueous channel pathways for passive and active transport. Thereafter, a sink on the serosal side follows.

The rate of disappearance of a drug from the intestinal lumen and appearance in the blood is given by:

$$\frac{dC_b}{dt} = -\frac{A}{V}P_{app}(C_b - C_{blood}) \tag{2}$$

when there is no accumulation of drug in the blood side, i.e., sink conditions

$$\frac{dC_b}{dt} = -\frac{A}{V}P_{app}C_b = -K_uC_b \tag{3}$$

where C_b is the total drug concentration in the lumen; $K_u = (\frac{A}{V})$; P_{app}, the apparent first-order absorption rate

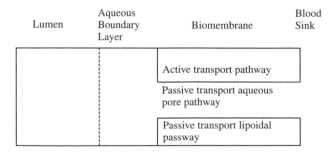

Lumen	Aqueous Boundary Layer	Biomembrane	Blood Sink
		Active transport pathway	
		Passive transport aqueous pore pathway	
		Passive transport lipoidal passway	

Fig. 7 The physical model for the simultaneous passive and active membrane transport of drugs in the intestinal lumen.

constant; A is the surface area; and V is the lumenal solution volume.

Assuming no significant aqueous boundary layer on the blood side, the apparent permeability coefficient (P_{app}) in Eq. 1 is expressed by:

$$P_{app} = \cfrac{1}{\cfrac{1}{P_{aq}} + \cfrac{1}{P_{membrane}}} \tag{4}$$

With the use of Eq. 4, the absorption rate constant can be expressed as:

$$K_u = \frac{A}{V} \cdot \cfrac{1}{\cfrac{1}{P_{aq}} + \cfrac{1}{P_{membrane}}} \tag{5}$$

For highly lipophilic drugs ($\sim$log PC >3.0), the absorption rate constant will be dependent on the diffusion rate across the aqueous boundary layer in front of the membrane, and is expressed by:

$$K_u = \left(\frac{A}{V}\right) \cdot P_{aq} \tag{6}$$

and is also shown in illustration:

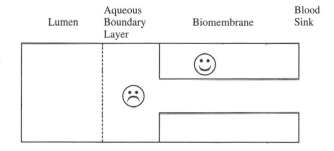

For the hydrophilic drugs such as peptides and proteins, the absorption rate constant will be dependent on the diffusion across the membrane ($P_{aq} \gg P_{membrane}$).

$$K_u = \left(\frac{A}{V}\right) \cdot P_{membrane} \tag{7}$$

Table 1 includes additional mathematical definitions of effective membrane permeability coefficient for various transport mechanisms.

During the past 10 years, it has been reported that the 170-kDa P-glycoprotein, which is known as the principal component of pleiotropic (multidrug) resistance (MDR) in tumor cells, works as an apically polarized efflux transporter (also known as an efflux pump). This efflux transporter opposes the transcellular movement of drugs in the epithelial cells. P-glycoprotein is known to be present in the apical region of epithelial cells in the kidney, liver, and GI tract. Many drugs are known to be substrates for this efflux transporter including cyclosporin A (16) and other peptides (17). The existence of efflux pumps for peptides is demonstrated by measuring the apparent permeability coefficient (P_{app}) values of peptides (e.g., cyclosporin A) using the Caco-2 cell culture model with and without efflux pump inhibitors. With efflux pump inhibitors (chlorpromazine and progesterone), the P_{app} value of apical to basalateral transport for both cyclosporin A increases significantly compared with the control (without inhibitors). In contrast, the basolateral to apical transport is decreased with an inhibitor. Cyclosporin A is a substrate for the efflux transporter P-glycoprotein, and the efflux pump is located on the apical side of the intestinal epithelial cells. Whenever unexplainable poor absorption of peptides is seen, the role of these efflux pumps should be examined.

Table 1 Effective membrane permeability coefficients for various transport mechanisms

Mechanism	$P_{membrane} =$
Passive diffusion of small electrolytes	$P_L X_s + P_p$
Passive diffusion of small nonelectrolytes	$P_L + P_p$
Passive diffusion of large nonelectrolytes	P_L
Passive transport of ampholytes	$P_L^{\pm} X_s^{\pm} + P_p^+ X_s^+ + P_p^- X_s^-$
Passive diffusion coupled with active transport	$P_L X_s + P_L^*(1-X_s)$ where $P_L^* = J_{max}^*/K_L^*$

P_L is the permeability coefficient of the lipoidal membrane; P_p is the permeability coefficient of the aqueous pore; X_s is the fraction of unionized species; $P_L^{\pm}$ is the permeability coefficient of the lipoidal membrane of neutally charged species; P_p^+, P_p^- is the permeability coefficient of aqueous pore of positively and negatively charged species, respectively; $X_s^{\pm}, X_s^+, X_s^-$ is the fraction of neutrally, positively, and negatively charged species at the membrane surface, respectively; P_L^* is the permeability coefficient of the membrane for active transport; J_{max}^* is the maximum flux for active transport; K_L^* is the Michaelis constant for active transport.

Paracellular transport

The primary barrier to paracellular transport is the tight junction (also known as *zonula occludens*), which plays a central role in sealing the intercellular space in epithelial cells (18). These tight junctions are located just under the brush border and form a seal between adjacent epithelial cells. Tight junctions act as a gate and fence to control the intercellular movement of molecules. In addition, tight junctions prevent free diffusion and intermixing of certain apical and basolateral plasma membrane proteins, resulting in polarization of the epithelial cell layers. These junctions are composed of paired intramembrane strands, which consist of lipid molecules and several protein components such as occuludin, claudin-1, and claudin-2. Based on coexpression studies, it appears that claudin-1 and claudin-2 are more likely involved in sealing the tight junctions, and occuldin plays a supporting role for coordinating and modulating functions of tight junctions (19). The strands are thought to contain multiple and discrete aqueous pores (12). The tight junctions are lined with fixed negative charges such as COO^-, SO_4^{2-}, and PO_4^{3-} ions present on the surface of glycoproteins and proteoglycans on neighboring cell membranes (20). Because the tight junctions are negatively charged, this barrier has cation selectivity. In general, cations diffuse through the tight junctions faster than anions (21). The radius of the tight junctions of the intestinal mucosa can be a critical factor for the paracellular transport of peptide and protein drugs. The radius of the tight junction is about 12 Å (22). Because of the size limit of the tight junction, only small molecules and ions are capable of diffusing through the paracellular route. Amino acids, dipeptides, and tripeptides may be small enough to be absorbed across the intestinal wall through the paracellular route, but polypeptides and proteins are restricted because of their size.

One approach for overcoming this diffusion restriction is to change the aqueous pore radius of tight junctions by coadministering drugs with enhancers. Numerous enhancers have been investigated to increase the permeability of the intestinal membrane. They can be categorized into two groups: anionic surfactants such as long-chain acylcarnitines, bile acids, disodium dodecyl sulfate, and sodium caprate, and calcium-chelating agents such as EDTA and citrate (17). The calcium-chelating agents reduce the levels of calcium and induce opening of tight junctions. The anionic surfactants open up the tight junctions by interacting with the cell membrane. It is very important to weigh the benefits versus the toxic risks of enhancers with respect to causing long-term, irreversible damage to the membrane. Very little work has been reported on the toxicological effects of enhancers. It is generally known

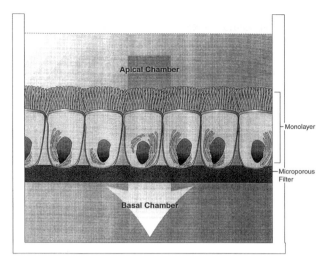

Fig. 8 Schematic representation of Caco-2 cell. (Illustration by Leigh A. Rondano, Boehringer Ingelheim Pharmaceuticals, Inc.)

that nonionic surfactants exhibit lower levels of toxicity than do ionic surfactants; however, the ionic surfactants are considered much more potent enhancers.

TECHNIQUES FOR ASSESSING THE INTESTINAL MEMBRANE PERMEABILITY

Various techniques have been used for assessing the permeability of drug molecules across the intestinal membrane including as everted sacs (23), brush border membrane vesicles (24), intestinal rings (24), recirculation method (25), modified in situ Doluisio technique (4), through-and-through in situ method (26), Caco-2 cell culture model (17), and human intubation method (27). During the last 10 years, the Caco-2 cell culture model (Fig. 8) has gained the most attention in the pharmaceutical industry. This human colon carcinoma cell line model has been shown to mimic the intestinal epithelial cells and is used for assessing the permeability of molecule (17). This Caco-2 cell model has been used as a routine screening tool for compounds produced by combinatorial chemistry.

In the Caco-2 cell experiment, the apparent permeability coefficient (P_{app}) is determined by the following equation:

$$P_{app} = \frac{1}{AC_d} \cdot \frac{dM}{dt} \tag{8}$$

where $C_{d,0}$ is the initial concentration of drug in the donor side, and M is the mass of the drug in the receiver side at the time t.

The apparent permeability coefficient is further defined in Eq. 9:

$$\frac{1}{P_{app}} = \frac{1}{P_{aq}} + \frac{1}{P_{mono}} + \frac{1}{P_F} \tag{9}$$

where P_F is the permeability coefficient of the filter support and P_{mono} is the permeability coefficient of the Caco-2 cell monolayer.

INTESTINAL ABSORPTION OF AMINO ACIDS, PEPTIDES, AND PROTEINS

Much is known regarding the uptake of food-derived amino acids and peptides from the GI tract. This is useful information to review because it gives insight into how peptide and protein drugs are likely to be absorbed.

Absorption of Amino Acids

The uptake of single amino acids is more active in the ileum than in the jejunum. The intestinal cell membrane contains many different amino acid transporters. Amino acids are absorbed across the brush border plasma membrane into the epithelial cell by certain specific amino acid transporters. Transporter types B, $B^{0,+}$, IMINO, β, and X_{AG}^- are sodium-dependent, and types $b^{0,+}$ and y^+ are sodium-independent transporters (1). The sodium-dependent transporters bind amino acids only after binding sodium. The amino acid-bonded transporter then undergoes a conformational change that dumps sodium and the amino acid inside the cell, followed by its reorienta-tion back to the original form. The basolateral membrane of the absorptive cell contains additional transporters that carry amino acids from the cell into the blood. The amino acid transporters of the basolateral membrane are categorized as sodium-dependent types A and ASC and sodium-independent types asc, L, and y^+ (1).

Transporter type X_{AG}^- is for the transport of acidic amino acids, and basic amino acids are preferred substrates for transporter type y^+. The transporter types A and IMINO help the transport of amino acids such as proline and hydroxy-proline. The remaining transporters (B, $B^{0,+}$, β, $b^{0,+}$, ASC, asc, L) are for the transport of neutral amino acids. The intestinal absorption of amino acids is a stereochemically specific mechanism. The rate of absorption of the L-isomer is greater than that of the corresponding D-isomer when racemic mixtures of the amino acid are introduced in the small intestine (28).

Absorption of Small Peptides

After the break down of proteins by proteolytic enzymes, the pancreas, and brush border peptidases, the di- and tripeptides are absorbed through the epithelial cell membrane. Many studies have shown that intact di- and tripeptides are absorbed across the epithelial cell membrane by active transport via specific carrier systems. The absorption process is mediated by the hydrogen-coupled peptide transporter (PEPT1) located in the intestinal apical cell membrane (29). Because there are 20 amino acids, there may be 400 dipeptides and 8000 tripeptides with different molecular sizes and charges. This means that a single membrane transport system has a high affinity for di- and tripeptides but very low affinities for tetra- or higher oligopeptides. Peptide-like drugs such as angiotensin-converting enzyme (ACE) inhibitors, bestatin, cephalosporins, beta-lactam antibiotics, and renin inhibitors are recognized by peptide transporter because of their structural similarities with small peptides. Once inside the enterocyte, the vast majority of di- and tripeptides are digested into amino acids by intracellular peptidases and are exported from the cell into the blood. Only a very small number of these small peptides enter the blood intact. Peptides that are resistant to hydrolysis by cytoplasmic peptidases exit across the basolateral cell membrane by less well-studied basolateral peptide transporters. The sodium/hydrogen exchanger maintains the incoming proton gradient on the apical membrane side, whereas the sodium/potassium-ATPase in the basolateral

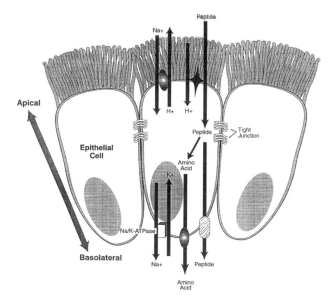

Fig. 9 Model of peptide transport across intestinal epithelial cells. (Illustration by Leigh A. Rondano, Boehringer Ingelheim Pharmaceuticals, Inc.)

Table 2 GI Absorption of peptides and peptidelike drugs

Compound	MW[a]	Extent of absorption (%)	Reference
Dietary di- and tripeptides	200–300	5–50	(30)
Aminocephalosporins	350	>50	(31)
Enalapril	377	>50	(32)
Dietary tetrapeptides	≈400	≈5	(28)
Thyrotropin-releasing hormone (TRH) analogs	≈400	≈5	(28)
Talampicillin	482	>50	(33)
Enkephalins	600	<2	(28)
Pepstatinyl glycine	740	<2	(28)
Cyclic somatostatin	806	<5	(34)
Bradykinin	1060	<2	(28)
Vasopressin	1200	<2	(28)
Cyclosporine	1203	>50	(35)
Leuprolide	1208	<5	(36)

[a] Molecular weight.

membrane maintains a low intracellular sodium concentration. Thus, the sodium/hydrogen exchanger coupled with the sodium/potassium-ATPase drives the transport of di- and tripeptides across the epithelial cells (Fig. 9). The intestinal peptide transporter PEPT1 can transport di- and tripeptides but not free amino acids or tetrapeptides.

The intestinal absorption of dipeptides is a stereochemically specific mechanism. Dipeptides of L-L forms are transported more easily than are their isomers with a D-Amino acid. Dipeptide isomers of the L-L form have the highest absorption rates, followed by L-D and D-L isomers, and then D-D isomers.

The intestinal absorption mechanisms of amino acids and di- and tripeptides are characterized relatively well, as described above. However, only a limited amount of

work has been published for the absorption of tetra- and higher peptides, and the results are somewhat mixed. In general, it appears that tetra- or higher peptides are not well absorbed from the GI tract. Table 2 shows the oral bioavaiability of peptides and peptide-like drugs (molecular weight <1500).

Absorption of Polypeptides and Proteins

Enterocytes of the intestinal membrane do not have transporters to carry polypeptides and proteins across the intestinal membrane, and they certainly cannot permeate through tight junctions because of their size. Also, polypeptides and proteins are substrates for luminal, brush border, and cytolytic enzymes. Therefore, as

Table 3 GI Absorption of polypeptide and protein drugs

Compound	MW[a]	Extent of absorption (%)	Reference
Beta-endorphin	≈3500	<2	(28)
Calcitonin	≈3500	<2	(28)
Corticotropin (ACTH)	≈4700	<2	(28)
Insulin	5700	0.5	(36)
Growth hormone	22,600	<2	(28)
Horseradish peroxidase (HRP)	40,000	3	(37)
Bovine serum albumin (BSA)	50,000	4.5	(38)

[a] Molecular weight.

illustrated in Table 3, peptide/protein drugs are poorly absorbed across the GI tract.

One exception to the poor absorption of intact proteins is that neonates have the ability to absorb intact proteins for a few days after birth. Absorption cells of the neonatal mammalian intestine are functionally and morphologically specialized for the uptake and transport of milk macromolecules (39). The newborn has low levels of proteolytic enzymes in the intestinal lumen, and this highly unique endocytic mechanism allows intact proteins to adhere to the epithelial cell membrane and transport across the cell membrane. This function is very important for newborns to acquire passive immunity by absorbing immunoglobulins in colostral milk. In contrast to humans and rodents, many animals such as cattle, sheep, horses, and pigs do not provide enough antibodies across the placenta, and the young are born without circulating antibodies. Therefore, for these animals, the acquisition of passive immunity after birth depends primarily or entirely on the uptake of immunoglobulins in the small intestine by the endocytic mechanism. In addition, the highly endocytic nature of the small intestine provides no protection to invasion of bacterial proteins and antigens. At maturation, there is an abrupt change in the epithelial morphology of the small intestine that results in the cessation of the highly endocytic nature of the epithelium and in the corresponding loss in the capacity to absorb intact proteins.

Although the adult intestine provides a more effective epithelial barrier than that in newborns, evidence indicates that small quantities of intact proteins are transported across intestinal epithelial cells. There are two possible mechanisms associated with the absorption of intact proteins: endocytosis and transport through the epithelium of Peyer's patches.

Endocytosis

The epithelial membrane of the GI tract consists of a continuous barrier of cells, which allows the transport of low-molecular-weight molecules by simple diffusion or various carrier processes. Macromolecules such as proteins may be absorbed from the intestinal lumen by cellular vesicular processes, through fluid-phase endocytosis (pinocytosis), or by receptor-mediated endocytosis or transcytosis (Fig. 6). In pinocytosis, extracellular fluid is captured within an epithelial membrane vesicle. It begins with the formation of a pocket when a localized region of the epithelial membrane sinks inwardly. As the pocket deepens, it pinches into the cytoplasm, forming a vesicle containing the macromolecule that had been outside the cell. As a consequence, the majority of macromolecules taken into the cell by the vesicle do not find their way into the underlying tissues and thence to the blood circulation.

Rather, the vesicle shuttles the macromolecule to an endosome, which fuses with a lysosome where the membrane is recycled back to the epithelial membrane and the macromolecule is degraded. For example, HRP is taken up by the cell through the endocytosis process in the rabbit jejunum, and approximately 97% of these molecules are degraded during passage through the lysosomal system (37). Pinocytosis is unspecific in the substances it transports. Certain viruses and micro-organisms get into the cells by the endocytic mechanism, but they are not broken down within the lysosomal system. Some parasites and micro-organisms actually live within the lysosomal system, whereas others can find their way into the cytoplasm through mechanisms that may involve the presence of certain structures on membrane surfaces or changes in lysosomal pH.

In contrast, receptor-mediated endocytosis is very specific. Embedded in the membrane are proteins with specific receptor sites exposed to the extracellular fluid. The receptor proteins are usually clustered in regions of the membrane called coated pits, which are lined on their cytoplasmic side by a fuzzy layer consisting of a protein called clathrin. When ligands bind to the receptor sites, they are carried into the cell by the inward budding of a coated pit to form a coated vesicle. Clathrin-coated vesicles become uncoated and fuse to form an endosome. Ligand and receptor dissociate within the endosome, and the receptor shuttles back to the cell surface. The endosome fuses with the lysosome on which ligand degradation occurs.

Transcytosis is a process by which an endocytic vesicle (endosome) carries its contents across the epithelial cell without fusion with a lysosome (Fig. 6). The majority of endocytosed proteins are degraded, indicating that the transcytotic pathway is a minor one, with most endocytosed protein being routed to lysosomes. According to careful measurement (37), only 3% of horseradish peroxidase (HRP) avoids fusion with the lysosomal compartments to reach the blood circulation. However, it is interesting to note that immunoglobulin A (molecular weight ≈160 kDa) and immunoglobulin M (molecular weight ≈970 kDa) internalize into the cell by receptor-mediated endocytosis and are conveyed from one side of the cell to the other without fusing with the lysosome. It would be very interesting to explore whether the transcytosis process of immunoglobulins and the above-mentioned endocytosis processes of microorganisms and parasites, in which no degradation by the lysosomes occurs, could be harnessed for the delivery of peptides and proteins.

Transport through the epithelium of Peyer's patches

Although the GI tract has effective barrier properties, the mucous membrane is one of the major sites of entry for most pathogens. The defense of these vulnerable membrane surfaces is provided by organized structures of lymphoid follicles known as Peyer's patches. Peyer's patches were discovered by Johanni Peyeri in 1677 and consist of 30 to 40 lymphoid nodules on the outer wall of the intestines (40). They are most prominent in the ileum of the small intestine in humans and are characterized by the presence of specialized epithelial cells called M (microfold or membranous) cells. Morphologically, M cells are quite different from absorptive cells. Their apical luminal surface contains numerous microfolds, truncated microvilli, and low levels of membrane-bound enzymes. In addition, M cells possess a relatively sparse glycocalyx and almost no lysosomes. Furthermore, the basolateral membrane surfaces of M cells are deeply invaginated toward the luminal side to form a pocket that is filled with a cluster of B cells, T cells, and macrophages (Fig. 10). All these unique structural characteristics of M cells are specialized for endocytosis of macromolecules or particles and transport to the lymphatic system. Several proteins such as native ferritin, HRP, and lectins are taken up by a pinocytosis process and traverse across M cells from the lumen to the extracellular space. This is in contrast to immunoglobulin A, which is internalized by a receptor-mediated endocytosis process, as described in the previous section. In addition to macromolecules, viruses and bacteria have been shown to gain entry via the Peyer's patches. The HRP concentration affects the transport process from the lumen to the lymph system; low levels of HRP are predominantly taken up by M cells, but higher levels are simultaneously taken up by M cells as well as by absorptive cells (39). HRP is transported through the intestinal segments containing Peyer's patches more quickly in the intact form than through neighboring patch-free segments. The apparent permeability coefficient (P_{app}) of HRP in the segment containing Peyer's patches is approximately seven-fold larger than in the segment without Peyer's patches (41).

APPROACHES TO IMPROVE THE ORAL ABSORPTION OF PEPTIDES AND PROTEINS

As noted in the introduction to this article, the oral absorption of peptides (>3 amino acids) and proteins is very poor because of their potential degradation by the strong acidic environment and enzymes in the GI tract. Also, peptides and proteins have a very low permeability across the GI membrane.

Various formulation concepts have been introduced as potential ways to protect peptide and protein drugs from the hostile GI environment to increase their oral absorption such as use particulate drug carriers (microspheres, lipo-somes, and lectins), coadministration of enzyme inhibitors and absorption enhancers, use of chemical modification (prodrug), and site-specific delivery to the colon or rectum. Some of these approaches are discussed later.

Proteinoid Microspheres

Protenoids are thermally condensed amino acids and spontaneously form microspheres when exposed to an acidic medium (42). The microsphere size is approximately 1–5 μm in diameter. The protenoid microspheres are very stable at lower pH conditions of 1 to 3 but unstable at the pH range of 6 to 7. Therefore, the proteinoid microspheres are able to protect the peptide and protein drugs from the gastric acids and enzymes while in the stomach and to release the encapsulated drug in the small intestine to be available for absorption. The proteinoids are also able to inhibit the activity of peptidases such as trypsin and chymotrypsin. Oral administration of proteinoid encapsulated insulin in diabetic rats has shown a significant hypoglycemic effect and provided a longer duration of action than when administered subcutaneously. Also, proteinoid-encapsulated calcitonin has been shown to significantly decrease serum calcium levels in treated rats compared with rats in a placebo control group. Both results demonstrate that proteinoid encapsulation can enhance the oral absorption of peptide and protein drugs (42).

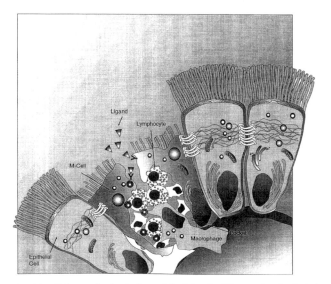

Fig. 10 Schematic depiction of the M cell. (Illustration by Leigh A. Rondano, Boehringer Ingelheim Pharmaceuticals, Inc.)

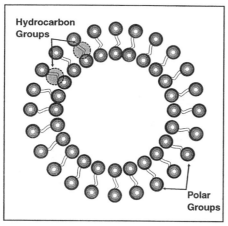

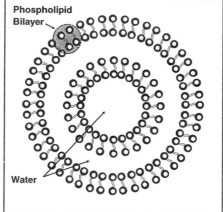

Fig. 11 Types of liposome: unilamellar liposome and multilamellar liposome. (Illustration by Leigh A. Rondano, Boehringer Ingelheim Pharmaceuticals, Inc.)

Liposomes

Liposomes have received considerable attention as a possible delivery tool for peptide and protein drugs by protecting labile compounds from degradation or by enhancing the uptake of poorly absorbed compounds. Liposomes have been studied extensively as a potential oral delivery system for proteins, especially insulin, and the oral administration of liposome-entrapped insulin into diabetic rats has produced a significant fall in blood glucose levels (43). There are three types of liposomes: multilamellar liposomes (MLV), 0.05–10 μm small unilamellar liposomes (SUV), 0.025–0.05 μm and large unilamellar liposomes (LUV), 0.2—2 μm (Fig. 11).

Liposomes are defined as vesicular lipid bilayers that enclose a volume of aqueous solution. Liposomes can be formed from a variety of phospholipids. The most widely used lipid is phosphatidylcholine. The liposome's outer membrane is semipermeable, and its permeability can be altered by varying the types of lipids used in preparing the liposomes. Liposomes can be made with a high permeability by using unsaturated lipids that will make a more fluid membrane. However, liposome with low permeability can be obtained by using a mix of phospholipids and cholesterol. Cholesterol is known to condense the packing of the phospholipids, thereby reducing their permeability and increasing the stability of the phospholipid bilayers. Negatively charged liposomes can be prepared by using phosphatidylserine or phosphotidylglycerol, and positively charged liposomes are made using stearylamine. Three possible mechanisms in the membrane transport of liposome-entrapped drugs

have been proposed (44): free molecule mechanism, simultaneous free molecule and direct liposome/membrane mechanism, and direct liposome/membrane mechanism. The free molecule model is for water-soluble drugs and includes the diffusion of a drug molecule from the liposome into the lumen first and then by membrane transport of the free molecule. The simultaneous free molecule and direct liposome/membrane mechanism is the sum of the permeations attributed to the drug molecule in the lumen and the direct transfer of molecule between liposome and membrane. The last mechanism, the direct liposome/membrane mechanism, is for water-insoluble drugs. This mechanism likely occurs because the release kinetics from a liposome system into the lumen is negligible.

Since 1970, there have been numerous reports detailing the advantages of liposomes as drug-delivery systems. However, in general these systems have not been successful for oral delivery. Some of the reasons may be related to: 1) their lack of stability in the GI tract and 2) their susceptibility to changes in pH, bile salts, and lipases. In addition, it has been shown that liposome systems are immunogenic.

Lectins

Lectins are known to have specific binding properties to the epithelial cell surface and have been tested as a possible oral delivery system for peptide and protein drugs. The lectin-coated nanoparticles that contain peptide or protein drugs can protect against degradation in the lumen of the small intestine and facilitate the uptake of peptide or protein drugs across M cells by acting as a specific targeting ligand.

Coadministration of Enzyme Inhibitors

To promote the oral absorption of polypeptide and protein drugs from the GI tract, the enzyme barrier must be overcome. Various protease/peptidase inhibitors have been tested to enhance the oral bioavailability of peptide and protein drugs. To date, the known inhibitors are aprotinin, bacitracin, Bowman–Birk inhibitor, camostat mesilate, soybean trypsin inhibitor, sodium glycocholate, and chymotrypsin inhibitor (FK-448). Some of these inhibitors have absorption-enhancing activity in addition to enzymatic inhibition activity. As an example, insulin has often been used as a model protein drug in studies on enzymatic inhibition activity. Trypsin inhibitor and aprotinin have shown a marginal effect on increasing insulin absorption in rats. However, a significant hypoglycemic effect has been observed after administration of insulin with sodium glycocholate, camostat mesilate, and bacitracin (45), which may be related to the fact that these compounds act not only as enzymatic inhibitors but also as absorption enhancers. Although various potential candidates for enzyme inhibition and absorption enhancers have been identified, the long-term safety of these compounds in humans must be evaluated further.

Coadministration of Absorption Enhancers

Most polypeptide and protein drugs show low permeability across the intestinal membrane because of their polarity and size. Therefore, one approach to increase the permeability of these drugs is to coadminister with absorption enhancers. Thus far, the known enhancers tested for the oral delivery of peptide and protein drugs are bile salts, nonionic surfactants, anionic surfactants, lysolecithin, amines, medium chain glycerides, and salicylates. Although their mechanisms of action are not well understood, several possible mechanisms have been proposed, especially for insulin absorption, which include: 1) that some enhancers, such as bile salts, act not only as an absorption enhancer but also as an enzyme inhibitor; 2) that the enhancers act as a kind of dispersing agent to prevent aggregation of peptide and protein molecules in solution, resulting in increased solubility of the drugs; 3) that the enhancers reduce the viscosity of the membrane mucous layer and increase the membrane fluidity, resulting in increased absorption by opening up the aqueous channel on the cell membrane; and 4) that the positively charged enhancers may interact with the negatively charged epithelial cell membrane and neutralize the membrane surface, resulting in increased absorption of the protein. Most enhancers are known to cause membrane irritation, and their long-term toxicity has not been well characterized and must be established (46).

Chemical Modifications

The reasons for poor absorption of most natural peptides and proteins from the GI tract are that most natural peptides and proteins are hydrophilic compounds and have a low partition coefficient (log of octanol/water partition coefficient, log P) on the order of -1. For example, the log P values of TRH and vasopressin are -1.43 and -2.15, respectively. There are some exceptions such as cyclosporine. Cyclosporine is a lipophilic peptide (log P = 3.0) and exposes very few polar groups on the surface. Medicinal chemists have routinely applied three types of chemical modification to improve the absorption of peptide and protein drugs including analogs, irreversible derivatives, and prodrugs. The irreversible derivative and the analog approaches are usually applied when compounds exhibit poor absorption because of in vivo metabolism. Peptide drug examples include enkephalins, TRH, and vasopressin, and insulin can be a model for protein drugs. The chemical modifications by the irreversible derivative and the analog approaches can prevent hydrolysis of peptides or proteins; however, these modifications may also reduce biological activity. For example, chymotrypsin, one of the major peptidases secreted by the pancreas into the intestinal lumen, is known to cleave at five bonds within the insulin molecule in a very short time. Four of these five residues play an important role in maintaining the biological activity of insulin and are essential for receptor binding ability (47). A number of chemical modifications at these sites could produce greater chemical stability; however, such changes in the insulin molecule could result in a loss in activity because of possible alterations of the three-dimensional structure of the protein.

The prodrug approach is the most widely applied chemical modification for improving the absorption of peptides. The unique feature of the prodrug approach is that the optimum physicochemical properties required for the drug with respect to lipophilicity and degradation can be achieved without altering the intrinsic biological activity of the parent drug. The prodrug itself is inactive. However, once the peptide prodrug is absorbed, it is converted to an active peptide, usually by an enzyme. A good example is an ACE inhibitor, enalapril, which was found to be orally well absorbed and metabolized to the active form, enanaprilat, in the liver. In contrast, the parent drug, enanaprilat, is very poorly absorbed via the oral route.

Colon Delivery

The colon has received considerable attention as a possible delivery site for peptide and protein drugs because enzymatic activities, especially peptidases, are significantly lower in the colon compared with the small intestine, and the residence time in the colon is longer than in the small intestine. However, there are some drawbacks for site-specific delivery of peptide and protein drugs in the colon as follows:

1. The colonic mucosa does not have the villi and microvilli of the small intestine. Therefore, the surface area available for absorption in the colon is considerably less than that in the small intestine.
2. Peptidases such as aminopeptidases and diaminopeptidases are at lower concentrations in the colon than in the small intestine. However, it has been shown that prolyl endoprotease and collagenase activities are five to six times higher in the colon than in the small intestine. TRH is more readily hydrolyzed to deaminated TRH in colonic homogenates compared with small intestine and rectum. Therefore, peptide drugs that are substrates for prolyl endoprotease and collagenase will likely be degraded in the colon and may not be suitable for colon delivery.
3. The concentration of bacteria in the colon, largely anerobic species, is much higher than that in the small intestine. This high concentration of bacteria may lead to faster degradation of certain drugs such as digoxin, which is degraded to dihydrodigoxin by the microflora in the colon.

The microflora degradation mechanism has been exploited as a possible tool for the site-specific delivery of peptide and protein drugs. Peptide and protein drugs are coated with azoaromatic groups to form an impermeable film to protect them from digestion in the stomach and small intestine. When the polymer-coated peptide and protein drugs reach the colon, the colonic bacteria cleaves the azo bonds and breaks the polymer film, releasing the drugs into the lumen of the colon for absorption. This polymeric system was demonstrated to protect and deliver orally administered insulin and vasopressin (7) in rats.

Rectum Delivery

In general, oral delivery of polypeptide and protein drugs is limited because of degradation in the GI tract and poor absorption through the membrane. Rectal administration offers some advantages compared with oral delivery, such as low enzymatic activity, neutral pH, and partial avoidance of first-pass metabolism. Even though the rectal route has long been known as a specific absorption site for the delivery of small lipophilic molecules, rectal delivery of large hydrophilic molecules is problematic because of poor absorption, and absorption enhancers may be required. Increased absorption of peptides, such as des-enkephalin-gamma-endorphin and desglycinamide arginine vasopressin, and proteins, e.g., albumin, insulin, and a somastatin analog, has been demonstrated by coadministration with enhancers. The enhancers used for the rectal absorption of insulin are surface active agents; bile acids; EDTA; and phospholipids such as lecithin, saponins, sodium salicylate, organic alcohols, acids, amines, and fats. Their mechanisms of action are generally not fully understood. Some of the possible enhancing mechanisms are described in "Coadministration of Enzyme Inhibitors," previously.

CONCLUSION

Rapid developments in biotechnology have led to the production of large quantities of pure potent and highly specific polypeptide and protein drugs. To date, they have been administered primarily by the parenteral route, even though the oral route is the patient's preferred choice. The oral route offers many advantages over parenteral administration, such as ease of administration and increased patient compliance. However, in general the peptide and protein drugs are very difficult to administer orally because they are of large molecular weight, hydrophilic in nature, and substrates for peptidases and proteases in the GI tract. There are many different locations where peptide and protein drugs can be hydrolyzed after oral administration. Their exposure to the strong hostile acidic environment of the stomach may cause partial degradation. Further degradation occurs in the lumen of the small intestine by the peptidases secreted by the pancreas, and then additional degradation by enzymes on the brush border and inside the epithelial cells follows. Even if some of the peptide and protein drugs survive and enter the cell, as they diffuse across the cell, they are taken up by lysosome where most of them are hydrolyzed by the lysosomal enzymes. Finally, those peptide and protein drugs that get through the epithelial cell into the portal vein could still be metabolized by the liver. In addition, they usually show poor permeability across the intestinal membrane because of their molecular size and polar nature.

To minimize degradation and improve absorption of peptide and protein drugs administered orally, several factors are significant. First, peptide and protein drugs have to be protected from the acidic environment in the stomach and from enzyme degradation in the lumen and on the brush border of the small intestine. This may be accomplished by coadministration of peptidase inhibitors or by chemical modifications, such as analogs or prodrug approaches, or formulation approaches, such as microspheres and liposomes.

Second, because of their molecular size and hydrophilic nature, peptide and protein drugs are poorly absorbed through the intestinal membrane, and absorption has to be improved. This may be accomplished by coadministration of penetration enhancers or by chemical modifications such as increasing lipophilicity.

Finally, all these approaches may be possible; however, there is still a major hurdle to overcome: how intact peptide and protein drugs may pass across the inside of the epithelial cell without being taken up by the lysosome and also bypass first-pass metabolism in the liver. The best chance of avoiding lysosomal uptake and first-pass metabolism is by diffusion through the M cells on the Peyer's patches, which contain almost no lysosomes, and unloading the diffusates directly into the lymphatic system. This may be accomplished by exploring whether the transcytosis mechanism of antigens or microparticulates across the intestinal wall could be applied for the delivery of peptide and protein drugs.

In conclusion, although oral delivery is the preferred route for peptide and protein drugs, there are many drawbacks, as addressed previously. Successful oral delivery of peptide and protein drugs is likely to remain a formidable challenge for some time.

ACKNOWLEDGMENTS

We gratefully acknowledge Leigh Rondano of Boehringer Ingelheim Pharmaceuticals Inc., for her preparation of all the figures in this article. In addition, we thank Dr. Martha Brown, Mayur Dudhedia, and Mary Tanenbaum of Boehringer Ingelheim Pharmaceuticals, Inc. for their kind comments.

REFERENCES

1. Kutchai, H.C. The Gastrointestinal System. *Physiology*, 4th Ed.; Berne, R.M., Levy, M.N., Eds.; Mosby: St. Louis, MO, 1998.
2. Egberts, H.J.; Koninkx, J.F.; Dijk, J.; Mouwen, J.M. Biological and Pathobiological Aspects of the Glycocalyx of the Small Intestinal Epithelium. A review. Vet. Q. **1984**, *6* (4), 186–199.
3. Russell-Jones, G.J.; Aizpurua, H.J. Vitamin B$_{12}$: A Novel Carrier for Orally Presented Antigens. Proceedings of the International Symposium on Controlled Release of Bioactive Materials, 1988; *15*, 142–143.
4. Park, J.Y. Biophysical Model Approach to the Mechanistic Studies of Intestinal Absorption of Drugs. The University of Michigan: Ann Arbor, 1977; Thesis.
5. Sallee, Y.L.; Wilson, F.A.; Dietschy, J.M. Determination of Unidirectional Uptake Rates for Lipids Across the Intestinal Brush Border. J. Lipid Res. **1972**, *13* (2), 184–192.
6. Ugolov, A.M. Physiology and Pathology of Membrane Digestion. Plenum Press: New York, 1968.
7. Saffran, M.; Kumar, G.S.; Savariar, C.; Burnham, J.C.; Williams, F.; Neckers, D.C. A New Approach to the Oral Administration of Insulin and Other Peptide Drugs. Science **1986**, *233* (4768), 1081–1084.
8. McNally, E.J. Protein Formulation and Delivery. *Drugs and the Pharmaceutical Sciencies*; Marcel Dekker, Inc.: New York, 2000; 99.
9. Campbell, N.A. Structure and Function of Macromolecules. *Biology*, 2nd Ed.; The Benjamin/Cummings Publishing Co.: Redwood City, CA, 1990.
10. Lehninger, A.L.; Nelson, D.L.; Cox, M.M. Amino Acid Oxidation and the Production of Urea. *Principle of Biochemistry*, 2nd Ed.; Worth Publishers: New York, 1993; 510.
11. Adibi, S.A.; Moore, E.L. The Number of Glycine Residues Which Limit Intact Absorption of Glycine Oligopeptides in Human Jejunum. J. Clin. Invest. **1977**, *60* (5), 1008–1016.
12. Tsukita, S.; Furuse, M. Pores in the Wall: Claudins Constitute Tight Junction Strands Containing Aqueous Pores. J. Cell. Biol. **2000**, *149* (1), 13–16.
13. Ho, N.F.H.; Higuchi, W.I.; Turi, J. Theoretical Model Studies of Drug Absorption and Transport in the GI Tract III. J. Pharm. Sci. **1972**, *61* (2), 192–197.
14. Ho, N.F.H.; Higuchi, W.I. Theoretical Model Studies of Intestinal Drug Absorption. IV. Bile Acid Transport at Premicellar Concentrations Across Diffusion Layer-Membrane Barrier. J. Pharm. Sci. **1974**, *63* (5), 686–690.
15. Ho, N.F.H.; Park, J.Y.; Morozowich, W.; Higuchi, W.I. Physical Model Approach to the Design of Drugs with Improved Intestinal Absorption. *Design of Biopharmaceutical Properties Through Prodrugs and Analogs*; Roche, E.B., Ed.; American Pharmaceutical Association: Washington, DC, 1977; 136–227.
16. Augustijns, P.F.; Bradshaw, T.P.; Gan, L.-S.L.; Hendren, R.W.; Thakker, D.R. Evidence for a Polarized Efflux System in Caco-2 Cells Capable of Modulating Cyclosporin a Transport. Biochem. Biophys. Res. Commun. **1993**, *197* (2), 360–365.
17. Burton, P.S.; Conradi, R.A.; Hilgers, A.R.; Ho, N.F.H. Evidence for a Polarized Efflux System for Peptides in the Apical Membrane of Caco-2 cells. Biochem. Biophys. Res. Commun. **1993**, *190* (3), 760–766.
18. Anderson, J.M.; van Itallie, C.M. Tight Junctions and the Molecular Basis for Regulation of Paracellular Permeability. Am. J. Physiol. **1995**, *269* (32), G467–G475.
19. Daugherty, A.L.; Mrsny, R.J. Regulation of the Intestinal Epithelial Paracellular Barrier. Pharmaceutical Science & Technology Today **1999**, *2* (7), 281–287.
20. Lutz, K.L.; Siahaan, T.J. Molecular Structure of the Apical Junction Complex and Its Contribution to the Paracellular Barrier. J. Pharm. Sci. **1997**, *86* (9), 977–984.

21. Knipp, G.T.; Ho, N.F.; Barsuhn, C.L.; Borchardt, R.T. Paracellular Diffusion in Caco-2 Cell Monolayers: Effect of Perturbation on the Transport of Hydrophilic Compounds that Vary in Charge and Size. J. Pharm. Sci. **1997**, *86* (10), 1105–1110.

22. Adson, A.; Raub, T.J.; Burton, P.S.; Barsuhn, C.L.; Hilgers, A.R.; Audus, K.L.; Ho, N.F.H. Quantitative Approaches to Delineate Paracellular Diffusion in Cultured Epithelial Cell Monolayers. J. Pharm. Sci. **1994**, *83* (11), 1529–1536.

23. Lukie, B.E.; Westergaard, H.; Dietschy, J.M. Validation of a Chamber that Allows Measurement of Both Tissue Uptake Rates and Unstirred Layer Thicknesses in the Intestine Under Conditions of Controlled Stirring. Gastroenterology **1974**, *67* (4), 652–661.

24. Osiecka, I.; Porter, P.A.; Borchardt, R.T.; Fix, J.A.; Gardner, C.R. In Vitro Drug Absorption Models. I. Brush Border Membrane Vesicles, Isolated Mucosal Cells and Everted Intestinal Rings: Characterization and Salicylate Accumulation. Pharm. Res. **1985**, *2* (6), 284–292.

25. Kakemi, K.; Arita, T.; Muranishi, S. Absorption and Excretion of Drugs. XXV. On the Mechanism of Rectal Absorption of Sulfonamides. Chem. Pharm. Bull. **1965**, *13* (7), 861–869.

26. Ho, N.F.H.; Park, J.Y.; Ni, P.; Higuchi, W.I. Advancing Quantitative and Mechanistic Approaches in Interfacing Gastrointestinal Drug Absorption Studies in Animals and Humans. *Animal Models for Oral Drug Delivery in Man: In Situ and In Vivo Approaches*; Crouthamel, W., Sarapu, A.C., Eds.; American Pharmaceutical Association: Washington, DC, 1983; 27–106.

27. Schedl, H.P.; Clifton, J.A. Cortisol Absorption in Man. Gastroenterology **1963**, *44* (2), 134–145.

28. TenHoor, C.N.; Dressman, J.B. Oral Absorption of Peptides and Proteins. Sciences Technologies Pratiques Pharma. Sci. **1992**, *2* (4), 301–312.

29. Liang, R.; Fei, Y.-J.; Prasad, P.D.; Ramamoorthy, S.; Han, H.; Yang-Feng, T.L.; Hediger, M.A.; Ganapathy, V.; Leibach, F.H. Human Intestinal H+/Peptide Cotransporter. Cloning, Functional Expression, and Chromosomal Localization. J. Biol. Chem. **1995**, *270* (12), 6456–6463.

30. Nightingale, C.H.; Greene, D.S.; Quintiliani, R. Pharmacokinetics and Clinical Use of Cephalosporin Antibiotics. J. Pharm. Sci. **1975**, *64* (12), 1899–1927.

31. Ganapathy, V.; Leibach, F.H. Is Intestinal Peptide Transport Energized by a Proton Gradient. Am. J. Physiol. **1985**, *249* (12), G153–G160.

32. Yokohama, S.; Yamashita, K.; Toguchi, H.; Takeuchi, J.; Kitamori, N. Absorption of Thyrotropin-Releasing Hormone After Oral Administration of TRH Tartrate Monohydrate in the Rat, Dog and Human. J. Pharm. Dyn. **1984**, *7* (2), 101–111.

33. Bell, J.; Peters, G.E.; McMartin, C.; Thomas, N.W.; Wilson, C.G. Estimation of Gut Absorption of Peptides by Biliary Sampling. J. Pharm. Pharmacol. **1984**, *36* (Suppl.), 88.

34. Wood, A.J.; Lemaire, M. Pharmacologic Aspects of Cyclosporine Therapy: Pharmacokinetics. Transplant. Proc. **1985**, *17* (4 Suppl 1), 27–32, Review.

35. Okada, H.; Yamazaki, I.; Ogawa, Y.; Hirai, S.; Yashiki, T.; Mima, H. Vaginal Absorption of a Potent Luteinizing Hormone-Releasing Hormone Analog (Leuprolide) in Rats I: Absorption by Various Routes and Absorption Enhancement. J. Pharm. Sci. **1982**, *71* (12), 1367–1371.

36. Crane, C.W.; Luntz, G.R. Absorption of Insulin from the Human Small Intestine. Diabetes **1968**, *17* (10), 625–627.

37. Heyman, M.; Ducroc, R.; Desjeux, J.F.; Morgat, J.L. Horseradish Peroxidase Transport Across Adult Rabbit Jejunum in Vitro. Am.J.Physiol. **1982**, *242* (5), G558–G564.

38. Kimm, M.H.; Curtis, G.H.; Hardin, J.A.; Gall, D.G. Transport of Bovine Serum Albumin Across Rat Jejunum: Role of Enteric Nervous System. Am. J. Physiol. **1994**, *266* (29), G186–G193.

39. Gornellia, P.A.; Walker, W.A. Macromolecular Absorption in the Gastrointestinal Tract. Adv. Drug Del. Rev. **1987**, *1*, 235–248.

40. Kuby, J. *Immmunology*, 2nd Ed.; Feeman, W.H., Ed.; W.H. and Company: New York, 1994; 76–77.

41. Ho, N.F.H.; Day, J.S.; Barsuhn, C.L.; Raub, T.J. Biophysical Model Approaches to Mechanistic Transepithelial Studies of Peptides. J. Controlled Rel. **1990**, *11*, 3–24.

42. Steiner, S.; Rosen, R. Delivery Systems for Pharmacological Agents Encapsulated with Proteinoids. US. Patent 4925673, 1990.

43. Patel, H.M.; Ryman, B.E. Oral Administration of Insulin by Encapsulation Within Liposomes. FEBS Lett. **1976**, *62* (1), 60–63.

44. Ganesan, M.G.; Weiner, N.D.; Flynn, G.L.; Ho, N.F.H. Influence of Liposomal Drug Entrapment on Percutaneous Absorption. Int. J. Pharm. **1984**, *20*, 139–154.

45. Bernkop-Schnürch, A.; Marschütz, M.K. Development and In Vitro Evaluation of Systems to Protect Peptide Drugs from Aminopeptidase. N. Pharm. Res. **1997**, *14* (2), 181–185.

46. Zhou, X.H. Overcoming Enzymatic and Absorption Barriers to Non-Parenterally Administered Protein and Peptide Drugs. J. Controlled Rel. **1994**, *29*, 239–252.

47. Pullen, R.A.; Linsay, D.G.; Wood, S.P.; Tickle, I.J.; Blundell, T.L.; Wormer, A.; Krail, G.; Brandenburg, D.; Zahn, H.; Glieman, J.; Gammeltoft, S. Receptor-Binding Region of Insulin. Nature **1976**, *259* (5542), 369–373.

FURTHER READING

Amidon, G.L.; Wolfgang, S. Membrane Transporters as Drug Targets. *Pharmaceutical Biotechnology*; Kluwer/Plenum Publishers: New York, 1999; 12.

Bai, J.P.F.; Chang, L.-L.; Guo, J.-H. Targeting of Peptide and Protein Drugs to Specific Sites in the Oral Route. Crit. Rev. Ther. Drug Carrier Syst. **1995**, *12* (4), 339–371.

Davis, S.S.; Illum, L.; Tomlinson, E. NATO ASI Series. Series A: Life Sciences. *Delivery Systems for Peptide Drugs*; Plenum Press: New York, 1986; 125.

Lee, V.H.L. Peptide and Protein Drug Delivery. *Advances in Parenteral Sciences*; Marcel Dekker, Inc.: New York, 1991; 4.

Woodley, J.F. Enzymatic Barriers for GI Peptide and Protein Delivery. Crit. Rev. Ther. Drug Carrier Syst. **1994**, *11* (2,3), 61–95.

PEPTIDES AND PROTEINS—PULMONARY ABSORPTION

Igor Gonda

Aradigm Corporation, Hayward, California

INTRODUCTION

The human respiratory tract has the potential to provide the means for noninvasive drug delivery of molecules that could not be efficiently and reproducibly, or rapidly, delivered without injecting them into the body. From the early parts of the 20th century, there have been many attempts to use inhalation to deliver insulin for the treatment of diabetes (1). These early approaches failed because the aerosol generators (jet nebulizers and metered dose inhalers) had low and variable delivery to the lung. Inhalation therapy for the treatment of diseases of the respiratory tract, especially asthma, underwent spectacular growth in the last three decades of the 20th century (2). The discovery of potent drugs that could be administered in one or two puffs from a low cost hand-held device, such as a metered dose inhaler or dry powder inhaler, led to the acceptance of aerosols as the preferred mode of therapy of asthma. One of the main advantages of targeting the lung was the minimization of systemic side effects of these drugs. Nevertheless, it was observed already in the early development of these asthma products that systemic absorption of the inhaled drugs did occur (3).

The biotechnology revolution resulted in the production of many potentially valuable therapeutic proteins. However, it was recognized that these molecules had properties that necessitated the use of injections for their administration. Intensive research in noninvasive drug delivery accompanied the dawn of recombinant biologics, but it met with somewhat limited success. Early work on peptides such as insulin (1) and some proteins (4) certainly indicated that such molecules were absorbed from the lung. Mackay et al. (5) reported in 1994 a summary of extensive studies in which the absolute bioavailabilities of several proteins and peptides were measured in rat models of pulmonary, nasal, and colonic absorption. The compounds were human and salmon calcitonins, the human parathyroid hormone and its 34-peptide fragment, hirudin, and a hybrid alpha interferon. All routes of administration exhibited general reduction of bioavailability with increasing molecular weight. However, the pulmonary route (via intratracheal administration) resulted in much higher values than the other two routes. Thus, pulmonary delivery was known to be exceptionally promising among the noninvasive routes of delivery of delivery of peptides and proteins, but the key reasons for its poor delivery efficiency and variability needed to be investigated and removed. Industrial and academic research in the latter part of the last century demonstrated the need for targeting of the drug into "deep lung" to increase the efficiency of delivery and in particular to avoid the highly variable deposition in the oropharyngeal cavity (6). The conventional therapeutic aerosol generators used for delivery of asthma drugs to the airways were not designed with these requirements in mind. New types of delivery systems had to be developed that could generate very fine particles with aerodynamic properties suitable for drug delivery to the distal part of the respiratory tract with large highly absorptive surfaces.

SAFETY OF PROTEINS AND PEPTIDES DELIVERED TO THE LUNG

Satisfactory efficiency of delivery is only meaningful when it goes hand-in-hand with adequate safety. The inhalation route in general has been associated with a very good safety record for the delivery of asthma drugs evidenced both during the development stages and by their wide acceptance postapproval. The experience with inhaled protein and peptide drugs is so far relatively limited. Overall, the pulmonary safety of inhaled proteins and peptides has been good (7). The most extensive preclinical and clinical experience thus far is available for the recombinant human deoxyribonuclease (rhDNase) approved by inhalation for the treatment of cystic fibrosis in 1993 (8, 9). Inhaled leuprolide, a small peptide, was extensively studied with "clean" preclinical and clinical safety findings (10). A new large safety data base is being generated in conjunction with late stage development of insulin by several companies (11, 12).

Encyclopedia of Pharmaceutical Technology

ABSORPTION AND OTHER CLEARANCE MECHANISMS IN THE RESPIRATORY TRACT

Absorption of the protein and peptide molecules delivered to the respiratory tract competes against various other clearance mechanisms. When a particle containing a therapeutic substance is deposited in the respiratory tract, the following mechanisms of the drug-containing particle clearance can take place:

Removal of particulates from the respiratory tract:

- Mucociliary clearance
- Phagocytosis
- Clearance of the phagocytosed particles

After the drug is released from the particle (e.g., by dissolution, diffusion, or erosion), the three above listed mechanisms can also clear the free drug. Additional clearance of the released drug can take place as follows:

Removal of molecules deposited in the respiratory tract:

- Metabolism
- Chemical (non-enzymatic) decomposition
- Binding to fluid and tissue components in the respiratory tract
- Lymphatic uptake
- Absorption into blood stream

Absorption, Phagocytosis, and Mucociliary Clearance

These clearance pathways are not distributed uniformly throughout the lung. The gas-exchange areas, for example, do not have the mucociliary clearance but they have alveolar macrophages that can phagocytose "foreign" materials. These alveolated regions also have a much greater and more permeable environment than the upper and conducting airways. The main barrier in the deep lung to transport into blood stream appears to be the alveolar epithelium rather than the endothelial cells. While the majority of the cells lining the alveoli are Type II, most of the surface area (~95%) is covered by Type I cells. Alveolar cell monolayers resembling Type I cells are therefore thought to be representative of the barrier for pulmonary absorption.

Several authors reported on the biphasic nature of peptide and protein absorption from the lung (13, 14). The rapid component was proposed to be representing paracellular absorption through water-filled pores. The origins of the slower absorption phase into the blood circulation are not well understood. The respiratory tract has a rich lymphatic system, and, in addition to transcellular

and paracellular transport into the blood circulation, it is possible that a significant portion of macromolecules ends up first in the lymphatic system and is only then slowly released into the blood circulation. The molecular weight dependence of transfer of materials into the intra-pulmonary lymph nodes following intratracheal administration in the rat was investigated with a series of labeled dextrans. It was found that the threshold for increased ratio of blood/lymph transfer was between 10 and 20 kDa, similar to the large intestine. Certain absorption enhancers were found to increase this ratio, suggesting that the use of such materials could be exploited in the future to target therapeutics into the pulmonary lymph nodes (15).

The clearance mechanisms have been modeled quantitatively to get a better understanding of the effects of interplay of the complex kinetics on the magnitude and duration of residence in the lung (Fig. 1) (16). This model can be significantly simplified if only a few of the pathways dominate the transport and a only low-resolution compartmental analysis is experimentally feasible (17).

Colthorpe et al. (17) showed that the mucociliary clearance is the elimination pathway that contributes most to the reduction of bioavailability of insulin, at least in the rabbit model they studied. Thus, the less insulin is deposited on the conducting airways and the more that gets into the nonciliated gas exchange spaces, the higher is the bioavailability. Similar conclusions were reached studying the pulmonary absorption of growth hormone in the same model (18). The pulmonary to blood transfer rate constants were found to be also somewhat higher for the aerosol delivery compared with intratracheal administration. This is consistent with the pioneering work of Schanker's group (19), who showed in experiments with inhibited mucociliary clearance that the aerosol technique results in faster absorption rates presumably associated with the coverage of a bigger surface area of the respiratory tract and better penetration into the permeable lung periphery. This was confirmed more recently also in the work of Niven et al. (20) in which they compared instillation of liquid formulations, powder insufflation, and aerosol delivery of recombinant human granulocyte colony stimulating factor (rhG-CSF) and its pegylated derivatives in several species. They highlighted the fact that the nature of the distribution of the drug in the respiratory tract has a far greater impact on the rate and extent of absorption than even the molecular modifications. Similarly, it was shown (21) that the bioavailability of leuprolide administered to dogs increased with the downstream distance from epiglottis. In humans, Newman et al. (22) compared the bioavailability of a peptide molecule delivered to human volunteers in the form of inhaled "coarse" and "fine" aerosols. The ratio of

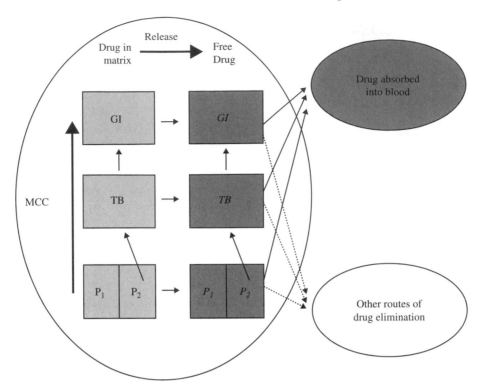

Fig. 1 Inhaled drug in a carrier can exist in the slow clearing pulmonary compartment (P_1) without mucociliary clearance or in the faster clearing pulmonary compartment with mucociliary clearance (P_2), tracheobronchial compartment (TB) or gastrointestinal tract (GI). When the drug is released into these compartment (the released drug is represented by italicized letters P_1, P_2, *TB*, *GI*), it can be absorbed into the bloodstream, or it can be removed by non-productive pathways such as mucociliary clearance represented by the vertical arrows, or chemical and enzymatic decomposition. Large molecules may also enter lymphatics before they appear in the blood stream. (The detailed model was described in Ref. 16 while the simplified three-compartment model represented by the ellipses is from Ref. 17.)

the bioavailabilies was almost identical to the ratio of the mass of the drug delivered to alveoli (as assessed by external gamma scintigraphic measurement). Getting protein deeper into the lung to access greater and more permeable surface areas that are not cleared by the mucociliary escalator thus results in better bioavailability.

Recent work with insulin provides evidence that the total lung volume at the end of the delivery impacts the kinetics of absorption of this peptide: delivery of fine particle insulin aerosol resulted in faster absorption with a higher plasma peak level in humans when the inhalation was done with a deep breath (close to vital capacity), as compared with a more shallow breath (about 50% of the vital capacity) (14, 23). The kinetics following the latter was similar to subcutaneous absorption of insulin. The exact reasons for this observation are unknown. However, the lung does have the above-described water channels that could expand during breathing. If the size of the peptide or protein molecule approaches the diameter of these channels, it would be expected that the channel expansion would lead to faster absorption. For molecules whose size

exceeds the channel diameter, the lung volume does not play a role in their pulmonary absorption rate (24).

Age, Disease, and Smoking Effects on Protein and Peptide Absorption

The effect of age on pulmonary absorption of three macromolecular markers, bovine IgG (BigG, MW = 150 kDa), bovine serum albumin (BSA, MW = 67 kDa), and 1-deamino-cysteine-8-D-arginine vasopressin (dDAVP, MW=1.067 kDa) was studied following intratracheal instillation in young and adult rats. The bioavailabilies for the three compounds were approximately 1.5, 5, and 20% in the adult rats. Low bioavailabilies were also found in the young rats for BigG and BSA but the absorption of dDAVP was significantly increased to 45% (25). Smoking profoundly increases the rate of absorption of insulin (26).

In experiments with aerosolized BSA and dDAVP in the rat (27), acute inflammation markedly increased the bioavailabilies.

Absorption Enhancers

The use of absorption enhancers for pulmonary delivery of peptides and proteins has been investigated in animal models but has not found commercial applications yet. This is presumably out of concern for potential safety impact from the use of such excipients. For example, Yamamoto et al. (28) showed that bacitracin and N-lauryl-beta-D-maltopyronoside in particular enhanced pulmonary absorption of insulin in a rat model but the toxicity of these enhancers was not investigated. The mechanism of "absorption enhancement" by bacitracin could have been in fact suppression of enzymatic degradation. Protease inhibitors were also found to improve the pulmonary absorption of a calcitonin analog (29) in a rat model but the mechanisms of this enhancement, or the potential pulmonary toxicity, were not studied. Changes to the barrier properties ranging from transient effects to complete stripping of epithelial cells have been among proposed mechanisms of pulmonary absorption enhancement.

Metabolism of Proteins and Peptides

There does not appear to be any significant proteolytic degradation by enzymes in the extracellular fluid in normal human airways and alveoli. However, the presence of peptidases makes absorption of small peptides variable and difficult to predict. Peptidase-resistant peptides generally show better bioavailabilities than other peptides with comparable molecular weights (30). Difference in metabolism and absorption of D and L forms of peptides glycyl-D-phenylalanine and glycyl-L-phenylalanine was demonstrated by Morimoto et al. (31). The L peptide was subject to metabolism, and it had significant paracellular transport with a smaller transcellular component. In contrast, the D peptide was not metabolized and it was only transported by passive diffusion via the paracellular route.

Given the complexity of the clearance mechanisms and the differences in the anatomy and physiology of the respiratory tract among various animal species, it is not surprising to find that the absorption rate constants for proteins and peptides are difficult to predict with any degree of accuracy. Fig. 2 shows the dependence of the apparent absorption rate constants as a function of molecular weight in dogs, rabbits, rats, and humans. While it is clear that generally the rate of pulmonary absorption is reduced for bigger molecules, the actual rate for a macromolecule in humans can be reliably determined at present only through direct experimentation.

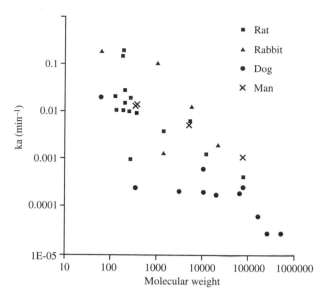

Fig. 2 Apparent pulmonary absorption rate constants as a function of molecular weight calculated from data in Refs. 17, 18, 32–34. (From Dr. Glyn Taylor, University of Wales, Cardiff, UK, and Dr. Stephen Farr, Aradigm Corporation, Hayward, CA.)

REGIONAL DEPOSITION OF INHALED PARTICLES AND DROPLETS IN THE HUMAN RESPIRATORY TRACT

Since the human respiratory tract is anatomically and physiologically a very heterogeneous system, the rate and extent of absorption of macromolecules as well as their potential adverse reactions depend on the regional doses. The most convenient method to deliver drugs to the respiratory tract is by inhalation. Other methods of delivery such as intratracheal instillation are used in experimental settings but are generally unsuitable for real-life therapeutic products. This section describes the basics underlying the deposition dosimetry following inhalation of particles.

Aerodynamic Particle Size

The probability of deposition of particles in the various parts of the human respiratory tract depends on their aerodynamic diameter, D_{ae}. This parameter in turn is a function of the physical dimensions, shape, and density of the particles. For spherical particles, the aerodynamic diameter is simply

$$D_{ae} = D \times \sqrt{(\rho/\rho_o)}$$

where D is the physical diameter, ρ is the density of the particle, and ρ_o is unit density (in the old cgs units, it was

$1 \, g/cm^3$). For droplets containing dilute aqueous solutions, the aerodynamic diameter is therefore equal to the geometric diameter of the droplet. For porous particles, the ratio of densities can be less than one, in which case the geometric diameter is larger than the effective aerodynamic diameter.

Mechanisms of Deposition

Particle deposition in the human respiratory tract takes place primarily by three mechanisms. Inertial impaction causes filtering of particles according to their aerodynamic size and velocity. This mechanism of deposition is especially important in the upper and central airways. In particular, oropharyngeal deposition increases approximately in proportion to the particle velocity and the square of its aerodynamic size. Therefore, particles with large aerodynamic diameters, especially if they are inhaled rapidly, will not be delivered to the lung for absorption. Gravitational sedimentation and diffusion are important for deposition of particles in airways and the alveolated regions. The extent of deposition by both of these mechanisms increases with breath-holding. Particles with aerodynamic diameters around $0.5 \, \mu m$ are neither small enough to deposit rapidly by diffusion, nor large enough to be deposited without prolonged breath-holding by sedimentation. It would be also practically quite difficult to produce submicron size aerosols containing proteins and peptides. The aim is therefore to produce a slow, moving aerosol cloud with drug containing particles in the size range $1–3 \, \mu m$ to minimize oropharyngeal deposition since peptides or protein are poorly absorbed from this region. Indeed, deposition of inhaled particles in this part of the human respiratory tract has been the primary cause of inefficiency and poor reproducibility of pulmonary delivery in the past (6).

Importance of the Mode of Inhalation on Deposition

The nose is a much better particle filter than the mouth, and oral inhalation is therefore preferred for more efficient and reproducible delivery to the lung.

We have already discussed the impact of inspiratory flow rate on deposition: the faster the subject inhales, the more material is deposited at bends and bifurcations in the upper and central airways, and the less material reaches the deep lung. Inspiratory flow rate may also affect the performance of inhalation systems; this is particularly important in passive dry powder inhalers in which the energy of breathing is utilized to deagglomerate the formulation (35). Thus, for such systems, there is a contradictory requirement for the need to use high inspiratory flow rate to achieve fine particle size for deep lung delivery and yet to have sufficiently low inspiratory flow rate to avoid impaction before the drug entry to the absorptive surfaces devoid of mucociliary clearance.

It would be also expected that to get to the deep lung, the drug containing aerosol needs to be inhaled at the beginning of the inspiration, starting from "empty" lung since there is relatively little mixing of an inhaled "bolus" with the rest of the inhaled air (36). Therefore, the preferable maneuver is a full exhalation followed by a slow, deep inspiration, and finally a breath-holding period. In practice, a few seconds appears to be adequate for practically complete deposition of particles in the optimum size range for "deep lung" delivery.

Recurrent training of patients taking inhalation therapy is required to achieve reproducible delivery of inhalation therapy. Electronic systems with visual feedback to the patients have been developed to assist the patients to use their drug product correctly (36–38).

DETERMINATION OF PULMONARY ABSORPTION

The structural and functional heterogeneity of the respiratory tract also leads to the finding that generalization of results of pulmonary absorption experiments can only be made if the regional deposition of the materials in the respiratory tract is also determined. Intratracheal administration facilitates quantitative deposition of the material whose absorption properties are being studied. Several variants of this technique exist: some of them require surgical procedure (e.g., incision that exposes the rodent trachea through which a needle with the drug formulation is injected), some utilize the insertion of a cannula or a microspray nozzle into the animal's trachea. However, the material thus deposited is not distributed to the same extent throughout the respiratory tract as when given by inhalation of aerosols (17–20).

Lung cell cultures can provide mechanistic insights (39) but they do not represent the complexity in the delivery and disposition of drugs in the human respiratory tract. Perfused lung organ studies provide the next level in complexity (40). Various animal models have been used with the view to predict quantitatively absorption of peptides and proteins from the human lungs. However, due to the major differences in the anatomy and physiology of respiration in primates, the predictive power of these models is quite limited as evidenced by the data in Fig. 2. (Animal models are, of course, essential in the assessment of safety and they can provide valuable mechanistic information.)

The use of drugs in conjunction with gamma radiation emitting radiolabels that facilitate noninvasive measurement of regional doses is the favorite way to investigate mechanistic aspects of pulmonary absorption. The drug can be radiolabeled directly, or, more often, the radiolabel and drug are physically mixed. It is important to prove that the radiolabel does not affect the performance of the drug product either chemically or in terms of its emitted dose (ED) and particle size distribution (PSD). Further, the functional perfomance, ED and PSD, measured in vitro with the drug assay and the radiolabel assay should be the same. This method can thus determine both the total dose to the lung as well as its distribution in various parts of the respiratory tract, both in animal (17, 18, 41–42) and humans (22, 43).

STABILITY ISSUES

A key issue for effective protein and peptide absorption is the preservation of biochemical and structural integrity during the preparation, storage, and aerosolization of the drug molecule. Many proteins and peptides are available as stable aqueous formulations for delivery by injection. However, the process of aerosolization can cause damage to the active molecule. The generation of small droplets provides a vast increase in the air-liquid interfacial area, which may cause unfolding of proteins followed by aggregation. This is particularly likely to happen for hydrophobic proteins that undergo multiple recirculation in jet nebulizers (44) or during spray-drying (45) and may be prevented by addition of suitable surfactants (42). Single-pass systems that form aerosol by extrusion of the solution through a fine nozzle (46) do not appear to cause protein denaturation, in contrast to conventional nebulizers that involve multiple recirculation of the solutions. Thermal denaturation can occur also during the high temperature spray-drying or with some ultrasonic nebulizers that warm the solution for nebulization during their operation (47). Freeze-dried parenteral protein preparations are typically unsuitable for delivery by inhalation for at least two reasons: they often contain excipients such as citrate that could cause irritation if inhaled in sufficient quantities. The freeze-dried materials form cohesive powders that do not lend themselves to be dispersed into respirable particles. Spray-drying has been employed to make respirable protein powders (48, 49). Judicious choice of the quality and quantity of excipients used in dry powders is required to minimize the potential

for adverse reactions, especially in subjects with compromised airways (50, 51). Avoidance of excessive temperature and the use of excipients such as certain sugars in spray-dried formulations may prevent the formation of potentially immunogenic protein aggregates and loss of activity. The nature of the formulation can also affect the quality and physical stability of the particles carrying the peptide or protein. These particles need to flow well during the filling operation and to provide high emitted doses, and they also have to disperse readily into particles with the right aerodynamic diameters. The appropriate balance thus needs to be struck between the chemical stability of the biologic and the physical stability on storage that preserves the solid state form and protects the particles against aggregation and loss of dispersibility into respirable particles (48, 51).

CASE STUDIES WITH SPECIFIC MOLECULES

Insulin

Pulmonary delivery of insulin for systemic absorption in the treatment of diabetes has been studied extensively since the early days of insulin discovery almost a century ago (1). Colthorpe et al. (17) and Pillai et al. (42) demonstrated in rabbit and monkey models, respectively, that the deeper into lung the dose of insulin was delivered, the higher was the bioavailability. The work of Laube et al. (43) showed the need to achieve deep pulmonary deposition of this molecule for efficient absorption in humans. Hand-held liquid and dry powder delivery systems have been developed to generate insulin-containing aerosols with the majority of the particles in the aerodynamic size range 1–3 μm. The relative bioavailability compared with subcutaneous injection based on the insulin contained in the dosage form was ~11% (52) for the dry powder system and ~16% (53) for the aqueous-based bolus delivery system. The reproducibility of pharmacokinetic and pharmacodynamic parameters following pulmonary administration was reported to be similar to subcutaneous delivery. The total lung volume at the end of inspiration was reported to have a major effect on insulin absorption, with deep breath leading to a significantly faster absorption than a more shallow inhalation (14, 23). This suggests that in addition to the inspiratory flow rate and inspired volume at the time of insulin delivery by inhalation, total lung volume may need to be controlled, too, for efficient and reproducible delivery of this molecule that has a rather narrow therapeutic index.

Human Growth Hormone

Wall and Smith (54) reviewed the literature data on pulmonary absorption of recombinant human growth hormone (rhGH) in animal models. A wide range of absolute bioavailability ranging from 3–36% was found. Bioavailability of hGH delivered to the lung increases dramatically the deeper into the lung the formulation reaches (18). Since rhGH is a growth factor, at least theoretically there is a possibility that its delivery to the lung could cause unwanted growth of some lung tissues. Aerosolized delivery of rhGH for 11 days induced body growth of hypophysectomized ("hypox") rats but caused no abnormal lung growth in these animals. A mild immune reaction was seen in the lung, which was not present, when aerosolized bovine growth hormone (bGH) was used instead of hGH. bGH has a much closer amino acid sequence to rat growth hormone than hGH and is thus not significantly immunogenic in this species. Interestingly, IgG titers following subcutaneous administration of hGH were higher than those in the inhalation group and no IgE antibodies were found in the course of inhalation treatment in rats. While total body weight increased in the hypox rats treated with aerosolized hGH, the ratio of lung weight to total body weight did not change. GH receptors are present in many types of cells, but no GH receptor message was found on the "air side" of rabbit lung (55).

Luteinizing Hormone Releasing Hormone (LH-RH)

LH-RH analogs were extensively researched (10). The nonapeptide leuprolide in particular underwent extensive development. Absorption was very significantly dependent upon the depth of deposition of the material in animal models: essentially quantitative absorption was found when the intratracheal adminstration in beagle dogs was done 20–25 cm downstream from epiglottis. Leuprolide acetate suspension aerosols were prepared in chlorofluorocarbon propellants. No adverse reactions were found in association with multiple dosing of these formulations in beagle dogs. Bioavailabilities ranging from ~7–26% found in human studies with these metered dose inhalers, in good agreement with the general fraction of the nominal metered dose that reaches the lung from this type of aerosol delivery system (56).

Soluble Recombinant Interleukine-4 Receptor

(IL-4R) was delivered by nebulization to Cynomolgus primates (41). The peak serum levels were reached after 9.5 h. Absolute bioavailabities close to 30% were measured.

Interferons

Niven et al. (13) studied the absorption of consensus interferon in rodent models. Absolute bioavailabilities approaching 70% were found for the pulmonary route, with evidence of biologically active molecules being absorbed. Mackay et al. (5) compared the absolute bioavailabilities of a hybrid BDBB alpha-interferon in the rat following different routes of administration and found 0.75% for colon, 0.014% for buccal, 0.5% for nasal, and 4.5% for the lung (via intratracheal instillation). Pharmacokinetics of inhaled alpha-interferon was followed in several human studies: Kinnula et al. (57) reported detectable levels with high doses and systemic adverse reactions indicative of biological activity of the absorbed cytokine. In a related study (58), it was observed that the recombinant version of the molecule seems to be less well absorbed than the natural interferon. Differences in metabolism between the natural and recombinant alpha-interferon were also found in a perfused rabbit lung model (59).

Calcitonin

The salmon form of this 32-amino acid non-glycosylated polypeptide is available as a nasal spray with a biovailability in humans of ~3% (60). Mackay et al. (5) reported that the absolute bioavailabilities of human calcitonin across the colon of rat and man, and the lung (via intratracheal instillation) of rat, were 0.9, 0.15 and 36%.

Human Recombinant Granulocyte Colony Stimulating Factor

The systemic bioavailability of recombinant human granulocyte colony stimulating factor (rhG-CSF) based on the amount reaching the lung lobes following intratracheal instillation to the hamster was estimated to be 62% relative to intracardiac administration. Remarkably, about 20% of the absorbable dose of this 18.8-kDa protein was present in serum within 6 min postadministration. The biological activity of the absorbed material was confirmed by the increase of the circulating white blood cells (20). No apparent toxicity was found even on repeated dosing in animals with this protein. Pegylated forms of this molecule were also found to be well absorbed. The rate of and extent of absorption were very much affected by the mode of administration (instillation, powder insufflation, and aerosol administration), reflecting

Table 1

Physiological parameter	Breathing maneuver for optimum peptide and protein absorption
Lung volume prior to inhalation	Full exhalation
Volume inhaled at the time of actuation of aerosol delivery	Minimum volume inhaled prior to actuation of drug delivery
Inspiratory flow rate	The minimum flow rate consistent with acceptable performance of the aerosol delivery device
Total volume inhaled during delivery	Close to vital capacity (shown to be important for insulin)
Respiratory pause between inspiration and exhalation	Several seconds (minimum time to be determined by experimentation)

the differences in the penetration of the material into the deep lung.

PULMONARY ABSORPTION OF PEPTIDES AND PROTEINS INTENDED FOR LOCAL EFFECTS IN THE LUNG

Numerous proteins have been investigated for administration to the respiratory tract to treat local disease (61). In some of these investigations, absorption into the systemic circulation was also followed. These results have their utility when absorption of similar molecules is being considered for the purpose of systemic delivery or to estimate the systemic exposure of locally delivered macromolecules for safety purposes.

Cyclosporine

Cyclosporine is an endecapeptide isolated from fungi. It is an immunosuppressive used to prevent rejection in organ transplantation. Studies have been carried out to investigate the effectiveness of inhalation of this compound in patients receiving lung transplants. Very rapid peak plasma levels were observed followed by a slow phase but the interpretation of this behavior is compromised by the low aqueous solubility of this compound (62).

Alpha-1 Antitrypsin

(A1AT) has been used in injectable form for the treatment of hereditary A1AT deficiency that markedly increases the risk of development of emphysema. Absorption of aerosolized human plasma and recombinant A1AT into the lymph and blood was studied in sheep and humans (63). Human plasma A1AT was found in the sheep blood and interstitial lymph at concentrations ~1/1000 of that in the

alveolar epithelial lining fluid (ELF). The recombinant human A1AT is nonglycosylated and has a terminal methionine residue. In the sheep model, this molecule disappears from the alveolar fluid faster than the human plasma A1AT, with the lymph levels around 10% of ELF and blood levels about 10% of the lymph. The recombinant form was also detected in the blood 24 h after administration to humans.

Recombinant Human Deoxyribonuclease

(rhDNase) has been approved for administration by inhalation for the treatment of cystic fibrosis (9). Bioavailability <15 and <2% in rodents and monkeys respectively was found with this molecule in single-dose studies. In humans, the serum levels of rhDNase following nebulization did not lead to a significant increase above the baseline levels of the endogenous rhDNase.

Anti-IgE

Elevated levels of immunoglobulin E (IgE) in the respiratory lumen and blood are associated with allergic asthma. Sweeney et al. measured concentrations of a monoclonal humanized antibody against IgE (E25) in the blood and bronchoalveolar lavage of different animal species and humans following administration into the respiratory tract. Only small quantities of the antibody were absorbed over a period of several days. The authors suggested that the mechanism of uptake was nonspecific (64).

SUMMARY

While there are no currently approved therapeutic protein or peptide products for delivery via the pulmonary route into the systemic circulation, the data on the efficiency, reproducibility, and safety of molecules such as insulin are particularly encouraging. From a molecular perspective, there is a general trend in the reduction of the rate and extent of absorption with increasing molecular weight, but predictive theories are lacking due to our poor understanding of the complexity and multitude of channels of entry of drugs from the respiratory tract into the systemic circulation. The aerodynamic size distribution is a key parameter affecting the regional distribution, and hence the absorption, of macromolecular drugs from the lung. The synchronization of optimum breathing and aerosol delivery appears to be a prerequisite for efficient and reproducible delivery; the key parameters to control are listed in Table 1.

Relatively little work has been done so far on the control of the rate of absorption of macromolecules from the lung with modified release formulations. Slow pulmonary absorption of insulin in the rat was reported when the drug was encapsulated in polylactic glycolic acid spheres (65). The long-term safety of such long-acting excipients needs to be investigated: in contrast to small molecules, it would be expected that significant accumulation of these materials could occur on multiple dosing (16).

REFERENCES

1. Farr, S.J.; Taylor, G. Insulin Inhalation. Its Potential as a Nonparenteral Method of Administration. *Inhalation Delivery of Therapeutic Peptides and Proteins*; Adjei, L.A., Gupta, P.K., Eds.; Ch. 13; New York, 1997; 371–378.
2. Gonda, I. The Ascent of Pulmonary Drug Delivery. J. Pharm. Sci. **2000**, *89*, 940–945.
3. Moss, G.F.; Jones, K.M.; Ritchie, J.T.; Cox, J.S.G. Plasma Levels and Urinary Excretion of Disodium Cromoglycate After Inhalation by Human Volunteers. Toxicol. Appl. Pharmacol **1971**, *20*, 147–156.
4. Takada, K.; Yamamoto, M.; Asada, S. Evidence for the Pulmonary Absorption of Fluorescent Labelled Macromolecular Compounds. J. Pharm. Dyn. **1978**, *1*, 281–287.
5. Mackay, M.; Phillips, J.; Steward, A.; Hastewell, J. Pulmonary Absorption of Therapeutic Peptides and Proteins. *Respiratory Drug Delivery IV*; Byron, P.R., Dalby, R.N., Farr, S.J., Eds.; Interpharm Press, Inc.: Buffalo Grove, IL, 1994; 31–37.
6. Gonda, I. Targeting by Deposition. *Pharmaceutical Inhalation Aerosol Technology*; Hickey, A.J., Ed.; Marcel Dekker, Inc.: New York, 1992; 61–82.
7. Adjei, A.L., Gupta, P.R., Eds.; *Inhalation Delivery of Therapeutic Peptides and Proteins* Marcel Dekker, Inc.: New York, 1997.
8. Green, J.D. Pharmaco-Toxicological Expert Report Pulmozyme™ RhDNAse Genentech, Inc.: Human Exptl. Toxicol. **1994**, *13*(suppl. 1), S1–S42, 7.
9. Gonda, I. Deoxyribonuclease Inhalation. *Inhalation Delivery of Therapeutic Peptides and Proteins*; Adjei, A.L., Gupta, P.R., Eds.; Ch. 12; Marcel Dekker, Inc.: New York, 1997; 355–365.
10. Adjei, L.A.; Lu, F.M-Y. LH-RH Analogs. *Inhalation Delivery of Therapeutic Peptides and Proteins*; Adjei, A.L., Gupta, P.R., Eds.; Ch. 14; Marcel Dekker, Inc.: New York, 1997; 389–412.
11. Berelowitz, M.; Becker, G. Inhaled Insulin—Clinical Pharmacology and Clinical Study Results. *Respiratory Drug Delivery VII*; Dalby, R.N., Byron, P.R., Farr, S.J., Peart, J., Eds.; Serentec Press, Inc.: Raleigh, NC, 2000; 151–154.
12. Clauson, P.G.; Balent, B.; Brunner, G.A.; Sendlhofer, G.; Jendle, J.H.; Hatorp, V.; Dahl, U.L.; Okikawa, J.; Pieber, T.R. PK-PD of Four Different Doses of Pulmonary Insulin Delivered with the AERx® Diabetes Management System. *Respiratory Drug Delivery VII*; Dalby, R.N., Byron, P.R., Farr, S.J., Peart, J., Eds.; Serentec Press, Inc.: Raleigh NC, 2000, 155–161.
13. Niven, R.W.; Whitcomb, K.L.; Woodward, M.; Liu, J.; Jornacion, C. Systemic Absorption and Activity of Recombinant Consensus Interferon After Intratracheal and Aerosol Administration. Pharm. Res. **1995**, *12*, 1889–1995.
14. Farr, S.J.; McElduff, A.; Mather, L.E.; Okikawa, J.; Ward, M.E.; Gonda, I.; Licko, V.; Rubsamen, R.M. Pulmonary Insulin Administration Using the AERx® System: Physiological and Physicochemical Factors Influencing Insulin Effectiveness in Healthy Fasting Volunteers. Diabetes Technol. Ther. **2000**, *2*, 185–197.
15. Hanatani, K.; Takada, K.; Yoshida, N.; Nakasuji, M.; Morishita, Y.; Yasako, K.; Fujita, T.; Yamamoto, A.; Muranishi, S. Molecular Weight-Dependent Lymphatic Transfer of Fluorescein Isothiocyanate-Labeled Dextrans After Intrapulmonary Administration and Effects of Various Absorption Enhancers on the Lymphatic Transfer of Drugs in Rats. J. Drug Targeting **1995**, *3*, 263–271.
16. Gonda, I. Drugs Administered Directly into the Respiratory Tract: Modeling of the Duration of Effective Drug Levels. J. Pharm. Sci. **1988**, *77*, 340–346.
17. Colthorpe, P.; Farr, S.J.; Taylor, G.; Smith, I.J.; Wyatt, D. The Pharmacokinetics of Pulmonary-Delivered Insulin: A Comparison of Intratracheal and Aerosol Administration to the Rabbit. Pharm. Res. **1992**, *9*, 764–768.
18. Colthorpe, P.; Farr, S.J.; Smith, I.J.; Wyatt, D.; Taylor, G. The Influence of Regional Deposition on the Pharmacokinetics of Pulmonary-Delivered Human Growth Hormone in Rabbits. Pharm. Res. **1995**, *12*, 356–359.
19. Brown, R.A., Jr.; Schanker, L.W. Absorption of Aerosolized Drugs from the Rat Lung. Drug Metab. Disp. **1983**, *11*, 355–360.
20. Niven, R.W. Feasibility Studies with Recombinant Human Granulocyte Colony-Stimulating Factor. *Inhalation Delivery of Therapeutic Peptides and Proteins*; Adjei, A.L., Gupta, P.R., Eds.; Ch. 15; Marcel Dekker, Inc.: New York, 1997; 413–452.
21. Qui, Y.; Gupta, P.K.; Adjei, A.L. Absorption and Bioavailability of Inhaled Peptides and Proteins. *Inhalation Delivery of Therapeutic Peptides and Proteins*; Adjei, A.L., Gupta, P.R., Eds.; Ch. 4; Marcel Dekker, Inc.: New York, 1997; 89–131.

22. Newman, S.P.; Hirst, P.H.; Pitcairn, G.R.; Clark, A.R. Understanding Regional Lung Deposition Data in Gamma Scintigraphy, Pulmonary Absorption of Therapeutic Peptides and Proteins. *Respiratory Drug Delivery VI*; Dalby, R.N., Byron, P.R., Farr, S.J., Eds.; Interpharm Press: Buffalo Grove, 1998; 9–16.

23. Farr, S.J.; Gonda, I.; Licko, V. Physicochemical and Physiological Factors Influencing the Effectiveness of Inhaled Insulin, Pulmonary Absorption of Therapeutic Peptides and Proteins. *Respiratory Drug Delivery VI*; Dalby, R.N., Byron, P.R., Farr, S.J., Eds.; Interpharm Press, Inc.: Buffalo Grove, IL, 1998; 25–33.

24. Egan, E. Lung Inflation, Lung Solute Permeability, and Alveolar Edema. J. Appl. Physiol.: Respirat. Environ. Exercise Physiol. **1982**, *53*, 121–125.

25. Folkesson, H.G.; Westrom, B.R.; Karlsson, B.W. Permeability of the Respiratory Tract to Different-Sized Macromolecules After Intratracheal Instillation in Young and Adult Rats. Acta. Physiol. Scand. **1990**, *139*, 347–354.

26. Kohler, D. Aerosols for Systemic Treatment. Lung **1990**, *168* (suppl.), 677–684.

27. Folkesson, H.G.; Westrom, B.R.; Dahlback, M.; Lundin, S.; Karlsson, B.W. Passage of Aerosolized BSA and the Nona-Peptide DDAVP via the Respiratory Tract in Young and Adult Rats. Exp. Lung Res. **1992**, *18*, 595–614.

28. Yamamoto, A.; Umemori, S.; Muranishi, S. Absorption Enhancement of Intrapulmonary Administered Insulin by Various Absorption Enhancers and Protease Inhibitors in Rats. J. Pharm. Pharmacol. **1994**, *46*, 14–18.

29. Morita, T.; Yamamoto, A.; Takakura, T.; Hashida, M.; Sezaki, H. Improvement of the Pulmonary Absorption of (Asu 1, 7)-eel Calcitonin by Various Protease Inhibitors in Rats. Pharm. Res. **1994**, *11*, 909–913.

30. Patton, J.S.; Nagarajan, S.; Clark, A.R. Pulmonary Absorptioin and Metabolism of Peptides and Proteins. *Respiratory Drug Delivery VI*; Dalby, R.N., Byron, P.R., Farr, S.J., Eds.; Interpharm Press, Inc.: Buffalo Grove, IL, 1998; 17–24.

31. Morimoto, K.; Yamahara, H.; Lee, V.H.L.; Kim, K.J. Dipeptide Transport Across Rat Alveolar Epithelial Cell Monolayers. Pharm. Res. **1993**, *10*, 1668–1674.

32. Taylor, G.; Colthorpe, P.; Farr, S.J. Pulmonary Absorption of Proteins: Influence of Deposition Site and Competitive Elimination Processes. *Respiratory Drug Delivery IV*; Byron, P.R., Dalby, R.N., Farr, S.J., Eds.; Interpharm Press, Inc.: Buffalo Grove, IL, 1994, 25–30.

33. Huchon, G.J.; Montgomery, A.B.; Lipavsky, A.; Hoeffel, J.M.; Murray, J.F. Respiratory Clearance of Aerosolized Radioactive Solutes of Varying Molecular Weight. J. Nucl. Med. **1987**, *28*, 894–902.

34. Effros, R.M.; Mason, G.R. Measurements of Pulmonary Epithelial Permeability In Vivo. Am. Rev. Resp. Dis. **1984**, *129* (Suppl.), S59–S65.

35. Gonda, I. Physico-Chemical Principles in Aerosol Delivery. *Topics in Pharmaceutical Sciences 1991*; Crommelin, D.J.A., Middha, K.K., Eds.; Ch. 7; Medpharm Scientific Publishers: Stuttgart, 1992; 95–115.

36. Farr, S.J.; Rowe, A.M.; Rubsamen, R.; Taylor, G. Aerosol Deposition in the Human Lung Following Administration from a Microprocessor Controlled Pressurised Metered Dose Inhaler. Thorax **1995**, *50*, 639–644.

37. Phipps, P.R.; Gonda, I.; Anderson, S.D. Apparatus for the Control of Breathing Patterns During Aerosol Inhalation. J. Aerosol Med. **1992**, *5*, 155–170.

38. Gonda, I.; Schuster, J.A.; Rubsamen, R.M.; Lloyd, P.; Cipolla, D.; Farr, S.J. Inhalation Delivery Systems with Compliance and Disease Management Capabilities. J. Contr. Rel. **1998**, *53*, 269–274.

39. Mathias, N.R.; Yamashita, F.; Lee, V.H.L.Respiratory Epithelial Cell Culture Models for Evaluation of Ion and Drug Transport. Adv. Drug Del. Rev. **1996**, *22*, 215–249.

40. Byron, P.R.; Roberts, N.S.; Clark, A.R. An Isolated Perfused Rat Lung Preparation for the Study of Aerosolized Drug Deposition and Absorption. J. Pharm. Sci. **1986**, *75*, 168–171.

41. Pettit, D.K.; Moutvic, R.; Maliszewski, C.F.; Abbott, N.M.; Gombotz, W.R.; Smith, P.B.; Zhusti, A.; Slauter, R.W. Pharmacokinetics of Interleukin-4 Receptor Delivered to Primates by Nebulization and Intravenous Injection. *Respiratory Drug Delivery VII*; Dalby, R.N., Byron, P.R., Farr, S.J., Peart, J., Eds.; Serentec Press Inc.: Raleigh, NC, 2000; 405–406.

42. Pillai, R.S.; Hughes, B.L.; Wolff, R.K.; Heisserman, J.A.; Dorato, M.A. The Effect of Pulmonary-Delivered Insulin on Blood Glucose Levels Using Two Nebulizer Systems. J. Aerosol Med. **1996**, *9*, 227–240.

43. Laube, B.L.; Benedict, G.W.; Dobs, A.S. Time to Peak Insulin Level, Relative Bioavailability, and Effect of Site of Deposition of Nebulized Insulin in Patients with Noninsulin-Dependent Diabetes Mellitus. J. Aerosol Med. **1998**, *11*, 153–173.

44. Niven, R.W.; Ip, A.Y.; Mittelman, S.D.; Farrar, C.; Arakawa, T.; Prestrelski, S.J. Protein Nebulization: I. Stability of Lactate Dehydrogenase and Recombinant Granulocyte-Colony Stimulating Factor to Air-Jet Nebulization. Int. J. Pharm. **1994**, *109*, 17–26.

45. Mumenthaler, M.; Hsu, C.C.; Pearlman, R. Feasibility Study on Spray-Drying Protein Pharmaceuticals: Recombinant Human Growth Hormone and Tissue-Type Plasminogen Activator. Pharm. Res. **1994**, *11*, 12–20.

46. Schuster, J.A.; Rubsamen, R.M.; Lloyd, P.; Lloyd, J. The AERx™ Aerosol Delivery System. Pharm. Res. **1997**, *14*, 354–357.

47. Cipolla, D.C.; Clark, A.R.; Chan, H.-K.; Gonda, I.; Shire, S.J. Assessment of Aerosol Delivery Systems for the Recombinant Human Deoxyribonuclease I (rhDNase). STP Pharma Sciences **1994**, *4*, 50–62.

48. Clark, A.R.; Dasovich, N.; Gonda, I.; Chan, H.-K. The Balance between Biochemical and Physical Stability for Inhalation Protein Powders. *Respiratory Drug Delivery V*; Byron, P.R., Dalby, R.N., Farr, S.J., Eds.; Interpharm Press, Inc.: Buffalo IL, 1996; 167–174.

49. Chan, H.K.; Gonda, I. Solid State Characterization of Spray-Dried Powders of Recombinant Human Deoxyribonuclease (rhDNase). J. Pharm. Sci. **1998**, *87*, 647–654.

50. Anderson, S.D.; Brannan, J.; Spring, J.; Spalding, N.; Rodwell, L.T.; Chan, K.; Gonda, I.; Walsh, A.; Clark, A.R. A New Method for Bronchial-Provocation Testing in Asthmatic Subjects Using a Dry Powder of Mannitol. Am. J. Respir. Crit. Care Med. **1997**, *156*, 758–765.

51. Clark, A.R.; Shire, S.J. Formulation of Proteins for Pulmonary Delivery. *Protein Formulation and Delivery*;

McNally, E.J., Ed.; Ch. 7; Marcel Dekker, Inc.: New York, 2000; 201–234.

52. Gelfand, R.A.; Schwartz, S.L.; Horton, M.; Law, C.G.; Pun, P.F. Pharmacological Reproducibility of Inhaled Human Insulin Pre-Meal Dosing in Patients with Type 2 Diabetes Mellitus. Diabetes **1998**, *47*, A99.

53. Kipnes, M.; Otulana, B.; Okikawa, J.; Farr, S.; Jendle, J.; Thipphawong, J.; Schwartz, S. Pharmacokinetics and Pharmacodynamics of Pulmonary Insulin Delivered Via the AERx Diabetes Management System in Type 1 Diabetics. Abstr. EASD, Jerusalem, Sept. 2000.

54. Wall, D.A.; Smith, P.L. Inhalation Therapy for Growth Hormone Deficiency. *Inhalation Delivery of Therapeutic Peptides and Proteins*; Adjei, A.L., Gupta, P.R., Eds.; Ch. 16, Marcel Dekker, Inc.: New York, 1997; 453–469.

55. Patton, J.S.; Platz, R.M. Routes of Delivery: Case Studies (2): Pulmonary Delivery of Peptides and Proteins for Systemic Action. Adv. Drug Deli. Rev. **1992**, *8*, 179–186.

56. Laube, B.L. In Vivo Measurements of Aerosol Dose and Distribution: Clinical Relevance. J. Aerosol. Med. **1996**, *9*(Suppl. 1), S77–S91.

57. Kinnula, V.; Mattson, K.; Cantell, K. Pharmacokinetics and Toxicity of Inhaled Human Interferon-Alpha in Patients with Lung Cancer. J. Interferon Res. **1989**, *9*, 419–423.

58. Maasilta, P.; Halme, J.; Mattson, K.; Cantell, K. Pharmacokinetics of Inhaled Recombinant and Natural Alpha Interferon. Lancet **1991**, *337*, 371.

59. Bocci, V.; Pessina, G.P.; Pacini, A.; Paulesu, L.; Muscettola, M.; Mogensen, K.E. Pulmonary Catabolism of Interferons: Alveolar Absorption of 125 I-Labeled Human Interferon Alpha is Accompanied by Partial Loss of Biological Activity. Antiviral Res. **1984**, *4*, 211–220.

60. Physicians' Desk Reference, PDR Electronic Library, Release 2000; Medical Economics Company.

61. Adjei, A.L. Part Three: Localized Delivery of Peptides and Proteins to the Lung: Case Studies. *Inhalation Delivery of Therapeutic Peptides and Proteins*; Adjei, A.L., Gupta, P.R., Eds.; Marcel Dekker, Inc.: New York, 1997; 277–279.

62. Burckart, G.J.; Keenan, R.; Griffith, B.P.; Iacono, A.T. Cyclosporine. *Inhalation Delivery of Therapeutic Peptides and Proteins*; Adjei, A.L., Gupta, P.R., Eds.; Ch. 8, Marcel Dekker, Inc.: New York, 1997; 281–299.

63. Hubbard, R.C. Alpha-1 Antitrypsin. *Inhalation Delivery of Therapeutic Peptides and Proteins*; Adjei, A.L., Gupta, P.R., Eds.; Ch. 10, Marcel Dekker, Inc.: New York, 1997; 315–330.

64. Sweeney, T.D.; Marian, M.; Achilles, K.; Bussiere, J.; Ruppel, J.; Shoenhoff, M.; Mrsny, R. Biopharmaceutics of Immunoglobulin Transport Across Lung Epithelium. *Respiratory Drug Delivery VII*; Dalby, R.N., Byron, P.R., Farr, S.J., Peart, J., Eds.; Serentec Press, Inc.: Raleigh, NC, 2000; 59–66.

65. Edwards, D.A.; Hanes, J.; Caponnetti, G.; Hrkac, J.; Lotan, N.; Ben-Jebria, A.; Langer, R. Large Porous Biodegradable Particles for Pulmonary Drug Delivery. Science **1997**, *276*, 1868–1871.

PEPTIDES AND PROTEINS—TRANSDERMAL ABSORPTION

Richard H. Guy
M. Begoña Delgado-Charro
Diego Marro
Centre Interuniversitaire de Recherche et d'Enseignement, Archamps, France
University of Geneva, Switzerland

INTEREST AND RATIONALE

An increasing number of peptides and proteins will be introduced into therapeutics in the forthcoming years. The gradual maturation of the biotechnology industry has led to many advances, not the least of which is that it is now possible, for the first time, to produce large quantities of highly pure peptides and proteins. However, their potential usefulness as therapeutic agents will be much enhanced if constraints imposed by the parenteral route of delivery, the only one currently available for most of these agents, can be overcome. The design of successful dosage forms for the delivery of these complex biotechnology products by alternative routes is a challenging objective for the pharmaceutical scientist.

Possible nonparenteral routes for the delivery of peptide and protein drugs include the nasal, oral, transdermal, buccal, ocular, rectal, and vaginal pathways (1–3). In general, the primary advantages of these strategies over parenteral delivery are the relatively noninvasive nature and simplicity of administration. However, it goes without saying that these alternative routes are generally much less efficient than an injection (whether intravenous, intramuscular, or subcutaneous) with frequently very low bioavailabilities.

Transdermal delivery has attracted considerable interest as a route for administering peptides and proteins. Among its appealing features, the transdermal path a) avoids the hepatic first-pass effect and gastrointestinal breakdown, a very important factor for these metabolically very fragile drugs; b) provides controlled and sustained administration, particularly suitable for the treatment of chronic disease; c) reduces side-effects, often related to the peak concentrations of the circulating agent; d) enables self-administration and improves patient compliance, due to its convenience and ease of use; and d) permits abrupt termination of drug effect by simply removing the delivery system from the skin surface (3).

Because the skin has a relatively low proteolytic activity compared with other tissues, the poor inherent skin permeability of the peptide drugs is the prime limiting factor for their delivery by the transdermal route (1). Generally speaking, peptide and protein drugs are polar and compared with "normal" drugs, of high molecular weight. Such molecules diffuse poorly, as a result, across the skin, making the use of an appropriate enhancement strategy (as we shall see) obligatory. Several approaches being investigated to enhance the transdermal absorption of peptide and protein drugs are reviewed in this chapter. These include the use of chemical penetration enhancers, iontophoresis, the application of transient high-voltage pulses (electroporation), the use of ultrasound (sonophoresis), and various, so-called minimally invasive strategies.

SKIN BARRIER FUNCTION

Stratum Corneum and Routes of Passive Permeation

The remarkable barrier function of the skin is primarily located in the stratum corneum (SC), the thin, outermost layer of the epidermis (4). The SC consists of several layers of protein-filled corneocytes (i.e., terminally differentiated keratinocytes) embedded in an extracellular lipid matrix. Attached to the outer corneocyte envelope are long-chain covalently bound ceramides that interact with the lipids of the extracellular space. These lipids are composed primarily of free fatty acids, ceramides, and cholesterol arranged in multiple lamellae (5). Passive permeation across the SC is believed to occur primarily via the intercellular lipid pathway (Fig. 1a), which constitutes the only continuous phase through the SC (6). Evidence for this deduction is provided by the temperature dependence of SC water permeability (7) and the remarkable correlation between water transport and the degree of disorder of the intercellular lipids (4). In addition, several imaging techniques, using various different tracers have been used to directly visualize permeation via the intercellular path (6, 8). Further, it has recently been concluded that the

Encyclopedia of Pharmaceutial Technology

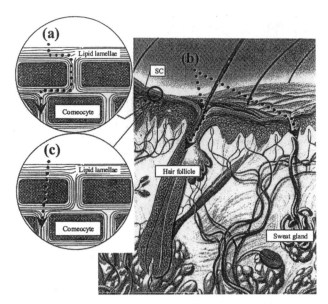

Fig. 1 Routes of passive permeation across the stratum corneum (SC): (a) intercellular lipid pathway; (b) appendageal transport; and (c) transcellular path.

barrier function of the SC is rather uniformly distributed across its entire thickness (9). Appendageal transport through hair follicles and sweat glands is another potential route, these structures offering "shunt" pathways across the continuity of the SC (Fig. 1b). Visualization of appendageal transport has been accomplished both for passive diffusion and for percutaneous transport enhanced by one means or another (e.g., iontophoresis) (6, 10). Passively, while it has been postulated that the appendageal structures dominate initially, their contribution to total steady-state transport is believed to be rather small due to the small area available relative to the entire surface of the skin (10, 11). A third possible route across the SC is the transcellular path (Fig. 1c). However, despite its favorable surface area and short pathlength (compared with the tortuous intercellular route), no evidence exists in support of molecular permeation by this way; indeed, the implausibility of the route has been demonstrated by certain authors (8, 12).

Structure–Permeation Relationships: Application to Peptide Absorption

Most structure–permeation evaluations of transdermal transport indicate the strong relationship between a chemical's permeability coefficient across the skin (K_p) and its lipophilicity (13–15). Potts and Guy (14) analyzed a diverse database of skin penetration data, comprising 91 compounds (15) and developed a simple relation indicating that K_p depended only on lipophilicity, as measured by the chemical's octanol–water partition coefficient (P), and molecular weight (MW):

$$logKp(cm/sec) = -6.3 + 0.71logP - 0.0061xMW$$

However, for compounds of high lipophilicity, the algorithm needs to be modified (16) to account for the fact that these substances may become transport-limited not by their diffusion through the SC, but rather by their ability to partition out of this membrane into the underlying aqueous, viable epidermis. At the opposite end of the lipophilicity scale, the very small log P values of polar compounds, including peptide and proteins, of course, many of which retain a charge (or multiple charges) over a broad pH range, mean that their K_p values are extremely small and, hence, their inherent transdermal fluxes, without a suitable enhancement technique, are not therapeutically useful. As a general point, it must be emphasized that no matter what one might do to enhance transdermal delivery, the route remains useful exclusively for compounds of high potency (including peptides).

STRATEGIES FOR THE TRANSDERMAL DELIVERY OF PEPTIDES AND PROTEINS

Passive Delivery and Chemical Enhancement

It is widely accepted that the two most important physicochemical parameters that determine a molecule's skin permeability are a) its lipophilicity, with a log (octanol/water partition coefficient) value of 2 being quite favorable, and b) its molecular size—smaller compounds permeating better than big ones (14). Thus, it is no surprise that the passive transdermal delivery of peptides and proteins, which are typically either very polar (or charged) and/or of high molecular weight (>1000 Da), is extremely inefficient and rarely results in fluxes, which would elicit significant therapeutic effect.

Consequently, a number of enhancer formulations have been considered in an attempt to improve peptide transport across the skin. These vehicles include, as we shall briefly discuss, either well-known chemical promoters or combinations thereof, peptide metabolism inhibitors, or colloidal (principally liposomal) structures. Table 1 summarizes much of the available literature. Before addressing specifically certain examples of the results obtained, it is worth noting that, although increased peptide transport has been possible, little attention has been focused upon the effects of the enhancer formulations on the skin (such as irritation and, in consequence, long-term tolerability) nor

Table 1 Effect of chemical enhancers and vehicle composition on the transdermal passive delivery of peptide drugs

Peptide	Vehicle	Skin model	Comments	Ref.
A. Passive + chemical enhancer				
Octreotide	40% EtOH; 1% Decylmethyl sulfoxide in 40% EtOH; 50% Dimethyl sulfoxide	Hairless mouse skin; heat-separated human epidermis	In vitro; clinically relevant delivery	(17)
[NLe^4, D-Phe^7]-α-MSH (melanotropic peptide analog)	26% PEG 400; 74% PEG 3350	Mice shaved skin	In vivo; follicular melanogenesis induction	(18)
		Mouse skin; rat skin	In vitro; delivery through mouse but not through rat skin	(19)
		Dermatomed human skin	In vitro; delivery measured	(20)
Des-enkephalin-γ-endorphin (1300 Da)	Azone; PEG	Human SC and de-glycerinized dermatomed skins (Dutch Burns Society)	In vitro; enhancers required for relevant delivery	(21)
Leu-enkephalin	n-Decylmethyl sulfoxide (10 mM) + metabolism inhibitors (piromycin, amastatin)	Hairless mouse skin	In vitro; study of the metabolism; coadministration of inhibitors to increase flux	(22)
Vasopressin (1084 Da)	Sodium laurylsulphate (0.9 to 19.2 × 10^{-3}M)	Rat shaved skin	In vitro; effect of pH and peptide concentration; no effect of enhancer found	(23)
	Azone (3–25%); dimethyl sulfoxide; DMAC; NNDMT; transcutol; labrafil	In vitro hairless mouse/rats; in vivo rats; "clipping" hair shaved	Best results with Azone (clinical effect in vivo: reduction of urine volume and increase in urine osmolality)	(24)
Elcatonin ([Asu^{17}] eel-calcitonin) (3363 Da)	Carbopol gel + different enhancers and protease inhibitors: e.g., bile salts, gabexate, bestaline, OG, OTG.	Shaved rat	In vivo; effect of protease inhibitors; observation of the hypocalcemic effect	(25)
	Carbopol gel; vitamine D3 + Estradiol + OTG + aurocholate	Rats (suffering experimental osteoporosis); shaved skin	In vivo; efficiency in treating experimental osteoporosis in rats	(26)
Leuprolide (1209 Da)	2% HPMC; EtOH:water (4:1) + enhancer: menthol (1–2%); camphor (2%); methyl salicilate; (2%); lauric acid (2%); decanoic acid (2%); 20–80% ethylalcohol; 10% urea	Nude mouse; dermatomed human skin; snake skin	In vitro	(27)
Nafarelin	PG, azone; glyceryl mono-oleate; EtOH; β-cyclodextrin	Dermatomed human and monkey skin	In vitro; 80 h permeation time	(28)
Tetragastrin	In PBS solution	Rat shaved skin	Prodrug approach: Permeation of parent compound and acylated derivatives.	(29)
B. Passive + colloidal vehicle				
Cyclosporin	Oil/water emulsion liposomes	Hairless mouse skin	In vitro; stripping procedure; cyclosporin accumulated; high cyclosporin into the skin	(30)
Interferon-γ	Liposomes	Human skin grafted in nude mice	In vitro; measurement of ICAM-1 induction	(31)
	Liposomes	Dermatomed human skin	In vitro; measurement of bio-activity of the transported peptide (10% active)	(32)
Enkephalin	Liposomes + iontophoresis	Human skin	In vitro	(33)
Tyrosine	Microemulsion liquid crystals	Stripped rat skin	In vitro	(34)

Abbreviations: EtOH (ethanol); PEG (polyethylene glycol); SC (stratum corneum); DMAC (dimethyl acetamide); NNDMT (*N*,*N*-dimethyl-*m*-toluamide); OG (*n*-Octyl-β-D-glucoside); OTG (*n*-Octyl-β-D-thioglucoside); HPMC (hydroxipropylmethylcellulose); PG (propylene glycol); PBS (phosphate buffer solution); ICAM-1 (intercellular adhesion molecule-1).

has the fact that animal models of questionable relevance (e.g., the shaved skin of hairy rats, notorious for their higher skin permeability relative to man even in the absence of penetration enhancer) have been used. To illustrate the "gap" between laboratory and reality, with respect to the feasibility of some enhancer vehicles proposed, one can cite the delivery of octreotide from a formulation containing 40% ethanol and 50% dimethyl-sulphoxide (17) and the delivery of leuprolide from a 4:1 v/v ethanol–water solution to which various known chemical skin permeation enhancers had been added (27). It is not foolhardy to predict that both these approaches would cause local irritation of the skin in vivo in man and that their chronic use would be precluded.

Among the more interesting and reasonable results published are a series of studies demonstrating the delivery of the melanotropic peptide [Nle^4, D-Phe^7]-α-MSH across mouse and human skin from a relatively mild formulation consisting of 1:3 v/v PEG 400-PEG 3350 (18–20). In vivo across shaved mouse skin, in fact, it was possible to show induction of melanogenesis (18). Unfortunately, however, these data remain at best semiquantitative: no actual flux values were measured precluding comparison with other work in the field.

Positive pharmacological results have also been observed following the delivery of the relatively high molecular weight peptide, elcatonin (3363 Da, a calcitonin analog) across shaved rat skin in vivo (25, 26). Hypocalcemia was documented together with a beneficial effect on this animal model of osteoporosis. Successful formulations included taurocholate and peptidase inhibitors, such as gabexate and bestatine. Another approach has involved the use of lipophilic prodrugs of the peptide tetragastrin but, in this case, one has to ask whether the improvement in delivery is sufficient to warrant the additional regulatory complexities concomitant with the prodrug strategy (29).

The largest body of recent work in this area has involved the use of colloidal carriers, in particular liposomes (see Table 1); comprehensive reviews of this research can be found elsewhere (35–37). A general observation on the information published to-date is that the amount of lipid formulation applied is often very high when compared with the quantity of intercellular SC lipid in the treated area of the skin. That such liposomal formulations can significantly perturb (or, perhaps, overwhelm is a better word) normal barrier function is not too surprising, especially if the exogenous lipids employed can mix efficiently with their endogenous counterparts (30, 32, 38); this may explain why liposomes based upon lipid mixtures that mimic the composition of those in the SC are sometimes useful.

These lipid-based systems have been used to deliver peptides for both dermatological and systemic therapy. In the former case, the administration of cyclosporin (CSA) to treat psoriasis has been considered, with the idealistic objective of somehow localizing the drug in the skin while minimizing its entry into the systemic circulation (30). In vitro, from the lipid-based vehicles, almost no CSA permeated into the receptor phase in conventional diffusion cell experiments. However, this result was not different from the "control" formulation, which simply contained CSA in 40% ethanol. Much of the drug (>60%), and the lipids from the liposomal-based formulation, were actually found in the SC at the end of the experiment. In the same category, a particularly well-conducted study considered the delivery of γ-interferon from liposomes across human skin in vitro (32); topical application of γ-interferon has been proposed for the treatment of atopic dermatitis and keloidal scarring. Initial investigation with γ-interferon suggested a quite short lag-time (on the order of an hour) but that the liposomally delivered peptide had lost most of its biological activity (32). In a subsequent series of experiments, the work was extended to an in vivo model of human-skin grafted nude (athymic) mice (31). It was found that the γ-interferon delivered in this case retained its biological activity and promoted epidermal ICAM-1 induction (Fig. 2).

With respect to systemic delivery of peptide and protein drugs encapsulated in lipid-based carriers, Cevc et al. (39) have investigated the transdermal delivery of insulin encapsulated in "elastic" liposomes (Transfersomes^{TM}), which differ from conventional liposomes in that a surfactant is added to the formulation (e.g., sodium cholate, sodium dodecyl sulfate, or bile salts). A dose-dependent systemic hypoglycemia has been reported in human volunteers following topical application of such an insulin formulation, over an area of 45–90 cm^2; the effect was typically 25–45% of that following a subcutaneous injection of the same formulation. The authors claim that this outcome is not the result of the disrupting effect of the ethanolic (10%), surfactant-rich formulation on the integrity of the skin barrier, since "rigid" liposomes (ethanolic liposomes without bile salt) and insulin/mixed micelles (which contain the highest bile salt concentration of all formulations studied) had no significant hypoglycemic effect. On the contrary, they argue that the specifically elastic properties of thetransfersomes are the crucial features that allow the lipid vesicle to carry the encapsulated agent across the skin (39).

Finally, the topical application of proteins to intact skin as a noninvasive method for immunization and vaccination has been described recently. The cholera toxin (86 kDa) has been shown to induce significant antibody production when topically applied to shaved, previously hydrated, mouse skin (40). The cholera toxin has also been shown to act as an immunizing adjuvant, that is, it enhances immune responses against less potent antigens, such as diphtheria toxoid, and tetanus toxoid, when coadministered topically (40). A subsequent report identified several other bacterial products that also elicit adjuvant properties, but having less risk of toxicity and reduced secondary effects than cholera toxin (41). Transdermal immunization has also been obtained in mice with large proteins, such as the gap junction protein, encapsulated in lipid vesicles (42, 43). A more sophisticated approach, the transdermal delivery of an antigen-encoding plasmid, which induces in vivo the production of the antigen protein, has also been investigated and will be discussed later in this chapter. Overall, the future development of noninvasive, easily administered vaccines is of much interest, particularly for massive immunization programs in developing countries, where the lack of trained personnel capable of performing accurately repeated injections (which are far from welcomed) poses a significant barrier to prophylactic health care.

Iontophoresis

Iontophoresis is a noninvasive technique that uses a mild electric current (<0.5 mA/cm^2) to facilitate the transfer of molecules across the skin (Fig. 3). The frequently polar and/or charged nature of biotechnology drugs makes them

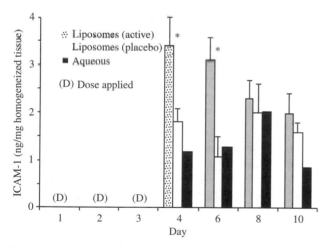

Fig. 2 ICAM-1 production after topical application of gamma interferon to a human skin graft on nude mice. One dose (100 μl) of a liposomal (20 mg/ml lipid) or aqueous (phosphate buffered saline) formulation was applied daily for three days. Active formulation contained 0.51 mg/ml gamma interferon. Placebo liposomal formulations contained no added protein. Significant differences (active versus placebo) are indicated by asterisks (*). (Redrawn from data in Ref. 31.)

potentially well-suited candidates for electrically controlled drug delivery across the skin (44, 45). Indeed, as we shall see, human studies using iontophoresis have already demonstrated the safe, effective, and reproducible delivery of intact peptides to the systemic circulation. Specific accomplishments for certain peptide iontophoretic applications of particular note to date are: a) that steady-state plasma levels can be achieved relatively rapidly and then maintained for reasonably prolonged periods of time, until the current is stopped and b) that the current profile can be adjusted to change the delivery profile, and hence to preprogram perhaps the more complex dosing regimes required. In addition, for two small nonpeptide drugs, at least, small easily portable and integrated iontophoretic devices are in advanced stages (Phase III) of development.

Iontophoresis enhances drug delivery across the skin by two principal mechanisms: electrorepulsion and electroosmosis (46) (Fig. 4). Electrorepulsion is the direct effect of the applied electric field on a charged permeant. Practically speaking, this means, for example, that a positively-charged (cationic) drug is formulated at the anode and, upon applying the electric field, is repelled toward and through the skin. The drug ion acts, therefore, as a charge carrier in the electric circuit. However, the fraction of the total charge delivered by the power supply that is carried by the drug may be quite small and, for larger peptides, rarely approaches even a few percent. This is because there may be competing (e.g., buffer, electrolyte) cations in the formulation and there are always competing anions (especially Cl$^-$) carrying a significant amount of charge out of the skin toward the anode (Fig. 3). Formulations must therefore be optimized to minimize the presence of competing ions, at least in the direction from the skin surface into the body. The second mechanism, electroosmosis, results from the fact that the skin supports a net negative charge at physiological pH (47, 48) [the pI of the human skin has been shown to be within the range 4.5–5 (47)]. Imposing an electrical potential gradient across a charged membrane produces a convective solvent flow in the direction of counterion transport (i.e., from anode-to-cathode in the case of skin). This solvent flow therefore augments the electrotransport of cationic, and very polar, yet neutral, compounds, while acting against the electromigration of anions (Fig. 4).

The relative importance of electrorepulsion and electroosmosis has been the subject of much investigation (49–58). It is generally agreed that small, highly mobile ions (e.g., Na$^+$, Cl$^-$, small charged amino acids) are principally moved across the skin by electrorepulsion, whereas large, bulky species carrying only a fraction of the charge passing across the skin can only be transported by electroosmosis (Fig. 5). As molecular size increases for

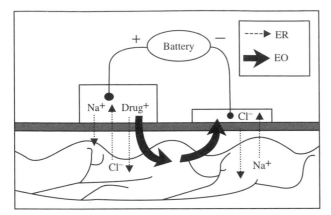

Fig. 3 Schematic representation of iontophoresis. Two electrode chambers, connected to a power source, are placed in contact with the skin. Upon application of the electric field, drug ions are repelled from the electrode of similar polarity (in this case, cations are repelled from the anode). This electrorepulsion (ER) also imposes "inward" motion on i) other cations present in the anode formulation, and ii) the "outward" transport of anions (e.g., Cl⁻) from within the skin. At the 'non-working' electrode (in this case, the cathode), negative anions from the electrolyte are driven into and through the skin, while cations (e.g., Na⁺) are "extracted" from the tissue. The direction of the electroosmotic flow (EO) is also shown (see text for details).

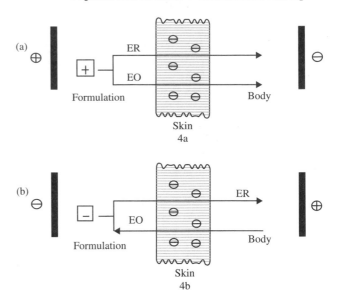

Fig. 4 Imposing an electrical potential gradient across a charged membrane produces a convective solvent flow in the direction of counter-ion transport (i.e., from anode-to-cathode in the case of skin). This electroosmotic effect (EO) adds to electrorepulsion (ER) to enhance the transport of cationic compounds during iontophoresis (4a) while acting against the electromigration of anions (4b).

cations, therefore, there will be a transition in the dominant mechanism from electrorepulsion to electroosmosis (50) (however, it should be said that where this transition occurs has not been fully defined); for anions, on the other hand, as molecular size increases, it is clear that, at the transition, the electrorepulsive contribution will be cancelled by electroosmotic convective flow going in the opposite direction (a fact that explains, at least in part, why insulin has proved a futile candidate for iontophoresis, see later). It should also be noted that there are examples of lipophilic cations (including peptides such as the LHRH analogs, nafarelin, and leuprolide) that can apparently associate strongly with the net negatively charged lipophilic skin, thereby neutralizing the anionic membrane, reducing its permselectivity and "turning off" electroosmotic flow, that is, the principal mechanism for the transport of such species (52–54, 58, 59).

The principal parameters controlling the iontophoresis of peptides/proteins can be summarized as follows:

a. *Charge and pH*: As discussed above, in general, cationic species are delivered more efficiently than anions because they can take advantage of both electrorepulsive and electroosmotic mechanisms. Neutral species can also be enhanced if formulated appropriately at the anode. Increasing charge does not necessarily lead to better delivery (all other parameters remaining equal) primarily due, it is believed, to increased association with the membrane and, once again, reduced electro-osmosis (48). The pH can be adjusted to optimize peptide stability, and sometimes to elicit better transport (because, e.g., the peptide swifts from being zwitterionic to cationic). However, pH cannot be adjusted too far i) because of concerns about irritation; ii) as this alters the inherent charge on the skin and, in consequence, its permselectivity properties.

b. *Molecular size*: Simplistically, small charged molecules are better delivered than larger ones for reasons already articulated (Fig. 5). The absolute relationship is probably complex and may be difficult to deduce. For molecules delivered only by electroosmosis, transport should be somewhat independent of size (assuming that the dimensions of the drug never approach that of the pathway). Few studies have addressed this issue with respect to peptides/proteins specifically, although one investigation with poly-L-lysines of increasing molecular weight clearly indicated that a 4-kDa oligomer was more easily transported than the higher molecular weight (7- and 26-kDa) species (59).

c. *Formulation*: The basic principles that apply generally to iontophoresis are especially relevant to peptides/

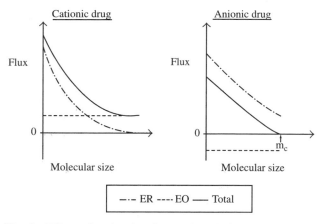

Fig. 5 Effect of molecular size on the relative importance of electrorepulsion (ER) and electroosmosis (EO) to the overall iontophoretic transport of cations and anions. Small, highly mobile cations are principally moved across the skin by ER. But, as molecular size increases, the fraction of charge carried by a cationic drug decreases, and the principal mechanism of transport becomes EO. For anions, on the other hand, EO is a negative contribution to the total flux and, once the molecular size reaches a critical value, (m_c, completely cancels out the ER contribution to electrotransport (resulting in no net flux).

proteins. If the drug carries a measurable fraction of the charge being passed, then it makes sense to minimize the presence of competing ions in the formulation. Generally speaking, lower electrolyte levels also mean that electroosmosis is slightly higher too (49, 60). Moreover, stability issues may demand at least some level of background electrolyte and/or buffer; thus, polymeric buffers, for example, which are not necessarily competitive for charge-carrying, have been used to improve peptide delivery (61). Peptide stability during storage of an iontophoresis device has also been addressed (44, 62). Because iontophoretic formulations employ aqueous-based gels, there are, in particular, potential problems of hydrolysis. This issue has been attacked recently in the case of calcitonin by making a dry reservoir disc for iontophoresis (via compression of a mixture of freeze-dried peptide and gelatin), which is hydrated at the moment of use (62). Proof-of-concept of the idea has been achieved via the observation of a hypocalcemic response in rabbits (62). The other crucial component of the formulation, of course, is the electrode. In general, reversible, and especially Ag/AgCl, electrodes are preferred (63). These very stable and reproducible electrodes are well suited to iontophoresis and avoid the problems inherent in bare metal electrodes such as those made of platinum (in particular, the hydrolysis of water that leads to very

large changes in pH in the electrode formulations and/or demands the presence of a strong buffer) (64–67). A potential problem with the use of Ag/AgCl electrodes for peptide/protein delivery is that these drugs may be inactivated/degraded at the silver chloride surface (52, 68). It may be necessary, therefore, to devise a means to keep the drug away from the electrode (e.g., use of a semipermeable membrane or a salt bridge) (52, 68–70).

Now, we can summarize the principal teachings of the field with respect to peptide and protein delivery by iontophoresis. First, we consider the major results reported in vivo in different animal models. The tripeptide Thr-Lys-Pro has been iontophoresed into hairless rats (71). The apparent urinary excretion rate of the peptide following in vivo delivery was shown to be completely consistent with the measured flux in vitro. Pretreatment of rats with an iontophoretic current followed by passive application of the peptide, also resulted in enhanced delivery. No histological changes were detected following current passage in vivo, only slight reddening at the skin area under the electrodes. Notable delivery rates of octreotide (a somatostatin analog) were obtained following application of mild current densities (50–150 $\mu A/cm^2$) in vivo in rabbits (72). Increasing the intensity of the applied current elicited a proportional increase in peptide plasma levels, and drug input declined quickly upon current termination. On the other hand, another study, in which human calcitonin was delivered into hairless rats, showed that the lowering of serum calcium was not linearly dependent upon either current density or time of current application (73). Iontophoresis of LHRH has been investigated in vivo in pigs (74). Elevated LHRH concentrations were measured in the blood and concomitant increases in LH (luteinizing hormone) and FSH (follicle stimulating hormone) levels were observed, demonstrating that the hormone was delivered as the pharmacologically active species. Circulating levels of LHRH fell rapidly upon termination of iontophoresis. A larger peptide, growth hormone releasing factor, GRF (1–44) (MW 5040), was delivered by iontophoresis into hairless guinea pigs, resulting in steady-state plasma levels of ∼0.2 ng/ml, which, in terms of flux, signifies that an input rate of ∼3.16 $\mu g/h$ was achieved (75).

Secondly, we survey briefly the published findings on peptide/protein delivery by iontophoresis in man. Delivery of calcitonin gene-related peptide (CGRP) and vasoactive intestinal polypeptide (VIP) has proven useful in the clinical treatment of venous stasis ulcers (76). In 66 patients, 40 cm^2 iontophoretic patches were applied to intact skin in the proximity of the ulcer. Pulsed electric current was delivered for 20 min. It was found that CGRP and VIP delivery was enhanced, as deduced from the clinical results, and that the electric current passing close to the ulcer area had a positive influence on the healing process. The iontophoretic delivery of leuprolide, a LHRH analog, has also been investigated in human subjects (77, 78). It was shown, following iontophoresis, that the observed increases in LH levels were comparable with those obtained after subcutaneous injection (77). The result was particularly remarkable considering the low current density delivered: that is, 0.2 mA over 70 cm^2 (~3.1 µA/cm^2). Only 2/13 volunteers reported a tingling sensation during current passage while some erythema (which, nevertheless, resolved quickly after current termination) was observed at the electrode sites in 6/13 subjects. In a further report in human volunteers, the effect of formulation variables on the iontophoretic delivery of leuprolide (78) was examined. Highest transport was observed with the lowest leuprolide concentration investigated (Fig. 6). Changes in the ionic strength of the donor formulation had a greater effect on circulating leuprolide than on LH and testosterone levels, an observation that can be partially explained in terms of interindividual differences in the pharmacological response.

Lastly, we address insulin delivery to which much effort has been dedicated. While the insulin "spikes" required postprandially may be difficult to achieve with iontophoresis, the method may have the potential to mimic the physiological, nearly constant, basal secretion (1 IU/h) of the hormone, which is observed in the nondiabetic adult (i.e., a requirement that is not provided by intermittent subcutaneous injections) (79). A recent, excellent review (80) of the work performed (almost exclusively in animal models) concludes that while insulin iontophoresis can be sufficient to treat a small diabetic animal, the best deliveries achieved are still 1–2 orders of magnitude below that necessary to meet the basal secretion level in humans. It seems unlikely, therefore, that we will see an insulin iontophoretic delivery system on the market in the foreseeable future.

Electroporation

The application of high-voltage electrical pulses to the skin (so-called electroporation) is another approach that has also been used to increase peptide delivery across the epidermal barrier. Several reviews of the application of electroporation to increase transdermal delivery have been published within the last few years (81–85). Unlike iontophoresis, which employs small currents (0.5 mA/cm^2) for relatively long periods of time (many minutes to hours), electroporation involves exposure of the skin to

relatively high voltages (on the order of 30–100 V imposed across the skin) for rather short times, typically one to several hundred milliseconds (85–87).

Mechanistically, as well, electroporation almost certainly differs from iontophoresis and an important effect involves the creation of new, low-resistance pathways through the stratum corneum. However, a detailed discussion of the physical impact of electroporation on skin barrier function is beyond the scope of this chapter, and the reader is referred to the literature for specific details (84, 86, 88).

In terms of peptide/protein delivery using electroporation, the most systematic work has been performed with the decapeptide LHRH (89, 90), and the ability of electroporation to induce its rapid delivery relative to "conventional" iontophoresis, in particular, has been clearly demonstrated (89). Specifically, using human skin in vitro, it was shown that a single electroporative pulse applied for 5 ms, followed by 30 min of iontophoresis at "normal" current densities, induced significantly higher delivery of LHRH than iontophoresis alone (89) (Fig. 7). An obvious allusion to an intravenous bolus followed by an infusion can be drawn from this work. Subsequently, in a sophisticated ex vivo model (the isolated perfused porcine skin flap), the pulsatile input of LHRH by electroporation was again examined, with the

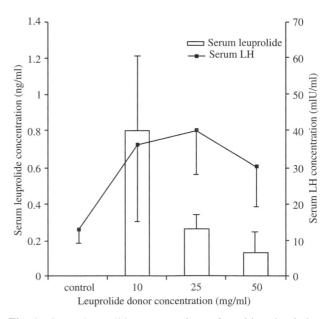

Fig. 6 Serum leuprolide concentration and resulting circulating levels of luteinizing hormone (LH) in human volunteers following iontophoresis, as a function of drug donor concentration. Constant current (0.2 mA) was applied for 10–12 h. (Redrawn from data in Ref. 78.)

reproducibility of input following a second pulse of particular interest (90).

Another recent pair of investigations have examined the application of electroporation to enhance the delivery of cyclosporin for the treatment of psoriasis (91, 92). Compared to passive transport, single electroporative pulses resulted in up to a 60-fold enhancement in hairless rat skin permeability depending upon the vehicle used.

It must be said, however, that practical questions pertaining to electroporation are important barriers to its further development. Use of the high voltages required raises significant questions about safety, and how exactly electroporation would be practised in reality—only in hospital, or a doctor's office? What are the effects of electroporation on the skin? Acutely, within certain limits, the results are cautiously optimistic but, chronically, no one knows. And, from a marketing standpoint, electroporation must be grouped with other so-called "minimally invasive" technologies, which effectively remove the SC from the delivery equation. Under these circumstances, will electroporation compete with microneedles or "painless" injections? In short, electroporation has a long way to go before it can ever be perceived as a serious challenge to a simple injection.

Sonophoresis

The use of ultrasound (US) to enhance percutaneous absorption (so-called sonophoresis or phonophoresis) has been studied over many years, and is the basis of US propagation and US effects on tissue, and the use of US in transdermal delivery have been reviewed in detail (93–96). The proposed mechanisms by which US enhances skin penetration include cavitation, thermal effects and mechanical perturbation of the SC; that is, US acts on the barrier function of the membrane (96).

Sonophoresis has employed three distinct categories of US: "high-frequency" or diagnostic US (2–10 MHz), "mid-frequency" or therapeutic US (0.7–3 MHz), and "low-frequency" US (5–100 kHz). It appears, from a general overview of the literature, that the efficiency of US-mediated drug delivery depends on several factors, including US frequency, intensity (i.e., power per unit area), continuous versus pulsed mode, duty cycle, duration, coupling medium, and so on. The fact that very few studies have used common values for some or any of these parameters almost certainly accounts for the different and sometimes contradictory results in the public domain.

It should be noted that the US beam is made up of two components: the field closest to the transducer, and the field further away (the final, diverging conical part) (93). The relative size of these two zones, and their separation,

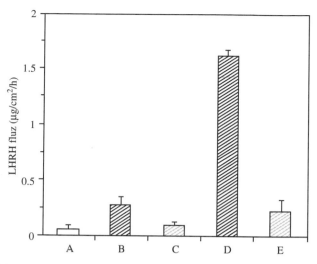

Fig. 7 Transport of LHRH (mean ± SD) across human epidermis in vitro. A) passive flux, B) transport after 30 min of iontophoresis at 0.5 mA/cm^2; D) transport after a single electroporative pulse (1000 V, 5 msec) followed by 30 min of iontophoresis at 0.5 mA/cm^2. The passive fluxes 2 h after termination of treatments B and D (columns C and E, respectively) are also shown. (Redrawn from data in Ref. 89.)

is a function of a) the US wavelength (i.e., frequency) and b) the transducer radius. The distribution of energy across these two regions is not uniform; indeed, near the transducer, it becomes quite complex, emphasizing again how small changes in experimental protocol between studies can lead to significantly different results.

Form a practical standpoint, unlike the situation with iontophoresis, the transition from laboratory-size US equipment to a small, user friendly, and compatible device remains a challenging "scale-down" problem. Furthermore, as mentioned above, it appears that US acts on the skin barrier per se (while iontophoresis seems to exert its effects more specifically on the substance targeted for delivery) implying, therefore, that control of the enhancement technology continues to be an issue for the long-term, safe, and effective application of this method.

With respect to US-enhanced peptide and protein delivery, the most impressive results have been seen in the "low-frequency" domain. Tachibana et al. were the first to report the increased delivery of insulin across the skin of hairless mice (97) and rabbits (98) in vivo. Using US at 105 kHz (90 min, "pulsed": 5 s on, 5 s off), significant insulin delivery and concomitant lowering of blood sugar were seen in diabetic rabbits (98) (Fig. 8). At a slightly lower frequency (48 kHz), a similar glucose-lowering effect was observed in the hairless mouse (97). Subsequently, Mitragotri et al. (99) described similar results in hairless rats; in this case, the US frequency was 20 kHz, with a duration of application of up to 4 h, using 100 ms pulses at US intensities between 12.5 and 225 mW/cm^2 [lately, this intensity range has been corrected to 1.6–14 W/cm^2 (100)]. The same authors also reported that this low frequency US approach could be used to significantly enhance the delivery of interferon-γ (MW ~17 kDa) and erythropoietin (MW ~48 kDa) in vitro, that is, that macromolecules of much greater size could now be deliverable across the skin. It should be said, however, that no further data on these proteins has been reported since the initial publication in 1995 (99).

Additional work, however, has addressed mechanistic aspects of the effects of low-frequency US. Cavitation and thermal effects have been postulated and, to a certain extent, characterized (101–104), but further work is clearly needed to define exactly how US interacts with the skin barrier to increase its permeability.

Only one publication has presented data to support the idea that higher frequency (1 MHz) US can be used to increase peptide delivery across the skin (105). The enhanced transport of poly-L-lysine (MW = 4-kDa) across human epidermis has been reported, a finding completely at odds with the relatively modest action of US at this frequency on the percutaneous penetration of several "small" molecular weight substances (96).

Finally, in a related approach, Lee et al. have used photomechanical waves to enhance the skin delivery of 5-aminolevulinic acid (ALA), a δ-amino acid used in photodynamic therapy (106). The broadband, compressive waves appear to interact with tissues uniquely via mechanical forces. ALA delivery was shown to be proportional to the peak stress (388–503 bar) of the photomechanical wave applied.

In conclusion, despite the exciting low-frequency US results obtained, there remain important questions about mechanism, local skin effects and tolerability, reversibility, and ultimate practicability. These issues must be addressed before sonophoresis can move from research to development mode.

Gene and DNA Delivery to the Skin

The goal of gene therapy is to modify in some way the synthetic capability of a target cell, or population of cells, to provoke in situ the desired "therapeutic response" (107). While conceptually attractive, gene therapy is presently limited by problems associated with delivery; that is, how does one get the gene to the place where it can elicit its effect, and then how does one appropriately regulate the expression of the gene introduced?

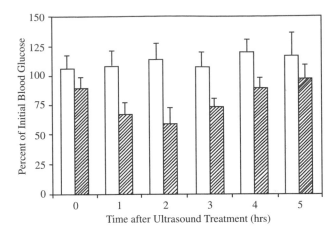

Fig. 8 Change in blood glucose level following insulin delivery by ultrasound exposure to alloxan-diabetic rabbits. Filled bars (mean ± SD) show the relative blood glucose level following ultrasound treatment for 1.5 h. The area of skin exposed was 7 cm^2; the ultrasound frequency used was 105 kHz. Open bars indicate the corresponding control values. (Redrawn from Ref. 98.)

Gene delivery to, or via, the skin has three principal objectives (108): a) the treatment of primary cutaneous diseases and wounds, b) inducing skin cells to encode a protein which is subsequently released into the systemic circulation in a controlled fashion, and c) immunization. The first two instances involve a chronic delivery challenge, whereas immunization requires only acute exposure to the DNA involved.

Chronic delivery can be achieved, at least theoretically, either ex vivo or in vivo. In the former approach, cells are harvested from the skin by biopsy and cultured in vitro. Gene transfer is then effected in this in vitro setting (e.g., by electroporation) and the transfected cells are finally grafted back into the host (108). Clearly, this is a labor-intensive, complex, and expensive procedure. In the latter case, genetic material has been administered directly to intact skin, using either viral or nonviral vectors (e.g., adenovirus or modified herpes virus and DNA complexed with liposomes, respectively). In addition, a variety of physical methods have been investigated for DNA transfer into skin including direct injection (of both the naked DNA and plasmid associated with different vectors), particle bombardment (the "gene gun"), ultrasound, electroporation, and other so-called minimally invasive techniques (108–110). However, direct gene transfer in vivo, while attractive conceptually and technically easier to perform, has proven to-date to be rather inefficient and to result in only low and transient levels of gene expression (108).

DNA immunization consists of encoding an antigen in a plasmid, which is then transfected into cells in vivo. This results in expression of the antigen and the subsequent induction of an immune response to the expressed protein (111). As the protein antigen is produced "naturally" in vivo, both cellular and humoral responses are developed. Skin has been proposed as an attractive site of immunization, and several skin cell types can become involved in DNA uptake, antigen expression and presentation. Quite recently, for example, in a mouse model, immunization has been reported following topical application of an aqueous solution of naked DNA (112). Given what one knows about the skin's passive permeability to macromolecules, it is clear that only a very small quantity of DNA vaccine is required for immunization.

In summary, while the field of gene therapy in general is attracting widespread interest at this time, real successes at the level of the skin (beyond those positive results obtained in various model systems) are few and far between. It is clear, then, that considerably more work needs to be done. Detailed, and current, overviews of the state-of-the-art in cutaneous gene delivery can be found in Refs. (108) and (111).

Minimally Invasive Delivery Technologies

Finally, we consider the delivery of peptides and proteins across the skin by methods that physically circumvent the stratum corneum barrier in ways designed to be less invasive than the use of a classic needle and syringe. In these approaches, therefore, the excellent barrier function of the SC is acknowledged, and one turns one's attention to bypassing this membrane in as least offensive a fashion as possible. This strategy for peptide delivery into the systemic circulation has been known for some time, however. The Matse Indians from Peru use one variation of this idea in shamanic hunting practices (113). Having obtained an extract from the skin of the frog Phyllomedusa bicolor (which contains ~7 wt% active peptides), a formulation is prepared and then applied to a small area of skin the epidermal barrier of which is first burned away with a smouldering twig. Within minutes of application, the treated individual experiences violent peripheral, gastrointestinal, and cardiovascular effects, followed by further remarkable central responses (increase in physical strength, resistance to hunger, thirst, stress, and so on).

Back in the world of intellectual property and patent protection, a number of sophisticated technologies have evolved in recent years and have often been applied to peptide and protein delivery objectives. Among the approaches used, one can cite ablation of the SC by laser radiation, by heat, and by erosion, as well as the use of particle bombardment and microneedles of various configuration. Some approaches are even suggested for

use in combination with other transdermal technologies, such as iontophoresis. As yet, none of these methods are approved clinically for peptide/protein delivery and all have yet to show real superiority over the gold standard injection via a conventional needle and syringe. An excellent review of the field has recently been written by Down et al. (114).

Mid-infrared laser ablation of the SC has been used to allow the transdermal delivery of interferon-γ (115). The mechanism by which this laser beam "explodes" away the SC is complex, yet quite reproducible and controllable, in that the number of laser pulses is correlated to the degree of SC damage (and hence to the peptide's permeability through the tissue). Tissue destruction below the SC appeared to be minimal.

The MicroPors^{TM} technology (114, 116) consists of directing tightly focused thermal energy into the SC to create micropores. The skin is contacted by a wire mesh through which a current is passed that causes local heating sufficient to burn small holes in the barrier. Delivery of insulin by this approach has been suggested (116). A more macroscopic method to create an erosion in the SC is via "suction de-epithelialization" (117). Using a vacuum, a small blister (6 mm diameter) is formed on the skin; the tissue separates at the dermal–epidermal junction. The roof of the blister is then removed ("guillotined," as it were) exposing a small area of dermis to which a drug solution can be directly applied. Feasibility, in vivo in man, was demonstrated using the antidiuretic peptide 1-deamino-8-D-arginine vasopressin (dDAVP) and stable, therapeutically active plasma levels were achieved rather quickly (117). The successful delivery of an oxytocin analog has also been shown (118). The authors claim that the dermal microcirculation remains intact and functional following creation of the erosion. Mild inflammation is observed and the erosion self-heals over time with, apparently, minimal scarring. However, practical applications of this approach, especially for chronic disease treatment, appears unlikely, and issues related to local infections will have to be addressed.

High-velocity particle delivery across the skin is the technology of a major drug delivery operation based in the UK and USA (PowderJect, Inc.) (119). Once a drug has been formulated as an appropriate and well-characterized powder, it is then introduced into a compact hand-held device in which a supersonic flow of gas accelerates the particles to a speed high enough that they can collide with the skin having enough energy to penetrate the outer layers and effect drug delivery. The depth and extent of delivery depends on the speed, diameter, and density of the drug particles. Again, insulin has been a peptide of choice for study by this method (120).

Finally, with the explosion of interest in micromachining and microfabrication, it is not surprising that drug delivery afficionados have turned their attention to the production of arrays of micron-sized microneedles capable of creating transport pathways across the SC without eliciting disagreeable perception on the part of the patient (121, 122). Various configurations and forms of these devices have been evolved, the majority of which involve extremely sharp tips and needle lengths on the order of 100 μm. At the time of writing, no specific publications detailing peptide/protein delivery using this technology have appeared.

Overall, then, the minimally invasive field is an active and imaginative one, of much perceived promise. However, it remains to be seen, as this technology matures and as it moves closer to real clinical testing against known effective methodologies, whether the current level of excitement (and investment) will be rewarded by the realization of successful and marketable products.

CONCLUSIONS

The relatively noninvasive nature of transdermal drug delivery, and the fact that this route can simultaneously avoid problems associated with presystemic metabolism and mimic (at least, to some extent) parenteral input profiles, are significant advantages. There have been, therefore, diverse attempts to exploit the skin for peptide and protein delivery. As we have noted before, transdermal administration, with or without one or more enhancement technologies, will always be limited to potent drugs and this accounts, once more, for the effort devoted to peptide and protein (i.e., typically very active substances) administration via this route.

Even the simplest structure–permeation relationships for percutaneous transport (no matter their limitations) indicate that the bigger a molecule, the poorer its diffusivity across the skin. Thus, larger molecules cannot be considered as transdermal candidates unless they are extremely potent. Vaccines are one such example and, given the skin's role as an immunological organ, represent a potentially very interesting opportunity for the transdermal route. For other peptides and proteins, at least to-date, an enhancement strategy appears to be obligatory in order that the skin's barrier function can be overcome.

The different approaches used have all yielded *some* effect, in that increased peptide/protein delivery has been achieved. However, with the possible exception of iontophoresis, few of the various technologies employed have achieved an advanced state of maturity. Even in the case of iontophoresis, despite considerable activity and many publications in the literature, there are no peptide delivery systems on the immediate horizon (although there are products with "normal" drugs in the later steps of development). Typically, in the biotech era of the last 20 years, the newer technologies, including the "minimally invasive" methods (i.e., those about which we know the least and whose associated problems are poorly, or have yet to be, characterized!) are now attracting most attention and the highest level of investment.

It remains to be seen, therefore, whether the transdermal route will eventually yield a marketable delivery system for one or more peptides and/or proteins. For some of the enhancement technologies available, considerably more work needs to be done to establish that there is a distinct advantage over a needle and syringe (e.g., ultrasound, electroporation, and all "minimally invasive" methods); for iontophoresis, much of the groundwork has been done and the basic, mechanistic principles are becoming clearer—the challenge now is to identify the right peptide candidates and to initiate a serious development effort. Vaccine delivery appears to be an intriguing opportunity and of much interest; time will tell if the transdermal route will prove compatible with this important goal.

REFERENCES

1. Audus, K.L.; Raub, T.J. Biological Barriers to Protein Delivery. *Pharmaceutical Biotechnology*; Plenum Press: New York, 1993; 4.
2. Wearley, L.L.; Banga, A.K. Peptide and Protein Drug Delivery. *Encyclopedia of Pharmaceutical Technology*, 1st Ed.; Swarbrick, J., Boylan, J.C., Eds.; Marcel Dekker, Inc.: New York, 1995; 11, 395–411.
3. Hadgraft, J.; Guy, R.H. *Transdermal Drug Delivery—Development Issues and Research Initiatives*; Marcel Dekker, Inc.: New York, 1989; 35.
4. Potts, R.O.; Francoeur, M.L. The Influence of Stratum Corneum Morphology on Water Permeability. J. Invest. Dermatol. **1991**, *96*, 495–499.
5. Wertz, P.W. The Nature of the Epidermal Barrier: Biochemical Aspects. Adv. Drug Deliv. Rev. **1996**, *18*, 283–294.
6. Turner, N.G.; Nonato, L.B. Visualization of Stratum Corneum and Transdermal Permeation Pathways. *Mechanisms of Transdermal Drug Delivery*; Potts, R.O., Guy, R.H., Eds.; Marcel Dekker, Inc.: New York, 1997; 83, 1–40.

7. Potts, R.O.; Francoeur, M.L. Lipid Biophysics of Water Loss Through the Skin. Proc. Natl. Acad. Sci. **1990**, *87*, 3871–3873.

8. Boddé, H.E.; Van den Brink, I.; Koerten, H.K.; Haan, F.H.N. Visualization of In Vitro Percutaneous Penetration of Mercuric Chloride; Transport Through Intercellular Space Versus Uptake Through Desmosomes. J. Controlled Release **1991**, *15*, 227–236.

9. Kalia, Y.N.; Pirot, F.; Guy, R.H. Homogeneous Transport in a Heterogeneous Membrane: Water Diffusion Across Human Stratum Corneum in Vivo. Biophys. J. **1996**, *71*, 2692–2700.

10. Grimnes, S. Pathways of Ionic Flow Through Human Skin in Vivo. Acta Derm. Venereol. (Stockh.) **1984**, *64*, 93–98.

11. Keister, J.C.; Kasting, G.B. The Use of Transient Diffusion to Investigate Transport Pathways Through Skin. J. Controlled Release **1986**, *4*, 111–117.

12. Albery, W.J.; Hadgraft, J. Percutaneous Absorption: In Vivo Experiments. J. Pharm. Pharmacol. **1979**, *31*, 140–147.

13. El Tayar, N.; Tsai, R.S.; Testa, B.; Carrupt, P.A.; Hansch, C.; Leo, A. Percutaneous Penetration of Drugs: A Quantitative Structure–Permeability Relationship Study. J. Pharm. Sci. **1991**, *80*, 744–749.

14. Potts, R.O.; Guy, R.H. Predicting Skin Permeability. Pharm. Res. **1992**, *9*, 663–669.

15. Flynn, G.L. Physicochemical Determinants of Skin Absorption. *Principles of Route-to-Route Extrapolation for Risk Assessment*; Gerrity, T.R., Henry, C.J. Eds.; Elsevier: New York, 1990; 93–127.

16. Cleek, R.L.; Bunge, A.L. A New Method for Estimating Dermal Absorption from Chemical Exposure. I. General Approach. Pharm. Res. **1993**, *10*, 497–506.

17. Weber, C.J.; Jicha, D.; Matz, S.; Siverly, J.; O'Dorisio, T.; Strausberg, L.; Laurencot, J.; McLarty, A.; Norton, J.; Kazim, M.; Reemtsma, K. Passage of Somatostatin Analogue Across Human and Mouse Skin. Surgery **1987**, *102*, 974–981.

18. Hadley, M.E.; Wood, S.H.; Lemus-Wilson, A.M.; Dawson, B.V.; Levine, N.; Dorr, R.T.; Hruby, V.J. Topical Application of a Melanotropic Peptide Induces Systemic Follicular Melanogenesis. Life Sciences **1987**, *40*, 1889–1895.

19. Dawson, B.V.; Hadley, M.E.; Kreutzfeld, K.; Dorr, R.T.; Hruby, V.J.; Al-Obeidi, F.; Don, S. Transdermal Delivery of a Melanotropic Peptide Hormone Analogue. Life Sciences **1988**, *43*, 1111–1117.

20. Dawson, B.V.; Hadley, M.E.; Levine, N.; Kreutzfeld, K.L.; Don, S.; Eytan, T.; Hruby, V.J. In Vitro Transdermal Delivery of a Melanotropic Peptide Through Human Skin. J. Invest. Dermatol. **1990**, *94*, 432–435.

21. Boddé, H.E.; Verhoef, J.C.; Ponec, M. Transdermal Peptide Delivery. Biochem. Soc. Trans. **1989**, *17*, 943–945.

22. Choi, H.K.; Flynn, G.L.; Amidon, G.L. Transdermal Delivery of Bioactive Peptides: The Effect of *n*-Decylmethyl Sulfoxide, pH, and Inhibitors on Enkephalin Metabolism and Transport. Pharm. Res. **1990**, *7*, 1099–1106.

23. Banarjee, P.S.; Ritschel, W.A. Transdermal Permeation of Vasopressin. I. Influence of pH, Concentration, Shaving and Surfactant on In Vitro Permeation. Int. J. Pharm. **1989**, *49*, 189–197.

24. Banarjee, P.S.; Ritschel, W.A. Transdermal Permeation of Vasopressin. II. Influence of Azone on In Vitro and In Vivo Permeation. Int. J. Pharm **1989**, *49*, 199–204.

25. Ogiso, T.; Iwaki, M.; Yoneda, I.; Horinouchi, M.; Yamashita, K. Percutaneous Absorption of Elcatonin and Hypocalcemic Effect in Rat. Chem. Pharm. Bull. **1991**, *39*, 449–453.

26. Ogiso, T.; Iwaki, M.; Tanino, T.; Paku, T. Effectiveness of the Elcatonin Transdermal System for the Treatment of Osteoporosis and the Effect of the Combination of Elcatonin and Active Vitamin d_3 In Rat. Biol. Pharm. Bull. **1993**, *16*, 895–898.

27. Lu, M.F.; Lee, D.; Rao, G.S. Percutaneous Absorption Enhancement of Leuprolide. Pharm. Res. **1992**, *9*, 1575–1579.

28. Roy, S.D.; de Groot, J.S. Percutaneous Absorption of Nafarelin Acetate, an LHRH Analog, Through Human Cadaver Skin and Monkey Skin. Int. J. Pharm. **1994**, *110*, 137–145.

29. Setoh, K.; Murakami, M.; Araki, N.; Fujita, R.; Yamamoto, A.; Muranishi, S. Improvement of Transdermal Delivery of Tetragastrin by Lipophilic Modification with Fatty Acids. J. Pharm. Pharmacol **1995**, *47*, 808–811.

30. Egbaria, K.; Ramachandran, C.; Weiner, N. Topical Delivery of Ciclosporin: Evaluation of Various Formulations Using In Vitro Diffusion Studies In Hairless Mouse Skin. Skin Pharmacol. **1990**, *3*, 21–28.

31. Short, S.M.; Paasch, B.D.; Turner, J.H.; Weiner, N.; Daugherty, A.L.; Mrsny, R.J. Percutaneous Absorption of Biologically-Active Interferon-Gamma in a Human Skin Graft-Nude Mouse Model. Pharm. Res. **1996**, *13*, 1020–1027.

32. Short, M.S.; Rubas, W.; Paasch, B.D.; Mrsny, R.J. Transport of Biologically Active Interferon-Gamma Across Human Skin In Vitro. Pharm. Res. **1995**, *12*, 1140–1145.

33. Vutla, N.B.; Betageri, G.V.; Banga, A.K. Transdermal Iontophoretic Delivery of Enkephalin Formulated in Liposomes. J. Pharm. Sci. **1996**, *85*, 5–8.

34. Février, F.; Bobin, M.F.; Lafforgue, C.; Martini, M.C. Advances in Microemulsions and Transepidermal Penetration of Tyrosine. S.T.P. Pharma. Sci. **1991**, *1*, 60–63.

35. Rolland, A.; *Pharmaceutical Particulate Carriers: Therapeutic Applications*; Rolland, A., Ed.; Marcel Dekker, Inc.: New York, 1993; 367–421.

36. Schreier, H.; Bouwstra, J. Liposomes and Niosomes as Topical Drug Carriers, Dermal and Transdermal Drug Delivery. J. Controlled Release **1994**, *30*, 1–15.

37. Cevc, G.; Blume, G.; Schätzlein, A.; Gebauer, D.; Paul, A. The Skin: A Pathway for Systemic Treatment with Patches and Lipid-Based Agent Carriers. Adv. Drug Deliv. Rev. **1996**, *18*, 349–378.

38. Weiner, N.; Williams, N.; Birch, G.; Ramachandran, C.; Shipman, C., Jr.; Flynn, G. Topical Delivery of Liposomally Encapsulated Interferon Evaluated in a Cutaneous Herpes Guinea Pig Model. Antimicrob. Agents Chemother. **1989**, *33*, 1217–1221.

39. Cevc, G.; Gebauer, D.; Stieber, J.; Schätzlein, A.; Blume, G. Ultraflexible Vesicles, Transfersomes, Have an Extremely Low Pore Penetration Resistance and Transport Therapeutic Amounts of Insulin Across the Intact Mammalian Skin. Biochim. Biophys. Acta **1998**, *1368*, 201–215.

40. Glenn, G.M.; Rao, M.; Matyas, G.R.; Alving, C.R. Skin Immunization Made Possible by Cholera Toxin. Nature **1998**, *391*, 851.

41. Scharton-Kersten, T.; Yu, J.M.; Vassell, R.; O'Hagan, D.; Alving, C.R.; Glenn, G.M. Transcutaneous Immunization with Bacterial ADP-Ribosylating Exotoxins, Subunits, and Unrelated Adjuvants. Infect. Immun. **2000**, *68*, 5306–5313.

42. Paul, A.; Cevc, G.; Bachhawat, B.K. Transdermal Immunization with Large Proteins by Means of Ultradeformable Drug Carriers. Eur. J. Immunol. **1995**, *25*, 3521–3524.

43. Paul, A.; Cevc, G.; Bachhawat, B.K. Transdermal Immunisation with an Integral Membrane Component, Gap Junction Protein, by Means of Ultradeformable Drug Carriers, Transfersomes. Vaccine **1998**, *16*, 188–195.

44. Green, P.G. Iontophoretic Delivery of Peptide Drugs. J. Controlled Release **1996**, *41*, 33–48.

45. Delgado-Charro, M.B.; Guy, R.H. Iontophoresis of Peptides. *Electronically Controlled Drug Delivery*; Berner, B., Dinh, S.M., Eds.; CRC Press: Boca Raton, 1998; 129–157.

46. Kim, A.; Green, P.G.; Rao, G.; Guy, R.H. Convective Solvent Flow Across the Skin During Iontophoresis. Pharm. Res. **1993**, *10*, 1315–1320.

47. Marro, D.; Guy, R.H.; Delgado-Charro, M.B. Characterization of the Iontophoretic Perselectivity Properties of Human and Pig Skin. J. Controlled Release **2000**, *70*, 213–217.

48. Burnette, R.R.; Ongpipattanakul, B. Characterization of the Permselective Properties of Excised Human Skin During Iontophoresis. J. Pharm. Sci. **1987**, *76*, 765–773.

49. Pikal, M.J. The Role of Electroosmotic Flow in Transdermal Iontophoresis. Adv. Drug Deliv. Rev. **1992**, *9*, 201–237.

50. Guy, R.H.; Kalia, Y.N.; Delgado-Charro, M.B.; Merino, V.; López, A.; Marro, D. Iontophoresis: Electrorepulsion and Electroosmosis. J. Controlled Release **2000**, *64*, 129–132.

51. Delgado-Charro, M.B.; Kalia, Y.N.; Guy, R.H. The Relative Contributions of Electrorepulsion and Electroosmosis to Iontophoretic Transport. Proc. Int. Symp. Controlled Rel. Bioact. Mater. **1998**, *25*, 599–600.

52. Delgado-Charro, M.B.; Guy, R.H. Characterization of Convective Solvent Flow During Iontophoresis. Pharm. Res. **1994**, *11*, 929–935.

53. Hoogstraate, A.J.; Srinivasan, V.; Sims, S.M.; Higuchi, W.I. Iontophoretic Enhancement of Peptides: Behaviour of Leuprolide Versus Model Permeants. J. Controlled Release **1994**, *31*, 41–47.

54. Hirvonen, J.; Kalia, Y.N.; Guy, R.H. Transdermal Delivery of Peptides by Iontophoresis. Nature Biotech. **1996**, *14*, 1710–1713.

55. Green, P.G.; Hinz, R.S.; Cullander, C.; Yamane, G.; Guy, R.H. Iontophoretic Delivery of Amino Acids and Amino Acid Derivatives Across the Skin "In Vitro". Pharm. Res. **1991**, *8*, 1113–1120.

56. Green, P.G.; Hinz, R.S.; Kim, A.; Szoka, F.C.; Guy, R.H. Iontophoretic Delivery of a Series of Tripeptides Across the Skin In-Vitro. Pharm. Res. **1991**, *8*, 1121–1127.

57. DelTerzo, S.; Behl, C.R.; Nash, R.A. Iontophoretic Transport of a Homologous Series of Ionized and Nonionized Model Compounds: Influence of Hydrophobicity and Mechanistic Interpretation. Pharm. Res. **1989**, *6*, 85–90.

58. Hirvonen, J.; Guy, R.H. Transdermal Iontophoresis: Modulation of Electroosmosis by Polypeptides. J. Controlled Release **1998**, *50*, 283–289.

59. Turner, N.G.; Ferry, L.; Price, M.; Cullander, C.; Guy, R.H. Iontophoresis of Poly-L-Lysines: The Role of Molecular Weight. Pharm. Res. **1997**, *14*, 1322–1331.

60. Santi, P.; Guy, R.H. Reverse Iontophoresis—Parameters Determining Electroosmotic Flow. I. PH and Ionic Strength. J. Controlled Release **1996**, *38*, 159–165.

61. Sarpotdar, P.P.; Daniels, C.R. Use of Polymeric Buffers to Facilitate Iontophoretic Transport of Drugs. Pharm. Res. **1990**, *7* (Suppl.), S-185.

62. Santi, P.; Colombo, P.; Bettini, R.; Catellani, P.L.; Minutello, A.; Volpato, N.M. Drug Reservoir Composition and Transport of Salmon Calcitonin in Transdermal Iontophoresis. Pharm. Res. **1997**, *14*, 63–66.

63. Cullander, C.; Rao, G.; Guy, R.H. Why Silver/Silver Chloride? Criteria for Iontophoresis Electrodes. *Prediction of Percutaneous Penetration*; Brain, K.R., James, V.J., Walters, K.A., Eds.; STS Publishing: Cardiff, U.K., 1993; 3b, 381–390.

64. Knoblauch, P.; Moll, F. In Vitro Pulsatile and Continuous Transdermal Delivery of Buserelin by Iontophoresis. J. Controlled Release **1993**, *26*, 203–212.

65. Gupta, S.K.; Kumar, S.; Bolton, S.; Behl, C.R.; Malick, A.W. Optimization of Iontophoretic Transdermal Delivery of a Peptide and a Non-Peptide Drug. J. Controlled Release **1994**, *30*, 253–261.

66. Kumar, S.; Char, H.; Patel, S.; Piemontese, D.; Iqbal, K.; Malick, A.W.; Neugroschel, E.; Behl, C.R. Effect of Iontophoresis on In Vitro Skin Permeation of an Analogue of Growth Hormone Releasing Hormone Factor in the Hairless Guinea Pig Model. J. Pharm. Sci. **1992**, *81*, 635–639.

67. Brady, A.B.; Corish, J.; Corrigan, O.I. Passive and Electrically Assisted Transdermal Delivery of Desamino-8-D-Arginine Vasopressin In Vitro from a Gel Matrix. *Prediction of Percutaneous Penetration*; Scott, R.C., Guy, R.H., Hadgraft, J., Boddé, H.E. Eds.; STS Publishing: Cardiff, U.K., 1991; 2, 401–409.

68. Hager, D.F.; Mancuso, F.A.; Nazareno, J.P.; Sharkey, J.W.; Siverly, J.R. Evaluation of a Cultured Skin Equivalent as a Model Membrane for Iontophoretic Transport. J. Controlled Release **1994**, *30*, 117–123.

69. Delgado-Charro, M.B.; Guy, R.H. Iontophoretic Delivery of Nafarelin Across the Skin. Int. J. Pharm. **1995**, *117*, 165–172.

70. Delgado-Charro, M.B.; Rodriguez-Bayón, A.M.; Guy, R.H. Iontophoresis of Nafarelin: Effects of Current Density and Concentration on Electrotransport In Vitro. J. Controlled Release **1995**, *35*, 35–40.

71. Green, P.G.; Shroot, B.; Bernerd, F.; Pilgrim, W.R.; Guy, R.H. In Vitro and In Vivo Iontophoresis of a Tripeptide Across Nude Rat Skin. J. Controlled Release **1992**, *20*, 209.

72. Lau, D.T.W.; Sharkey, J.W.; Petryk, L.; Mancuso, F.A.; Yu, Z.; Tse, F.L.S. Effect of Current Magnitude and Drug Concentration on Iontophoretic Delivery of Octreotide Acetate (Sandostatin®) in the Rabbit. Pharm. Res. **1994**, *11*, 1742–1746.

73. Thysman, S.; Hanchard, C.; Préat, V. Human Calcitonin Delivery in Rats by Iontophoresis. J. Pharm. Pharmacol. **1994**, *46*, 725–730.

74. Heit, M.C.; Williams, P.L.; Jayes, F.L.; Chang, S.K.; Riviere, J.E. Transdermal Iontophoretic Peptide Delivery: In Vitro and In Vivo Studies with Luteinizing Hormone Releasing Hormone. J. Pharm. Sci. **1993**, *83*, 240–243.

75. Kumar, S.; Char, H.; Patel, S.; Piemontese, D.; Malick, A.W.; Iqbal, K.; Neugroschel, E.; Behl, C.R. In Vivo Transdermal Iontophoretic Delivery of Growth Hormone Releasing Factor GRF (1–44) in Hairless Guinea Pigs. J. Controlled Release **1992**, *18*, 213–220.

76. Gherardini, G.; Gürlek, A.; Evans, G.R.D.; Milner, S.M.; Matarasso, A.; Wassler, M.; Jernbeck, J.; Lundeberg, T. Venous Ulcers: Improved Healing by Iontophoretic Administration of Calcitonin Gene-Related Peptide and Vasoactive Intestinal Polypeptide. Plast. Reconstr. Surg. **1998**, *101*, 90–93.

77. Meyer, B.R.; Kreis, W.; Eschbah, J.; O'Mara, V.; Rosen, S.; Sibalis, D. Transdermal Versus Subcutaneous Leuprolide: A Comparison of Acute Pharmacodynamic Effect. Clin. Pharmacol. Ther. **1990**, *48*, 340–345.

78. Lu, M.F.; Lee, D.; Carlson, R.; Rao, G.S.; Hui, H.W.; Adjei, L.; Herrin, M.; Sundberg, D.; Hsu, L. The Effects of Formulation Variables on Iontophoretic Transdermal Delivery of Leuprolide to Humans. Drug. Dev. Ind. Pharm. **1993**, *19*, 1557–1571.

79. Guy, R.H. Current Status and Future Prospects of Transdermal Drug Delivery. Pharm. Res. **1996**, *13*, 1765–1769.

80. Sage, B.H., Jr. Insulin Iontophoresis. *Protein Delivery—Physical Systems*; Sanders, L.M., Hendren, R.W., Eds.; Plenum Publishing Corp.: New York, 1997; 319–341.

81. Vanbever, R.; Préat, V. In Vivo Efficacy and Safety of Skin Electroporation. Adv. Drug Deliv. Rev. **1999**, *35*, 77–88.

82. Weaver, J.C.; Vaughan, T.E.; Chizmadzhev, Y. Theory of Electrical Creation of Aqueous Pathways Across Skin Transport Barriers. Adv. Drug Deliv. Rev. **1999**, *35*, 21–39.

83. Prausnitz, M.R. A Practical Assessment of Transdermal Drug Delivery by Skin Electroporation. Adv. Drug Deliv. Rev. **1999**, *35*, 61–76.

84. Jadoul, A.; Bouwstra, J.; Préat, V. Effects of Iontophoresis and Electroporation on the Stratum Corneum: Review of the Biophysical Studies. Adv. Drug Deliv. Rev. **1999**, *35*, 89–105.

85. Pliquett, U. Mechanistic Studies of Molecular Transdermal Transport Due to Skin Electroporation. Adv. Drug Deliv. Rev. **1999**, *35*, 41–60.

86. Vanbever, R.; Pliquett, U.F.; Préat, V.; Weaver, J.C. Comparison of the Effects of Short, High-Voltage and Long, Medium-Voltage Pulses on Skin Electrical and Transport Properties. J. Controlled Release **1999**, *69*, 35–47.

87. Chen, T.; Segall, E.M.; Langer, R.; Weaver, J.C. Skin Electroporation: Rapid Measurements of the Transdermal Voltage and Flux of Four Fluorescent Molecules Show a Transition to Large Fluxes Near 50 V. J. Pharm. Sci. **1998**, *87*, 1368–1374.

88. Vanbever, R.; Préat, V. In Vivo Efficacy and Safety of Skin Electroporation. Adv. Drug Deliv. Rev. **1999**, *35*, 77–88.

89. Bommannan, D.B.; Tamada, J.; Leung, L.; Potts, R.O. Effect of Electroporation on Transdermal Iontophoretic Delivery of Luteinizing Hormone Releasing Hormone (LHRH) in Vitro. Pharm. Res. **1994**, *11*, 1809–1814.

90. Riviere, J.E.; Monteiro-Riviere, N.A.; Rogers, R.A.; Bommannan, D.; Tamada, J.A.; Potts, R.O. Pulsatile Transdermal Delivery of LHRH Using Electroporation: Drug Delivery and Skin Toxicology. J. Controlled Release **1995**, *36*, 229–233.

91. Wang, S.; Kara, M.; Krishnan, T.R. Transdermal Delivery of Cyclosporin-A Using Electroporation. J. Controlled Release **1998**, *50*, 61–70.

92. Wang, S.; Kara, M.; Krishnan, T.R. Topical Delivery of Cyclosporin a Coevaporate Using Electroporation Technique. Drug Dev. Ind. Pharm. **1997**, *23*, 657–663.

93. Weiman, A.E. Physical Principles of Ultrasound. *Principles and Practice of Echocardiography*; Weiman, A.E. Ed.; Lea & Febiger: Philadelphia, 1994; 3–28.

94. Meidan, V.M.; Walmsley, A.D.; Irwin, W.J. Phonophoresis —Is it a Reality. Int. J. Pharm. **1995**, *118*, 129–149.

95. Camel, E. Ultrasound. *Percutaneous Penetration Enhancers*; Smith, E.W., Maibach, H.I. Eds.; CRC Press: Boca Raton, 1995; 369–382.

96. Mitragotri, S.; Blankschtein, D.; Langer, R. Sonophoresis: Enhanced Transdermal Drug Delivery by Application of Ultrasound. *Encyclopedia of Pharmaceutical Technology*, 1st Ed.; Swarbrick, J., Boylan, J.C. Eds.; Marcel Dekker, Inc.: New York, 1996; 14, 103–122.

97. Tachibana, K.; Tachibana, S. Transdermal Delivery of Insulin by Ultrasonic Vibration. J. Pharm. Pharmacol. **1991**, *43*, 270–271.

98. Tachibana, K. Transdermal Delivery of Insulin to Alloxan-Diabetic Rabbits by Ultrasound Exposure. Pharm. Res. **1992**, *9*, 952–954.

99. Mitragotri, S.; Blankschtein, D.; Langer, R. Ultrasound-Mediated Transdermal Protein Delivery. Science **1995**, *269*, 850–853.

100. Mitragotri, S.; Farrell, J.; Tang, H.; Terahara, T.; Kost, J.; Langer, R. Determination of Threshold Energy Dose for Ultrasound-Induced Transdermal Drug Transport. J. Controlled Release **2000**, *63*, 41–52.

101. Mitragotri, S.; Edwards, D.A.; Blankschtein, D.; Langer, R. A Mechanistic Study of Ultrasonically-Enhanced Transdermal Drug Delivery. J. Pharm. Sci. **1995**, *84*, 697–706.

102. Menon, G.K.; Bommannan, D.B.; Elias, P.M. High-Frequency Sonophoresis: Permeation Pathways and Structural Basis for Enhanced Permeability. Skin Pharmacol. **1994**, *7*, 130–139.

103. Meidan, V.M.; Docker, M.; Walmsley, A.D.; Irwin, W.J. Low Intensity Ultrasound as a Probe to Elucidate the

Relative Follicular Contribution to Total Transdermal Absorption. Pharm. Res. **1998**, *15*, 85–92.

104. Merino, G.; Delgado-Charro, M.B.; Kalia, Y.N.; Guy, R.H. Mechanism of Enhanced Transdermal Transport by Low-Frequency Ultrasound: The Role of Local Heating. Proc. Int. Symp. Controlled Release Bioact. Mater. **2000**, *27*, 942–943.

105. Weimann, L.J.; Wu, J. Enhancement of Skin Penetration of Poly-L-Lisine by Ultrasound. Proc. Int. Symp. Controlled Release Bioact. Mater. **1999**, *26*, 417–418.

106. Lee, S.; Kollias, N.; McAuliffe, D.J.; Flotte, T.J.; Doukas, A.G. Topical Drug Delivery in Humans with a Single Photomechanical Wave. Pharm. Res. **1999**, *16*, 1717–1721.

107. Blau, H.M.; Springer, M.L. Gene Therapy—A Novel Form of Drug Delivery. N. Engl. J. Med. **1995**, *333*, 1204–1207.

108. Khavari, P.A. Therapeutic Gene Delivery to the Skin. Mol. Med. Today **1997**, December,533–538.

109. Jaroszeski, M.J.; Gilbert, R.; Nicolau, C.; Heller, R. In Vivo Gene Delivery by Electroporation. Adv. Drug Deliv. Rev. **1999**, *35*, 131–137.

110. Lin, M.T.; Pulkkinen, L.; Vitto, J.; Yoon, K. The Gene Gun: Current Applications in Cutaneous Gene Therapy. Int. J. Dermatol. **2000**, *39*, 161–176.

111. Babiuk, S.; Baca-Estrada, M.; Babiuk, L.A.; Ewen, C.; Foldvari, M. Cutaneous Vaccination: The Skin as an Immunologically Active Tissue and the Challenge of Antigen Delivery. J. Controlled Release **2000**, *66*, 199–214.

112. Fan, H.; Lin, Q.; Morrissey, G.R.; Khavari, P.A. Immunization Via Hair Follicles by Topical Application of Naked DNA to Normal Skin. Nature Biotech. **1999**, *17*, 870–872.

113. Erspamer, V.; Falconieri-Erspamer, G.; Severini, C.; Potenza, R.L.; Barra, D.; Mignogna, G.; Bianchi, A. Pharmacological Studies of 'Sapo' From the Frog *Phyllomedusa Bicolor* Skin: A Drug Used by the Peruvian

Matses Indians in Shamanic Hunting Practices. Toxicon **1993**, *31*, 1099–1111.

114. Down, J.A.; Harvey, N.G. Minimally Invasive Systems for Transdermal Drug Delivery. in press.

115. Nelson, J.S.; McCullough, J.L.; Glenn, T.; Wright, W.H.; Liaw, L.L.; Jacques, S.L. Mid-Infrared Laser Ablation of Stratum Corneum Enhances In Vitro Percutaneous Transport of Drugs. J. Invest. Dermatol. **1991**, *97*, 874–879.

116. Eppstein, J.A.; Delcher, H.K.; Hatch, M.R.; McRae, M.S.; Papp, J.; Woods, T.J. Insulin Infusion Via Thermal Micropores. Proc. Int. Symp. Controlled Release Bioact. Mater. **2000**, *27*, 1010–1011.

117. Svedman, P.; Lundin, S.; Svedman, C. Administration of Antidiuretic Peptide (DDAVP) by Way of Suction De-epithelialised Skin. Lancet **1991**, *337*, 1506–1509.

118. Lundin, S.; Svedman, P.; Höglund, P.; Jönsson, K.; Broeders, A.; Melin, P. Absorption of an Oxytocin Antagonist (Antocin) and a Vasopressin Analogue (dDAVP) Through a Standardized Skin Erosion in Volunteers. Pharm. Res. **1995**, *12*, 2024–2029.

119. Sarphie, D.F.; Johnson, B.; Cormier, M.; Burkoth, T.L.; Bellhouse, B.J. Bioavailability Following Transdermal Powdered Delivery (TPD) of Radiolabeled Insulin to Hairless Guinea Pigs. J. Controlled Release **1997**, *47*, 61–69.

120. Sarphie, D.F.; Varadi, A.; Bellhouse, B.J.; Ashcroft, S. Transdermal Delivery of Powdered Bovine Insulin to Diabetic and Non-Diabetic Wistar Rats. Diabetes **1995**, *44* (Suppl. 1), 129a.

121. Henry, S.; McAllister, D.V.; Allen, M.G.; Prausnitz, M.R. Microfabricated Microneedles: A Novel Approach to Transdermal Drug Delivery. J. Pharm. Sci. **1998**, *87*, 922–925.

122. McAllister, D.V.; Kaushik, S.; Patel, P.N.; Mayberry, J.L.; Allen, M.G.; Prausnitz, M.R. Solid and Hollow Microneedles for Transdermal Protein Delivery. Proc. Intl. Symp. Controlled Release Bioact. Mater. **1999**, *26*, 192–193.

PHARMACEUTICAL EXCIPIENT TESTING—A REGULATORY AND PRECLINICAL PERSPECTIVE[a]

Paul Baldrick

Regulatory Affairs-Pharmaceuticals, Covance Laboratories Ltd., Harrogate, England

INTRODUCTION

Pharmaceutical excipients are additives used in the formulation of pharmacologically active drugs and can be viewed as any ingredient of a medicinal product other than the active ingredient. Excipients include diluents, fillers and bulking agents, binders and adhesives, propellants, disintegrants, lubricants and glidants, colors, flavors, coating agents, polishing agents, fragrances, sweetening agents, polymers, and waxes. A review of the literature indicates approximately 1300 excipients used in the pharmaceutical industry. Chemical and manufacturing (quality) data can be found for many of these excipients in European, U.S., and Japanese pharmacopoeias (1–3) or in a range of other publications (4–6), but safety (preclinical) data are limited. General safety data can be found in some publications (5, 7). Reference to excipients included in drug submissions is given in the FDA *Inactive Ingredients Guide* (8), the *National Formulary* (9), and the U.K. *ABPI Data Sheets* (10). It is assumed that reference to an excipient in these publications is a guarantee of acceptance by a regulatory body of the excipient in a new drug formulation. Although this is often the case, there may be gaps in the available data that may necessitate additional preclinical evaluation. The use of a novel excipient in a drug formulation necessitates preclinical testing and evaluation. This article addresses strategies for preclinical assessment of completely novel, essentially similar, and established excipients in view of current difficulties posed by the lack of a concerted international guideline relating directly to pharmaceutical excipients. In addition, the active role of excipients in producing adverse patient effects and in modulating active drug release is presented.

[a]Updated from Pharmaceutical Excipient Testing—A Regulatory and Preclinical Perspective. In *Encyclopedia of Pharmaceutical Technology*; Swarbrick, J.; Boylan, J.C. (Eds.), 1st Ed., Marcel Dekker, Inc., New York, 2000, Vol. 19, 289–310.

REGULATIONS AND GUIDELINES

From an international regulatory point of view, there is currently little help to address the question of registration of an excipient as a separate entity. Furthermore, there is no such thing as an approved excipient (11). In Europe, it is assumed that novel excipients need to be evaluated as new chemical entities (12–14). Established excipients are included in marketing authorization applications (MAAs) for new drugs, with the assumption that their presence and characterization in pharmacopoeias will not cause concern with European regulators. Information on excipients is expected in MAA applications (15). In the United States, the Food and Drug Administration (FDA) assesses and permits use of excipients as part of a new drug application (NDA). As in Europe, it is assumed that the use of an "approved" excipient ensures its acceptance in the new drug formulation. Thus, the FDA favors commercially established excipients (16). Interestingly, in the U.S. guideline relating to preclinical data for NDA submission, excipients are not mentioned (17). Although excipients per se are not mentioned in the Japanese guidelines (18), the situation with regard to such materials is similar to that in Europe and the United States. Under the new Japanese Ministry of Health and Welfare (JMHW) evaluation system (operational since 1997), the assessment of pharmaceutical products containing excipients with prior use in Japan is performed at the Pharmaceuticals and Medical Devices Evaluation Center (PMDE). Approval of a product that contains an excipient with no prior use in Japan has to be evaluated by the Subcommittee on Pharmaceutical Excipients of the Central Pharmaceutical Affairs Council (CPAC) concurrently with the approval process undertaken through the PMDE Center (19). Reasons for inclusion of the excipient; precedents of use; and quality, stability, and safety data are all needed.

The lack of international regulatory guidelines led to the formation of the International Pharmaceutical Excipients Council (IPEC) in 1991. This industry association, with European, U.S., and Japanese membership, has championed the international standardization of excipients, the introduction of useful new excipients, and the development of safety evaluation guidelines. These guidelines, addressing all the primary routes of drug administration, have been published (16). These proposed safety guidelines has been given to the FDA by the IPEC, with a request for an evaluation procedure, independent of the NDA process, for new pharmaceutical excipients (20).

In Europe, the need for companies to fully consider the types of excipients in new drug formulations has been the focus of a guideline released recently by the European commission on drug label and package leaflet excipient information for all MAAs (14). This guideline indicates that all excipients must be listed on the drug label for parenteral, topical, inhalation, and ophthalmic products. For other medicinal products, only those excipients with a defined and recognized action of effect, as listed in the guidance document (over 40 materials are mentioned), need to be declared on the label. In drug package leaflets, all excipients must be included. European regulations and guidelines (12, 13, 21) also require that a full statement of the excipients used be given in the Summary of Product Characteristics (SPC) document for new drug formulations. In Japan, the identity and quantity of the inactive components must be indicated on package inserts and similar materials for medicines for oral use, injection, and applications on the skin and mucosal surfaces (22).

The situation is different in the United States, where labeling of inactive ingredients remains voluntary (23), although such labeling has been adopted by two major pharmaceutical industry trade associations (the Proprietary Association and the Pharmaceutical Manufacturers Association). It may be that companies are reluctant to give details on their products because the excipients will not have patent protection. Thus, full disclosure of excipients is still not a general practice and can lead to opposition (24). The FDA indicated, however, that inactive ingredients (that have the same meaning as excipients) that present an increased risk of toxic effects to neonates or other pediatric subgroups need to be noted in the contraindications, warning, or precautions section of labels on prescription drugs for humans (25).

In Europe, in the preclinical area stage, reference is made (but without any details) to the suitable demonstration of safety of any new propellant (26, 27). Vaccine guidelines group excipients (identified as inactive components including stabilizers) with adjuvants and preservatives as additives and indicate that safety appraisal is needed, again without details (28). A recent European regulatory guidance on the development of pharmaceutics has stated that, "A new substance introduced as a constituent will be regarded in the same way as a new active ingredient H unless it is already approved for use in

food for orally administered products, or in cosmetics for topical administration. Additional data may still be required where an excipient is administered via an unconventional route, or in high doses" (29). However, although this wording may allow for some reduced data for commonly used nonpharmaceutical materials, it is unlikely that in the meantime in Europe, novel excipients will be treated as other than new chemical entities.

CATEGORIES

New (Novel) Recipients

A new excipient is a compound that has not been used previously or permitted for use in a pharmaceutical preparation (16). The need to develop an excipient as a new chemical entity, leading to expense and potential time delay (the excipient would be of low regulatory priority compared with active new drug formulations), has resulted in a reluctance in the pharmaceutical industry to introduce new materials. Indeed, it is likely that if there is doubt about the safety of an excipient, pharmaceutical manufacturers would rather reformulate than incur registration delays (11). Furthermore, despite the possibility that greater effectiveness of pharmaceutical products containing new excipients exists, a desire to avoid regulatory delays has resulted in a lack of research in this area (19). A review of the 12 most common excipients (water, magnesium stearate, starch, lactose, microcrystalline cellulose, stearic acid, sucrose, talc, silicon dioxide, gelatin, acacia, and dibasic calcium phosphate, respectively) in NDAs from 1964 to 1984 shows that six were being used in 1904, increasing to the majority of these materials by 1949 (30). A review of the most common excipients in U.K.-licenced medicines showed the following materials: water, magnesiun stearate, povidone, sodium chloride, stearic acid, and dextrose (31). In 1992, Strattan reported that no truly new excipients have become available for general use in the past 50 years (32). The appearance of the cyclodextrins in the 1990s and the recent approval of the inhalation propellant hydrofluoroalkane (HFA) have only slightly changed this fact. The U.S. pharmaceutical companies have primarily used "grandfathering" for their new substances (using old "unapproved" drug formulations), thus preventing advancement in the use of excipients.

As noted above, the IPEC has proposed guidelines for the safety assessment of new excipients. It is hoped that implementation of these guidelines would expedite the review of a proposed new excipient by regulatory agencies

Table 1 Summary of excipient guideline[a]

Tests	Oral	Mucosal	Transdermal	Topical	Parenteral	Inhalation/intranasal	Ocular
						Routes of exposure for humans	
Appendix 1 (Base set):							
Acute oral toxicity	R	R	R	R	R	R	R
Acute dermal toxicity	R	R	R	R	R	R	R
Acute inhalation toxicity	C	C	C	C	C	R	C
Eye irritation	R	R	R	R	R	R	R
Skin irritation	R	R	R	R	R	R	R
Skin sensitization	R	R	R	R	R	R	R
Acute parenteral toxicity	—	—	—	—	R	—	—
Application site evaluation	—	R	R	R	R	R	—
Pulmonary sensitization	—	—	—	—	—	R	—
Phototoxicity/photoallergy	—	—	R	R	—	—	R
Bacterial gene mutation	R	R	R	R	R	R	R
Chromosomal damage	R	R	R	R	R	R	R
ADME-intended route	R	R	R	R	R	R	R
28-day toxicity (two species) intended route	R	R	R	R	R	R	R
Appendix 2							
90-day toxicity (most appropriate species)	R	R	R	R	R	R	R
Teratology (rat and/or rabbit)	R	R	R	R	R	R	R
Additional assays	C	C	C	C	C	C	C
Genotoxicity assays	R	R	R	R	R	R	R
Appendix 3							
Chronic toxicity (rodent, nonrodent)	C	C	C	C	C	C	C
One-generation reproduction	R	R	R	R	R	R	R
Photocarcinogenicity	—	—	C	C	—	—	—
Carcinogenicity	C	C	C	C	C	C	—

[a] Extent of testing is dependent on conditions and duration of exposure: Appendix 1 for exposures of less than 2 weeks, Appendix 2 for exposures of 2 to 6 weeks, and Appendix 3 for exposures of greater than 6 weeks.
(From Ref. 16.)
R, required; C, Conditional.

(16). A summary of the IPEC guidelines is given in Table 1. This organization has defined a testing strategy for human exposure to single or limited dosing (less than 2 weeks), limited and repeated dosing (2–6 weeks), and long-term dosing (longer than 6 weeks). Different tests for oral, mucosal, transdermal, topical, parenteral, inhalation/intranasal, and ocular routes in humans are described. Common recommended toxicity studies for longer term use in humans include acute oral and dermal toxicity studies, eye and skin irritation studies, a skin sensitization study, genotoxicity and ADME studies, subacute and chronic studies, and reproduction studies. These guidelines are useful as a basis for the development of a new excipient, although they raise some questions. The basis for the guidance is that because of the defined inert nature of excipients, the safety assessment procedure should not be as complex or as extensive as that for an active drug. However, the program described is not dissimilar to the strategy used for an active drug. Furthermore, acute dermal, irritation, and skin sensitization studies are not routinely performed in new drug assessment unless there are specific issues or questions about the drug class. Finally, and most important, if a drug company was developing a drug with a completely new excipient in the formulation, it is possible to include the excipient alone as an extra dose group in the preclinical studies. These studies would presumably use the clinical formulation (containing the excipient). It is vital that kinetics studies identify any drug-excipient interaction. As for active drug, a sensitive analytical method is needed to measure levels of excipient (if possible) in plasma samples from toxicology studies. If the impurity profile of the new excipient causes concern, addition toxicological evaluation of each impurity has to be carried out as well. It is crucial to clarify the excipient impurity profile because even established pharmacopoeia-listed materials such as magnesium stearate can raise questions as to the safety and toxicity of its impurities (33).

In Japan, Uchiyama has recently published requirements for the safety evaluation of new excipients (19). These requirements include studies on acute, subacute, and chronic toxicity, mutagenicity, effects on reproduction, dependency, antigenicity, carcinogenicity, and local irritation (human patch test). The first five of these tests are mandatory. With the exception of the local irritation test, for which a domestic trial is required, non-Japanese data are acceptable for these studies. Even if a material has been used in a pharmaceutical product outside Japan, the material is treated as a new excipient if there has been no prior use in Japan, although relevant overseas data for the material are acceptable for regulatory submission. A material is treated as a new excipient

when the route of administration differs or the dose level exceeds that of prior use even after approval for the Japanese market (19).

Although not viewed as a typical excipient, the inhalation propellant HFA has been approved in both the United States and Europe in recent years. Because of concerns about ozone layer depletion defined in the Montreal protocol, the need for a replacement for chlorofluorocarbonates (CFCs) in metered-dose inhalers (MDIs) used by patients with asthmas led to the development of two types of HFA (134a and 227) in Europe (34, 35). Both compounds underwent extensive preclinical testing in the early to mid-1990s. The change from established CFC-containing drugs to those with HFA requires toxicity-bridging studies. From a regulatory point of view, these studies can vary from 1 month to lifetime in duration. A recent U.S. publication has revealed a number of preclinical studies, including those for carcinogenicity, using hydrochlorofluorocarbons (HCFCs) and hydrofluorocarbons (HFCs) as replacements for CFCs (36). The data show that the new HFA-134a and -227 excipients are as safe for use in humans as the CFCs they are replacing (37, 38). Using the example of HFA, it can be seen that even with government pressure to change a formulation, considerable time and effort are needed for the development of a new excipient.

Finally, with regard to the development of new materials for inhalation products, Wolff and Dorato suggest acute or short-term toxicology studies of a number of possible excipients in different formulations (34). This process will allow the narrowing to one or two acceptable possibilities that can then undergo more complete toxicological testing. The testing of new inhalation excipients is also addressed in a guidance from the FDA's Center for Drug Evaluation and Research (CDER) (39). A complete toxicological evaluation is recommended for a new excipient with unknown inhalation toxicology potential (such as a new propellant) alone as well as bridging studies in animals with the new complete formulation. Such studies are generally sufficient for regulatory approval.

Essentially New Excipients

Essentially new excipients can be thought of as substances resulting from a structural modification of an "approved" excipient, a recognized food additive, a structurally modified food additive, or a constituent of an over-the-counter (OTC) medicine. Food additives are similar to excipients in that they are used to impart specific functional characteristics and are usually added in low levels (16). International organizations including the Joint Food and Agriculture Organisation (FAO) and the World Health Organization (WHO) Expert Committee (JECFA) have established safety standards such as an acceptable daily intake (ADI) or "generally recognized as safe" (GRAS) for a number of food additives, including materials that have applications as excipients. Safety evaluation of these additives involves a detailed risk-assessment process, with ADI calculations having factors such as 100-fold-above-animal data as safety margins.

Although not covered by any regulatory guidance, the safety of many food additives determined through JECFA evaluation and long-term human exposure allows for approval of these materials as new excipients in drug formulations without the need for extensive preclinical testing. Indeed, the FDA favors commercially established food additives and GRAS substances (16). However, limitations and possible significant financial investment exist because of the possibility of long waiting periods for approval and the fact that food additive data relate to oral administration and are of little use for nonoral products (11).

Additionally, problems may arise if the preclinical data on which the assessment is made are old and unreliable and raise specific toxicological concerns. Considering all these factors, it is probable that a robust expert review of available preclinical and human exposure data for a food additive may satisfy a regulatory body. As noted above, there is an indication in Europe that new pharmaceutical excipients already used in food for orally administered products or for topical cosmetics may not have to be considered new chemical entities, and therefore full evaluation may be bypassed (29).

Other problems may arise if the level of the food additive to be used as a proposed new excipient is higher than the ADI value or if a food additive or an established excipient are structurally (albeit simply) modified. The new material may have a different or more toxic profile. There are no easy solutions to these

situations for pharmaceutical companies. The regulatory answer will be that each material is assessed on a case-by-case basis. However, some form of preclinical testing will probably be required, and a possible minimal program is given in Fig. 1. In this program, an Ames study determines that the new excipient has no genotoxicity potential, and a single-dose toxicity study shows that there are no adverse effects after administration of the material at the limit (high) dose generally used in the pharmaceutical industry. An investigative mass, balance, whole-body autoradiography study provides information on absorption, distribution, metabolism, and excretion. This study also involves an investigation of suitable labeling of the material. An in vitro metabolism study (e.g., in rat versus human hepatocytes) may also be useful for modified food additives and excipients to compare the break-down process and to show possible differences between rat and human in these processes.

A 1-month toxicity study will establish whether the limit dose is causing any form of high-dose toxicity or metabolic overload. It may be useful to include toxicokinetic satellite animals in this study to demonstrate what level of exposure to the excipient occurs in the blood. Favorable findings from these studies can be presented to the regulatory bodies and advice sought as to whether additional testing is recommended. As with other preclinical studies in drug development, all these investigations should be performed according to good laboratory practice (GLP).

In the United States, OTC products do not need regulatory approval of submission of an NDA. Thus, if an excipient has a record of safe use in an OTC medicine, the FDA may accept the material, provided the product manufacturer can demonstrate evidence that the excipient is safe to use (11). However, this manner of approval is not guaranteed to be successful and may not be useful for nonoral administration routes.

In Japan, all these pathways to reduce ease the burden of introducing new excipients are more complex. If not already approved as a pharmaceutical excipient in Japan, food additives for oral administration or cosmetic substances for external application in drug formulations requires that they be treated as new excipients (19). For excipients already used in orally or intravenously administered products, a change to an externally applied product necessitates additional safety testing. Studies include acute and subacute toxicity (including adsorption through the skin) and local irritation investigations (19).

Many excipients used by the pharmaceutical industry in the last 15 years in sugar-free medical preparations

Test
Ames test
Acute oral toxicity study
Mass/balance/whole body autoradiography
(WBA) study and/or in-vitro metabolism
study
One-month repeat dose toxicity study

Fig. 1 Minimal preclinical testing strategy for an essentially new excipient.

probably come under the category of essentially new excipients. Pressure for their introduction has been encouraged by the definite relationship between the dietary consumption of sucrose and the incidence of dental caries (40, 41). These materials include intense sweeteners such as saccharin and cyclamate plus bulk sweeteners such as the polyols sorbitol, xylitol, and lactitol. These materials are all either approved for food use or have pharmacopoeia monographs in existence or in draft (42). Literature reviews show number of preclinical safety studies for these excipients. Many of these studies are related to specific toxicological concerns such as bladder tumor formation with saccharin use and adrenal glands and testes proliferation with polyol use (Table 2).

The cyclodextrins (CDs) fall into the categories of new and essentially new excipients. CDs are enzymatically modified starches with many favorable properties as excipients. The use of CDs in food products in the late 1970s and 1980s, together with extensive preclinical testing, has resulted in the inclusion of these materials in marketed drugs (32, 62). Various companies now market forms of CDs as safe and efficient delivery systems for active drugs.

Established ("Approved") Excipients

The presence of well known established excipients in a new drug formulation does not necessarily mean that regulatory authorities question will not their inclusion. However, issues can be avoided if the excipient is clearly characterized in the quality section of the documentation and addressed sufficiently in the preclinical section. The preclinical assessment can take the form of an expert review of available safety data that defines safety margins between values reported in the literature and the level(s) used in the new drug formulation. This process is becoming easier for toxicologists as more data on established excipients become available through published literature reviews and/or publication of in-house studies. Examples include lactose (58), povidone or polyvinylpyrrolidone (PVP) (50, 63), saccharin (64), polyethylene glycols (PEGs) (65), HFA-134a (66), and vaccine adjuvants/excipients (67). Similarly, the establishment of global standardized monographs in major pharmacopoeias is helpful. However, it is surprising how little useful toxicology data are available for many well known materials such as maltodextrin, peppermint oil, and menthol.

Problems can arise when the currently available published data suggest that there may be potential toxicity concerns, especially when an excipient approved for one dose route is applied to another route with a different systemic exposure and target site. Scientific discussions of the data on the relevance of animal findings to humans, together with the establishment of safety margins, are necessary. The absence of toxicity findings in the new drug preclinical program that includes the excipient can also be used in these discussions. Examples of established excipients with reported toxicological concerns and the relevance of these findings to humans are given in Table 2. Another potential issue for discussion arises if the level of excipient in the new drug formulation exceeds that already known to the regulatory agency for prior use.

A less important but interesting point is that many of the established and pharmacopoeia-listed excipients are not accompanied by strict standardized assay methods. In this situation, a "new" assay needs to be established by the company with the new drug formulation for characterization and/or plasma measurement of the excipient.

The discussion above indicates that little or no extra preclinical studies are required for well known excipients. From an unofficial FDA regulatory perspective, this view is supported for inhalation excipients by De George et al. (39), who state that no additional toxicology information is generally needed for qualitative or quantitative changes of well characterized, nontoxic excipients used in approved inhalation drug products. A case-by-case assessment, however, will be used for reformulations because excipient toxicity may change. In addition, for excipients with previous use in humans but limited inhalation toxicity information, evaluation of inhalation toxic potential of the excipient after repeated dosing is recommended.

ADVERSE EFFECTS OF EXCIPIENTS

By traditional definition, excipients should be inert and display no pharmacological activity. However, a number of clinically relevant adverse reactions are known for various established excipients, albeit of low occurrence and uncommon compared with the overall prevalence of adverse drug reactions. This area is covered extensively in the literature (e.g., 7, 14, 23, 40, 68–71). Some examples are given in Table 3. Groups susceptible to excipient toxicity include low-birth-weight infants (particularly during the first 2 weeks of life) and patients

Table 2 Toxicological issues with various excipients

Excipient	Toxicological finding	Relevance to humans	Reference
Lactose and polyols	Adrenal medullary proliferative changes/tumors in rats	Considered to be rat-specific and caused by altered calcium homeostasis attributable to high dose levels given and not relevant to humans	43–45
Lactose and polyols	Hyperplastic/neoplastic changes in rat testes	See above	46
Saccharin	Proliferative changes in male rat bladder epithelium	Considered to be species-specific with large doses used. Mechanism of action may involve urinary proteins not normally found in humans	23, 40, 47–49
PVP	Accumulation in the reticuloendothelial system in rodents, with the occurrence of "foam cells"	Toxicological significance is unclear from the literature, but findings may be related to high-dose regimens used. No adverse effects from long-term storage in humans. There is also over 50 years of safe use for PVP in humans	50–52
Menthol	Limited sensitization reaction in guinea pigs	Toxicological significance is not clear from the literature, although very infrequent human allergy reactions are reported in the presence of menthol (8)	53
Limonene	Hyaline droplet formation in male rat kidney	Considered to be male rat-specific and related to the presence/accumulation of alpha 2 μ-globulin	54–56
Talc	Lung tumors in female rats	Related to high dose level and resulting chronic toxicity	57
Talc	Adrenal gland neoplasms (pheochromocytomas) in rats	Review of data indicates that tumors were not treatment-related	57
Maltodextrin	Minimal reversible laryngeal irritation (squamous metaplasia) with 4% maltodextrin in chronic rat inhalation study	Considered to be a background finding of no consequence to humans. May be related to the presence of peppermint oil (1%) in dosing preparation.[a,b] Local irritation of the mouth and oesophagus can occur in patients taking peppermint oil preparations (7, 10)	Personal observation
CFCs	Cardiac arrhythmias, notably in the dog	Relatively good safety margins and long/wide use of CFC propellants in MDIs has shown these compounds to be safe	34

[a] Minimal laryngeal squamous metaplasia has also been reported in a chronic rat study with lactose (58) and may be related to a physiological adaptive response attributable to the inhalation of particulate dust at high levels over long periods. Certain histological changes in the respiratory epithelium have been defined as adaptive and not toxic (59, 60).

[b] Peppermint oil contains a large percentage of menthol (30–55%) (1). Any question that the laryngeal irritation may be related to the presence of menthol within peppermint oil is doubtful because a recent chronic rat inhalation study has shown that 5000 ppm of menthol had no substantial effect on the histopathological changes in the respiratory tract normally associated with inhalation of mainstream cigarette smoke (61).

Table 3   Adverse effects encountered with various pharmaceutical excipients

Excipient (purpose)	Major adverse event(s)	Reference
Benzalkonium chloride (bacterial preservative)	Irritant known to discolor soft contact lens; rare hypersensitivity, bronchoconstriction	7, 14, 23
CFCs (propellent)	Bronchospasm	23
Aspartame (artificial sweetener)	Headache, various neuropsychiatric disorders, seizures, rare hypersensitivity reactions. Contraindicated for patients with phenylketonuria	7, 23, 40, 70
Saccharin (artificial sweetener)	Rare hypersensitivity, photosensitivity (with cross-sensitivity in patients with sulfonamide allergy)	7, 23, 40, 70
Benzyl alcohol (preservative)	Rare hypersensitivity reactions including contact dermatitis. Contraindicated for infants and young children because of high dose level toxicity	7, 14, 23, 70
Lactose (filler/bulking agent)	Contraindicated for patients with lactose insufficiency (diarrhea, abdominal pain)	14, 58
Propylene glycol (solubilizer)	CNS toxicity, hyperosmolality, lactic acidosis, hypersensitivity including contact dermatitis	7, 23, 70
Benzoic acid (preservative)	Irritant; may have role in asthma, urticaria, anaphylaxis, vasculitis	7, 14, 70
Ethanol (vehicle)	Irritation/dry skin. Contraindicated at high dose levels with liver disease, epilepsy, alcoholism, pregnant women, children	14
Polyols (artificial sweeteners)	Diarrhea	14, 58
Glycerol (vehicle)	Headache, stomach upset, diarrhea, increased serum osmolality, cardiac arrhythmias	7, 14
Sodium and potassium (supplement)	Adverse in cases of low sodium/potassium diet, stomach upset, diarrhea. Phlebitis and injection pain with potassium	7, 14
Sulphites (antioxidants)	Allergic hypereactions, e.g., anaphylaxis, bronchospasm, gastrointestinal irritation/upset	7, 14, 23, 40, 70
Gums, e.g., arabic, tragacanth (emulsifying agents)	Rare hypersensitivity reactions	7, 70
Cremophor EL–Polyoxyethylated castor oil (solvent)	Anaphylactic reactions, nausea, vomiting, colic, hyperlipidaemias	7, 14, 70
Azo dyes e.g., tartrazine (dyes)	Anaphylactoid reaction. Contraindicated for aspirin-intolerant individuals	7, 23, 70
Chlorobutanol (preservative)	Anaphylactic shock/hypersensitivity reactions, CNS toxicity	7, 70
Formaldehyde (preservative)	Allergic reactions, stomach upset, diarrhea, irritant, role in asthma	7, 14, 70
Aluminium hydroxide (adjuvant/adsorbant)	Aluminium allergy, skin nodules	7, 70
Methylcellulose (stabilizer/suspending agent)	Intestinal upset	7
Hydroxyethylcellulose (stabilizer/suspending agent)	Ocular irritation	7
Gluten/wheat starches (binders)	Intolerance for patients with coliac disease	14, 40

with asthma (69). It is interesting that, as for many adverse effects, most of the reported excipient-related findings in patients were not or could not be predicted by the preclinical data.

In Europe, it is now a requirement to include adverse excipient effects in the product leaflet in a consumer-friendly manner (14); information on ingredient content is also required in Japan (22). The fact that the labeling of inactive ingredients remains voluntary in the United States means that excipient-related adverse reactions will continue to be reported. Wong (24) highlights a worst-case scenario by showing that a drug can be marketed in various formulated dosage forms such as tablets, injections, and oral solutions, with each of these forms containing a different set of excipients that are not disclosed on the package label. Because the choice of excipients for any pharmaceutical preparation is decided by each company, different manufacturers producing the same drug may use different excipients in different proportions. Another potential issue is the quality of the excipients used in the drug formulation. Inferior grades of excipients may seriously jeopardize the quality and thus the potential safety and efficacy of the final product (24). Fortunately, standardization of the quality of excipients in pharmacopoeias reduces the significance of efficacy as an issue, although the example of the use of counterfeit excipients resulting in 90 pediatric fatalities in Haiti in the mid-1990s should not be forgotten (71).

Chowhan (33) points out the increasing awareness of excipient manufacturers and users of the importance and consequences of process changes. From a medical perspective for drugs with technically inert ingredients that are not necessarily pharmacologically inactive, full information is needed to facilitate the assessment and treatment of patient symptoms. Most excipient-related toxicity is preventable when the formulation is known (69, 72). However, difficulty in obtaining such information from U.S. manufacturers continues to be a problem (73). Literature on the occurrence of well known excipients in pharmaceutical products is available as an aid to physicians in selecting preparations containing different excipients when an adverse reaction occurs (74, 75).

Overall, even in early drug development, a consideration of the excipient profile of the final product is important. If use of the established excipients is planned, an awareness of potential adverse effects in humans is necessary. Development should use pharmacopoeia-listed materials. For new excipients, this information is not available, and safety will be assessed in the preclinical evaluation. Extrapolation may only be possible if the new excipient is in the same class or is structurally similar to

established materials, but such a comparison would not necessarily be reliable.

DRUG-EXCIPIENT INTERACTIONS AND AN ACTIVE ROLE FOR EXCIPIENTS

That all excipients are neither truly inert nor inactive is shown by the fact that drug-excipient interactions can considerably affect the physiological availability of many drug products (76). By either accelerating or retarding the release of the active ingredients, excipients can affect the therapeutic performance of the drug by increased or reduced bioavailability (24, 69). Indeed, relatively small variations in the physical properties of an excipient can produce a significant difference in the behavior of formulated products (5). In turn, the modified bioavailability may also result in adverse reactions. For modern drug-delivery systems, certain excipients can have a well defined function associated with the need to achieve a specific drug bioavailability profile or therapeutic effect (11). Liposomes (phospholipid-based vesicles) have been increasingly explored as novel drug-delivery systems, and there are examples of active excipient involvement, such as that with PVP- and PEG-liposomes, in development (77, 78). Review of the literature shows a surge in interest in using excipients in sustained-release formulations in the 1990s. Various selective functional regions are identified, such as colonic targeting. Currently, many of these new formulations with an active role for the excipient have only been tested using in vitro pharmaceutical systems to establish release patterns, although the role of materials such as methylcellulose in tablet formulations for sustained release has been well established (5). It is beyond the scope of this article to review the progress of these developments, but Naidoo (79) has discussed the effect of excipients on controlled drug-release properties of dosage forms. Reports on controlled delivery of peptide drugs and vaccines using active excipient properties are also available (80, 81). Such roles may reflect the definition of an excipient in the U.K. legislation on medicines as "any substance which does not contribute directly to the pharmacological action of the medicinal product otherwise than by regulation of the release of the active ingredients" (82).

Preclinical and clinical pharmacokinetics studies with a new drug indicate systemic exposure after administration of the therapeutic dose formulation. Thus, even if there is an interaction from an established or new excipient, adequate safety evaluation can be assessed. However, it would be useful to demonstrate to a regulator that possible interference of the active drug by the rest of the formulation had been considered. If an excipient is added to the new drug form for an active role, the proposed mechanism of action will need to be discussed carefully.

OVERALL SUMMARY AND CONCLUSION

Pharmaceutical excipients have a vital role in drug formulations, a role that has tended to be neglected as evidenced by the lack of mechanisms to assess excipient safety outside a new drug application process. Currently, it is assumed that an excipient is "approved" when the new drug formulation of which it is a constituent receives regulatory acceptance. The existing system works for well known excipients that are listed in international pharmacopoeias and for which there are published safety data. However, drug companies are faced with a lack of information on the testing needed for completely or essentially new excipients (the latter category comprising recognized food additives, structurally altered approved excipients or food additives, or constituents of OTC medicines). Existing regulations and guidelines indicate that new excipients be treated as new chemical entities and therefore, by inference, undergo full toxicological evaluation. Other drug requirements in Europe and Japan require that information on excipients appear in patient literature, although there is no similar legal requirement in the United States.

For new (novel) excipients, drug companies need to carefully assess the benefits of using the new substance in consideration of the extra workload, costs, and possible regulatory delays or rejection. However, now that an active role for excipients is recognized in the form of sustained-release or drug-delivery systems, there is more need for companies to use new excipients. The replacement of CFCs with HFAs in inhalation therapy, although driven by necessary government demands, still involved extensive preclinical evaluation of the new excipient propellants and the usual regulatory approval times. Old CFC formulations with either HFA-134a or -227 as the new excipient are still being submitted and/or are under regulatory review and need to include bridging toxicity studies. The change from CFC has also meant modifications in MDI structure that, in turn, can result in the need for other formulation changes (and additional excipients). The publication of

the IPEC recommendations for safety evaluation of new excipients is helpful, although there is still no official response from the FDA. The suggested evaluation is not dissimilar to the full preclinical program necessary for a new chemical entity. If a drug company decides to introduce a new excipient, extensive preclinical data are probably necessary. However, if preliminary investigations, such as those given in Fig. 1, show that the material is safe at high dose levels, the excipient can enter the full drug development program as part of the formulation and/or in the form of an extra dose group. Expert evaluation of the data should identify any potential problems.

The situation for developing essentially new excipients is different inasmuch as some data on the material or a related material are available. Provided that these data are expertly evaluated and/or supported by some preliminary studies (as given in Fig. 1), along with the usual new drug studies, regulators should not raise disapproval. Each excipient, however, will be assessed on a case-by-case basis, with issues such as toxicological findings in the "old" data and duration of use of the excipient carefully assessed. As with new excipients, the increased workload and costs, along with regulatory approval time, will need to be considered. The cyclodextrins have entered pharmaceutical use by means of being present in food products. However, this process has taken many years and has involved extensive preclinical testing. Other materials such as saccharin have been established from food use, but they have had to undergo severe regulatory challenge over whether preclinical findings of bladder tumors are relevant in human use.

Established excipients pose some issues for regulatory consideration. Such issues include the use of a well known excipient by an "unapproved" route, for example, inhalation of a material that has been used in oral formulations. In these cases, some preliminary toxicity studies may be necessary. Additionally, a well designed scientific review of safety data on the excipient will be necessary, with old findings fully evaluated.

The acceptance that excipients are neither inert nor inactive substance and may affect drug bioavailability and cause adverse reactions (commonly hypersensitivity) means that even more consideration of these materials is needed when formulating new drugs. With these facts in mind, regulators will expend greater efforts to examine the ingredients in drug formulations. Furthermore, because there is no international requirement to provide details of drug formulations to health professionals (notably in the United States), adverse reactions will continue to be reported, putting extra pressure both on drug companies and on regulators. Overall, the lack of regulatory guidance for excipient development leads to confusion for drug companies. In view of international agreement in other areas of drug development, an excipient-testing strategy would be an excellent topic for International Conference on Harmonization (ICH) consideration. Furthermore, with more standardization of pharmacopoeia materials, it may be possible to have excipients reviewed by a committee of an international pharmacopoeia. Safety data would be assessed by elected experts and published. Hopefully, these data would be acceptable to international regulatory bodies.

REFERENCES

1. *European Pharmacopoeia*, 3rd Ed.; European Pharmacopoeia Commission, Council of Europe: Strasbourg, France, 1997; 1299–1300.

2. *United States Pharmacopeia*, 23rd Edn.; United States Pharmacopeial Convention, Inc.: Rockville MD, 1995.

3. *Japanese Pharmacopoeia*, 13th Ed. The Society of Japanese Pharmacopoeia, Yakuji Nippo Ltd.: Tokyo, 1996.

4. *U.S. Physicians Desk Reference*, 50th Ed.; Medical Economics Company, Inc.: Montvale, NJ, 1996.

5. Kibbe, A.H. *Handbook of Pharmaceutical Excipients*, 3rd.; The American Pharmaceutical Association, Washington DC; The Pharmaceutical Press: London, 2000; 336.

6. Smolinske, S.C. *Handbook of Food, Drug and Cosmetic Excipients*, CRC Press: Boca Raton, FL, 1992.

7. Reynolds, J.E.F. *Martindale. The Extra Pharmacopoeia*, 31st Ed.; Royal Pharmaceutical Society: London, 1996.

8. *Inactive Ingredients Guide*; U.S. Food and Drug Administration, Division of Drug Information Resources: Rockville, MD, 1996.

9. *The National Formulary*, United States Pharmacopeial Convention, Inc.: Rockville, MD, 1995.

10. *ABPI Compendium of Data Sheets and Summaries of Product Characteristics 1998–1999*; (For Irrigation with Peppermint Oil, See p.981) Datapharm Publications Ltd: Whitehall, London, 1998.

11. Wotton, P.K.; Khosla, R. Acceptability of Excipients in the European Community and USA. BIRA J. **1991**, *10* (7), 11–13.

12. *Rules Relating to Marketing Authorisation of Medicinal Products for Human Use and Related Council Directives 81/852/EEC, 91/507/EEC and 92/18/EEC plus Council Recommendations 83/571/EEC and 87/176/EEC*; Office for Official Publications of the European Communities: Luxembourg, 1998.

13. Medicinal Products for Human Use, Presentation and Content of the Dossier. *The Rules Governing Medicinal Products in the European Union Notice to Applicants*; Office for Official Publications of the European Communities: Luxembourg, 1998; 2B.

14. Medicinal Products for Human Use, Safety, Environment and Information. *The Rules Governing Medicinal Products in the European Union, Guidelines*; Office for Official Publications of the European Communities: Luxembourg, 1998; 3B.

15. *Note for Guidance: EC Application Format*; CPMP and DGIII Guideline III/3038/91, Commission of the European Communities: Brussels, adopted March 1992.

16. Steinberg, M.; Borzelleca, J.F.; Enters, E.K.; Kinoshita, F.K.; Loper, A.; Mitchell, D.B.; Tamulinas, C.B.; Weiner, M.L. A New Approach to the Safety Assessment of Pharmaceutical Excipients. Regul. Toxicol. Pharm. **1996**, *24*, 149–154.

17. Center for Drug Evaluation and Research (CDER). Guidance for Industry, Guidelines for the Format and Content of the Nonclinical Pharmacology/Toxicology Section of an Application. FDA: Rockville, MD, 1987.

18. *Japanese Technical Requirements for New Drug Registration*; Yakuji Nippo Ltd.: Tokyo, 1997.

19. Uchiyama, M. Regulatory Status of Excipients in Japan. Drug Inform. J. **1999**, *33*, 27–32.

20. *British Institute of Regulatory Affairs BIRA News*; Institute Update 84, 1992.

21. *Note for Guidance: Summary of the Product Characteristics*; Adopted October 1991 Commission of the European Communities, Brussels, adopted October 1991.

22. Japanese Ministry of Health and Welfare. *Notice on the Indication of the Inactive Ingredients in Prescription Drugs*; Pharmaceutical Affairs Bureau, Ministry of Health and Welfare, Yakuji Nippo Ltd: Tokyo, 1988.

23. American Academy of Pediatrics, Committee on Drugs. "Inactive" Ingredients in Pharmaceutical Products: Update. Pediatrics **1997**, *99* (2), 268–278.

24. Wong, Y.L. Adverse Effects of Pharmaceutical Excipients in Drug Therapy. Ann. Acad. Med. Singapore **1993**, *22* (1), 99–102.

25. Specific Requirements on Content and Format of Labelling for Human Prescription Drugs; Revision of "Pediatric" Subsection in the Labelling. Federal Register: , 1994.

26. *Note for Guidance: Replacement of Chlorofluorocarbons (CFCs) in Metered Dose Inhalation Products*, CPMP and DGIII Guideline III/537/93, Commission of the European Communities, Brussels, adopted December 1993.

27. *Matters Relating to the Replacement of CFCs in Medicinal Products*, CPMP and DGIII Guideline III/5462/93, Commission of the European Communities, Brussels, adopted December 1993.

28. *Note for Guidance on Preclinical Pharmacological and Toxicological Testing of Vaccines*, CPMP/SWP/465/95, EMEA: Canary Wharf, London, adopted December 1997.

29. *Note for Guidance on Development Pharmaceutics*, CPMP/QWP/155/96, EMEA, Canary Wharf, London, adopted January 1998.

30. Shangraw, R. Developments in Tablet Excipients Since 1960. Manufact. Chem. **1986**, (December), 22–23.

31. Robertson, M.I. Regulatory Issues with Excipients. Int. J. Pharm. **1999**, *187*, 273–276.

32. Strattan, C.E. 2-Hydroxypropyl- β-Cyclodextrin. I. Patents and Regulatory Issues. Pharm. Technol. Int. **1992**, *4* (4), 45–49.

33. Chowhan, Z.T. A Rational Approach to Setting Limit Tests and Standards on Impurities in Excipients. Pharm. Tech. Europe **1995**, *7* (10), 66–75.

34. Wolff, R.K.; Dorato, M.A. Toxicologic Testing of Inhaled Pharmaceutical Aerosols. Crit. Rev. Toxicol. **1993**, *23* (4), 343–369.

35. Maginley, R. The Transition to CFC-Free Metered Dose Inhalers (MDIs): Regulatory Process, Implications and Conundrum. BIRA, Regul. Rev. **1998**, *7*, 11–18.

36. Bakshi, K.S. Toxicity of Alternatives to Chlorofluorocarbons: HFC-134a and HCFC-123. Inhal. Toxicol. **1998**, *10*, 963–967.

37. Harrison, L.I.; Donnell, D.; Simmons, J.L.; Ekholm, B.P.; Cooper, K.M.; Wyld, P.J. Twenty-Eight-Day Double-Blind Safety Study of an HFA-134a Inhalation Aerosol System in Healthy Subjects. J. Pharm. Pharmacol. **1996**, *48* (6), 595–600.

38. Blumenthal, M.N.; Casale, T.B.; Fink, J.N.; Uryniak, T.; Casty, F.E. Evaluation of a Nonchlorofluorocarbon Formulation of Cromolyn Sodium (Intal) Metered-Dose Inhaler Versus the Chlorofluorocarbon Formulation in the Treatment of Adult Patients with Asthma: A Controlled Trial. J. Allergy Clin. Immunol. **1998**, *101* (1), 7–13.

39. De George; et al. Considerations for Toxicology Studies of Respiratory Drug Products. Reg. Toxicol. Pharmacol. **1997**, *25* (2), 189–193.

40. Golightly, L.K.; Smolinske, S.S.; Bennett, M.L.; Sutherland, E.W., III; Rumack, B.H. Pharmaceutical Excipients. II. Adverse Effects Associated with "Inactive" Ingredients in Drug Products. Med. Toxicol. **1998**, *3*, 209–240.

41. Kinghorn, A.D.; Kaneda, N.; Baek, N.I.; Kennelly, E.J.; Soejarto, D.D. Noncariogenic Intense Natural Sweeteners. Med. Res. Rev. **1998**, *18* (5), 347–360.

42. Herbert, K. Novel Excipients for Sugar-Free Preparations—Functionality and Performance. *European Pharmaceutical Contractor*, Ballantyne Ross Ltd: London, 1998; 132–139.

43. Bär, A. Sugars and Adrenomedullary Proliferative Lesions: The Effects of Lactose and Various Polyalcohols. J. Am. Coll. Toxicol. **1988**, *7* (1), 71–81.

44. Roe, F.J.C. Relevance for Man of the Effects of Lactose, Polyols and Other Carbohydrates on Calcium Metabolism Seen in Rats: A Review. Hum. Toxicol. **1989**, *8*, 87–98.

45. Lynch, B.S.; Tischler, A.S.; Capen, C.; Munro, I.C.; McGirr, L.M.; McClain, R.M. Low Digestible Carbohydrates (Polyols and Lactose): Significance of Adrenal Medullary Proliferative Lesions in the Rat. Regul. Toxicol. Pharmac. **1996**, *23*, 256–297.

46. Bär, A. Significance of Leydig Cell Neoplasia in Rats Fed Lactitol or Lactose. J. Am. Coll. Toxicol. **1992**, *11* (2), 189–207.

47. Cohen, S.M. Human Relevance of Animal Carcinogenicity Studies. Regul. Toxicol. Pharmacol. **1995**, *21* (1), 75–80.

48. Cohen, S.M. Cell Proliferation and Carcinogenesis. Drug Metab. Rev. **1998**, *30* (2), 339–357.

49. Wysner, J.; Williams, G.M. Saccharin Mechanistic Data and Risk Assessment: Urine Composition, Enhanced Cell Proliferation, and Tumour Promotion. Pharmacol. Ther. **1996**, *71* (1–2), 225–252.

50. Robinson, B.V.; Sullivan, F.M.; Borzelleca, J.F.; Schwartz, S.L. *PVP: A Critical Review of the Kinetics and Toxicology of Polyvinylpyrrolidone (Povidone)*, Lewis Publishers, Inc.: Chelsea MI, 1990.

51. Frommer, J. The Pathogenesis of Reticulo-Endothelial Foam Cells. Effect of Polyvinylpyrrolidone on the Liver of the Mouse. Am. J. Path. **1956**, *32*, 433–453.

52. Nelson, A.A.; Lusky, L.M. Pathological Changes in Rabbits from Repeated Intravenous Injections of Periston (Polyvinyl Pyrrolidone) or Dextran. Proc. Soc. Exp. Biol. Med. **1951**, *76*, 765–767.

53. Sharp, D.W. The Sensitisation Potential of Some Perfume Ingredients Tested Using a Modified Draize Procedure. Toxicology **1978**, *9*, 261–271.

54. Alden, C.L. A Review of Unique Male Rat Hydrocarbon Nephropathy. Toxicol. Pathol. **1986**, *14* (1), 109–111.

55. Lehman-McKeeman, L.D.; Rodriguez, P.A.; Takigiku, R.; Caudill, D.; Fey, M.L. D-Limonene-Induced Male Rat-Specific Nephrotoxicity: Evaluation of the Association Between D-Limonene And $\alpha_{2\mu}$-Globulin. Toxicol. Appl. Pharmacol. **1989**, *99*, 250–259.

56. Flamm, W.G.; Lehman-McKeeman, L.D. The Human Relevance of the Renal Tumor-Inducing Potential of D-Limonene in Male Rats: Implications for Risk Assessment. Regul. Toxicol. Pharmacol. **1991**, *13*, 70–86.

57. Goodman, J.I. An Analysis of the National Toxicology Program's (NTP) Technical Report (NTP TR 421) on the Toxicology and Carcinogenesis Studies of Talc. Regul. Toxicol. Pharmacol. **1995**, *21* (2), 244–249.

58. Baldrick, P.; Bamford, D.G. A Toxicological Review of Lactose to Support Clinical Administration by Inhalation. Food Chem. Toxicol. **1997**, *35*, 719–733.

59. Gopinath, C.; Prentice, D.E.; Lewis, D.L. *Atlas of Experimental Toxicological Pathology*; Gresham, G., Ed.; MTP Press Ltd.: Lancaster, 1987; 24–42.

60. Burger, G.T.; Renne, R.A.; Sagartz, J.W.; Ayres, P.H.; Coggins, C.R.E.; Mosberg, A.T.; Hayes, A.W. Histologic Changes in the Respiratory Tract Induced by Inhalation of Xenobiotics: Physiologic Adaptation or Toxicity? Toxicol. Appl. Pharmacol. **1989**, *101*, 521–542.

61. Gaworski, C.L.; Dozier, M.M.; Gerhart, J.M.; Rajendran, N.; Brennecke, L.H.; Aranyi, C.; Heck, J.D. Thirteenth-Week Inhalation Toxicity Study of Menthol Cigarette Smoke. Food Chem. Toxicol. **1997**, *35* (7), 683–92.

62. Thompson, D.O. Cyclodextrins-Enabling Excipients: Their Present and Future Use in Pharmaceuticals in Drug Formulations. Crit. Rev. Ther. Drug Carrier Syst. **1997**, *14* (1), 1–104.

63. Adeyeye, C.M.; Barabas, E. Povidone. *Analytical Profiles of Drug Substances and Excipients*; Brittain, H.G., Ed.; Academic Press: San Diego, 1993; 22, 555–683.

64. Renwick, A.G. Saccharin: A Toxicological Evaluation. Comments Toxicol. **1998**, *3* (4), 289–305.

65. Rowe, V.K.; Wolf, M.A. *Patty's Industrial Hygiene and Toxicology*; Clayton, G.D., Clayton, F.E., Eds.; Interscience: New York, 1982; 3844–3852.

66. Alexander, D.J.; Libretto, S.E. An Overview of the Toxicology of HFA-134a (1,1,1,2-Tetrafluoroethane). Hum. Exp. Toxicol. **1995**, *14* (9), 715–720.

67. Vogel, F.R.; Powell, M.F. A Compedium of Vaccine Adjuvant and Excipients. Pharm. Biotechnol. **1995**, *6*, 141–228.

68. Napke, E.; Stevens, D.G.H. Excipients and Additives: Hidden Hazards in Drug Products and in Product Substitution. Can. Med. Assoc. J. **1984**, *131*, 1449–1452.

69. Golightly, L.K.; Smolinske, S.S.; Bennett, M.L.; Sutherland, E.W., III; Rumack, B.H. Pharmaceutical Excipients. I. Adverse Effects Associated with Inactive Ingredients in Drug Products. Med. Toxicol. **1988**, *3*, 128–165.

70. Barband, A. Place of Excipients in Drug-Related Allergy. Clin. Rev. Allergy. Immunol. **1995**, *13*, 253–263.

71. Gebhart, F. Drugs' Inactive Ingredients Drawing Government Attention. Drug Top. **1997**, *141*, 18S–20S.

72. Scott, A.W. Non-Medicinal Ingredients. Drug Safety **1990**, *5* (1), 95–100.

73. Johnston, K.R.; Govel, L.A.; Andritz, M. Gastrointestinal Effects of Sorbitol as an Additive in Liquid Medications. Am. J. Med. **1994**, *97* (2), 185–191.

74. Kumar, A.; Aitas, A.T.; Hunter, A.G.; Beaman, D.C. Sweeteners, Dyes and Other Excipients in Vitamin and Mineral Preparations. Clin. Pediatr. **1996**, *35* (9), 443–450.

75. Altimaras, J.; Nieto-Hernandez, T.; Buitrago, F. Presence of Excipients in Pharmaceutical Products in Three Sources of Therapeutic Information. Aten. Primaris. **1996**, *18* (4), 190–193.

76. Monkhouse, D.C.; Lach, J.L. Drug-Excipient Interactions. Can. J. Pharm. Sci. **1972**, *7* (2), 29–46.

77. Reimer, K.; Fleischer, W.; Brogmann, B.; Schreier, H.; Burkhard, P.; Lanzendorfer, A.; Gumbel, H.; Hoekstra, H. Povidone-Iodine Liposomes—An Overview. Dermatology **1997**, *195* (Suppl 2), 93–99.

78. Ishida, O.; Maruyama, K. Transferring Conjugated PEG-Liposomes as Intracellular Targeting Carrier for Tumor Therapy. Nippon Rinsho **1998**, *56* (3), 657–662.

79. Naidoo, R. Examining Excipients. Pharm. Cosmet. Rev. **1997**, *24*, 23 25–27.

80. Zhao, Z.; Leong, K.W. Controlled Delivery of Antigens and Adjuvants in Vaccine Development. J. Pharm. Sci. **1996**, *85*, 1261–1270.

81. Rubinstein, A.; Tirosh, B.; Baluom, M.; Nassar, T.; Friedman, M. Rationale for Peptide Drug Delivery to the Colon and the Potential of Polymeric Carriers as Effective Tools. J. Controlled Rel. **1997**, *46*, 59–73.

82. Medicines Order. *The Medicines (General Sale List) Order*, The Stationery Office Ltd.: London, 1997.

P

PHARMACEUTICAL QUALITY ASSURANCE MICROBIOLOGY

Anthony M. Cundell
Wyeth-Ayerst Pharmaceuticals, Pearl River, New York

INTRODUCTION

The pharmaceutical microbiologist has an important role in product development, manufacturing process development, ensuring control of microorganisms in the manufacturing environment and routine raw material, inprocess material, and product testing. The involvement of experienced microbiologists in each stage of the product life cycle is important to maintain product quality. Typically, microbiologists are involved in formulation, manufacturing process development, and specification-setting decisions that can prevent microbial contamination of pharmaceutical products. In this chapter, the appropriate level of involvement of microbiologists in establishing the quality, purity, efficacy, and safety of pharmaceutical and over-the-counter drug products is discussed, and areas of future challenge to the pharmaceutical microbiologist are explored.

A review of the regulations governing the pharmaceutical industry outlines some of the formal responsibilities of the microbiologist. The U.S. Federal Regulations that govern the pharmaceutical industry are called Current Good Manufacturing Practices (cGMPs). The U.S. Federal Food and Drug Administration (FDA) was mandated by the 1962 New Drug Amendments to the U.S. Federal Food, Drug, and Cosmetics Act to promulgated regulations that had the force of law to ensure that drug manufacturers maintain the safety, identity, strength, quality, and purity of their products. These official regulations were published in the Federal Register, September 29, 1978, as 21 C.F.R. Parts 211 through 226 (1) as they pertain to drugs. The regulations are considered minimum requirements, and failure to comply with any part of the regulations during the manufacture, processing, packaging, or holding of a drug renders that product to be adulterated under section 501(a) (2) (B) of the Federal Food, Drug, and Cosmetics Act. The drug product as well as the persons who are responsible for the failure to comply with the regulations may be subject to regulatory action.

Sections of the cGMPs most pertinent to the pharmaceutical microbiologist include Subpart B Organization and Personnel: 211.22 Responsibilities of the Quality Control Unit and 211.25 Personnel Qualifications; 211.113 Control of Microbiological Contamination; and Subpart I Laboratory Controls: 211.167 Special Testing.

The cGMP regulations require that a pharmaceutical manufacturer have an independent quality control unit responsible for approval or rejection of all components, drug product containers, closures, in-process materials, packaging materials, labels and drug products, review of production records for possible error, and investigation of manufacturing deviations. The quality control unit also reviews and approves all specifications and procedures impacting on the products and leads the investigation of manufacturing deviations and product failures.

The quality control unit must have access to an adequate testing laboratory to aid in the approval of the materials under its control. One of these laboratory facilities would be suitably equipped and staffed to conduct microbiological testing. The quality control unit need not manage the microbiology laboratory. The laboratory could be run by quality control, research and development, even manufacturing or could be a contract testing laboratory, provided it meets cGMP requirements and is responsive to the needs of the quality control unit. Although not a regulatory requirement, it is industry practice to use the audit process as a tool to ensure that the microbiology laboratory meets all regulatory requirements and internal company policies.

The 211.25 Personnel Qualifications requirement is that all persons engaged in all phases of pharmaceutical manufacture have the education, training, and experience to enable them to do their job and have a working knowledge of the cGMP regulations that applies equally to laboratory personnel. For example, bench microbiologists should have a bachelor of microbiology or allied life sciences degree and be adequately trained in the laboratory procedures and testing documentation conducted in the microbiology laboratory. They need to be assigned responsibilities in keeping with their level of skill and experience. Microbiologists with supervisory or managerial responsibilities need training in supervisory skills, scheduling, budgeting, laboratory investigations, technical report writing, pharmaceutical products, and the manufacturing processes. They need to understand the requirements of the quality control unit and ensure that

Encyclopedia Pharmaceutical Technology

the unit is supplied with quality test results in a timely and cost-effective manner. Since the pressures to manufacture, test, and release products in a timely manner can be considerable, they need to work well under pressure and enjoy team work.

The educational background of bench microbiologists, supervisors, and managers is now even more important, given, the current transition from classic to nucleic acid-based testing methods.

The demands of microbiological testing require that the core educational background of the staff, supervisors, and managers be in microbiology. Training and experience in aseptic techniques are necessary. According to the author, the skill sets of chemists, pharmacists, and even biologists do not allow them to readily act effectively as microbiologists without extensive training. Course work invaluable to the pharmaceutical microbiologist includes:

- Isolation, enumeration, and identification of bacteria and fungi;
- Pathogenic microbiology;
- Microbial physiology and biochemistry;
- Introductory chemistry including organic, inorganic, and physical chemistry and quantitative analysis;
- Introductory physics;
- Introductory mathematics;
- Introductory pharmaceutical manufacturing;
- Introductory statistics and probability; and
- Written and oral expression with emphasis on technical report writing.

According to 211.113, Control of Microbiological Contamination, pharmaceutical manufacturers need written procedures describing the systems designed to prevent objectionable microorganisms in both nonsterile and sterile drug products. All sterilization processes used to manufacture parenteral drugs need to be validated.

There needs to be a laboratory test for each batch of drug product to determine that the product conforms to specification, including the identity and strength of each active ingredient, before release. Where sterility and/or pyrogen testing are conducted on specific batches of short-lived radiopharmaceuticals, such batches may be released before completion of this testing, provided such testing is completed as soon as possible. The 211.165 Testing and Release for Distribution regulation states that there be appropriate laboratory testing, as necessary, of each batch of drug product required to be free of objectionable microorganisms. This implies that each and every batch of product need not undergo microbial evaluation.

The pharmaceutical microbiologist in product development plays a major role in bring safe products to the market. Typically, the Research & Development (R&D)

microbiologist is found in the analytical development group. The role of the R&D microbiologist is to develop and validate the microbial tests that may be applied to the new pharmaceutical products to confirm that they are not contaminated with an excessive number of microorganisms or objectionable microorganisms that may infect patients or degrade the quality of the product during its shelf life.

These tests include compendial tests for microbial limits, sterility, bacterial endotoxins, and antimicrobial effectiveness.

These compendial tests need to be developed and qualified for each new products before the phase II clinical trials, which involve 100–200 subjects. Considering the large investment to bring a new pharmaceutical drug product to market, i.e., an estimated U.S. $ 250–500 million, it is important not to jeopardize the future of a new product or the subjects in the clinical trial by administering a drug product that may be contaminated with objectionable microorganisms. However, for the results of microbial testing to have any meaning, the microbial test needs to be qualified as suitable for use with each product.

Many dosage forms have active pharmaceutical ingredients or contain preservative systems that may inhibit the recovery of any bioburden associated with the product. This inhibition may be overcome by inactivating the active ingredient or preservative system with neutralizing agents, dilution to overcome the inhibition, or a combination of both strategies. U.S. Pharmacopoeia chapters 51, Antimicrobial Effectiveness Test; 61 Microbial Limit Tests; and 71 Sterility Testing (2) contain specific instructions on how to qualify the test for use with specific pharmaceutical drug products and the microorganisms to use during this process.

A major concern for Pharmaceutical Operations, i.e., Materials Management, Manufacturing, and QA, is whether the R&D microbiologists develop microbial tests that meet the QA requirements of robustness, simplicity, and standard for ease of testing for the routine release testing of pharmaceutical products. Good communications between the two microbiology groups will ensure the smooth technology transfer of the most appropriate tests from R&D to QA.

During development of the manufacturing process, an experienced microbiologist should be consulted as to the potential for microbial contamination of the product. Issues may include the selection of appropriate pharmaceutical ingredients, the ability of the manufacturing steps to control microbial contamination, the validation of sterilization processes, the cleaning and sanitization of process equipment, the adequacy of the water system, the holding times for intermediates, the training of personnel, and the design of the packaging.

CURRENT MICROBIOLOGICAL TESTING PRACTICES

The compendial microbial methods currently used for the routine testing of pharmaceutical products are generally conservative and may be used to referee disputes concerning the microbial contamination of pharmaceutical products. The USP is recognized as an official compendium by the U.S. Federal Food, Drug and Cosmetic (FDC) Act. USP standards are used to determine the identity, strength, quality, and purity of pharmaceutical articles. The "General Chapters" section of the USP includes requirements for tests and assays and is numbered from 1 to 999, whereas general information include chapters 1000 and above. Of particular interest to the pharmaceutical microbiologist are USP 24 Informational Chapters 1116, Microbiological Evaluation of Clean Rooms and other Controlled Environments; 1111 Microbiological Attributes of Pharmaceutical Articles; 1225, Validation of Compendial Methods; and 1231, Water for Pharmaceutical Purposes (3). Testing chapters pertinent to pharmaceutical microbiology and their JP and Ph. Eur. counterparts are as follows:

USP Chapter 51, Antimicrobial Effectiveness Test

Antimicrobial preservatives are substances added to multiuse nonsterile liquids, ointments, and creams and sterile injectable products to protect them from microbial contamination that may be introduced inadvertently during use of the product (postmanufacturing).

The test for antimicrobial effectiveness is used to demonstrate the effectiveness of any added antimicrobial preservative(s). Compendial references include USP 24 Chapter 51, Antimicrobial Effectiveness Test; JP XIII, General Information 3, Preservatives-Effectiveness Tests; and Ph. Eur. 3rd Ed., Biological Tests, 5.1.3., Efficacy of Antimicrobial Preservation.

USP Chapter 61, Microbial Limits Tests

The tests for microbial limits and recommendations for microbial quality criteria of raw materials, excipients, drug substances, and pharmaceutical products have been established in pharmacopoeial compendia for over 30 years. These tests are listed in USP 24, Chapter 61, Microbial Limits Tests; Ph. Eur. 3rd Ed., Biological Tests

2.6.12 and 2.6.13, Microbial Contamination of Products not Required to Comply with the Test for Sterility (Total Viable Count, Tests for Specified Micro-Organisms); and JP XIII 30, Microbial Limit Test.

USP Chapter 71, Sterility Test

The sterility test is applicable for determining whether drug substances, preparations, or other pharmacopeial articles are sterile as defined by the compendial method. A satisfactory result indicates only that no contaminating microorganisms have been found in the sample examined according to the conditions of the test. Therefore, the result is a function of the efficiency of the adopted sampling plan. Compendial references to sterility testing include USP 24, Chapter 71, Sterility Tests; Ph. Eur. 3rd Ed., Biological Tests 2.6.1., Sterility; and JP XIII 45, Sterility Test.

General Informational Chapter 1116, Microbiological Evaluation of Clean Rooms and Other Controlled Environments

The microbiological monitoring of air, surfaces, and personnel in facilities used for sterile pharmaceutical manufacturing is discussed in the USP 24 Informational Chapter 1116, Microbiological Evaluation of Clean Rooms and Other Controlled Environments. The chapter also covers the design and implementation of a microbiological monitoring program and suggests monitoring frequencies and microbiological acceptance criteria.

USP Informational Chapter 1231, Water for Pharmaceutical Purposes

Types of water and methods and specifications for testing them are listed in USP Informational Chapter 1231, Water for Pharmaceutical Purposes. The USP also references Standard Methods for the Examination of Water and Waste Water (APHA), 19th Ed., for information on specific test methods (4).

Other Testing Methods

New microbial testing methods are being introduced in the marketplace based on advanced technologies. These new tests represent improvements in the timeliness and qualify of testing.

The USP 24 General Notices states that alternative methods may be used to determine that products comply with the pharmacopeial standards for advantages in accuracy, sensitivity, precision, selectivity, and adaptability to automation or computerized data reduction or for any other special circumstances. Such alternative or automated methods must be validated; however, when disputed, the compendial method is conclusive because it is the official or referee test. In addition, USP Chapter 61, Microbial Limit Tests, states that automated methods may be substituted, provided they are validated and give equivalent or better results, whereas USP Chapter 71, Sterility Tests, states that alternative procedures may be used to demonstrate that an article is sterile, provided the results obtained are at least of equivalent reliability.

It is not required to have prior FDA approval to use an alternate method to a compendial test. According to 21 CFR 314.70, "Supplements and Other Changes to an Approved Application," the addition or deletion of an alternate analytical method does not require prior approval and may be filed in the Annual Product Report. However, we would need to document the equivalency of the alternate method to the regulatory or compendial test method and the validation report must be available for an FDA investigator to inspect at our manufacturing site. Where the test method is particularly novel it may be advisable to include the test in an NDA supplement so the FDA can review the new method and your company can get prior FDA approval before the new test method is implemented.

ORGANIZATION OF THE PHARMACEUTICAL QUALITY ASSURANCE MICROBIOLOGICAL TESTING LABORATORY

The microbiology manager has three major roles in the QA organization. They are: 1) establishing, staffing, and running the microbiological testing laboratory; 2) monitoring pharmaceutical ingredients, water for pharmaceutical purposes, the manufacturing environment, and finished products submitted to the laboratory to demonstrate control of microbial contamination of the pharmaceutical products manufacturing at the site; and 3) providing microbiological expertise to the QA organization to prevent microbial contamination.

The microbiology manager is responsible for the establishment of a suitably constructed and equipped laboratory; recruiting and retaining an appropriately educated, skilled, and experienced staff; and operating the laboratory in compliance with all company policies and cGMP regulations. The needs of business require that microbial testing be conducted in a timely manner so that products can be released to the market.

The microbiological monitoring program established at a pharmaceutical manufacturing site will depend on the range of products manufactured there. Typical microbiological monitoring programs for release testing and environmental monitoring for nonsterile and sterile product manufacturing sites are given in Table 1.

The general procedures to be followed when selecting a microbial testing strategy a Marketed Product Stability Program for pharmaceutical drug products based on cGMP and compendial requirements and commitments made in regulatory filings are tabulated.

These approaches are in general accord with C.F.R. 21, Parts 211.113 Control of Microbiological Contamination, Section (b); 211.137, Expiration dating; 211.167, Special Testing Requirements Section (a); U.S.P. 24 51, Antimicrobial Effectiveness Testing, 61, Microbial Limit Tests, 71, Sterility Tests, 85, Bacterial Endotoxin Tests, General Informational Chapter 1151, Pharmaceutical Dosage Forms and the June,1998, Draft FDA Stability Testing of Drug Substances and Drug Products guidance document (5). The tests that may be included in the program include: 1) antimicrobial effectiveness testing, 2) Microbial Limit Testing, 3) Sterility Testing, 4) Bacterial Endotoxin Testing, and 5) Container-closure Integrity Testing.

Table 2 outlines a possible testing policy.

Antimicrobial Effectiveness Testing

The following principles apply to preservative effectiveness testing in a pre- and postmarketed product stability program.

1. The selection of the preservative system for multiuse new products is the responsibility of the R&D formulation group. Typical shelf specifications are 80 to 120% LS. The appropriate preservative system for the particular formulation should be demonstrated to be effective by microbial challenge down to at least 75% and preferably to 50% of the target concentration. It is recommended that during development, the product be formulated with preservative concentrations of 100, 75, and 50% of the labeled amount and be subjected to Antimicrobial Effectiveness Testing to determine the lowest effective preservative concentration.

2. The release and shelf-life specifications are established based on both the premarketed stability data for the preservative system concentration and the Antimicrobial Effectiveness Test results.

3. If the study outlined in item 1 was not conducted during product development, it is recommended that QA and/or the Technical Services groups undertake a study

Table 1 Sample microbiological monitoring programs

Dosage form	Monitoring	Frequency
Tablets and capsules	Pharmaceutical ingredients	Periodic after history is established; rule accept on supplier certificate of analysis
	Purified water	Loop daily and taps weekly
	Manufacturing environment	Quarterly
	Products	Periodic after history is established owing to low water activities of tablets and capsules
Topicals, otics, vaginal and rectal products	Pharmaceutical ingredients	As above
	Purified water	Loop daily and taps weekly
	Manufacturing environment	Weekly or monthly
	Products	Routine for products with high water activity; periodic after history is established for product with low water activity
Nasal sprays and inhalants	Pharmaceutical ingredients	As above
	Purified water	Loop daily and taps weekly
	Manufacturing environment	Daily or weekly
	Products	Routine for products with high water activity; periodic after history is established for product with low water activity
Injectable products, ophthalmic products, and inhalation solutions	Pharmaceutical ingredients	As above
	Purified water	Loop and taps daily
	Manufacturing environment	Every shift in critical aseptic processing areas
	Products	Every batch with the exception of terminally sterilized products approved for parametric release

Table 2 Sample testing policy

Dosage form	Microbial test	Testing plan	Test intervals[a]
Tablets, powder-, and liquid-filled capsules	Microbial Limit Test (TAMC and TCYMC only)	Test development, scale-up, and validation batches only	0, 6, 12, 24, and 36 months.
Topical liquids, ointment, and creams	Microbial Limit Test (TAMC and TCYMC only); USP Antimicrobial Effectiveness Test (AET) for multi use products	Aw <0.75 test development, scale-up and validation batches only; Aw >0.75 all batches on stability for Microbial Limit and first three batches for Antimicrobial Effectiveness (AE)[b]	0, 6, 12, 24, and 36 months; 0, middle of stability period and expiry
Vaginal creams and suppositories	Microbial Limit Test (TAMC and TCYMC only) and AET	As above	0, 6, 12, 24, and 36 months
Rectal creams and suppositories	As above	As above	0, 6, 12, 24, and 36 months
Nasal sprays	As above	As above	0, 6, 12, 24, and 36 months
Inhalation sprays and aerosols	As above	As above	0, 6, 12, 24, and 36 months
Ophthalmic ointments and solutions	Sterility Test, Container-Closure Integrity (CCI) and AET	Test all batches on stability with the exception of the first three batches for AE[b]	0, 12, 24, and 36 months
Injectables and Inhalation solutions	Sterility Test; CCI and AET; Bacterial Endotoxin Test	Test all batches on stability with the exception of the first three batches for AE[b]	0 only; 0, 12, 24, and 36 months; 0 and expiry only

[a]Time intervals suggested in the 1998 Draft FDA Stability Guide. Add additional annual test intervals if the expiration dating exceeds 36 months.
[b]Justify using a stability-indicating preservative assay only at all time intervals as a substitute for the USP Antimicrobial Effectiveness Test by confirming preservative efficacy at 50, 75, and 100% of label claim.

to justify the current specifications and the elimination of routine Antimicrobial Effectiveness Testing in the Stability Program.

4. All preservative systems for both parenteral and nonsterile dosage forms should meet the 3 log reduction at 14 days for bacteria., i.e., USP category I requirements. EP/BP Antimicrobial Effectiveness Testing would be run only if requested by the Marketing Group.

5. Preservative effectiveness testing should be included at the 3-, 12-, 24- and 36-month intervals for pilot validation batches or of the first three commercial batches of a new product only.

6. With subsequent batches, chemical assays would be used only to confirm the preservative level, because the effectiveness during shelf life is being demonstrated. If the formulation is changed, the preservative effectiveness must be verified with at least one batch throughout the shelf life.

7. The choice of additional challenge organism used in formulation development will be determined by 1) the range of activity of the preservative system, i.e., if a preservative system has reduced activity against *Pseudomonas* spp., additional organisms from these genera or related genera could be added to the challenge organisms; 2) the organisms considered objectionable for that product and dosage form; and 3) the frequency of isolation of organisms from the manufacturing environmental and product monitoring.

8. Repeat challenges should be limited to the evaluation of preservative systems that cannot be improved because of formulation difficulties and limitation owing to the intended site of use and products that may be misused during multiple consumer use.

Microbial Limit Test

The following principles apply to microbial limit testing within a pre- and post marketed product stability program.

1. The inclusion of a routine Microbial Limit Test in a marketed product stability protocol willl depend on the pharmaceutical dosage form. Typically, the test would be used for only nonsterile products, particularly oral liquids, nasal sprays; and topical liquids, lotions and creams that have a sufficient water activity to support the growth of microorganisms. In contrast, tablets, powder and liquid-filled capsules, topical ointments, vaginal and rectal suppositories, nonaqueous liquids, and inhalation aerosols with a water activity too low to allow for the product to support the growth of microorganisms would not be routinely tested.

2. To establish a Microbial Limit Testing history, all development, clinical, scale-up, and process validation batches of new nonsterile dosage forms would be tested to verify that the pharmaceutical ingredients, manufacturing process, and packaging do not contribute the bioburden of the product. After the testing history has been established, products with a water activity below 0.75 should not include Microbial Limit Testing in the stability protocol.

Sterility Testing

The following principles apply to sterility testing within a pre- and postmarketed product stability program.

1. All injectable and ophthalmic products with the exception of terminally sterilized product subject to parametric release should undergo Sterility Testing at release.

2. Because the sterility assurance of an injectable or ophthalmic product is established through media fill or sterilization validation for aseptically filled and terminally sterilized products, respectively, Sterility Testing has been included in past stability protocols as a measure of container-closure integrity of the product throughout its shelf life. If there is a continued need because of previous regulatory commitments to include Sterility Testing in a protocol, then testing at release and expiry is recommended.

3. Whenever possible, Container-Closure Integrity Testing should be substituted for Sterility Testing as recommended in the draft FDA Stability Guide.

Bacterial Endotoxin Test

The following principles apply to Endotoxin Testing in a pre- and postmarketed product stability program.

1. All injectable products should be tested for endotoxin at release.

2. Because, in the absence of bacterial growth in the product, the endotoxin level will not increase on storage during shelf life Bacterial Endotoxin Testing is not indicated in the stability protocol. If there is a continued need to include Endotoxin Testing in a protocol, then testing at release and at expiry is recommended

Container-Closure Integrity Test

The following principles apply to integrity testing a pre- and postmarketed product stability program.

1. The integrity of the container-closure system as a microbial barrier should be assessed using an appropriately sensitive and adequately validated Container-closure Integrity Test.
2. One of a number of physical Container-closure Integrity tests may be selected and validated against the Bacterial Liquid Immersion Test. The Physical Leak Test should be correlated to bacterial ingress.
3. The selection of the physical Container-closure Integrity Test method should be made after consideration of the container-closure type, the performance criteria, and the available validated test methods.
4. Test methods described in the literature include bubble, helium mass spectrometry, liquid trace (dye), head space analysis, vacuum/pressure decay, weight loss/-gain, and high-voltage leak detection (6).
5. The number of samples tested should reflect the sampling requirements provided in the USP 71 Sterility Tests.
6. The testing should be performed annually and at expiry.

The third role of supplying microbiological expertise to the Manufacturing and Quality Assurance is important because depth of experience in microbiology may be lacking in these organizations in some companies.

Typically, the management of these organizations is trained in chemistry, engineering, business, or pharmacy. Microbiologists should assist management to exercise the best judgment on microbiological issues. Given that the ultimate objective is to prevent microbial contamination of pharmaceutical and OTC drug products, it is important that pharmaceutical microbiologists be knowledgeable in the areas of microbiological testing, infectious diseases, compendial changes, regulatory issues, product formulation, and manufacturing processes so they can give credible advice.

A common practice in microbiological testing is that pharmaceutical ingredients and products are tested without full consideration of their significance. Sometimes, all raw materials purchased and product manufactured are submitted to the microbiology laboratory and tested, or if materials for testing are selected, insufficient judgment is made with respect to whereas materials are tested, i.e., materials with a low risk of microbial contamination are tested whereas materials with a high risk are not tested. Testing should always reflect the risk of microbial contamination. An important managerial tool to rationalize the microbial testing is the reduced testing program. An important aspect of a reduced pharmaceutical ingredient monitoring program, after supplier audit and an evaluation of the equivalency of results from the supplier's certificate of analysis and the manufacturing site microbiological testing laboratory, is an understanding of the potential risk of the microbial contamination of a pharmaceutical ingredient, manufacturing environment, or pharmaceutical product. The microbiologist needs to make a judgment based on the source of the ingredient, how it is processed, its water activity and testing history, and how it is used in formulations to determine whether periodic microbial monitoring to ensure that the testing laboratory confirms the microbial results reported on the supplier certificate of analysis is justified.

IMPLEMENTATION OF NEW MICROBIOLOGICAL TESTING METHODS

Opportunities exist to implement new microbiological testing methods as alternatives to the compendial methods to improve the quality of the test results and reduce the product-release cycle time. Selection of candidate test methods, proof of concept studies, assay development and validation, regulatory approval, and implementation of the new microbiological testing methods are major issues that need to be addressed to take advantage of the new technologies. These new methodologies offer significant improvements in terms of the speed, accuracy, precision, specificity, etc., with which testing can be performed.

The majority of testing performed today relies on century-old methods based on the recovery and growth of microorganisms using solid or liquid microbiological growth media. This is true in part because these methods can be very effective and have a long history of application. However, they are often limited by slow microbial growth rates, unintended selectivity for microorganisms that grow in nutrient-rich culture media, and the inherent variability of microorganisms in their response to culture methods. Despite the limitations of current methods, acceptance of new and potentially superior methods is often slow because of the understandable conservative tendency of microbiologists.

This may be in part attributable to a lack of clear guidance regarding the demonstration of their equivalence to existing methods acceptable to regulatory agencies and validation of the equipment associated with the new methods.

Considerable guidance can be found regarding the validation of chemical methods that is applicable to microbial testing. Examples include USP Chapter 1225, "Validation of Compendial Methods," and a recent publication by the International Conference on Harmonization (ICH), "Validation of Analytical Methods." These publications provide very specific instructions regarding the demonstration of new analytical chemistry methods and their equivalence to existing methods.

When instrumentation is developed for existing microbiological methods to automate sample handling, result reading, or data management, it is not difficult to demonstrate the equivalency of the alternate method using guidelines developed for chemical assays because the test remains essentially the same. In a similar manner, when a new technology continues to rely on the measurement of microbial growth (e.g., impedance, ATP bioluminescence, or other metabolic changes in a microbial culture), equivalence can be readily demonstrated. However, when a new method is based on novel technology without direct ties to the existing method (e.g., microbial identification by rRNA amplification versus patterns of biochemical reactions, or counting fluorescent-labeled bacterial cells instead of colony-forming units on an agar plate), demonstration of equivalency may require a new application of the validation principles, although the method provides higher quality results. The principles that can be applied to the validation of new microbiological testing methods are found in the recently published PDA Technical Report (7).

For convenience, the technologies are divided into growth-based technologies, viability-based technologies, cellular component or artifact-based technologies, and nucleic acid-based technologies as shown in Table 3.

IMPLEMENTATION OF A RISK-BASED MICROBIOLOGICAL TESTING PROGRAM

A testing program to be both cost-effective and to control microbial contamination must reflect the potential risks of microbial contamination of pharmaceutical drug products. A knowledge of product formulation, manufacturing processes, packaging, and ability of product to support microbial growth can be applied to develop rational specifications and a monitoring program that reflects the potential risk to the consumer of each dosage form. This emphasis on potential risk will require that the pharmaceutical microbiologist most closely addresses products having a higher potential for microbial contamination to best serve the needs of pharmaceutical companies and end-user of products.

A recall is a removal or correction of a marketed product by the pharmaceutical manufacturer when that product violates the laws enforced by the FDA. Unlike the FDA's other methods for achieving compliance such as seizures and court-ordered injunctions, recalls are almost always voluntary. The FDA cannot order a company to recall a product, except in some cases involving infant formulas, biological products, and devices that present a serious health hazard. A class I recall occurs when there is a reasonable probability that the use of or exposure to a violative product will cause serious adverse health consequences or death. A class II recall occurs when use of or exposure to a violative

Table 3 Classification of new biological testing methods

Testing method	Example technologies
Growth-based technologies	ATP bioluminescence Impedance/conductivity Hydrophobic grid membrane filter methods
Viability-based technologies	Direct epifluorescent filter Microscopy membrane laser Scanning fluorescence cytometry Fluorescence flow cytometry
Cellular component or artifact-based technologies	GL chromatographic fatty acid profiles MALDI-TOF mass spectrometry Fluorescence antibody techniques Enzyme-linked immunosorbent assay *Limulus* amebocyte lysate-endotoxin assay
Nucleic acid-based technologies	Nucleic acid probe Polymerase chain reaction–DNA amplification 16S rRNA sequencing techniques Automated riboprinting

Table 4 Summary of the nonsterile pharmaceutical and OTC products recalled, 1991–1998, by the FDA because of microbial contamination problems as to class of recall ($n = 46$)

Year	Recalls	Class I	Class II	Class III	% Pseudomonads
1998	7	2	3	2	57
1997	5	1	2	2	60
1996	4	1	2	1	75
1995	4	0	3	1	0
1994	8	1	4	3	38
1993	9	0	6	3	44
1992	6	1	5	0	33
1991	3	0	0	3	0
1991–98	46	6	25	15	38

(From Ref. 8.)

product may cause temporary or medically reversible adverse health consequences or in which the probability of serious adverse health consequences is remote. A class III recall occurs when use of or exposure to a violative product is not likely to cause adverse health consequences. When the center receives the Recall Report from the FDA district office, it evaluates the health hazard presented by the product and categorizes it as class I, II, or III. The classification is determined by an ad hoc Health Hazard Evaluation Committee made up of FDA scientists chosen for their expertise. Classification is done on a case-by-case basis, considering the potential consequences of a violation.

The average number of recalls per annum for microbial contamination of nonsterile pharmaceutical and OTC drug products is six (Table 4). The emphasis on waterborne Gram-negative bacteria of the species *Bulkholderia (Pseudomonas) cepacia* (nine recalls), *P. putida* (three recalls), *P. aeruginosa* (three recalls), *Pseudomonas* spp. (two recalls), and *Ralstonia (P.) pickettii* (one recall) is notable and reflects the concern for bacteria capable of growth in liquid oral dosage forms that overwhelm the preservative system.

Analyses of the underlying probable cause of the microbial contamination of nonsterile products suggest to this researcher that they are the result of: 1) microbial contamination of water for pharmaceutical purposes, 2) the use of pharmaceutical ingredients with higher microbial counts, 3) failure of preservative systems to protect liquid products, 4) microbial contamination during the manufacturing process, or 5) improper use and/or storage of the products during shelf life.

The suitable water systems, the appropriate management of the equipment, and the appropriate monitoring programs were emphasized during past regulatory inspections so that manufacturers have no excuse for using unsuitable ingredient water during the manufacture of products. In most cases, pharmaceutical ingredients of high microbial quality can be selected for pharmaceutical manufacturing. More emphasis must be placed on preservative systems during formulation development, especially on opportunities to optimize a preservative system by manipulating the pH, surfactant properties, and water activity of formulations to make them unsuitable for microbial growth. A comprehensive discussion of the application of water activity determination in product formulation and the development of microbial monitoring programs has appeared recently in the literature (9).

A greater appreciation of the ability of different manufacturing steps to affect the microbial content of a formulation by formulators, microbiologists, and manufacturing personnel would be helpful. Exposure of pharmaceutical products to high humidity during shelf life may increase the water activity of a liquid, ointment, cream, or tablet, allowing for the growth of microorganisms on the surface of the product. Thus suitable packaging and appropriate patient handling of the drug product are important.

FUTURE TRENDS IN THE MICROBIOLOGICAL TESTING LABORATORY

The four major trends in the pharmaceutical microbiological testing laboratory are: 1) the drive to introduce new microbiological testing technologies, 2) the organization of the laboratory based on work stations, 3) the use of computerized information management systems, and

4) the change of emphasis from testing to prevention of microbial contamination.

If the pioneering German bacteriologist Robert Koch visited a routine microbiological testing laboratory in the pharmaceutical, biotechnology, or medical device industry, he would recognize that most of our techniques were first developed or used in his laboratory during the last three decades of the 19th century.

These methods include the fixing and staining of bacterial cells on glass slides for microscopic examination and photomicroscopy; growth of colonies in solid media; streaking for isolation of pure cultures in solid media; the use of agar-agar as a support for microbiological media in Petri dishes; serial dilution and plating in solid media to enumerate the microbial population in water; monitoring bacteria in the air; the classification of bacteria by their cellular morphology and differential staining; sterilization of microbiological media by filtration or steam sterilization; disinfectant testing; and aerobic and anaerobic incubation. A major trend is under way in the pharmaceutical QA microbiological testing laboratory in which the classic microbiological cultural methods developed in the late 19th century will be replaced for routine testing by biochemical, fluorescent cytometric, and nucleic acid-based techniques. Although many companies have developed instruments to automate the running or miniaturizing of existing test methods, technological improvements are progressing rapidly, with new methods based on fluorescent laser detection and nucleic acid-based detection. The future of microbiological testing is in the commercialization of automated specific detection methods that will reduce our reliance on cultural methods. This should result in routine testing with significantly shorter test cycle times and higher quality results.

Organization of the microbiology laboratory is more and more frequently based on self-directed work teams, with the widespread use of workstations based on the newer testing technologies. The workstations will reflect the product mix manufactured by the pharmaceutical company. This will rationalize the deployment of lab personnel and the flow of materials and information through the laboratory. Common workstations include: 1) sample receipt and distribution, 2) water for pharmaceutical monitoring, 3) microbial limits of pharmaceutical ingredients and nonsterile products, 4) antimicrobial effectiveness testing, 5) microbial identification, 6) environmental monitoring, 7) growth promotion, 8) sterility testing, 9) microbial assay of antibiotics and vitamins, and 10) information management.

Each testing workstation manned by trained laboratory personnel who will rotate through the laboratory contain dedicated testing equipment interfaced to LIMS, media, reagents, and supplies, with accompanying SOPs, training documents, and calibration and preventative maintenance logs. Test specimens would be received, inspected, and entered into the information management system via keyboard or by bar code scanning and distributed to the appropriate workstation. The results would be generated at the workstations, and test results will be reviewed and transferred from the workstation into LIMS.

In conclusion, the important role of the microbiologists in the pharmaceutical industry must be reinforced. The need to involve experienced microbiologists in each stage of the product life cycle to maintain product quality, safety, and efficacy is highlighted in this chapter.

REFERENCES

1. Current Good Manufacturing Practices in Manufacturing, Processing, Packaging of Drugs. *21 C.F.R. §211 through §226.*
2. Testing Chapters: Antimicrobial Effectiveness Testing, Ch. 51; Microbial Limit Tests; Ch. 61; Sterility Tests, Ch. 71. *U.S.P. 24.*
3. Informational Chapters: Microbiological Evaluation of Clean Rooms and Other Controlled Environments, Ch. 1116; Microbiological Attributes of Pharmaceutical Articles, Ch. 1111; Pharmaceutical Dosage Forms, Ch. 1151; Validation of Compendial Methods, Ch. 1225; Water for Pharmaceutical Purposes, Ch. 1231. *U.S.P. 24.*
4. Eaton, A.; Clesceri, L.S.; Greenberg, A.E. *Standard Methods for the Examination of Water and Wastewater*, 19th Ed.; American Public Health Association, 1998.
5. FDA Draft Guidance for Industry. *Stability Testing of Drug Substances and Drug Products*; FDA: Washington, DC, June 1998.
6. *Pharmaceutical Packaging Integrity.* PDA Technical Report No. 27, April 1998.
7. *The Evaluation, Validation and Implementation of New Microbiological Testing Methods.* PDA Technical Report No. 33, April 2000.
8. *The Gold Sheet;* FDC Reports, Inc.: Chevy Chase, MD, Jan. 1991.
9. Friedel, R.R.; Cundell, A.M. The Application of Water Activity Measurement to the Microbiological Attributes Testing of Nonsterile OTC Drug Products. Pharm. Forum **1998**, *25* (2), 6087–6090.

BIBLIOGRAPHY

Baird, R.M. *Microbial Quality Assurance in Cosmetics, Toiletries and Nonsterile Pharmaceuticals*; Taylor and Francis: London, 1996.

Clontz, L. *Microbial Limit and Bioburden Tests*; Interpharm Press: Buffalo Grove, IL, 1998.

Denyer, S.; Baird, R. *Guide to Microbiological Control in Pharmaceuticals*; Ellis Horwood: London, 1990.

Difco Laboratories. *Difco Manual*, 11th Ed.; Division of Becton Dickinson & Company: Sparks, MD, 1998.

FDA Bacteriological Analytical Manual, 8th Ed.; AOAC International: 1998.

FDA Guide to Inspections of Microbiological Quality Control Laboratories, July 1993.

Murray, P.R. *Manual of Clinical Microbiology*; ASM Press: Washington, DC, 1995.

Olson, W.P. *Automated Microbial Identification and Quantation*; Interpharm Press: Buffalo Grove, IL, 1998.

Russell, A.D.; Hugo, W.B.; Ayliffe, G.A.J. *Principles and Practices of Disinfection, Preservation and Sterilization*, 3rd Ed.; Blackwell Science Ltd.: Oxford, U.K., 1999.

Willig, S.H.; Tuckerman, M.M.; Hitchings, W.S. *Good Manufacturing Practices for Pharmaceutiucals*; Marcel Dekker, Inc.: New York, 1982.

PHARMACOPEIA STANDARDS: *EUROPEAN PHARMACOPOEIA* [a]

Agnès Artiges

European Directorate for the Quality of Medicines (EDQM), Council of Europe, Strasbourg, France

INTRODUCTION

The purpose of a pharmacopoeia and particularly of the *European Pharmacopoeia* is to promote public health by providing common standards recognized by health authorities and all those concerned with the quality of medicines. Such standards are to be of appropriate quality as a basis for the safe use of medicines by patients and consumers. Their existence facilitates the free movement of medicinal products in Europe and ensures the quality of medicinal products exported from Europe.

As noted previously (1), the status of the *European Pharmacopoeia* is based on the existence of an international convention created under the aegis of the Council of Europe (2). The primary characteristics and goals of the *European Pharmacopoeia* are described in this convention. The following chapters present its evolution in the area of the quality of medicines to fullfil the needs of European and International Harmonisation for both regulatory authorities and industries.

THE THIRD EDITION AND ITS CHARACTERISTICS

The *European Pharmacopoeia* plays an important role, not only for well known products manufactured for many years but also for new types of medicines by:

1. elaborating unified specifications for substances from different sources;
2. publishing validated methods;
3. providing common reference substances;
4. producing monographs that are clear (description of impurities controlled by the monograph); and
5. providing a forum for users and other organizations.

The 3rd Edition was published in 1996, and an annual supplement is published in midyear (supplement 1998 in 1997, supplement 1999 in 1998, supplement 2000 in 1999).

[a] Throughout the text of this article, the European spelling *pharmacopoeia* is used

All new editions of the *European Pharmacopoeia* now include the year their texts entered into force in their titles; this should make them easier to use. Each supplement is cumulative and replaces the previous one and includes on average approximately 100 new monographs and more than 150 revised texts.

It is available in both print and electronic versions that are published by the European Directorate for the Quality of Medicines (EDQM) of the Council of Europe (3).

Content

The 3rd Edition includes an introductory chapter (General Notices), a chapter on general methods and texts and reagents, followed by monographs in alphabetical order on all type of substances used in the preparation of drug products including excipients (4) and herbal drugs (5). A few monographs on preparations such as radiopharmaceuticals, vaccines, and some hormone preparations (e.g., insulin) are included. There is also a monograph on homeopathic preparations.

The last chapter of the book is focused on general monographs for dosage forms.

We comment here on the main categories of monographs.

General notices

This introductory chapter summaries the characteristics of the legalities of the *European Pharmacopoeia* and gives the principal definitions. It explains the legal significance of each part of the *Pharmacopoeia* and the role of each section of a monograph. This chapter is essential reading when reference must to be made to a monograph of the *European Pharmacopoeia*.

Monographs on chemical substances

All such monographs are presented in the same format, which is described in the "Technical Guide for the Elaboration of Monographs of the European Pharmacopoeia" (6). This guide contains the same concepts as those defined in Community guidelines, which themselves contain the guidelines adopted jointly at the international level, via the International Conference on Harmonisation (ICH). Hence, the two guidelines on analytical validation

P

are integrated into this technical guide and are even supplemented by specific chapters on the principal methods of analysis (such as spectrophotometry and liquid chromatography, etc.).

The ICH guideline on impurities is also integrated into the technical guide, and the guideline on residual solvents has been integrated into a general chapter of the *European Pharmacopoeia*.

European Pharmacopoeia monographs on chemical substances have therefore been modified in connection with these changes for better control of the impurity profile of substances produced by numerous manufacturers using diverse methods of synthesis. Each revised or new monograph now contains an impurities section at the end that describes the list of impurities known to be detectable by the monograph. Whenever necessary, this impurities section consists of two parts: the list of qualified impurities and the list of impurities that can be detected analytically by the monograph but that are not qualified according to the ICH guideline. The list of impurities includes both the chemical nomenclature and the graphic formula, which makes the section easier to use.

In addition, the presentation of monographs has now been supplemented by the establishment of a procedure for Certification of Suitability of Monographs (see later), thus fully satisfying the requirements of Directives 75/318/EEC for medicines for human use (7) and 81/852/EEC for medicines for veterinary use (8), and the EU note for guidance, "Summary of Requirements on Active Substances in Part II of the Dossier" (9).

Finally, the identification section of these monographs has also been modified to clarify the presentation of monographs that give alternative series of identification tests. The status of this section is clearly defined in the general notices. They specify that when there are two identification series, the first, more complete series will be fully implemented by manufacturers of active substances; the second series is an alternative with less sophisticated analytical methods, but its use requires that the product be traceable from the manufacturer (which carried out all the methods described in the first series) to the user.

Monographs on biological substances

All types of biological medicines such as hormones (10), vaccines for human use (11–13), vaccines for veterinary use (14), and blood products (15) are covered in specific monographs.

Important conceptual changes have also been made to the establishment of this type of monograph to satisfy the needs of Community licensing and to keep up with progress in that field. The following changes merit special attention:

1. the introduction of a production section;
2. the replacement, whenever possible, of tests involving the use of laboratory animals; and
3. the elimination of the test for abnormal toxicity and its replacement by the test for endotoxins (LAL).

The role of the production section is described in the General Notices. The requirement described in this section applies primarily to the manufacturers of the substance in question and to the body of inspectors responsible for checking compliance with the prescriptions of the *European Pharmacopoeia* or with the information given in the licensing dossier.

The tests described in this section cannot necessarily be carried out on the finished product by outside analysts, as with the tests described in the sections on identification, tests, and assay. Nevertheless, they play a major role to guarantee the quality of the substances in question.

In recent years, the European Pharmacopoeia Commission has elaborated a policy of replacing the use of animals in quality control testing of medicines in parallel with the application of the corresponding Convention of the Council of Europe. A sizeable program has been set up to apply the 3-R concept (refine, reduce, replace). To this end, the Council of Europe, represented by the EDQM, and the Commission of the European Communities are now working on an extensive standardization programme (16) to set up collaborative studies to:

1. evaluate, develop, and improve the standardization of test methods for biologicals;
2. prepare European working standards;
3. apply the 3-R concept to replace the use of laboratory animals; and
4. continue the harmonization of test methods for biologicals in Europe and, if possible, the world, in collaboration with the World Health Organization (WHO).

These collaborative studies have led to the establishment of European working standards. Consequently, the titers and potencies of biological products will be expressed with respect to the same reference standard. The existence of reference standards recognized throughout Europe enables national control agencies and manufacturers to avoid costly duplications of work on secondary standards that could otherwise lead to disagreements.

Collaborative studies are also aimed at the validation of alternative reference methods. Comparative tests of various analytical or operating procedures can be used to validate a method of choice or even to establish a close correlation among a method involving tests on animals, an in vitro biological method, and a method based on physicochemical analysis, thus facilitating the replacement of one method by another in the future.

To facilitate communication and understanding among partners, the results of collaborative studies are published in special issues of *Pharmeuropa* (17).

Monographs on dosage forms

A new chapter has been introduced that brings together all the monographs describing dosage forms, and whenever necessary, the monographs have been supplemented by technological tests and harmonized so that the chapter constitutes a coherent whole.

It should be noted that this chapter and the previous EEC guideline published in 1991 on "authorised terms for dosage forms, routes of administration and containers" were revised together by the European Pharmacopoeia Commission at the request of the Commission of the European Communities.

Thus, both tasks were carried out in parallel and coherently: on the one hand, the revision of all the monographs of the *European Pharmacopoeia* and on the other hand, the revision of the Community guideline on authorized terms.

This guideline has been replaced by a revised version elaborated in the *European Pharmacopoeia* called "Standard Terms" (18); it has been translated into all the languages of the Community. Indeed, not only does this document give the terms in the languages of the Community, but it also includes terms in the national languages of several delegations to the *European Pharmacopoeia* that are not members of the European Union but that also wish to provide a translation in their language. The revised document will therefore list terms in 21 European languages (Bulgarian, Croatian, Czech, Danish, Dutch, English, Finnish, French, German, Greek, Hungarian, Icelandic, Norwegian, Italian, Polish, Portuguese, Slovak, Slovenian, Spanish, Swedish, and Turkish).

This relatively large document, which covers both human and veterinary medicines, is published as a special issue of *Pharmeuropa*. The first version was published in November 1996, then revised yearly; the next revised version was published in February 2000. This will produce a harmonious and coherent whole that can be used throughout Europe. The terms are mandatory for applications and summaries of product characteristics for EU centrally and decentrally authorized products.

The list can be extended on request if justification is provided. A specific procedure has been set up (18). Forms are also available on the EDQM Web site.

General monograph on methods of manufacture

Another way to address the quality of the monograph is to apply the concept developed in the 1980s and 1990s, which is that one cannot control the quality of a product simply by testing the finished product. One is controlling only what is being sought. The quality of a product has to be included from the very beginning and maintained throughout the manufacturing process.

To avoid repeating key points of policy in its texts, the European Pharmacopoeia Commission's current approach is to prepare general monographs that cover all the specific monographs but that can also be referred to for substances that have no monograph in the *European Pharmacopoeia*. Thus, new general monographs on the method of production have been prepared, such as the monograph "Products of Fermentation" (19), "Products of r-DNA Technology" (20), and "Products with Risk of Transmitting Spongiform Encephalopathy" (21).

In addition, compilers of the *European Pharmacopoeia* have been asked to add a production section to the monographs for specific substances. The production section gives key points but not all the details that refer to a specific manufacturer. In addition to the production section in specific monographs, general concepts in line with new ICH guidelines are also identified. Such details are described in the application for a Certificate of Suitability by each manufacturer (see above).

Revision of Monographs

The European Pharmacopoeia Commission is very attentive to updating its monographs. Revisions can be made at any time if a pharmacopeial or licensing authority requests a particular change. The European Pharmacopoeia Commission has defined its criteria for revision of monographs when:

1. poor quality products appear on the market;
2. a request is made in connection with the certification procedure;
3. there is a public health risk (presence of nonqualified impurities, risk of falsification, etc.);
4. the analytical methods are no longer adequate;
5. certain tests in a monograph are no longer applicable;
6. reagents are unavailable; and
7. the patent is close to the expiry date.

In addition, a more extensive program of revisions corresponding to new developments in methods is carried out every 5 years. Such revisions take account of new guidelines from the licensing authorities and the need for harmonization within families of substances.

How and by Whom Are Texts Elaborated?

The *European Pharmacopoeia* is elaborated by a Commission made up of national delegations from regulatory authorities, with decisions requiring a unanimous vote by the delegations (2). (Today, the Convention has been signed by 27 European countries[b] including all EU members and by the EU Commission itself. Nine other European[c] and eight Non-European countries are also observers.)

The monographs are elaborated by the groups of experts appointed by the European Pharmacopoeia Commission based on proposals by the national delegations. The experts participating in this work are from industry, universities, and national control laboratories.

The *European Pharmacopoeia* has progressively been replacing the national pharmacopoeias. Nevertheless, we need to emphasize the major role played by the national pharmacopoeia secretariats in the elaboration of the common European work. Indeed, they are in the best position to identify national needs and to organize:

1. consultation with the pharmaceutical, chemical, and biological industries that manufacture in their territories (consolidated comments sent to the secretariats of the *European Pharmacopoeia*);
2. consultation with other governmental organizations impacted by the work (e.g., ministries of industry or agriculture); and
3. collaboration with other departments in medicine-related agencies such as licensing authorities, national control laboratories, and inspection.

Finally, the national secretariats play an important role in providing information at the national level on how European rules are elaborated, and any national text is prepared and revised in compliance with the *European Pharmacopoeia*.

Before final adoption, all texts and monographs are published in *Pharmeuropa* for 4 months of public inquiry. For European countries, comments should be sent through the national secretariat; for non-European companies, comments should be sent directly to the EDQM-Council of Europe (B.P. 907, F-67029 Strasbourg Cedex, France). *Pharmeuropa*, the users's forum is a quarterly publication prepared and published by the EDQM.

[b]Austria, Belgium, Bosnia-Herzegovina, Croatia, Cyprus, Czech Republic, Denmark, Finland, France, The Former Yugoslav Republic of Macedonia, Germany, Greece, Hungary, Iceland, Ireland, Italy, Luxembourg, the Netherlands, Norway, Portugal, Slovakia, Slovenia, Spain, Sweden, Switzerland, Turkey, the United Kingdom of Great Britain and Northern Ireland and the European Union.
[c]Albania, Bulgaria, Estonia, Latvia, Lituania, Malta, Poland, Rumania, Ukraine.

Implementation by the Parties

The *European Pharmacopoeia* is a common supranational document that supersedes any national texts for the signatory parties. A common implementation date is adopted by the European Pharmacopoiea Commission for each supplement/edition (or individual text for rapid revision) that enters into force by means of a resolution of the Council of Europe/Public Health Committee.

Although the signatory parties are bound by the texts and specifications of the *European Pharmacopoeia* published by the Council of Europe, they are free to implement then in ways that are compatible with their technical, legal, and administrative regulations. Thus, different procedures are used in different countries.

A majority of members implement directly the volume published by the Council of Europe; others continue to issue a national pharmacopoeia that republishes all or some of the harmonized European texts translated if necessary into the national language or style (Austria, Bulgaria, the Czech Republic, Germany, Greece, Hungary, Portugal, Spain, Switzerland, and the United Kingdom). In all cases, it is the European text that is implemented and made legally binding, superseding any translation in cases of doubt.

CERTIFICATION OF SUITABILITY OF MONOGRAPHS

This unprecedented procedure for Certification of Suitability of Monographs of the *European Pharmacopoeia* was established a few years ago (22). Why? For centuries, pharmacopeias were designed to be references that were complete and obligatory in themselves. However, in the 20th century, with the growth of world trade, the EU licensing authorities found that they increasingly had to ask manufacturers to provide in their licensing applications complete details on the synthesis of their product to demonstrate that the product was suitably controlled by the *European Pharmacopoeia* monograph. Thus, it then became apparent that it was absolutely necessary to reconsider how this essential information could be made available to those who needed it without duplication of work by the *Pharmacopoeia* compilers and licensing authorities.

To solve this problem, it was necessary not only to adapt the content of monographs to new needs but also to set up a procedure for Certification of Suitability that would establish a link between licensing and the *Pharmacopoeia* in this area.

As noted above, the content of monographs was supplemented where relevant by production and impurities sections to make these monographs more complete and clear (23).

The certification procedure is a complement and bridge between the public standards described in the *European Pharmacopoeia* and the need to prepare a file for licensing. This procedure is a result of much common discussion and agreement among the partners concerned. It was in fact made to measure its collaboration not only with the European regulatory authorities so that they could rely on it totally and recognize unreservedly its validity but also with the industries so that they could be absolutely sure of the protection of industrial property.

On the basis of the data collected during the elaboration of the monograph and the specific data provided by a specific manufacturer on a specific substance, the Certificate of Suitability certifies that both types of data make it possible to conclude that the quality of the substance corresponds to the quality defined in the *European Pharmacopoeia* monograph.

In principle, a certificate can be granted for any substance (active substances, excipients) such as organic or inorganic substances, substances produced by fermentation as indirect gene products, and products with risk of TSE for which a monograph published in the *European Pharmacopoeia* exists. Excluded, however, are biological substances such as proteins, products obtained from human tissues, vaccines, blood products, and preparations.

The certificate, granted for 5 years, may include additional specifications (methods and limits) when monograph specifications do not fully control the purity of the substance (e.g., control of residual solvents, specific impurities, etc.).

The procedure is described in Resolution AP-CSP (99) 4, together with the content of the file to be submitted (24). This procedure, lists of certificates granted (420 at the end of January 2000), and lists of assessors are published regularly in *Pharmeuropa* and on the EDQM Web site (http://www.pheur.org, direct link with the Certification Unit: cert@pheur.org).

Certificate of Suitability Versus European Drug Master File

Although both procedures have the same aim and require dossiers with exactly the same contents, the certification procedure is especially designed to cover substances for which there is a monograph in the *European Pharmacopoeia,* whereas the European Drug Master File procedure is aimed at substances for which there is no *European Pharmacopoeia* monograph.

In conclusion, a procedure makes it possible to avoid duplication of work not only by manufacturers of raw materials and manufacturers of medicines (finished products) when they prepare licensing dossiers but also by the licensing authorities and pharmacopoeia authorities when they assess these dossiers. Differences among the various European licensing authorities in approach and assessment of compliance with *European Pharmacopoeia* monographs are also avoided, and clearer communications are facilitated. Finally, the procedure allows *European Pharmacopoeia* monographs to be constantly updated to keep up with new developments in the world market.

TOWARD THE 4TH EDITION

European Pharmacopoeia authorities have decided to publish a fourth edition. For this purpose, both the technical guide and the style guide have been revised, and more general monographs have been or will be elaborated.

Technical Guide

This guide (6) is intended for the experts who participate in the elaboration of *European Pharmacopoeia* monographs; it establishes the general rules to be followed. This document specifies the philosophy behind the choice of techniques for identification testing of a substance and for the determination of the limit contents of impurities and the methods used to detect them.

The 2nd Edition had been revised particularly to be in line with the ICH guideline. The 3rd Edition was published in February 2000.

Style Guide

This is an internal guide for professionals of the *European Pharmacopoeia* and for the secretariat to make the monograph style more uniform in English and French, the two official languages of the Council of Europe. The aim is to provide the means of drafting clear, unambiguous texts. The style, which will appear in the 4th Edition, is more telegraphic than that used in the 3rd Edition.

General Monographs

The fundamental goal of the *European Pharmacopoeia* is to promote the harmonization of standards for medicinal products in the member states and in view of this, the European Pharmacopoeia Commission considers that it is desirable and possible to extend the scope of general monographs to encourage a convergence of approach by licensing authorities and thus avoid future difficulties in harmonization.

The *European Pharmacopoeia* contains a number of general monographs that cover categories of products defined by the:

1. presentation of the medicinal product (dosage form monographs such as "Tablets," "Eyedrops," etc.);
2. nature of the product (radiopharmaceutical preparations, vaccines for human use, etc.); and
3. methods of production (products of fermentation, products of rDNA technology, products with TSE risks).

New general monograph on substances for pharmaceutical use (active substances and excipients) (25) had been prepared to include in the *European Pharmacopoeia* the ICH guideline for residual solvents and the ICH qualification threshold for new impurities without revising each individual monograph concerned. In addition, the monographs are used to simplify the *Pharmacopoeia* requirements concerning sterility, bacterial endotoxins, and pyrogens tests contained in individual monographs. However, because it is the policy of the Commission to add these requirements whenever it is considered to be appropriate, a general regulation will now replace the regulations in individual monographs.

Furthermore, the monograph gives a definition of the terms "active substance" and "excipients"; it explains the policy of the Commission concerning polymorphic forms, active substances of special grade, processing of active substances with and without the addition of excipients, and the two sets of identification tests that may be contained in a monograph.

The status of these general monographs will be defined in the chapter, "General Notices."

International Harmonization with USP and JP

This review will not be completed without highlighting the close relationship that has developed since 1990 among the European, Japanese, and U.S. pharmacopoeias. They cofounded the Pharmacopoeial Discussion Group, which is working diligently for harmonization at the world level and which participates in the ICH program (26–28). This group meets regularly (twice a year) in Europe, Japan, and the United States. Approximately 50 monographs on excipients and 20 general methods of analysis proposed by national associations of manufacturers of pharmaceutical products have been selected for convergence and harmonization in the three pharmacopoeias.

A special section of the *European Pharmacopoeia* quarterly journal *Pharmeuropa* is now dedicated to this activity. Joint open conferences organized by the five pharmacopoeias, in Verona, Italy (on biotechnology products in April 1993); St. Petersburg, FL (on excipients in 1994); Barcelona, Spain (on microbiological tests in 1996); Seville, Spain (on dosage-form pharmacotechnological tests in 1998); and Strasbourg, France (on new trends in biologicals in 1999) regularly brought together specialists from all over the world.

REFERENCES

1. Artiges, A. Pharmacopoeial Standards: European Pharmacopoeia. *Encyclopedia of Pharmaceutical Technology*, 1st Ed.; Swarbick, J., Boylan, J., Eds.; Marcel Dekker, Inc.: New York, 1995; 12, 53–71.
2. Convention on the Elaboration of a European Pharmacopoeia. *European Treaty*; Series No. 50, Council of Europe: Strasbourg, France.
3. *European Pharmacopoeia*, 3rd Ed., Council of Europe: Strasbourg, France.
4. Artiges, A. Excipients: Aspects Réglementaires. Thérapie **1999**, *54*, 15–19.
5. Artiges, A. Pharmacopoeial Standards for Herbal Medicinal Products in Europe, Proceedings of the 5th ESCOP International Symposium.
6. *Technical Guide for the Elaboration of Monographs*, 3rd Ed.; Council of Europe: Strasbourg, France, December 1999; Pharmeuropa Special Issue.
7. *The Rules Governing Medicinal Products in the European Union*, 5, Council Directive 75/318/EEC, Amended.
8. *The Rules Governing Medicinal Products in the European Union*, 5, Council Directive 81/852/EEC, Amended.
9. *The Rules Governing Medicinal Products in the European Union*, Guidelines on Medicinal Products for Human Use, 3.
10. Charton, E. Hormones: The Role of the European Pharmacopoeia. Alternatives to Animals in the Development and Control of Biological Products for Human and Veterinary Use. Dev. Biol. Standardisation (Basel, Karger) **1999**, *101*, 159–167.
11. Castle, P. Policy and Progress of the European Pharmacopoeia in the Use of Alternatives of Animal Testing in Vaccine Production and Quality Control. *Alternatives to Animal Testing in the Production and Quality Control of Vaccines: Present Practice and Prospectives*; RIVM: Bilthoven, 1992; 41–52.
12. Castle, P. Alternatives to Animal Testing: Achievements and Recent Developments in the European Pharmacopoeia. *Development in Biological Standardization*; PEI: Langen, 1994; 86, 21–29.
13. Castle, P. The European Pharmacopoeia and Humane End Points, International Conference on the Use of Humane Endpoints in Animal Experiments for Biomedical Research, Zeist, NL, November, 23–25, 1998; 86.

14. Artiges, A. The Role of Pharmacopoeias. *Veterinary Vaccinology*; Part. 9, Pastoret, et al. Eds.; 708–711.

15. Artiges, A. Quality and Safety of Plasma Products: Control Authority Batch Release Within the Countries of the European Union and Economic Area, Proceedings of EPFA-EAPPI, 5th Annual European Regulatory Affairs Symposium, Vienna, Austria, September, 29–30, 1998, 108–110

16. The Biological Standardisation Programme. *Pharmeuropa Bio*; Council of Europe: Strasbourg France, July 1996; Special Issue 96–1.

17. *Pharmeuropa Bio* Council of Europe: Strasbourg, France, Special Issues 96-1, 96.2; Special Issues 97-1, 97.2; Special Issue 98.1; Special Issues 99–1, 99.2.

18. Standard Terms: Pharmaceutical Dosage Forms, Routes of Administration, Containers. *Pharmeuropa*; Council of Europe: Strasbourg, France, January 2000; Special Issue.

19. *European Pharmacopoeia,* 3rd Ed.; Monograph No. 1468, 1111–1112, Supplement 2000.

20. *European Pharmacopoeia,* 3rd Ed.; Monograph No. 0784, 1435–1438.

21. *European Pharmacopoeia,* 3rd Ed.; Rapid Implementation Monograph No. 1483, Resolution AP-CSP (99) 5, Pharmeuropa 12 (2).

22. Helboe, P. Certification Procedure: Purposes and Procedure The Feed-Back Mechanism, Proceedings of the International Conference on the Vision of the European Pharmacopoeia in the 21st Century, July, 1997, Pharmeuropa, Special Issue, Workshop Session II.

23. Artiges, A. Certification of Suitability of Monographs of the European Pharmacopoeia: Summary of Objectives and Scope of the Procedure, Proceedings of the International Conference, Berlin, Germany, November 11–12, 1999, Pharmeuropa Special Issue 2000.

24. Certification of Suitability of Monographs of the European Pharmacopoeia. Pharmeuropa **2000**, *12* (2), Resolution AP-CSP (99) 4.

25. Monographs on "Active Substances" And "Excipients." Pharmeuropa **1999**, *11* (3).

26. Artiges, A. International Harmonisation of Pharmacopoeias ICH, Proceedings of the First International Conference on Harmonisation, Brussels, 1991, 143–152, Topic 3: Pharmacopoeias.

27. Halperin, J.A. Session 5, Harmonisation of Pharmacopoeial Monographs and Methods, Proceedings of the Second International Conference on Harmonization (ICH), Orlando, 195–217.

28. ICH Guideline on Specification on Drug Substances and Drug Products, (Q6A-paragraph 2.8).

PHARMACOPEIAL STANDARD: *JAPANESE PHARMACOPOEIA*[a]

Mitsuru Uchiyama
Japan Pharmacists Education Center, Tokyo, Japan

INTRODUCTION

The *Pharmacopoeia of Japan* (JP), which dates back to 1886, provides the official standards and test methods for regulating the properties and quality of drugs important for medical treatment. In general, the standards set forth in the JP affect not only those articles included in the JP but all drugs and drug products in circulation in Japan. The JP has played an important role in ensuring and improving drug quality through all phases of development, application, evaluation, distribution, inspection, and consumption before and after manufacture. Thus, revision of the Pharmacopoeia must occur within a structure and system that are unaffected by bias and undue influence of any party for its standards to be recognized as credible and reliable for ensuring drug quality.

FRAMEWORK

The JP is currently published by the Ministry of Health and Welfare through the Committee on the JP of the Central Pharmaceutical Affairs Council (CPAC), pursuant to the Pharmaceutical Affairs Law. The Committee on the JP includes a subcommittee consisting of 12 advisory panels, each concentrating on one of the following subject areas: principles of revision; selection of articles; medicinal chemicals; biologics and biologicals; general test methods; physical test methods; biological test methods; preparations; crude drugs; nomenclature; and pharmaceutical excipients.

The panel members are scientists from national institutes, universities, and prefectural laboratories, who are appointed every 2 years by the Minister of Health and Welfare. As a rule, a panel member is not appointed for more than 8 consecutive years. A certain number of liaison members from industry serve on 10 of the 12 panels. In contrast, the panels responsible for nomenclature and selection of articles do not include liaison members from industry.

[a]Throughout the text of this article, the European spelling *pharmacopoeia* is used.

The JP secretariat is part of the Evaluation and Licensing Division of the Pharmaceutical and Medical Safety Bureau of the Ministry. The secretariat works under the scientific and technical support of the National Institute of Health Sciences (NIHS). The Pharmaceutical and Medical Safety Bureau is a new organization, established in July 1998, as a result of a reorganization of the former Pharmaceutical Affairs Bureau. The CPAC itself will be terminated in January 2001 in response to further reorganization of government offices and will resume operation as the council responsible for both pharmaceutical and food sanitation affairs.

REVISION PROCESS

Revision Cycle

The Pharmaceutical Affairs Law stipulates that the JP be revised at least once every 10 years. However, beginning in 1967, because of the rapid progress and changes in medicinal and pharmaceutical research and development, the revision cycle of the JP has been reduced to once every 5 years. Thus, the 11th and 12th editions were published in 1986 and 1991, respectively, and the most recent edition, the 13th, was published in April 1996. An English version has subsequently been released. In the event of a discrepancy between the Japanese original and its English translation, the former is considered official. The English version of the JP is available through Yakuji Nippo, Ltd. (Kanda Izumicho 1, Chiyoda, Tokyo 101-8648, Japan) (1).

A supplement, the first in JP history, was published in October 1988, 2 years after publication of the 11th edition. The Ministry published two supplements to the 12th edition in October 1993 and December 1994, respectively. The first and second supplements to the 13th edition became available in December 1997 and December 1999, respectively. The 14th edition will be published in April 2001.

Principle of Revision

The current fundamental goal and most important consideration of the JP revision, to which the evaluation of new drug quality also conforms, is to obtain pharmaceuticals of consistent quality, but not necessarily of higher purity, to provide maximum benefit to the consumer. The specification should be sufficient to at least identify and ensure adequate quality, and the analytical procedures should be accurate and easy to perform. However, a proper balance between accuracy and ease of use needs to be maintained to allow for this analysis. Although extremely high accuracy is not necessary, the limit of detection or the limit of quantitation, as well as the recovery in purity tests, should be validated by sufficient data. Hazardous chemicals should be avoided, and experimental testing on animals should be minimized.

Revision Process

Proposals for revision of the JP monographs or test methods can be submitted through the JP secretariat in the Pharmaceutical and Medical Safety Bureau by any concerned individual or organization. The proposed monograph, either for a new entry or for a revision, is then drafted by a panel member or an industry professional. New or revised test methods are handled in a similar manner. To accomplish this, panels are assisted by the Japanese Pharmaceutical Manufacturers' Associations of Tokyo and of Osaka, the Japan Pharmaceutical Excipients Council, the Crude Drugs Association of Tokyo, the Federation of Crude Drugs Association of Japan, and the Japanese Society of Hospital Pharmacists.

The draft monograph is reviewed by the two panels on Medicinal Chemicals. The Panel on Medicinal Chemicals I adopts new entries, whereas the Panel on Medicinal Chemicals II revises existing monographs. The drafts for traditional medicines and pharmaceutical excipients are reviewed by the Panel on Crude Drugs and the Panel on Pharmaceutical Excipients, respectively. Nomenclature and chemical structures are examined by the Panel on Nomenclature once the draft monograph has been finalized. Additions or changes to the three general test methods (chemical, physical, and biological) and reagents are addressed by the corresponding panel for each test method.

The establishment of reference standards is adopted at the suggestion of the related panels after due consideration of the opinion of the NIHS, which is directly responsible for establishing those reference standards in cooperation with the Society of Japanese Pharmacopoeia. The Society of Japanese Pharmacopoeia (Shibuya 2-12-19, Shibuya, Tokyo 150-0002, Japan) is a nonprofit private organization that carries out activities in support of MHW administration and regulation of pharmaceuticals. The Society plays several roles and, in particular, makes reference standards available including a part of the pharmacopoeial reference standards. It also distributes *Pharmacopoeia* and related informative documents, such as the *JP Forum*, and convenes public meetings and symposia.

JP Forum

After finalization by each panel, all drafts for revision are opened for public comment through the *JP Forum*, a vehicle for notification and commentary (2). The *JP Forum* is published quarterly by the Society of Japanese Pharmacopoeia under the auspices of the JP secretariat. The *JP Forum* was first published in January 1992 as a medium for both local and international communication. It will continue to provide a more open revision process for the JP and announce revisions and future directions of the JP committees. The *JP Forum* is issued in Japanese, primarily for domestic users, but articles related to the international community and commentary will be issued in English concurrently with the Japanese version. Therefore, we anticipate that the *JP Forum* will aid in the process of international harmonization and will promote a better understanding of and increased trust in the JP.

After comments are reviewed and changes are made, the revised draft is reviewed by the Committee on the Japanese Pharmacopoeia and then by the Executive Committee of the Central Pharmaceutical Affairs Council before it is submitted for publication in the JP.

Time Frame

Regarding the interval between new drug approval and the adoption of a pharmacopoeial monograph in Japan, the first monograph generally does not appear in the JP until publication of the outcome of its reevaluation. The term of current reevaluation for a new active ingredient is generally 6 years after approval. The reevaluation period is needed to ensure the safety and efficacy of new drugs. For a particular drug, such as an orphan drug, the reevaluation period is 10 years after approval.

In addition, not all new drugs are listed in the JP, and the Panel on the Selection of Articles decides which drugs should be listed based on their importance in terms of medical treatment. The innovators sometimes do not want their drugs to be listed in the JP, concerned that such listings will trigger the introduction of generic brands. As a result, the JP contains fewer monographs than does the *U.S. Pharmacopeia–National Formulary* (USP–NF). The JP 13 contains 1292 monographs, which is approximately one-third the number included in the USP–NF.

SIZE, SCOPE, AND PRESENTATION OF JP 13

The JP 13 is a single volume comprising two parts. Part 1 includes 824 monographs of widely used drug substances and their preparations, for 532 organic and inorganic chemical ingredients, 187 preparations (single-ingredient dosage forms), 91 antibiotics, 11 radiopharmaceuticals, and 3 medicinal gases. Part 2 includes 468 articles, for 106 mixed preparations, 132 pharmaceutical excipients, 172 traditional (crude) drugs, 30 biologics, 21 miscellaneous substances of plant or animal origin, and 7 surgical dressings. In addition to the monographs, the JP contains sections on notices of importance, rules, standards, test methods, and apparatus commonly applicable to any of its articles. There are 131 JP Reference Standards.

The General Notices in the JP provide specific definitions. Some examples are:

1. definitions of standard temperature, ordinary temperature, room temperature, and lukewarm as 20, 15–25, 1–30, and 30–40°C, respectively;
2. the term "in vacuum" indicating, unless otherwise specified, a pressure not exceeding 15 mm Hg;
3. the tabulation of the degree of coarseness or fineness of a powdered medicine; and
4. that in the monograph, if the upper limit of the content of an ingredient determined by assay is not specified but expressed simply as not less than a certain percentage, 101.0% should be understood as the upper limit.

The dosage form monograph in the JP has a section on methods of preparation that refers to the General Rules for Preparations, which gives definitions, methods of preparation, storage, and other information on 28 different dosage forms. The insoluble particulate matter test, included as a subsection in the section Injection, is currently under discussion among pharmacopoeia compilers for the purpose of establishing international harmonization.

The General Tests, Processes, and Apparatus section contains 60 test methods, such as fluorometry and electrometric titration, dissolution and disintegration tests, content uniformity, and a bacterial endotoxin test. Qualitative tests, reagents and test solutions, and standard solutions are also included. The Infrared Reference Spectra of 124 chemical entities are included in an appendix and will be updated in subsequent editions. The JP monographs consist of the drug name, description, identification, rational values, and purity, as well as special tests if any, tests for preparation, and assay. No specifications are given in the JP 13 under monographs for antibiotics, biologics, and radiopharmaceuticals. Howerer, they may be found in Requirements for Antibiotic Products of Japan 1993 (formerly the Japanese Minimum Requirements of Antibiotic Products) and other corresponding compendia.

NONPHARMACOPOEIAL STANDARDS FOR PHARMACEUTICALS IN JAPAN

In addition to the *Pharmacopoeia of Japan*, there are several compendia, standards, and guides in which Japanese standards for pharmaceuticals are published. The following are standards determined for drugs under the provisions noted above, although the specifications and standards included in these compendia are mandatory. As presented above, some of the monographs in the following compendia are quoted in the JP:

- Requirements for Antibiotic Products of Japan 1993 (to be combined with the JP; antibiotic substance will be included in JP 14, due for release in 2001, and antibiotic products will be compiled in the Japanese Pharmaceutical Codex)
- Minimum Requirements for Biological Products
- Minimum Requirements for Blood Grouping Sera
- Radiopharmaceutical Standards

Several standards are published as advisements from the Pharmaceutical Affairs Bureau that set voluntary standards for various pharmaceuticals to ensure and improve their quality. Because the standards and specifications in these guides are voluntary, there is no overlap with the JP monographs.

- Japanese Pharmaceutical Codex, which contains monographs for 682 active ingredients and 175 pharmaceutical preparations (3)
- Japanese Pharmaceutical Excipients, which has 206 monographs for pharmaceutical excipient
- Standards for Crude Drugs
- Standards for Raw Materials for Clinical Diagnostics
- Guideline for Radiopharmaceuticals for In Vitro Diagnostics
- Insecticide Standards

IMPLICATIONS OF PHARMACOPOEIA IN THE REGULATORY PROCEDURES

Given that ensuring drug quality, efficacy, and consumer safety is a common objective for both pharmacopoeial standards and drug quality regulation, the basic policy of one is not inconsistent in principle with that of the other. The JP Committee and regulatory agencies will enjoy a more harmonious relationship as they continue to develop closer contacts, both legal and otherwise. The JP secretariat belongs to the same Pharmaceutical and Medical Safety Bureau of the Ministry that oversees new drug approvals. Furthermore, several members of the JP Committee are also members of the NIHS, which shares some responsibility for reviewing new drug applications (NDAs) and for establishing guidelines for the technical requirements governing NDAs. These guidelines are updated whenever the JP is revised. History suggests that the revision of the JP and the revision of guidelines can be easily synchronized by the regulatory agencies that work closely together (4, 5).

Conformity of NDA Dossier with Pharmacopoeia

In the NDA procedures, specifications and methodologies should be based, as much as possible, on the entries in the JP, and careful attention must be given to the terminology used in the JP. In principle, reagents, test solutions, and testing apparatus used in proposed methodologies should be the same as those in the JP. When those used are not in the JP, their quality, formulas, schematics, and dimensions, etc. are to be entered on an attached sheet in accordance with the entries for such items in the JP. If the reference standards used are not specified in the JP or by the NIHS, details of the specifications and test methods must still be attached.

How Revisions of the JP Affect Drugs in a Market

As noted above, pharmacopoeial descriptions are mandatory for all drugs, regardless of whether they are listed in the JP or are in the process of being evaluated as a new drug. It follows, therefore, that revisions of the JP will greatly influence the standards for those pharmaceuticals. Revisions of the JP affects three areas of products already on the market:

1. In cases in which a new pharmacopoeial monograph is established, the NDA holder of a particular drug is required to apply for permission to change approved items, such as specifications and test methods, to ensure that the drug satisfies the pharmacopoeial monograph. A grace period of 1.5 years is allowed under current regulations for those products already on the market to comply with new pharmacopoeial standards.

2. Whenever the standards in a monograph governing content, properties, testing, and purity limits for purity are revised, all related drug products currently in circulation must be changed to comply with the new standards in the JP. Manufacturers are responsible for ensuring that their products comply with the new standards. If these products do not comply, manufacturers are required to standardize the quality of their products to the level of the new standards within the grace period of 1.5 years.

3. When there are changes in the general notice, general rules for preparations, and specified test apparatus and test conditions in the General Tests, Processes, and Apparatus, previously approved drug products in some cases no longer conform to the specifications for which they were originally approved. For example, if the pH value of the medium in a disintegration test for a solid preparation changes, some products may yield different results under the new pH value requirement. In such a case, changing part of the formulation is recommended so that the product can comply with the specifications under the new test conditions. These situations occasionally present obstacles for later international harmonization of general test methods. It is necessary to overcome such obstacles by taking regulatory measures.

INTERNATIONAL HARMONIZATION

Role of Pharmacopoeia in the International Conference on Harmonization (ICH) Activities

The JP compilers are now part of an international harmonization effort with compilers of the *U.S. Pharmacopoeia* and the *European Pharmacopoeia*. Pharmacopoeias were taken up as an Expert Working Group (EWG) subject at an earlier stage of the ICH. However, pharmacopoeial harmonization should attempt to facilitate the international circulation of drugs and to improve drug quality rather than to simply facilitate the approval of new drugs. Furthermore, the Pharmacopoeial Discussion Group (PDG), which consists of European, U.S. and Japanese pharmacopoeia compilers and which was established in 1989 before the ICH, has held meetings periodically in parallel with the ICH to investigate a wide range of problems related to pharmacopoeia and to work on the harmonization of all the monograph specifications and general test methods according to a long-term schedule. The PDG agreed with the ICH Steering Committee in that it felt it more appropriate to present a regular progress report at each ICH meeting from the PDG rather than to retain it as an EWG topic.

PDG Policy

To date, in its action plan for harmonization, the PDG has placed a high priority on the monographs of major excipients that can be used for a number of new drug products as well as on important general test methods. The PDG has established its general policy for harmonization, in which it is shown that the goal of harmonization is to bring the policies, standards, monograph specifications, analytical methods, and acceptance criteria of pharmacopoeias into agreement. Nonetheless, the PDG recognizes that such unity may not always be obtained. Where unity cannot be achieved, harmonization means agreement based on objective comparability and a clear statement of any differences. The goal, therefore, is harmony, not unison (6).

In harmonization of analytical methods, the ideal approach is to establish a single method that satisfies the criteria for validation of all pharmacopoeias. However, this is not always possible because of a number of unavoidable differences in the technical circumstances of each nation. When different tests or methods yield the same results, provisions have already been made in the three pharmacopoeias to allow for alternative methods. In such cases, alternative methods should be subjected to validation via a comparison with the standard analytical procedure.

It is undoubtedly impossible to achieve harmonization of quality for new drugs without harmonization of compendial standards and methodology. The PDG will continue to proceed with what it believes to be the correct approach to pharmacopoeial harmonization and to contribute to advancing effective harmonization for the quality of new drugs and products.

Mutual Agreement

In the licensing process, it is essential for each regulatory authority to recognize as equivalent those test procedures that have been harmonized and adopted as validated methods by the PDG. This concept is already included in the Japanese *Guidelines for Preparation of Section B of the Documents Accompanying New Drug Applications* as of September 1995; in its assertion that, "The analytical

procedures in the Japanese Pharmacopoeia and other compendia and those which are accepted through international harmonization are considered to be validated methods."

The ICH step 4 guidelines on specifications, Q6A, October 6, 1999, notes in the item concerning pharmacopoeia that:

> References to certain procedures are found in pharmacopoeias in each region. Wherever they are appropriate, pharmacopoeial procedures should be utilized. Whereas differences in pharmacopoeial procedures and/or acceptance criteria have existed among the regions, a harmonized specification is possible only if the procedures and acceptance criteria defined are acceptable to regulatory authorities in all regions. The full utility of this guideline is dependent on the successful completion of harmonization of pharmacopoeial procedures for several attributes commonly considered in the specification for new drug substances or new drug products (7).

In this manner, key objectives of harmonization will be attained only when the PDG is able to achieve mutually agreeable standards and test methods, which provide the same conclusions when performed on the same specimens, even if they use different specifications, procedures, or reagents. We should continue to take necessary steps to deepen international cooperation and to obtain harmonized compendial standards and methodology, using the PDG as the forum for harmonization of drug quality.

CONCLUSION

This article describes the development of JP standards and their international harmonization and the relationship of the JP with drug regulatory procedures in Japan. It also notes that the JP has been playing a basic and leading role in ensuring and improving the quality of drugs in Japan. The pharmacopoeias of every country must constitute the basic technical foundation for the nation's drug quality standards and contribute to the promotion of public health by providing better pharmaceuticals to the public in the most efficient manner. The role of any pharmacopoeia is not only to define objectives for drug quality control based on the establishment of standards, test methods, and acceptance criteria, but also to provide means to implement the international harmonization of pharmaceutical regulation.

REFERENCES

1. Society of Japanese Pharmacopoeia. *The Japanese Pharmacopoeia*, 13th Ed.; Yakuji Nippo, Ltd., Tokyo, 1996; http://www.yakuji.co.jp.

2. Society of Japanese Pharmacopoeia. *Japanese Pharmacopoeial Forum*; Society of Japanese Pharmacopoeia: Tokyo, http://www.sjp.or.jp.

3. Society of Japanese Pharmacopoeia. *Japanese Pharmaceutical Codex 1997*; Jiho, Inc.: Tokyo, http://www.jiho.co.jp.

4. Pharmaceutical Review System Study Group, Ministry of Health and Welfare. *Pharmaceutical Administration in Japan*, 9th Ed.; Yakuji Nippo, Ltd.: Tokyo, 2000; http://www.yakuji.co.jp.

5. English Regulatory-Information Working Group. *Pharmaceutical Administration and Regulation in Japan (1999-12)*; Japanese Pharmaceutical Manufacturers Association: Tokyo, 1999; http://www.nihs.go.jp/mhw/koukai/1999/yakuzi/version5e.pdf.

6. Pharmacopeial Discussion Group. Policies for Harmonization of the Three Pharmacopoeias. Japanese Pharmacopoeial Forum **1995**, *4* (4), 65–67.

7. ICH Expert Working Group, *Specifications: Test Procedures and Acceptance Criteria for New Drug Substances and New Drug Products: Chemical Substances*; ICH Steering Committee: October 6, 1999; http://www.nihs.go.jp/dig/ich/qindex-e.html.

PHARMACOPOEIAL STANDARDS: THE *UNITED STATES PHARMACOPEIA* AND THE *NATIONAL FORMULARY*[a]

Lee T. Grady
United States Pharmacopoeia, Rockville, Maryland

INTRODUCTION

United States Pharmacopeia (USP) and *National Formulary* (NF) standards and specifications relate to the quality, purity and strength, packaging, and labeling of medicines and related articles. The standards are public standards, and new and revised standards are published regularly. Official drug names and definitions are established, as well as tests or assay procedures that allow determination of compliance with the standards. But do the compendia reflect the state of pharmaceutical technology?

Resolutions adopted by the 1995 USP Convention are indicative of the interest and professional expertise shown by delegates. The General Committee of Revision elected by the Convention included categories of expertise critical to a modern pharmacopoeia. From the 138 standards-related members, 20 Division of Standards Development subcommittees were organized, along with a joint standards-information Nomenclature Committee, to carry out the continuous revision process.

The USP24-NF19 contains 3777 monographs and 164 general chapters (1). There are 543 new monographs, 504 in the USP and 39 in the NF. Continuous revision led to many new or improved requirements; 3941 individual revisions were processed through *Pharmacopeial Forum* (PF) during the 5-year cycle. Obsolete material deleted during the preparation of this volume included 130 USP and 12 NF monographs, and 4 general chapters.

USP and Legal Recognition

Unlike all other pharmacopeias, the USP and NF are not produced by government. The USP and NF are published by the U.S. Pharmacopeial Convention, Inc., a voluntary, not-for-profit institution that holds the public trust. Standards established in the USP and the NF are recognized by law and can be enforced by federal and state authorities. References to the USP and NF occur in numerous statutes regulating articles used in medical and pharmacy practice. The most significant is recognition of the official compendia in the Federal Food, Drug, and Cosmetic Act. These statutes usually empower the governmental agency to enforce the law using certain defined aspects of the compendia. Most commonly recognized are USP and NF standards for determining the identity, strength, quality, and purity of the articles and specifications for packaging and labeling. The Pure Food and Drug Law enacted by Congress in 1906 is a landmark in U.S. history. At that time, the USP-NF standards were given legal status, and the federal government was empowered, now resident in the FDA, to enforce USP requirements.

Congress reaffirmed this authority in 1938, and even the sweeping 1962 amendments did not alter this essential fact. During the 1995–2000 cycle, two statutes, the Dietary Supplements for Health and Education Act of 1994 (DSHEA) and the Food and Drug Administration Modernization Act of 1997 (FDAMA), extended the use of the USP and NF by amending the Federal Food, Drug, and Cosmetic Act. DSHEA specifically provided that a dietary supplement represented as conforming to the specifications of an official compendium will be deemed misbranded if it fails to do so. FDAMA requires pharmacists compounding drug products to use bulk drug substances that comply with the standards contained in a USP or NF monograph and the General Chapter on Pharmacy Compounding. Thus, the USP and NF are not published in response to any statute, but statutory recognition places burdens on the USP and NF with regard to clarity and precision of presentation.

Separate from recognition by drug laws of the various nations and use by registration or related authorities, pharmacopeial requirements are used by commercial codes in that a request for a standardized article should be satisfied only by the article that meets those standards.

---

[a]Throughout this article, the abbreviation USP, when used alone, signifies the U.S. Pharmacopeial Convention, Inc. The abbreviation USP followed by Roman numerals signifies a particular revision of the *Pharmacopeia*. The abbreviation USP-NF is used to signify the *U.S. Pharmacopeia-National Formulary* and are taken to be USP24 and NF19, unless otherwise specified.

Pharmacopeias historically came before government regulations because rules or specifications had to be established before they could be supervised and enforced by the government. In recent decades, however, governments will not permit marketing of drugs unless these are duly registered or scrutinized for quality. Approval of new drugs is most widely appreciated, but international commerce also places such demands on a continuing basis. Compendial standards are a regular feature of all these governmental processes, usually by way of reference in one document or another.

Mission

The mission of the USP is to promote the public health through establishing and disseminating legally recognized standards of quality and information for the use of medicines and related articles by healthcare professionals, patients, and consumers.

U.S. Pharmacopeial Convention

The U.S. Pharmacopeial Convention (USPC) consists of delegates of nearly 400 organizations, including colleges of pharmacy and medicine, professional associations, and some federal agencies. The Convention arose from a national convention called by Dr. Lyman Spalding in 1817 to develop national drug standards for the polyglot, rapidly expanding developing nation. It met in 1820 and published that year the first U.S. Pharmacopeia (Fig. 1). The present revision is USP24 and NF19 (1). Between 1888 and 1975, the NF had been published separately by the American Pharmaceutical Association. It was acquired by the USPC

in 1975, along with the assets of the Drug Standards Laboratory that was a joint body funded by USP, the American Pharmaceutical Association, and the American Medical Association.

Essential aspects of compendial standards are intrinsic in the history and composition of the Convention. USP standards are meant to describe an acceptable article from the point of view of the physician–pharmacist–patient interfaces; and they are inherently time-of-use (that is, shelf life) requirements. Another outcome of this focus is that practical, medically significant aspects are dominant in assigning requirements and the limits therein. Compendial standards are always established from the viewpoints of the medical and pharmaceutical professions, which in the United States are represented by the USPC.

General Committee of Revision

The Quinquennial USP Convention in 1995 elected a Committee of Revision of 138 outstanding scientists and practitioners in the various disciplines relating to quality standards and drug information. Approximately 1000 prospective experts made themselves available when both standards and information programs are considered. These experts are volunteers from industry, academia, and government. Of these, 100 were experts in public standards. The other 38 accepted assignments in the Drug Information Division. Each elected standards-setting expert was assigned to one or more of 20 subcommittees (Table 1). The 20 subcommittee chairpersons and the chair of the Committee of Revision make up the Division of Standards Development Executive Committee. The entire Committee adopts "Rules and Procedures" (2, 3) by which

---

THE FIRST U.S. PHARMACOPEIA, 1820

Preface Statement

It is the object of a Pharmacopeia to select from among substances which possess medicinal power, those, the utility of which is most fully established and best understood; and to form from them preparations and compositions, in which their powers may be exerted to the greatest advantage. It should likewise distinguish those articles by convenient and definite names, such as may prevent trouble or uncertainty in the intercourse of physicians and apothecaries.

The value of a Pharmacopeia depends upon the fidelity with which it conforms to the best state of medical knowledge of the day. Its usefulness depends upon the sanction it receives from the medical community and the public; and the extent to which it governs the language and practice of those for whose use it is intended.

Fig. 1   *U.S. Pharmacopeia* Preface Statement, 1820.

Table 1 USP Subcommittees and chairs, 1995–2000

Subcommittee	Chairperson
Antibiotics	Henry S.I. Tan, Ph.D.
Biopolymers, Bioproducts, and Vaccines	Everett Flanigan, Ph.D.
Biotechnology and Gene Therapy	Robert L. Garnick, Ph.D.
Chemistry 1	Stanley L. Hem, Ph.D.
Chemistry 2	Dennis K.J. Gorecki, Ph.D.
Chemistry 3	Judy P. Boehlert, Ph.D.
Chemistry 4	Elliott T. Weisman
Chemistry 5	Edward G. Lovering, Ph.D.
Dissolution and Bioavailability	Thomas S. Foster, Pharm.D.
Excipients 1 (Monographs)	Zak T. Chowhan, Ph.D.
Excipients 2 (Methods)	Gregory E. Amidon, Ph.D.
General Chapters	Thomas P. Layloff, Ph.D.
Microbiology	Joseph E. Knapp, Ph.D.
Multisource Products Issues	James T. Stewart, Ph.D.
Natural Products	Paul Kucera, Ph.D.
Nonprescription Drugs and Nutritional Supplements	David B. Roll, Ph.D.
Packaging, Storage, and Distribution	Thomas Medwick, Ph.D.
Radiopharmaceuticals	Dennis P. Swanson, M.S., R.Ph.
Toxicity, Biocompatability, and Cell Culture	Sharon J. Northup, Ph.D.
Water and Parenterals	James C. Boylan, Ph.D.

revision proceeds. A portion of the compendia is delegated to each subcommittee and, in agreement with its chairman, to each subcommittee member. Responsibilities are distributed for the more than 3700 monographs and the more than 160 general tests and information chapters. Every sentence in the USP and NF and every standard and its recognition are reexamined during each revision cycle. And every addition or change is given advance public notice and opportunity for comment.

The listing of subcommittee titles in Table 1 indicates the present scope of Committee interest and activity. The simple fact that a subcommittee has been created to deal with a subject area is a statement of its importance and implies that there are priorities in that area on the agenda of the Committee. As these interests change, the alterations are reflected in the USP periodical, *Pharmacopeial Forum*, discussed below. As outlined in the "Rules and Procedures" and noted above, any actions of subcommittees, or considered revisions to or adoptions of standards, are published for public evaluation and comment and are subject to mechanisms for appeal or request for postponement.

Council of Experts

The year 2000 USP Convention has adopted new structures and processes for setting public standards. The Council of Experts replaces the historic General Committee of Revision. The resultant array of expert bodies and responsibilities is not available at this writing but may be found in *Pharmacopeial Forum* in 2000.

Headquarters

The USPC occupies several headquarters buildings complete with laboratories in Rockville, MD. It employs a staff of approximately 300 scientists, editors, and other employees to support the work of the Committee of Revision (Council of Experts). November 1998 saw the opening of the *Reference Standards Center*, a facility housing the *Reference Standards Laboratory* and the *Reference Standards Operations* unit. The USP Research and Development Laboratory remains in the 1989 headquarters building. As a publisher, the USPC performs its own phototypesetting, and its extensive in-house editing and production capability have been important to the timely publication of the standards. A modernization program is in progress to take advantage of the rapidly changing world of information-based products and technologies.

Financial Aspects

Independent standards setting is possible only because support for the program is undistorted by the impact of standards on the governing bodies that ensure adequate funds. Funding is not dependent on those elements on which the standards impinge. Direct and narrow-based economic support from either government or industry would place standards setting in a less free or dampened environment. Opposed priorities or response to adverse impacts cannot be isolated from direct support. Financial independence is the component on which the USP program turns. Neither government nor industry gives direct supporting funds to the USPC for standards-setting activities or programs. Because these two are the major sources of funds for most nonprofit institutions, the corollary is that the USPC lacks immense reserves on which to draw and must be prudent in its expenditures. The USPC generates adequate income to meet its challenge as a public trust and to support growth and some ancillary programs noted here. Revenues for the USPC come from the following significant sources: sale of Reference Standards and publications. The committee members, advisory panelists, trustees, and convention delegates serve without monetary compensation, out of their sense of public service and professional responsibility.

PROGRAMS AND PUBLICATIONS

Pharmacopeial Forum and Continuous Revision

Pharmacopeial Forum, with the ability to publish official supplements twice yearly, has brought to fruition a dominant feature of the USP continuous revision. Only in this way can the USP keep pace with the progress of pharmaceutical technology and thereby escape the doom of continuing obsolescence. As the art of pharmacy, whether in design, manufacturing, or testing, became ever more the science of pharmacy, the compendia kept pace. An electronic, web-based product became available in 2000.

The bimonthly *Pharmacopeial Forum*, called "the journal of drug standards development and official compendia revision," presents proposed new or revised USP and NF standards for public review and comment. *Pharmacopeial Forum* enables the reviewer to see at a glance both the text that is proposed for deletion and the text that is proposed for addition or modification. *Pharmacopeial Forum is* offered by subscription to all interested parties. Thus, interested scientists and practitioners from the general public other than the Committee of Revision and its advisory panels have access to the latest proposed revisions in the official standards and tests and can readily transmit their comments, suggestions, and data to USP headquarters for consideration by the Revision Committee.

In addition to presenting proposals recommended by the Committee of Revision in a section entitled "In-process Revision," the *Pharmacopeial Forum* contains several other sections. The "Headquarters Column" gives information on publication deadlines, news, or statements of the Pharmacopeial Convention and the Committee of Revision, summaries of issues discussed by the Drug Standards Division Executive Committee, and various tabulations or lists that aid in keeping track of the multifaceted revision program. A section called "Stimuli to the Revision Process" publishes reports or statements of authoritative committees, scientific articles relevant to compendial issues, general commentaries by interested parties, and collations of comments received in response to policy initiatives. A recent addition is a section on International Harmonization.

Pharmacopeial Forum is intended to promote public comment at the earliest possible stage in standards development. Industry is the largest single participant in that activity. This periodical has been shown to stimulate comment and therefore can be credited with increasing the pace of revision. What comes to mind is an analogy of USP revision to a thixotropic gel—as the pressure is increased, so is the flow. This periodical operates in tandem with the program of Open Conferences to ensure vigorous participation in standards setting.

Related Publications

Efforts are under way to make the USP-NF more useful worldwide. Incorporation of monographs for multivitamin products, biotechnology-derived products, veterinary drugs, and botanicals and other dietary supplements help. The USAN and *USP Dictionary of Drug Names* has wide international applicability, thereby making it a repository of International Names & Nomenclature (INN) and British Adopted Names (BAN), as well as U.S. Adopted Names (USAN). *Pharmacopeial Forum* now contains announcements of proposals from the *Japanese Pharmacopoeia* and *European Pharmacopoeia* for revision of standards for international harmonization.

Open Conferences and Meetings

Consistent with the USP policy of emphasis on public participation in standards setting, open conferences and meetings are held to allow interactive examination of selected topics. Twenty-five of these conferences were held between 1980 and 1999, with an average attendance of approximately 150. Roundtable format is used to get maximum participation policy initiatives as well as proposed standards revisions on the table.

International Training and Outreach Programs

USP standards and information are recognized and used by many countries (19, 21), and the USP seeks to encourage, enhance, and facilitate their use. Examples of USP programs to train non-U.S. scientists and to seek their advice on how USP programs and products can be made more useful to other countries include sponsorship of visiting scientists and scholars, supporting doctoral and postdoctoral fellowships, cosponsorship of meetings and conferences, and formation of the International Health Advisory Panel.

Visiting Scientists and Scholars Program

Since 1990, the USP has substantially expanded its program for visiting scientists and scholars. Originally conceived as a program to train scientists from pharmacopeias and official control laboratories, the program has been expanded to include scientists who spend up to 4 months in the USP Drug Research and Testing Laboratory or in the secretariat for the USP-NF within the standards development divisions to gain experience in laboratory techniques or pharmacopoeial revision procedures, as well as scholars from regulatory agencies and drug information centers around the world interested in the work of the information-development divisions in compiling and updating the USP DI database and USP information products.

Since 1990, the USP has hosted visiting scientists and scholars from China (13), Indonesia (2), Argentina (5), Nigeria (3), Poland (2), Romania (2), Turkey (2), Russia (2), and 1 each from Germany, Japan, Thailand, Korea, Kenya, Italy, and Kyrghyzstan.

Fellowship Program

The Fellowship Program is directed primarily at pre- and postdoctoral U.S. students. The USP has awarded 160 fellowships since 1981. The USP Fellowship Program also grants awards to non-U.S. students and postdoctoral fellows at U.S. universities and at universities outside the United States, provided the criteria for award can be satisfied. Currently the USP grants 10 fellowships annually: 6 in drug standards and 4 in drug information. Stipends are $15,000 per year, and a fellow may compete for support for a second year. Eligibility criteria require, among other factors, that the fellowship application be signed by a member of the USP Committee of Revision, an advisory panel, or the board of trustees at the institution where the applicant is studying. Applications are reviewed for technical merit and relevance to USP standards and information programs by committees of members of the Committee of Revision from the standards and information divisions.

Asian edition

In response to globalization and increasing use of the USP-NF abroad and to the foreign exchange picture, USP23-NF18 and USP24-NF19 both were published in Mumbai (Bombay) India simultaneous with the main publication in the United States.

Spanish language version of the USP-NF

The Spanish language edition of USP 23-NF 18 was published in 1995 as a DOS-based electronic product. In 1998, the product was converted to a Windows-based electronic product. Work on the translation of USP-NF text began in 1993 with the exploration of machine translation software suitable for use in the translation of the characteristic text of the USP-NF. The software selected was ENG-SPAN-AM^{SM} from the Pan American Health Organization. This was fortified by a microdictionary and software macros specific to the compendia. Since the initial release in 1995, the USP has released Supplements for the Spanish language edition concurrent with the release of the English language Supplements. The database continues to be kept abreast of revisions to the USP and NF, but it was not marketed after 1998.

NATURE OF COMPENDIAL STANDARDS

Scope

The first USP begins, "It is the object of a Pharmacopeia to select from among substances H those, the utility of which is most fully established and best understood" (Fig. 1). Subsequent USP Conventions have broadened that to encompass all safe and effective medicines and some related articles. Recognition by the USP is not based on the identity of the manufacturer, the environment in which used, or the existence of borders or restrictions on commerce. Articles are adopted into the USP and receive standards scientifically appropriate to the articles, irrespective of whether the article is over-the-counter or prescription only and whether the article is used at home, in the practitioner's facility, in the hospital, or even in a licensed facility. The same modern standards are applied, and the public is offered the same parameters of strength, quality, and purity. Also, the same opportunities exist for analytical challenge or regulatory compliance.

USP and NF Standards Are Public Standards

This distinction was expressed well by the late C.A. Johnson of the *British Pharmacopoeia* (4):

> The first point to be underlined is that the pharmacopoeia provides a collection of publicly available standards that are open for inspection and challenge by all—a fundamental right in any civilized society. The standards are established only after wide public consultation—a procedure that deserves to be maintained and supported. Because of the public availability of standards for medicines any authority or, indeed, any individual, may cause a random sample of a medicine on the market to be challenged.

As noted previously, compendial standards arose from the professions on behalf of the public. There are no attempts at regulation by the USP of the daily application of pharmaceutical technology. USP standards are not to be confused with such concepts as the "product description." As addressed below, compendial standards are not manufacturing directions as such and do not constitute the manufacturers' release criteria. They define the acceptable article as and when used.

Functions and Responsibilities of Compendial Standards (5)

What are the functions of USP standards? First, remember the nature of any standard. A standard is a rule, a principle of orderliness, that implies: 1) an element of agreement or acquiescence of most concerned, 2) some authority, and 3) some benefit to be gained by all concerned. To obtain this agreement in a reasonably democratic way, as opposed by way of authoritarian edict, there must be an element of compromise. However, one fact cannot be ignored: adoption of one rule implies rejection of alternative rules. In a real sense, this is loss of freedom of choice. The question comes—what do we get in trade? Why standardize? Why go through the occasionally wrenching experience of compromise? We get orderliness instead of chaos, and where there is orderliness, and only then, we get predictability. The essence of a USP standard is predictable drug product quality. The benefits of that predictability are settled on all concerned: the public, the professionals, the manufacturers of quality products. Without predictability in use, drugs would not have won the fullness of their position in society today. Physical and chemical tests and specifications are given for measurable quality parameters. Official drug names and definitions are established, which give a common vocabulary and a clear understanding to communications within and among the professions.

Why do we persist in saying "public" standards? Because compendial standards, proposed and adopted, are published and circulated in public. The standards state to the public, manufacturers, and professions what constitutes predictable drug product quality from lot to lot and from manufacturer to manufacturer. The parameters of that predictability are published for all to see, for all to discuss, for all to grant their element of agreement, or for that matter, for all to contest publicly. Other agreements and other compromises, however reasonable and neatly filed away and for whatever reason not available, cannot fill that simple, rightful need of public information.

Codifying an element of predictability is not the only function of public standards. The USP-NF standards are enforceable by law, and are enforced strongly. This is the second function of USP standards: providing a basis for active protection of the public from unacceptable articles, not merely establishing ideals to be ignored when convenient. The USP and NF give detailed tests or assay procedures that allow determination of compliance with the standards; indeed, to call for a quality level without supplying a proof test would be unenforceable. Third, the quality manufacturer knows that other manufacturers of the same article must pass muster as well. Two less obvious purposes should be noted. The participants in the revision process also focus timely attention of industry and government on important problems or new technologies. Also, to a large measure the compendia define the state of the art of pharmaceutical analysis and therefore have impact as well on general drug registration and nonofficial articles both here and abroad.

Beyond defining acceptable articles, what are the responsibilities of USP and NF standards? The USP must strike a balance between the right of all concerned parties to act independently and efficiently and the need to preserve the rights of the patient to safety and quality. The USP and NF are responsible first to the public. These compendia can encourage the experts to make the quality judgments that the public cannot. The USP and NF are responsible to the practitioners of medicine and pharmacy who understand and are bound by the need for standards. The USP and NF are responsible to put forth standards that are meaningful to government and that can be enforced. The USP and NF are responsible to industry to put forth standards that are meaningful, practical, and affordable. The goal of the USP and NF is to set standards that are equal to the need, that can be enforced, that can be met by capable manufacturers, and that, at least for the moment, satisfy pharmaceutical scientists and practitioners.

Drug product quality in the United States is more reliable, more predictable than other aspects of the system of healthcare delivery as a whole. Adding tests or tightening specifications at the manufacturer level that does not help patients or professionals derive further benefits from drugs does little except increase patient or taxpayer drug bills. There is something to be said for knowing when to stop. We must be able to recognize diminishing return!

Drug product quality stands out in sharpest detail and is most highly visible to those of us in this technical community. Our concerns are those of the specialist for his or her field. In contrast, consider the heavy mist through which we gaze at problems of predictable therapy—not of differences in predictability resulting from variations in lots or brands, but of differences in pharmacogenetics; dietary habits such as preferences in beverages or entrees; metabolism as a function of disease, age, or sex; or, on a larger scale, failures in patient compliance or drug interactions.

General Approaches to Standards (5)

We can recognize three distinct but interdependent, effective standards: 1) USP-NF standards, 2) current good manufacturing practices, and 3) in-house quality assurance or process validation protocols. The three programs are different but have the same objective: drug product quality. The official standards are developed to be meaningful in this multiple context. In recent years, a similar array has occurred in most developed nations, and this is rightfully seen as a measure of success.

Currently, public standards tend to be performance rather than design standards. To illustrate: Are only automobile exhaust emissions measured as proof of success in reducing pollution or is an "official engine," complete with engineering drawings, promulgated? In performance tests, desired attributes are tested for postmanufacture. This is end-product testing. These answer the fundamental question: How did it turn out? Older monographs, with prescription-like formulas but few tests, were essentially design standards. Only a few such appear in USP24. The resurgence of pharmacy dispensing now will result in more design-type standards. The trend toward performance tests has been the case in all standards except, notably, plumbing codes. One can imagine the difficulty of converting a visit of the plumbing inspector from an examination of allowable joints, angles, and materials to an experiment in which recovery of a test specimen of a hamburger slurry is a pass/fail criterion. Pharmaceutical technology now takes this one step further

and recasts the design standard as a "validated process" when the demonstration by end-product testing can lead to sufficient confidence in both the design and the process off carrying out the design.

Design standards intrinsically must be more detailed, more complex, more arbitrary, and more authoritarian than performance standards. Specific formulas can be specified by USP-NF, as can methods of compounding or processes of manufacture if necessary. However, end-product testing is believed by most pharmaceutical scientists to be adequate public standardization. That is what the patient does—end product testing!

USP-NF standards are established with the specific intent of serving as instruments of enforcement. Because these standards may be the common ground in a legal contest, the compendia publish both the experimental details and the limits within which the results must fall. Pass or fail—not how well, or by how much. Is it or is it not an acceptable article? Claims that a product "exceeds" USP specifications distort standards concepts. The compendial standard is that which any specimen of that article must meet at any time during its valid life. Although not a criterion aimed at use as a release standard, it is clearly the ultimate element in assigning expiration dates. It is the door at the end of a long hallway, not an immediate opening to the marketplace.

Limitations of Standards

Let us start with a truism. Quality is built into a product; it cannot be tested into it. It is also true that failure to build quality into a product can be tested for, as can variations from a good norm. The last century coped with a problem and a paradox: a redefinition of what was good and, most significantly, what was good enough (6). In this way, statistical quality control developed. We accepted the idea that even if absolute precision in manufacturing were possible (and it is not), it would be superfluous. When we strive for product uniformity, we still remember that quality will vary, so that what we really aim for is standardization of quality within limits. That is why "quality" requires control. The object of control is to enable us to do what we want to do, with economic limits (6).

We accept the inevitability of imperfection, thus we must accept the inevitable need for quality standards. Thus must we also accept the imperfection of those same quality standards. Compendial standards must be what can be done; failure to publish a standard because it is imperfect can be failure to serve the public. I submit that a willingness to move forward in the face of imperfections is consistent with the second maxim stated by Descartes (7), which applies to any uncertain situation, to move resolutely and unswervingly in the most promising direction.

TECHNICAL FEATURES OF COMPENDIAL STANDARDS

Pharmacopoeias always have been as much statements of current technology as of current therapy. Examination of an older pharmacopoeia from any time or place gives a fair measure of the contemporary drugs available, therapeutic strategies, and medical knowledge. No less does such examination give a fair measure of the contemporary pharmaceutical technology. Pharmacopoeial standards arise from the contemporary, controlling concepts of what constitutes good quality and, further, how one achieves or demonstrates that quality. However, selection requirements can come only from processes and equipment in general use. Available technology determines what is to be required or standardized, just as it determines what can be made.

A rough correlation existed between pharmacopoeias and pharmaceutical technology. At least that was so until the modern drug era, when new drug discoveries proceeded at rates that, in one generation, rendered many pharmacopoeias obsolete, especially those that could not revise as frequently as is done by the USP. Increased international trade and acceptance undercut the need for large numbers of national pharmacopoeias. Technology forged ahead on many fronts in manufacturing processes and equipment, dosage form design, new kinds of excipients, and new analytical capabilities. Only a few pharmacopoeias continue to publish specifications of practical import consistent with the state of pharmaceutical technology, and these are primarily regional or international in scope. Different adaptations to rapidly changing therapy and technology account for some of the unevenness in and among pharmacopoeias and a consequent need for harmonization. We report here on current compendial specifications, what they are, by whom and where they are established, and how and why they are created.

Official Names

Pharmacopoeias are an accumulation of responses to problems in medicine, pharmacy, or pharmaceutical technology as these presented themselves over the years, even over centuries. From the beginning of pharmacopoeias, a fundamental function has been the establishment of names "such as may prevent trouble or uncertainty in the intercourse of physicians and apothecaries" (Fig. 1). Different things should have different names; that is a fundamental principle of compendial standards. This applies to dosage forms as to well as to molecules. This deeply rooted function seldom gets much attention until someone wants to change something. A recent case is the desire to change the capability of consumers to identify the ingredients of products through product labeling of all inactive ingredients. The need for concise, unambiguous names for these ingredients as well is inescapable of notice.

A cooperative effort since 1961 between the American Medical Association and the USPC was augmented in 1964 by the addition of the American Pharmaceutical Association, then the publisher of the NF, to form what has been known since as the U.S. Adopted Names (USAN) Council. The U.S. Food and Drug Administration (FDA) was invited to join the Council in 1967, and the FDA refers to USAN names in its regulations. The Council consists of persons conversant with the needs and problems of naming drugs and an appeals body. The names determined by the Council are incorporated, along with other names for drugs (including public, proprietary, chemical, and code-designated names), in an annual book, USAN *and the USP Dictionary of Drug Names*, published by the USPC.

Method and Specification Selection

The selection of USP methods and specifications can be concluded to be practical consequences of what has been successful in detecting drug product quality variability and what can ensure demonstration that variations in quality remain within acceptable limits. USP methods are selected for their fitness for use for that monograph application, just as USP Reference Standards are adopted on the basis of suitability for intended use in that monograph.

Tests and specifications, and reagents as such, were introduced into the USP in the 1890s. The first truly instrumental determination used was the Wild polaristrobometer for natural oils in 1890. Trends were established in USP XV (1955) toward decreased monograph prescriptions, or design standards, and, separately, toward the increasing range of General Tests. The USP now has more than 160 general chapters. There are few analytical methods used in modern pharmaceutical analysis that are not used by the compendia.

An interesting historical change in the orientation of the USP is implicit in this discussion. Until the age of instrumentation, there was an expectation that compendial methods could be performed in a community pharmacy. What became possible decided where it could be done, and the focus moved out of the pharmacy and into the central analytical laboratory.

Tremendous changes in the selection of compendial methods have occurred in recent decades. Classic physical and chemical measurements had long been established as objective criteria for quality assurance and for compliance testing, but these had significant limitations for dosage forms, both as assays and as limit tests. As recent decades have witnessed a torrent of instrumental developments, it should be no surprise that the compendia have experienced a resultant flood of applications that use those instrumental methods popular in the industry. The previous limiting factors, the availability of instruments their and reliability (or certainty of repair) ceased to be a problem even before the revolution in microelectronics.

The USP placed emphasis in the last 20 years on stability-consciousness and impurity-consciousness in preparing monographs. See 1086, *Impurities in Official Articles* (1). These major trends explain the prominence of chromatography. It is obvious that the major portion of recent revision revolves around chromatography: high-pressure liquid chromatography (HPLC), gas-liquid chromatography (GLC), and thin-layer chromatography (TLC) for identity tests and reference standard evaluation; HPLC, GLC, and TLC for purity or limit tests; and HPLC and GLC for assays. Much effort is spent in evaluating chromatographic systems and identifying System Suitability Tests (see discussion below) to make these methods more reliable. The amazing speed with which HPLC was adopted as mature scientific measurement is nowhere more evident than in drug analysis and, therefore, in the USP. The USP 24/NF 19 contains 1800 HPLC/GLC and 740 TLC initial references. Because of cross-referencing of substance methods in dosage form monographs, the total number of chromatography-based requirements is much, much higher.

To a large extent, modern separation science has solved a previous significant problem in compendial method selection, that of interfering substances. The USP does not lock all manufacturers into the same formulation and manufacturing procedure, and the USP allows considerable freedom as long as the substances added in dosage forms do not interfere, which these must not do (8), with the official tests and assays. Because the manufacturer can change the formula or introduce new products, it is unreasonable to assume that the USP would have tested every conceived and about-to-be conceived product. Thus, in exchange for the freedom of formulating, the individual manufacturers have the responsibility of keeping up with

proposals in the *Pharmacopeial Forum* and assessing the applicability of proposed methods to their specific existing products and their contemplated new products, i.e., validation for their formulations. Separation science now available makes it likely that a method workable for all can be identified.

Automated Methods

In considering the introduction of new test methods, it has been necessary for the USP to recognize the appropriateness of automating compendial assays and tests. The Committee of Revision prefers to adopt automatable procedures, especially for multiple-unit specimens such as those arising from dissolution or content uniformity requirements. Thus, since the publication of the USP XVIII in 1970, the General Notices to the USP has included automated procedures in discussions on the use of suitable alternative methods. The General Notices to the USP24 state (9):

Automated procedures employing the same basic chemistry as those assay and test procedures given in the monograph are recognized as being equivalent in their suitability for determining compliance. Compliance may be shown also by the use of alternative methods, chosen for advantages in accuracy, sensitivity, precision, selectivity, or adaptability to automation or computerized data reduction or in other special circumstances. Since Pharmacopeial standards and procedures are interrelated, only the result obtained by the procedure given in this Pharmacopeia is conclusive where a difference appears or in the event of dispute.

Thus, the USP states explicitly what is to be done and in what sequence but not by whom or by what.

Stability

Monographs do not include a specific section that deals directly with this major aspect of drug product quality, primarily because stability is related to a number of factors including chemical structure, formulation ingredients and processing, bioburden, packaging materials and storage, repackaging, and geography. Concern for stability is manifest in the Pharmacopeia in at least seven ways: 1) the general requirement for expiration dates, 2) monograph packaging and storage requirements, 3) standards for packaging materials and containers, 4) standards for repackaging and storage, 5) limit tests for decomposition products, 6) stability-indicating tests or assays, and 7) the informational General Chapter, "Stability Considerations in Dispensing Practice." Underlying these standards are standard definitions of storage conditions. An emerging establishment of requirements for Labile preparations will add an eighth stability-resultant category. New informational chapters are likely to expand this list. Stability is not causal—it is the effect of choices during formulation development, packaging, and storage instructions.

Test Results, Statistics, and Standards (10)

Confusion of compendial standards with release tests and with statistical sampling plans occasionally occurs. Interpretation of results from official tests and assays requires an understanding of the nature and style of compendial standards. Tests and assays given in the USP prescribe operation on a single specimen; that is, the singlet determination. This is the minimum sample on which the attributes of a compendial article should be measured. Some tests, such as those for dissolution and uniformity of dosage units, require multiple-dosage units in conjunction with a decision scheme. It is to be understood that these tests, albeit using a number of dosage units, are in fact the singlet determinations of those particular attributes of the specimen. These quantities should not be confused with statistical sampling plans. The compendial procedures demonstrate compliance of the attributes of an article with compendial standards only for that specimen (of one or more dosage units) that is subjected to analysis. Repeats, replications, and extrapolation of results to larger populations are neither specified nor proscribed by the compendia; such decisions are dependent on the objectives of the testing.

Commercial or regulatory compliance testing, or manufacturer's release testing, may or may not require examination of additional specimens, in accordance with predetermined guidelines or sampling strategies. Moreover, a statistical plan may be necessary to relate the shelf life of the product, test results, and release specifications to the ultimate compendial specifications.

System Suitability Tests

System Suitability Tests are now characteristic of USP methods (10, 11). They are based on the concept proposed by this author in early 1971 that the instrument, reagents, packings, conditions, procedural details, detectors, electronic accessories, and even the analyst constitute a single system that is therefore amenable to an overall test of system function. Reliable chromatographic performance, for example, may require specifications for resolution,

column efficiency, peak tailing, precision of replications, or extremes of conditions. Such tests obviate the necessity of specifying a multitude of instrumental settings, model numbers, names of manufacturers, packings and lot numbers, and other physical-chemical and engineering characteristics. Also avoided is the distribution of official lots of chromatographic packings through the compendial headquarters. System suitability tests were first made official in the USP XIX and have come into general application.

New Technology and USP Contents

During the revision cycle, the USP introduced a Web site that contains up-to-date information about the USP and its program as well as ordering instructions. The USP home page is located at www.usp.org.

Law and regulations ensure the adequacy of the premises, practices, and documentation of the manufacture of drug substances and preparations expected to result in articles that comply with pharmacopoeial standards. It was the practice of previous USP revisions to publish and update the FDA Good Manufacturing Practices (GMPs) in a general information chapter *Good Manufacturing Practices* (1077). This was perceived to be a service to those in manufacturing establishments and pharmacists. Rapid expansion of the Internet and almost universal establishment of Web sites by all institutions abrogates, in general, the perceived need that necessitates this service. Therefore, this revision cycle culminated in the deletion of federal and other texts now reliably available at no cost through the new technology. Federal documents can be found on the U.S. Food and Drug Administration Web site at www.fda.gov. Along with *Good Manufacturing Practices* (1077), two other general information chapters based on federal regulations are deleted: *Federal Food Drug and Cosmetic Act Requirements Relating to Drugs for Human Use* (1076) and the frequently revised *Controlled Substance Act* (1071).

Drug Release

Nowhere have the value and failures (and political pressure) of pharmaceutical technology been more apparent than in the complex of processes that amount to release of active ingredient from its pharmaceutical presentation. A major concern, now a generation old, was reliable release of drug from solid oral dosage forms (11). The USP and NF each introduced dissolution tests in six monographs in 1970. For some drugs, absorption is dissolution-rate controlled, reduction in bioavailability results. This is precisely a reduction in strength and has no additional resulting in medical significance. The problem arises when two formulations of such a drug are compared where dissolution rates are substantially different—this is known as bioinequivalence. This led to much commercial mischief and distortion of scientific facts to achieve protection of existing products from competition. Some scientists emphasized drug chemical properties as the central factor—particle size or solubility, for example. Others pointed to the inactive ingredients used in the processing of compressed tablets—lubricants and disintegrants, for example. Or there was emphasis on the process itself, as in overcompression. Pragmatists noted the continued use of hydrophobic tablet coatings—shellac, for example.

A drug release test, dissolution, was a satisfactory standard every time there was a problem of any practical consequence. Of equal significance was the recognition of the strength of dissolution testing as a tool for quality control. Thus, equivalence in dissolution behavior was sought in light of both bioavailability and quality control considerations. The USP 24 has more than 600 monographs for tablets and capsules: 500 have an official dissolution requirement; 100 others have a different performance test considered appropriate for acceptable drug product quality.

For USP tablet and capsule monographs, we know of none where two articles, fully in conformance, have clinically significant inequivalence. Experience has demonstrated that when a medically significant difference in bioavailability has been found among supposedly identical articles, a dissolution test has been efficacious in discriminating among these articles. Because the USP sets forth attributes of an acceptable article, such a discriminating test is satisfactory because the dissolution standard can exclude definitively any unacceptable article. Therefore, no compendial requirements for animal or human tests of bioavailability were necessary. The practical problem has been the obverse; that is, dissolution tests are so discriminating of formulation factors that may only sometimes affect bioavailability not uncommon for a clinically acceptable article to perform poorly in a typical dissolution test. In such cases, the Committee of Revision has been mindful to include as many acceptable articles as possible but, at the same time, to exclude dissolution specifications so generous as to raise reasonable scientific concern for bioinequivalence.

There is no known medically significant bioinequivalence problem with articles of which 75% is dissolved in water at 37°C for 45 minutes with the use of either official apparatus at usual speed. A majority of monographs have that as the requirement, and this is called "First Case" in the *Pharmacopeial Forum*. Other articles for which there are no known or likely medically significant bioavailability problems have required some adjustment of medium or apparatus.

Details of tests and specifications can be found in the USP. For ordinary tablets and capsules, the apparatus used (basket and paddle) affords low levels of agitation appropriate for challenging drug products with a significant potential for diminished physiologic availability. Similarly, only the most discriminating solvents are selected. See 1088, *In Vitro and In Vivo Evaluation of Dosage Forms*. Extended-release formulations present different standards problems. Pharmacologically sound judgment that a drug is acceptable as an extended-release product obviates the necessarily conservative choice of apparatus and conditions applied to ordinary articles. Either the drug does not have a significant absorption problem or its metabolites are active, in which case a higher agitation apparatus may be necessary. A new apparatus is presently under consideration to handle those cases in which the current apparatus is unworkable.

Dietary Supplements

Dietary supplements are now covered by federal legislation (see DSHEA under Legal Status of the Official Compendia, above). They are a rapidly growing aspect of consumer choice. The USP and NF made great progress in this field in the years after the 1995 Convention. The Convention debated vigorously on the proper placement in the compendia, if any, necessitated by the resurgence in the United States of the use of botanicals, amino acids, and other substances. These had fallen into disuse earlier in the century (see *1995–2000 Resolutions* in the *Proceedings*). The feasibility of standards was established quickly, and there developed a broad support for USP-NF monographs. The area of information for consumers and practitioners has been the more contentious. The first task was to identify the most widely used botanicals having no counteracting safety concerns.

Dietary supplements are on a different legal footing from drugs, being regulated as foods or under food statutes. In contrast to drugs, supplements are not required to comply with compendial requirements unless labeled to be the official article, in which case it is necessary to use compendial methods. Labels that specify USP or NF in supplements are gaining momentum. Although there is extensive analytical experience with vitamins and minerals, problems in the analysis of botanicals are likely to arise because a tradition of testing is not widespread.

Very complex mixtures are the rule, and there is uncertainty as to the critical components.

In response to a resolution adopted at the USPC's 1995 Quinquennial Meeting, the Committee of Revision addressed issues concerning natural products of plant origin used as dietary supplements. The Subcommittee on Natural Products, assisted by the Advisory Panel on Analytical Methods for Identification and Characterization of Natural Products, set priorities for 21 botanicals for standards development. The criteria underlying the selection included absence of safety risk; extent of use as reported by trade sources; positive assessment by recognized pharmacognosists, usually on a presumption of beneficial pharmacological action and history of use in traditional medicine; and the ability of the article to be able to meet typical USP-NF monograph requirements.

A new admission policy addresses botanicals used as dietary supplements recommended for their official adoption by the USP Committee of Revision. When the FDA has approved a use or a USP DID advisory panel has accepted a use, it is to the USP. If neither condition is met, and there is no safety concern, the article is admitted into the NF. If there is a safety concern for an article, then no NF monograph is published, and USP DID will publish a monograph that is negative on the use of this article. The first official monograph resulting from the 1995 USPC appeared in the Seventh Supplement to the USP in 1997. That was Ginger, USP. A total of 18 monographs were published through the First Supplement to the USP24-NF19.

Compounding Pharmacy Monographs

A corresponding resurgence in compounding practice has arisen from the unavailability of strengths or forms suitable for special populations, especially pediatric patients, and for short-life preparations such as a buffered, diluted solution of sodium hydrochlorite. The Advisory Panel on Pharmacy Compounding was installed. Pharmacists from this Panel advised the Subcommittee on Packaging, Storage, and Distribution where most scientific questions on prescription stability, packaging, and storage could best be resolved.

The USP laboratory evaluated all the monographs, and its findings were published in *PF*. Ten official monographs were published through the USP24-NF19 Second Supplement. The International Association of Compounding Pharmacists is playing a key role in selecting among the many known formulas to identify those of more medical merit and wider usage. Additional monographs are expected to appear in subsequent supplements. If a commercial article is available, no compounding USP monograph is needed. As noted above (see Legal Status of the Official Compendia), recent legislation supports and guides pharmacy compounding.

Excipients

Standards for more than 350 excipients are published by the USPC, primarily in the NF (approximate 270 versus 80 in the USP). Before 1975, the USP and NF were published by different organizations; each had monographs for drug substances, dosage forms, and excipients. The USP adopted the medically best, and the NF adopted those widely used. With the 1975 merger, it was decided to publish the so-called inactive ingredients in the NF and, in addition, that both the USP and NF publications would be bound together in a single volume and have joint supplements.

The advance of pharmaceutical technology ever forces forward new or refined excipients, some with heretofore unexploited properties. Polymers are a case in point and have been central to many of the technological advances of recent years. New and different challenges for compendial standards are offered by materials used in new wave formulations. Modern analytical chemistry allows rather thorough evaluation of materials.

Excipients were a major, and the initial, component of programs for international harmonization. The USP focuses on functionality tests, such as for that compressibility. These are available for many excipients. Why incorporate functionality requirements into the NF that assess parameters that are critical to a minority of purchasers, thus restricting the channels of commerce and probably raising everyone's costs? If viscosity range or degree of crystallinity is critical to one formulation, isn't that the problem for that formulation? One solution would be to adopt a standard test but to require that the product labeling state the specification to be applied to the contents. The product label would state the definitive parameter(s). The NF is satisfied at present with an array of standards of identity, purity, assay, moisture, packaging, storage and labeling, and so forth that supports the name and labeling of materials.

Reference Standards

In support of its program for public standards for drugs, the USPC supplies the Reference Standards required by the monograph standards, tests, and assays of both the USP and the NF. Biologic assays in the USP were the first to require use of reference materials. Authoritative sources of these were needed, and the first were adopted in 1926. As an index of the growth of analytical science, 45 were needed in 1950 for the USP and NF and 438 in 1980. As of 2000, there are 1400.

One cannot fail to note the vast expansion of the collection in the last few decades. Surely this was not fueled by additional biologic assays. Underlying the initial growth phase was the widespread utilization of spectrophotometry for identification and assay. Separation science was the second phase in pharmaceutical industry control laboratories. As a corollary, USP and NF method selection moved in the same direction. Spectrophotometric identity tests and assays are more reliable, especially for compliance testing, when performed in the relative mode, which uses a reference standard, rather than the absolute mode, which is the norm in titrimetry. There is some residual difference of opinion in other countries on this point, but that is rendered moot by the widespread adoption of separation science by the pharmaceutical industry and, thus, by the compendia. It is a characteristic of chromatographic methods that a reference standard be required, sometimes more than one for a procedure. The accumulation of modern tests and assays results in 5 to 10 uses for many reference standards.

Two critical features of this program should be remembered: all USP Reference Standards are subjected to collaborative testing to generate a purity profile and then must be approved by the USP Reference Standards Committee, which is composed of members from the Division of Standards Development Executive Committee. Three or more laboratories test each one. For this purpose, reference standard purity is defined as known composition with respect to intended use. Adoption of a chemical batch demands a known purity profile, which is obtained by meaningful experiments. Although the USP or NF monograph requirements are met, testing usually ranges beyond the monograph tests to construct a purity profile, particularly in the accumulation of more extensive chromatographic characterization. In contrast to the highly purified synthetic organic medicinals, heterogeneous substances of natural origin continue to be used in addition to the highly purified products of chemical syntheses. Biotechnology-based products in particular are chemically complex. These usually have counterparts in international standards, but the inherent heterogeneity makes direct interchange unworkable. In these cases, careful characterization of the compositional and biologic profile allows for lot-to-lot consistency.

Existence of a reference standard used in a compendial procedure can in effect transfer the quality standard from print to the contents of the reference standard vial. Specifically, the content of the drug product is assayed relative to the USP Reference Standard, which is taken to be 100%. The late C.A. Johnson was fond of stating that the printed standard turning yellow was not the same as a yellowing reference standard.

The Committee of Revision takes steps relative to the continuing acceptability of any specific lot of a USP Reference Standard. Publication of a list of current items in each *Pharmacopeial Forum* keeps the collection up to date in this regard, as well as indicates which are new, have been deleted, or are unavailable.

PARTICIPATION

Food and Drug Administration

Close working relations with the FDA continued as a hallmark of the revision program, both with individual scientists and with FDA laboratories and centers. Formal liaison efforts were conducted primarily through the Compendial Operations Staff in the Center for Drug Evaluation and Research of the FDA. Staff are responsible for obtaining and coordinating agency comments on proposals appearing in the *PF* and for serving as an official point of contact with the Center. They have been effective in contributing many suggestions for improvement as well as a greater degree of consistency between FDA and compendial requirements. Each subcommittee has an ad hoc reviewer assigned by the FDA to ensure communications.

The National Center for Drug Analysis in St. Louis, MO, was a constant, valued, and cooperative participant in the revision process for nearly 3 decades. This laboratory continued from past cycles to do extensive development and review of tests and assays. During this cycle, it continued as the primary FDA participant in the ongoing evaluation of established and proposed new USP Reference Standards. Moreover, careful review was given to many General Chapters and issues in harmonization. The FDA is the single most productive outside source of scientific data and information.

Industrial Cooperation

The *U.S. Pharmacopeia* and scientists in industry interact in a number of important ways (13). The pharmaceutical industry is highly quality conscious; thus the program of a standards-setting body is of pervasive interest. Many interfaces with industrial scientists can be discerned: they use USP standards; serve as members on the General Committee of Revision; serve as members on the Board of Trustees and on appeals bodies and as delegates to the USP Convention; they propose revision and review revision proposals; they serve on USP Advisory Panels, cooperating organization committees, and panels; they help develop USP Reference Standards; and they purchase USP publications and reference standards. Of these, the most important is that they observe the standards, consistent with the original intent (Fig. 1) of the *U.S. Pharmacopeia*.

Participation by individual

Nearly equal numbers of industrial and academic scientists are involved with USP and NF standards determinations, and 10 of 20 DSD Executive Committee members are industrial. An average of half of the DSD Executive Committee consisted of industrial scientists during the last three cycles. The DSD Executive Committee is the policy-setting body and addresses all broad-interest topics. Pharmaceutical technology is the predominant category of information discussed. Other participants include government scientists and medical and pharmacy practitioners.

Participation by manufacturers

Industrial participation on advisory panels, or the General Committee of Revision itself, in addition to industrial interaction on scientific proposals to and from the USP, represents a substantial time demand for any single company. The enormous amount of laboratory work that supports the pharmaceutical and analytical technology incorporated in USP and NF monographs should be emphasized. In terms of economic value, all other participation does not match the cost of laboratory experiments performed by the industry. Indeed, it is what can be done at the bench and on the manufacturing floor that determines what can or cannot appear in the *U.S. Pharmacopeia*.

It should not be concluded that the USP relies entirely on comments from a single manufacturer. There are other interested parties. Testing may be performed as deemed necessary to supplement or corroborate results reported by or disputed among manufacturers. USP laboratories develop data to enable the Committee of Revision to decide on standards establishment and revision. Note that commercial products are not tested by the USP to determine compliance with official standards. Rather, USP testing is called on as necessary to 1) test methods that are considered for new or revised standards in monographs, 2) test products to generate data for the USP Committee of Revision when information needed for standards development and improvement is not forthcoming from other sources, 3) participate in collaborative studies, 4) test materials considered for use as USP Reference Standards, and 5) test USP Reference Standards periodically for degradation.

Industrial Organizations

Revision of the *U.S. Pharmacopeia*, particularly in development of new General Chapters and tests and assays for specialized products, continues to progress through the strong and proactive participation by industry.

No recent pharmacopoeia was issued without notable contributions by the Pharmaceutical Research Manufacturers of America through its standing technical committees in quality control, statistics, and biologicals. Careful reference to the *PF* also will reveal many contributions by scientists from individual member companies.

The Council for Responsible Nutrition (CRN) and the Consumer Health Products Association (CHPA) contribute to new standards for over-the-counter articles. Growth continued on the multiple vitamin-mineral combinations described by class monographs for cough and cold remedies, which include a very large number of products.

Parenteral Drug Association (PDA) members and committees focus on standards for sterile products, testing, and environments.

Self-Regulation

A continuing element of the USP seldom remarked on (13) is the fact that our program of public standards represents the substantial realization of self-regulation by the pharmaceutical industry. Self-regulation is an ideal. It is a natural ideal for free peoples and a historic impulse in our national life. However, it is not directly achievable as a uniform or practical principle. Pressures of money and competition and differing relative values get in the way. What is an obvious improvement to one is an inconvenience or an unreasonable expense to another. Unpopular causes are not written into most corporate job descriptions, especially when the employer suffers the costs of that employee's self-regulatory campaign and, more starkly, sees competition that gets a free ride. In this regard, one should recall the extensive industrial cooperation described above. This fact is remarkable, and it is so important that all understand this characteristic of the *U.S. Pharmacopeia* repeated here.

What is necessary to achieve the ideal of self-regulation is an instrument to transform individual efforts.

Table 2 1990 to 2000 Committees of Revision

870	New monographs adopted
23	New general chapters adopted
270	Deleted monographs
9240	Individual revision actions proposed in *Pharmacopeial Forum*

That instrument is a neutral but authoritative institution. It can insulate individuals and diffuse responsibility while maintaining necessary accountability. The truly knowledgeable can act on their natural inclinations to self-regulate but remain insulated from all negative counter-forces. That is one primary reason the USP is so productive, even though it is a small organization.

The ideal of self-regulation realized through institutional transformation has another consequence. It explains why USP standards are not limited in practice to the "lowest common denominator" but are the "acceptable common denominator." Although our sub-committees strive for consensus when a number of parties are involved, or acquiescence of one party, USP standards are held to the more idealistic level of knowledgeable self-regulation. Consensus is not prerequisite.

Often quoted is de Tocqueville's observation that Americans like to form associations to accomplish mutual purposes without the burden of additional government. This is fueled by our spirit of voluntarism. The USP effort, starting in 1820, certainly fits that description (14). However, why can't trade associations be the vehicles of effective self-regulation? All who have worked with these know it cannot be done readily when any member's vested interest is seriously threatened. Consensus in the strictest sense applies. The same type of experts, if elected to the USP Committee of Revision, can take that last essential step in self-regulation: they can set meaningful end-product standards free of strict consensus. It is the majority vote that decides. It is the unique nature of the USPC that effects that transformation. It does what deserves to be done, but without all the baggage that comes with more government.

To appreciate the impact of this element, consider the sheer magnitude of the USP revision effort. Table 2 gives summary facts about the magnitude of recent USP activity. Each of these pharmacopeial revisions involved industrial participation. Ask yourself: How could so many things get done unless participants of all types were willing or at least favorably disposed? They are so disposed because in this quality-conscious industry, people want standards and because most would be willing to regulate themselves.

INTERNATIONAL RELATIONSHIPS

International Harmonization

The phenomenon of globalization of pharmaceutical manufacturing and distribution, already evident in the excipient monographs of the NF 18, continued throughout the revision cycle leading to the USP 24-NF 19.

Although originally founded as an organization to standardize medicines in the United States, the USP and its products and services are now known and used throughout the world. In today's transnational and multinational economy for pharmaceuticals, the USP needs a strong international presence and influence for its survival as well as for continued growth and recognized leadership. Economic forces are driving major trading parties to affiliate to reduce trade barriers. Integral to this process is harmonization of requirements, regulations, and standards governing the approval and marketing of drugs, devices, etc., by governments. (See also *Harmonization of Pharmacopeial Standards* in the second edition of this Encyclopedia.) In view of the contemporaneous publication of that chapter, also prepared here, only formal publication agreements are discussed herein.

Two organizations account for harmonization of new and revised standards: the Pharmacopeial Discussion Group (PDG) and the International Conference on Harmonisation (ICH). Primary impact is attributed in this cycle again to the PDG consisting of the USP with the Japanese and European pharmacopoeias. Joint open conferences held on an international basis were crucial to any progress here because these ensured direct contact among experts from the three pharmacopoeias (see "Open Conferences and Meetings," earlier).

Harmonization is not a one-time event, and it does not imply superimposability of texts. Residual disharmony can exist at the end of any specific attempt to harmonize standards. Iterations of harmonization, already evident, will be the norm in the future. Refer to the *PF* as the essential source of any future understanding or tracking of harmonization topics or sequences.

One serious discrepancy exists between requirements in this Pharmacopoeia and ICH guidelines beyond the relative mandatory status. USP-NF requirements are enforceable by U.S. federal and state laws and regulations. The standards give the attributes of acceptable articles already used in healthcare. A key contrast can be seen in the strict focus of the ICH, which is explicit in treating new drugs, that is, those not yet in use. The situations differ dramatically in practical consequences and breadth of application. Therefore, the goal of harmonization in some cases is not currently achievable because justification does not exist to disturb many established products in favor of the most recent new drug approval practices.

Foreign Use of the USP and NF

Evidence of the utility of the USP beyond North America is found in the many orders received for USPC publications (USP, Supplements, *Pharmacopeial Forum*) and reference standards. In return, the contributions of foreign scientists in questioning existing standards and in commenting on *Pharmacopeial Forum* proposals frequently reveal insights not otherwise focused in domestic queries and comments. Although many of these insights that originate in foreign countries are passed to the USP through domestic affiliates, committee members usually are aware of the originator's contribution. Foreign scientific input is extensive and receives the same consideration on merit as does domestic comment.

Limitations on foreign use of USP standards arise from that same high technological level of the standards. Instruments cost, availability, and maintenance prospects set high barriers where foreign exchange is a problem for a country. Arranging for training of pharmaceutical scientists, and then keeping them, is also a limiting factor.

The Drug Information Division selects the person from a large pool of candidates for nomination in the particular class of service. For example, the nominating committees for the 1990–1995 Committee of Revision screened a pool of over 1200 candidates before they agreed on 228 nominees for 114 positions, representing 45 classes of service.

The advisory panels have an even more active program to identify highly qualified persons from other countries. As the USP DI database becomes more widely known and used outside the United States, the USP seeks qualified persons from countries using USP drug information to provide advice on the utility of the information in those countries and advice on how the drugs in the database are used in those countries. In this way, the database can be enriched and made more useful to a greater number of countries.

OTHER PHARMACOPEIAS

International Pharmacopoeia

The USP has established formal arrangements with individual countries or pharmacopeias that are not direct participants in harmonization, although the practical effects may be the same. As noted above, harmonization per se is the subject of a separate chapter in the second edition of this Encyclopedia.

Canada

Canada has a special relationship with the USP. The USP-NF has been officially recognized by statute as a legal compendium in Canada since 1954. Approximately 95% of drugs claiming compliance with compendial standards in Canada follow the USP-NF. The USP is proud of its status in Canada and values the contributions of its Canadian members. Representatives of the Therapeutic Products Programme (TPP) of Health Canada and the Canadian Pharmaceutical Association are members-at-large of the U.S. Pharmacopeial Convention. Relations between the Health Protection Branch and the USP are cordial; the USP seeks to work closely with the TPP, as it does with the FDA. Six Canadians were elected to the USP Committee of Revision for the 1995–2000 period, and 45 Canadians have been appointed to USP advisory panels. Canadian pharmaceutical scientists, physicians, pharmacists, and other healthcare professionals take an active interest in the USP. In addition to the USP-NF being official in Canada, the USP drug information database *USP DI* covers all drugs on the Canadian market as well as on the U.S. market.

Argentina, Mexico, and Brazil

The USP initiated discussions with compilers of the three other active pharmacopeias in the Western Hemisphere. USP scientists, practitioners, and staff have been intimately involved in meetings and programs, both in standards and in information. These successful efforts put down the groundwork for the first agreement with Argentina and subsequently with Brazil and Mexico between the USP and other Western Hemisphere pharmacopeias that allows use of any part of the USP or NF, in English or Spanish, as an aid to elaboration of a national pharmacopeia. Establishment of the same standards obviates the less desirable effort of harmonization. Adoption of the NAFTA pact within Canada, Mexico, and the United States stimulated progress on this bilateral basis.

The *Farmacopea de los Estados Unidos Mexicanos* (FEUM) is the Mexican Pharmacopoeia. Stimulated by the signing of the North American Free Trade Agreement (NAFTA), the USP and the FEUM initiated a dialogue in January 1993 to explore opportunities for harmonization. Originally conceived as a semiannual meeting after the Pharmacopeial Discussion Group (PDG) model, the USP has hosted five visiting scientists from Latin America.

China

The *Pharmacopoeia of China* contains volumes dealing with both Western and traditional Chinese medicines. A series of informal visits has taken place at the initiation of the Chinese Pharmacopoeia Commission (ChPC). The USP has been host to visiting scientists from China and has had seven scientists from the Chinese Pharmacopoeia in residence for periods up to 4 months each.

International Pharmacopoeia

The World Health Organization (WHO) took over the programs begun by the League of Nations, based on the work of the Brussels conferences in the early 1900s. Special emphasis was directed at the establishment of the *International Pharmacopoeia* (IP). The IP differs from national and regional pharmacopoeias in that it is not directly mandatory in few countries. Focus is on the needs of developing countries where acquisition and use of modern, automated analytical technologies may be difficult. The IP provides analytical methodologies that can be used where more advanced technologies are not readily available. The WHO program for International Non-proprietary Names is coordinated with the U.S. Adopted Names Council. Over the years, members of the Committee of Revision and members of the USP staff have served on the Expert Committees on Specifications for Pharmaceutical Preparations and Antibiotics, continuing the USP's long-standing commitment to WHO drug quality programs.

In accordance with Article 41 of its Constitution, the WHO published a first edition of the *International Pharmacopoeia* in 1952. Because no official national representatives were part of the Commission, the *International Pharmacopoeia* was considered not to have legal force. That legal characteristic has continued. Nevertheless, the *International Pharmacopoeia* continues to attract the energies of pharmaceutical scientists from many countries. The *International Pharmacopoeia* has been positioned to address national needs not satisfied by the large regional pharmacopoeias such as the USP. The USP must be in accord with well-equipped analytical laboratories, technologically advanced manufacturers, highly varied and competitive markets, and therapeutic strategies and expectations characteristic of our intensive, personalized medical care. In contrast, the *International Pharmacopoeia* seeks to publish standards using technology appropriate to some small- and medium-sized quality control laboratories (20). Basic tests to check drug identity and to exclude substantial decomposition are notable and extensive achievements by WHO experts. A scheme for certification of suppliers is also published.

Color tests have fallen into disuse in North America as convenient but analytically powerful instruments have come in the budgetary range for control laboratories. This condition does not yet pertain to much of the world. Attention to the provisions of the *International Pharmacopoeia* in those countries can make important contributions to the drug product quality received by their populations. To help realize this, the WHO has supplied detailed guidance for staffing and equipping small, medium, and large analytical laboratories with increasing degrees of technology and instrumentation (20).

The present scope of the *International Pharmacopoeia* continues to be that defined by Wieniawski (21), that of furnishing quality specifications for drug substances and general requirements for dosage forms. Thus, no monographs for individual dosage forms are published in the *International Pharmacopoeia*. WHO leadership may intend to include dosage forms in the future, but a more definitive statement cannot be made at this writing. The three volumes of the third edition give standards for "essential" drug substances (22).

European Pharmacopoeia

European Pharmacopoeia provisions now take precedence over all European national pharmacopoeias.

British Pharmacopoeia

Many similarities existed between the *British Pharmacopoeia* and the USP. Common elements of origin, continuing commerce, and a long history of cooperation have resulted in close correspondence in critical details. Both are legal instruments, both are recognized in the laws of countries other than those of origin, both establish standards for dosage forms as well as for bulk pharmaceutical chemicals. Both use experts from industry, academia, and government at all stages of standards development. Also, for most of its history, the *British Pharmacopoeia* was not a direct government effort.

Other National Pharmacopoeias

There are national pharmacopoeias established by governments to meet perceived needs for compendial standards for locally produced articles. A number of these have published recent editions as evidence of continuing commitment, but it is often difficult to locate a U.S. bookseller for these. Cities of publication are Berlin, Paris, Prague, Rome, Tokyo, Peking, Seoul, Stuttgart, and Taipei. Most countries require imported articles to conform to one or another widely recognized pharmacopoeia, such as the USP or the *British Pharmacopoeia*.

USP Products and Services in Other Countries

Since 1982, the USP has developed distributorships in other countries to meet the needs of customers more directly. The Zentrallaboratorium Deutscher Apotheker [Central Laboratory of the German Pharmacists Association (ZL)] in Eschborn, Germany, was the first distributor and now serves clients in Europe and in the Middle East. The largest distributor is Promochem GmbH, with headquarters in Wesel, Germany, and branches throughout Europe. The British Pharmaceutical Society distributes Reference Standards throughout the United Kingdom. The Society for the Japanese Pharmacopoeia became a distributor in 1991. In Canada, at least two firms distribute Reference Standards. Distributor information appears in each bimonthly Reference Standard Catalog published in *Pharmacopeial Forum*.

Agency for International Development

The USP had a cooperative agreement with the U.S. Agency for International Development (USAID) since 1992 to assist developing countries in establishing programs of pharmaceutical management (including procurement, storage, and distribution) and control (including country-specific formularies and drug information resources). This program is jointly funded by the USAID and the USP.

U.S. Department of Commerce

In 1992, the Department of Commerce (DOC) established the Special American Business Internship and Training (SABIT) program to train scientists from the newly independent states (NIS). The USP secured an agreement whereby the DOC sponsors travel expenses for six Russian scientists under the USP Visiting Scientists Program to learn techniques in drug analysis at the USP Drug Research and Testing Laboratory. To date, two scientists have each completed 4-month training programs. The laboratory in which these scientists will work will be established in Moscow and funded by the World Bank. The International Foundation for Drug Efficacy and Safety (IFDES), a not-for-profit group chartered under Russian, Swiss, German, and U.S. laws, is a voluntary group working with the NIS to assist in restoring their programs of drug supply regulation and quality control.

REFERENCES

1. *The United States Pharmacopoeia*, 24th Rev. The National Formutary, 19th Ed.; The United States Pharmacopeial Convention, Inc.: Rockville, MD, 1999; Both Official from January 1, 2000.
2. Rules and Procedures of the General and Executive Committees of Revision for 1995–2000. Pharmacopoeial Forum **1995**, *21*, 1619.
3. USP, 24th Rev., xxxvii–xiii.
4. Johnson, C.A. The Purposes and Limitations of a Pharmacopoeia. International Symposium on the Compendia and Industry, Montreal 1985; Pharmazeut. Ind.: 1986; 48, 760.
5. Grady, L.T.; J. A. Pharm. Assoc. **1976**, *16*, 603, NS.
6. Boorstin, DanielJ. *The Americans—The Democratic Experience*; Chap. 22, Random House: New York, 1973.
7. Descartes, R. *Discourse on the Method*; [L. J. Lafleur transl. 1637.
8. Added Substances. *Ingredients and Processes*; USP, 24th Rev., General Notices.
9. *Tests and Assays—Procedures*; USP, 24th Rev., 7General Notices.
10. USP, 24th Rev., General Notices.
11. Grady, L.T.; Pharmazeut. Ind. **1983**, *45*, 640.
12. King, R.H.; Grady, L.T.; Reamer, J.T. J. Pharm. Sci. **1974**, *63*, 1571.
13. Grady, L.T. Cooperation between USP and Industry [see Ref. 5].
14. Heller, W.M. Private Communication.
15. Florey, K. Reflections of a Quality Control Watcher. *Progress in the Quality Control of Medicines*; Deasey and Timonesy, Ed.; Elsevier Biomedical Press: Amsterdam, 1981; 15.
16. Stainer, C. *Ceremony of the Presentation of the European Pharmacopoeia*; Council of Europe: Strasbourg, France, 1969; 1, 5–71.
17. Schorn, P.J. International Harmonization of Pharmacopoeial Standards [see Ref 5].
18. *European Pharmacopoeia*, 2nd Ed.; II. 10th Fascile.; Council of Europe: Strasbourg, France, 1986.
19. Sagath, J. Proceedings of the International Meeting on Pharmacopoeias and Quality Control of Drugs, Cingolani, E., Ed.; 228 Annali Istit. Super. Sanita **1975**, 11, 228
20. World Health Organization. *WHO Technical Report Series*; World Health Organization: Geneva, 1984.
21. Wieniawski, W. Proceedings of the International Meeting on Pharmacopoeias and Quality Control of Drugs, 204–210.
22. World Health Organization. *The International Pharmacopoeia*, 3rd Ed.; World Health Organization: Geneva, 1988.

PHOTODECOMPOSITION OF DRUGS

Hanne Hjorth Tønnesen

University of Oslo, Oslo, Norway

INTRODUCTION

Numerous compounds degrade when exposed to light. Some light-sensitive drugs are rapidly affected, either by natural light (particularly ultraviolet) or by artificial light (e.g., fluorescent light). This may lead to a change in the physicochemical properties of the product, e.g., a precipitate is formed, the product becomes discolored or cloudy, a loss in viscosity is observed, or the active ingredient undergoes photodegradation, which may not be visually detectable. The most obvious result of drug photodecomposition is a loss of potency of the product. Consequently, this can result in a drug preparation that is therapeutically inactive. Although this does not occur often, the study of photodegradation is important because the decomposition products that might occur in the formulation during storage may be toxic. Such products may also develop by the action of sunlight on the epidermal layers of the skin or in the eye of patients receiving the drug and may thereby cause photosensitivity reactions. Photostability testing is therefore an essential part of product development and is needed to ensure that satisfactory product quality is maintained during practical usage.

In this chapter, various aspects of drug photoreactivity are presented. Common photochemical reactions by which drugs have been found to decompose are described. The influence of formulation factors, e.g., excipients, on product stability is discussed. Finally, variables that have to be considered in photostability studies are noted.

PHOTOREACTIVITY OF DRUG SUBSTANCES

The photochemical reaction is a complex process. During the last decade, a body of data relating to drug degradation pathways has been accumulated and recently reported (1–3). The light-sensitive drug molecules may be affected directly or indirectly by irradiation, depending on how the radiant energy is tranferred to the drug molecules. Primary photochemical reactions occur when the drug molecule itself absorbs energy, i.e., when there is a certain overlap between the absorption spectrum of the molecule and the incident radiation. Many drug substances are white, and thus the degradation depends primarily on the amount of UV radiation absorbed by the material. Colored substances absorb light in the visible region of the spectrum. Degradation products formed during shelf life can be colored and thereby change the overall absorption characteristics of the formulation. Any overlap of the product absorption spectrum with the photon source impinging on it has the potential to cause a photochemical change. One consequence may be that a drug substance with an absorption spectrum that does not overlap with the photon source still photodecomposes in a formulated product. This takes place in a process called photsensitization. The energy absorbed by the nondrug molecule is imparted to the active ingredient, which subsequently degrades. The absorbing component is called a photosensitizer. The sensitizer may transfer the absorbed energy completely and not be altered itself in the process, but in many cases it will undergo some degradation. Photochemical stability of a drug compound in a formulation therefore cannot be predicted from only the absorption spectrum/stability studies of the drug in a pure solvent. Stability studies of the drug substance in the final product must also be considered.

Light acts as a reactant and never as a catalyst in a photochemical reaction. Light energy (a photon) is absorbed by the promotion of an electron from an initially occupied, low-energy orbital to a high-energy, previously unoccupied orbital. The result is an electronically excited molecule. In the singlet state, the electron spins are paired (antiparallel), whereas in the triplet state, the electron spins are unpaired (parallel). Excited states are both better donors and better acceptors of electrons than are ground states. They are unstable and often return to the ground state by dissipating their energy as heat and/or light. In many cases, the excited state leads to the formation of high-energy products such as free radicals or radical ions. Photochemical processes usually occur in two stages. The primary reaction is the reaction directly attributable to the absorption of a photon, i.e., it involves the excited state. This reaction does not depend on temperature for activation of the molecules. The primary photochemical reaction, however, will often be followed by secondary (thermal) reactions occurring from the intermediates produced by the primary photochemical process (e.g., radicals, radical ions). These intermediates can eventually react through "dark" reactions to form the final, stable products. In some cases, the final products may resemble the products of the purely thermal reaction (dark reaction from the molecular ground state), but this similarity is coincidental.

Drugs are usually stored in contact with atmospheric oxygen and are always in contact with dissolved oxygen in circulating blood and living tissues. Energy transfer from an excited drug molecule will often lead to the formation of reactive oxygen species (ROS)(4). A type I photosensitized reaction proceeds through the transfer of electrons or protons. The resulting cation or neutral radical is likely to undergo further reactions. In the absence of oxygen, dimerization or recombination can result. When oxygen is available in sufficient concentrations, molecular oxygen will rapidly add to the radical, leading to the formation of peroxy radicals. These radicals are highly reactive and tend to abstract a proton from neighboring molecules. This sequence is often described as a chain reaction. In another photosensitization mechanism, an electron is transferred from an excited drug molecule to ground-state oxygen to give an anion radical known as superoxide. Superoxide is a powerful oxidizing agent and very toxic to biological systems.

Most molecules are singlet in the ground state. The oxygen molecule is unusual in that it is a triplet. In a type II photosensitized reaction, energy transfer from an excited drug molecule to ground state oxygen gives excited oxygen in the singlet state. Singlet oxygen is very reactive toward organic molecules and can lead to the formation of hydroperoxides by addition to olefinic bonds.

A relationship between structure and photoreactivity can be difficult to predict, but certain structural types are

known to have a high possibility of photodecomposition. Examples are shown in Table 1. Olefinic carbon–carbon double bonds can undergo *cis-trans* isomerization and may cyclize as a result; arylacetic acids are likely to decarboxylate; and some amines *N*-Dealkylate and haloaromatic compounds tend to dehalogenate. A drug can also sensitize its own degradation or drugs in a mixture can undergo cross-sensitization (5). Unfortunately, several pathways are reported for many drugs, complicating the elucidation of mechanisms. An extensive list of common photoreactions of drug substances was compiled by Greenhill and McLelland (1).

A drug that displays photochemical reactivity in vivo may cause adverse photosensitivity effects in patients. Sunlight penetrates the skin to a sufficient depth to reach molecules circulating in the surface capillaries, or it can react with compounds accumulated in the eye. In both cases, sunlight may convert the drug to a toxic decomposition product or induce the formation of ROS. Singlet oxygen and superoxide are both toxic to human tissues. Cutaneous photosensitization can be classified as phototoxicity, in which the skin reactions derive directly from photosensitized damage to the cellular components of the skin, and photoallergy, in which the mechanisms of the immune system are activated. Phototoxic reactions may be oxygen-dependent (photodynamic) or oxygen-independent (nonphotodynamic). In some cases, photodegradation products can circulate in the blood stream and cause damage to deep-seated organs. However, it should be noted that a combination of drugs and light can be beneficial, such as in the treatment of vitiligo, psoriasis, and skin cancer and in the development of site-specific drug-delivery systems.

The rate of a photochemical reaction is in general dependent on the rate at which light is absorbed by the system (i.e., the number of photons absorbed per second) and the efficiency of the photochemical process (i.e., the quantum yield for the reaction). The quantum yield is usually independent of wavelength. A primary photochemical reaction follows first-order kinetics in a formulation that contains the drug substance in a low concentration (6). The kinetics is more complicated at higher concentrations. Most of the light will then be absorbed close to the sample surface. The drug molecules inside the volume become protected from irradiation and do not participate in the primary reaction (inner filter effect). If the concentration of the active compound is high (absorbance approaches 2), the degradation kinetics may follow a pseudo-zero-order rate. In this case, essentially all the light is absorbed by the drug, and the rate-limiting factor is the light intensity. It is, however, the overlap integral that determines the rate of the reaction. Because of a small overlap integral, first-order kinetics can be

Table 1 Chemical functions that are expected to introduce photoreactivity

Carbonyl group
Nitroaromatic group
N-oxide function
Carbon-carbon double bond
Aryl halide
C   H bond α to an amine nitrogen
C—II bond at a benzylic position
Reactions with singlet oxygen
Alkenes
Polyenes
Phenol
Sulfides

observed even if the product contains a large amount of the absorbing species. The rate of disappearance of the drug in a sensitized reaction may be dependent on both the drug and the sensitizer concentrations, i.e., the degradation process follows second-order kinetics. It is difficult to use reaction order to characterize photodegradation in the solid state. The photochemical processes take place on the product surface, and the change in total concentration measured as a function of irradiation time does not necessarily follow any particular reaction order model (7).

INFLUENCE OF PRODUCT FORMULATION ON DRUG PHOTOSTABILITY

Most photochemical reactions are affected by the medium, i.e., both by excipients and by the type of formulation (8). Examples of formulation factors influencing product photostability are given in Table 2. A drug substance in an intravenous infusion product is likely to be presented as a dilute solution, whereas the active compound of a topical preparation represents a situation part way between the solution phase and the solid state. Parenteral solutions ensure high light impingement on the drug molecules owing to a large surface-to-volume ratio and usually a low drug concentration. In the solid state; the depth of light penetration is determined by the characteristics of the sample surface. For example, a capsule and a tablet have different light-scattering characteristics and different surface area-to-volume ratios.

Cosolvents, such as ethanol or higher alcohols, and surfactants are often used in a formulation to enhance the solubility of sparingly soluble compounds or to modify the stability of the drug molecule. Cosolvents will change the polarity and, in some cases, the viscosity of the medium. This may influence the photochemical reactivity of a compound. An increase in solubility will change the sample absorbance. Dissolution of particle aggregates leads to an increase in light impingement on the separate drug molecules. Surfactants will form micelles that can interact with drug molecules. This can lead to a change in drug molar absorptivity or in reactivity owing to a micro-environmental effect. Cosolvents and surfactants can have a photostabilizing or photodestabilizing effect on the product, as demonstrated for phenobarbital and nitro-furazone, respectively (9, 10).

For many drug substances, the photodegradation process is highly dependent on the ionization form of the molecule (e.g., ciprofloxacin, midazolam, and chloro-quine) (11–13). The dicationic form of the antimalarial drug mefloquine is almost not photolyzed, whereas the monocationic and neutral forms of the molecule readily undergo photodecomposition (14). The oxygen concentration plays an important role in the process. Flushing the mefloquine samples with helium during irradiation leads to a substantial increase in the degradation rate. Destabilization by removal of oxygen is also demonstrated for other drugs such as nitrazepam (15). For oxygen-sensitive compounds, a stabilizing effect would ordinarily be obtained by purging the solution and headspace with an inert gas. However, it should be recalled that for reactions

Table 2 Formulation factors that may influence the photostability of drugs

Solutions	Solid preparations	Miscellaneous
Drug concentration	Crystal modification	Cyclodextrins (type)
Solvent system	Particle size	Liposomes (type, charge)
Cosolvents	Particle surface (porous, smooth)	Micelles (type, charge)
Surfactants		Emulsifying agent
pH	Color	Partition coefficient
Oxygen concentration	Coating	
Buffer salt (type, concentration)	Thickness of powder bed	
Ionic strength	Container	
Metal ions		
Chelating agents		
Antioxidants		
Preservatives		
Sweetening agents		
Tonicity adjustors		
Colors		
Container		

in which oxygen participates only catalytically, even trace amounts of residual oxygen may render the product unstable. An increase in ionic strength is reported to have a photostabilizing effect on certain drugs by providing a protective film of solvated ions around the reacting molecule (16). This effect is not observed in mefloquine (14). On the other hand, an increase in degradation rate was measured as a function of phosphate ion concentration in the buffer system used. The phosphate ion is known to influence the photochemical properties of compounds (e.g., tyrosine) by facilitating proton transfer from the excited state of the reacting species (17). Various types of buffer salts exert different effects on the photodegradation process, as demonstrated for the drug daunorubicin (18). Buffer salts such as citrate can also change the absorption characteristics of the formulation by forming complexes with other components present, leading to products that absorb in the visible part of the spectrum.

In many cases, the degradation rate is highly dependent on the presence of trace metals. A variety of chelating agents and antioxidants is available for use in pharmaceutical preparations. The most commonly used in aqueous systems are bisulfite and EDTA. Many drugs have shown reactivity toward bisulfite. A significant photodestabilizing effect on epinephrine has been demonstrated (19). Fe(III)-EDTA chelates are reduced by superoxide quite rapidly. EDTA therefore will not inhibit degradation of drugs in systems in which the iron-catalyzed Haber-Weiss reaction plays an important role. The effect of antioxidants and chelating agents on drug instability must be carefully evaluated before use. Other excipients such as tonicity adjustors, colors (see below), and sweetening agents could further interact with commonly used stabilizers or influence the photoreactivity of the drug substance (20–23).

Photoprotection by spectral overlay with suitable excipients can stabilize various drugs and preparations. Incorporation of the yellow compound curcumin in the shell of soft gelatin capsules was demonstrated to have a protective effect on drugs such as nifedipine, chloramfenicol, frusemide, and clonazepam (24). The addition of colors is further shown to stabilize drugs in tablets, solution, and topical preparations (25). A mixture of colors or pigments, however, can undergo catalytic fading (26) or induce degradation of other components in the formulations by radical formation (27, 28).

Photodegradation in the solid state takes place only at the sample surface. The degradation rate is therefore dependent on factors that will influence the depth of light penetration, i.e., change the absorption and reflection at the surface (e.g., particle size, crystal modification, color, thickness of powder bed, and coating of the individual particles or the dosage form). Mefloquine, chloroquine, carbamazepine, and furosemide are examples of drug substances that show different decomposition rates dependent on their polymorphous modification (29–32).

A change in drug photoreactivity by complexation with suitable carriers can be observed both in solution and in the solid state. Metronidazole was found to be less sensitive to irradiation after complex formation with sodium urate (33). The extent of photodegradation of various drugs including phenothiazine has been reduced by inclusion complexation with cyclodextrins (34–36). There are marked differences in stabilizing effect among various types of cyclodextrin. Liposomes or a combination of liposomes and cyclodextrins are also demonstrated to improve drug photostability (37, 38).

The method used most commonly to protect photosensitive drugs is to place the preparation in a protective market pack or in a colored or amber immediate container. During storage and use, the protective market pack may be removed. In cases in which the immediate container is made of transparent glass or plastic material, little protection against radiation is obtained. Amber containers offer better protection but vary in thickness, chemical nature (plastic), and degree of coloration, which may influence their photoprotective properties. The stabilizing effect of amber glass as the only means of photoprotection is not satisfactory for highly photolabile drugs such as molsidomine (39). Even brown glass can offer inadequate protection, as demonstrated for drugs like epinephrine, isoprenaline, and levarterenol (40). The destabilizing effect of the container was attributed to release of alkali and traces of heavy metal ions that import color to the glass.

PHOTOSTABILITY STUDIES

It is essential to obtain information about the photoreactivity of a drug molecule as early as possible in the formulation process (41). Knowledge about the photochemical and photophysical properties of a drug substance is important for the handling, packaging, and labeling of the product. One approach to evaluate overall photosensitivity is to design a photoassay, as noted in an earlier report (42). A basic protocol for testing new drug substances and products for first submissions is described in the ICH Guideline for photostability testing, which has been implemented since January 1998 (43). The Guideline notes that photostability testing should be an integral part of stress testing. Although the proposed test is reasonably simple to conduct, there are some variables that have to be controlled carefully during photostability studies.

Problems related to the application of the current guideline are discussed in a recent review (44). Important factors to consider are irradiation source, irradiation level, calibration, and presentation of the samples (45–48).

Various irradiation sources can be used in the stability studies of drugs and drug products. The source(s) selected should be comparable in spectral distribution with those to which products are exposed in practical use. The portion of radiant energy from the sun reaching the Earth includes the UVB (290–320 nm), UVA (320–400 nm), and visible (VIS) light (400–700 nm) ranges. It may be difficult, however, to predict the exact amount of UV and VIS irradiation to which the product is exposed during shelf life. The irradiation conditions therefore should provide a "worst-case" exposure. The ICH Guideline gives two options for the selection of irradiation source. Option 1 addresses exposure to outdoor daylight or window glass-filtered daylight. In most cases, a source providing glass-filtered daylight (ID65 according to ISO 10977) would be appropriate. Option 1 can be achieved by use of a fluorescent lamp that combines UV and VIS outputs or by use of a xenon or metal halide lamp. To simulate indoor conditions, it is necessary to use a window glass filter in combination with sources producing significant radiation below 320 nm (e.g., xenon and metal halide lamps, near-UV fluorescent tubes). Option 2 in the ICH Guideline addresses exposure to indoor fluorescent light (cool white). During shelf life the product is likely to be exposed to a mixture of natural light through window glass and artificial light (e.g., light from a fluorescent tube). A UV source is therefore added in Option 2 to cover the spectral region of natural light that may reach the sample. According to this option, the test is more severe than that for indoor fluorescent light alone, but it does not adequately simulate daylight through window glass.

The ICH Guideline recommends a total exposure of 200 Wh/m^{-2} in the UV range of 320 to 400 nm and 1.2 million lux hours in the VIS range (400–700 nm). For an average source simulating window glass-filtered daylight, a total irradiance of 200 Wh/m^{-2} in the UV region corresponds to approximately 0.45 million lux hours in the visible region. A test run with the end criterion of 1.2 million lux hours is therefore likely to exceed the requirement of 200 Wh/m^{-2} with a factor of up to 2.5 to 3 when a lamp according to Option 1 is selected, unless precautions are taken (44). In this context, Option 2 may be easier to handle because the UV lamp can be turned off when the desired UV exposure is obtained.

The ICH Guideline offers no guidance for the choice of Option 1 or 2. Although the options are not scientifically equivalent, they could be regarded as equivalent for purposes of a confirmatory study. It is important, however, to combine the results with knowledge already obtained from other tests before labeling decisions are made.

The overall illumination is specified in the ICH Guideline, whereas the irradiance level is not indicated. An irradiance level that is high enough to accelerate the test without causing unwanted temperature effects must be selected. Tests conducted at significantly different irradiance levels could not be compared unless correlation has been established. The distance between the source and the sample surface should be defined to keep the radiant intensity constant. The irradiance at the specimen surface may also change as a function of the sample location inside the test chamber. The UV and visible levels should therefore be measured across the test chamber to ensure that the samples are placed at points of equal irradiance.

Even though the lamps are changed at defined intervals as specified by the producer, it is essential to calibrate the light source and periodically monitor its irradiance to obtain the predetermined exposure value. For instrumentation without a build-in sensor, calibration can be performed manually. The ICH Guideline recomends the use of a calibrated radiometer or a validated actinometric system to monitor the exposure in the UV region and a calibrated luxmeter to determine the overall illumination in the visible range. Neither will provide any information about the spectral distribution of the irradiation source. A UV filter radiometer is a broad-band meter designed to measure incident radiation in the UV region. An optical filter limits the spectral responsivity to a certain band (e.g., UVB and UVA). Unfortunately, there are no international standards for the filters and radiometers from different manufacturers, and therefore they may measure different fractions of radiant energy. A luxmeter will measure light as perceived by the human eye, i.e., it has a photopic response curve. The phototopic sensitivity range of the human eye is approximately 380 to 780 nm, with the highest sensitivity at 555 nm. Neither the radiometer nor the luxmeter have a constant spectral responsivity over the actual wavelength range (i.e., the relative weighting given to the different wavelengths is not constant). The devices should be calibrated by the manufacturer at regular intervals. If the meters are used as received, they are well suited for measuring evenness of irradiance across the sample area and changes in total output with time. However, they cannot be used to give an absolute measurement of irradiance or to compare irradiance between sources unless they are calibrated specifically for each source (44). The ICH Guideline proposes quinine actinometry as an alternative to the radiometer for calibration in the UV range. The total irradiance is then determined by using a reaction of known photochemical efficiency (47, 49).

Samples may be placed in clear or amber glass, in plastic, in marketed containers, or in a Petri dish during exposure. The spectral transmittance characteristics of the container will influence the results. For example, the illuminance inside clear glass is higher than that inside amber, blue, or green glass, and the spectral distribution is different. Other factors to consider are the orientation of the sample container (upright, inverted, or sideways), thickness of the container material, and surface area/volume (weight) ratio. It is recommended in the ICH Guideline that the sample thickness should not exceed 3 mm for drug substances in the solid form. Preparations such as tablets or capsules should be spread in a single layer. The primary disadvantage in using a protective container is that a significant increase in temperature can be expected. Therefore, dark controls should be placed alongside the authentic sample. Stirring or shaking of samples during exposure is not recommended for the purpose of photostability testing, according to the ICH Guideline.

REFERENCES

1. Greenhill, J.V.; McLelland, M.A. Photodecomposition of Drugs. Prog. Med. Chem. **1990**, *27*, 51–121.
2. Greenhill, J.V. Is the Photodecomposition of Drugs Predictable? *Photostability of Drugs and Drug Formulations*; Tønnesen, H.H., Ed.; Taylor & Francis: London, 1996; 83–110.
3. Albini, A.; Fasani, E. Photochemistry of Drugs: An Overview and Practical Problems. *Drugs. Photochemistry and Photostability*; Albini, A., Fasani, E., Eds.; The Royal Society of Chemistry: Cambridge, 1998; 1–74.
4. Moore, D.E. Photophysical and Photochemical Aspects of Drug Stability. *Photostability of Drugs and Drug Formulations*; Tønnesen, H.H., Ed.; Taylor & Francis: London, 1996; 9–38.
5. Moore, D.E.; Mallesch, J.L. Photochemical Interaction between Triamterene and Hydrochlorthiazide. Int. J. Pharm. **1991**, *76*, 187–190.
6. Tønnesen, H.H. Photochemical Degradation of Components in Drug Formulations. I. An Approach to the Standardization of Degradation Studies. Pharmazie **1991**, *46*, 263–265.
7. Sande, S.A. Mathematical Models for Studies of Photochemical Reactions. *Photostability of Drugs and Drug Formulations*; Tønnesen, H.H., Ed.; Taylor & Francis: London, 1996; 323–340.
8. Kerker, R. Untersuchungen zur Photostabilität von Nifedipin, Glococorticoiden, Mosidomin und Ihren Zubereitungen, München, 1991, Dissertation.
9. Shahjahan, M.; Enever, R.P. Photolability of Nitrofurazone in Aqueous Solution. II. Kinetic Studies. Int. J. Pharm. **1996**, *143*, 83–92.
10. Asker, A.F.; Islam, M.S. Effect of Sodium Thiosulphate on the Photolysis of Phenobarbital: Evidence of Complex Formation. PDA J. Pharm. Sci. Technol. **1994**, *48*, 205–210.
11. Torniainen, K.; Tammilehto, S.; Ulvi, V. The Effect of pH, Buffer-Type and Drug Concentration on the Photodegradation of Ciprofloxacin. Int. J. Pharm. **1996**, *132*, 53–61.
12. Andresin, R.; Tammilehto, S. Photochemical Decomposition of Midazolam. IV. Study of pH-Dependent Stability by High-Performance Liquid Chromatography. Int. J. Pharm. **1995**, *123*, 229–235.
13. Nord, K.; Orsteen, A.-L.; Karlsen, J.; Tønnesen, H.H. Photoreactivity of Biologically Active Compounds. X. Photoreactivity of Chloroquine in Aqueous Solution. Pharmazie **1997**, *52*, 598–603.
14. Tønnesen, H.H. Photoreactivity of Biologically Active Compounds. XV. Photochemical Behaviour of Mefloquine in Aqueous Solution. Pharmazie **1999**, *54*, 590–594.
15. Cornelissen, P.J.G. Beijersbergen van Henegouwen, G.M.J. Photochemical Decomposition of 1,4-Benzodiazepines. Nitrazepam. Photochem. Photobiol. **1979**, *30*, 337–341.
16. Chinnian, D.; Asker, A.F. Photostability Profiles of Minoxidil Solutions. PDA J. Pharm. Sci. Technol. **1996**, *50*, 94–98.
17. Lakowicz, J.R. *Principles of Fluorescence Spectroscopy*; Plenum Press: New York, 1983; 360.
18. Islam, M.S.; Asker, A.F. Photoprotection of Daunorubicin Hydrochloride with Sodium Sulfite. PDA J. Pharm. Sci. Technol. **1995**, *49*, 122–126.
19. Brustugun, J.; Tønnesen, H.H.; Klem, W.; Kjønniksen, I. Photodestabilization of Epinephrine by Sodium Metabisulfite. PDA J. Pharm. Sci. Technol. **2000**, *50*, 136–143.
20. Asker, A.F.; Canady, D. Influence of Certain Additives on the Photostabilizing Effect of Dimethylsulfoxide for Sodium Nitroprusside Solutions. Drug Dev. Ind. Pharm. **1984**, *10*, 1025–1039.
21. Asker, A.F.; Harris, C.W. Influence of Certain Additives on the Photostability of Physostigmine Sulfate Solutions. Drug Dev. Ind. Pharm. **1988**, *14*, 733–746.
22. Ho, A.H.L.; Puri, A.; Sugden, J.K. Effect of Sweetening Agents on the Light Stability of Aqueous Solutions of L-Ascorbic Acid. Int. J. Pharm. **1994**, *107*, 199–203.
23. Asker, A.F.; Colbert, D.Y. Influence of Certain Additives on the Photostabilizing Effect of Uric Acid for Solutions of FD&C Blue No. 2. Drug Dev. Ind. Pharm. **1982**, *8*, 759–774.
24. Tønnesen, H.H.; Karlsen, J. Studies on Curcumin and Curcuminoids. X. The Use of Curcumin as a Formulation Aid to Protect Light-Sensitive Drugs in Soft Gelatin Capsules. Int. J. Pharm. **1987**, *38*, 247–249.
25. Thoma, K. Photodecomposition and Stabilization of Compounds in Dosage Forms. *Photostability of Drugs and Drug Formulations*; Tønnesen, H.H., Ed.; Taylor & Francis: London, 1996; 111–140.
26. Kuramoto, N.; Kitao, T. Mechanism of the Photofading of Dye. Contribution of Singlet Oxygen in the Catalytic Fading of Anthraquinone Dye Mixtures. J. Chem. Technol. Biotechnol. **1980**, *30*, 129–135.
27. Skowronski, T.A.; Rabek, J.F.; Rånby, B. The Role of Commercial Pigments in the Photodegradation of Poly (Vinyl Chloride) (PVC). Polym. Degrad. Stab. **1984**, *8*, 37–53.
28. Sidhu, D.S.; Sugden, J.K. Effect of Food Dyes on the Photostability of Aqueous Solutions of L-Ascorbic Acid. Int. J. Pharm. **1992**, *83*, 263–266.

29. Nord, K.; Andersen, H.; Tønnesen, H.H. Photoreactivity of Biologically Active Compounds. XII. Photostability of Polymorphic Modifications of Chloroquine Diphosphate. Drug Stab. **1997**, *1*, 243–248.

30. Tønnesen, H.H.; Skrede, G.; Martinsen, B.K. Photoreactivity of Biologically Active Compounds. XIII. Photostability of Mefloquine Hydrochloride in the Solid State. Drug Stab. **1997**, *1*, 249–253.

31. Matsuda, Y.; Akazawa, R.; Teraoka, R.; Otsuka, M. Pharmaceutical Evaluation of Carbamazepine Modifications: Comparative Study for Photostability of Carbamazepine Polymorphs by Using Fourier-Transformed Reflection-Absorption Infrared Spectroscopy and Colorimetric Measurement. J. Pharm. Pharmacol. **1994**, *46*, 162–167.

32. de Villiers, M.M.; van der Watt, J.G.; Lötter, A.P. Kinetic Study of the Solid State Photolytic Degradation of Two Polymorphic Forms of Furosemide. Int. J. Pharm. **1992**, *88*, 275–283.

33. Habib, M.J.; Asker, A.F. Complex Formation Between Metronidazole and Sodium Urate: Effect on Photodegradation of Metronidazole. Pharm. Res. **1989**, *6*, 58–61.

34. Lutka, A. Effect of Cyclodextrin Complexation on Aqueous Solubility and Photostability of Phenothiazine. Pharmazie **2000**, *55*, 120–123.

35. Mielcarek, J. Photochemical Stability of the Inclusion Complexes of Nicardipine with α-, γ-Cyclodextrin, Methyl-β-Cyclodextrin and Hydroxypropyl-β-Cyclodextrin in the Solid State and in Solution. Pharmazie **1996**, *51*, 477–479.

36. Thoma, K.; Kübler, N. Einfluss von Hilfsstoffen auf die Photozersetzung von Arzneistoffen. Pharmazie **1997**, *52*, 122–129.

37. Habib, M.J.; Asker, A.F. Photostabilization of Riboflavin by Incorporation into Liposomes. J. Parent. Sci. Technol. **1991**, *45*, 124–127.

38. Loukas, Y.L.; Jayasekera, P.; Gregoriadis, G. Novel Liposome-Based Multicomponent System for the Protection of Photolabile Agents. Int. J. Pharm. **1995**, *117*, 85–94.

39. Thoma, K.; Kübler, N. Einfluss der Wellenlänge auf die Photozersetzung von Arzneistoffen. Pharmazie **1996**, *51*, 660–664.

40. Wollmann, H.; Grünert, R. Einfluss des Sichtbaren Lichtes auf die Haltbarkeit von Isoprenalin-, Epinephrin- und Levaterenollösungen in Unterschiedlichen Behältnissen. Pharmazie **1984**, *39*, 161–163.

41. Merrifield, D.R.; Carter, P.L.; Clapham, D.; Sanderson, F.D. Addressing the Problem of Light Instability During Formulation Development. *Photostability of Drugs and Drug Formulations*; Tønnesen, H.H., Ed.; Taylor & Francis: London, 1996; 141–154.

42. Tønnesen, H.H.; Kristensen, S.; Nord, K. In Vitro Screening of the Photoreactivity of Antimalarials: A Test Case. *Photostability of Drugs and Drug Formulations*; Tønnesen, H.H. Ed.; Taylor & Francis: London, 1996; 267–285.

43. ICH Harmonised Tripartite Guideline. Q1B: Photostability Testing of New Drug Substances and Products. Federal Register **1997**, *62*, 27115–27122.

44. Tønnesen, H.H. The ICH Photostability Guideline. A Discussion of Experimental Conditions. *Pharmaceutical Photostability and Stabilization Technology*; Thoma, K., Piechocki, J.T., Eds.; Marcel Dekker, Inc.: New York, In press.

45. Piechocki, J.T. Selecting the Right Source for Pharmaceutical Photostability Testing. *Drugs. Photochemistry and Photostability*; Albini, A., Fasani, E., Eds.; The Royal Society of Chemistry: Cambridge, UK, 1998; 247–271.

46. Boxhammer, J.; Willwoldt, C. Design and Validation Characterisitcs of Environmental Chambers for Photostability Testing. *Drugs. Photochemistry and Photostability*; Albini, A., Fasani, E., Eds.; The Royal Society of Chemistry; Cambridge, UK, 1998; 272–287.

47. Favaro, G. Actinometry: Concepts and Experiments. *Drugs. Photochemistry and Photostability*; Albini, A., Fasani, E., Eds.; The Royal Society of Chemistry: Cambridge, UK, 1998; 295–304.

48. Moore, D.E. Standardization of Photodegradation Studies and Kinetic Treatment of Photochemical Reactions. *Photostability of Drugs and Drug Formulations*; Tønnesen, H.H. Ed.; Taylor & Francis: London, 1996; 63–82.

49. Baertschi, S.W. Commentary on the Quinine Actinometry System Described in the ICH Draft Guideline on Photostability Testing of New Drug Substances and Products. Drug Stab. **1997**, *1*, 193–195.

PHYSIOLOGICAL FACTORS AFFECTING ORAL DRUG DELIVERY

Clive G. Wilson
Bridget O'Mahony
Blythe Lindsay
University of Strathclyde, Glasgow, United Kingdom

INTRODUCTION

Thirty years on from the explosion of commercially successful applications of targeted and controlled release pharmaceutical formulations, it is evident that there remains a need for further refinements and innovations in the field of drug delivery. Many of the larger corporations focus on the use of novel technology for extension of a product life cycle; however, in many cases solubility and permeability issues limit the application of such technologies. Additional complications arise due to inter- and intrasubject variability, compliance, and chronobiological variation in disease incidence.

Variability has many causes and an understanding of the factors that predict that certain therapeutic approaches will work better for some individuals than in others is key. This article will consider a few such examples from the literature and our own studies, which we hope will illustrate how physiological factors impact on disease treatment.

ORAL DRUG DELIVERY

In most cases, oral drug delivery is the cheapest and most convenient method of dosing. Unfortunately, it is difficult to achieve a precise control of the plasma-concentration-time profile by this route due to marked intra- and intersubject variation in gastrointestinal transit even under the rigidly controlled conditions of the clinical trial. Daily patterns of food intake, activity, and posture are large contributors to this variation. Drugs that are only absorbed from specific areas of the gastrointestinal tract, i.e., have a narrow "window of absorption," will be most affected by alterations in transit. The major determinants of this variation will be the amount of food and drink consumed.

In the western world, the average adult consumes and excretes between 1.5 and 2.5 L of fluid per day. The liquid is consumed as beverages whose intake is closely linked to the level of salt in the diet or as water in the fluid component of food. In addition, metabolic processes generate approximately 350 ml of water per day. Water turnover in the epithelial tissues of the gut (secretion and absorption) is estimated at 9 L per day and in view of this prodigious flux, we might expect that most of the internal cavities of the body have water in excess.

This is however, not true and certain environments of the gut might be regarded as moist rather than wet: for example, the oropharynx, the esophagus, and most of the large bowel. This lack of water increases the variability of drug delivery to these areas.

ESOPHAGEAL TRANSIT

For dosage forms to reach the stomach they must first pass through the oesophagus, a 25–30 cm long moist hollow tube. It is commonly assumed that swallowed dosage forms pass without hindrance into the stomach unless an underlying oesophageal condition is present. Up to 60% of healthy subjects over the age of 60 years report a problem in swallowing intact tablets (1). To assist swallowing of a tablet, patients are instructed to take a dosage form with plenty of water. It might be expected that simple encouragement and education could encourage compliance. In practice, when patients are presented with a 240-ml glass of water and instructed to swallow a tablet "*according to normal practice*," they imbibe only two to three mouthfuls (between 50 and 100 ml). Fig. 1 shows the variation in water volume imbibed with a placebo tablet under these conditions. These data suggest that patients are unlikely to be concordant with physician's or pharmacist's instructions.

Water intake and posture are recognized as important factors in avoiding "pill-erosion" of the oesophagus. This condition is usually caused by drugs that are irritant, highly acidic or basic, e.g., NSAIDS, potassium chloride, ferrous salts, tetracycline, and rifampicin (2–4). If tablets are taken without water or when semirecumbent, there is a risk that they may remain lodged in the lower third of the oesophagus. This may result in mucosal damage as the formulation starts to dissolve, causing a high local

Encyclopedia of Pharmaceutical Technology

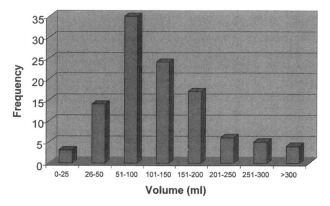

Fig. 1 Volume of water swallowed with a capsule when allowed water ad lib. (Data courtesy of Dr. Richard Dansereau, to be published.)

concentration of drug and dehydrating the surface epithelium. In addition, components of the formulation may help to form a strong bioadhesive bond between the unit and the tissue surface, aiding retention.

Esophageal retention frequently occurs even in clinical trials where correct dosing is carefully monitored. Figure 2 illustrates esophageal retention of a radiolabelled fast-dissolving analgesic hard gel formulation administered to a young volunteer. Subjects received two doses of the radiolabelled formulation. In this subject, the first dose cleared normally while the second adhered to the lower third of the oesophagus leading to significant reduction in peak plasma paracetamol concentration compared with other volunteers (Fig. 3).

As we get older, the ability to swallow certain kinds of formulations becomes problematic. In a series of studies conducted at the Queen's Medical Center, Nottingham, it was found that elderly patients had problems swallowing

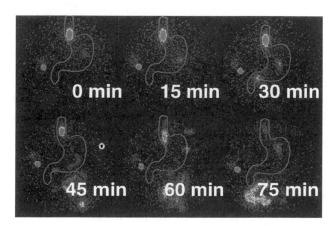

Fig. 2 Radiolabelled hard gelatin capsule lodged in the esophagus.

hard gelatin capsules. This appears to be due to an inability to coordinate the cricopharyngeal reflex to both water and capsule bolus (5, 6).

GASTRIC EMPTYING

The process of gastric emptying is extremely complex and is influenced by many factors such as presence of food, food content, pH, and posture. Most drugs are not absorbed from the stomach and are therefore dependent on the gastric emptying process to deliver them to their site of absorption. Consequently, the process and factors that affect it have been extensively studied with many conflicting views reported.

The stomach can exist in two states: fed and fasted. The empty stomach has a volume of approximately 50 ml, that increases to about 1 L when full. The fate of a dosage form is dependant on the state of the stomach at time of administration.

In the fed state, the environment within the stomach is infinitely variable in terms of food content. The nature of food intake is not only specific to race and geographic location but unique for each person and can vary significantly on a day-to-day basis. An average daily intake of 3–4 kg of food and drink is typical and some 5 L of fluids such as saliva, gastric juice, pancreatic juice, and other body liquids are added to the stomach contents during the day. The liquid–solid content within the stomach is a key factor in determining the fate of ingested material. Liquids and solids have separate and distinct emptying patterns.

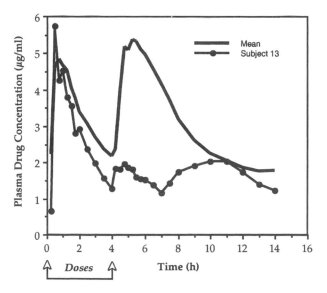

Fig. 3 Reduction in peak plasma-concentration on second dose.

Following a meal, liquids empty first in a monoexponential pattern, before the gastric emptying of solids is initiated.

The stomach acts as sieve and a calorie regulator for the small intestine: As a consequence, meals that contain large fragments of food or are nutrient-dense will take longer to empty and hence will delay the passage of dose forms to the small intestine. Small tablets and pellets mix and empty from the stomach with food, but large nondisintegrating tablets are reliant upon the migrating myoelectric complex (MMC, the patterns of motor activity that act to move food through the gastrointestinal tract) in the fasted pattern of motility to empty them from the stomach. If the stomach is maintained in the fed state by continuous feeding then large dosage forms are retained in the stomach for that period.

Often patients are instructed to take their medication "with a meal," but instructions are never precise and this can be interpreted by the patient as taking the medication immediately before, during the meal, or just after the food. O'Reilly and co-workers (7) demonstrated that the initial-gastric emptying rate of multiparticulates dosed before a meal was faster than for those dosed during and after food.

Gastric emptying follows a circadian rhythm with slower emptying occurring in the afternoon compared with the morning. Such variation can be very marked: In a study by Ghoo and colleagues emptying of the solid phase of the meal decreased by over 50% when it was consumed in the evening (8). The fasted pattern of motility establishes itself overnight, as this is generally the longest period in which no food intake occurs. MMC occur with the greatest frequency in the early hours of the morning. Changes in MMCs probably produce the largest physiological variability in oral drug delivery.

FAT AND GASTRIC HOMOGENEITY

The fat content of food is one of, if not the, most important influence on the rate of gastric emptying. Within the stomach, fat will separate and form layers exposing the pyloric–duodenal region to different amounts of fat according to posture of the individual: erect, supine, prone, or lying on one side. Since digested fat has a marked inhibitory effect on gastric emptying, retardation will occur to varying degrees. Brown and colleagues found that fat quickly layered in the proximal stomach away from the pylorus, thus delaying gastric emptying (9). The delaying effect of lipid on gastric emptying is increased in the elderly (10).

If a dispersing phase such as minced meat is present, the fat will spread more uniformly. Edelbroek and colleagues labelled the fat phase of a meal with Tc-99m-thiocyanate,

to compare the gastric emptying and intragastric distribution of oil in a soup, based meal with and without minced beef (11). The emptying rate of oil in the oil/soupmeal was about twice that for oil consumed in the oil–soup–minced beef meal. These results show that major differences in the intra-gastric distribution of oil occur following incorporation of predispersed solids into the meal.

The gastric residence of a meal with identical composition will be prolonged if the fat content is used to fry the food rather than be ingested as the cold oil. The behavior of oils within the stomach is also affected by other constituents of the meal that are present. The effect of fat on gastric emptying and absorption of nutrients depends on the relation to the other components of the meal when the fat is consumed.

CARBOHYDRATE AND GASTRIC HOMOGENEITY

A study conducted in our laboratories looking at the absorption of a drug from low-volume, oil-filled soft gelatin capsules resulted in a variable bioavailability profile. Labelling the capsule with Tc-99m showed that formulation emptied immediately to the duodenum when given with fluid after a carbohydrate-based meal (sandwich). This unusual behavior was also investigated using magnetic resonance imaging (MRI). In this case, it was not necessary to label the formulation as the oil can be discriminated from the gastric contents using a T1, weighted FLASH sequence.

In the clinical trial, oil filled gelatin capsules were given immediately following a sandwich meal and the subjects were imaged in the prone position. Fig. 4 shows a cross-section of the body at the level of the upper abdomen: the agglomeration of the sandwich by the pyloric antrum into a "doughball" can be clearly seen. Following ingestion the meal is softened by mastication to aid swallowing. Although the maximum rate of salivary secretion is less than 5 ml min^{-1}, the bread is sufficiently softened. This moistened bolus is swallowed and the subsequent action of the stomach consolidates the mass. Eventually, the material is hydrated and the ball disperses. A small, almost buoyant gelatin capsule taken after the meal virtually bounces off the carbohydrate mass and exits from the stomach. This was confirmed by the gamma scintigraphic imaging study.

EFFECT OF POSTURE AND GRAVITY ON GASTRIC EMPTYING

Many studies have provided evidence that changes in posture can affect both the gastric emptying rates of

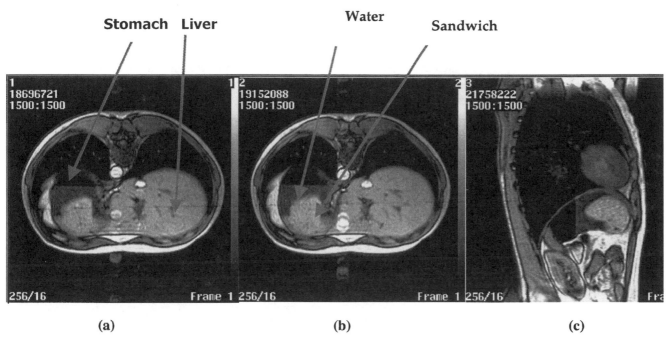

Fig. 4 MR images of the upper GI tract that show the compression of swallowed bread into a dough ball, viewed in (a) and (b) horizontal and (c) sagittal section.

materials and the absorption characteristics of drugs. Lying down decreases the rate of gastric emptying when compared with sitting and a combination of sitting and standing produces the most rapid gastric emptying. Bland, unbuffered liquids, and pellet formulations empty more slowly from the stomach when the subject is lying down compared with when he is upright or sitting erect. For floating formulations, such as raft-forming alginates, the buoyant raft empties faster than food in subjects lying on their left side or their backs and slower in subjects lying on their right side with the raft positioned in the greater curvature. When the subjects lay on their left side the raft was presented to the pylorus ahead of the meal and so emptied first.

The time to maximum plasma-concentration (T_{max}) of coadministered soluble paracetamol and nifedipine is significantly decreased when subjects are standing or lying on their right side compared with when they lie on their left side (12). These postures also resulted in a significantly higher peak plasma-concentration and area under the plasma-concentration–time curve of nifedipine.

GENDER AND PREGNANCY

Studies have examined the effect of gender and the menstrual cycle on gastrointestinal transit. Gastric

emptying of both solids and liquids is reported to be slower in women than men (13). Premenopausal women and postmenopausal women taking oestrogen and progesterone replacement were shown to have slower

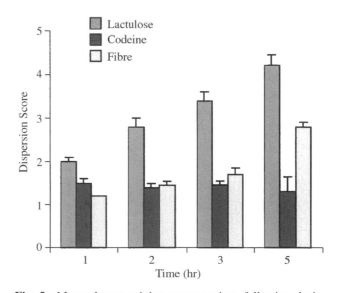

Fig. 5 Mean plasma quinine concentrations following dosing with 50 mg of the dihydrochloride salt in the Pulsincap after treatment with codeine or lactulose. Error bar shows standard deviation.

gastric emptying of liquids than men. However, while premenopausal women and postmenopausal women taking hormone replacement therapy showed slower gastric emptying of liquid, postmenopausal women not taking hormones had a similar rate to men (14). It has been shown that females have faster emptying times when in the ovular stage of the menstrual cycle.

In women, pregnancy can drastically alter transit of drugs in certain regions of the gastrointestinal tract, although gastric emptying is not delayed (15). Nausea and vomiting occurs in 50–90% of pregnant women and may be so severe that hospitalization is required to prevent dehydration. Often pregnant women suffer from heartburn and constipation, which is attributed to decreased oesophageal sphincter pressure and impaired colonic motility (16).

SOCIAL EFFECTS—SMOKING AND ALCOHOL

Scintigraphic studies do not clarify the effect of smoking on transit. One study reported that smoking or chewing nicotine gum did not appear to affect oesophageal transit or the rate of liquid emptying; however, solid emptying was delayed (17). Other studies reported delayed emptying on both liquids and solids, which was associated with increased periods of retrograde intragastric movement of solids from distal to proximal stomach (18, 19). This suggests an initial impairment of antral function and/or a lack of antropyloroduodenal coordination once a contraction is initiated.

Strong alcoholic drinks such as whisky delay gastric emptying. A study showed that administration of beer or white wine significantly accelerated gastric emptying compared with ethanol of the same concentration (20). This suggests that the observed effect is due to compounds in the beer and white wine other than alcohol. Gastric emptying is delayed in 24% of chronic alcoholics (21). Finally, smoking delays the gastric emptying of alcohol indicating the possibilities of complex interactions due to social activities (22).

SMALL INTESTINAL ABSORPTION, FOOD, AND EXCIPIENTS

The small intestine is the main organ of digestion with specialized sites of nutrient uptake and drug absorption. The small intestine is a convoluted tube about 5 m in length with three regions: duodenum, jejunum, and ileum. During the fed phase the contractions serve to mix chyme with enzymes and digestive secretions, circulate the contents to

facilitate contact with the intestinal mucosa, and finally propel the contents towards the large bowel. The major areas in which digestion occurs are the jejunum and ileum, and digestion of proteins and fats is largely complete as the chyme enters the caecum. Small intestinal transit in man has been measured by a wide variety of techniques and is generally accepted to be around 4 h.

Components of food can alter drug absorption by affecting drug solubility. Recent findings suggest that drinks such as grapefruit juice can increase the bioavailability of certain drugs, by reducing presystemic intestinal metabolism (23). The solubility of the drug in the GI tract can also be enhanced when the drug is highly soluble in a coadministered food component. The solubility of dicumarol is five times higher in defatted milk than in buffer at 37°C. This increase in solubility and bioavailability is due to the main milk protein casein. Griseofulvin absorption is also enhanced by concomitant food intake, especially after ingestion of heavy fat meals. This enhanced bioavailability is probably due to the increased bile output and the prolonged gastric emptying.

Excipients such as mannitol can affect small intestinal transit, which in turn can affect the absorption of certain drugs. Oral solutions are rarely likely to fall short of bioequivalence relative to solid oral formulations, although during the development of a ranitidine effervescent oral solution dosage form containing sodium acid pyrophosphate (SAPP), a marked decrease in absorption was observed in the extent of ranitidine absorption from the liquid formulation relative to the conventional oral tablet. The formulation contained 150 mg ranitidine with 1132 mg SAPP together with 1.5 MBq [111]indium chloride solutions. Small intestinal transit time was decreased to 56% in the presence of the excipient. The rapid small intestinal transit associated with an excipient of a solution dosage form resulted in a decreased extent of ranitidine absorption (24).

Intestinal transit rate is highly dependent on the motility state of the GI tract either fasted or fed partly due to the higher viscosity of chyme in the fed state. Blair and co-workers conducted a study in 20 men (energy intake 1272–5342 kcal/day) and found that higher calorific intake was associated with faster transit (25). Exercise in moderation appears to have no effect on transit.

THE COLONIC ENVIRONMENT

By the end of the small intestine, deposition is almost complete and there is no need for intestinal secretions to aid assimilation. The principal role of the colon is to resorb water and reclaim sodium; however, complex carbohydrate components of vegetable origin have nutritional value but are relatively resistant to attack from intestinal secretion. In the caecum, a complex bacterial environment digests the soluble, fermentable carbohydrates to yield short-chain fatty acids, which are assimilated into the systemic circulation by the colon, together with vitamin K released from the plant material.

The presence of the complex carbohydrates provides the environment with a viscous hydrogel structure; water removal gradually yields a mass of bacteria bound by undigested carbohydrates (celluloses) to form the stool. The presence of a hydrogel softens the mass and also provides water for dissolution. Carbon dioxide release is also a fermentation product, and if the redox potential is sufficiently low, bacteria can produce methane and hydrogen that can be detected in the breath particularly after the ingestion of pulses. In the upright position, the gas will rise to the transverse colon: It is estimated that an adult produces approximately 2–3 L per day on 20 g fermentable fibre (most of which is eliminated in the breath) (26). The presence of large volumes of gas appears to restrict the availability of water past the hepatic flexure, and the consequences of this must be carefully considered.

Residence of dosage forms is approximately 10–12 h in the proximal colon and 12 h in the descending and rectosigmoid colon regions, giving a whole colon transit time of 24–48 h. The relative residence time in the segments of the large bowel is highly dependent upon feeding pattern. Administration of a midday meal to a previously fasted subject may produce dramatic movement, shifting dosage forms from the ascending to the descending colon. Dietary fibre in the form of bran, wholemeal bread, and fruit and vegetables reduces colonic transit time but increases faecal weight by acting as a substrate for colonic bacterial metabolism. For example, an additional 20 g/day of bran increases faecal weight by 127% and decreases mean transit time from 73 ± 24 to 43 ± 7 h (27). However, the same quantity of fibre given in the form of cabbage, carrot, or apple produced a smaller effect.

EFFECTS OF CHANGES TO THE COLONIC ENVIRONMENT

Administration of osmotic laxatives such as lactulose to healthy subjects increases defaecation frequency, producing a reversible syndrome that mimics irritable bowel syndrome. Administration of 20 ml lactulose three times per day creates a more fluid environment as indicated by increased stool water content (28). To examine the effect

of such an environment on drug delivery we administered pulse release units (Pulsincap) containing quinine dihydrochloride (50 mg) following treatment with lactulose for 3 days (29).

Plasma-concentration-time profiles following lactulose treatment showed a faster T_{max}, a higher C_{max}, and an increased AUC indicating significantly improved absorption. These data correlated with a higher dispersion score for the marker indicating that the water content of the colon plays an important part in determining the extent of absorption in man. This will be especially important for pulsed release systems in which the exterior is covered by an impermeable coat. The sluggish mixing and the low availability of water past the ascending colon could compromise efficient release of the drug encapsulated in the system.

EFFECTS OF DISEASE ON GASTROINTESTINAL TRANSIT

Esophageal transit time is adversely affected by various disease states, for example, achalasia (30) scleroderma, oesophageal carcinoma, Barrett's oesophagus, cervical vertebropathy (31), left side heart enlargement, and reflux oesophagitis. Abnormalities in oesophageal function can occur as a result of a variety of disease such as chronic alcoholism and diabetes mellitus (32).

Diseases that affect gastric motility and emptying are predominantly diseases of the gastrointestinal tract itself, although diseases such as diabetes that produce neuropathy can also alter transit. Diseases associated with accelerated transit can reduce the bioavailability of drugs delivered in a controlled-release formulation and conversely diseases that slow transit can enhance absorption. Stasis or stagnation at a particular site is always of concern since high local concentrations of drug may result. Inhibition of motility, especially of the stomach, is widely recognized as a consequence of many acute illnesses such as severe pain of any origin, trauma, major infections, and metabolic disturbances.

Some diseases only affect one of the phases of gastric emptying. Generally, duodenal ulcers produce accelerated emptying while gastric ulcers reduce antral motility, producing normal emptying of liquids but delayed emptying of solids. Emptying of a solid meal is slowed in patients with pernicious anaemia and atrophic gastritis but in achlorhydric patients liquids empty rapidly.

Gastro-oesophageal reflux is an extremely common disease affecting between 10 and 20% of the general population, although it is speculated that the incidence is considerably higher since a large proportion of sufferers self-medicate. The effect of this disease on gastric emptying is unclear since some studies report no effect on the emptying of liquids or mixed meals whilst others demonstrate a delay. It is possible that the emptying of solids in a mixed meal is selectively delayed, suggesting impaired antral motility. This would lead to a greater difference in emptying among liquids, pellets, and tablets than in normal subjects.

There are conflicting reports as to the effect of obesity on gastrointestinal transit. Some studies show no effect, whilst others report delayed emptying of solids particularly in men. This phenomenon is not reversed after significant weight loss. The eating disorders anorexia nervosa produces both delayed solid and liquid emptying (33). Voluntary suppression of defecation also decreases gastric emptying rate (34). The effects of gastrointestinal disease on dosage form performance have recently been reviewed by Milovic and Stein; the reader is referred to this review for further information (35).

Diarrhea and constipation are associated with many illnesses and always produce concern to the effectiveness of therapeutic agents. Like gastro-oesophageal reflux, the aetiology of these conditions is diverse and hence the effect on transit will vary. For example, in a group of constipated patients, a scintigraphic study using a water-soluble marker demonstrated a rapid and diffuse spread through the colon, 5/37 showed normal transit, 26/37 showed that the major site of hold-up was the transverse colon, and the splenic flexure and 6/37 the hold-up was in the descending and rectosigmoid colon (36). Prodrugs such as sulphasalazine, which rely on colonic bacteria to release the active moiety, will be affected by diarrhea (37).

Diseases such as diabetes, which have diverse complications, can produce different changes in gastrointestinal motility in different patients. Delayed oesophageal transit is common, although it does not tend to produce clinically significant problems. However, diabetic gastroparesis is a problem. These patients demonstrate reduced postprandial antral times compared with diabetic-without this complication, although overall transit is not different. There was no correlation among disturbed gastric clearance, impaired gall bladder contraction, and prolonged colonic transit time in the patients with cardiovascular autonomic neuropathy nor was there a correlation between any disturbed motor function and age or duration of diabetes (38).

Patients with cystic fibrosis require pancreatic enzyme supplements to aid food digestion. A recent investigation in which enteric coated enzyme pellets were labelled with [111]indium and given to patients with a pancake meal labelled with Tc-99m tin colloid showed that the pellets passed through the intestine ahead of food (39). These data suggest that the incorrect delivery of this enzyme might be responsible for malabsorption and the development of strictures in the proximal colon caused by the high-dose supplements reaching this region before the food.

pH IN HEALTH AND DISEASE

Food affects bulk pH in the stomach by dilution, buffering, and stimulating acid secretion. In the colon, pH is affected by meals containing a high proportion of fermentable fibre. The greatest secretory activity occurs in the stomach within the first hour of eating and the volume of gastric juices produced may be up to twice that of the meal. Studies using a triple pH electrode show that the peak buffering effects of food occurs within 30 min of eating with recorded variations in the stomach varying from pH 2 to around 4.5 (40). Even small volumes of water taken with medications can cause a temporary rise in pH due to neutralization effects on the residual acid.

Content of the meal also affects gastric pH. For example, a pure carbohydrate meal has no detectable effect on acidity (41), whereas a high protein meal matched for calorific content confirming that it is not the protein but its digestion products, the peptides, and amino acids, which are the potent stimulators of acid secretion. A liquid meal, rather than a mixed phase meal, with a balance of carbohydrate and protein has a strong buffering effect but the pH falls rapidly as the liquid is emptied.

Some research workers have found that the basal gastric pH can be surprisingly high. Spontaneous achlorhydria has been observed in healthy subjects during which they have temporary periods of profound reduction in acid secretion and may have complete anacidity (42, 43).

The pH in the small intestine is less variable than the stomach or colon and is in the region of 5.0–6.5, rising slowly along its length. The mean pH in the right colon is 6.4 rising to 6.6 and 7.0 in the transverse, and descending colon, respectively. The presence of fermentable dietary fibre produces a reduction in both viscosity and pH in the colon (44). Recent studies in Japan suggest that patients with Crohn's disease, whether active or in remission, have wider fluctuations in colonic pH, and values in the right and left colon are much lower than would be expected on the basis of control subjects (45).

A circadian rhythm of basal gastric acidity is known to occur with acid output being highest in the evening and lowest in the morning. The daytime patterns of gastric pH vary greatly between individuals, in part due to the differences in the composition of meals, the physiological responses of acid secretion and gastric emptying provoked postprandially; however, it has been found that the nocturnal patterns of gastric acidity are very similar with very low pH between midnight and early morning (41). The later in the day the evening meal is taken, the later the nocturnal peak of acidity occurs (46). It is, therefore, important to standardize the time for the evening meal when comparing the nocturnal effects of antisecretory drugs.

pH AND GENDER

There is a sex-related difference in human gastric acid secretion. Healthy women secrete significantly less basal and pentagastrin-stimulated acid then men with a median 24 h integrated acidity of 485 mmol h^{-1} versus 842 mmol h^{-1}. In a sample of 365 healthy subjects, the average basal pH was 2.16 ± 0.09 for men and 2.79 ± 0.18 in women (47).

pH AND AGE

It has always been assumed that gastric acid secretion decreased with age, however, a recent study has demonstrated that a group of healthy subjects with a mean age of 51 years (range 44–71 years) had a higher basal acid production than a group with a mean age of 33 years (range 23–42 years) (48). The age, related increase in secretion was greater in men than women but it was not correlated with height, weight, body surface area, or fat-free body mass or by the increased incidence of *Helicobacter pylori* infection.

Very few data are available on gastrointestinal pH in children. In 12 healthy subjects aged 8–14 years, the mean gastric pH was 1.5 and duodenal pH was 6.4, but this gradually rose in the small intestine reaching a peak value of 7.4 in the distal ileum (49). The pH dropped to 5.9 as the pH radiotelemetry capsule entered the caecum but increased to 6.5 in the rectum. The median gastric residence time of the telemetry capsule was 1.1 h, small intestinal transit time was 7.5 h, and colonic transit time was 17.2 h.

CONCLUDING REMARKS

It is clear that numerous physiological factors and disease states alter the gastrointestinal environment and affect the transit and absorption of a formulation through the gastrointestinal tract. An appreciation of these physiological factors is essential for the optimization of clinical studies. However, high individual variability will remain the major challenge in clinical trial design.

ACKNOWLEDGMENTS

The authors gratefully acknowledge the permission to use data generated in clinical trials in association with industry and clinical services. In particular, we thank Dr. M Frier and Professor A.C. Perkins (Queen's Medical Centre Nottingham), Dr. Tim Grattan (SB Healthcare), Dr. Richard Dansereau (Proctor & Gamble Pharmaceuticals Inc.), and Dr. J. Foster (Western Infirmary, Glasgow).

REFERENCES

1. Hey, H.; Jorgensen, F.; Sorensen, K.; Hasselbalch, H.; Wamberg, T. Esophageal Transit of Six Commonly Used Tablets and Capsules. Br. Med. J. **1982**, *285*, 1717–1719.
2. Pemberton, J. Esophageal Obstruction and Ulceration Caused by Oral Potassium Therapy. Br. Heart J. **1970**, *32*, 267–268.
3. Eng, J.; Sabanathan, S. Drug-Induced Esophagitis. Am. J. Gastroenterol. **1991**, *86*, 1127–1133.
4. Smith, S.J.; Lee, A.J.; Maddix, D.S.; Chow, A.W. Pill-Induced Esophagitis Caused by Oral Rifampin. Ann. Pharmacother. **1999**, *33* (1), 27–31.
5. Perkins, A.C.; Wilson, C.G.; Blackshaw, P.E.; Vincent, R.M.; Dansereau, R.J.; Juhlin, K.D.; Bekker, P.J.; Spiller, R. Impaired Esophageal Transit of Capsule Versus Tablet Formulation in the Elderly. Gut. **1994**, *35*, 1363–1367.
6. Perkins, A.C.; Wilson, C.G.; Frier, M.; Vincent, R.M.; Blackshaw, P.E.; Dansereau, R.J.; Juhlin, K.D.; Bekker, P.J.; Spiller, R.C. Esophageal Transit of Risedronate Cellulose-Coated Tablet and Gelatin Capsule Formulations. Int. J. Pharm. **1999**, *186*, 169–175.
7. O'Reilly, S.; Hardy, J.G.; Wilson, C.G. The Influence of Food on the Gastric Emptying of Multiparticulate Dosage Forms. Int. J. Pharm. **1987**, *34*, 213–216.
8. Ghoo, R.H.; Moore, J.G.; Greenberg, E.; Alazraki, N.P. Circadian Variation in Gastric Emptying of Meals in Humans. Gastroenterology **1987**, *93*, 515–518.
9. Brown, B.P.; Gross, J.; Schulzedelrieu, K.; Carmichael, D.C.; Barloon, T.J.; Abuyousef, M.M. Layering of Fat and Intermittent Cessation of Antral Contractions Delay Liquid Fat Emptying in the Human Stomach. Gastroenterology **1994**, *106* (4 SS), A472.
10. Nakae, Y.; Onouchi, H.; Kagaya, M.; Kondo, T. Effects of Aging and Gastric Lipolysis on Gastric Emptying of Lipid in Liquid Meal. J. Gastroenterol. **1999**, *34* (4), 445–449.
11. Edelbroek, M.; Horowitz, M.; Maddox, A.; Bellen, J. Gastric Emptying and Intragastric Distribution of Oil in

the Presence of a Liquid or a Solid Meal. J. Nuc. Med. **1992**, *33* (7), 1283–1290.

12. Renwick, A.G.; Ahsan, C.H.; Challenor, V.F.; Daniels, R.; Macklin, B.S.; Waller, D.G.; George, C. The Influence of Posture on the Pharmacokinetics of Orally Administered Nifedipine. Br. J. Clin. Pharmacol. **1992**, *34* (4), 332–336.

13. Datz, F.L. Considerations for Accurately Measuring Gastric-Emptying. J. Nuc. Med. **1991**, *32* (5), 881–884.

14. Hutson, W.R.; Roehrkasse, R.L.; Wald, A. Influence of Gender and Menopause on Gastric-Emptying and Motility. Gastroenterol. **1989**, *96* (1), 11–17.

15. Magides, A.D.; Macfie, A.G.; Richmond, M.N.; Reilly, C.S. Gastric-Emptying in Pregnancy. Brit. J. Anaesth. **1990**, *65* (4), 580P–581P.

16. Wald, A.; Van Thiel, D.H.; Hoechstetter, L.; Gavaler, J.S.; Egler, K.M.; Verm, R.; Scott, L.; Lester, R. Gastrointestinal Transit: The Effect of the Menstrual Cycle. Gastroenterol. **1980**, *80*, 1497–1500.

17. Miller, G.; Palmer, K.R.; Smith, B.; Ferrington, C.; Merrick, M.V. Smoking Delays Gastric Emptying of Solids. Gut **1989**, *30* (1), 50–53.

18. Scott, A.M.; Kellow, J.E.; Eckersley, G.M.; Nolan, J.M.; Jones, M.P. Cigarette Smoking and Nicotine Delay Postprandial Mouth-Cecum Transit Time. Dig. Dis. Sci. **1992**, *37*, 1544–1547.

19. Scott, A.M.; Kellow, J.E.; Shuter, B.; Nolan, J.M.; Hoschl, R.; Jones, M.P. Effects of Cigarette Smoking on Solid and Liquid Intragastric Distribution and Gastric Emptying. Gastroenterol. **1993**, *104*, 410–416.

20. Pfeiffer, A.; Hogl, B.; Kaess, H. Effect of Ethanol and Commonly Ingested Alcoholic Beverages on Gastric Emptying and Gastrointestinal Transit. Clin. Investig. **1992**, *70* (6), 487–491.

21. Wegener, M.; Schaffstein, J.; Dilger, U.; Coenen, C.; Wedmann, B.; Schmidt, G. Gastrointestinal Transit of Solid Liquid Meal in Chronic-Alcoholics. Dig. Dis. Sci. **1991**, *36* (7), 917–923.

22. Johnson, R.D.; Horowitz, M.; Maddox, A.F.; Wishart, J.M.; Shearman, D.J.C. Cigarette Smoking and Rate of Gastric Emptying: Effect on Alcohol Absorption. Br. Med. J. **1991**, *302* (67), 20–23.

23. Evans, A.M. Influence of Dietary Components on the Gastrointestinal Metabolism and Transport of Drugs. Ther. Drug Monitoring **2000**, *22* (1), 131–136.

24. Koch, K.M.; Parr, A.F.; Tomlinson, J.J.; Sandefer, E.P.; Digenis, G.A.; Donn, K.H.; Powell, J.R. Effect of Sodium Acid Pyrophosphate on Ranitidine Bioavailability and Gastrointestinal Transit Time. Pharm. Res. **1993**, *10* (7), 1027–1030.

25. Blair, E.H.; Wing, R.R.; Wald, A. Rapid Orocecal Transit in Chronically Active Persons with High Energy Intake. J. App. Physiol. **1991**, *70* (4), 1550–1553.

26. Campbell, J.M.; Fahey, G.C. Psyllium and Methylcellulose Fermentation Properties in Relation to Insoluble and Soluble Fiber Standards. Nutr. Res. **1997**, *17* (4), 619–629.

27. Cummings, J.H.; Branch, W.; Jenkins, D.J.A.; Southgate, D.A.T.; Houston, H.; James, W.P.T. Colonic Response to Dietary Fibre from Carrot, Cabbage, Apple, Bran and Guar Gum. Lancet **1978**, *1*, 5–9.

28. Barrow, L.; Spiller, R.C.; Wilson, C.G. Pathological Influences on Colonic Motility—Implications for Drug Delivery. Adv. Drug Delivery Rev. **1991**, *7* (1), 201–218.

29. Hebden, J.M.; Gilchrist, P.J.; Perkins, A.C.; Wilson, C.G.; Spiller, R.C. Stool Water Content and Colonic Drug Absorption: Contrasting Effects of Lactulose and Codiene. Pharm. Res. **1999**, *16* (8), 1254–1259.

30. Mearin, F.; Papo, M.; Malagelada, J.R. Impaired Gastric Relaxation in Patients With Achalasia. Gut **1995**, *36* (3), 363–368.

31. Hep, A.; Vanaskova, E.; Tosnerova, V.; Prasek, J.; Vizda, J.; Dite, P.; Ondrousek, L.; Dolina, J. Radionuclide Esophageal Transit Scintigraphy—A Useful Method for Verification of Esophageal Dysmotility by Cervical Vertebropathy. Dis. Esophagus **1999**, *12* (1), 47–50.

32. Holloway, R.H.; Tippett, M.D.; Horowitz, M.; Maddox, A.F.; Moten, J.; Russo, A. Relationship Between Esophageal Motility and Transit in Patients with Type I Diabetes Mellitus. Am. J. Gastroenterol. **1999**, *94* (11), 3150–3157.

33. Hutson, W.R.; Wald, A. Gastric-Mmptying in Patients with Bulimia Nervosa and Anorexia-Nervosa. Am. J. Gastroenterol. **1990**, *85* (1), 41–46.

34. Tjeerdsma, H.C.; Smout, A.; Akkermans, L. Voluntary Suppression of Defecation Delays Gastric-Emptying. Dig. Dis. Sci. **1993**, *38* (5), 832–836.

35. Milovic, V.; Stein, J. Gastrointestinal Disease and Osage Form Performance. *Oral Drug Absorption: Prediction and Assessment*; Dressman, J.B., Lennernas, H., Eds.; Marcel Dekker, Inc.: New York, 2000; 17–30.

36. Roberts, J.P.; Newell, M.S.; Deeks, J.J.; Waldron, D.W.; Garvie, N.W.; Williams, N.S. Oral [in-111] Dtpa Scintigraphic Assessment of Colonic Transit in Constipated Subjects. Dig. Dis. Sci. **1993**, *38* (6), 1032–1039.

37. Rijk, M.C.M.; Vanhogezand, R.A.; Vanschaik, A.; Vantongeren, J.H.M. Disposition of 5-Aminosalicylic Acid from 5-Aminosalicylic Acid-Delivering Drugs During Accelerated Intestinal Transit in Healthy Volunteers. Scand. J. Gastroenterol. **1989**, *24* (10), 1179–1185.

38. Werth, B.; MeyerWyss, B.; Spinas, G.A.; Drewe, J.; Beglinger, C. Non-Invasive Assessment of Gastrointestinal Motility Disorders in Diabetic Patients with and without Cardiovascular Signs of Autonomic Neuropathy. Gut **1992**, *33* (9), 1199–1203.

39. Hillel, P.G.; Tindale, W.B.; Taylor, C.J.; Frier, M.; Senior, S.; Ghosal, S. The Use of Dual-Isotope Imaging to Compare the Gastrointestinal Transit of Food and Pancreatic Enzyme Pellets in Cystic Fibrosis Patients. Nuc. Med. Communi. **1998**, *19* (8), 761–769.

40. Washington, N.; Washington, C.; Wilson, C.G. *Physiological Pharmaceutics*; Rubenstein, M., Wilson, C.G., Eds.; Taylor Francis Series in Pharmaceutical Technology, Taylor & Francis: London, 2001.

41. Bumm, R.; Blum, A.L. Lessons from Prolonged Gastric pH Monitoring. Aliment. Pharmacol. Therap. **1987**, *1*, 518S–526S.

42. Desai, H.G.; Zaveri, M.P.; Anita, F.P. Spontaneous and Persisting Decrease in Maximal Acid Output. Br. Med. J. **1971**, *ii*, 313–315.

43. Waterfall, W.E. Spontaneous Decrease in Gastric Secretory Response to Humoral Stimuli. Br. Med. J. **1969**, *4*, 459–461.

44. Tomlin, J.; Read, N.W. Comparison of the Effects on Colonic Function Caused by Feeding Rice Bran and Wheat Bran. Eur. J. Clin. Nutr. **1988**, *42* (10), 857–861.

45. Sasaki, Y.; Hada, R.; Nakajima, H.; Fukuda, S.; Munakata, A. Improved Localizing Method of Radiopill in Measurement of Entire Gastrointestinal pH Profiles: Colonic Luminal pH in Normal Subjects and Patients with Crohn's Disease. Am. J. Gastroenterol. **1997**, *92* (1), 114–118.

46. Lanzon-Miller, S.; Pounder, R.E.; McIsaac, R.I.; Wood, J.R. Does the Timing of the Evening meal Affect the Pattern of 24 Hour Intragastric Acidity. Gut **1988**, *29*, A1472.

47. Feldman, M.; Barnett, C. Fasting Gastric pH and Its Relationship to True Hypochlorhydria in Humans. Dig. Dis. Sci. **1991**, *36*, 866–869.

48. Goldschmiedt, M.; Barnett, C.C.; Schwarz, B.E. Effect of Age on Gastric Acid Secretion and Serum Gastric Concentrations in Healthy Men and Women. Gastroenterology **1991**, *101*, 977–990.

49. Dantas, R.O.; Dodds, W.J. Measurement of Gastrointestinal pH and Regional Transit Times in Normal Children. J. Pediatr. Gastroenterol. Nutr. **1990**, *11* (2), 211–214.

PLANTS AS DRUGS

Christine K. O'Neil
Duquesne University, Pittsburgh, Pennsylvania

Charles W. Fetrow
St. Francis Medical Center, Pittsburgh, Pennsylvania

HISTORY OF PLANTS AS DRUGS

Phytomedicine, the use of plants or plant parts to evoke a therapeutic cure or to treat an ailment, has been part of humankind's attempt to free itself of disease for several thousand years. Some references suggest that Neanderthals may have been one of the first phytomedicinal practitioners. Archeologists exhuming relics from lake beds in the Middle East have found evidence suggesting that early human's carried plant parts for more than just food or clothing. Some of the earliest writings found in Babylonian clay tablets from 3000 B.C. are about plants used for ceremonies, magic, and medicine. During the next thousand years, parallel cultures in China, India, and Egypt developed written records of medicinal herbs. Among other early historical documentation, the ancient Middle Easterners appear to have been the one of the first to rigorously document the use of plants for various diseases, compiling the first known pharmacopoeia, entitled the *Materia Medica*. The Greek historian Herodotus recounts how the Egyptians worshiped certain plants, believing that the some plants held the secret to a healthy life and longevity. Not to be outdone by the Egyptian peoples, the Greeks incorporated various plants and flowers into various aspects of Greek mythology. One of the largest compilations, dating approximately 600 B.C., is credited to a series of Chinese emperors and provides detailed instructions about the use, benefits, and preparation of herbs.

Scholars throughout the centuries have made valiant attempts to demystify herbs; however, people continued to hold deep beliefs about the significance of plants. The Doctrine of Signatures, dating from the first century A.D., suggests that some aspect of the plant's appearance provided clues to its medicinal properties. This belief remained popular for 15 centuries and is noted in many Asian and Western cultures, including that of the Native Americans.

In the beginning, these primitive medicinals were used primarily in their natural form and incorporated into compresses and poultices. Much of the knowledge obtained from these first pharmaceuticals was put to use by Native Americans and early American colonists. Not surprisingly, plants were manipulated into somewhat more complex formulations known as decoctions and infusions, the fundamental herbal preparations resembling modern-day teas. Typically, these botanical remedies were given to folks suffering from illness without regard to prior investigation. Formulas for various ailments were passed down from household to household much like recipes in a cookbook.

As science emerged after the 17th century, plants were classified and demystified. New technical skills permitted analysis of the plant's components so that standardized tinctures and extract could be prepared. Extraction of the relevant chemicals from these plants became popular around the turn of the 19th century. Active principal components such as opium and digitalis were isolated and applied therapeutically, although still lacking much in the way of formal prior investigation. As science advanced, medicines were synthesized and herbalism declined. Newly developed principles of organic chemistry made it possible to replicate plant-produced chemicals, paving the way for creative manipulation of these molecular entities, leading to the synthesis of new compounds that preserved the beneficial properties of the natural chemical, but minimized its toxic effects. The conception of local anesthetic agents from the naturally occurring alkaloid cocaine and the creation of the aspirin from natural salicylic acid in willow bark are important hallmarks that characterize the beginning of the era of "allopathic" medicines.

Many medicines that we use today were isolated from plant sources (Table 1). Examination of today's allopathic medications reveals that approximately 25–33% of currently available modern medicines in the United States have their origin in plants, animal, or mineral systems. These include aspirin, digoxin, quinine, colchicine, and vinca alkaloids, to name a few.

The focus on synthesized and biotechnolgy medicines has continued. However, in the latter part of the 20th century, there has been an intense renewed interest in

Table 1 Some contemporary pharmaceuticals of plant origin

Modern drug name	Therapeutic indications	Botanical name	Common plant name
Capsaicin	Topical analgesic	*Capsicum annum*	Red pepper plant
Cascara sagrada	Laxative	*Rhamnus purshiana*	Cascara sagrada
Colchicine	Gout; anti-inflammatory	*Colchicum autumnale*	Autumn crocus
Digoxin	Cardiac inotroph for heart failure/arrythmia	*Digitalis purpurea*	Foxglove
Ephedrine and pseudoephedrine	Sympathomimetic/decongestant	*Ephedra sinica*	Mahuang
Methysergide	Vasoconstrictor for headaches	*Claviceps purpurea*	Ergot
Opiates (i.e., morphine, codeine)	Narcotic analgesics	*Papaver somniferum*	Poppy
Pilocarpine	Cholinergic agent used for glaucoma	*Pilocarpus jaborandi*	Jaborandi tree
Podophyllum	Antimitotic for venereal warts	*Podophyllum peltatum*	Mayapple
Qunidine and quinine	Antiarrythmic/antimalarial agent	*Cinchona pubescens*	Quinine tree
Reserpine	Antidepressant	*Rauvolfia serpentina*	Rauwolfia
Senna concentrate	Laxative	*Cassia senna*	Senna
Taxol	Chemotherapeutic drug	*Taxus brevifolia*	Pacific yew
Vincristine and vinblastine	Chemotherapeutic drug	*Catharanthus roseus*	Madagascar periwinkle
Warfarin	Blood thinner for clots	*Melilotus officinalis*	Sweet clover
Yohimbine	Treatment of impotence	*Pausinystalia johimbe*	Yohimbe

herbalism. The United States, however, appears to be one of the last countries to embrace this practice of phytomedicine. The practice of phytomedicine has remained primarily outside the mainstrean of contemporary American medical practice. Germany, the Orient, and several European countries (Italy, Spain, the Netherlands, Belgium, and others) have taken a more aggressive approach. Eighty percent of the world's population reportedly uses herbs for medicinal purposes (1). One of the most famous countries for this is Germany, which, by recent estimates, has allowed some 600–700 herbal products to be marketed in that country. Approximately 70% of German physicians now prescribe phytopharmaceuticals to their patients, which serves to maintain one of the worlds' largest markets for herbal drugs (2). Furthermore, the Commision E, a branch of German government somewhat similar to the U.S. Food and Drug Administration (FDA), has compiled therapeutic monographs for several hundred herbal medicines that discuss their general safety and efficacy.

Despite a sluggish start, the commercialized herbal industry is now blossoming in the United States. More than 500 different herbs are currently marketed in the United States, responsible for over 3.2 billion in sales in 1997(3). Limited regulatory guidelines and direct-to-consumer advertising have created a booming herbal market. Products are readily available in health food stores, supermarkets, and pharmacies, through mail-order catalogs, and via the Internet. Safety and efficacy data for these products are extremely limited. Varro E. Tyler, a well known author and researcher once said, "More misinformation regarding the efficacy of herbs is currently being placed before consumers than at any previous time, including the turn-of-the century heyday of patent medicines." With the exceptions of the German Commission E monographs and some emerging studies, a critical evaluation of these entities is lacking. This presents both opportunities for research and challenges to modern science, medicine, and pharmacy.

TERMINOLOGY

Herbal products are considered a type of alternative medicine (e.g., herbal medicines, Chinese herbs, homeopathy, acupuncture, biofeedback, color therapy, music therapy, hypnotherapy, aromatherapy, Ayurvedic medicine, massage, therapeutic touch, Bach flower remedies, chiropractic, reflexology, naturopathy, and more). According to the Office of Alternative Medicine of the National Institutes of Health (NIH), characteristics of alternatives medicine include treatments that lack sufficient documentation in the United States for safety and effectiveness against specific disease and conditions and are not generally taught in U.S. medical schools or reimbursable by health insurance providers. Although uncertainty exists about the safety and efficacy of herbal products, there is even confusion about the terms used to describe such products. Some products are not herbs (i.e, saw palmetto is a tree) or botanicals (melatonin, glucosamine). Thus, further clarification is necessary.

Herbs are specifically defined as nonwoody, low-growing plants such as basil and parsley. Herbal medicine is considered to be the use of crude drugs of plant origin to treat illness or to promote health. A more correct term for this would be botanical medicine. Phytomedicinals are those common preparations, including capsules, tablets, tinctures, and fluidextracts that have been prepared from plant sources. This should be distinguished from plant-derived drugs that have been isolated, purified, and standardized from plant sources.

The words "natural" and "organic" are quite appealing to the consumer. Synthetic is often considered less desirable. Many believe that natural is better, safer, or not foreign to the body, but quite the opposite may exist. Native is identical to what is produced by or present in the body. Natural products refers to substances that are use to promote health or treat illness derived from plant, mineral, or animal sources. Organic refers to the level of pesticides or chemicals used in the growing process. For example, insulin from pork or beef sources is natural, but not native. Recombinant insulin is synthetic, but native. Thus, synthetic, as in synthetic insulin or estrogen, does not necessarily mean foreign or less desirable.

Two other broad terms that are used quite frequently are nutraceuticals and dietary supplements. Nutraceuticals include food, dietary supplements, and medical or functional foods that have a health or medical benefit including the prevention or treatment of disease. The newest term, introduced by the Dietary Supplement Health and Education Act of 1994 (DSHEA) is dietary supplement. A dietary supplement is neither a food nor a drug, according to the FDA. This term encompasses vitamins, minerals, herbs or other botanicals, amino acids, and any other dietary substance for use by humans to supplement the diet and promote health.

TRENDS IN HERBAL USE

The prevalence of alternative medicine use in the United States is steadily increasing. One may even describe the phenomenon as an explosion. A landmark survey published in 1993 estimated that 33.8% of Americans used one type of alternative therapy (4). A follow-up survey released in 1997 reported that frequency to be 42.1%, with 12.1% taking herbal medicine (5). In over 50% of the cases, use of alternative medicine was not supervised by the primary medical physician, and only 38.5% of consumers reported such use to their physicians.

Why do individuals seek alternative medicine? Many individuals are seeking health promotion and disease prevention and believe that the "natural" way may be the best. For many people, conventional therapies may not be available or ineffective or may carry significant risk that the user may not be willing to accept. Some have tried several conventional therapies without relief and look to alternative medicine as the only remaining option. Additionally, extensive direct to consumer advertising and limited regulatory oversight have fueled the expansion of the alternative medicine industry.

Recent surveys have revealed some characteristics of alternative medicine consumers (5). Approximately 50% of consumers are between the ages of 35 and 49 and have a college-level education. Income levels exceeded $50,000 for 48.1% of alternative medicine consumers. This may not be surprising because most insurance companies do not reimburse for such products. There appears to be a regional difference with use of alternative medicine, with over 50% of consumers living in the western portion of the United States. An earlier survey revealed that alternative medicine consumers were more likely to have one or more health conditions and less likely to be enrolled in an HMO. Furthermore, they had twice as many visits to traditional medicine providers and had a higher level of unmet medical need.

REGULATORY ISSUES REGARDING HERBALS

A major contention of the herbal medicine advocacy is the notion that because these entities are natural products, they are somehow safer and better for human consumption. However, the vast majority of alternative medicine products are essentially unregulated and not yet required to demonstrate efficacy, safety, or quality before becoming commercially available (6, 7). Currently, in the United States, there exists continued debate on what role the FDA should have in regulating and approving alternative medicines (7, 8).

The regulatory status of herbal medicine has changed over the past century. At one time, the United States Pharmacopeia, (USP), 1st Edition contained mostly herbal medicines. The first attempt by the U.S. government to regulate any "medicine" was the Food and Drugs Act of 1906, which simply prohibited the adulteration and/or misbranding of drugs. The act focused primarily on the quality of products being marketed but neglected the safety and efficacy of the medicines themselves. The Food and Drugs Act itself arose from public pressure imposed on the government after a series of fraudulent incidents involving patent medicine manufacturers and meat-packing firms were exposed and widely publicized.

The FDA was established by Congress in 1928, but it had been granted little authority and even less guidance with regard to how to proceed. The issue of product safety was finally addressed in the late 1930s after Elixir of Sulfanilamide contributed to the deaths of more than 100 people. With the 1938 Food, Drug and Cosmetic Act (FDCA), drugs were required to demonstrate safety before marketing. The FDCA defined drugs as substances, other than foods, that are recognized in *USP/National Formulary* and are intended to treat or prevent disease or affect body structure. In effect, herbs not included in the *USP/NF* were now considered food substances. Herbs that had been in the *USP/NF* were viewed as exempt and held official drug status until more recently.

As a result of Kefauver–Harris Amendment in 1962, drugs were required to demonstrate efficacy before marketing. The FDA presently regulates the pharmaceutical industry by requiring new product manufacturers to file a New Drug Application (NDA) for each new entity, which must include scientifically sound laboratory and clinical trials that demonstrate a drug product's safety and efficacy. Herbals and other products that lacked safety and efficacy data were considered over-the-counter agents. In 1972, panels were formed to evaluate the active components of these over-the-counter agents. The results of this effort were released in 1990. Products were classified as category I, II, or III. Category I products were generally recognized as safe and effective and were not misbranded. Category II and III substances were considered to be unsafe, ineffective, misbranded, or lacking sufficient data (7). Only a few herbals, such as senna, earned category I status. Because it was not cost-effective for most companies to present data, most substances now were considered foods of food additives that could not present labeling claims.

Although most herbals packaging could not be labeled with therapeutic claims, products continued to be sold with be readily available literature, pamphlets, and advertisements touting the benefits of these substances. The Nutrition Labeling and Education Act of 1990 sought to improve labeling and education about food products and dietary supplements. At one point, there was even some consideration given to removing such products from the market. Concern over the ability to market herbal products led to extensive lobbying in Congress, which resulted in the Dietary Supplement, Health and Education Act of 1994 (DSHEA).

The DSHEA classified herbal products as dietary supplements intended to supplement the diet. Also included in the definition of dietary supplement were vitamins, minerals, botanicals, amino acids, and other substances intended to supplement the diet. Dietary supplements were not considered foods or drugs and therefore were exempt for FDA oversight and the pre-market approval process. For all products introduced before October 1994, the burden of proof to demonstrate safety was now in the hands of the FDA and not in the hands of the manufacturer. Products introduced after October 1994 must be proven safe by the manufacturer. Manufacturers are currently not required to submit safety and efficacy data, and there are no good manufacturing standards (GMP) in place. However, the FDA does have the authority to establish GMP standards, and they are currently under development. Preliminary proposals indicate these GMP standards will more likely reflect GMP for food rather than for drugs.

The Office of Alternative Medicines (OAM) was also established at this time for the study and compilation of data on alternative medicines. The OAM functions within the NIH, and it is hoped that the OAM can further clarify the role of alternative medicines such as herbal remedies in this country. In other countries, similar committees (such as Commission E in Germany) have reviewed the safety and efficacy of herbs and published the results so that product debates can be resolved.

Although there is limited information regarding the therapeutic efficacy and standards for herbals some resources do exist. The most widely recognized source is the German E Commission E monographs, which contain information on more than 300 herbal products. Other well referenced resources include the *American Herbal Pharmacopeia*, the *British Herbal Pharmacopeia* (BHP), the *British Herbal Compendium*, the European Scientific Cooperative for Phytomedicines (ESCOP), the *U.S. Pharmacopeia*, and the World Health Organization (WHO).

At this time, consumers cannot be assured of purchasing a product that meets any regulatory standard, despite what may be listed on the label. Because they are derived from plant sources, the ability to standardizes herbal content from lot to lot is confounded by many variables. Growing conditions, storage, harvesting, preparation, and processing all may affect the quality of the final product. Additionally, the actual active ingredient of many of these plant products may be unknown.

In review, alternative medicines have been exempted from demonstrating efficacy (Kefauver-Harris Amendment) by being classified as dietary supplements (Dietary Supplement Health and Education Act). This means that herbal products cannot make therapeutic claims on the label or package but may distribute third-party information regarding therapeutic claims, as long as this information is not misleading or product-specific.

LABELING ISSUES REGARDING HERBALS

Although the FDA lists many herbs as safe, herbal manufacturers cannot legally claim therapeutic efficacy of their product for a disease state without the evidence to support this claim. Dietary supplements may claim effects on structure and function of the body and may have authorized health claims. They cannot be labeled as intending to treat, prevent, mitigate, cure, or diagnose any disease. Dietary supplements may not be represented as food and cannot use the term "significant scientific agreement" when making a claim. Supplement manufacturers are required to have data on file to substantiate any "structure/function" claims that the manufacturer makes about the product. Examples of structure/function claims might include statements such as "helps you relax," "supports prostate health," "for liver maintenance," or "helps promote cardiovascular health." Claims that would not be allowed include such statements as "lowers cholesterol," "improves benign prostatic hypertrophy," or "treats immunodeficiency." The FDA may ban dietary supplements if they pose an imminent hazard and may ban claims that are inherently misleading. Although the FDA regulates labeling, advertising of dietary supplements fall under the purview of the Federal Trade Commission. The FDA has suggested that manufacturers not make any claims with respect to their products and use in pregnancy. Additional rulings from the FDA are expected in the near future with respect to dietary supplements and their use in pregnancy.

THE MAKING OF A CRUDE DRUG

Approximately 250,000 species of flowering plants exist in the world today. Only a small percentage has been studied adequately for pharmacological activity. Based on past performance, it is reasonable to suggest that many valuable agents await being discovered in plants that we have not yet screened for therapeutic potential. Anecdotal reports of therapeutic efficacy and local folk medicine lore are a means to identify potentially valuable plant entities.

The term "pharmacognosy" refers to the study of chemicals from "natural" sources for medicinal application. Although this frequently refers to the study of chemical entities in higher plants, lower plants (fungi, molds, and yeast); animals; marine animals; fish; insects; and minerals are also fair game for evaluation of potential medicinal agents. In most industrialized nations, crude drugs (natural substances that are only collected and dried before manufacturing) are seldom used as the chief therapeutic agent. Usually, important chemical constituents of the plant are identified, removed, derived, or modified and applied therapeutically in a consistent pharmaceutical vehicle in an effort to enhance the "natural" benefits and reduce any inherent risk.

Many plants can be grown in similar climates that resemble the plant's native land. Compatibility of the plant to a particular region and the cost of harvesting the plant in that same area are two criteria that determine the availability of crude drugs in a particular country. Additionally, national and international restrictions on the collection of wild plants tend to limit availability of plant resources and escalate cost of production. These factors also force countries to specialize in producing only certain types of phytomedicinal resources.

Despite the tendency for a country to produce only certain phytosubstrates, the quality of crude drugs is often suspect. By the time a crude drug arrives at the manufacturing process, it has been exposed to various opportunities for adulteration, deterioration, and contamination.

During the collection or harvesting phase, skilled labor can be an important factor that influences quality of the harvest of wild plants. Deliberate adulteration most frequently occurs with expensive natural substances or natural substances in short supply. Mechanical devices may be more economical in the collection of some plants but may be of little use when only particular parts of another plant are desired. Cultivated plants ensure a more reliable source of the desired plant with less risk of substitution. Environmental conditions (temperature, rainfall, day length and sunlight, altitude, atmosphere, and soil) can dramatically affect quality, concentration, and presence of active constituents in plants. The age of the plant can also be an important determinant of the quality of active constituents in a crude drug.

At this stage, before drying, any insect-infested or disease-infested part of the plant should be removed. "Garbling" is the term for this semiskilled process of removing unwanted material (dirt, debris, and unnecessary plant parts) from the plant before drying and again before packaging and storage.

Drying can take from a few hours to a few weeks. This depends on the relative humidity of the local climate and the physical nature of the plant constituents. Drying by artificial heat (hot water pipes, stoves, and continuous belt dryers) carries the advantage of shorter drying times. Veterans of the process have learned when to stop the drying phase to prevent plant parts from becoming too brittle and overdried.

Deterioration of the dried product can occur as moisture from the surrounding air (usually approximately 10–15%)

and light return to the plant after drying. Return of moisture to the product provides a more favorable environment for contamination from molds, bacteria, and insects. Some processes introduce sterilization as a way to minimize microbial contamination. Proper storage and preservation must take place to ensure that quality of the product is maintained until delivery to the manufacturing facility where the crude drug undergoes a variety of grinding, crushing, extraction, and distillation procedures before being formed into an herbal pharmaceutical.

STANDARDIZATION OF DIETARY SUPPLEMENTS

Official standards are absolutely necessary to ensure the quality, reliability, and homogeneity of herbal products for consumers. Standardized products are paramount to those in healthcare planning to conduct clinical research with these products. Independent laboratories and university-affiliated research reports have documented the considerable variation that exists in terms of quality and reliability in these products. Abroad, the ESCOP, composed of manufacturers of herbal medicines and herbal associations, is working with European research groups to develop quality-control standards for the production of natural products. This committee is developing monographs for incorporation into such references as the *British Herbal Pharmacopoeia* and the *British Herbal Compendium.*

Likewise, in 1995, the USP commissioned an advisory panel on natural products whose mission was to establish standards and develop information concerning herbal or "dietary" supplements. Supplement monographs created by this endeavor address various issues associated with the standardization of individual herbals. The following list of section headings outlines the information found in each of the monographs:

1. Title—identifies the most commonly accepted name of the entity.
2. Definition—describes plant parts used, genus, species, authority, and family of the botanical.
3. Packaging and storage—cites appropriate packaging and storing conditions designed to promote integrity of the product.
4. Labeling—states requirements for label nomenclature.
5. Reference standards—identifies appropriate reference standards.
6. Botanic characteristics—describes visible and microscopic shape and structure characteristics of the whole plant or plant parts.

7. Identification—describes pharmacognostic tests useful in the identification of the entity.
8. Total ash—sets limits for the amount of inorganic residue remaining after incineration.
9. Acid-insoluble ash—sets limits for the amount of foreign inorganic residue remaining after boiling the total ash with 3N hydrochloric acid (an indication of how much dirt and soil remain in sample).
10. Water-soluble ash—sets limits for the residue remaining after boiling the total ash with water.
11. Foreign organic matter—limits the amount of nondrug-containing matter.
12. Loss on drying—sets criteria for loss limits of water, volatile oils, or other volatile chemical compounds.
13. Water content—limits variation in the water content of dried botanicals.
14. Alcohol-soluble/water-soluble extractives—sets thresholds for minimum acceptable amount of aqueous-, alcohol-, or aqueous alcohol-soluble extractives.
15. Volatile oil—describes the quantity of volatile oil present in the botanical.
16. Heavy metals—limits heavy metals present in the botanical.
17. Pesticide residue—sets strict limits of pesticide content.
18. Microbial limits—sets limits of total bacteria and mold count.
19. Marker substances and content tests—establish standards for quantitative chemical analysis of botanical for the presence of certain marker substances that aid in proper identification.

RISKS AND REALITIES OF HERBAL MEDICINES

Herbal drugs have many unknown and undocumented risks, side effects, and drug interactions. Like contemporary, rigorously tested pharmaceuticals, herbal medicines have some risk associated with their consumption. The fact that a plant is completely "natural" does not necessarily make that plant entirely risk-free. Several plants, when consumed in their most natural form, can cause grave illness or even death to humans and animals. A partial list of some of these natural herbal agents with the potential to harm is listed in Table 2. Herbalists, scientists, and the general public routinely avoid many of the plants listed in Table 2 because of their impending risks. However, hundreds of additional herbs and alternative medicines exist, much of their toxicologic profiles untested and undescribed. Adverse reactions with

Table 2 Examples of plants with the potential to harm

Common name	Botanical name	Reported toxic events
American mistletoe	*Phoradendron flavescens*	Hypertension and hypertensive crisis
American yew	*Taxus canadensis*	Cytotoxic
Arnica	*Arnica montana*	Violent gastroenteritis, nervous disorders, muscle weakness, collapse
Autumn crocus	*Colchicum autumnale*	GI toxicity, vomiting, neurologic toxicity, kidney failure
Belladonna	*Atropa beladonna*	Anticholinergic toxicity
Betal palm	*Areca catechu*	Teratogen
Bird's foot trefoil	*Lotus corniculatus*	Cyanide poisoning, convulsions, paralysis, coma, death
Bittersweet nightshade	*Solanum dulcamara*	Cardiac toxicity
Black nightshade	*Solanum americanum*	Cardiac toxicity
Black locust	*Robina pseudoacacia*	Bradycardia, nausea, vomiting, dizziness
Bloodroot	*Sanquinaria canadensis*	Destroys tissue on application
Blue flag	*Iris versicolor*	Nausea, vomiting, and diarrhea
Broom	*Cytisus scoparius*	Diarrhea, GI toxicity/dehydration
Calabar bean	*Physostigma venenosum*	Cholinergic toxicity
Castor oil plant	*Ricinus communis*	GI toxicity/dehydration
Celandine	*Chelidonium majus*	
Chapparral	*Larrea trindentata*	Fulminant hepatic failure
Chinese lantern	*Physalis alkekengi*	
Comfrey	*Symphytum officinale*	Hepatotoxicity
Cotton	*Gossypium hirsutum*	Hypokalemia, male sterility, heart failure at high doses
Daffodil	*Narcissus pseudonarcissus*	CNS depression, miotic, coma, salivation, vomiting, death
Death camas	*Zigadenus elegans*	
Desert plume	*Stanleya pinnata*	
Ergot	*Claviceps purpurea*	Hallucinations, hypertension, tissue ischemia, St. Anthony's fire
Figwort	*Scrophularia nodosa*	
Foxglove	*Digitalis purpurea*	Bradycardia, heart block, arrythmia
Goldenseal	*Hydrastis candensis*	Hyperreflexia, hypertension, convulsions, respiratory failure
Green false hellebore	*Veratrum viride*	
Heliotrope	*Heliotropium europaeum*	Hepatotoxicity
Hedge mustard	*Sisymbrium officinale*	Cardiac toxicity, heart failure
Hemp dogbane	*Apocynum cannabinum*	Cardiac stimulant, arrythmias
Henbane	*Hyoscyamus niger*	Anticholinergic toxicity
Horse chestnut	*Aesculus hippocastanum*	Bleeding
Indian pink	*Spigelia marilandica*	Overdoses have caused fatalities
Indian tobacco	*Lobelia inflata*	Vomiting, paralysis, hypothermia, collapse, coma, death
Jalap root	*Exagonium purga*	Dramatic purgative cathartic
Jimsonweed	*Daturia stramonium*	Anticholinergic toxicity, hallucinations
Larkspur	*Delphinium ajacis*	
Life root	*Senecio longilobus*	Hepatic failure from hepatic veno-occlusive disease
Lily of the valley	*Convallaria majalis*	Cardiac toxicity
Marsh marigold	*Caltha palustris*	Second most common killer of livestock (accidental ingestion)
Mayapple	*Podophyllum peltatum*	Severe GI irritation
Monkshood, wolfsbane	*Aconitum* spp.	Cardiotoxicity, neurotoxicity, hypotension, arrythmias
Moonseed	*Menispermum canadense*	Tachycardia, severe vomiting, purging
Morning glory	*Ipomoea purpurea*	Potential for hallucinations/psychosis
Mountain laurel	*Kalmia latifolia*	
Periwinkle	*Vinca major, vinca minor*	Cytotoxicity, renal failure, hepatic failure, neurological damage
Poison hemlock	*Conicum maculatum*	Birth defects, "crooked calf disease"
Pokeweed	*Phytolacca americana*	
Queen's delight	*Stillingia sylvatica*	GI toxicity, mutagenic
Red baneberry	*Actea rubra*	

(Continued)

Table 2 Examples of plants with the potential to harm (*Continued*)

Common name	Botanical name	Reported toxic events
Rosebay rhododendron	*Rhododendron maximum*	
Strychnine tree	*Strychnos nux-vomica*	CNS stimulation leading to seizures and cardiac arrest
Tall buttercup	*Ranunculus acris*	
Wallflower	*Cheiranthus cheiri*	Cardiac toxicity, heart failure, bradycardia
White false hellebore	*Veratrum album*	
Wild cherry	*Prunus virginiana*	Dyspnea, vertigo, convulsions
Wild licorice	*Glycyrrhiza lepidota*	Hypotension, hypernatremia, hypertension, muscle weakness
Wintercress	*Barbarea vulgaris*	Renal damage in animals
Wormseed	*Chenopodium ambrosioides*	Nausea, dizziness, convulsions, paralysis
Wormwood	*Artemisia absinthium*	Rhabdomyolysis, renal failure, seizures, "absinthism," mental doze
Yellow jessamine	*Gelsemium sempervirens*	Paralysis and death

herbal medicines can be directly related to exposure of chemical components of the plant (intrinsic) or to inappropriate or incorrect manufacturing/production procedures during preparation of a dietary or herbal supplement (extrinsic)(9). Drug interactions, toxicity from high concentrations, or undesirable effects from simple ingestion of the chemicals of the herbal supplement are considered typical intrinsic misadventures.

Although laws do not require reporting of adverse events of dietary supplements to the FDA at this time, many untoward events have been documented. The FDA has created MEDWATCH [(800) FDA-1088] to receive and compile reports of adverse reactions from pharmaceuticals. Healthcare providers are encouraged to report to this organization any and all adverse events related to dietary supplements and their consumption.

A review of adverse events related to herbal medicines reported in the medical literature from 1992 to 1996 has been compiled (10). This report highlights cases of hypersensitivity reactions, hepatotoxic reactions, and various types of renal damage associated with various herbal products. Some Chinese herbal preparations appear to be notorious for causing nephropathy (11–13). One of the more infamous adverse events related to the consumption of a dietary supplement was associated with the amino-acid L-tryptophan, touted for it's ability to reduce pain and promote sleep. During the late 1980s, it was discovered that excipients or tablet "fillers" contained in a few L-tryptophan products caused a rare, but reportedly fatal, syndrome (eosinophilia-myalgia syndrome). Additionally, popular dietary supplements and weight-loss products containing ephedra alkaloids have become a recent cause of adverse effects (e.g., increased blood pressure, tremor, arrhythmia, seizure, stroke, heart attack, and death), as supported

by several hundred incident reports to the FDA between 1993 and 1997 (14). Furthermore, a study designed to assess the prevalence of herbal product use and it's associated morbidity in a population of adults with asthma found an increase in the number of hospitalizations attributed to patients who self-medicated with herbal products and black coffee or tea (15). In a large retrospective study of admissions to a Taiwan hospital, 4% were found to be drug-related. Herbal medications ranked third as the drug category most responsible for adverse effects (16).

Herbal-Drug Interactions

Potential drug interactions are usually either unknown or unconsidered. Many herbs contain naturally occurring coumarins and cardiac glycosides, chemicals that potentiate hypoglycemia or hyperglycemia and promote sedation, or various other actions that can endanger the lives of patients taking prescription medications. Recently, two reports strongly suggest that a potential drug interaction exists between some drugs when used in combination with St. John's Wort (17, 18). It appears that St. John's Wort may act as an enzyme inducer of the cytochrome P-450 system. Subsequently, drugs that undergo metabolism by the CYP-450 3A isoenzyme must be used more cautiously when taken in combination with St. John's Wort. Not surprisingly, metabolism-oriented interactions are not the only type of drug interactions reported with herbal medicines. A case report of malabsorption of levothyroxine has been reported because of the ingestion of a combination herbal remedy (19). Some recent reviews cite potential risks related to herb-anesthesia interactions and other preoperative concerns with herbal medicines (20).

Propagation of Herbal Medicine Misinformation

Inadequate or inappropriate dissemination of information to the lay public, combined with less-than-stringent regulation, leads unwary consumers down the path of dangerous adverse events related to the consumption of herbal medicines. Successful dietary supplement and herbal manufacturers spend several million dollars each year on advertising. Existing regulations and product labeling of herbal supplements fail to provide ample warning of risks to consumers. In many cases, product advertising could be considered misleading, or at least questionable, despite FDA restrictions to limit manufacturer claims that relate only to proper health maintenance (10). The awesome marketing power of the Internet has by far the greatest potential to magnify and express the unknown dangers of herbs, if information regarding commercialization and marketing of alternative medicines is left unreviewed. Herbal products otherwise unobtainable in the United States have been purchased over the Internet and have been associated with substantial morbidity in uninformed consumers (21).

Misbranding, Substitution, Contamination, and Adulteration

Generally, dietary supplement and herbal medicine manufacturers are not required to meet the same standards and regulations that apply to the pharmaceutical superpowers.

In the spring of 1998, the FDA issued a warning regarding an herbal medicine called Sleeping Buddha. Apparently, the product contained an unlabeled sedative, the benzodiazepine estazolam. Fortunately, no misadventures with this product were reported. At about the same time, the FDA issued another warning regarding an herb called plantain. This plant contains digitalis-like glycosides and, therefore, consumption could be problematic for elderly patients or patients with cardiac disease. Potential dangers of this sort fall in the category of extrinsic misadventures. These are usually related to a lack of standardization, contamination, adulteration, or substitution of the products, in addition to either misidentification or misbranding of the supplement. Additionally, adulteration of Chinese herbs with mefenamic acid has been responsible for cases of herbal nephropathy (12). A more detailed discussion of misbranding, adulteration, and the like has already been published (9).

Many plants can vary considerably as to their quantities of active chemical constituents. This variability may depend on the time of year of harvest; age of the plant; method of pollination; and/or conditions of watering, wind, weather, and soil. These variables can lead to considerable differences in the finished product after manufacturing.

Additionally, consumers are often exposed to a variety of compounds when they ingest herbal supplements. Supplement manufacturers do not always separate out the active chemical ingredients of the plant; subsequently consumers ingest many different chemicals that occur "naturally" in the plant along with the reportedly active constituent.

Additional concerns arise from the notable lack of stability testing of the product, because these data are usually not available on the label or otherwise. Various contaminants (i.e., heavy metals, aspirin, caffeine, theophylline, diuretics, corticosteroids, benzodiazepines, atropine, and others) have been discovered in reportedly "pure" herbal products (10).

Lack of Consensus on Usage and Monitoring

There exists an overwhelming lack of consensus as to how an herbal medicine should be ingested or applied therapeutically. Recommended doses vary considerably from source to source, even among noted advocates in the field. No standards exist for monitoring adverse events or effectiveness.

Delay in Time to Proven Therapy

The time an individual spends evaluating a desired response from an herbal supplement could be spent seeking professional medical advice and proven pharmacotherapy. In cases such as severe depression, extreme mental illness, or other life-threatening diseases, the delay in seeking professional help could be the difference between life and death.

Abuse of Herbal Medicines

Unlike their prescription-only counterparts, herbal medicines can be purchased and consumed freely by virtually anyone. This can take place without forethought or advice, without restriction or limitation, without even something as insignificant as confirming a person's age or identification. Yet, in stark contrast, we require that individuals be of a certain age before purchasing cigarettes or alcohol. Individuals wishing to purchase these chemicals must be able to demonstrate proof of the minimum age requirement by displaying a valid identification card. This is likely required of minors because society believes they are not mature enough and perhaps lack "sufficient education" before the designated age to handle the potential dangers and responsibilities that accompany use of chemicals (cigarettes and alcohol) that can intoxicate, addict, or even cause physiological damage. Herbal medicines, like cigarettes and alcohol, are not without the potential for abuse, the potential to harm, and in some cases, the potential to addict or intoxicate. A similar corollary to the minor purchasing cigarettes or alcohol can be envisioned, analogous to a uninformed or misinformed consumer purchasing herbal medicines.

One such example is the opium poppy plant, which has been used to treat pain for centuries. Its derivatives continue to be used in modern medicine, yet its potential for abuse is also well documented. No one would argue that this plant should be regulated because of its potential for abuse. The same can be said of the leaves of the coca shrub, which have been chewed by the Incas and their descendants for countless generations to help them work in the high altitudes of the Andes Mountains. In many cultures, traditional healers and religious leaders have used psychoactive plants as part of their rituals, yet the perception remains that plants are safe and pose no danger for abuse or dependence. Many plants may have been safely used for hundreds of years in controlled settings such as religious rituals, but when used indiscriminately by the general public, they can lead to problems. A good example is the herbal anxiolytic kava, which is currently being promoted heavily. It has been used traditionally in Polynesia for hundreds of years without any reported adverse consequences, yet it is now known to increase the effects of alcohol and even by itself can lead to intoxicating effects (22–24). Its users continue to consume kava even after they develop adverse effects such as the skin reaction, which can occur from chronic use. Like many drugs with abuse potential, not everyone abuses a substance to the same degree. However, as its use becomes more prevalent, more and more cases of misuse will continue to appear. The abuse potential of many drugs is not identified immediately but rather after controlled clinical trials. Unfortunately, as noted above, herbal products do not have to undergo these rigorous trials before being marketed and thus problems can be identified only after many people experience an adverse effect such as dependence.

Cost

Although herbal medicines tend to be less expensive than their FDA-labeled counterparts, the cost can still be substantial if examined over several weeks to months. Costs related to delayed effective therapy, side effects, drug interactions, and hospital admissions might also be considered in this regard. As herbal medicine becomes more popular and as herbal medicine manufacturers spend more and more on advertising, the margin of cost difference between the two types of drugs will diminish.

SPEAKING THE LANGUAGE—A BRIEF LOOK AT SOME "ALTERNATIVE" TERMINOLOGY

In this section, we define some terminology commonly used when discussing alternative medications. Throughout the Encyclopedia, we have attempted to replace this terminology with more readily recognizable medical terms. However, in the event that the reader comes across an unfamiliar term, we hope to have included the definition for that term here in this section. We have made some assumptions as to what we thought might be unknown by the average healthcare practitioner not skilled in alternative medicine. *The information contained in this section is purely informative and not meant to be instructional or considered factual in any way.*

Alternative Remedy Formulations

Compresses and poultices

A compress is clean linen soaked in an infusion or decoction, whereas a poultice is a solid material (powdered or fresh dried herb, often fashioned into a paste), that is then typically placed over a wound in an effort to accelerate the healing process. In some cases, a covering of wax paper and warmth from a hot water bottle is thought to be beneficial.

Decoctions

A decoction is a water-based preparation, much like a tea. Its use is thought to be more potent with hard, woody plants that require higher heat to release their active constituents. Dried herb is placed into boiling water for 10–15 min and then strained before consuming.

Extracts

Extracts are concentrated solutions—occasionally concentrated solid or powdered extracts are produced—of chemical constituents of the plant. These are obtained using alcohol-based (organic) or water-based (aqueous) solvent extraction of the plant, after which the solvent is partially or completely removed from the solution.

Infusions

Making an infusion is essentially synonymous with making a tea. Infusions can be hot or cold and are particularly favored for chemical compounds that are thought to be heat-labile. Leaves, flowers, or tender stalks are often prepared for consumption using this process. The solution is typically strained free of debris before consumption. This type of infusion is not be confused with a sterile intravenous infusion administered in contemporary medicine.

Tinctures

These are a form of weakly concentrated alcoholic extract of a plant. Occasionally, vinegar or glycerin extracts have been used. Tinctures typically do not need heat to help extract active constituents of the plant, but they do need the solvent and a longer period to extract the active ingredients.

Alternative remedy therapeutic effects (not necessarily proven) include:

1. Alteratives—otherwise known as "blood cleansers," which promote health and vitality.
2. Adaptogens—enable the body to deal with stress more effectively.
3. Anticatarrhals—help the body remove edema, congestion, and mucous, typically associated with sinus and respiratory infections/conditions.
4. Astringents—shrink and toughen skin cells, reduce secretions and discharges.
5. Bitters—Supposedly stimulate digestion through "taste sensation."
6. Carminatives—serve to promote normal bowel function by stimulating peristalsis and "relaxing" the gastrointestinal tract.
7. Cholagogues—stimulate secretion of bile from gallbladder, also produce a laxative effect.
8. Demulcents—internal use soothes and protects inflamed/irritated tissue.
9. Emmenagogues—promote normal menstrual flow.
10. Emollients—external application soothes and protects inflamed/irritated skin.
11. Galactogogues—increase lactation in breastfeeding women.
12. Sialagogues—stimulate flow of saliva.
13. Styptics—stops external bleeding through "astringent" properties.
14. Tonics—agents that "strengthen" an organ or organ system.

Chemical Constituents of Plants

Alkaloids

These naturally occurring nitrogen-containing chemicals (amines) have very diverse in pharmacological effects. Examples include codeine, morphine, caffeine, and emetine.

Anthraquinones

Constituents that typically exhibit laxative effects. Examples are alloin, emodin, barrbaloin, rhein, and chrysophanol.

Bitter principles

Diverse in structure, these include iridoids and terpenes thought to promote normal bowel function.

Coumarins

These are naturally occurring anticoagulants.

Flavonoids

Examples include vitamin P and hesperidin. They perform a wide range of activities.

Glycosides

Sugar-containing compounds, glycosides perform various activities. Examples include digitalis glycosides, sennosides, and cascarosides.

Phenols

Phenols are weak acids that exhibit analgesic and antiseptic properties. Examples are salicylic acid and eugenol.

Saponins

These are constituents that form foams when agitated in water-based solutions. They are thought to have antiinflammatory, hemolytic, and expectorant effects. Saponins are found in extracts of yucca, sarsaparilla, alfalfa, fenugreek, licorice, and ginseng.

Tannins

Tannins have astringent properties but have the potential to produce liver damage at high concentrations. They are thought to be useful in the treatment of burns and wounds.

Volatile oils (essential oils)

Composed of complex organic compounds (phenols, acids, alcohols, ethers, ketones, and aldehydes), volatile oils evaporate when exposed to air. Volatile oils are found in many plants and may produce the aroma of the plant. Volatile oils exhibit various properties; but some common oils are antiseptic or local irritants, or sedative. Oils of peppermint, clove, cinnamon, garlic, and thyme are volatile oils.

SUMMARY

Precedent suggests it may be foolish to ignore promising chemical constituents in the herbal compendium. Experts in pharmacognosy (the study of drugs that originate from plant and animal systems) suggest that only a small percentage of plants have been thoroughly investigated for pharmacological activity. Today's major pharmaceutical companies appear to have forgotten this fertile reservoir of unique chemical entities in favor of spin-offs of existing successful agents and new compounds in biotechnology. Our previous practice of developing new medicines from plants has helped many people and, in some cases, brought about the synthesis of even more valuable compounds than those taken directly from the plant itself. With global public interest in the area of alternative and complementary medicine at an all-time high, it is imperative for the safety of patients that we investigate these compounds thoroughly and provide relevant clinical data with respect to herbal medicines and their derivatives. Pharmaceutical companies may wish to redirect some attention toward these botanical chemicals. Patients can only make informed decisions about theirhealth care if indeed healthcare providers themselves are truly informed.

REFERENCES

1. Atherton, D. Towards the Safer Use of Traditional Remedies. Br. Med. J. **1994**, *308*, 673–674.
2. Alschuler, L.; et al. Herbal Medicine: What Works, What's Safe. Patient Care **1997**, (October), 49–68.
3. Bartels, C.L.; Miller, S.J. Herbal and Related Remedies. Nut. Clin. Pract. **1998**, *17*, 5–19.
4. Eisenberg, D.M.; Kessler, R.C.; Foster, C.; et al. Unconventional Medicine in the United States: Prevalence, Costs, and Patterns of Use. N. Engl. J. Med. **1993**, *328*, 246–252.
5. Eisenberg, D.M.; Davis, R.B.; Ettner, S.L.; et al. Trends in Alternative Medicine Use in the United States, 1990–1997: Results of a Follow-Up National Survey. J. Am. Med. Assoc. **1998**, *280*, 1569–1575.
6. Tyler, V.E. The Honest Herbal. *A Sensible Guide to the Use of Herbs and Related Remedies*, 3rd Ed.; Pharmaceutical Product Press: New York, 1993.
7. Castleman, M. *The Healing Herbs: The Ultimate Guide to the Curative Power of Nature's Medicine*; Rodale Press: Emmau, PA, 1991.
8. Sale, J.D. *Overview of Legislative Developments Concerning Alternative Health Care in the United States*; John E. Fetzer Institutes: Kalamazoo, MI, 1994.
9. Drew, A.K.; Myers, S.P. Safety Issues in Herbal Medicine: Implications for the Health Professions. Med. J. Aust. **1997**, *166*, 538–541.
10. Ernst, E. Harmless Herbs. A Review of the Recent Literature. Am. J. Med. **1998**, *104*, 170–178.
11. Lord, G.M.; Tagore, R.; Cook, T.; et al. Nephropathy Caused by Chinese Herbs in the UK. Lancet **1999**, *354*, 481–482.
12. Abt, A.B.; Oh, J.Y.; Huntington, R.A.; et al. Chinese Herbal Medicine Induced Acute Renal Failure. Arch. Intern. Med. **1995**, *155*, 211–212.
13. Vanherweghem, J.L. Aristolochia Nephropathy in Humans: An Outbreak in Belgium. J. Am. Soc. Nephrol. **1993**, *4*, 327.
14. Nightingale, S.L. New Safety Measures are Proposed for Dietary Supplements Containing Ephedrine Alkaloids. J. Am. Med. Assoc. **1997**, *278*, 15.
15. Blanc, P.D.; et al. Use of Herbal Products, Coffee or Black Tea and Over the Counter Medications as Self-Treatments Among Adults with Asthma. J. Allergy. Clin. Immunol. **1997**, *100*, 789–791.
16. Lin, S.H.; Lin, M.S. A Survey on Drug-Related Hospitalization in a Community Teaching Hospital. Int. J. Clin. Pharmacol. Ther. Toxicol. **1993**, *31*, 66–69.
17. Piscatelli, S.C.; Burnstein, A.H.; Chaitt, D.; et al. Indinavir Concentration and St. John's Wort. Lancet **2000**, *355*, 547–548.
18. Ruschitzka, F.; Meier, P.; Turina, M.; et al. Acute Heart Transplant Rejection Due to St. John's Wort. Lancet **2000**, *355*, 548–549.
19. Geatti, O.; Barkan, A.; Turrin, D.; et al. L-Thyroxine Malabsorption Due to the Ingestion of Herbal Remedies. Thyroidol. Clin. Exp. **1993**, *5*, 97–102.
20. Murphy, J.M. Preoperative Considerations with Herbal Medicines. AORNJ **1999**, *69* (1), 173–183.
21. Weisbord, S.D.; et al. Poison on Line: Acute Renal Failure Caused by Oil of Wormwood Purchased Through the Internet. N. Engl. J. Med. **1997**, *337*, 825–827.
22. Cantor, C. Kava and Alcohol. Med. J. Aust. **1997**, *167* (10), 560.
23. Spillane, P.K.; et al. Neurological Manifestations of Kava Intoxication. Med. J. Aust. **1997**, *167* (3), 172–173.
24. Heiligenstein, E.; et al. Over-the-Counter Psychotropics: A Review of Melatonin, St. John's Wort, Valerian and Kava-Kava. J. Am. Coll. Health **1998**, *46* (6), 271–276.

POLAROGRAPHY AND VOLTAMMETRY

A. David Woolfson

The Queen's University of Belfast, Belfast, United Kingdom

INTRODUCTION

Voltammetry is a term that encompasses all measurements based on controlled electrolysis at a microelectrode. Polarography, first introduced by the Czech electrochemist Jaroslav Heyrovsky in 1922, is voltammetry at a special form of mercury microelectrode, the dropping mercury electrode (DME). Mercury electrodes can only be driven to negative potentials because otherwise, the metal dissolves in aqueous solutions as Hg^{2+}. Consequently, polarography is an electroanalytical method based on the cathodic reduction of electroactive species, either metal cations or electroreducible organic species, in an electrically conducting solution. By contrast, voltammetry is based on electroanalysis involving anodic oxidation, preferably in a flowing system in which a self-cleaning action prevents fouling of the solid electrode surface by the products of the electrochemical reaction, thereby leading to nonreproducible current/voltage curves.

HISTORICAL BACKGROUND OF POLAROGRAPHY AND VOLTAMMETRY

The determination of electrocapillary curves for mercury, a phenomenon attributable to changes in the surface tension of the liquid metal as a function of applied potential in an electrolyte solution, was known from the beginning of the 20th century. An electrode consisting of mercury dropping from a fine glass capillary was devised for this purpose. However, secondary maxima appeared at certain points on the electrocapillary curves. The origin of these distortions to the electrocapillary curve was unknown at that time, and it was this phenomenon that Heyrovsky originally sought to investigate and explain. He noted that when certain cations were added to an electrolyte solution, kinks appeared on the electrocapillary curves at potentials close to the values for known electrochemical processes at the DME. The applied voltage between the DME and a mercury pool formed at the bottom of a cell containing an aqueous metal ion solution was gradually increased. Under these conditions,

the resulting current had a small initial value that began to rise rapidly in a reproducible manner as the voltage scan progressed. The point at which this rapid rise in current occurred, the threshold potential, depended only on the species of metal ion present in the test solution. The rapid current rise increased linearly with an increasing applied voltage until the current eventually became constant again. This constant current value, which was found to be proportional to the concentration of metal ion in solution, forms the quantitative basis of polarographic/voltammetric analysis. The method by which Heyrovsky obtained the current voltage curve at the DME involved gradually increasing the applied external voltage (the voltage scan), measuring the corresponding mean current, and plotting this current against the applied voltage. This method constitutes analytical polarography, sometimes referred to as classic or direct current (d.c.) polarography to distinguish it from more modern variants. Heyrovsky was awarded the Nobel Prize in 1959 for his work on the discovery and development of polarographic analysis.

Classic d.c. polarography was limited in its development by the unreliability of early polarographs (instruments used to record current versus applied voltage curves), and the difficulties inherent in operating what were, at that time, relatively complex instruments. Although the method was suitable for metal cations, analytical applications in the field of electroactive organic compounds were restricted by the problem of the higher electrical resistance of nonaqueous solvent systems. Thus, only a water or water-alcohol system could be used with a conventional polarographic cell making up a two-electrode system of DME and reference electrode. Furthermore, determination of metals could be achieved at great sensitivity with spectroscopic methods such as flame emission and atomic absorption spectroscopy. This situation generally remained unchanged until the late 1950s, when modified polarographic techniques, such as square-wave, pulse, and a.c. polarography, began to appear, facilitated by the development of solid-state electronics. The development of a three-electrode system, linked to an electrical circuit known as a potentiostat, overcame the high resistance associated with the use of nonaqueous systems and widened the analytical applicability of the polarography. These developments,

Encyclopedia of Pharmaceutical Technology

which form the basis of modern polarographic and voltammetric analysis, including their applications to the pharmaceutical sciences, have been referred to as the "renaissance" in polarography (1).

THEORY OF POLAROGRAPHY AND VOLTAMMETRY

In a simple electrolysis experiment in which an electrolyte solution is electrolyzed between two platinum plate electrodes, an anode and a cathode, efficient stirring of the solution is necessary to drive ions toward the electrodes. When the potential difference between the two electrodes, which is a function of the applied external voltage, is sufficiently high, ions are discharged at the electrode surfaces. Such electrodes are working electrodes. The current flowing caused by ion discharge is an electron transfer or faradaic current, i.e., a current attributable to transfer of electrons to the electrode (anodic oxidation) or gain of electrons from the electrode (cathodic reduction). This faradaic current continues to flow until all of the electroactive species is consumed by electrolysis (Fig. 1A). Replacement of a platinum plate electrode with a platinum wire microelectrode and use of a quiet (unstirred) solution result in the electrolysis current reaching a limiting value (Fig. 1B).

The current interest in polarography is attributable to electron transfer between the electrode and the electroactive species. Therefore, the limiting current must be proportional to the concentration of the electroactive species in the bulk solution. This remains true provided the electroactive species can only reach the electrode surface by diffusion along a concentration gradient. The concept of a limiting diffusion current is central to quantitative analysis by polarography or voltammetry. However, the magnitude of this limiting current is nonreproducible because the electrode surface becomes fouled easily by the products of the electrochemical reaction. To overcome this problem, a microelectrode with a renewable surface is required. Use of a microelectrode ensures that an infinitesimally small proportion of the bulk electroactive species is consumed in a single polarographic run, making the technique essentially nondestructive of the analate.

Suitable working electrodes for voltammetry are those that can be driven to take up a new potential in response to an applied external voltage, a process known as electrode polarization. Reduction or oxidation of an electrochemically active species at a working electrode results in depolarization of the electrode. The word depolarizer is therefore sometimes used to describe an electrochemically active species. In voltammetry, the working electrode may

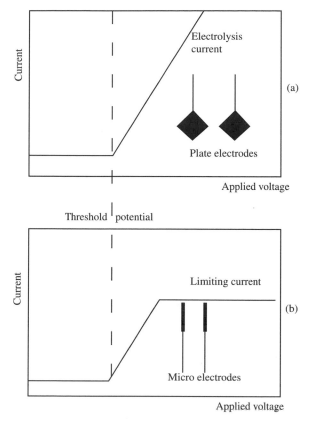

Fig. 1 Comparison between electrolysis and limiting currents. (A) A faradaic electrolysis current between platinum plate electrodes at an applied voltage beyond the threshold potential of the electroactive species. (B) Effect of replacing the platinum plate electrodes with platinum wire microelectrodes. In the absence of stirring, the current reaches a limiting value rather than increasing linearly with an increasing applied voltage.

be fabricated from metals such as gold or platinum, various forms of carbon, or metallic mercury.

The use of mercury dropping from the tip of a fine glass capillary (the DME) as the polarizable electrode has certain specific advantages. Most important, however, the electrode surface is reproducibly renewed as each succeeding drop is formed at the capillary tip. Electrical connection to the DME can be made using a brass post projecting through the glass capillary and contacting the liquid mercury column. The primary disadvantages of mercury as an electrode relate to environmental and safety concerns, difficulties in using mercury in flowing systems (although this is now possible to some extent), and its restriction to electroactive species amenable to cathodic reduction rather than to anodic oxidation. Problems of safety and practicality can be solved through the use of a multimode electrode polarographic/voltammetric electrode assembly. This replaces the classic DME and can also generate a hanging mercury drop electrode (HMDE.) for use in stripping analysis, in addition to the intermediate static mercury drop electrode (SMDE). Multimode electrodes also offer replacement electrode assemblies for non-DME voltammetric applications in both quiet and stirred solutions. Rotating electrode designs can also be accommodated. For mercury electrodes, the multimode electrode is compact and does not require the gravitational force of the mercury column to extrude the drop. Rather, the drop is formed pneumatically, using nitrogen gas pressure. The mercury is hermetically sealed, an important safety consideration, and only a few milliliters are required for up to 200,000 drops without the need for refilling.

Classic d.c. Polarography

In classic polarography at the DME, as with classical electrolysis, the electrochemical reduction occurs when the applied potential becomes sufficiently negative, i.e., when the applied potential exceeds the threshold value for a given depolarizer. The applied potential is in the form of a linearly increasing voltage ramp with a typical slope of between 2 and 10 mV s^{-1}. Unlike electrolysis, however, the current resulting from application of the ramp voltage does not continue to increase indefinitely until all the electroactive material is consumed. Rather, the current reaches a limiting value represented by the plateau in Fig. 2. This current is limited because when the applied potential is sufficiently negative, the rate of electron transfer becomes instantaneous and exceeds the rate of supply of the depolarizer to the electrode surface. Because the depolarizer can reach the electrode surface only by diffusion along a concentration gradient, the process is said to be diffusion-limited, and the resulting electron-transfer current is the limiting diffusion current, i_d (Fig. 2). The limiting diffusion current is directly proportional to the analyte concentration in the bulk solution.

The electroactive species can also reach the electrode surface by migration under the influence of the electrical field between the electrodes. This gives rise to a migration current that is not diffusion- and, therefore, concentration-dependent. This migration current must be eliminated by providing an excess of charge carriers in the solution that are not discharged within the working potential range of the experiment. Various salt solutions may be used for this purpose. More conveniently, because electrochemical reactions are often pH-dependent, a buffer solution may be used. This solution is variously referred to as the base, inert, or supporting electrolyte. Therefore, although the ions of the supporting electrolyte will move through the solution and carry charge, no current will flow in the external circuit because no faradaic process will occur in the absence of a depolarizer.

The electroactive species can also reach the electrode surface by convection, giving rise to a convection current that is, again, nonconcentration-dependent. Convection effects are attributable to stirring of the solution or, less frequently, to thermal currents. Thus, polarography and voltammetry are carried out in quiet (unstirred) solutions.

The concentration-dependent mass transport process, when other mass transport processes have been eliminated, is diffusion of the electroactive species toward the electrode surface along a concentration gradient. As the electroactive species approaches the surface of the DME, it will be electrochemically reduced. Thus, in a narrow solution layer, the diffusion layer, immediately adjacent to the drop surface, there will be a lower concentration of the electroactive species than that present in the bulk solution, giving rise to the concentration gradient. It may be shown from Fick's law of diffusion that for an electroactive species diffusing across a thin diffusion layer of thickness d, the diffusion current, i_d, will be given by Eq. 1.

$$i_d = n \cdot F \cdot A \cdot D \cdot (C - C_i)/d \qquad (1)$$

where D is the diffusion coefficient of the electroactive species, F is Faraday's Constant, A is the drop surface area, n is the number of electrons transferred per molecule of depolarizer, C is the bulk concentration of the depolarizer, and C_i is its concentration in the diffusion layer.

As C_i approaches zero, the rate of diffusion becomes proportional to the concentration of depolarizer in the bulk solution. Beyond the threshold potential, the electron transfer reaction will be initiated, and, as the potential is gradually increased, the rate of this reaction will continue to increase until it exceeds the rate of supply of the depolarizer to the electrode surface by diffusion, with all other mass transport processes having been suppressed. Under these conditions, the diffusion process becomes the rate-limiting step, and the resulting faradaic current, i_d, is now said to be the limiting diffusion current. Because i_d is measured over many individual drop lifetimes, it is properly described as the average limiting diffusion current and is given by Eq. 2, where i_d and C are the only variables.

$$i_d = n \cdot F \cdot A \cdot D \cdot C/d \qquad (2)$$

The limiting diffusion current is described quantitatively by the Ilkovic equation (Eq. 3).

$$i_d = 708 \cdot n \cdot D^{1/2} \cdot m^{2/3} \cdot t^{1/6} \cdot C \qquad (3)$$

where m is the rate of flow of mercury from the DME in mg s^{-1} and t is the drop lifetime in seconds. D has units of cm^2 s^{-1}, C is expressed as mM l^{-1}, and i_d is expressed in mA.

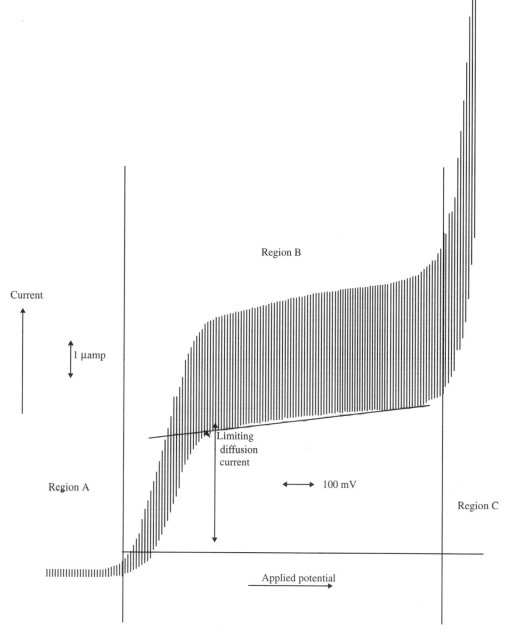

Fig. 2 Classic d.c. polarogram of diazepam (20 mg ml^{-1}) in 0.1 M sulfuric acid as the supporting electrolyte. Region A is the background current attributable to the supporting electrolyte, region B shows the rising faradaic current as it reaches a limiting value, and region C is the cut-off point at which the current goes off scale caused by the reduction of hydrogen ions.

Electrical Double Layer

When only the inert electrolyte is present in the polarographic cell a residual current will still flow. This current, which is nonfaradaic, is attributable to the formation of an electrical double layer in the solution adjacent to the electrode surface (Fig. 3). At all applied potentials, a current flows to develop this double layer, and the process may be considered analogous to the charging of a parallel plate capacitor. Therefore, the charging current is a capacitance current and varies during the drop lifetime, i.e., with the size of the mercury drop. When the drop surface area is increasing rapidly from the start of the drop lifetime, the capacitance current is a maximum, falling to a

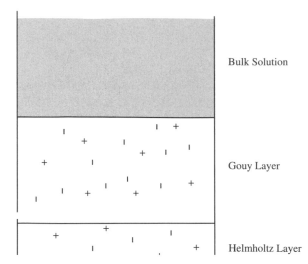

Fig. 3 The electrical double layer at a mercury drop shorted to a reference electrode and with no external applied potential.

minimum near the end of the drop lifetime when the drop size is at a maximum and the surface area of the drop is momentarily constant. The magnitude and direction of the capacitance current vary with the applied potential because of the variation in the surface tension of mercury with electrode potential. When the mercury drop is at its maximum surface tension, there is effectively no electrical double layer at the drop surface and, therefore, no capacitance current, a point known as the electrocapillary maximum. Beyond this potential, the capacitance current changes direction as the double layer is reversed, with the mercury drop now possessing a negative charge. The practical consequence of this is to impose the familiar serrated pattern on the polarographic wave (Fig. 2).

Mechanisms of Electrode Processes

The shape of the polarographic wave is further influenced by the nature of the electrode process occurring at the drop surface. Polarographic waves may be reversible, irreversible, or quasireversible. The overall electrode process comprises the diffusion, electron transfer, and electrochemical reaction steps.

Reversible processes are those that attain thermodynamic equilibrium at every instant of the drop life owing to rapid electron transfer. Reversible processes give rise to well-defined d.c. polarograms, and diffusion control is always the determining factor. Irreversible processes are so slow that equilibrium is not attained during the drop lifetime, and d.c. polarograms dependent on such processes often show poor definition. The rate-controlling step may be either the electron transfer process or the

subsequent chemical reaction. Many organic reductions at the DME, however, fall into an intermediate category, quasireversible processes. Whereas the rate constant for the reverse reaction will be negligible for a wholly irreversible reaction, it has an intermediate value for quasireversible reactions. Such reactions are normally seen only with longer drop times of at least 3 s.

The reversibility, or otherwise, of an electrode process is best investigated using the technique of cyclic voltammetry (2), in which a rapid forward and reverse voltage ramp is applied in triangular form (Fig. 4A) to interact with both the electroactive substance and its reduction product that, for quasi- or fully reversible processes, may be oxidized back to the starting material, giving the characteristic waveform shown in Fig. 4B. The separation between anodic and cathodic peaks indicates whether the electrode process is quasi- or fully reversible. Additional mechanistic investigations can also be made in respect to the number of electrons involved per molecule

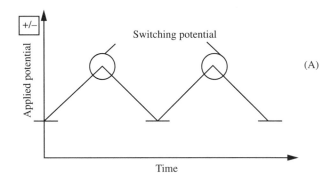

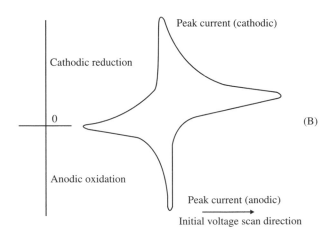

Fig. 4 Cyclic voltammetry. (A) Voltage waveform showing the rapid forward and reverse voltage sweeps. (B) Typical cyclic voltammogram for completely reversible system.

in the electron transfer process, a factor that can be determined by controlled-potential coulometry (3).

Effect of Oxygen in Polarography

In polarography, but not in anodic voltammetry, it is necessary to provide a facility for removing oxygen from the electrolyte solution in the polarographic cell. This is normally achieved by bubbling oxygen-free nitrogen through the solution for 10 min before starting the voltage scan. The surface of the solution is then blanketed by oxygen-free nitrogen during the polarographic run to prevent ingress of additional oxygen from the atmosphere. Removal of oxygen is necessary because the dissolved gas is polarographically active and can mask the analytical signal of interest in certain potential regions.

MODERN POLAROGRAPHIC AND VOLTAMMETRIC METHODS

In classic d.c. polarography, the actual current measured comprises the limiting diffusion current, together with current components, because of background electrical signals and, more important, the current charging the double layer capacitor at the electrode surface. Classic d.c. polarography is in many ways best suited to the elucidation of electrode processes. It lacks sensitivity for modern analytical purposes, and the sigmoidal current/voltage curves are difficult to measure. Modern polarographic and voltammetric methods are now available (Fig. 5) in which these problems have generally been resolved, producing an analytical technique with much enhanced sensitivity and a more easily interpretable current–voltage waveform.

Current-Sampled d.c. Polarography

Current-sampled polarography is a modern variant of the original *tast* (from the German "to touch") polarography, a method that involved the measurement of the polarographic current only at a fixed time interval during each drop lifetime. This was originally accomplished by the use of a mechanical touching contact (4) but is achieved in modern instruments using a digital approach in which the current is electronically sampled at a precise moment, typically 20 ms, near the end of the drop lifetime when the area of the drop is effectively constant. For this purpose, the drop lifetime is precisely and mechanically controlled by the instrument rather than being gravity-dependent, a feature shared by other modern methods. Current-sampled polarography produces a smooth polarogram by

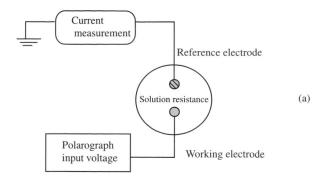

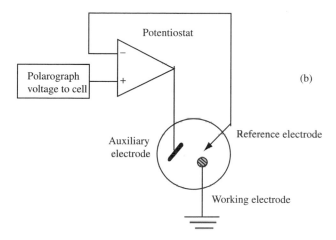

Fig. 5 Electrical circuitry for polarography/voltammetry. (A) A simple two-electrode system. (B) Illustrates a modern three-electrode system incorporating a potentiostat circuit.

elimination of the current variation during the drop lifetime (Fig. 6). However, although the typical serrations of the classic polarogram are gone, a slight staircase pattern can still be discerned on the current-sampled polarogram, a feature shared with many other modern voltammetric methods. The staircase pattern is attributable to the sampled current being held in the memory of the instrument and its value fed out continuously to the recording device until the next sampling period.

Current-sampled polarography offers only a marginal improvement on the sensitivity of the classic method because there is a more favorable faradaic-to-charging-current ratio at the end of the drop time when the drop is almost stationary. Thus, its only real benefit over the classic method is the clearer polarogram obtained.

Pulse Polarography

For routine quantitative analysis, pulse polarography and voltammetry are perhaps the most useful of the modern

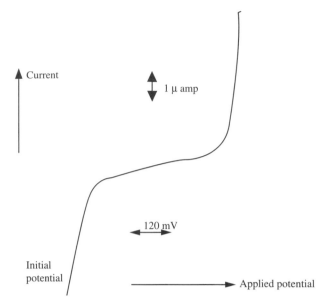

Fig. 6 A typical current-sampled polarogram. Note the staircase pattern indicating the individual current sampling periods.

variants on the classic method. Unlike d.c. and current-sampled polarography, the applied voltage is not a simple d.c. ramp but has a more complex format involving periodic application of the potential during short time intervals. There are two major pulse methods: normal (integral) pulse and differential pulse polarography/voltammetry, although many variations of these are now available.

The primary advantage of pulse methods is its significantly more favorable faradaic-to-charging-current ratio and, in the case of differential pulse methods, a more conventional Gaussian-shaped waveform for the current potential plot. In pulse methods, the initial charging current is increased when the pulse is applied, effectively giving a pulse charging current. If the pulse falls on the rising (faradaic) portion of the polarogram/voltammogram, there will be a large increase in current, over and above the value of the pulse charging current. Provided the pulse has been applied at the end of the drop lifetime, when the drop surface area of the DME is briefly constant, or if a solid electrode is used, then both currents will decay from the point of the initial pulse application, the current decay being a function of time. However, the charging current component of the total measured current decays much more rapidly than does the faradaic component. Thus, if the current is measured (sampled) at the end of the pulse application period, it will consist primarily of the faradaic component, thus yielding a marked sensitivity increase over d.c. methods. Sensitivity is also greater because the boundary diffusion layer at the electrode-solution interface

is narrower than is that when the potential is applied continuously. Therefore, the rate of diffusion of the electroactive species toward the electrode is increased, with a concomitant increase in the diffusion current.

Normal (Integral) Pulse Polarography/Voltammetry (NPP/NPV)

In NPP/NPV (5), the voltage is applied in a series of increasing voltage pulses (Fig. 7) from a baseline voltage selected by the analyst. Between pulses, the baseline voltage is restored. The pulse amplitude increases linearly with time, depending on the conditions set by the operator. The voltage pulse is applied at the end of the drop lifetime in polarography. Although precise timings vary with different instruments, typically the voltage pulse is applied for the last 60 ms of the drop. As with current-sampled polarography, the resulting current is sampled over only the final 20 ms of the drop lifetime, producing a polarogram/voltammogram identical in appearance to that of the current-sampled technique but with a greater current yield. The appearance of the polarogram is perceived to be the primary disadvantage of NPP/NPV because analysts tend to prefer a more conventional Gaussian-shaped graphic output of data, the sigmoidal shape being difficult to quantify.

Differential Pulse Polarography/Voltammetry (DPP/DPV)

DPP and DPV are probably the most analytically useful of all the voltammetric methods. DPP and DPV produce current-potential plots in the typical peak form familiar to,

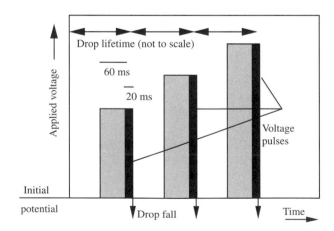

Fig. 7 Applied voltage waveform for normal pulse polarography.

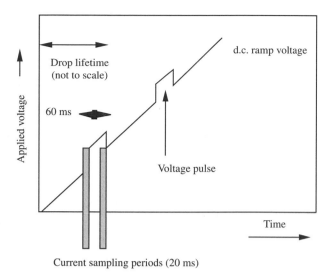

Fig. 8 Applied voltage waveform for differential pulse polarography.

and readily interpretable by, the analyst. DPP and DPV result from a variation in the pattern of the applied voltage.

In DPP/DPV, a small fixed voltage pulse of between 5 and 100 mV is superimposed on a slow linear voltage ramp (Fig. 8). When the ramp voltage coincides with the faradaic process, a faradaic current occurs continuously, along with the charging current. When the small pulse voltage is applied, in addition to the ramp voltage, at a given time, then both a new faradaic and a new charging current will be generated. As with NPP/NPV, the faradaic component decays during the pulse application, which, for polarography, is at the end of the drop lifetime. The charging current owing to the pulse also decays, but much more rapidly than the faradaic component so that if the current is sampled at the end of the pulse application, there is maximum separation between faradaic and charging currents and, thus, maximum sensitivity. In fact, in DPP/DPV the current is sampled twice, typically for 20 ms immediately before application of the pulse and again for the last 20 ms of the pulse application. The differential signal thus recorded results from the small increase in current (di) because of the small increase in the applied voltage pulse (dE). This further reduces the charging current contribution before the pulse and leads to an additional sensitivity increase over NPP/NPV. Effectively, it is the derivative (di/dE) of the classic polarographic wave that is produced (Fig. 13). This quantity, when plotted against the applied potential, yields a peak-shaped output because the change in the faradaic component when the constant voltage pulse is applied reaches a maximum on the steepest part of the polarogram and falls to almost zero in the baseline and plateau regions.

The sensitivity of DPP/DPV exceeds even that of the normal pulse method by approximately a single order of magnitude, being approximately equivalent to that of gas chromatography with F.I.D. (approximately 10^{-8} M). It may, therefore, be used for the determination of drugs in biological matrices. In addition, DPP and DPV have excellent resolving power, being able to differentiate peaks, which are no more than 50 mV apart, owing to different electroactive species in the same solution. Both normal and differential pulse techniques are suitable for use with solid working electrodes such as glassy carbon. The various instrumental timings remain the same, even though the constraint imposed by the variable area of the DME has been removed. The $E_{1/2}$ value is, of course, not discernible from DPP/DPV and is replaced by the near-identical quantity E_p, the peak potential.

The magnitude of the peak current (i_p) in DPP/DPV is given by Eq. 4 (6).

$$i_p = \frac{n^2 F^2}{RT} \cdot E \cdot A \cdot C \cdot \frac{D}{\sqrt{\pi t}}$$
$$\cdot \frac{\exp(E - E_{12} + 0.5\,E) \cdot CnF/RT}{\{1 + [\exp(E - E_{1/2} + 0.5\,E) \cdot nF/RT]\}^2} \quad (4)$$

where n is the number of electrons transferred in the electrode reaction, F is Faraday's constant, R is the universal gas constant, T is the absolute temperature, DE is the pulse amplitude or modulation, A is the electrode surface area, C is the concentration of the electroactive species, D is the diffusion coefficient of the electroactive species, t is the time elapsed from pulse application to current measurement, E is the ramp potential just before application of the pulse, and $E_{1/2}$ is the half-wave potential.

Equation 4 indicates that a linear relationship exists between peak current in DPP/DPV and peak potential and that the peak current will increase with pulse amplitude. However, the charging current also increases with pulse amplitude so that the value for DE must be chosen to maximize i_p but must not be too large; otherwise, resolution of the peak will be diminished. Typical values for DE are 50 or 100 mV.

Linear Sweep Voltammetry (LSV)

Linear sweep voltammetry involves the application of a rapid voltage scan, 100 mV s^{-1} or higher, to a stationary electrode such as the HMDE or a solid electrode such as glassy carbon. The theoretical treatment is based on the Randles-Sevcik equation (2, 7). At slow scan rates, the magnitude of the concentration gradient across the diffusion layer is governed by the rate of depletion of the electroactive species across this layer. With the fast scan rates used in LSV, the diffusion layer is narrower, the concentration gradient is consequently larger, and the resulting diffusion current is greater. As the depolarizer is used up by reaction at the electrode surface, the diffusion layer widens as it extends further into the bulk solution, and, unlike the DME, equilibrium conditions are not periodically restored by the stirring effect of the falling drop. Thus, there is a gradual decay in the diffusion current, giving a peak-like appearance to the LSV output (Fig. 9). The rapidly increasing potential in LSV results in nonequilibrium conditions at the electrode surface throughout the period of the voltage scan.

Alternating Current Polarography/Voltammetry (ACP/ACV)

Alternating current polarography and voltammetry encompass a wide range of polarographic and voltammetric modes characterized by a periodic applied voltage waveform, such as a square-wave, pulsed, or sawtooth pattern. The production of such waveforms may require a voltage function generator in addition to the normal polarograph, although some instruments have the function generator built in and can therefore perform ACP/ACV as a standard technique.

The most common applications of ACP/ACV involve the application of a small-amplitude sinusoidal alternating

potential superimposed onto a ramp voltage. The resulting current is an alternating current, the d.c. component being filtered out by use of a phase-sensitive current detector. This is possible because the faradaic and charging components of the current, respectively, have phase angles of 45 and 90° with reference to the applied sinusoidal potential. The detector rejects the 90° component and measures only the faradaic current.

The applied sinusoidal voltage has a typical amplitude range of ±50 mV, and the polarogram is a plot of the fundamental harmonic alternating current (a.c.) against the ramp voltage. Because the d.c. current component is filtered out, the current values before and after the rising portion of the d.c. polarogram are close to zero in the a.c. mode, and therefore, the resulting polarogram has a peak shape that approximately follows the rising portion of the d.c. wave. The use of a fast voltage scan, analogous to LSV, is possible with ACV at a solid (stationary) electrode.

The special case of square-wave voltammetry (SWV) is worth noting separately from other alternating current techniques because it is both more rapid and more sensitive than DPP/DPV. In SWV, the applied potential waveform is a staircase with constant step height on which is superimposed an asymmetrical forward and reverse voltage pulse of constant amplitude and very short duration, typically less than 10 ms. Thus, the entire polarogram may be run in about approximately 1 s, with the enhanced sensitivity of the method owing to sampling of the current at the end of both the forward and reverse directions of the pulse.

Stripping Voltammetry

This is an ultrasensitive technique most widely used in the trace determination of metals and, increasingly, for organic compounds, including pharmaceuticals. The outstanding sensitivity of the method is due to an initial preconcentration (accumulation) step that can result in a 1000-fold increase in the available analyte concentration compared with the bulk solution. The most commonly used working electrode design for stripping analysis has a single mercury drop hanging from the electrode tip during the course of the stripping experiment. Such an electrode is the HMDE, although other designs such as the mercury film electrode (MFE), in which the mercury is supported as a thin film on a carbon electrode support (8), and SMDE have become increasingly important (9). The SMDE allows faster stirring rates during the deposition step than are possible with the HMDE, the limiting factor in the latter case being the dislodgement of the mercury drop by vigorous stirring. In addition to mercury, nonplated solid

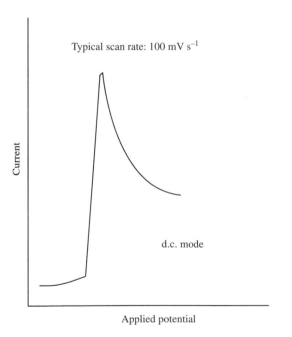

Typical scan rate: 100 mV s^{-1}

Current

d.c. mode

Applied potential

Fig. 9 Typical appearance of a linear sweep voltammogram at a fast-scan rate of 100 mV s^{-1}.

electrodes fabricated from a noble metal (gold or platinum) or from carbon (glassy carbon, carbon paste) have also been used for stripping analysis, typically for the determination of metals that are insoluble in mercury that have very positive redox potentials. For most pharmaceutical applications of stripping analysis that involve organic compounds, mercury electrodes are used. Stripping analysis can then be performed using a conventional modern polarograph linked to a specific working electrode suitable for the chosen analysis.

Stripping analysis for compounds of pharmaceutical interest consists of two steps. First, the electroactive material is deposited onto a mercury electrode, thus concentrating the analate by extracting it from the bulk solution. This controlled deposition, which may be electrolytic, is carried out for a defined time period, with constant stirring of the bulk solution because, in this case, it is necessary to drive the analyte toward the electrode surface as efficiently as possible. Second, there is the stripping step. This involves stripping (removing) the analyte from the electrode surface back into the solution by application of a suitable potential. This second step is the measurement step, the resulting faradaic current being quantitative in respect to the amount of analate present in the bulk solution. The applied potential can be a simple ramp voltage, pulse, or periodic waveform. Thus, most of the modern polarographic modes can be coupled to the stripping step to give additional increases in both sensitivity and selectivity. Fast stripping steps such as the use of the semidifferential mode (10) have become increasing popular, although differential pulse and linear sweep modes remain prevalent.

Anodic stripping voltammetry (ASV) has been the most widely used stripping variant, typically for the trace analysis of metals in solution. Thus, an electrolytic deposition step onto a mercury cathode, possibly lasting several minutes, is followed by an anodic stripping step in which the potential scan goes toward positive values. The deposition step itself results in the formation of a metal amalgam. As with all stripping variants, hydrodynamic parameters (stirring rate, deposition time, solution composition, electrode location) must be carefully controlled and reproducible to obtain a quantitative response to changing bulk concentrations. The process may be summarized as:

$$\text{Cathodic deposition:} \quad M^{n+} + ne \; \rightleftharpoons \; M(Hg)\downarrow$$
$$\text{Anodic stripping:} \quad M(Hg) \; \longrightarrow \; M^{n+} + ne + Hg$$

Cathodic stripping voltammetry (CSV) may be considered the reverse of ASV in that the electrolytic

deposition step is carried out at a positive (anodic) applied potential, the deposited analate then being stripped by application of a cathodic voltage scan. CSV has been used for the determination of various anions (11) and for certain drug molecules such as organosulfur compounds (12). CSV may be summarized as:

$$\text{Anodic deposition:} \quad 2\,Hg \; \rightleftharpoons \; Hg_2^{2+} + 2e$$
$$Hg_2^{2+} + 2A^- \; \rightleftharpoons \; Hg_2A_2\downarrow$$
$$\text{Cathodic stripping:} \quad Hg_2A_2 + 2e \; \longrightarrow \; 2Hg + 2A^-$$

Adsorptive stripping voltammetry (AdSV) is of increasing importance in trace determinations of pharmaceutical compounds. In this method, the preconcentration step is adsorptive rather than electrolytic, resulting in an adsorbed film of the analate on the electrode surface (13). The stripping step typically uses LSV or the differential pulse mode in either the cathodic or anodic direction, as required. The HMDE is typically used for cathodic reductive stripping, whereas carbon or noble metal electrodes are used in the adsorptive mode.

Factors affecting the adsorptive process in AdSV include the solvent, solution pH, mass-transport processes, stirring rate, deposition time, and applied potential. The sensitivity advantage of AdSV over conventional polarography/voltammetry using an equivalent mode may be up to 100-fold. However, the primary advantage of AdSV is its ability to simplify sample preparation when the analyte is in a complex matrix, such as the determination of a drug or its metabolite in body fluids. Having adsorbed the analyte to the electrode directly from the complex medium, the electrode with the adsorbed analate film may then be transferred to a blank electrolyte solution before the stripping step. This method, known as medium exchange (14), has considerable potential, particularly in a flow analysis mode (15) for both pharmaceutical and clinical analyses. Its value is perhaps not yet fully realized because of a preference for, and greater familiarity with, chromatographic methods.

Electrochemical Detection for High-Performance Liquid Chromatography (ELCD) and Flow-Injection Analysis (ED-FIA)

Pharmaceutical analysts often have no experience in direct polarographic or voltammetric methods, but almost all will have used high-performance liquid chromatography (HPLC) for the determination of drugs and/or metabolites in biological matrices or drugs and/or their degradation products in pharmaceutical formulations. Spectroscopy (ultraviolet and fluorescence) is the most common detection method in HPLC, but for molecules that do not possess a suitable chromophore or when increased sensitivity or specificity is required, electrochemical detection offers a suitable alternative. ELCD is applicable to any molecular species capable of electrochemical oxidation or reduction at an electrode. Most detectors are based on solid electrodes, notably carbon paste and, particularly, glassy carbon. These detectors are best operated in the anodic mode, but they can also be used for reductive processes. Alternatively, mercury films on a noble metal electrode can be used for cathodic reduction.

The principle of ELCD is described in Fig. 10 and has been addressed in detail by Stulik and Pacakova (16). The detector is set to an applied voltage large enough to cause the electrochemical reaction of interest to occur, i.e., the applied voltage is on the plateau of the polarographic wave. Thus, when the species of interest is eluted from the column, a faradaic current is produced in the detector and results in the usual chromatographic signal. This is an example of amperometric detection because an electrical current is responsible for the analytical signal. With a solid electrode, the detector may be described as a voltammetric detector. Various detector cell designs are available. The most common configuration is the wall-jet cell (Fig. 11), in which the eluent is sprayed against an internal wall of the detector cell. The wall is fabricated from glassy carbon, a highly polished and impermeable material. The flowing eluent spray ensures that any products from the electrochemical oxidation reaction are

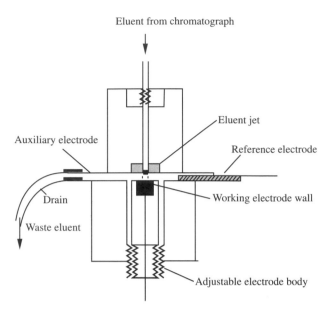

Fig. 11   Wall-jet electrochemical detector cell for HPLC.

removed from the electrode surface, thus ensuring signal reproducibility.

In conjunction with the various designs of electrochemical detector cells, a range of applied voltage waveforms may be used for ELCD (Fig. 12). The

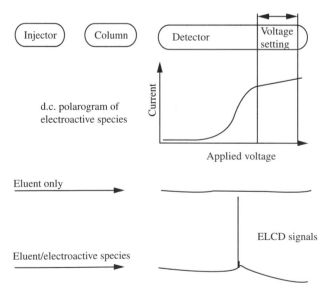

Fig. 10   Principle of electrochemical detection for HPLC.

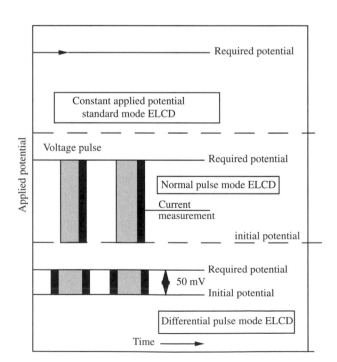

Fig. 12   Applied voltage waveforms for various modes of electrochemical detection in HPLC.

Additional information can also be obtained using a rapid-scan square-wave detector. As the name implies, this mode uses very fast voltage scans so that a three-dimensional output can be obtained. In effect, many voltammograms are run of a component as it elutes from the column, giving an output of current versus applied potential versus time. Thus, peak purity can be checked, and the device is analogous in its applications to the better known diode array spectrophotometric detector. Voltammetric detectors may also be used in a flow-injection mode (17), effectively omitting the chromatographic step, for drug analysis. Again, a wide range of detector cell designs and polarographic/voltammetric modes are available.

APPLICATIONS OF POLAROGRAPHY AND VOLTAMMETRY TO PHARMACEUTICAL ANALYSIS

A comprehensive review of the use of polarography and voltammetry for drug analysis is beyond the scope of this article. (See Bibliography for reviews on the subject.) The analytical range of the methods is also well illustrated in the references (18–28).

CONCLUSIONS

The availability of a wide range of modern polarographic and voltammetric modes, together with the use of ELCD and stripping analysis, offers the analyst powerful analytical tools for performing drug assays. The decision as to whether an electroanalytical method should be used for a given assay and the selection of a particular polarographic/voltammetric technique will depend on the drug of interest, the analytical matrix, and the type of data that are required. Given the advances in analytical instrumentation, polarography/voltammetry may now be used with confidence, when necessary, by all pharmaceutical analysts.

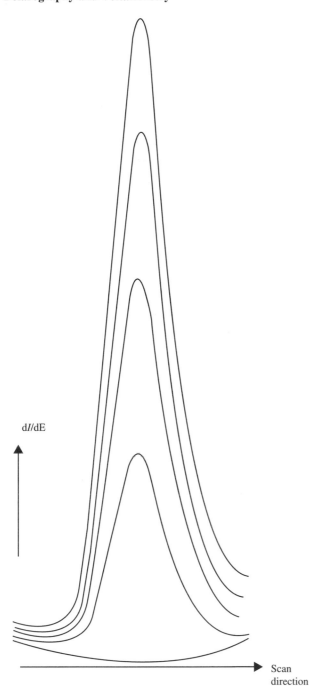

dI/dE

Scan direction

Fig. 13 Differential pulse voltammograms of pyridoxine hydrochloride at the glassy carbon electrode obtained by adding successive aliqouts (0.1 ml) of an aqueous solution (0.1M) of the vitamin to pH 4 citric acid as the supporting electrolyte.

differential pulse mode (Fig. 13) is particularly suited to ELCD because it can further enhance the separability of components by selectively setting the detector to the peak potential of an individual component in a mixture.

REFERENCES

1. Flato, J.B. Renaissance in Polarographic and Voltammetric Analysis. Anal. Chem. **1972**, *44*, 75a–85a.
2. Sevcik, A. Oscillographic Polarography with Periodical Triangular Voltage. Coll. Czech. Chem. Commum. **1948**, *13*, 349–354.
3. Hickling, A. Automatic Control of the Potential of a Working Electrode. Trans. Faraday Soc. **1942**, *38*, 27–33.

4. Kronenberger, K.; Strehlow, H.; Elbel, A.W. Intermittent Polarography. Leybolds Polarogr. Berlin **1957**, *5*, 62–77.

5. Barker, G.C.; Gardner, A.W. Pulse Polarography. Z. Anal. Chem. **1960**, *173*, 79–83.

6. Vire, J.C.; Patriarche, G.J.; Pharm. Int. **1981**, (May), 119–123.

7. Randles, J.E.B. Cathode Ray Polarograph. Trans. Faraday Soc. **1948**, *44*, 322–327.

8. Florence, T.M. Anodic Stripping Voltammetry with a Glassy Carbon Electrode Mercury-Plated In Situ. J. Electroanal. Chem. **1970**, *27*, 273–281.

9. Peterson, W.R. Static Mercury Drop Electrode. Am. Lab. **1979**, *12*, 69–74.

10. Goto, M.; Ikenoya, K.; Kajihara, M.; Ishii, D. Application of Semi-Differential Analysis to Anodic Stripping Voltammetry. Anal. Chim. Acta **1978**, *101*, 131–138.

11. Brainina, K.Z. Film Stripping Voltammetry. Talanta **1971**, *18*, 513–539.

12. Davidson, I.E.; Smyth, W.F. Cathodic Stripping Voltammetry of Some Sulfur-Containing Organic Compounds in Biological Fluids. Anal. Chem. **1977**, *49*, 1195–1198.

13. Wang, J. Adsorptive Stripping Voltammetry. Int. Lab. **1985**, *15*, 68–70.

14. Neeb, R.; Kiehnast, I.Z. Effect of Salts on the Anodic Peak Height in Inverse Voltammetry. Anal. Chem. **1967**, *241*, 142–155.

15. Wang, J.; Dewald, H.D.; Greene, B. Anodic-Stripping Voltammetry of Heavy-Metals with a Flow-Injection System. Anal. Chim. Acta **1983**, *146*, 45–50.

16. Stulik, K.; Pacakova, V. *Electroanalytical Measurements in Flowing Liquids*; Ellis Horwood: Chichester, UK, 1987.

17. Tougas, T.P. Recent Developments in Electrochemical Detection for Flow Injection Analysis. Int. Lab. **1988**, *18*, 17–28.

18. Smith, W.F.; Ivaska, A. A Study of the Electrochemical Oxidation of Some 1,4-Benzodiazepines. Analyst **1985**, *110*, 1377–1379.

19. Forsman, U. Cathodic Stripping Voltammetric Determination of Trace Amounts of Penicillins. Anal. Chim. Acta **1983**, *146*, 71–86.

20. Sithole, B.B.; Guy, R.D. Separation of Nitroimidazoles by Reversed-Phase High-Pressure Liquid Chromatography. Talanta **1986**, *33*, 95–97.

21. Wang, J.; Peng, T.; Lin, M.S. Trace Measurements of Tetracyclines Using Adsorptive Stripping Voltammetry. Bioelectrochem. Bioenerg. **1986**, *15*, 147–156.

22. Wang, J.; Bonakdar, M.; Morgan, C. Voltammetric Measurement of Tricyclic Antidepressants Following Interfacial Accumulation at Carbon Electrodes. Anal. Chem. **1986**, *58*, 1024–1028.

23. Wang, J.; Freiha, B.A.; Deshmukh, B.K. Adsorptive Extractive Stripping Voltammetry of Phenothiazine Compounds at Carbon Paste Electrodes. Bioelectrochem. Bioenerg. **1985**, *14*, 457–467.

24. Ballantine, J.; Woolfson, A.D. The Application of Differential Pulse Voltammetry at the Glassy Carbon Electrode to Multivitamin Analysis. J. Pharm. Pharmacol. **1980**, *32*, 353–356.

25. Kontoyannis, C.G.; Antimisiaris, S.G.; Douroumis, D. Simultaneous Quantitative Determination of Diazepam and Liposomes Using Differential Pulse Polarography. Anal. Chim. Acta **1999**, *391*, 83–88.

26. Zapardiel, A.; Bermejo, E.; Lopez, J.; Hernandez, L.; Gil, E. Electroanalytical Determinations of Halazepam—Study of Interaction with Human, Serum Albumin. Microchem. J. **1995**, *52*, 41–52.

27. Fernandez-Marcote, M.S.M.; Mochon, M.C.; Sanchez, J.C.J.; Perez, A.G. Electrochemical Reduction of Prilocaine as Its *N*-Nitrosamine Derivative At the Mercury Electrode. Electroanalysis **1998**, *10*, 492–496.

28. Reddy, G.V.S.; Reddy, S.J. Estimation of Cephalosporin Antibiotics by Differential Pulse Polarography. Talanta **1997**, *44*, 627–631.

BIBLIOGRAPHY

Bersier, P.M.; Bersier, J. Polarographic, Voltammetric, and HPLC-EC of Pharmaceutically Relevant Cyclic Compounds. Electroanalysis **1994**, *6*, 171–191.

Bond, A.M. *Modern Polarographic Methods in Analytical Chemistry*; Marcel Dekker, Inc.: New York, 1980.

Hart, J.P. *Electroanalysis of Biologically Important Compounds*; Ellis Horwood: Chichester, UK, 1990.

Hoffmann, H.; Volke, J. Polarographic Analysis in Pharmacy. In *Electroanalytical Chemistry*; Nurnberger, H.W., Ed.; John Wiley & Sons: New York, 1974.

Smyth, W.F. *Polarography of Molecules of Biological Significance*; Academic Press: London, 1979.

Smyth, W.F.; Woolfson, A.D. Drug Assays: The Role of Modern Voltammetric Techniques. J. Clin. Pharm. Ther. **1987**, *12*, 117–134.

Wang, J. *Stripping Analysis*; Verlag Chemie: Deerfield Beach, 1985.

POLYMORPHISM: PHARMACEUTICAL ASPECTS

Harry G. Brittain
Center for Pharmaceutical Physics, Milford, New Jersey

INTRODUCTION

It had been known since the middle of the 18th century that many substances could be obtained in more than one crystal form, and so the properties of these solids were studied to the fullest extent possible with the characterization tools (e.g., crystal morphology and melting phenomena) available at that time (1). Eventually the work of von Laue and Bragg on the diffraction of X-rays by crystalline solids led to the development of technology that could be used to directly study the structures of such materials and to provide the structural justification for the phenomenon that became known as polymorphism.

Among other things, it became established that the nature of the structure adopted by a given compound on crystallization would then exert a profound effect on the solid-state properties of that system. For a given material, the heat capacity, conductivity, volume, density, viscosity, surface tension, diffusivity, crystal hardness, crystal shape and color, refractive index, electrolytic conductivity, melting or sublimation properties, latent heat of fusion, heat of solution, solubility, dissolution rate, enthalpy of transitions, phase diagrams, stability, hygroscopicity, and rates of reactions were all affected by the nature of the crystal structure.

Subsequently, workers in pharmaceutically related fields realized that the solid-state property differences derived from the existence of alternate crystal forms could translate into measurable differences in properties of pharmaceutical importance (2). For instance, it was found that various polymorphs could exhibit different solubilities and dissolution rates, and these differences sometimes led to the existence of nonequivalent bioavailabilities for the different forms. Since then, it has become recognized that an evaluation of the possible polymorphism available to a drug substance must be thoroughly investigated early during the stages of development. In various compilations, it has been reported that polymorphic species are known for most drug substances (3, 4) and that one should be surprised to encounter a compound for which only one structural type can be formed.

THEORETICAL CONCEPTS

The full specification of a polymorphic system is specified by the thermodynamic properties of the phases involved. A solid phase has a uniform structure and composition throughout, is separated by other phases by defined boundaries, and undergoes a phase transition when a particular solid phase becomes unstable under a given set of environmental conditions. The course of these phase changes is dictated by differences in free energy at the transition that are associated with structural or compositional changes. Classical thermodynamics provides a basis for understanding the nature of these transitions.

During a phase transition, the free energy of the system remains continuous, while the entropy, volume, and heat capacity undergo discontinuous changes. Phase transitions are classified as being of the same order as the derivative of the Gibbs free energy that exhibits a discontinuous change at the transition. Gibbs free energy (G) is defined from enthalpy (H) and entropy (S) by

$$G = H - TS$$
$$= E + PV - TS$$

where T is the absolute temperature, P is the pressure, V is the volume, and E is the energy. It can easily be shown that transformations in which a discontinuous change occurs in volume or entropy (i.e., requiring a latent heat of transformation) will belong to the first order, while those involving a discontinuous change in heat capacity, thermal expansivity, or compressibility will belong to the second order.

The classical Clapeyron equation adequately predicts the features of first-order phase transitions, and this has been established for a number of examples of first-order transitions effected by the deliberate variation of temperature or pressure (5). Second- or higher-order transitions are not readily explained by classical thermodynamics. Unlike the case of first-order transitions, where the free-energy surfaces of the two phases intersect sharply at the transition temperatures, it is difficult to visualize the nature of the free-energy surfaces in second- or higher-order transitions. In second-order transitions, changes in heat capacity as well as compressibility and thermal expansivity can be detected at the transition temperature, complicating the analysis.

Under a given set of environmental conditions, the most stable polymorph will be the one having the lowest free energy ($G'_{metastable} > G_{stable}$), and all metastable forms must eventually transform to the most stable form. If some combination of P and T exists so that $G'_{metastable} = G_{stable}$, then a reversible phase transition may take place and one terms this situation *enantiotropy*. If however, $G'_{metastable} > G_{stable}$ at all values of P and T, then any process that converts the metastable form into the stable form must be irreversible. This situation is termed *monotropy*.

One generally finds, therefore, that absolute values for thermodynamic parameters are less important than are relationships that predict the relative stability of the various phases of a polymorphic system. Although it is possible to calculate such energy differences from considerations of the lattice energies of the different structures (6), most workers instead employ the time-honored empirical rules that have been developed over time (7). For instance, since $G'_{metastable} > G_{stable}$, then the vapor pressure of the stable form must be less than the vapor pressure of the metastable form.

A number of empirical rules have been proposed to deduce the relative order of stability of polymorphs and the nature of the process that interconverts these (i.e., enantiotropy vs. monotropy). Among the better known are the *Heat of Transition Rule*, which states that if an endothermic transition is observed at some temperature, it may be assumed that there must be a transition point located at a lower temperature where the two forms bear an enantiotropic relationship. Conversely, if an exothermic transition is noted at some temperature, it may be assumed that there is no transition point located at a lower temperature. This in turn implies that either the two forms bear a monotropic relationship to each other or that the transition temperature is higher than the temperature of the exotherm.

Another empirical rule is the *Heat of Fusion Rule*, which states that if the higher melting form has a lower heat of fusion relative to the lower melting form, then the two forms bear an enantiotropic relationship. Less well obeyed is the *Density Rule*, which states that the most dense form will be the most stable at absolute zero. Strictly speaking, the Density Rule is only properly applied to polymorphs of molecular solids where intramolecular hydrogen bonding is not a significant factor.

STRUCTURAL ASPECTS

An ideal crystal is constructed by the regular spatial repetition of identical structural units. One defines the symmetry properties of crystals in terms of a periodic *lattice*, or a 3D grid of lines connecting points in a given structure. The repetitive motif is termed the *unit cell* (which will typically contain a group of molecules), each of which is located at a lattice point. The unit cell is defined by the magnitude of its projections (a, b, and c) along the crystal axes and the angles between the cell axes (α, β, and γ). The symmetry of a crystal is ultimately summed up in its crystallographic *space group*, which is the entire set of symmetry operations that define the periodic structure of the crystal.

When considering the structures of organic molecules, one finds that different modifications can arise in two main distinguishable ways. Should the molecule be constrained to exist as a rigid grouping of atoms, these may be stacked in different motifs to occupy the points of different lattices. This type of polymorphism is then attributable to packing phenomena and so is termed *packing polymorphism*. On the other hand, if the molecule in question is not rigidly constructed and can exist in distinct conformational states, then it can happen that each of these conformationally distinct modifications may crystallize in its own lattice structure. This latter behavior has been termed *conformational polymorphism* (8).

Packing Polymorphism

During the very first series of studies using single-crystal X-ray crystallography to determine the structures of organic molecules, Robertson reported the structure of resorcinol (1,3-dihydroxybenzene) (9). This crystalline material corresponded to that ordinarily obtained at room temperature, and was later termed the α-form. Shortly thereafter, it was found that the α-form underwent a transformation into a denser crystalline modification (denoted as the β-form) when heated at about 74°C and that the structure of this newer form was completely different (10). The crystal structures of the α- and β-forms (viewed down the c-axis, or (001) crystal plane) are found in Fig. 1.

By its nature, resorcinol is locked into a single conformation, and it is immediately evident from a comparison of the structures in Fig. 1 that each form is characterized by a different motif of hydrogen bonding. In particular, the α-form features a relative open architecture that is maintained by a spiraling array of hydrogen bonding that ascends through the various planes of

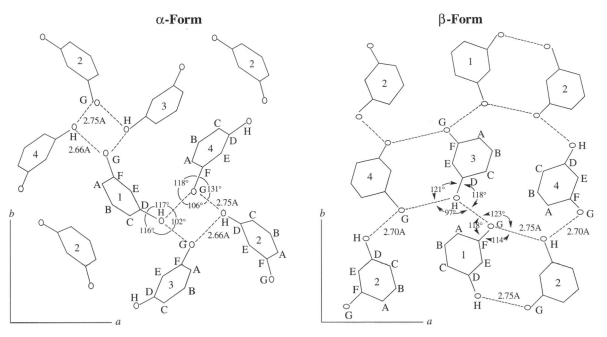

Fig. 1 Crystal structures of the α- and β-forms of resorcinol, as viewed down the *c*-axis (001 plane). (Adapted from Refs. 9 and 10.)

the crystal. In the view illustrated (defined by the *ab*-plane), the apparent closed tetramic grouping of hydroxyl groups is actually a slice through the ascending spiral. The effect of the thermally induced phase transformation is to collapse the open arrangement of the α-form by a more compact and parallel arrangement of the molecules in the β-form. This structural change causes an increase in crystal density on passing from the α-form (1.278 g/cm^3) to the β-form (1.327 g/cm^3). In fact, the molecular packing existing in the β-form was described as being more typical of hydrocarbons than of a hydroxylic compound (10).

Conformational Polymorphism

Probucol(4,4′-[(1-methylethylidene)bis(thio)]-bis-[2,6-bis(1,1-dimethylethyl)phenol]) is a cholesterol-lowering drug that has been reported to exist in two forms (11). Form II has been found to exhibit a lower melting point onset relative to Form I, and samples of Form II spontaneously transform to Form I upon long-term storage. The structures of these two polymorphic forms have been reported, and detailed views of the crystal structures are given in Fig. 2.

The conformations of the probucol molecule in the two forms were found to be quite different. In Form II, the CSCSC chain is extended, and the molecular symmetry

approximates C_{2v}. This molecular symmetry is lost in the structure of Form I, where now the torsional angles around the two CS bonds deviate significantly from 180°. Steric crowding of the phenolic groups by the *t*-butyl groups was evident from deviations from trigonal geometry at two phenolic carbons in both forms. Using a computational model, the authors found that the energy of Form II was 26.4 kJ/mol higher than the energy of Form I, indicating the less symmetrical conformer to be more stable. The crystal density of Form I was found to be approximately 5% higher than that of Form II, indicating that the conformational state of the Probucol molecules in Form I yielded more efficient space filling.

Solvatomorphism

One may define a solvatomorph as a crystalline solid in which solvent molecules have become included in the structure through the existence of positional substitution at positions that are site specific and that are related to other solvent molecules through translational symmetry. Other types of structural solvation exist (12) but will not be discussed here. Since water is such a ubiquitous substance, it is not surprising that the most important type of solvatomorphism involves the incorporation of water into a crystal lattice.

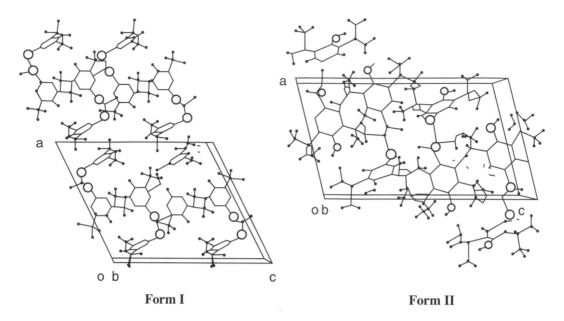

Fig. 2   Crystal structures of Forms I and II of Probucol. (Adapted from Ref. 11.)

Ampicillin (4-thia-1-azobicyclo[3.2.0]heptane-2-carboxylic acid) is an antibacterial agent that has been found to crystallize in one trihydrate and at least two anhydrate forms, and the structures of these have been critically compared (13). The transition temperature for the two forms in the presence of water has been found to be 42°C, where the trihydrate forms when crystallization is conducted below this value, and the anhydrate forms when the crystallization is effected at temperatures exceeding 42°C. Structures for the two solvatomorphs are shown in Fig. 3.

The ampicillin molecule exists as a zwitterion in both forms, with the overall molecular configuration being fairly similar as well. The structural differences induced by the presence of the water molecules in the trihydrate phase are evident in the differing configurations of the respective thiazolidine rings, where more planarity is found for the trihydrate phase than is found for the anhydrate phase. It was deduced that the three water molecules were extensively involved in the hydrogen bonding, and that they were located in a channel that lay parallel to one of the molecular screw axes. The intricate network of hydrogen bonding was invoked to explain the relative difficulty associated with dehydration of the trihydrate phase. Finally, the molecular packing of the two forms was judged to be so completely different that the authors concluded that there would be no way for the trihydrate phase to convert to the anhydrate phase as a pure solid–solid transition.

GENERATION OF POLYMORPHS

It is essential to determine the range of crystalline forms that are accessible to a potential drug substance and to determine which of the various forms will be the one used in products used in pivotal trials. To answer this question, investigators must conduct whatever studies might be required to evaluate the full range of possible polymorphs and solvatomorphs. The situation can be further complicated by the phenomenon of disappearing polymorphs, where metastable crystal forms become impossible to produce once more stable forms are uncovered (14).

Ideally, development programs devise a screening protocol for the discovery and preparation of any and all solid-state forms of chemical entities that may exist. Such protocols do not absolutely exclude the discovery of additional forms at later stages of development (i.e., during scale-up), but such approaches provide a comfort level regarding the level of knowledge and awareness regarding the scope of crystalline forms that may exist. A detailed exposition of the means available for the generation of polymorphs and solvates is available (15).

The first and primary method for production of polymorphs entails slow solvent evaporation of saturated solutions, with the rate of evaporation being adjusted by empirical means. Examples of solvents routinely used for such work are listed in Table 1 together with their boiling

Anhydrate   **Trihydrate**

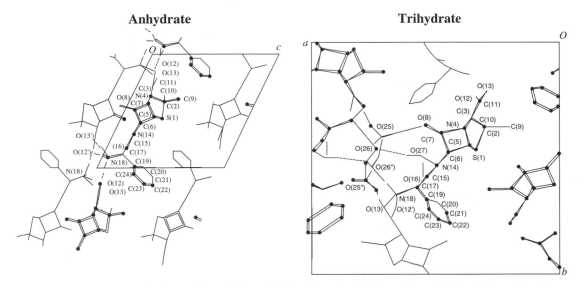

Fig. 3 Crystal structures of the anhydrate (viewed down the *b*-axis) and trihydrate (viewed down the *c*-axis) solvatomorphs of ampicillin. (Adapted from Ref. 13.)

Table 1 Solvents routinely used to isolate compound polymorphs and solvates

Solvent	Boiling point (°C)
Dipolar aprotic	
Dimethyl formamide	153
Acetonitrile	81
Dimethyl sulfoxide	189
N-methyl pyrolidinone	80
Protic	
Water (various pH values)	100
Methanol	65
Acetic acid	115
Ethanol	78
i-Propanol	82
n-Propanol	97
n-Butanol	118
Lewis acidic	
Dichloromethane	40
Chloroform	61
Lewis basic	
Acetone	56
2-Butanone	80
Tetrahydrofuran	66
Ethyl acetate	77
Methyl butyl ether	56
Aromatic	
Toluene	111
Xylene	140
Pyridine	115
Nonpolar	
Hexane	69
Cyclohexane	81

points. The process of solution-mediated transformation can be considered the result of two separate events, beginning with dissolution of the initial phase, and completing with nucleation and growth of the final, stable phase. If two polymorphs differ in their melting points by 25–50°C, for monotropic polymorphs the lower melting, more soluble, form will be difficult to crystallize. The smaller the difference between the two melting points, the easier can it be to obtain the unstable or metastable forms.

Another commonly used crystallization method involves controlled changes in temperature. Slow cooling of a hot, saturated solution can be effective in producing crystals if the compound is more soluble at higher temperatures, while slow warming can be used if the compound is less soluble at higher temperatures. Sometimes it is preferable to heat the solution to boiling, filter to remove excess solute, then quench cool using an ice bath or even a dry ice-acetone bath.

There are situations where kinetics determines the course of crystallization, and thermodynamics becomes of secondary consideration. For example, Ostwald's Law of Stages states that, "when leaving an unstable state, a system does not seek out the most stable state, rather the nearest metastable state which can be reached with loss of free energy." This form then transforms to the next most soluble form through a process of dissolution and crystallization. For crystals whose formation is dominated by kinetic factors, it is essential to isolate the metastable form from the crystallization solvent by rapid filtration so that subsequent phase transformation would not occur.

During the characterization of solids obtained from solvent crystallization studies, one finds that thermal treatment may be a means to produce new crystal forms. For instance, when using differential scanning calorimetry as an analysis technique, one can observe an endothermic peak corresponding to a phase transition, followed by a second endothermic peak corresponding to melting. Sometimes there is an exothermic peak between the two endotherms, representing a crystallization step. In these cases it is often possible to prepare the higher melting polymorph by thermal treatment.

In accordance with Ostwald's rule, the cooling of melts of polymorphic substances ordinarily yields the least stable modification, which subsequently rearranges into the stable modification in steps. Since the metastable form will have the lower melting point, it follows that supercooling is necessary to crystallize it from the melt. After melting, the system must be supercooled below the melting point of the metastable form, while at the same time the crystallization of the more stable form or forms must be prevented. Quench cooling a melt can sometimes result in formation of an amorphous solid that on subsequent heating undergoes a glass transition followed by crystallization.

Substances often crystallize containing water or solvent molecules located at specific sites in the crystal lattice, defining new crystalline forms known as solvatomorphs. Since water is a pharmaceutically acceptable solvent, hydrate species are of primary importance to drug development. The variety of hydrates that can exist has been summarized (12). Most solvatomorphs form with an integral number for the solvent/molecule ratio, but this is not always the case.

In the simplest type, water is bound to inorganic cations as part of a coordination complex. This type of water is denoted as water of crystallization and is common for inorganic compounds. For example, nickel sulfate forms a well-defined hexahydrate, where the waters of hydration are bound directly to the Ni(II) ion. Well-defined multiple hydrate species can also form with organic molecules, where the water molecules bridge unit cells in the overall structure. Finally, water molecules can exist in a semispecific manner, lining cavities within the crystal structure. This last hydrate type is often termed a channel hydrate.

Typically, hydrates are obtained by recrystallization from water. For example, trazodone hydrochloride tetrahydrate was prepared by dissolving the anhydrate in hot distilled water, allowing the solution to remain at room temperature overnight, and storing the collected crystals at 75% relative humidity and 25°C until they reached constant weight (16). Hydrates can sometimes be obtained by suspending the anhydrous material in water, a process that is analogous to Ostwald ripening. For instance, aqueous suspensions of anhydrous metronidazole benzoate are metastable, and storage at temperatures lower then 38°C leads to monohydrate formation accompanied by crystal growth (17). The exposure of an anhydrous powder to high relative humidity often yields the formation of new hydrate forms. For example, the experimental anti-cholesterol compound SQ-33600 was found to form a multitude of hydrate forms on exposure to various relative humidity environments (18).

METHODS OF CHARACTERIZATION

Once a variety of crystalline solids have been produced using a suitable polymorph protocol, it is very important to characterize these by proper techniques so that the system can become better defined. Fortunately, extensive discussions of the techniques suitable for the characterization of pharmaceutical solids are available (19, 20). The fruits of the most important characterization technique, single-crystal X-ray diffraction, have already been discussed in connection with the phenomenon of polymorphism in an earlier section. Certainly the determination of the crystal structures of all possible polymorphs and solvatomorphs would constitute the ultimate in characterization, especially if one could also conduct spectroscopic and thermal investigations on the same crystals used for the structural determination. This situation is rarely realized, so a series of additional techniques are ordinarily brought into use.

Of all the methods available for the physical characterization of solid materials, it is generally agreed that crystallography, microscopy, thermal analysis, solubility studies, vibrational spectroscopy, and nuclear magnetic resonance are the most useful for characterization of polymorphs and solvates. However, it cannot be overemphasized that the defining criterion for the existence of polymorphic types must always be a nonequivalence of crystal structures. For compounds of pharmaceutical interest, this ordinarily implies that a nonequivalent X-ray powder diffraction pattern is observed for each suspected polymorphic variation. All other methodologies must be considered as sources of supporting and ancillary information, but cannot be taken as definitive proof for the existence of polymorphism by themselves.

A correctly prepared sample of a powdered solid will present an entirely random selection of all possible crystal faces at the powder interface, and the diffraction off this surface provides information on all possible atomic spacings in the crystal lattice (21). The relationship between observed scattering angles and the spacings between planes of molecules in the lattice consists of Bragg's Law:

$$n\lambda = 2d \sin \theta z$$

where n is the order of the diffraction line, λ is the wavelength of the incident X-ray beam, d is the distance between the planes in the crystal, and θ is the observed angle of beam diffraction. To measure a powder pattern, a randomly oriented sample is prepared so as to expose all the planes of a sample, irradiated with monochromatic X-ray radiation, and the angles measured at which coherent scattering of X-rays is observed.

An extremely important tool for the characterization of polymorphs and solvates is that of microscopy, since the observable habits of differing crystal structures must necessarily be different and therefore useful for the characterization of such systems (22). Clearly, visual observation of materials suspected of being polymorphs or solvatomorphs would immediately follow their crystallographic study, which in turn would make the science of optical crystallography (23) an essential aspect of any program of study. Both optical and electron microscopies have found widespread use for the characterization of polymorphs and solvates. Although optical microscopy is more limited in the range of magnification suitable for routine work (working beyond 600× being difficult when observing microcrystalline materials), the use of polarizing optics introduces enormous power into the technique not available with other methods. Electron microscopy work can be performed at extraordinarily high magnification levels (up to 90,000× on most units), and the images that can be obtained contain a considerable degree of 3D information.

Often referred to as fusion microscopy or hot-stage microscopy, thermal microscopy can be an extremely valuable tool for the characterization of polymorphic or solvate systems. The technique requires that one make observations during the heating and cooling of a few milligrams of substance on a microscope slide, as well as observations on the crystallized material (24). It is therefore possible to conduct a very rapid analysis using only small quantities of material, and the entire phase diagram of a drug material can be deduced upon the conduct of suitably designed experiments. The most widely used device in the conduct of thermal microscopic studies is the hot state of Kofler, which has facilitated the conduct of an extraordinary number of studies (25).

Thermal analysis methods are defined as those techniques in which a property of the analyte is determined as a function of an externally applied temperature. Regardless of the observable parameter

measured, the usual practice requires that the physical property and the sample temperature are recorded continually and automatically and that the sample temperature is altered at a predetermined rate. Thermal reactions can be endothermic (melting, boiling, sublimation, vaporization, desolvation, solid–solid phase transitions, chemical degradation, etc.) or exothermic (crystallization, oxidative decomposition, etc.) in nature. Such methodology has found widespread use in the pharmaceutical industry for the characterization of compound purity, polymorphism, solvation, degradation, and excipient compatibility (26).

Although a large number of thermal analysis techniques have been developed, the most commonly applied are those of thermogravimetry (TG, the measure of thermally induced weight loss of a material as a function of applied temperature), differential thermal analysis (DTA, the difference in temperature existing between a sample and a reference as a function of temperature), and differential scanning calorimetry (DSC, the difference in heat capacity between the sample and a reference as a function of temperature). The primary applicability of DTA and DSC analysis to the study of polymorphs and solvatomorphs has been to obtain information about any phase transformations that take place as a function of temperature.

The simplest and most straightforward application of thermal analysis is concerned with studies of the relative stability of polymorphic forms. For example, DTA thermograms enabled the deduction that one commercially available form of chloroquine diphosphate was phase pure, while another consisted of a mixture of two polymorphs (27). DTA analysis was used to demonstrate that in spite of the fact that different crystal habits of sulfamethazine could be obtained, these in fact consisted of the same anhydrous polymorph (28). In a study aimed at profiling the dissolution behavior of the three polymorphs and five solvates of spironlactone, DTA analysis was used in conjunction with powder X-ray diffraction to establish the character of the various materials (29).

DSC analysis can also be used to obtain temperatures of compound melting, and such information can be of value in establishing the relative orders of stability in polymorphic systems. In addition, for suitable systems the technique can be used to study any phase interconversion that takes place during the DSC study. For instance, Form I of iopanoic acid yielded a single melting endotherm at 154°C, but the thermogram obtained on Form II was much more complicated (30). Form II was found to exhibit one endotherm at 133°C (the melting transition of Form I), an exotherm at 141°C (crystallization to Form II), and another endotherm at 153°C (melting of the recrystallized Form II).

DSC analysis represents a superior method of thermal analysis, in that the area under a DSC peak is directly proportional to the heat absorbed or evolved by the thermal event, and integration of these peak areas yields the enthalpy of reaction (in units of calories/gram or Joules/gram). Even though conclusions reached on the basis of enthalpies of fusion are possibly compromised by their omission of the entropy contribution, an indication of the thermodynamic trends inherent in the system is often possible. For instance, the same polymorphic form of moricizine hydrochloride was deduced on the basis of thermal analysis and equilibrium solubility measurements (31). On the other hand, auranofin represents a compound for which one anhydrous polymorphic form is predicted to be the most stable by virtue of its melting point and heat of fusion but for which solubility measurements demonstrate that the other polymorph was in fact the thermodynamically stable form (32).

The energies associated with the vibrational modes of a chemical compound can be observed directly through their absorbance in the infrared region of the spectrum or through the observation of the low-energy scattered bands that accompany the passage of an intense beam of light through the sample (the Raman effect). When the vibrational modes associated with the molecules in a polymorphic system are perturbed by features of the different crystal structures, these methods can be used in the spectroscopic investigation of polymorphs and solvates (33).

When the FTIR spectra of polymorph systems differ substantially, the results may readily permit the identification of a particular form. For instance, the two forms of ranitidine hydrochloride yielded spectra that differed in the region above 3000 cm^{-1} and in the regions spanning 2300–2700 cm^{-1} and 1570–1620 cm^{-1} (34). Zanoterone has been found to crystallize in a number of different forms, each of which yields a characteristic infrared spectrum (35). When solvent molecules are incorporated in a crystal lattice, the new structure is often sufficiently different from that of the anhydrous phase so that many of the molecular vibrational modes are altered.

The vibrational modes of a compound may also be studied using Raman spectroscopy, where one measures the inelastic scattering of radiation by a nonabsorbing medium (36). Although both infrared absorption and Raman scattering yield information on the energies of the same vibrational bands, the different selection rules governing the band intensities for each type of spectroscopy can be exploited by the skillful worker. For instance, both types of vibrational spectroscopy were used to investigate the polymorphism of nimodipine, and it was evident from the intensity relations that, although each

technique yielded a summary of the vibrational transitions, substantial differences in band intensity were readily discernible (37).

One technique that is becoming increasingly important for the characterization of materials is that of solid-state nuclear magnetic resonance (NMR) spectroscopy, and the application of this methodology to topics of pharmaceutical interest has been amply demonstrated (33, 38). The NMR spectra of polymorphs or solvatomorphs often contains nonequivalent resonance peaks for analogous nuclei since the intimate details of the molecular environments associated with differing crystal structures can lead to perturbations in nuclear resonance energies.

In its simplest application, solid-state NMR spectra can be used to qualitatively differentiate between polymorphs or solvates, much in the manner described for vibrational spectroscopy. When detailed assignments of solid-state spectra have been made, the technique can be used to deduce differences in molecular conformation, which cause crystallographic variations to exist. During the development of fosinopril sodium, a crystal structure was solved for the most stable phase, but no such structure could be obtained for its metastable phase (39). Studies of the solid-state vibrational and NMR spectroscopies permitted the deduction that the solid-state polymorphism was associated with different conformations of an acetal sidechain. The NMR data also suggested that additional conformational differences between the two polymorphs were associated with *cis–trans* isomerization along the peptide bond, which in turn resulted in the presence of non-equivalent molecules existing in the unit cell.

The solid-state NMR technique can be used to deduce quantitative measurements of phase composition, as has been reported for the anhydrate and dihydrate phases of carbamazepine (40). The applications of solid-state ^{13}C-NMR spectra for the study of polymorphs and solvates can go beyond evaluations of resonance band positions, making use of additional spectral characteristics. For instance, studies of T_{1p} relaxation times of furosemide polymorphs were used to show the presence of more molecular mobility and disorder in Form II, while the structure of Form I was judged to be more rigid and uniformly ordered (41).

POLYMORPHISM AND SOLUBILITY

Since the different lattice energies (and entropies) associated with different polymorphs or solvatomorphs give rise to measurable differences in a large variety of physical properties, it is hardly surprising that a family of different forms should exhibit different solubilities and dissolution rates (42). These varying solubilities can in turn be very important during the processing of drug substances into drug products (43) and may have implications for the adsorption of the active drug from its dosage form (44). A solid having a higher lattice free energy (i.e., a less stable polymorph) will tend to dissolve faster, since the release of a higher amount of stored lattice free energy will increase the solubility and hence the driving force for dissolution. At the same time, each species would liberate (or consume) the same amount of solvation energy, since all dissolved species (of the same chemical identity) must be thermodynamically equivalent. The varying dissolution rates possible for different structures of the same drug entity can in turn lead to varying degrees of bioavailability for different polymorphs or solvates.

Solubility determinations were used to characterize the polymorphism of 3-(((3-(2-(7-chloro-2-quinolinyl)-(E)-ethenyl)-phenyl)-((3-dimethylamino-3-oxopropyl)-thio)-methyl)-thio)-propanoic acid (45). The solubility of Form II was found to be higher than that of Form I in both isopropyl alcohol (IPA, solubility ratio equal to 1.7 over the range of 5–55°C) and methyl ethyl ketone (MEK, solubility ratio equal to 1.9 over the range of 5–55°C), indicating that Form I is the thermodynamically stable form over this temperature range. An analysis of the entropy contributions to the free energy of solution from the solubility results implied that the saturated IPA solutions were more disordered than were the corresponding MEK solutions, in turn indicating the existence of stronger solute–solvent interactions in the MEK solution.

Phenylbutazone has been found to be capable of existing in five different polymorphic structures, characterized by different X-ray powder diffraction patterns and melting points (46). While Form I exhibited the highest melting point (suggesting the least energetic structure at the elevated temperature), its equilibrium solubility was the lowest in each of the three solvent systems studied (demonstrating the lowest free energy). These findings indicate that Form I is the thermodynamically most stable polymorph both at room temperature and at the melting point (105°C). Identification of the sequence of stability for the other forms at any particular temperature was not straightforward, and it was concluded that the order of stability at room temperature was not the same as that at 100°C. This clearly indicates that some of the forms are enantiotropically related and that others are related by monotropism.

When the hydrates or solvates of a given compound are stable with respect to phase conversion in a solvent, the equilibrium solubility of these species can be used to characterize these systems. For instance, the equilibrium solubility of the trihydrate phase of ampicillin at 50°C is approximately 1.3 times that of the more stable anhydrate phase at room temperature (47). However, below the transition temperature of 42°C, the anhydrate phase is more soluble and is therefore less stable.

Solution calorimetry can be used on one level to merely obtain the enthalpy of solution for a given solute, or can be used in a deeper sense to obtain a full thermodynamic description of a system. The determination of solubility data over a defined temperature range can be used to calculate the differential heat of solution of a given polymorphic form. One can subtract the differential heats of solution obtained for the two polymorphs to deduce the heat of transition (ΔH_{Trans}) between the two forms:

$$\Delta H_{Trans} = \Delta H_S{}^B - \Delta H_S{}^A$$

where ΔH_S^a and ΔH_S^b denote the differential heats of solution for polymorphs A and B, respectively. The validity of the assumption regarding constancy in the heats of solution for a given substance with respect to temperature can be made by determining the enthalpy of fusion (ΔH_F) for the two forms, and then taking the difference between these:

$$\Delta H_{Trans} = \Delta H_F{}^B - \Delta H_F{}^A$$

where $\Delta H_{Trans'}$ represents the heat of transition between forms A and B at the melting point. When a sufficient number of assumptions are made, one deduces that ΔH_{Trans} and $\Delta H_{Trans'}$ should be equal, and thus DSC results can be used to verify the solution calorimetry results. For example, the heats of fusion and solution have been reported for the polymorphs of auranofin (32). The similarity of the heats of transition deduced in 95% ethanol (2.90 kcal/mol) and dimethylformamide (2.85 kcal/mol) with the heat of transition calculated at the melting point (3.20 kcal/mol) provides a fair estimation of the thermodynamics associated with this polymorphic system.

To illustrate the importance of free energy changes, consider the solvate system formed by paroxetine hydrochloride, which can exist as a nonhygroscopic hemihydrate or as a hygroscopic anhydrate (48). The heat of transition between these two forms was evaluated both by DSC ($\Delta H_{Trans'} = 0.0$ kJ/mol) and by solution calorimetry ($\Delta H_{Trans} = 0.1$ kJ/mol), which indicates that both forms are isoenthalpic. However, the free energy of transition (-1.25 kJ/mol) favors conversion of the anhydrate to the hemihydrate, and such phase conversion can be initiated by crystal compression or by seeding techniques. Since the two forms are essentially isoenthalpic, the entropy increase that accompanies the phase transformation is responsible for the decrease in free energy and may therefore be viewed as the driving force for the transition.

A basic thermodynamic understanding of a polymorphic system requires a determination of the free energy difference between the various forms. The two polymorphs of 3-amino-1-(m-trifluoromethlyphenyl)-6-methyl-1H-pyridazin-4-one have been characterized by a variety of methods, among which solubility studies were used to evaluate the thermodynamics of the transition from Form I to Form II (49). At a temperature of 30°C, the enthalpy change for the phase transformation was determined to be −5.64 kJ/mol. From the solubility ratio of the two polymorphs, the free energy change was then calculated as −3.67 kJ/mol, which implies that the entropy change accompanying the transformation was −6.48 cal/Kmol. In this system, one encounters a phase change that is favored by the enthalpy term but not favored by the entropy term. However, since the overall free energy change (ΔG_{Trans}) is negative, the process takes place spontaneously, provided that the molecules can overcome the activation energy barrier at a significant rate.

In other cases, an unfavorable enthalpy term was found to be compensated by a favorable entropy term, thus rendering negative the free energy change associated with a particular phase transformation. Lamivudine can be obtained in two forms, one of which is a 0.2-hydrate obtained from water or from methanol that contains water and the other of which is nonsolvated and is obtained from many nonaqueous solvents (50). Form II was determined to be thermodynamically favored in the solid state. Solubility studies of both forms as a function of solvent and temperature were used to determine whether entropy of enthalpy was the driving force for solubility. Solution calorimetric data indicated that Form I would be favored in all solvents studied on the basis of enthalpy alone. In higher alcohols and other organic solvents, Form I exhibited a larger entropy of solution than did Form II, compensating for the unfavorable enthalpic factors and yielding an overall negative freez energy for the phase change.

It is generally recognized that studies of dissolution rate are best conducted on compacted materials, where the process of forming the compact regulates the particle size and surface area of the solid. Such work yields the intrinsic dissolution rate, the trends of which usually parallel those deduced from studies of equilibrium solubility. Since under constant hydrodynamic conditions the intrinsic dissolution rate is proportional to the solubility of the dissolving solid, the most stable polymorphic form will exhibit the slowest intrinsic dissolution rate.

REFERENCES

1. Verma, A.R.; Krishna, P. *Polymorphism and Polytypism in Crystals*; John Wiley & Sons: New York, 1966; 1–7.
2. Brittain, H.G. *Polymorphism in Pharmaceutical Solids*; Marcel Dekker, Inc.: New York, 1999; 331–361.
3. Borka, L.; Haleblian, J.K. Crystal Polymorphism of Pharmaceuticals. Acta Pharm. Jugosl. **1990**, *40*, 71–94.
4. Borka, L. Review on Crystal Polymorphism of Substances in the European Pharmacopoeia. Pharm. Acta Helv. **1991**, *66*, 16–22.
5. Ubbelohde, A.R. *Reactivity of Solids*; de Boer, J.H., Ed.; Elsevier: Amsterdam, 1961; 141–168.
6. Mooij, W.T.M.; van Eijck, B.P.; Kroon, J. Ab Initio Crystal Structure Predictions for Flexible Hydrogen-Bonded Molecules. J. Am. Chem. Soc. **2000**, *122*, 3500–3505.
7. Burger, A.; Ramberger, R. On the Polymorphism of Pharmaceuticals and Other Molecular Crystals. I. Theory of Thermodynamic Rules. Mikrochim. Acta (Wien) II **1979**, 259–271, II. Applicability of Thermodynamic Rules. Ibid. 1979, 273–316.
8. Bernstein, J. Conformational Polymorphism. *Organic Solid State Chemistry*; Desiraju, G.R., Ed.; Elsevier: Amsterdam, 1987; 471–518.
9. Robertson, J.M. The Structure of Resorcinol: A Quantitative X-Ray Investigation. Proc. R. Soc. London **1936**, A*157*, 79–99.
10. Robertson, J.M.; Ubbelohde, A.R. A New Form of Resorcinol. I. Structure Determination by X-Rays. Proc. R. Soc. London 1938; 122–135.
11. Gerber, J.J.; Caira, M.R.; Lötter, A.P. Structures of Two Conformational Polymorphs of the Cholesterol-Lowering Drug Probucol. J. Cryst. Spect. Res. **1993**, *23*, 863–869.
12. Morris, K.R.; Rodriguez-Hornado; Hydrates, N. *Encyclopedia of Pharmaceutical Technology*; Swarbrick, J., Boylan, J., Eds.; Marcel Dekker, Inc.: New York, 1993; 7, 393–440.
13. Boles, M.O.; Girven, R.J. The Structures of Ampicillin: A Comparison of the Anhydrate and Trihydrate Forms. Acta Cryst. **1976**, B*32*, 2279–2284.
14. Dunitz, J.D.; Bernstein, J. Disappearing Polymorphs. Acc. Chem. Res. **1995**, *28*, 193–200.
15. Guillory, J.K. Generation of Polymorphs, Hydrates, Solvates, and Amorphous Solids. *Polymorphism in Pharmaceutical Solids*; Brittain, H.G., Ed.; Marcel Dekker, Inc.: New York, 1999; 183–226.
16. Sasaki, K.; Suzuki, H.; Nakagawa, H. Physicochemical Characterization of Trazodone Hydrochloride Tetrahydrate. Chem. Pharm. Bull. **1993**, *41*, 325–328.
17. Caira, M.R.; Nassimbeni, L.R.; van Oudtshoorn, B. X-Ray Structural Characterization of Anhydrous Metronidazole Benzoate and Metronidazole Benzoate Monohydrate. J. Pharm. Sci. **1993**, *82*, 1006–1009.
18. Morris, K.R.; Newman, A.W.; Bugay, D.E.; Ranadive, S.A.; Singh, A.K.; Szyper, M.; Varia, S.A.; Brittain, H.G.; Serajuddin, A.T.M. Characterization of Humidity-Dependent Changes in Crystal Properties of a New HMG-CoA Reductase Inhibitor in Support of Its Dosage Form Development. Int. J. Pharm. **1994**, *108*, 195–206.
19. Brittain, H.G. Methods for the Characterization of Polymorphs and Solvates. *Polymorphism in Pharmaceutical*

Solids; Brittain, H.G., Ed.; Marcel Dekker, Inc.: New York, 1999; 227–278.

20. Threlfall, T.L. Analysis of Organic Polymorphs. Analyst **1995**, *120*, 2435–2460.

21. Klug, H.P.; Alexander, L.E. *X-ray Diffraction Procedures*, 2nd Ed.; Wiley-Interscience: New York, 1974; 271–311.

22. Haleblian, J.K. Characterization of Habits and Crystalline Modifications of Solids and Their Pharmaceutical Applications. J. Pharm. Sci. **1975**, *64*, 1269–1288.

23. Wahlstrom, E.E. *Optical Crystallography*, 4th Ed.; John Wiley & Sons: New York, 1969.

24. McCrone, W.C. *Fusion Methods in Chemical Microscopy*; Interscience: New York, 1957.

25. Kuhnert-Brandstätter, M. *Thermomicroscopy in the Analysis of Pharmaceuticals*; Pergamon Press: Oxford, 1971.

26. Giron, D. Applications of Thermal Analysis in the Pharmaceutical Industry. J. Pharm. Biomed. Anal. **1986**, *4*, 755–770.

27. Van Aerde, Ph.; Remon, J.P.; De Rudder, D.; Van Severen, R.; Braeckman, P. Polymorphic Behavior of Chloroquine Diphosphate. J. Pharm. Pharmacol. **1984**, *36*, 190–191.

28. Maury, L.; Rambaud, J.; Pauvert, B.; Lasserre, Y.; Bergé, G. Physicochemical and Structural Study of Sulfamethazine. J. Pharm. Sci. **1985**, *74*, 422–426.

29. Salole, E.G.; Al-Sarraj, H. Spironolactone Crystal Forms. Drug Dev. Indust. Pharm. **1985**, *11*, 855–864.

30. Stagner, W.C.; Guillory, J.K. Physical Characterization of Solid Iopanoic Acid Forms. J. Pharm. Sci. **1979**, *68*, 1005–1009.

31. Wu, L.-S.; Torosian, G.; Sigvardson, K.; Gerard, C.; Hussain, M.A. Investigation of Moricizine Hydrochloride Polymorphs. J. Pharm. Sci. **1994**, *83*, 1404–1406.

32. Lindenbaum, S.; Rattie, E.S.; Zuber, G.E.; Miller, M.E.; Ravin, L.J. Polymorphism of Auranofin. Int. J. Pharm. **1985**, *26*, 123–132.

33. Brittain, H.G. Spectral Methods for the Characterization of Polymorphs and Solvates. J. Pharm. Sci. **1997**, *86*, 405–412.

34. Cholerton, T.J.; Hunt, J.H.; Klinkert, G.; Martin-Smith, M. Spectroscopic Studies on Ranitidine—Its Structure and the Influence of Temperature and pH. J. Chem. Soc. Perkin Trans. 2 **1984**, 1761–1766.

35. Rocco, W.L.; Morphet, C.; Laughlin, S.M. Solid-state Characterization of Zanoterone. Int. J. Pharm. **1995**, *122*, 17–25.

36. Grasselli, J.G.; Snavely, M.K.; Bulkin, B.J. *Chemical Applications of Raman Spectroscopy*; John Wiley & Sons: New York, 1981.

37. Grunenberg, A.; Keil, B.; Henck, J.-O. Polymorphism in Binary Mixtures, as Exemplified by Nimodipine. Int. J. Pharm. **1995**, *118*, 11–21.

38. Bugay, D.E. Solid-State Nuclear Magnetic Resonance Spectroscopy: Theory and Pharmaceutical Applications. Pharm. Res. **1993**, *10*, 317–327.

39. Brittain, H.G.; Morris, K.R.; Bugay, D.E.; Thakur, A.B.; Serajuddin, A.T.M. Solid State Characterization of Fosinopril Sodium Polymorphs. J. Pharm. Biomed. Anal. **1993**, *11*, 1063–1069.

40. Suryanarayanan, R.; Wiedmann, T.S. Quantitation of the Relative Amounts of Anhydrous Carbamazepine and Carbamazepine Dihydrate in a Mixture by Solid-State Nuclear Magnetic Resonance. Pharm. Res. **1990**, *7*, 184–187.

41. Doherty, C.; York, P. Frusemide Crystal Forms; Solid State and Physicochemical Analyses. Int. J. Pharm. **1988**, *47*, 141–155.

42. Grant, D.J.W.; Higuchi, T. Techniques of Chemistry. *Solubility Behavior of Organic Compounds*; Saunders, W.H., Jr. Ed.; Doctoral Thesis John Wiley and Sons: New York, 1947; 21.

43. Haleblian, J.K.; McCrone, W.C. Pharmaceutical Applications of Polymorphism. J. Pharm. Sci. **1969**, *58*, 911–929.

44. Higuchi, W.I.; Lau, P.K.; Higuchi, T.; Shell, J.W. Polymorphism and Drug Availability: Solubility Relationships in the Methylprednisolone System. J. Pharm. Sci. **1963**, *52*, 150–153.

45. Ghodbane, S.; McCauley, J.A. Study of the Polymorphism of 3-(((3-(2-(7-chloro-2-quinolinyl)-(*E*)-ethenyl)-phenyl)-((3-dimethylamino-3-oxopropyl)-thio)-methyl)-thio)-propanoic Acid by DSC, TG, XRPD, And Solubility Measurements. Int. J. Pharm. **1990**, *59*, 281–286.

46. Tuladhar, M.D.; Carless, J.E.; Summers, M.P. Thermal Behavior and Dissolution Properties of Phenylbutazone Polymorphs. J. Pharm. Pharmacol. **1983**, *35*, 208–214.

47. Poole, J.W.; Bahal, C.K. Dissolution Behavior and Solubility of Anhydrous and Trihydrate Forms of Ampicillin. J. Pharm. Sci. **1968**, *57*, 1945–1948.

48. Buxton, P.C.; Lynch, I.R.; Roe, J.A. Solid-state Forms of Paroxetine Hydrochloride. Int. J. Pharm. **1988**, *42*, 135–143.

49. Chauvet, A.; Masse, J.; Ribet, J.P.; Bigg, D.; Autin, J.M.; Maurel, J.M.; Patoiseau, J.F.; Jaud, J. Characterization of Polymorphs and Solvates of 3-Amino-1-(*m*-Trifluoromethlyphenyl)-6-Methyl-LH-Pyridazin-4-One. J. Pharm. Sci. **1992**, *81*, 836–841.

50. Jozwiakowski, M.J.; Nguyen, N.A.; Sisco, J.M.; Spancake, C.W. Solubility Behavior of Lamivudine Crystal Forms in Recrystallization Solvents. J. Pharm. Sci. **1996**, *85*, 193–199.

POTENTIOMETRY

Karel Vytras

University of Pardubice, Pardubice, Czech Republic

INTRODUCTION

Potentiometry is a method of electroanalytical measurement in which the equilibrium voltage of the cell consisting of an indicator electrode and a proper reference electrode is measured using a high-impedance voltmeter, i.e., effective at zero current. The potential of the indicator electrode is a function of particular species present in solutions and their concentration. By judicious choice of electrode material, the selectivity of the response to one of the species can be increased, and thus, interferences from other ions can be minimized. The method allows the determination of concentrations with detection limits of the order of 0.1 μmol per liter, although in some cases, as little as 10 pmol differences in concentration can be measured.

EQUILIBRIA AT INTERFACES

Electric potential is the electric work necessary to transfer the unit charge in vacuum from the infinite distance to a position, the potential of which is to be established. If this position is situated inside of a phase (metal, solution, etc.), it is called the inner electric potential and is denoted by ϕ. The chemical potential of an ion in the presence of an electric potential is called its electrochemical potential, $\tilde{\mu}$ expressed as in Eq. 1:

$$\tilde{\mu} = \mu + zF\phi \tag{1}$$

where μ is the chemical potential, z is the charge of the particle, and F is Faraday's constant (96.487 C mol^{-1}).

When two phases containing electrically charged particles come into contact, an electrical potential difference develops at their interface. A description of the interface is therefore essential when investigating the charge transfer. If the system is in equilibrium, the appropriate electrochemical potentials must be equal. Thus, for the charged particle i present in phases 1 and 2, Eq. 2 must be valid.

$$\tilde{\mu}_i(1) = \tilde{\mu}_i(2) \tag{2}$$

This equation can be rewritten as in Eq. 3 in terms of the standard chemical potentials, μ_i^0, and the activities, a_i,

$$\mu_i^0(1) + RT \ln a_i(1) + z_i F \phi(1)$$
$$= \mu_i^0(2) + RT \ln a_i(2) + z_i F \phi(2) \tag{3}$$

where R is the gas constant (8.313 J K^{-1} mol^{-1}) and T the absolute temperature (measured in K). Thus, Eq. 4 gives the potential difference at the interface,

$$\Delta\phi = \phi(2) - \phi(1)$$
$$= [\mu_i^0(1) - \mu_i^0(2)]/z_i F$$
$$+ RT/z_i F \ln[a_i(1)/a_i(2)] \tag{4}$$

which is the so-called Galvani potential difference, $\Delta\phi$.

ELECTRODE POTENTIALS

The potential difference $\Delta\phi$ given by Eq. 4 cannot be measured directly. An electrochemical cell is required, consisting of two electrode compartments (both first and second half-cells). Only in such a cell is the potential difference E measurable, as given by Eq. 5:

$$E = \Delta\phi_{st} - \Delta\phi_{nd} \tag{5}$$

If the second half-cell is taken as reference and combined with others, the same value $\Delta\phi_{2nd}$ occurs in all the differences in Eq. 5. This value can be chosen conventionally and set equal to zero (this amounts to a shift of the coordinate). The electrode for which the condition $\Delta\phi_{2nd} = 0$ is valid is the standard hydrogen electrode, in which hydrogen under the standard pressure $[p(H_2) = p^0 = 1.013 \times 10^5$ Pa] is bubbled over the surface of the platinum black through a solution of hydrogen ions of unit activity, schematically written as Pt(s)|H$_2$(g)|H$^+$(aq), where the vertical lines indicate the interphase. The reaction that determines the electrode potential is the so-called half-cell reaction, 2H$^+$(aq) + 2e = H$_2$(g). Owing to this convention, the first term of Eq. 5, $\Delta\phi_{1st}$, can be substituted by E and is called the electrode potential. In the same manner, the first

Encyclopedia of Pharmaceutical Technology

expression on the right in Eq. 4 can be replaced by Eq. 6:

$$E^0 = [\mu_i^0(1) - \mu_i^0(2)]/z_i F \tag{6}$$

and is called the standard electrode potential (values of selected standard electrode potentials are listed in Table 1).

The simplest situation occurs if a metal (phase 1) is immersed in an electrolyte solution (phase 2), for example, $Zn(s)|Zn^{2+}(aq)$. An electrode and its electrolyte make up a half-cell compartment or a so-called first-order electrode, the potential of which is given in Eq. 7:

$$E = E^0(Zn^{2+}/Zn) + RT/2F \ln a(Zn^{2+}) \tag{7}$$

known as the Nernst equation. The expression Zn^{2+}/Zn is used to shorten the half-cell reaction, which is $Zn^{2+}(aq) + 2 e = Zn(s)$; a zinc activity in pure zinc solid phase is equal to a unit. It follows from the text above that for a hydrogen electrode, the electrode potential can be written as in Eq. 8:

$$E = RT/2F \ln[a(H^+)]^2/p(H_{2,rel}) \tag{8}$$

where $p(H_{2,rel}) = p(H_2)/p^0$ is a partial pressure of hydrogen related to the standard pressure, and, in view of the convention, $E^0(H^+/H_2) = 0$. Thus, Eq. 8 can be rewritten as Eq. 9:

$$E = -0.05916 \, pH - 0.05916/2 \log p(H_{2,rel}) \tag{9}$$

because the term $RT/F \ln 10 = 0.05916$ V at 25°C. Thus, the hydrogen electrode can be considered a pH electrode (analytically, however, it has certain disadvantages compared with the glass electrode that now dominates pH measurements; see below).

Other half-cells that can be used as pH electrodes are metal–metal oxide electrodes. The most widely used is the antimony–antimony oxide electrode, which can be written as $Sb(s)|Sb_2O_3(s)|H^+$ or $Sb(s)|Sb_2O_3(s)|OH^-$ and with half-cell reactions assumed to be either $Sb_2O_3(s) + 6 H^+ + 6 e = 2 Sb(s) + 3 H_2O$ or $Sb_2O_3(s) + 3 H_2O + 6 e = 2 Sb(s) + 6 OH^-$. For example, the potential of the electrode can be expressed as Eq. 10, assuming unit activities of Sb, Sb_2O_3, and H_2O:

$$E = E^0(SbO/Sb) - 0.05916 \, pH \tag{10}$$

The electrode is favored for measurements in situations in which other electrodes are easily fouled, but because of its poor precision (0.1 pH unit when properly calibrated), it is mostly used as the pH indicator in titrations. Nevertheless, similar electrodes based on noble metals (for example, Pd|PdO) are still subjected to further development.

All electrodes depend on oxidation and reduction, but the term oxidation–reduction electrode, or redox electrode, is usually reserved for the case in which a species

exists in solution in two oxidation stages. This electrode is denoted M(s)|Ox, Red, where M is an inert metal (usually platinum) serving as an electron carrier and making electrical contact with the solution. The half-cell equilibrium can either be simple (e.g., $Fe^{3+} + e = Fe^{2+}$) or be affected by other ions (e.g., $MnO_4^- + 8 H^+ + 5 e = Mn^{2+} + 4 H_2O$). Corresponding electrode potentials are then expressed by Eq. (11):

$$E = E^0(Fe^{3+}/Fe^{2+}) + RT/F \ln a(Fe^{3+})/a(Fe^{2+}) \tag{11}$$

or Eq. 12, respectively:

$$E = E^0(MnO_4^-/Mn^{2+}) + RT/5F \ln a(MnO_4^-).[a(H^+)]^8/a(Mn^{2+}) \tag{12}$$

In the second case, the term of Eq. 13 can be isolated:

$$E^{0f} = E^0(MnO_4^-/Mn^{2+}) + 8RT/5F \ln a(H^+) \tag{13}$$

It expresses the formal redox potential and its pH dependence.

REFERENCE ELECTRODES

An insoluble salt electrode (also called a second-order electrode) consists of a metal covered by a porous layer of its insoluble salt. The whole assembly is immersed in a solution containing a corresponding anion. For example, a silver–silver chloride electrode is denoted $Ag(s)|AgCl(s)|Cl^-$; the electrode potential is a combination of the equation analogous to Eq. 7, and the solubility product of a sparingly soluble salt, $K_s(AgCl) = a(Ag^+).a(Cl^-)$, is shown in Eq. 14:

$$E = E^0(AgCl/Ag) - RT/F \ln a(Cl^-) \tag{14}$$

where a standard electrode potential for a half-cell reaction $AgCl(s) + e = Ag(s) + Cl^-$ is expressed by Eq. 15:

$$E^0(AgCl/Ag) = E^0(Ag^+/Ag) + RT/F \ln K_s(AgCl) \tag{15}$$

In potentiometric measurements, these electrodes are used as reference half-cells. For this purpose, their potential stability must be first guaranteed by the constant anion activity in the solution in contact. The usual arrangement is metal|insoluble salt|inner solution ⋮ test solution, where the vertical dashed line marks the diffusive barrier. The most frequently used reference electrodes are the silver–silver chloride electrode (preferred for its stable and reproducible potential, low tempetarure hysteresis, a wide useful temperature range, and easy preparation; when

Table 1 Selected standard electrode potentials

Half-cell reaction	E^0, V
$Ag^+ + e = Ag(s)$	+0.799
$AgBr(s) + e = Ag(s) + Br^-$	+0.073
$AgCl(s) + e = Ag(s) + Cl^-$	+0.222
$AgI(s) + e = Ag(s) + I^-$	−0.151
$Bi_2O_3(s) + 3 H_2O + 6e = 2 Bi(s) + 6 OH^-$	−0.44
$Br_2(l) + 2e = 2 Br^-$	+1.065
$BrO^{3-} + 6 H^+ + 6e = Br^- + 3 H_2O$	+1.44
$C_6H_4O_2$ [quinone] $+ 2 H^+ + 2e = C_6H_4(OH)_2$ [hydroquinone]	+0.699
$Ce^{4+} + e = Ce^{3+}$	+1.70
$Cl_2(g) + 2e = 2 Cl^-$	+1.359
$ClO^{3-} + 6 H^+ + 6e = Cl^- + 3 H_2O$	+1.45
$ClO_4^- + 2 H^+ + 2e = ClO_3^- + H_2O$	+1.19
$Cr_2O_7^{2-} + 14 H^+ + 6e = 2 Cr^{3+} + 7 H_2O$	+1.33
$Cu^{2+} + 2e = Cu(s)$	+0.337
$Cu^{2+} + e = Cu^+$	+0.153
$Cu^+ + e = Cu(s)$	+0.521
$CuI(s) + e = Cu(s) + I^-$	−0.185
$Fe^{3+} + e = Fe^{2+}$	+0.771
$Fe(CN)_6^{3-} + e = Fe(CN)_6^{4-}$	+0.36
$2 H^+ + 2e = H_2(g)$	0.000
$H_2O_2 + 2 H^+ + 2e = 2 H_2O$	+1.776
$Hg_2^{2+} + 2e = Hg(l)$	+0.788
$2 Hg^{2+} + 2e = Hg_2^{2+}$	+0.920
$Hg_2Cl_2(s) + 2e = 2 Hg(l) + 2 Cl^-$	+0.268
$Hg_2SO_4(s) + 2e = 2 Hg(l) + SO_4^{2-}$	+0.615
$HNO_2 + H^+ + e = NO(g) + H_2O$	+1.00
$I_3^- + 2e = 3 I^-$	+0.536
$IO_3^- + 6 H^+ + 6e = I^- + 3 H_2O$	+1.085
$K^+ + e = K(s)$	−2.925
$MnO_2(s) + 4 H^+ + 2e = Mn^{2+} + 2 H_2O$	+1.23
$MnO_4^- + 8 H^+ + 5e = Mn^{2+} + 4 H_2O$	+1.51
$MnO_4^- + 4 H^+ + 3e = MnO_2(s) + 2 H_2O$	+1.695
$MnO_4^- + e = MnO_4^{2-}$	+0.564
$Na^+ + e = Na(s)$	−2.714
$NO_3^- + 3 H^+ + 2e = HNO_2 + H_2O$	+0.94
$O_2(g) + 4 H^+ + 4e = 2 H_2O$	+1.229
$O_2(g) + 2 H^+ + 2e = H_2O_2$	+0.682
$O_2(g) + H_2O + 4e = 4 OH^-$	+0.401
$O_3(g) + 2 H^+ + 2e = O_2(g) + H_2O$	+2.07
$Pb^{2+} + 2e = Pb(s)$	−0.126
$PbO_2(s) + 4 H^+ + 2e = Pb^{2+} + 2 H_2O$	+1.455
$PbO_2(s) + SO_4^{2-} + 4 H^+ + 2e = PbSO_4(s) + 2 H_2O$	+1.685
$PbSO_4(s) + 2e = Pb(s) + SO_4^{2-}$	−0.350
$S(s) + 2 H^+ + 2e = H_2S(g)$	+0.141
$SO_4^{2-} + 4 H^+ + 2e = H_2SO_3 + H_2O$	+0.172
$S_2O_8^{2-} + 2e = 2 SO_4^{2-}$	+2.01
$S_4O_6^{2-} + 2e = 2 S_2O_3^{2-}$	+0.08
$Sb_2O_3(s) + 6 H^+ + 6e = 2 Sb(s) + 3 H_2O$	+0.152
$Sn^{2+} + 2e = Sn(s)$	−0.136
$Sn^{4+} + 2e = Sn^{2+}$	+0.154
$Ti^{3+} + e = Ti^{2+}$	−0.369

(Continued)

Table 1 Selected standard electrode potentials (*Continued*)

Half-cell reaction	E^0, V
$Tl^{3+} + 2e = Tl^+$	$+1.25$
$Tl^+ + e = Tl(s)$	-0.336
$TlCl(s) + e = Tl(s) + Cl^-$	-0.557
$UO_2^{2+} + 4 H^+ + 2e = U^{4+} + 2 H_2O$	$+0.334$
$Zn^{2+} + 2e = Zn(s)$	-0.763

s = solid; l = liquid; g = gas.

filled with saturated KCl solution, its potential is 0.198 V at 25°C) and the calomel (or mercury–mercurous chloride) electrodes (consisting of mercury covered with a paste of Hg and Hg_2Cl_2, which, when in contact with saturated KCl solution, the potential is 0.244 V at 25°C; a disadvantage of classic calomel electrodes is their considerable temperature hysteresis). Other reference electrodes are not often used.

The Ross reference electrode differs from the others and consists of a platinum wire immersed in a solution containing tri-iode and iodide ions. The Pt electrode responds to the redox potential established by the iodine(tri-iodide)-iodide couple. This solution is separated from the sample by a bridge electrolyte, which is 3 M KCl.

LIQUID JUNCTION

In a cell with two different electrolyte solutions in contact, as in the application of a reference electrode, there is an additional source of potential difference across the interface of the two miscible electrolytes, inner reference electrode solution : test solution. As noted above, the vertical dashed line is used in a cell scheme to denote such an interface and indicates the source of so-called liquid-junction potential, $\Delta\phi_L$. For example, if two HCl solutions of different concentrations are in such contact, the mobile H^+ ions diffuse into the more dilute solution. The bulkier Cl^- ions follow, but initially more slowly, which results in a potential difference at the junction. However, after the brief initial period, the potential reaches a value that the ions diffuse at the same rate.

Generally, the liquid-junction potential increases with increasing difference of the cation and anion mobilities at the interface. In an ideal situation, both ions are of the same mobility. Such salts are called equitransferent salts, or equitransferent mixtures. For that reason, KCl is commonly used as the inner electrolyte of reference electrodes; a mixture of 1.8 M KCl + 1.8 M KNO$_3$ serves

best. The liquid-junction potential, although not known, remains constant within limits, appears as a constant offset voltage, and is contained in the apparent (or formal) standard potential, E^{0f}. If both H^+ and OH^- do not participate at the border solutions, it usually does not exceed $\pm$ 10 mV. In direct potentiometric measurements, the liquid-junction potential can partially be reduced by the use of the reference electrode with a limited diffusion (the boundary between the two miscible electrolytes being a porous diaphragm) or by incorporating a salt bridge filled with a proper electrolyte solution that is equivalent to the use of a reference electrode with two bridge electrolytes (the so-called double-junction reference electrode) containing two porous diaphragms with limited diffusion, e.g., Ag(s)|AgCl(s)|KCl : a bridge electrolyte : a test solution. In the notation for cells, a double vertical line denotes an interface for which it is assumed that the junction potential has practically been eliminated, e.g., Ag(s)|AgCl(s)|KCl :: a test solution, which is equivalent to the previous scheme.

Some electroanalytical texts that contain sections with emphasis discussed in previous articles are given in Refs. 1 and 2.

MEMBRANE ELECTRODES

The difficulty that can arise with the cells comprising the first- and second-order electrodes noted above is whether oxidized and reduced species of more than one redox couple are present in solution so that they can contribute to the overall equilibrium potential that is thus a mixed potential. Such a measurement can have low selectivity in some real situations. This can be overcome by measuring the difference of potential across a membrane composed from a material that can selectively participate at ionic exchange equilibria.

A membrane separating medium 1 and medium 2 results in a three-phase system, medium 1|membrane|medium 2 because the membrane behaves as isolated phase (M).

Interfaces at which an ionic exchange occurs are geometric barriers between two phases. Membranes for potentiometric electrodes are as immiscible as conveniently possible with respect to the bathing solutions and solid contacts. They are usually constructed of hydrophobic organic liquids and solids or inorganic solids of low water solubility. Nevertheless, useful membranes are not electrical insulators. Porous membranes (organic liquids and solids, synthetic ion exchangers) absorb and become saturated by an external solvent, usually water. They also permit water from two bathing solutions with nonidentical ionic strengths to pass slowly from one side of the membrane to the other. However, many membranes are nonporous, and solvent transport is not an important process when considering membrane potential responses. Useful membranes are often solid or liquid electrolytes because they are composed of partially or completely ionized acids, bases, or salts or contain potentially ionizable species. A characteristic of these membranes is the presence of charged sites. A result of the ionic exchange occurring at both membrane interfaces is the membrane potential $\Delta\phi_M$, expressed as a difference of the inner electric potential of the two phases, which are separated by the membrane, as shown in Eq. 16:

$$\Delta\phi_M = \phi(2) - \phi(1) \tag{16}$$

Generally, the membrane potential is completed by three factors: the two potential differences at both inner and outer interfaces and a liquid-junction potential that can be formed across the membrane (especially in liquid membranes). Nevertheless, a galvanic half-cell, represented by a membrane electrode immersed in the sample test solution, usually consists of an ion-selective membrane, an internal electrolyte, and an internal reference electrode, e.g., Ag|AgCl|internal electrolyte Cl^-, Q^+|membrane selective to Q^+|test solution. This represents a conventional construction of the sensing half-cell; the other half-cell is represented by an external reference electrode. There are many factors to the experimentally observed voltage of a cell containing a membrane electrode that can be considered constant: the inner and outer reference electrode potentials, the potential difference at the inner membrane interface, and, at least in one instant, both liquid-junction potentials formed across the membrane and at the external reference electrode : test solution interface.

Thus, ion-selective membrane electrodes can be defined as electrochemical sensors that allow potentiometric measurements of the activity of particular species in aqueous and mixed solvents or partial pressures of dissolved gases in water. However, these sensors may respond to certain other ions in the sample in addition to the selected i ion; interferences by such j ions are usually expressed by the Nikolskii-Eisenman (Eq. 17):

$$E = \text{constant} + f(2.303\,RT/z_iF)\log\{a_i$$
$$+ \Sigma k_{ij}^{pot}\,a_j^{z_i/z_j}\} \tag{17}$$

where E is the voltage of the potentiometric cell in which an ion-selective membrane electrode participates, and the constant term includes all the constant potential contributions noted above; f is a correction for non-Nernstian response, terms z_i and z_j denote the charge of the ions i and j, and k_{ij}^{pot} is the potentiometric selectivity coefficient.

It should be noted that over the past 30 years, analytical methods utilizing ion-selective technology have been developed at an ever-increasing rate, and much additional information can be found in texts addressing the subject. Some are noted in the references (3–10).

Based on the membrane material, the ion-selective electrodes may be divided into the following groups.

Electrodes with Solid Membranes

These include membranes composed of solid salts that may be single crystals but are more often polycrystalline pellets pressed from powdered starting materials. These solid exchangers respond to species that exchange directly and rapidly and influence the activity of ions that exchange directly. For example, silver salt electrodes are believed to be rapid ion exchangers of both Ag^+ and component anions. In mixtures, Ag_2S holds the more soluble halides in a matrix and produces both electronic and ionic conductivities throughout the membrane. The electrode is also sensitive to other ions that can form sparingly soluble precipitates on the membrane surface, particularly if they have lower solubility products than those of the material of the membrane. As an example, the AgCl-based electrode responds to bromide and iodide; mercury(II) is always a serious interferent because HgS is less soluble than Ag_2S. For the same reason, membranes containing HgS instead of Ag_2S have the advantage of lower detection limits. Some examples of the membrane materials are LaF_3 for fluoride ions, $AgX + Ag_2S$ or $Hg_2X_2 + HgS$ for halide or pseudohalide (CN^-, SCN^-) ions, Ag_2S for both silver and sulfide ions, metal sulfide $+ Ag_2S$ for some metal ions (Cd^{2+}, Cu^{2+}, Pb^{2+}), and Cu_2Se $+ CuSe$ for copper(II) ions.

Glass Electrodes

These are the oldest and best investigated ion-selective electrodes, made of various multicomponent glasses (11).

The surface of a glass membrane must be hydrated to respond to pH. Hydration is accompanied by a reaction in which singly charged cations of the glass are exchanged for hydrogen ions of the solution $H^+(aq) + Na^+(glass) = Na^+(aq) + H^+(glass)$. The silicate structure $\equiv Si-O^-$ of a glass provides cation-bonding sites. A well soaked membrane is covered by a layer of silicic acid gel approximately 10^{-5} to 10^{-4} mm thick.

Glass electrodes respond to the activity of both the hydrogen ion and alkali metal ions in basic solution in which the former is small relative to the latter. At high pH, a negative pH error occurs that suggests that the electrode is responding to alkali metal ions as well as to hydrogen ions. The magnitude of the error varies according to the kind of singly charged cation and the glass composition. Because of this error in early glass electrodes, glasses were developed for which the alkaline error is negligible below a pH level of approximately 12. Other glasses have been developed that allow the determination of cations other than hydrogen ions such as Li^+, Na^+, K^+, and NH_4^+. Glass electrodes for H^+, Na^+, and K^+ are available commercially.

Electrodes with Liquid Membranes

These include membranes made of liquid electroactive substances or with electroactive substances dissolved in a suitable nonvolatile, water-immiscible solvent (mediator). In early designs, the organic phase was placed between two aqueous phases in bulk or with the support of a thin, porous cellulose sheet, sintered glass, or the like. As work with these sensors proceeded, more durable polymer supports were developed, most often poly(vinyl chloride)(PVC). An electroactive compound is dissolved in a solvent (usually tetrahydrofuran or cyclohexanone) together with the PVC and a suitable plasticizer. The solvent evaporates, leaving a plasticized PVC ion-selective membrane. Because the plasticized polymer behaves like a viscous liquid, the properties of the electrode are very similar to those of the original wet membrane. The electroactive materials used in these membranes fall into three main classes: ion exchangers, neutral carriers, and charged carriers.

In liquid ion-exchange electrodes, the electroactive material is usually the salt (ion pair) with a highly lipophilic cation or anion to guarantee oil solubility. For example, nitrate-, fluoroborate-, and perchlorate-selective electrodes are commercially available, based on corresponding ion pairs of an anion with tris(substituted 1,10-Phenanthroline)-metal(II) cations or a quaternary

ammonium salt containing at least one long-chain alkyl group. Selectivity over interferences is limited to ions less oil-soluble than the primary ion. In the case of the above-noted electrodes, the Hofmeister series is usually obeyed:

$$B(C_6H_5)^- > ClO_4^- > SCN^- > I^- > Br^-, NO_3^-$$
$$> Cl^- > HCO_3^- > F^-$$

and can serve as a rule for deciding possible interferences. Similarly, an organic anion such as tetraphenylborate is a suitable membrane counterion for cations (e.g., K^+, Rb^+, Cs^+, Tl^+, and univalent organic cations). A similar effect is seen because the electrodes are most selective for organic cations such as long-chain quaternary ammonium ions. These cation electrodes have frequently been used as sensors for clinically important molecules that are cationic at low pH levels (drugs).

Another category of liquid-membrane electrodes is based on neutral carriers. These are lipophilic, multifunctional compounds with active groups that are primarily alternating ether and/or keto oxygens that can form a cage for the positively charged ion. Cyclic polyethers and similar macrocyclic compounds, such as valinomycin and nonactin, are believed to discriminate among cations on the basis of size; cations that fit well in the complexing site are most strongly complexed. Potassium-selective electrodes based on valinomycin are the best examples of marketed sensors of this type. Various crown ethers, polyoxyethylene chain-containing compounds, or special selective carriers have been prepared and used in sodium-, barium-, and calcium-selective commercial electrodes.

A third class of ion-selective carriers consists of so-called charged carriers or associated ion exchangers. Unlike the simple ion exchangers, however, the selectivity of charged carriers is dictated by the degree of association of the analyte ion with the carrier as well as the partitioning of the analyte into the membrane solvent. The most notable examples of such agents are the alkyl phosphates originally used in Ca^{2+}-selective electrodes; calcium selectivity is further enhanced by using alkyl phosphonates as membrane mediators.

Gas-Sensing Electrodes

Gas-sensing electrodes are examples of multiple membrane sensors; these contain a gas-permeable membrane separating the test solution from an internal thin electrolyte film in which an ion-selective electrode is immersed. For example, for the ammonia sensor, the pH of the recipient layer is determined by the Henderson-Hasselbach equation (Eq. 18), derived from the chemical equilibrium between solvated ammonia and ammonium ions:

$$pH = pK_a(NH^+) + \log[NH_3]/[NH_4^+] \tag{18}$$

If the solution layer contains a large background concentration of ammonium salt (NH_4^+ picrate is often used), the pH of the immersed glass electrode is proportional to only one variable, $[NH_3]$, which is in turn dependent on the amount of NH_3 that diffuses across the gas-permeable membrane, as shown by Eq. 19:

$$E = \text{constant} + 0.05916 \log p(NH_3) \tag{19}$$

where $p(NH_3)$ is the partial pressure of NH_3 in the sample measured. Similarly, when the glass pH electrode is replaced by a polymeric membrane responsive to NH_4^+ (a nonactin-based NH_4^+-selective electrode), the signal is not dependent on the pH but on the equilibrium concentration of ammonium acquired from the sample. The ammonia gas-sensing electrode is primarily used for the determination of ammonium salts after the addition of NaOH, which releases ammonia from a sample under test. The total nitrogen can be determined after Kjeldahl decomposition of a sample.

The first gas-sensing electrode based on a similar principle was the carbon dioxide electrode, developed to determine CO_2 in blood. Later, sensors for other gases (e.g., SO_2, NO_x, and HCN, etc.) appeared on the market.

Electrodes with Biocatalytic Membranes

The gas-sensing configuration described above forms a very useful basic unit for potentiometric measurements of biologically important species (12–17). In principle, the immobilized or insolubilized biocatalyst is placed on a conventional ion-selective electrode used to measure the decrease in the reactants or the increase in products of the biochemical reaction. The biocatalyst include isolated enzymes, subcellular fractions, intact bacterial cells, and whole sections of mammalian or plant tissues. Because ions are usually formed during these reactions, it is possible to determine the substrate by monitoring the ion activity. For example, amygdalin can be degraded by β-Glucosidase to benzaldehyde, glucose, and HCN; the CN^--selective electrode is used as a inner sensor. Similarly, the NH_4^+-selective electrode can respond to NH_4^+ ions produced in the reaction of urea with urease.

In recent years, gas-sensing probes have been used most frequently because of their high selectivity over common cations and anions. Thus, the biocatalytic urea sensor noted above can be constructed by immobilizing urease onto the gas-permeable surface of an ammonia gas sensor; when the probe is inserted into a buffered sample containing urea, the enzyme catalyzes its conversion to NH_3, which is measured by the gas-sensing electrode described previously. By coupling the efficient and selective catalyzing powers of an enzyme to the selective detection of a gas-sensing electrode, it is possible to construct a sensitive tool for the measurement of many pharmaceutically important compounds. However, in general for biosensors, it should be noted that amperometric principles predominate in a majority of their recent constructions.

SELECTIVITY COEFFICIENTS

In measurements with ion-selective electrodes, interference by other ions is expressed by selectivity coefficients k_{ij}^{pot}, as in Eq. 17. If the nature of the ion-selective membrane is known, these interferences may easily be estimated. For example, in the determination of chloride with a Cl^--selective electrode containing AgCl as the electroactive component in its membrane, concentrations of bromides or iodides (generally X^-) must be controlled because they form less soluble silver salts than AgCl; the solubility products of corresponding silver halides are used in Eq. 20 to estimate the selectivity coefficient:

$$k_{Cl,X}^{pot} \cong K_s(AgCl)/K_s(AgX) \tag{20}$$

However, this estimation is approximate only. For exact determinations, two methods are primarily used.

In the separate-solution method, the cell voltage E_i is measured first in a solution of free determinant i, followed by E_j measured in a solution of interferant j. By applying Eq. 17 for these two solutions, Eq. 21 is obtained:

$$\log k_{i,j}^{pot} = (E_j - E_i)z_iF/2.303RT + \log a_i \\ - z_i/z_j \log a_j \tag{21}$$

This equation can be simplified further, assuming the main interferants are the ions of the same charge and considering solutions of the same activities.

In the simplest mixed-solution method, the cell voltage is measured in a series of solutions containing a range of activities of the primary ion and fixed activity of the interferant (Fig. 1). When a graph of E versus $\log a_i$ is constructed, the usual Nernstian slope changes

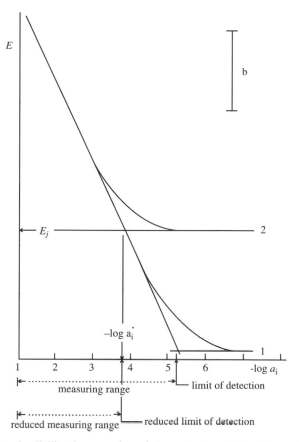

Fig. 1 Calibration graphs of ion-selective electrodes and evaluation of selectivity coefficients. 1) Calibration response against $-\log a_i$ in solution of free determinand i. The practical limit of detection may be taken as the activity (or the concentration) at the point of intersection of the extrapolated lines as shown. 2) Calibration against $-\log a_i$ in the presence of the interferant j, the activity of which is of a known and constant value. Response E_j is obtained for $-\log a_i^* = -\log k_{ij}^{pot} a_j^{zi/zj}$. The resulting interference can restrict the measuring range. b) The abscissa approximately equal to $60/z_i$ mV.

to an invariant E_j voltage at low a_i values, corresponding to the response to a constant a_j activity. The intersection of asymptots to this dependence gives a $\log a_i^*$ value, which is used to calculate k_{ij}^{pot} according to Eq. 22:

$$k_{ij}^{pot} = a_i^* / a_j^{zi/zj} \qquad (22)$$

The weakness of all the approaches is the assumption that the slope $2.303RT/z_iF$ is Nernstian or at least unaffected by the presence of interferants. In addition, for many electrodes, especially liquid-membrane systems, selectivity coefficients are not highly reproducible or precise quantities because they are time-dependent. This is why selectivity coefficients established by various methods can differ; nevertheless, they never differ by order of magnitude, and therefore they serve well to estimate measurement errors in the presence of interfering species.

EQUIPMENT

The selection of equipment for potentiometric measurements is guided primarily by the precision required and the application intended. An instrument must draw essentially no electricity from the cell being used. Historically, measurements (highly precise but tedious) were performed by compensation of the measured voltage with the aid of a reference cell, so that virtually no current passed through the measuring cell. This kind of potentiometer has by now been almost completely displaced by electronic voltmeters with very high internal resistances. This is particularly significant in measurements with membrane electrodes, which may have resistances of 1 to 100 MΩ or even more. These high-resistance instruments are usually called pH meters or ion-meters. A new generation of instruments is represented by microprocessor-controlled meters, making automatic evaluation of the measurements possible. They are produced by many companies (e.g., Orion Research, Radiometer, and Metrohm). Equipment for automated potentiometric titrations has also been developed; the apparatus is generally of the module type, and its individual components (ion-meter, autoburette, recorder, and computer unit) may be used separately.

EXPERIMENTAL TECHNIQUES

Direct Potentiometry

Direct potentiometric measurements are used to complete chemical analyses of species for which an indicator electrode is available. The technique is simple, requiring only a comparison of the voltage developed by the measuring cell in the test solution with its voltage when immersed in a standard solution of the analyte. If the electrode response is specific for the analyte and independent of the matrix, no preliminary steps are required. In addition, although discontinuous measurements are mainly carried out, direct potentiometry is readily adapted to continuous and automatic monitoring.

Table 2 Standard buffer solutions

Composition	pH Values at °C					
	0	20	25	30	38	60
0.1 m hydrochloric acid	1.187	1.194	1.197	1.200	1.202	1.213
0.05 m potassium tetraoxalate	1.666	1.675	1.679	1.683	1.691	1.723
Saturated (25°C) potassium hydrogen tartrate			3.557	3.552	3.548	3.560
0.05 m potassium dihydrogen citrate	3.863	3.788	3.776	3.766		
0.05 m potassium hydrogen phthalate	4.003	4.002	4.008	4.015	4.030	4.091
1+1 phosphate buffer (0.025 m KH_2PO_4 + 0.025 m Na_2HPO_4)	6.984	6.881	6.865	6.853	6.840	6.836
1+3.5 phosphate buffer (0.008695 m KH_2PO_4 + 0.03043 m Na_2HPO_4)	7.534	7.429	7.413	7.400	7.384	
0.01 m borax	9.464	9.225	9.180	9.139	9.081	8.962
1+1 carbonate buffer (0.025 m $NaHCO_3$ + 0.025 m Na_2CO_3)	10.317	10.062	10.012	9.966		
Saturated (25°C) calcium hydroxide	13.423	12.627	12.454	12.289	12.043	11.499

Measurement of pH

The electrochemical pH cell consists essentially of a measuring (or indicator) pH electrode, together with a reference electrode, both being in contact with the solution under investigation. Frequently, a pH glass and calomel electrodes are combined; then the pH meter measures the cell voltage E, given by Eq. 23, for example:

$$E = E_{ref} - E_{ind} + \Delta\phi \qquad (23)$$

where E_{ref} is the reference electrode potential, E_{ind} the indicator electrode potential, and $\Delta\phi_L$ is the liquid-junction potential arising at the boundary between the dissimilar liquids. For a cell with a pH-measuring electrode, Eq. 23 can be rewritten as Eq. 24:

$$E = \text{constant} - 2.303\,RT/F \log a(H^+) + \Delta\phi_L \qquad (24)$$

where the constant term (including E_{ref} and the constant substituting E^0 of the pH electrode) and $\Delta\phi_L$ are not available. These unknowns are eliminated by substracting the voltage $E(X)$ of the cell immersed into a test solution of pH(X) and that of $E(S)$ measured with the same cell immersed into a standard pH(S) solution (Table 2), as in Eq. 25:

$$E(X) - E(S) = -2.303\,RT/F[\log a(H^+)_x$$
$$- \log a(H^+)_s] \qquad (25)$$

and, subsequently, as in Eq. 26:

$$pH(X) = [E(X) - E(S)]F/2.303\,RT + pH(S) \qquad (26)$$

assuming that the difference $\Delta\phi_L(X) - \Delta\phi_L(S)$ is eliminated. It follows that the accuracy of the pH(X) value is partially dependent on how close in character

the tested solution is to the standardizing solution and how strictly Nerstian the cell response is; clearly, it is desirable to standardize as closely in pH as possible. For more accuracy measurements, it is suggested that two standard buffers be used, pH(S_1) and pH(S_2), which straddle the pH(X) value. The pH(X) is then given by Eq. 27:

$$[pH(X) - pH(S)]/[pH(S) - pH(S)]$$
$$= [E(X) - E(S)]/[E(S) - E(S)] \qquad (27)$$

Eq. 27 represents the so-called practical definition of the pH scale (18). Evidently, in practice the voltage differences expressed in Eqs. 26 and 27 are not measured inasmuch as the meters provide direct pH readings. Hence, instead of the $E(S)$ values, the pH(S) values are adjusted directly on the intrument scale. In the preparation of standard buffer solutions (see Table 2), it is essential to use high-purity materials and carbon dioxide-free freshly distilled water, the specific conductance of which should not exceed 2 $\mu S/cm$.

Frequently, it is necessary to measure pH at nonambient temperatures. Biological samples are often stored just above 0°C, clinical samples are measured at 38°C, buffers and gels used in media are measured at approximately 60°C, and many industrial processes take place at higher temperatures. The Nernst equation contains a temperature term that can be corrected by automatic temperature compensation; detailed instructions are attached to each pH meter. The glass Ross pH electrode, containing a Pt wire as a reference immersed in a solution based on iodine (tri-iodide) and potassium iodide, gives the best performace in terms of a fixed, reproducible contact potential that is thermodynamically reversible (the Pt wire potential does change with temperature, but the redox solution consists of a buffer with an equal and opposite temperature coefficient, which results in a reference system showing almost no potential change with temperature).

Measurement of pX

This includes direct activity (concentration) measurements using other than H^+-selective electrodes (19). Different methods are available, although none is as well organized as the pH measurement. The simplest procedure is to measure the voltage of the cell containing an ion-selective electrode in solutions of graduated concentrations, usually between 10^{-6} and 10^{-1} mol/L (or similarly on the pH scale, between pX 6 and 1). A typical calibration graph is linear between pX 1 and 5, defined for $pX = -\log a_i$ (Fig. 1). In practice, however, the determination of concentration is more frequently requested. In this case, the cell voltage values are plotted against the logarithms of the concentration of the ion determined, i.e., $pX = -\log c_i$. Such a calibration graph, however, differs from that obtained by measuring the activity at higher concentrations when the activity coefficients y_i are less than 1 (just to remember the relation between activity and concentration, which is $a_i = c_i\, y_i$). A series of standard solutions with a composition as close as possible to that of the sample is used, and the conditions are maintained identical to those used for the measurement on the sample (pH and ionic strength adjustments, screening of interferants, etc.). The best results are obtained with simulated standards, in which the effects of the other components of the sample solution are included in the calibration curve. As reported recently (20), dramatic improvement of the lower detection limit to phenomenal picomolar concentrations may be obtained by modifying the composition of the inner electrolyte of the ion-selective electrode.

The most frequently used mode (because it is the simplest mode) is calibration with two standard solutions. It is appropriate for any analysis by direct potentiometry in the Nernstian range of an ion-selective electrode, particularly for analyses carried out at varying temperatures. The calibration is performed with two standards in each sample batch. The first gives the value of the cell constant (or E^0 of the sensing electrode) and the second the calibration slope. The two standards should span the concentration range expected in the samples because any error is magnified by extrapolation. In the non-Nernstian region, the concentrations are obtained from a calibration graph rather than by calculation, and because the graph is curved, more (at least four) standard solutions are needed to define it.

Addition (as well as subtraction) methods may also be used. Both require a knowledge of the calibration slope but not of the cell constant. The simplest method includes two voltage readings, E_1 before and E_2 after the addition of a volume V_s of a standard solution to V_x volume of the sample, as shown in Eqs. 28 and 29:

$$E_1 = \text{constant} + \text{slope} \log c_x \tag{28}$$

$$E_2 = \text{constant} + \text{slope} \log\left(c_x V_x + c_s V_s\right)/(V_x + V_s) \tag{29}$$

where c_x denotes the concentration of the sample and c_s is the concentration of the standard solution. From the cell voltage change ($\Delta E = E_2 - E_1$), the unknown c_x concentration can be calculated as shown in Eq. 30:

$$c_x = c_s V_s/[(V_x + V_s)10^{\Delta E/\text{slope}} - V_x] \tag{30}$$

In the well-known addition method, the slope factor is determined simultaneously with the concentration by iterative calculation. If a multiaddition method is used, the unknown c_x concentration can be evaluated graphically (Fig. 2). For $(V_x + V_s)10^{E/\text{slope}} = 0$, the negative value of the volume equivalent to the unknown concentration is read from an intercept of the dependence with x-axis, $-V_e$, and the concentration calculated as shown in Eq. 31:

$$c_x = -c_s V_e/V_x \tag{31}$$

Flow measurements

A useful and rapid method of automated analysis is the technique of flow-injection analysis (FIA). The sample or a reagent is injected into the stream of a solution of constant composition. Calibration of FIA systems requires the injection of standard solutions, equal in volume to that of the sample, into the carrier stream. The background chemical composition of the standards should be equal, as nearly as possible, to that of the samples. Frequent standardization is not necessary because the measurement of peak height, albeit on a sloping base line, is relatively unaffected by cell voltage drift. Some difficulties can appear with peristaltic pumps, owing to extraneous potentials caused by pulsation of the stream. Cells with a small volume (<20 μl) or the cells of the wall-jet type are the most acceptable for continuous measurements (21, 22).

Potentiometric Titrations

In contrast to direct potentiometry, the potentiometric titration technique offers the advantage of high accuracy

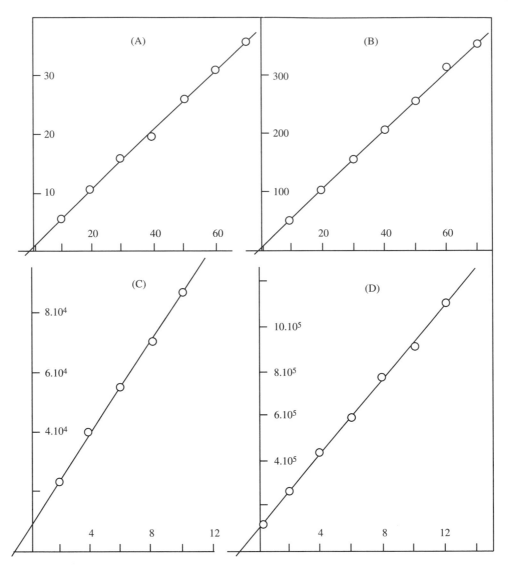

Fig. 2 Multiaddition method with graphic evaluation of the known ion concentration in a sample. Experimental data for the determination of tetrafluoroborate using a BF_4^--selective electrode. (A) $c_x = 10^{-4}$ mol/L, $c_s = 10^{-2}$ mol/L; (B) $c_x = 10^{-5}$ mol/L, $c_s = 10^{-3}$ mol/L; (C) $c_x = 10^{-3}$ mol/L, $c_s = 10^{-1}$ mol/L; (D) $c_x = 10^{-4}$ mol/L, $c_s = 10^{-2}$ mol/L; $V_x = 100$ mL in all cases. Values of $(V_x + V_s)10^{EF/2.303RT}$ are plotted on the y-axis against volume of the standard solution added, V_s, on x-axis. (Adapted from Sb. Ved. Pr., Vys. Sk. Chemickotechnol. Pardubice **1986**, *49*, 149.)

and precision, although at the cost of increased time and increased consumption of titrants. Another advantage is that the potential break at the titration endpoint must be well defined, but the slope of the sensing electrode response need be neither reproducible nor Nernstian, and the actual potential values at the endpoint are of secondary interest. In many cases, this allows for the use of simplified sensors.

For titrations to a fixed potential, the calibration slope is not needed, but the correct potential must be chosen by some means of calibration. In pH titrations, for example, this can be by means of a buffer solution. The errors involved are usually much smaller than those in direct potentiometry.

PHARMACEUTICAL APPLICATIONS

For analytical control of pharmaceuticals, most pharmacopoeias describe accurate methods, which, however, in some cases are lengthy and difficult. The ion-selective electrode techniques offer several advantages in terms of simplicity and rapidity over official methods (23–29). Generally, electrodes of all the types noted above can be used to analyze compounds of pharmaceutical significance. For example, halide ion-selective electrodes are often used in the determination of cationic compounds containing quaternary nitrogen and a counter-halide ion. Traditional titration techniques, such as potentiometric pH or redox titrations, are used to determine acids and bases or compounds containing groups that may be oxidized or reduced.

Most ion-selective electrodes, however, cannot be used for the direct determination of functional groups in organic compounds unless they are converted into ionic species. Thus, direct potentiometry is performed rarely with commercial ion-selective electrodes. For example, the CN^--selective electrode gives an almost Nernstian response in the determination of substituted phenylaceto-nitriles and benzonitriles. Thiols can be determined by direct measurement of the voltage of a cell with an Ag_2S-based electrode. Such examples are, however, not typical for applications of ion-selective electrodes.

Typical Drug Substance-Selective Electrode

The typical drug substance-selective electrodes are usually of the liquid-membrane type. It should be noted that virtually any ionic species can be detected and measured by liquid ion-exchange electrodes. The principle for design is as follows: To build a membrane responsive to anion X^-, for example, the salt Q^+X^- is dissolved in a nonvolatile solvent; the Q^+ cation must be highly lipophilic. Similarly, for an electrode responsive to cation Q^+, an oil-soluble salt Q^+X^- is used, where the X^- anion is lipophilic. Thus, the quaternary long-chain alkyl and aryl ammonium salts and high-molecular-weight cationic dyes etc. are known to behave as liquid anion exchangers suitable for the preparation of anion-selective liquid-membrane electrodes. Tetraphe-nylborate [or tetrakis(substituted phenyl)borates] and high-molecular anionic surfactants such as dodecylsul-fate show good selectivity for heavier univalent inorganic cations and are also often used in membrane electrodes for other "onium" ions. These rules are observed in the construction of drug substance electrodes; a few examples are given in Table 3.

Titrations Based on Ion-Pair Formation

In these titrations (28–31), a cationic (Q^+) or anionic (X^-) species is titrated with an oppositely charged titrant (X^- or Q^+), respectivelly. If the substance determined or the titrant (or both) has adequate lipophilic character, the poorly soluble ionpair precipi-tates, $Q^+ + X^- = QX$. Further, the same ion pairs can be used as active substances for liquid membrane-type electrodes because of their good extractability into organic water-immiscible solvents. For that reason, simplified sensors can be used to monitor such titrations. One strategy used with some success is that of coated-wire electrodes. Here, the membrane material is applied directly onto a metal wire (this assembly has no internal reference electrode, which is replaced by a direct contact). In addition, the membranes can be prepared from polymer solutions containing no active material. The organic phase (plasticizer) of a sensor, when immersed in a stirred aqueous suspension of the QX ion pair, becomes gradually saturated, and the concentration is given by Eq. 32:

$$[QX]_{org} = K_{ex}(QX)[Q^+]_{aq}[X^-]_{aq}$$
$$= K_{ex}(QX)K_s(QX) \quad (32)$$

where $K_{ex}(QX)$ and $K_s(QX)$ are the stoicheiometric extraction constant and the solubility product of QX, respectively. The $[QX]_{org}$ concentration indicates the number of ion-exchanging places in the membrane, although surface adsorption can also participate. This is why all liquid and/or plastic membrane electrodes sensitive to ions other than those to be determined can also be used to monitor titrations based on ion pair formation. Simple and inexpensive sensors of the coated-wire type, prepared by dipping the central conductor (Pt, carbon rod, but also aluminium wire can be used) into a solution containing dissolved polymer and plasticizer and allowing the solvent to evaporate, are sufficiently suitable.

Regarding titrants, cationic substances (for example, protonized alkaloids, compounds containing quaternary nitrogen, etc.) are usually titrated with sodium tetra-phenylborate, the exact concentration of which is determined titrimetrically against a standard substance such as thallium(I) nitrate or pure copper(II) or nickel(II) salts in the presence of 1,10-Phenanthroline. For titrations of anionics, substituted quaternary ammonium or pyr-idinium salts are applied (30). The procedures are simple and represent an ecologic alternative to so-called two-phase titrations (32).

Titrations Based on Complex Formation

Organic molecules containing atoms such as nitrogen, oxygen, and sulfur can donate pairs of electrons.

Table 3 Examples of drug substance-selective electrodes

Substance	Type	Electroactive compound in membrane	Mediator
Acetylcholine	PVC	Acridine orange reineckate	DOP
Amitriptyline	Liq	Eosin, tetraphenyl- or tetrakis(3-Chlorophenyl)-borates as counterions	NC, NT
Amphetamine	Liq	Amphetamine octadecylsulfate	NB
Atropine	Liq or PVC	Ion-pairs of atropine with tetraphenyl- or tetra-kis(3-chlorophenyl)borates, reineckate, dipicrylaminate, or tetraiodomercurate(II)	BA, NB, NT, OA or BEHP, DNP, DOP
Bamethan	PVC	Bamethan tetraphenylborate	Various
Brucine	PVC	Potassium tetraphenylborate	DBP
Bupivacaine	PVC	Bupivacaine dinonylnaphthalenesulfonate	
Butylscopolamine	PVC	N-Butylscopolamine tetraphenylborate	DBP
Cholic acid	Liq or PVC	Benzyldimethylammonium cholate or tributylcetylphosphonium benzoate	NB
Codeine	Liq	Codeine dipicrylaminate	NB
	PVC	Potassium tetraphenylborate	DBP
Ephedrine	Liq	Ephedrine 5-Nitrobarbiturate or flavianate	NB or OA
	PVC	Ephedrine tetraphenylborate	DOP
Glutamates	Liq	Methyltricaprylylammonium glutamate	DA
Lidocaine	Liq	Lidocaine dipicrylaminate or reineckate	NB
	PVC	Tetrakis(3-Chlorophenyl)borate or dinonyl-naphthalenesulfonate as counter ions	DNP or
Nicotine	Liq or PVC	Nicotine tetraphenyl- or tetrakis(3-Chloro-)phenyl)borates	NT, NB
Novocaine	Liq	Novocaine tetraphenylborate or dipicrylaminate	NB
Oxalate	Liq	Tricaprylylmethylammonium oxalate	DA
Papaverine	Liq	Ion-pairs with alkylsulfates, arenesulfonates, or tetraphenylborate	NB
Phencyclidine	PVC	Phencyclidine dinonylnaphthalenesulfonate	DOP
Pilocarpine	PVC	Pilocarpine reineckate or tetraphenylborate	DBP
Quinine	PVC	Quinine tetraphenylborate	DBP, DBS, NB, NPOE
Salicylate	Liq	Tricaprylylmethylammonium or tetrahexyl-ammonium salicylate	DA
	PVC	Ethyl violet as a counterion	
	Epoxy	Trioctylmethylammonium salicylate	
Strychnine	Liq	Strychnine picrolonate or tetrakis(3-Methyl-phenylborate	
Sulfamerazine	Liq	Tris(bathophenanthroline) iron(II) as a counterion	NB
Vitamins B$_1$, B$_6$	Liq	As for papaverine	

Liq = liquid membrane with ion-exchange solution into the porous diaphgragm; PVC = plasticized poly(vinyl chloride); Epoxy = conductive epoxy resin membrane. BA = benzyl alcohol; BEHP = bis(2-Ethylhexyl) phthalate; DA = 1-Decanol; DBP = dibutyl phthalate; DBS = dibutyl sebacate; DNP = dinonyl phthalate; DOP = dioctyl phthalate; NB = nitrobenzene; NPOE = 2-Nitrophenyl octyl ether; NT = 2-Nitrotoluene or 4-Nitrotoluene; OA = 1-octanol.

As electron donors, they can form complexes with metal ions (M), which are electron acceptors and are bound as unidentate or multidentate ligands (L). Depending on other groups of the organic molecule, these complexes can be charged or neutral and soluble or insoluble in water. Thus, the chemical reaction can be considered to be $nL + mM = M_mL_n$(charges are omitted). Experience has shown that the reaction noted above is affected by the pH value and by competitive side reactions caused by various substances usually present in the solution (such as other ligands from buffer constituents or counterions). Thus, if the conditional stability constant of the complex $\beta(M_mL_n)$ is sufficiently high, the ligand compound can be determined by titration with solutions of metal salts. Appropriate metal ion-selective electrodes are used to monitor these titrations. Regarding pharmaceuticals, many of them can be titrated with solutions of copper, lead, mercury, silver, and other metal salts (28, 29).

Titrations in Nonaqueous Media

Potentiometric measurements in nonaqueous media (33, 34) are performed in a similar manner and with similar apparatus as in aqueous media. There is a difference in the composition of the salt bridge established between the electrode and the solution being tested. In titrations in inert solvents, moreover, there are differences in the shielding and grounding of the titration vessel. Cell voltage is measured using a potentiometer of high internal resistance. Nonaqueous media are used because the substance has low water solubility or it acts as a weak acid or a weak base in aqueous solution. In solvents similar to water, the interactions between solute and solvent resemble the processes that take place in water, but differences owing to the smaller dielectric constants, the formation of different ion pairs by further associations, and the charge in the electrostatic field as a function of concentration can be observed. Potentiometric titrations in nonaqueous media can be applied over a wide area; the endpoint varies with the strength of the acid or base to be determined, the solvent, and the titrant. For the determination of water-insoluble weak bases, proton-donating acidic solvents (such as acetic or propionic acids) are used. A titrant is perchloric acid that, dissolved in the medium, gives acetacidium ions $CH_3COOH_2^+$. Proton-acceptor basic solvents, such as ethylenediamine, pyridine, butylamine, and dimethylformamide, are used for the solutions of acids and compounds with similar behavior (phenols, imides, sulfonamides, etc.). In this case, the conjugate base of the dissolved acid and the solvated proton are formed; tetrabutyl ammonium hydroxide or other basic titrants are used. In inert solvents such as hexane, benzene, carbon tetrachloride, etc., the highly variable strengths inherent in acids and bases are displayed. The solvent does not take part in the neutralization process, and the product formed is of an additive or associative character.

Titrations with Sodium Nitrite

This is a traditional titration that is still often used to determine compounds containing primary amino groups on the aromatic ring, with the endpoint being monitored with a Pt indicator electrode. This method, applied to the determination of pharmaceuticals (sulfonamide-based compounds, benzocaine, procaine, etc.), is rapid, and the results are in good agreement with official methods of analysis (35).

Titrations Based on Azo-Coupling Reactions

Aromatic diazonium salts, obtained in titrations with sodium nitrite, can be used in azo-coupling reactions (36). Various aromatic amines, phenols, and compounds containing active methylene groups can be titrated with arenediazonium salts, from which 4-Bromo-1-Naphthal-enediazonium chloride seems to be the most widely applicable titrant. Compounds that react slowly with arenediazonium salts can be determined by back-titration when the excess of arenediazonium salt is back-titrated with either sodium tetraphenylborate or 2,4-Diaminotol-uene. Indirect determination is useful for secondary amines, which react with arenediazonium ions to form triazenes. The determination of diazonium salts of ampholytic character is based on the reaction of these salts with 1-Phenyl-3-Methyl-5-Pyrazolone, the excess of which is titrated with 4-Bromo-1-naphthalenediazonium chloride solution.

Kinetic Methods

These have also been applied to the analysis of drug substances because they have advantages over equilibrium techniques, especially when mixtures of closely related compounds, compounds that react slowly, or catalytically acting compounds are to be analyzed. The selectivity and sensitivity of kinetic methods of analysis combined with the selectivity and sensitivity of ion-selective electrodes provide a versatile combination that may lead to new analytical schemes (37).

REFERENCES

1. Compton, R.G.; Sanders, H.W. *Electrode Potentials*; Oxford Univ. Press: Oxford, 1996.
2. Brett, M.A.; Oliveira Brett, A.M. *Electroanalysis*; Oxford Univ. Press: Oxford, 1998.
3. Bailey, P.L. *Analysis with Ion-Selective Eletrodes*; Heyden: London, 1976.
4. Lakshminarayanaiah, N. *Membrane Electrodes*; Academic Press: New York, 1976.
5. Veselý, J.; Weiss, D.; Štulík, K. *Analysis with Ion-Selective Electrodes*; Horwood: Chichester, 1978.
6. Koryta, J.; Štulík, K. *Ion-Selective Electrodes*; 2nd Ed.; Cambridge Univ. Press: Cambridge, 1983.
7. Buck, R.P. Electrochemical Methods: Ion-Selective Electrodes. *Water Analysis*; Minear, R.P., Keith, L.H. Eds.; Academic Press: Orlando, 1984; II, 250–321.
8. Janata, J. *Principles of Chemical Sensors*; Plenum Press: New York, 1989.
9. Midgley, D.; Torrance, K. *Potentiometric Water Analysis*, 2nd Ed.; Wiley: Chichester, 1991.

10. Cattrall, R.W. *Chemical Sensors*; Oxford Univ. Press: Oxford, 1997.

11. Eisenman, G. *Glass Electrodes for Hydrogen and Other Cations*; Marcel Dekker, Inc. New York, 1967.

12. Arnold, M.A. *An Introduction to Biocatalytic Membrane Electrodes*; Int. Lab., 1983; 13 (6), 24–32.

13. Guilbault, G.G.; Schmidt, R.D. Biosensors for the Determination of Drug Substances. Biotechnol. Appl. Biochem. **1991**, *14*, 133–145.

14. Kauffmann, J.M.; Guilbault, G.G. Enzyme Electrode Biosensors: Theory and Applications. *Bioanalytical Application of Enzymes*; Suetler, C.H., Ed.; Wiley: New York, 1992; 36, 63–113.

15. Pratinis, D.M.; Telting-Diaz, M.; Meyerhoff, M.E. Potentiometric Ion-, Gas-, and Bioselective Membrane Electrodes. Crit. Rev. Anal. Chem. **1992**, *23*, 163–186.

16. Buerk, D.G. *Biosensors, Theory and Applications*; Technomic Publ. Co. Lancaster, 1993.

17. Diamond, D. *Principles of Chemical and Biological Sensors*; Wiley: New York, 1998.

18. Bates, R.G. *Determination of pH, Theory and Practice*; Wiley: New York, 1964.

19. Buck, R.P.; Cosofret, V.V. Recommended Procedures for Calibration of Ion-Selective Electrodes (Technical Report). Pure Appl. Chem. **1993**, *65*, 1849–1858.

20. Bakker, E.; Bühlmann, P.; Pretsch, E. Polymer Membrane Ion-Selective Electrodes—What are the Limits? Electroanalysis **1999**, *11*, 915–933.

21. Ríoka, J.; Hansen, E.H. *Flow-Injection Analysis*; Wiley: New York, 1981.

22. Štulík, K.; Pacáková, V. *Electroanalytical Measurements in Flowing Liquids*; Horwood: Chichester, 1987.

23. Baiulescu, G.E.; Cosofret, V.V. *Applications of Ion-Selective Membrane Electrodes in Organic Analysis*; Horwood: Chichester, 1977.

24. Ma, T.S.; Hassan, S.S.M. *Organic Analysis Using Ion-Selective Electrodes*; Academic Press: London, 1982; 1/2.

25. Cosofret, V.V. *Membrane Electrodes in Drug-Substance Analysis*; Pergamon Press: Oxford, 1982.

26. Cunningham, L.; Freiser, H. Ion-Selective Electrodes for Basic Drugs. Anal. Chim. Acta **1982**, *139*, 97–103.

27. Cosofret, V.V.; Buck, R.P. Drug-Substances Analysis with Membrane Electrodes, Ion-Sel. Electrode Rev. **1984**, *6*, 59–121.

28. Vytas, K. The Use of Ion-Selective Electrodes in the Determination of Drug Substances. J. Pharm. Biomed. Anal. **1989**, *7*, 789–812.

29. Vytas, K. Contemporary Trends in the Use of Ion-Selective Electrodes in the Analysis of Organic Substances. *Advanced Instrumental Methods of Chemical Analysis*; Churáek, J., Ed.; Academia, Praha, and Horwood: Chichester, 1993, 142–164.

30. Vytas, K. Potentiometric Titrations Based on Ion-Pair Formations. Ion-Sel. Electrode Rev. **1985**, *7*, 77–164.

31. Schulz, R. *Titration von Tensiden und Pharmaka, Moderne Methoden für den Praktiker*; Verlag für chemische Industrie H. Ziolkowski: Augsburg, 1996.

32. Vytas, K.; Kalous, J.; Jeková, J. Automated Potentiometry as an Ecologic Alternative to Two-Phase Titrations of Surfactants. Egypt. J. Anal. Chem. **1997**, *6*, 107–123.

33. Gyenes, I. *Titrations in Non-Aqueous Media*; Akademiai Kiado: Budapest, 1967.

34. Šafařík, L.; Stránský, Z. *Titrimetric Analysis in Organic Solvents*; Elsevier: Amsterdam, 1986.

35. Šubert, J. Drug Analysis. VI. Studies of Conditions for Diazotizing Titrations of Drugs with Potentiometric Indication and Standardization of a Volumetric Sodium Nitrite Solution. Farm. Obz. **1981**, *50*, 273–278.

36. Vytas, K. Ion-Selective Electrodes in Titrations Involving Azo-Coupling Reactions, Parts 1–5. Anal. Chim. Acta **1982**, *141*, 163–171, (1984); 162, 141–151; (1984); 162, 373–377 (1985); 175, 309–312 (1985); 175, 313–317.

37. Efstathiou, C.E.; Kouparis, M.A.; Hadjiioannou, T.P. Application of Ion-Selective Electrodes in Reaction Kinetics and Kinetic Analysis Ion-Sel. Electrode Rev. **1985**, *7*, 203–259.

POWDERS AS DOSAGE FORMS

Jean-Marc Aiache
Erick Beyssac
Faculty of Pharmacy, Clermont-Ferrand, France

INTRODUCTION

Powders are both the simplest dosage forms and the basis of many other solid dosage forms, such as tablets, capsules, etc. Many drugs or ingredients are also in powder form before processing.

Powders were originally designed as a convenient mode of administering hard vegetable drugs such as roots, barks, and woods; powders were also found to be convenient for dispensing insoluble chemicals such as calomel, bismuth salts, mercury, and chalk.

Presentation in powder form permits drugs to be reduced to a very fine state of division, which often enhances their therapeutic activity or their efficacy by an increase of dissolution rate and/or absorption (1, 3–5). Divided powders are also found to be convenient for administering drugs that are excessively bitter, nauseous, or otherwise offensive to the taste.

This article describes the preparation of powders from bulk materials to finished products according to the administration routes, packaging, and storage conditions.

HISTORICAL BACKGROUND

In all the old books of Pharmacy were included powdered dosage forms resulting from the fine division of animal, vegetable, mineral, and synthetic solid substances (1).

Such powders can be administered singly (simple powders) or as a mixture of different medicinal powders (compound powders) (5). One of the most ancient compound powders was "Hiera Picra" (sacred bitters), a mixture of Aloe and Canella introduced in about 500 B.C. as a laxative (3). (A large number of bitter powders containing Aloe as the principal ingredient bore the name of Hiera.) This powder was listed in various Pharmacopoeias, and it was recognized up to the 4th edition of the *National Formulary* (official until 1926).

Other famous compound powders of the past (1–8) include:

- compound powder of Glycyrrhiza
- compound Senna powder
- Dover's powders introduced by the English physician Thomas Dover as Pulvis Diaphoreticus in the early Eighteenth century (and until recently in some Pharmacopoeias)
- aromatic powder of chalk (a simplified version of a complex confection devised by Sir Walter Raleigh during his imprisonment) known as The CONFECTIO RALEGHIANA (1721)
- Dr. James' antimonial powder (fever powder) patented in 1747
- SEIDLITZ powders (a saline cathartic originated and patented by Thomas Savory in 1815). They owed their value to the mineral properties of the Seidlitz springs in Germany (which contain magnesium sulfate).

DRUG POWDER FORMULATION

According to the European Pharmacopeia, powders as dosage forms are made of solid, dry, free, and more or less fine particles. They contain one or more active ingredients with or without excipients and if necessary, coloring or flavoring substances.

So, the formulation of powders as dosage forms is performed according to the following steps:

- obtention of powder as raw material from an original drug (animal, vegetable drugs, or animal or synthetic chemical entities) by different methods of division:
- mixing of various powders with or without excipients as a function of the powders' characteristics (e.g., flow properties)
- modification of their density (e.g., by granulation) if necessary
- packaging of the finished product for an easy patient's use

OBTENTION OF POWDERS AS RAW MATERIAL

Introduction

The main process is the mechanical (5) division that reduces lump drugs into fragment of different sizes (coarse division). To reduce the size, communition is then used.

Coarse division includes various operations such as cutting, chopping, crushing, grinding, milling, micronizing, and trituration, which depend on the type of equipment used, on the raw material to be treated (vegetable, synthetic, or mineral), and on the convenient particle size. These operations produce heat during processing, which makes it necessary to know certain physical and chemical properties of the drug itself, such as:

- liquefaction temperature
- melting point
- sticking properties
- thermolability
- hardness
- moisture content
- brittleness

Some physical aspects of fracture mechanisms are existing: Crushing or communition produces small-sized particles that present a new free surface area. This requires energy. With current knowledge, it is not possible to determine accurately the necessary energy for good communition, according to the particle size before and after treatment and their physical properties (e.g., brittle, elastic, viscous, plastic) (9).

Several fundamental laws have been suggested and they have been described previously (10–13).

Methods and Equipment

First, to decrease risks of contamination and deterioration, the equipment used in pharmaceuticals should be made of stainless steel, be easy to disassemble for cleaning, and be used in a closed room equipped with a dust removal system.

Coarse division

The devices are described in Table 1.

Comminution

Comminution gives particles smaller than that coarse division. The following factors may influence the choice of the appropriate device:

Physical properties of the drug (13)

Hardness: Hard substances must be subjected to compression, impact, and abrasion or milling, but equipment wear is severe. In some instances, mill wear may be so extensive that it leads to highly contaminated products.

Abrasiveness: This is measured on Moh's scale: 1–3 = soft substances, 8–10 = hard substances.

Elasticity

Friability

Fribrousness: Plant products require a cutting or a chopping action and cannot be subjected to pressure or impact techniques (9, 10).

Moisture content: Several Pharmacopoeias recommend drying (moisture content < 5%) the drug substances before communition (oven at 40–45°C) to avoid liquefaction or agglomeration. Hydrates that may release their water during the process require cooling or low-speed processing.

Initial feed particle size and degree of size reduction desired: Each device has a reduction ratio: it can accept materials of sizes in a certain range and will provide particle of a set size. The particle size distribution of the obtained powder must be as even as possible to obviate further treatment of the larger particles. It is therefore useful to combine, in the same equipment, a milling device with some type of classifier, such as a screen. The oversize particles are returned to the mill on a continuous basis while the particles of the desired size pass through the screen. This kind of equipment is very convenient for sensitive substances or to prevent overmilling and overproduction of fines.

Table 1 Different operations of a coarse division (with definition and devices used)

Operation	Definition	Devices used
Cutting	Obtention of coarse fragments (e.g., vegetable drugs)	Blades
Crushing	Division of coarse fragments	Mortar and pestles (Wedgwood ware, porcelain, glass, iron)
Attrition	Breaking down a substance by rubbing two surfaces together	Non-or stainless steel worn

Table 2 Different operations of comminution (with their devices)

Operation	Laboratory scale devices	Industrial scale devices[a]
Attrition	Mortar and pestles Grunding stones Cutter mills Sieves and screens	Jaw crushing device Mills (vertical or horizontal)

Rolling	Roller mills	Roller mills (smooth or saw-toothed cylinders)
		Attrition mills (diameter 1–2 mm)
		Cutter mills (diameter > 0.2 mm)
		Hammer mills (can be used in liquid
		   N_2 or CO_2 to decrease the milling temperature
		   and to protect the drug product)
		Pebble or ball mills (diameter
		   < 2 mm)(planetary pot or jarr
		   mills or vibration mills)
		Micronizers or jet mills (fluid-energy mills)
		   (diameter 1–10 μm)
		Centrifugal impact pulverizer (diameter 0.05–2 mm)

[a]All these devices have been described (see Ref. 13).

Particle shape desired (13): Different kinds of equipment produce different shapes (Table 2).

Quantity of material to be treated: The selected equipment must have the required capacity. The operation can be continuous or not.

All these operations are achieved by sieving to separate the coarse particles for grinding again if necessary.

It is to be noted that safety must be taken into account:

Noise: All equipment must be installed in a special sound-insulated room.

Toxicity: Due to particle air diffusion, protection of workers is compulsory. Cross-contamination must also be prevented.

Powder Characterization

Particle size

All these data must be introduced in the drug product registration file as well as for the raw material due to their impact on the drug bioavailability as for the powder dosage form as finished product.

A powder is characterized by its particle size, which is of importance in achieving optimum production of medicines (9). First of all, this parameter influences the dissolution rate of the drug in vivo, which in turn influences absorption rate and the onset of therapeutic activity. Particle size is important during the production of solid dosage forms in the manufacture of tablets and capsules. Appropriate equipment controls the mass of drug and other particles by volumetric filling. Any interference with the uniformity of fill volumes may therefore alter the mass of the drug incorporated into the dosage form (tablets or capsules) and so reduce the content uniformity. Powders with different particle sizes have different flow and packing properties, which alter the volume of powders during each event. To avoid such problems, the particle size of drugs should be defined during formulation and must be as uniform as possible (9).

However, it is not easy to evaluate the particle size of a powder. For a large lump, it is possible to measure it in three dimensions. But if the substance is milled, the resulting particles are irregular with different numbers of faces and it would be difficult or impracticable to determine more than a single dimension (14). For this reason, a solid particle is often considered to approximate to a sphere characterized by a diameter. The measurement is thus based on a hypothetical sphere that represents only an approximation to the true shape of the particle. The dimension is thus referred to as the equivalent diameter of the particle (14).

It is possible to generate more than one sphere that is equivalent to a given irregular particle shape. It is useful to evaluate Feret's or Martin's statistical diameter (12), which depends on both the orientation and shape of particle. Feret's diameter is determined from the mean distance between two parallel tangents to the projected particles perimeter, and the Martin's diameter is the mean chord length of the projected particle perimeter (Fig. 1). Instead of sphere equivalent diameter, it is possible to use equivalent

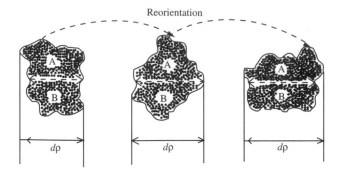

Fig. 1 Influence of particle orientation on statistical diameters. The change in Feret's diameter is shown by the distances, d_f: Martin's diameter (d_m) corresponds to the dashed lines.

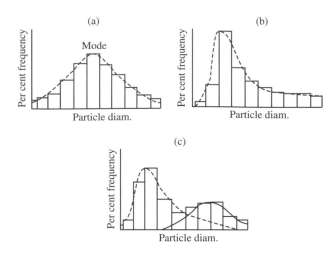

Fig. 2 Frequency distribution curves corresponding to (A) a normal distribution, (B) a positively skewed distribution, and (C) a bimodal distribution.

volume, sedimentation volume, mass, or sieve mass of a given particle to determine the particle size of a powder.

Finally, as powders contain particles of different diameters, it is necessary to present the results of size distribution in the form of histogram corresponding to each equivalent diameter evaluated. Such a histogram presents an interpretation of the particle size distribution, enabling the percentage of particles having a given equivalent diameter to be determined and allowing different particles size to be compared (Fig. 2A). An alternative to the histogram representation is obtained by sequentially adding the percent frequency values (Fig. 2B) to produce a cumulative percent frequency distribution (14). Finally, to summarize the data obtained in determining particle size, it is possible to use statistical methods (14).

Recently, some recommendations to include the following items in a particle sizing validation report have been published (15):

- the procedure (or reference to it)
- precision
- range (suitability assessment including microscopic comparison)
- robustness

Detection limit, quantification limit, accuracy, and specificity are not normally considered appropriate for validation of particle sizing methods.

The author of these recommendations added that the validation of particle sizing technique cannot be completed with the first batch of a sample, as data are insufficient to fully validate the procedure at this stage. It is not always important to know the absolute particle size of the first batch manufactured, but it is important to know how the second and subsequent batches compare with it. The validation of a particle size method should be in phases, with parts completed when the first sample is analyzed and other data completed or added later, for example, prior to the regulatory filing. Calibration or verification of an instrument being used is assumed to be normal part of GMP and may be used as a suitability assessment (15).

The different methods of particle size analysis can be grouped into several categories: size range analyses (sieve methods), wet or dry methods, and manual or automatic methods (laser-light). All these methods are described elsewhere (16, 17).

Flow properties (18, 19)

Flow properties of powders are important parameters in mixing and segregation phenomena, essentially during storage.

Depending on manufacturing and packaging processes, different flow characteristics are required that are essential for quality control and for the optimization formulation.

In fact a powder, as it has been said, can be made of one or many active powder drugs with or without excipients, and this final mixture will represent the dosage form to be packed and dispensed to patients. So, it is necessary in most of the cases to add excipients for diluting the active powder drug, to improve the packaging properties, and/or to insure a good compliance from the patient (e.g., taste masking). So, the excipients must present the following properties:

- optimal particle size distribution
- high flowability
- high compressibility
- optimal capacity for a drug

- sufficient reworkability
- physiologically inert
- resistant to heat, humidity, and oxidation
- tasteless and odorless

The bulk mixture obtained must present flow properties that are determined by

1. flow through an orifice
2. angle of repose
3. bulk density or bulk taped density (18)
4. shear cells

These methods are described quite in all the pharmacopeias and in an article elsewhere (20).

OBTENTION OF POWDERS AS DOSAGE FORMS

A powder as dosage form, as it has been said, is made of one or more drug powders, generally, with excipients. So, the mixing of all the components and the validation of this operation are very important.

Mixing of Powders

The aim of mixing is to obtain a homogeneous association of several solid products. Each fraction or dose randomly sampled must contain all the components in the same proportion as in the whole preparation (21). This is achieved because the different components "are treated so as to lie as nearly as possible in contact with a particle of each of the other components" (22).

Mixing has been described as a stochastic process by means of stationary and nonstationary MARKOV chains (10) in which the probabilities of particle movement from place to place in the bed are determined.

To obtain a good mixture, it is necessary to take into account the characteristics of the raw material, the finished mixture, the equipment used, and the operating conditions. The mixing process must be validated (discussed later).

Factors influencing the mixing of powders

Ideally, to avoid segregation, it is useful to mix powders with very close characteristics. Particle size is the most important factor. Normally, all the powders should have the same particle size. It is therefore necessary to mill and sieve them before mixing so that they present the same size. However, every substance has its own properties, and the same size does not mean the same shape and the same other properties.

The density of each component affects the stability of the mixture. The heavier particles have a tendency to fall to the bottom while the lighter ones rise to the top of the powder bed.

The amount (proportion) of each component is also another factor. Good homogeneity is more difficult to obtain if the proportion of one component is small. It is very important that this small amount is perfectly distributed throughout the whole mixture, for example, when a very active substance is diluted in a large amount of excipient to facilitate dosage form preparation and administration (same problem for coloring). So, it is recommended, first to mix together small quantities of constituents and then continue progressive additions. It is also possible to introduce small amounts of drug substances into the mixture, as a solution in a volatile solvent. After mixing, the solvent is evaporated.

Some mixtures need the addition of an adjuvant; thus, to mix magnesium oxide and charcoal, it is necessary to use alcohol or etheroxide, which are evaporated after mixing.

If these factors are not under control, segregation (demixing) can occur. Powder particles can be separated in a mixing device because their pathways depend on their size and density: this happens in rotating shell mixers. Segregation can also be seen when mixer is emptied, when powder is discharged, or during transport and storage. Due to vibrations, there are free spaces in which denser particles can slip and fall to the container's bottom. This separation is facilitated by the size and shape of the particles, which can slip more or less over each other. For very fine powders, density differences are more important than particle adhesion and friction. No segregation is seen for particles under 40 μm diameter. Three types of segregation have been described:

1. Percolation segregation is the movement of the small particles through the voids in the static powder bed.
2. Trajectory segregation occurs during mixing: particles are set in motion and kinetic energy is imparted to them. Larger particles have larger energies and tend to move a greater distance into a powder mass before they are brought to rest. This may result in preferential separation and can occur in both horizontal and vertical planes.
3. Densification segregation: density differences between particles may cause segregation. Large particles move upward through the mass. It seems that the small particles beneath dense large particles are slightly compacted, supporting the large particles. On vibration, the small particles move beneath the large particles and raise them upward in the bed.

The effect of mixing time on segregation is that nonsegregating mixtures continue to improve with an extended mixing time, but the reverse may be true for segregating mixes.

The factors promoting segregation require a longer time to establish a segregation mix that is needed to produce a reasonable degree of mixing. It is therefore counterproductive to prolong the mixing time beyond an optimum point.

Equipment

The three primary mechanisms responsible for mixing are (10) convective movement of relatively large portions of the bed, shear failure that primarily reduces the scale of segregation, and diffusive movement of individual particles.

Most efficient mixers operate by all three mechanisms. Thus, mixing can be considered a random shuffling-type operation, involving both large and small particle groups and even individual particles.

The ideal mixer should rapidly produce a complete blend with as gentle as possible a mixing action to avoid damage. It should be easily cleaned and discharged, be dust-tight, and require low maintenance and low power consumption.

Laboratory equipment: The pharmacist most often employs the mortar and pestle for the small-scale mixing usually required for prescription compounding. However, spatulas and sieves may also be used occasionally. The mortar and pestle method combines communition and mixing in a single operation.

Industrial equipment: Rotating-shell mixers or tumbling mixers are shown in Fig. 3. Drum-type, cubical-shaped, double-cone, and twin-shell blenders with their axis of rotation horizontal to the center of the drum on its axis increase crossflow and improve the mixing action. Cubical and polyhedron-shaped blenders with a rotating axis set at various angles are also available. Double-cone blenders or tumbling mixers have been developed; the Y-cone mixer (Fig. 3) is a good example

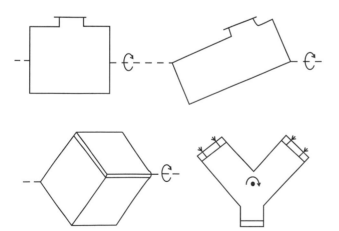

Fig. 3 Tumbling mixers.

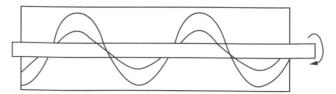

Fig. 4 Ribbon mixer.

(13). On rotation the charge flows into the top two arms of the Y and then back into the third arm. Mixing by shear and diffusion takes place when the streams mingle. Time must be allowed for the mix to flow into the arms, and there is an optimum speed rotation. The zigzag blender is an extension of the twin-shell blender.

A fixed-shell mixer or agitator mixer is shown in Fig. 4. Also called ribbon mixer, it consists of a relatively long throughlike shell with a semicircular bottom. The shell is fitted with a shaft on which are mounted spiral ribbons, paddles, or helical screws alone or in combination. These mixing blades produce a continuous cutting and shuffling of the charge by circulation the powder from end to end of the trough as well as rotationally. The shearing action that develops between the moving blade and the trough serves to break down powder agglomerates. A more recent type of agitator mixer is the Nautamixer (Fig. 5) that consists of a conical vessel fitted at the base with a rotating screw fastened to the end of a rotating arm at the top. The screw conveys material toward the top where it cascades back into the mass.

Sigma-blade and planetary-paddle mixers are used for solid blending and as a step prior to the introduction of liquids (Figs. 6 and 7). This type of mixer rapidly breaks down agglomerates.

Vertical impeller mixers employ a screw-type impeller, which constantly overturns the batch.

Motionless mixers are part of continuous-processing devices with no moving parts. They consist of a series of fixed flow-twisting or flow-splitting elements.

Validation of the Mixing Process

The mixing process is validated by the verification of the homogeneity of mixed powders, for instance, by taking three samples at three different levels of the mixer (top, middle, and bottom) and determining the amount of different active substances in these samples. Each sample must be of the same size as in the kind of dosage form to be used. A mixing index can also be used.

Other characteristics of the mixed powder such as particle size, flavor, flow rate, and bulk density before and after tapping have to be verified.

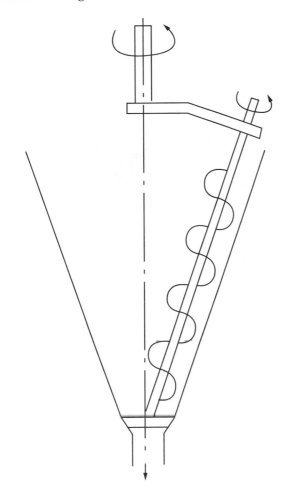

Fig. 5 Nautamixer.

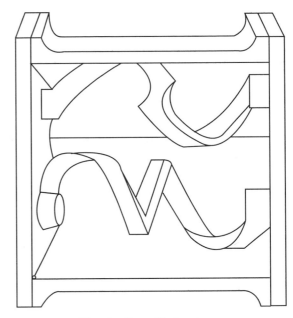

Fig. 6 Sigma-blade mixer.

The process reproducibility is assessed by performing operation and verification three times. The validation result is considered correct if the amount of each active substance found in each sample and all the other characteristics evaluated are within the set limits (22).

CLASSIFICATION AND EXAMPLES OF POWDERS AS DOSAGE FORMS

They can be classified as a function of their route of administration.

Oral Administration

Mode of administration and packaging

They are generally administered in or with water or with other appropriate liquids. In a few cases, they can be swallowed as they are. Both single and multiple doses are available.

Multiple-dose powders, presented in band or metal box, require a measure to deliver the prescribed dose. Initially, it was an ordinary spoon, but given the different sizes and shapes of the spoons used worldwide, powder density, humidity, degree of settling, fluffiness due to agitation, and personal judgment of patients (selecting a full or half spoon according to be patient's mood), it has been decided to use other devices. They are generally special measuring plastic spoons on which the volume is indicated and corresponds to a weight of powder as a function of its density (this volume corresponds to an adult or child dosage).

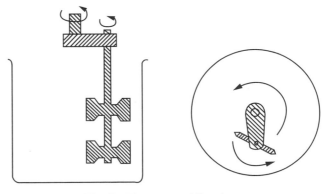

Fig. 7 Planetary-paddle mixer.

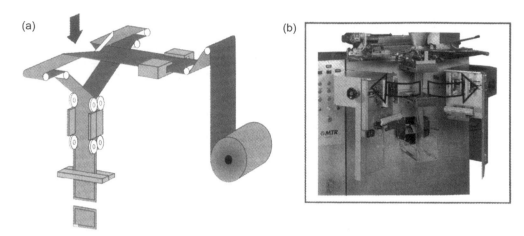

Fig. 8 (a) Foil preparation. (b) Multilane vertical sachet-filling machine. The hinged panels can be opened by 90° to allow complete access to the product dosing area, the film needed, and the sealing and cutting station.

Currently, the best way is to use single dose contained in a folded paper (in community pharmacy) or sachets filled with the same accuracy as a tablet or capsule by a fully automatic machine. The sachet is made of paper, aluminum, and/or complex mixtures that are a combination of aluminum and plastic substances. An aluminum or paper foil is covered on one or both sides (internal and/or external) with polyethylene, PVC, or PVDC (e.g., paper + polyethylene + aluminum + polyethylene). Generally, the foils are presented in rolls, printed on their outer face with the drug name, and assembled in automatic machines (Fig. 8) that use one or two rolls on which sachets are predrawn. First, the foils are cut longitudinally in a by-pass station and folded longitudinally. These folded paper webs are drawn off a roll, crosscut, and guided into presealed sachets. Powders are added by various devices (Fig. 9) such as micropiston, vacuum feeding, volumetric drawer slide filler, dosing plates (or telescopic cups), suction devices, and discharge and filling funnels for non-free-flowing powders. After filling, the sachets are sealed (three or four side sealed sachets) at 100–145°C for 0.5 s. During filling, the weight must be controlled. After filling, the sachets are submitted to different controls such as sealing, integrity of foils, opening ease as well as permeability to gases, and to humidity. These controls are generally performed on the raw foils and on the finished products.

Excipients and/or modification of powder density or flow characteristics

To obtain a good filling, the powders must be homogeneous during the whole filling time and must flow regularly to obtain similar volume. Homogeneity is

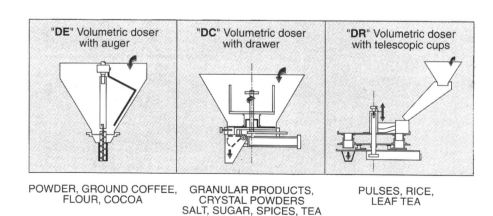

Fig. 9 Different types of volumetric dosers.

obtained by the help of the mixing devices described previously. The mixers are connected to the filling machine. If the duration of mixing is increased, it is absolutely necessary to prevent uncontrolled demixing during this last step.

For the second point, it is necessary to know the flow properties of the powders, and generally it is compulsory to add some excipients to modify these properties and adapt them to the filling device.

The excipients used are fillers, but the most important are lubricants, such as magnesium stearate, PEG 6000, calcium stearate, glycerol palmito stearate, and calcium behenate, which increase the flowability but at the same time modify the hydrophobic characteristics of powders. Their choice depends on compatibility with active ingredient and the flow properties of powders. The characteristics of the excipient have been described previously.

Sometimes, it is necessary to modify the density of the powder by granulation made by the ordinary way (23) as for tablet preparation or using new techniques such as rotogranulation (24). This transformation is sometimes quite necessary because it is easier to modify the taste using flavoring substances or flavor modifiers (25). In this last case, a recent article describes the taste masking as a consequence of the organization of powder mixture (26).

Examples of powders as dosage forms

Effervescent powders: Initialy these powders, described in the Pharmacopeia, consisted of sodium bicarbonate, tartaric acid, and potassium and sodium tartrate (wrapped in white paper). Each was separately dissolved in water and then mixed before drinking: they were called "English Seidleitz powders" (the Seltz or the English Soda powders are quite similar) (2).

Nowadays, effervescent powders are available in single or multiple units that contain acid substances and carbonates or bicarbonates, which quickly react in water by releasing carbon dioxide. They are dissolved or dispersed in water before being taken. This is a great advantage because the drug is then in solution, the pH of which is close to 7, which allows rapid passage through the pylorus. The drug absorption from the gut wall as well as the onset of therapeutic activity may thereby be hastened. Effervescent powders contain (27):

1. *Acid materials*

   Acids: citric (monohydrate or anhydrate), tartaric, ascorbic (drug or excipient), fumaric, nicotinic, acetylsalicylic (as drug or excipient), malic, and adipic acids (seldom used).

   Anhydrides: glutaric, citric.
   Salts: sodium dihydrogeno-citrate, sodium acid phosphate, sodium fumarate.

2. *Sources of carbon dioxide*

   Salts: sodium bicarbonate (the most widely used), sodium carbonate, potassium carbonate, calcium carbonate, sodium glycine carbonate (28).

3. *Other excipients* (main characteristic, solubility in water):

   Lubricants: PEG 6000 is most frequently used, alone or with sodium stearyl fumarate, sodium benzoate, sodium chloride, sodium acetate, or D,L-leucine.
   Binders: PVP, hydrogenated maltodextrin, maltodextrins, PEG 6000.
   Others: sweeteners, flavors, colors, surfactants, antifoaming agents (polydimethylsiloxane).

The manufacturing process requires a very low and controlled relative humidity (about 20% or less, if necessary) as well as a controlled ambient temperature close to 25°C. Generally, effervescent powders are made by classical wet granulation of the acid and carbonate part separately or mixed with water–ethanol or isopropanol. Special care must be taken in the case of total granulation to limit the effervescent reaction, except in case of use of the technique of granulation with a rotor (29).

The stability and shelf-life of effervescent powders are essentially assured by protection against external moisture. Single-dose sachets are manufactured with suitable complexes to prevent premature reaction caused by external moisture or excess internal moisture from the granulation process. Special stability studies under different conditions are required for these powders. The dissolution time must be less than 3 min; this is an index of stability.

Many drugs and drug compositions are used in effervescent products including aspirin, acetaminophen, ibupofen, nonsteroid-antiinflammatory drugs, cimetidine, antibiotics, mucolytic drugs, vitamins, and others. It has been demonstrated many times that drugs are rapidly, and sometimes better, absorbed in this form than in conventional dosage forms (30, 31).

Powders for Parenteral Use

For parenteral use, solid sterile substances are distributed in their final packages. A clear solution nearly free of particles or a uniform one is obtained after shaking with the prescribed volume of an appropriate sterile liquid. Freeze-dried substances for parenteral use are also used.

After dissolution or dispersion, preparations must comply with assay requirements for injectable preparations or injectable preparations for perfusion. Their preparation requires the same care as parenteral solutions, i.e. sterilization of raw material or finished product sterilization (32).

Powders for Cutaneous Applications

These are single- or multiple-unit powders free of agglomerated particles. They must be sterile for application on open wounds or damaged skin.

Multiple-unit powders for local application are preferably packaged in a dredger or a pressurized container (for skin, teeth, or vaginal douche use). These preparations consist of a dispersion of a solid phase (drug) in a liquid propellant (liquid phase). By action on the actuator, the suspension is released by gas pressure. The propellant in contact with ambient air is evaporated and the powder remains on the treated area. The particle size obtained depends on the powder particle size before the preparation of the suspension.

Many powders are presented in this special dosage form (e.g., antiseptics, antifungal drugs) as well as cosmetic preparations (dry shampoo, etc.). Generally, the drug is mixed with an inert diluent such as starch, magnesium carbonate, magnesium stearate, or silicon dioxide of particle size close to 50–60 μm. To increase the suspension stability and to prevent closure of the actuator,

lubricants and/or surfactants are added (mineral oils, isopropyl myristate, lecithin, sorbitane fatty acid esters). These last substances will also prevent agglomeration orcrystallization of drug substances (percentage about 0.1–1%).

The propellants used were some years ago chlorofluoro-carbons (CFCs) (11 and 12) in various proportions (65:35 or 50:50). The manufacturing process includes the suspension formation in liquid propellant 11 in a cooled and hermetically closed mixer containing drug and lubricants. This mixture is introduced in the cans that are closed by a special powder valve, and propellant 12 was then injected through the valve. The upper part of the valve has often a special aperture through which a gaseous phase cleans the valve as well as the actuator.

A major current issue is the suppression of the use of CFCs due to ozone depletion. Other liquid propellants (134a, 227, or dimethyl ether) are not used as easily as the CFCs and formulation is very difficult. So, many of these dosage forms disappeared or were substituted by "saltcellar" systems. The use of very volatile solvents, such as volatile silicone, can be proposed if their boiling point is close to room temperature (33), the use of butane is not recommended due to the explosion risks.

Powders for Pulmonary Application

As a consequence of the suppression or reduced use of CFC propellants, a new kind of dosage form is under

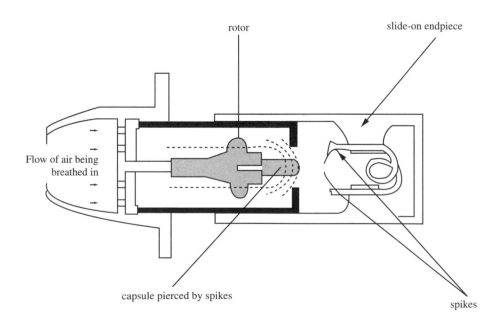

Fig. 10   Spinhaler.

worldwide development: drug powder inhalers (DPIs). The metered dose inhalers (MDIs) will probably be replaced by these. The MDIs were formulated several years ago. A drug in powder form (with a particle size close to 5 μm) was suspended in propellant 11 with a surfactant. Propellant 12 was added to the can after closure.

The metered valve delivers a fixed volume of suspension that after propellant evaporation, releases the active drug in the upper respiratory tract. Owing to its small diameter size, about 10% of the drug reaches the bronchopulmonary tract and provides therapeutic activity.

Currently, propellant issues have led companies to develop DPI. These consist of a very fine active drug (paricle size 5 μm or less) mixed with an inert excipient such as lactose. The mixture is administered through a special device.

Spinhaler (Fisons) (Fig. 10) and Rotahaler (Allen and Hanbury) (Fig. 11) were introduced more than 10 years ago for delivery of single metered doses of sodium cromogycate, salbutamol, or beclomethasone dipropionate in powder form, with the energy required to disperse the powder being derived from the patient's own inspiratory effort. Both the Spinhaler and Rotahaler (Ciba systems) are rather inconvenient to use because it is necessary to load a gelatin capsule containing the drug powder into the device immediately prior to use. However, a lot of new multidose dry powder inhalers have been recently introduced. The Diskhaler (Allen and Hanbury) contains eight doses of either salbutamol or beclomethasone dipropionate (2-day supply at normal dosing levels) in blisters around the periphery of a small disk. The Diskus is more interesting: it contains 60 doses of antiasthmatic drug

with a special counter, which indicates the number of delivered doses. The Turbuhaler (Astra) (Fig. 12) contains 200 metered doses of the bronchodilator terbutaline sulfate in the manner of a pressurized MDI, but without additives of any kind. The corticosteroid budesonide is available in a Turbuhaler in some countries.

The clickhaler is based on the same principle: a reservoir containing a number of doses releases one after an actuation.

It seems that all these devices are easy to use and are readily accepted by patients. According to some authors, they deliver a similar percentage of the drug dose to the lungs as a correctly used MDI and has an equivalent efficacy (34).

However, patients with low inspiratory flow rate (essentially children) have many difficulties to use them. Furthermore, when the particles are inhaled quickly, their inertia increases and there is an impaction in the throat. So, new devices are developed to improve the patient's compliance. They consist of a pump that compresses air in a special chamber so that the powder is expulsed as a cloud, owing to the pressure delivered by the compressed air (35). These systems are close to the old MDI.

CONCLUSION

The preparation of powders as dosage forms comprises many steps that are the same as for the preparation of powders used to manufacture other solid dosage forms such as tablets or hard gelatin capsules.

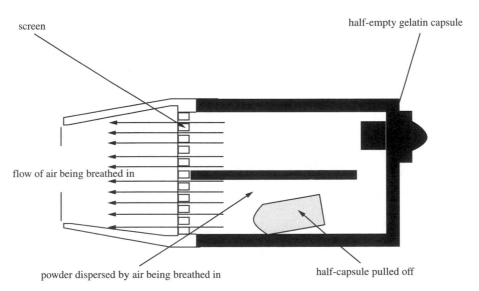

screen

half-empty gelatin capsule

flow of air being breathed in

powder dispersed by air being breathed in

half-capsule pulled off

Fig. 11   Rotahaler.

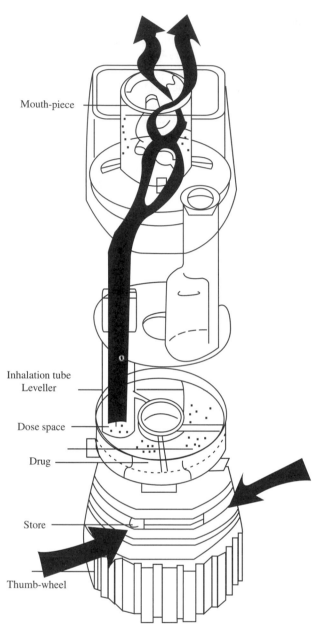

Mouth-piece

Inhalation tube
Leveller

Dose space

Drug

Store

Thumb-wheel

Fig. 12 Turbuhaler.

Years ago powders were used as dosage forms more frequently before the advent of more modern forms. However, biopharmaceutical problems arose with these new drug dosage forms, and companies have returned to powders and developed these further. Industrial sachet manufacturing considerably reduces handling and improves storage. Pressurized systems allow easy dispensation of disinfectants, which increases patients' compliance. It can be expected that powders will continue to be used in the future.

REFERENCES

1. Astruc, A. *Traité de Pharmacie Galénique*, 4th Ed.; Librairie Maloine: Paris, 1946.
2. Buerki, R.A.; Higby, G.J. History of Dosage Forms and Basic Preparations. *Encyclopedia of Pharmaceutical Technology*, 1st Ed.; Swarbrick, J., Boylan, J.C., Eds.; Marcel Dekker, Inc.: New York, 1993; 7, 299–338.
3. *Codex Medicamentarius, Pharmacopée Française*; Bechet Jeune: Paris, 1837.
4. *Codex Medicamentarius, Pharmacopée Française*; J.B. Baillière & Fils: Paris, 1866.
5. Henry, N.E.; Guibourt, C.B. *Traité de Pharmacie*; J.B. Baillière: Paris, 1847.
6. *Palestra Farmaceutica Chimico Galenica* : Madrid, 1706.
7. *Oficina Medicamentorom Valentiae MDCI* : Valence, 1601.
8. *Farmacopea Cathalana Sive Antidotarium Barcinonense*; Barcelona, 1686.
9. Le Hir, A. *Pharmacie Galénique*, 6th Ed.; Masson: Paris, 1992.
10. Ripple, E.G. Powders. *Remington's Pharmaceutical Sciences*; Gennaro, A.R., Ed.; Mack Pub. Co.: Easton, PA, 1980.
11. Parrot, E.L.; Milling, I.N.; Lachman, L.; Lieberman, H.A.; Kanig, J.L. *The Theory and Practice of Industrial Pharmacy*; Milling, I.N., Lachman, L., Lieberman, H.A., Kanig, J.L., Eds.; Lea & Febiger: Philadelphia, 1970; 100–119.
12. Perry, R.H. *Chemical Engineers' Handbook*, 4th Ed.; McGraw-Hill: New York, 1963.
13. Aiache, J.-M.; Beyssac, E. Powders as Dosage Forms. *Encyclopedia of Pharmaceutical Technology*, 1st Ed.; Swarbrick, J., Boylan, J.C., Eds.; Marcel Dekker, Inc.: New York, 1994; 12, 389–419.
14. Staniforth, J.N. Particle Size Analysis. *Pharmaceutics: The Science of Dosage Form Design*; Aulton, M.E., Ed.; Churchill Livingstone: Edinburgh, UK, 1988.
15. Bell, R.; Dennis, A.; Hendriksen, B.; North, N.; Sherwood, J. Position Paper on Particle Sizing: Sample Preparation, Method Validation and Data Presentation. Pharm. Technol. Eur. **1999**, *11* (11), 36–42.
16. Pharmeuropa **1993**, *5*, 89–91.
17. Staniforth, J.N. Particle Size Analysis. *Pharmaceutics: The Science of Dosage Form Design*; Aulton, M.E., Ed.; Churchill Livingstone: Edinburgh, UK, 1988.
18. Neumann, B.S. The Flow Properties of Powders. *Advances in Pharmaceutical Sciences*; Bean, H.S., Carless, J.E., Beckett, A.H., Eds.; Academic Press: London, UK, 1967; 2, 181–221.
19. Carr, R.L. Chem. Eng. **1965**, *7*, 163–167.
20. Neumann, B.S. The Flow Properties of Powders. *Advances in Pharmaceutical Sciences*; Bean, H.S., Carless, J.E., Beckett, A.H., Eds.; Academic Press: London, 1967; 2, 181–221.
21. Génie Pharmaceutique. *Galenica, Technique et Documentation*; Paris, 1982; 3.
22. Travers, D.N. Mixing. *Pharmaceutics: The Science of Dosage Form Design*; Churchill Livingston: Edinburgh, UK, 1988.

23. Kristensen, H.G. Granulations. *Encyclopedia of Pharmaceutical Technology*; 1st Ed.; Swarbrick, J., Boylan, J.C., Eds.; Marcel Dekker, Inc.: New York, 1993; 109–120.

24. *European Pharmacopeia*, 1999.

25. Adjei, A.L.; Doyle, R.; Reiland, T. Flavors and Flavor Modifiers. *Encyclopedia of Pharmaceutical Technology*, 1st Ed.; Swarbrick, J., Boylan, J.C., Eds.; Marcel Dekker, Inc.: New York, 1992; 6, 101–139.

26. Barra, J.; Lescure, F.; Doelker, E. Taste Masking as a Consequence of the Organisation of Powder Mixes. Pharm. Acta Helv. **1999**, *74*, 37–42.

27. Lindberg, N.O.; Engfors, H.; Ericsson, T. Effervescent Pharmaceuticals. *Encyclopedia of Pharmaceutical Technology*, 1st Ed.; Swarbrick, J., Boylan, J.C., Eds.; Marcel Dekker, Inc.: New York, 1992; 5, 45–71.

28. Aiache, J.-M. Les Comprimés Effervescents. Pharm. Acta Helv. **1974**, *49*, 169.

29. Gauthier, P.; Aiache, J.-M. Rotary Fluidized Bed Process and Its Possibilities. *Symposium Glatt*; Marseille: Octobre 1997.

30. Febvre, P.; Aiache, J.-M.; Bex, J.F. Etude En Continu In Vivo De La Salicylémie Du Lapin Après Ingestion D'aspirine Soluble Sous Différentes Formes Galéniques. C.R. Soc. Biol. **1969**, *163*, 1160.

31. Vatier, J.; Slama, A.; Vitre, M.T.; Mignon, M. Ranitidine 300 Mg Effervescente. Activité Antiacide Et Pouvoir Tampon Liés Au Complexe Effervescent. Med. Chir. Dig. **1992**, *21* (28).

32. Turco, S.J. Dosage Forms: Parenteral. *Encyclopedia of Pharmaceutical Technology*; Swarbrick, J., Boylan, J.C., Eds.; Marcel Dekker, Inc.: New York, 1991; 4, 231–247.

33. Beyssac, E.; Aiache, J.-M.; Grumel, J.-M. *Modification of the Impaction Device to Assess Particle Size Distribution of Nasal Sprays, 3th European Congress of Pharmaceutical Sciences*; Edinburgh, UK, September 1996.

34. Newman, S.P. Metered-Dose Pressurized Aerosols and the Ozone Layer. Eur. Resp. J. **1990**, *3*, 495–497.

35. Aiache, J.-M. The Ideal Drug Delivery System: A Look into the Future. J. Aer. Med. **1991**, *4*, 323–334.

PRESERVATION OF PHARMACEUTICAL PRODUCTS

Peter Gilbert
David G. Allison
University of Manchester, Manchester, United Kingdom

PRESERVATION

Microbial spoilage of pharmaceutical products has been known for many years. Spoilage may result in the deterioration of the product due to loss of potency or to the initiation of an infection in the user. Sterile pharmaceutical products (single dose or multiple dose forms) require the addition of an antimicrobial preservative when they have been manufactured under aseptic conditions from presterilized ingredients. Where the products are subject to a terminal sterilization process, only the multiple dose category requires the addition of an antimicrobial agent. In the latter instance, the preservative is added to protect the product and end user against the consequences of microbial entry during use. Chemical antimicrobial agents are thus added to all multidose sterile formulations and to aqueous and aqueous-based nonsterile pharmaceuticals. Their function is to reduce the microbial load to a level, which is safe for the designated use of the product, and to maintain the numbers of viable microorganisms at or below that value for the storage and use life of the product. Preservatives must, therefore, be stable within the formulation for the shelf life of the product and be capable of dealing with all the abuses made to it by the consumer and user (i.e. contamination during use, incorrect storage *etc*). Table 1 presents, in alphabetical order by chemical grouping, the agents most often employed for preservation of pharmaceutical products.

For multidose sterile products, the preservative must be capable of reestablishing sterility between each use, whereas for a nonsterile topical cosmetic the function of the preservative might simply be to prevent growth. The associated toxicity of preservatives often limits the concentrations at which they can be employed; thus, lower concentrations are generally employed for opthalmic products and injectables. In choosing a preservative the likely capacity required, the rate of killing desired, and the ingredients and pH of the formulation must be borne in mind.

The BP (1988) test for the "Efficacy of Preservatives in Pharmaceuticals" makes it quite clear that a preservative must in the first instance *kill* microorganisms and only accepts later that it will prevent growth. However, it does insist that there must be no outgrowth of the test organism, that is, the preservative possesses sufficient residual capacity to inhibit the growth of any survivors.

DEFINITION OF TERMS

Disinfectants, antiseptics, and preservatives are chemicals that have the ability to destroy or inhibit the growth of microorganisms, and are used for this purpose. These and other terms commonly employed are defined as follows:

- *Disinfectants*: Chemical agents or formulations that are too irritant or toxic on body surfaces, but are used to reduce the level of microorganisms from the surface of inanimate objects to one that is safe for a defined purpose.
- *Antiseptics*: Chemical agents or formulations that can be used as an antimicrobial agents on body surfaces.
- *Preservatives*: Chemical agents or formulations that are capable of reducing the number of viable microorganisms within an object or field to a level that is safe for its designated use and will maintain the numbers of viable microorganisms at or below a level for the use/shelf-life of the product.
- *Bacteriostasis*: A state in which the growth of microorganisms is halted or inhibited.
- *Bactericide*: A chemical antimicrobial agent that reduces the viability of a population of microorganisms exposed to it. This term is meaningless without specifying the concentration range over which this effect is obtained; such concentration ranges will vary between different species of microorganisms.
- *Bacteriostat*: A chemical antimicrobial agent that can prevent the growth of microorganisms within an otherwise nutritious environment. This term is meaningless without specifying the concentration at which this effect is achieved. Bacteriostatic concentrations do vary between different species of microorganisms.

Table 1 General properties of some widely used preservatives

Preservative	Advantages	Disadvantages	Application
Acids (organic): benzoic acid, parabens, sorbic acid	Active against bacteria and fungi	Highly pH dependent	Oral and topical formulations; gums and syrups
Alcohols: ethyl or isopropyl, chlorbutol, bronopol	Broad spectrum, including that against acid-fast bacteria	Volatile; poor penetration of organic matter	Solvent; eye drops and injections; synergistic properties
Aldehydes: formaldehyde, gluteraldehyde	Broad spectrum antibacterial, antifungal, and sporicidal activity	Acid solutions inactivated with temperature; toxic and carcinogenic	Chemical sterilization and storage of surgical instruments (e.g., endoscopes)
Biguanides: chlorhexidine, polyhexamethylene biguanide	Mainly active in cationic form against gram-positive bacteria	Water insoluble; inactivated by organic matter; limited antifungal activity	Solution for hard contact lenses and other opthalmic products
Halogens: hypochlorite, povidone-iodine, chloroform	Broad spectrum of antibacterial, fungal, and viral activity	Unstable; corrosive; inactivated by organic matter	Limited use nowadays
Organic mercurials: mercury, silver, thiomersal, phenylmercuric acetate	Broad spectrum of antibacterial activity	Low capacity to organic matter, ionic and some nonionic surfactants; toxicity	Eye drops; contact lens solutions
Phenolics: cresol, chlorocresol, bisphenol	Cheap, rapid activity against gram-positive bacteria and fungi	Low water solubility; adsorbed by rubber; volatile, irritant, pH dependent	Creams
Quaternary ammonium compounds: cetrimide, benzalkonium chloride	Narrow spectrum (gram-positive bacteria) of activity; surfactant properties	Low capacity to organic matter; low activity at acidic pH; incompatible with soaps, ionic and nonionic surfactants	Eye drops; surgical creams; ointments

It should be noted that terms such as bactericide and bacteriostat should be discouraged; in the USP and EP, the term "antimicrobial agent" has replaced these terms.

PRESERVATIVE IDEALS

At present there is no perfect preservative, and all materials are a compromise of a number of often contrary properties. The following are the properties of an ideal preservative compound and need to be considered when choosing a preservative.

1. *Definable in chemical terms*: Many of the existing preservatives, such as the quaternary ammonium compounds, are mixtures of various homologues. Often the activity obtained is a function of the mixture composition. Unless it is possible to define and control mixture composition, the performance of the agents will be variable, even if they conform to a pharmacopoeial specification.

2. *Broad spectrum of activity*: The compounds must possess a broad spectrum of antimicrobial activity against all species of microorganisms and also toward bacterial endospores. In practice, the only compounds that meet this requirement are formaldehyde, gluteraldehyde, hypochlorite, and ethylene oxide. All these compounds are highly irritant at sterilizing concentrations to be used in pharmaceutical products. Formaldehyde is, however, used at low concentrations in some shampoos; in these cases contact with the skin is short-lived and irritancy minimal. Agents such as quaternary ammonium compounds, phenolics, and the parabens group possess good activity against gram-positive bacteria but little or no activity toward spores. Certain gram-negative organisms such a *Pseudomonas aeruginosa* are virtually resistant to these agents. Generally, antifungal activity is difficult to obtain. Combinations of preservatives are sometimes employed to widen the spectrum of activity to include molds, bacteria, yeasts, and endospores.

3. *Effectiveness*: The compounds must be effective over a wide range of pH in order to be effective in all formulations. In practice, compounds are generally more active at either acid or alkaline pH. Thus, the pH of a formulation determines the types of preservative suitable for inclusion.

4. *Stability*: The compounds must be stable to light and elevated temperatures for the expected shelf life of the product. The effects of pH upon stability should be minimal. In this respect it is worth noting that the preservative Bronopol is stable only in the dark and at an acid pH. Under alkaline conditions or in the light it rapidly decomposes to give formaldehyde at concentrations that would be ineffective as a preservative. Instability to light can be protected against the packaging in a light-proof container. Storage tests must be performed on all formulations to ensure that adequate levels of preservative remain at the end of then expected shelf life of the product.

5. *Solubility*: Preservatives should ideally be used at concentrations much lower than that of the main constituents of the formulation. Their solubility ought to be such that it is possible to add them as a concentrated solution and where there is no danger of creating a saturated solution.

6. *Aesthetics*: Preservatives should have no perceptible odor, color, or taste, which might affect the aesthetic qualities of the final product. This can be of crucial importance for a cosmetic product but is less important for medical ones.

7. *Volatility*: Preservatives should be nonvolatile. Thus, chloroform is not an ideal preservative as it is lost from the formulation each time it is exposed to air.

8. *Product incompatibility*: Preservatives should not be incompatible with any of the likely excipients within the product formulation. This would include incompatibilities with the container material and also the active ingredients. In practice this is very difficult to achieve.

9. *Toxicity*: At the concentrations employed, the preservative should be nonirritant, not cause hypersensitivity reactions, and be nontoxic. In this respect, the site of application is critical. Relatively few compounds are approved for use in opthalmic products due to their high sensitivity towards xenobiotics. Also, compounds safe for use on intact skin might be hazardous for inclusion in parenteral products.

10. *Solubility in oil*: Preservatives must not be too oil soluble as this can produce problems in two- and three-phase systems where the preservative accumulates in the oil and micellar phases and is unavailable for antimicrobial action in the biological (aqueous) phase. It is worth noting that the oil:water partition coefficient can alter as a function of pH and also as a function of the nature of the oil.

11. *Cost*: The preservative must be cost-effective in the context of the overall product positioning (i.e., cost of goods ratio).

Although a very large number of antimicrobial compounds have been examined for their suitability for preservation of pharmaceuticals, only a few (<20) are currently used in the majority of pharmaceutical products. Moreover, in many cases, the "least unsuitable" rather than the "optimum" preservative is selected for a particular product.

DYNAMICS OF PRESERVATION

The critical lethal parameters of the effectiveness of antimicrobial agents are the concentrations of the agents employed, the time of exposure, the types and numbers of organisms exposed, the pH of the environment or formulation, and the temperature of application. An understanding of the effects of these conditions upon the killing process and of the terms that describe such dependence is important to rationalize the use of preservatives in different situations and formulations.

Time of Contact

When exposed to lethal concentrations of a chemical antimicrobial agent, the viability of a bacterial population decreases exponentially with time (Fig. 1). Such pseudo-first-order kinetics can be described by the equation

$$\frac{S}{S_0} = A\mathrm{e}^{-kt} \tag{1}$$

$$\log\frac{S}{S_0} = kt + \log A \tag{2}$$

where k is the rate constant, S is the number of surviving organisms at time t, and S_0 is the initial number of viable organisms within the population.

D-value is the time for 90% kill. That is,

$$\log S - \log S_0 = -1 \tag{3}$$

and

$$D\text{-value} = 1/k \tag{4}$$

In practice, such obedience to first-order kinetics is rare for chemical inactivation. More commonly, deviations from first-order kinetics are obtained, when there is either an initial lag in the rate of killing (Fig. 2A) or when the rate of killing decreases with time of exposure (Fig. 2B). The former is commonly observed when the concentrations of preservative are minimally bactericidal and reflects the time required for injuries caused to the bacterial cells to assume lethal proportions. Such plateauing therefore decreases as concentrations of agent employed become greater (Fig. 2A) and are inapparent at

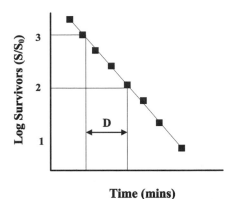

Fig. 1 Time survival kinetics for the inactivation of a bacterial population by treatment with a chemical agent. The D-value represents the time taken, at a given concentration of biocide, to reduce the surviving population by 90%.

very high concentrations. The second effect reflects the presence of resistant organisms within the population, capacity effects on the action of the preservative, or failure of the neutralizer. In such cases commonly observed with quaternary ammonium compounds and biguanides, the levels of kill at the plateau value increase with increasing concentration of preservative. From these relationships, an estimate of the initial rate of killing (k) or the D-value (actual time to effect a 90% reduction in viability) can be made, but their predictive value must be questioned.

Approximation to first-order kinetics implies that the sensitivity toward preservatives of a population of micro-organisms is normally distributed. Decreases in the rate of killing with time often results from adsorptive loss of the preservative onto and into the killed cells, causing a

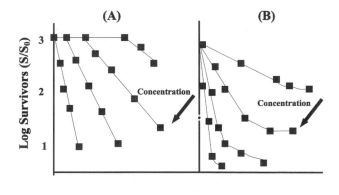

Fig. 2 Deviations from first-order kinetics of the inactivation of microbial populations by treatment with chemical agents due to (A) an initial lag in the rate of killing or (B) a decrease in the rate of killing with time of exposure.

decrease in the available concentration of the preservative for killing the surviving organisms. The susceptibility of preservatives to such adsorptive losses is described as its capacity.

Exponential decreases in viability with time mean that total elimination of all living cells cannot be guaranteed. Rather, knowing the initial size of the population and its susceptibility, the probability of having achieved sterility might be assigned to particular inactivation processes. Such assignments assume, often wrongly, that first-order kinetics are universally applicable.

Concentration of Preservative

The efficacy of an antimicrobial agent varies as a direct function of its concentration. At very low concentrations the antimicrobial effect might be negligible, at intermediate concentrations the effects might be growth-inhibitory, whereas only at relatively high concentrations might they be bactericidal. Often different mechanisms of action are involved to bring about these different effects. For example, chlorhexidene inhibits growth through direct effects upon respiratory enzymes and ATP synthesis, but kills through causing gross permeability changes to the bacterial cell envelope. The minimum growth inhibitory concentration (MIC) of an agent gives little or no information about its bactericidal activity, but might indicate weaknesses in the overall antimicrobial spectrum of activity. Minimum lethal concentrations can range from $2 \times$ MIC $- 20 \times$ MIC, dependent upon the antimicrobial substance and target organism. In the bactericidal range, the concentration exponent (η) describes the dependence of activity on concentration. This can be obtained as the slope of a graph of log D or k versus log concentration. Although these values vary slightly among organisms, they are fairly characteristic of compound groups and also often relate to mammalian toxicity. Thus, compounds with high concentration exponents more readily lose their biological activity when diluted upon parenteral administration than those with low exponents (Table 2).

The concentration exponent gives no indication as to the level of activity of a particular agent, It only indicates the degree of dependence of activity upon concentration. If the $\log_{10}$ of a death time is plotted against the $\log_{10}$ of the concentration, a straight line is usually obtained, the slope of which is the concentration exponent. Given the D-value for a single concentration and concentration exponent, it is possible to calculate (from Eq. 5) the activity at any other concentration. As different antimicrobial mechanisms are often involved in growth inhibition and killing, the use of concentration

Table 2 Some examples of preservative concentration exponents

Compound	Exponent
Organic mercurials	0.9–1.0
Iodine	0.9–1.0
Formaldehyde	1.0–1.1
Benzalkonium chloride	0.8–2.5
Bronopol	0.7–0.9
Parabens	2.5–3.0
Phenolics	4.0–9.9
Aliphatic alcohols	6.0–12.7

exponents to extrapolate MIC data to bactericidal situations should be avoided.

$$(\eta) = \frac{(\log DatC_2 - \log DatC_1)}{\log C_1 - \log C_2} \qquad (5)$$

The value of the concentration exponent also gives an indication of the susceptibility of the agent to inactivation by dilution and/or losses in activity through adsorption of the agent on organic debris or killed bacterial cells. The loss of an antimicrobial agent from solution in this manner relates to concentration in solution and absorptivity rather than to the inherent antimicrobial activity of the agent. The activity and concentration exponents of four hypothetical agents are described (Fig. 3). Agents A & B and C & D have similar concentration exponents

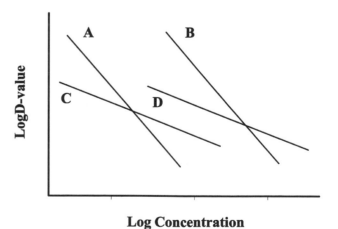

Log Concentration

Fig. 3 Comparisons of the activity and concentration exponents of four hypothetical preservatives. Agents A & B and C & D have similar concentration exponents but different activities, whereas A & C and B & D have similar activities yet different concentration exponents.

but different activities, whereas A & C and B & D have similar activities yet different concentration exponents.

If isotoxic concentrations of each agent (equivalent D-value) are employed, and undergo a uniform drop in concentration through adsorption, the compounds with the higher activity will undergo the greatest loss of activity (A & C > B & D). For compounds of similar activity, the one with the higher concentration exponent will have the greatest activity loss (A > C and B > D). This can be generalized in the statement that capacity is inversely related to both the concentration exponent and activity. Preservatives used in sterile products generally have high concentration exponents and high activity. Such considerations are also helpful in determining inactivation conditions for the preservatives prior to sterility and preservative effectiveness tests.

Temperature Effects

The rate of killing of an antimicrobial agent is directly dependent on the temperature of the interaction. This dependence is described by the temperature coefficient (Q or θ), which can be determined either from the slope of the graph relating the D-value or K and temperature, or from Eq. 6.

$$\text{Temp. Coefficient } [\theta_{t_1 - t_2}]$$
$$= \frac{D\text{-value } _{t_2(D_2)}}{D\text{-value } _{t_1(D_1)}} = \frac{kt_1}{kt_2} \tag{6}$$

The subscripts denote the temperature range over which the change in activity is defined. This is commonly given as the coefficient per 10°C rise (i.e., θ_{10} or Q_{10}), but is sometimes quoted for 1°C and 25°C changes.

Although the temperature coefficients vary a little between organisms, they are characteristic for particular preservative groups (Table 3). A high θ_{10} value renders a compound suitable for application at elevated temperatures but unsuitable for the preservation of formulations that might be stored over a wide temperature range.

It should be noted that the temperature will also affect the degree of ionization in some circumstances; therefore,

Table 3 Temperature coefficients (10°C) for some commonly used preservatives

Compound	θ_{10}
Aliphatic alcohols	30–50
Phenolics	3–5
Formaldehyde	1.5
Chlorocresol	6.0
Organic mercurials	1.0

the concentration exponent for some compounds will be apparently affected by temperature.

Effect of pH

The degree of ionization of acidic and basic antimicrobial agents depends on pH. Some compounds are active only in the unionized state (e.g., phenolics) whereas others are preferentially active as either the anion or cation. It therefore follows that the activity of a particular concentration of an agent will be enhanced at a pH that favors the formation of the active species. Thus, cationic antibacterials such as acridines and quaternary ammonium compounds are more active under alkaline conditions. Conversely, phenols and benzoic acid are more active in an acid medium. Chlorbutol is less active above pH 5 and unstable above pH 6. Phenylmercuric nitrate is only active at above pH 6 whereas thiomersal is more active under acid conditions. The sporicidal activity of glutaraldehyde is considerably enhanced under alkaline conditions whereas hypochlorites are virtually ineffective at above pH 8.

Knowledge of the pK_a of a preservative allows the calculation of the fraction undissociated at any particular pH and hence (via the concentration exponent) the level of activity at that pH.

$$\text{Fraction of undissociated biocide}$$
$$= \frac{1}{1} + \text{antilog } (pH - pK_a) \tag{7}$$

The pH also affects activity by altering the net surface charge on the microorganisms. Thus, as pH is decreased, the surface becomes less negative and adsorption and thereby activity of cationic agents is reduced. These effects are greater for gram-negative than gram-positive bacteria.

Presence of Interfering Substances

In most instances, before an antibacterial agent can act on a cell, they must first combine. The presence of other materials, commonly referred to as organic matter, may reduce the effect of such an agent by adsorbing or inactivating it and thus reducing the amount available for combining with target cells. Extraneous matter may be able to form a protective coat around the cell, thereby preventing the penetration of the active agent to its site of action.

PRESERVATIVE INTERACTIONS

Until the late 1930s, cosmetic and pharmaceutical formulations were stabilized with soaps. Although preservatives were often required, spoilage was only rarely a problem. With the advent of new materials for emulsion stabilization, preservation of the systems, or the lack of it, became a major problem. Nowadays we are aware of apparent incompatibilities between the new excipients and the established preservative agents and of the many interactions that can lead to preservative failure. No all-embracing set of rules have emerged to enable the "correct" preservative to be chosen for each formulation; only general guidelines exist.

The simplest form of interaction is one of adsorption/adsorption of the preservative from the formulation into and onto container and excipients. In this respect, it is convenient to divide these into colloidal excipients, suspensions, metal ions, and polymers.

Colloids

- *Gums*: Tragacanth, acacia, and plant polysaccharides such as agar and alginates are generally anionic in nature and will adsorb cationic preservatives such as chlorbutol, benzalkonium chloride, substituted phenols, phenylmercuric acetate, and merthiolates. Generally the adsorptive process increases with the increase in concentration of the gum or polysaccharide. Colloidal solutions of tragacanth and acacia, but not agar or alginates, can often be preserved with cationic agents by increasing the concentration of the preservative to saturate the colloid. For preservatives such as parabens, the problem is exacerbated at alkaline pH when the preservative becomes fully ionized.
- *Starches*: These bind substituted phenols but this can be overcome by increasing the concentration of the phenolic. Gelatin shows a slight interaction with the parabens group.
- *Proteins*: These interact both with cationic and anionic preservatives depending on to the pH of the formulation and the net charge of the protein.

- *Nonionic surfactants*: Interactions with a range of preservatives are unpredictable. Cationic and anionic surfactants interact and are contraindicated with anionic and cationic preservatives respectively.
- *Polyethylene glycols*: These interact particularly with the phenolic group of preservatives. The interaction increases with increase in molecular weight of the polymer. With increasing temperature, the extent of binding increases due to thermal desolving of the polymer and the creation of further binding sites.

Suspending Agents

These include clays, bentonite, kaolin, and talcs. They are generally anionic in nature and interact with most cationic agents. Inactivation depends on the pH of the system. Preservatives are only loosely associated with clays and therefore, desorb on dilution. The extent of these interactions are difficult to predict.

Container Materials

Nylon strongly adsorbs phenols and sorbic acid by covalent linkage. The degree of interaction depends on the pH, nature of the solvent, temperature, contact time, surface area, preservative concentration, and thickness of the nylon.

Acrylates and polyethylene affect most preservatives, including organic mercurials, phenolics, and benzoic acids. Leaching of hydroxyl ions from glass raises the pH and indirectly affects preservative activity. In this respect, glass must pass a "limit-test" for alkalinity.

Changing the container of a product from glass to plastic can alter its preservation. The container is as much a part of the formulation as is the product that is placed in it. Equally, adsorption and absorption into rubber closures can be significant, as exemplified by the phenolics (Table 4).

Table 4 Loss of preservative through absorption into rubber caps

Preservative	Initial concentration (% w/v)	Final concentration (% w/v)	Percentage loss
Phenol	0.5	0.39	22
Cresol	0.3	0.21	30
Chlorocresol	0.1	0.04	60
Phenyl mercuric nitrate	0.001	0.00005	95

PRESERVATION OF TWO-PHASE SYSTEMS

When preservatives are added to two-phase oil–water systems, depending upon the hydrophilicity of the agent, they partition between the two phases. Bacteria will only grow within the aqueous phase or at the oil–water interface. Thus, preservative lost to the oil is unavailable for antibacterial action. Hence the concentration in the water phase is reduced, affecting the rate of kill, but the capacity of the system is unaffected as preservative lost by adsorption onto organic debris and bacteria is replaced from that held in the oil.

The distribution between the oil and water phases is easily predicted from the oil–water partition coefficient, K_w^0 (Eq. 8)

$$K_w^0 = \frac{\text{Concentration in oil}}{\text{Concentration in water}} \qquad (8)$$

By knowing the concentration of preservative required for the necessary biological effect in the aqueous phase (C_W), the oil: water phase ratio (θ) and the K_w^0 for the system, C, the concentration needed in the formulation, may be calculated from the expression

$$C_W = \frac{C(\theta + 1)}{K_w^0 \theta + 1} \qquad (9)$$

It is also worth noting that altering the nature of the oil can affect partition coefficients quite dramatically, for example, the differences between vegetable and mineral oils (Table 5).

If the preservative favors the oil, increasing the oil: water ratio dramatically decreases available concentration; if it favors the aqueous phase, the reverse occurs and can cause solubility problems. Unfortunately, both temperature and pH also affect K_w^0, in addition to the effects of pH directly on the activity of the preservative.

Table 5 Partition data for various preservatives

Preservative	K_w^0	
	Mineral oil	**Vegetable oil**
Chlorocresol	0.5	11.7
Methyl parabens	0.02	7.5
Propyl parabens	0.5	80.0
Butyl parabens	3.0	280.0
Cetrimide USP	<1.0	<1.0
Bronopol	0.043	0.11
Phenonip	>1.0	>1.0
Phenyl mercuric nutrate	<1.0	<1.0

PRESERVATION OF THREE-PHASE SYSTEMS

Most oil–water systems contain surfactants as emulgens in order to provide a stable emulsion. Some preservatives may associate directly with the surfactants whereas others may partition into the micellar phase of the surfactant, treating it as a third phase for partitioning.

These effects can be calculated to some extent, where C_W depends not only on K_w^0 but also on surfactant concentration. Initially it is assumed that the surfactant micelles form part of the aqueous phase. Thus, if K_w^0 is the oil:aqueous phase partition coefficient and C_A the total aqueous concentration, then, as in Eq. 9,

$$C_A = \frac{C(\theta + 1)}{K_A^0 \theta + 1} \qquad (10)$$

Now

$$C_W = \frac{C_A}{R}$$

where

$$R = C_A/C_W \text{ that is } C_A = RC_W.$$

As

$$K_w^0 = C_A/C_W \text{ and } C_0 = K_w^0 C_W,$$

substitution in Eq. 9 gives

$$C_A^W = \frac{C(\theta + 1)}{C_0/C_A^{\theta + 1}} \qquad (11)$$

and substituting once again for C_0,

$$C_A = \frac{C(\theta + 1)}{(K_W^0 \frac{C_W}{C_A \theta} + 1)} \qquad (12)$$

Substituting in Eq. 12 for $C_A = RC_W$ gives

$$RC_W = \frac{C(\theta + 1)}{(K_W^0 C_W/RC_W \theta) + 1} \qquad (13)$$

which then reduces to

$$C_W = \frac{C(\theta + 1)}{[K_W^0 \theta + R]} \qquad (14)$$

Eq. 14 allows the active concentration in the water phase to be calculated from C, the phase ratio (θ), K_w^0 and R. This is useful as K_A^0 varies with the concentration of the surfactant. R can be found from a graph relating

C_A/C_W and surfactant concentration, where the slope of the line is k.

$$R = 1 + k[\text{surfactant concentration}]$$

All preservative manufacturers provide values of k for a range of surfactants.

TOXICITY AND SAFETY CONSIDERATIONS

There are certain limitations on the use of antimicrobial preservatives based on their toxicity and potential side effects. The British Pharmacopoeia recommends that the maximum quantity of an injection containing an antimicrobial preservative to be administered at a single occasion is 15 ml. The USP, on the other hand, recommends a maximum of 5 ml. These maximum volumes must be considered when toxicity data and concentrations of the agents included in the formulations are considered. The final concentration of any substance employed is a balance between its potential toxicity and antimicrobial activity. Additionally, because meninges are readily irritated, the inclusion of antimicrobial preservatives in any formulation that might gain access to the cerebrospinal fluid is precluded. Intracardiac and intraarterial injections must also not contain an antimicrobial preservative.

It is not surprising that preservatives sometimes prove toxic to humans. To assess the toxicity of any substance, it is necessary to know its acute and cumulative toxicity together with its "no effects levels" and also to be aware of its mutagenic, teratogenic, and carcinogenic potential. In addition, its local actions as well as its liability to cause hypersensitization might be important. Any new preservative must be subjected to a battery of such mandatory tests to provide these data as must a new application of an established biocide.

ACUTE TOXICITY

Preservatives, for the most part, are used at very low concentrations and the question of their acute toxicity rarely arises. The margin of safety is not always very high, however.

SUBACUTE AND CHRONIC TOXICITY

When substances are given repeatedly, manifestations of toxicity may differ, particularly if the compound is given at a rate faster than what the individual can detoxify or excrete. Some preservatives contain mercury and this may accumulate in the body.

REPRODUCTIVE TOXICITY

As part of the general safety testing of all preservatives, consideration is give to possible effects in higher animals on the fertility of either sex, the gestation or postnatal care, and development of the embryo. No direct causal relationships have been shown between any of the commonly used preservatives and reproductive toxicity. However, indirect reproductive toxicity has been suggested, for example, benzoic acid as a preservative, increases blood salicylate levels, and may cause a significant increase in the teratogenic potential of aspirin. Organic mercury has been shown to be responsible for a congenital form of Minimata disease, but not at levels likely to be taken into the body through mercury-containing preservatives.

CARCINOGENICITY AND MUTAGENICITY

Several preservatives have been scrutinized for being possible carcinogens, and their use regulated (e.g., chloroform and formaldehyde). Another possibility is that the preservative interacts with amines or amides to form carcinogenic nitrosamines. Published data on the mutagenicity of preservatives is limited as tests such as the Ames test can only be carried out at concentrations far less than those employed.

PRESERVATIVE COMBINATIONS

The ideal properties expected from preservatives are not met by any of the current, established agents. All chemical agents have their limitations in terms of their antimicrobial activity, resistance to organic matter, stability, incompatibility, irritancy, or toxicity. It is also unlikely that new preservatives will be developed because of high costs of putting a new compound through toxicity tests and the likelihood of a new compound being impossible to cover by patent. More likely preservative combinations will be employed in the future, possibly to give synergistic combinations (e.g., hydrogen peroxide and peroxygen compounds, chlorhexidine and cetrimide). In this manner,

Table 6   Examples of interactions between preservatives

Preservative A	Preservative B		
	Synergistic	Additive	Antagonistic
Benzalkonium	Phenylmercurics	3-Cresol	Hexachlorophane
Benzoic acid	Dehydroacetic acid	Parabens	Boric acids
Bronopol	Benzalkonium	Sorbic acid	—
Chlorbutanol	Phenylethanol	—	EDTA, EGTA
Chlorocresol	Phenylethanol	—	—
Phenylmercurics	3-Cresol	—	—
Parabens	Germall	Benzoic acid	Boric acid
Sorbic acid	Dehydroacetic acid	Benzoic Acid	Parabens

preservative combinations may be used to extend the range and spectrum of preservation (Table 6); for example, by combining a series of alkyl esters of 4-hydroxybenzoic acid, water solubility is decreased to such an extent that both the aqueous and oil phase of an emulsion are protected.

When acting simultaneously on a microbial population, combinations of preservatives may cause an increased, decreased, or unchanged antimicrobial response when compared with their summed individual effects. A minimum requirement of any combination should be that it achieves at least the same level of protection overall as the individual components do. Ill-considered preservative combinations may lead to inclusion of irrelevant agents. In general, agents from the same chemical group or those having the same mode of action are likely to produce merely additive efects whereas those exhibiting different mechanisms or sites of action may serve either to reinforce (synergize) or reduce (antagonize) their individual activities. Such effects may be evaluated by preparing mixtures of the two preservatives being investigated and determining their growth inhibitory power by an MIC determination. Results may then be plotted in the form of a graph, termed an isobologram, an example of which is shown in Fig. 4.

In general, synergistic effects can occur through three different mechanisms. The first mechanism is by inhibition of inactivation. Here, one compound increases the effective concentration of the other by inhibiting the microbial system responsible for its inactivation. To date, however, there are no reported observations of this mechanism with preservatives. The second synergistic mechanism is very common amongst preservatives and occurs when one compound increases the accessibility of targets to another. This usually occurs when one agent exerts its action by increasing the permeability of the cell wall or cell membrane. Besides damaging the cell in its own right, this can permit access (or increased access) of the second compound to targets that were previously concealed. An example of this type of synergy is seen in the cooperative action between benzalkonium chloride and thiomersal which disrupts the cytoplasmic membrane, thereby facilitating access of organomercurial agents that react with sulphydryl-containing enzymes in the cytoplasm. This type of synergy does not necessary require

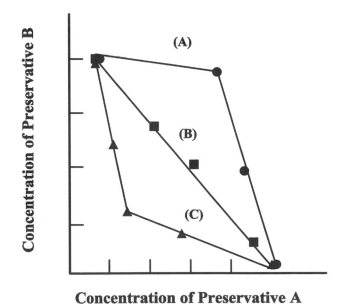

Fig. 4 Isobologram showing three possible outcomes of interaction between preservatives A and B, namely (A) antagonism, (B) additivity, and (C) synergy.

both compounds to possess significant antimicrobial activity. Finally, perhaps the broadest category of synergistic interactions is that in which two compounds act simultaneously at different targets, thereby significantly influencing the biochemistry of the cell. Although these targets must be different in order to produce synergy, they can be closely related. For example, the synergy between chlorocresol and 2-phenylethanol is thought to be through their respective effects on the generation and coupling of a proton gradient to active transport.

There are many significant practical benefits and advantages of preservative combinations. These include an increased spectrum of activity; the need for lower concentrations of each of the individual components, thereby possibly reducing potential toxicity; the prevention of resistance to individual preservatives; possible enhancement of antimicrobial activity beyond that expected by simple addition; an extended time course of preservation achieved by combining a labile, markedly biocidal preservative with a stable longer-acting ingredient. Furthermore, careful selection of individual agents for combination, based on their physicochemical properties, may serve to overcome microbiological problems created by the physical limitations of individual preservatives. In this respect, factors affecting preservative efficacy must be carefully considered.

PROCESS CHEMISTRY IN THE PHARMACEUTICAL INDUSTRY

Kumar G. Gadamasetti

ChemRx Advanced Technologies, Inc., San Francisco, California

Ambarish K. Singh

The Bristol-Myers Squibb Pharmaceutical Research Institute, New Brunswick, New Jersey

INTRODUCTION

In the pharmaceutical industry, identification of a development drug candidate (preclinical lead profile, PLP, or early candidate notification, ECN), filing of investigational new drug application (IND), and new drug application (NDA) are important milestones before the launch of a new drug. The IND and the NDA are the events where the industry interacts with the Food and Drug Administration (FDA) prior to launching. Various governmental departments play specific roles in furthering drug development programs. The medicinal or discovery chemists identify the new drug candidates to treat or prevent a particular medical indication, whereas the process chemists are responsible for devising a synthesis and supplying the active pharmaceutical ingredient (API) or bulk drug substance (BDS) in multigram quantities for various studies needed to file the IND and support other drug development programs. On approval of the IND, the compound can be administered to humans for the first time as part of the phase-I clinical studies, also known as first-in-man (FIM) trials. Studies that are reported in an IND include synthesis, animal toxicology, pharmaceutics and formulation, drug substance and drug product stability and safety, and metabolic and pharmacokinetics.

The clinical development is the most expensive and resource-intensive segment of the process. Process research and development play a key role in shortening the overall timeline from candidate identification to drug launch. On an average, it takes about 10–15 years from discovery to launch a drug into the market at a cost in excess of $400 million. The paradigm shift (in the 1990s) of increasing the number of compounds entering development has made a tremendous impact on chemists responsible for preparing supplies of these new drug candidates. Early and effective interaction of process research personnel with medicinal chemists and early innovations in process development are believed to shorten the IND and NDA timelines, respectively. These overall reduced timelines would allow for an early launch of the drug into the market (1).

PHARMACEUTICAL DRUG DEVELOPMENT EVENTS: THE CHEMIST'S VIEWPOINT

A simplified view of the pharmaceutical drug development events (not to the timescale) is given in Fig. 1.

Genomics to Lead Development Candidate (PLP)

During the past decade, the pharmaceutical industry has seen a paradigm shift in the drug discovery process. The driving force for such change, arguably, was propelled by a variety of factors, including

- Generation of new targets (for human diseases) from advances in genomics and functional genomics.
- Advances in combinatorial chemistry methods to increase the number of compounds for high throughput screening (HTS), and
- Advances in automation and high-throughput screening techniques for rapid identification of lead compounds.

Although these approaches promise to provide an increased number of novel drug candidates for evaluation in the treatment of a greater number of diverse diseases, successful realization of the potential benefit of these compounds is very much dependent on the ability of the pharmaceutical industry to develop suitable manufacturing processes.

PLP Development Candidate to IND and the Kilo Lab

The IND studies require relatively large amounts of the drug substance, substantially more than what was prepared during the course of the medicinal chemistry programs. Generally, it becomes the responsibility of the process research group to produce this material within the shortest feasible time frame (2). Most of the major pharmaceutical companies have kilo-lab facilities as an interface between the process research labs and the pilot plants. Pharmaceutical process groups are organized in different ways. In some companies, process research is responsible for

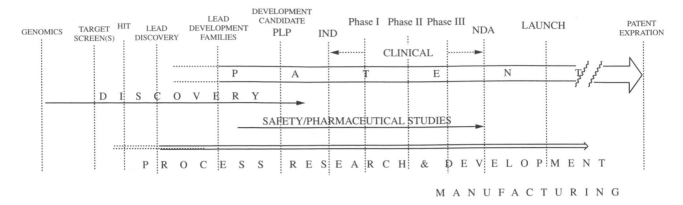

Fig. 1 Pharmaceutical drug development events, a simplified view. *Preclinical*: Medicinal chemistry, combinatorial chemistry, process research. *Clinical*: Process R&D & manufacturing (operations).

providing the supplies of BDS required for an IND filing, including the initial clinical batch (or batches). Typically, the initial supplies are prepared by the combination of modified medicinal chemistry synthesis and new, alternative synthetic processes more suitable for scale-up. In some companies, the chemists in process research labs and kilo labs share this responsibility. Kilo-lab scale-up work typically is performed in 22-L glassware and small reactors (50–100 L). The process development group, on the other hand, is responsible for further optimization and scale-up in the pilot plant and interfaces with the manufacturing.

Clinical Phase, NDA, and Launching of the Drug

The clinical phase (phase I) of the drug development begins after the IND where humans are subjected to the clinical trials. After a successful phase-I trial, efficacy of the drug is tested on a large number of patients as part of the phase-II/III clinical trials. Once the phase-II/III clinical trials are completed, the NDA is filed with the FDA. Clinical trials and NDA are prerequisites for launching the drug.

PROCESS RESEARCH AND DEVELOPMENT

The goal of the medicinal or drug discovery chemist is to identify a new lead to treat or prevent some particular medical indication and define a synthetic strategy to allow for the preparation of as many analogs as possible. The focus of process chemistry differs from routine organic chemistry. It emphasizes optimization and defines the controls to make the sequence of chemical reactions amenable to scale-up. A viable process should reliably yield

a high-purity product made by a process unencumbered by a patent. In short, the overall thrust of the scientists engaged in process chemistry is to develop the shortest, least expensive, safest, and most environmentally friendly processes to produce the API in multi-kilogram quantities.

The term "process" is, in general, misinterpreted as scale-up work by the overwhelming majority of the scientists and technologists involved with drug discovery and development programs in the pharmaceutical industry. Scientists and engineers engaged in the various aspects of pharmaceutical process research and development have a highly refined appreciation for the challenges of large-scale synthesis and the purification of the API. An algorithm for process research and development is shown in Fig. 2.

The mission of process chemistry in the pharmaceutical industry is to provide documented, controlled synthetic processes for the manufacture of the supplies to support the development programs and future commercial requirements of the API. The science and technology associated in accomplishing this mission provide a tremendous challenge to the individuals or the group of individuals for the drug supply progress from milligram to metric ton quantities.

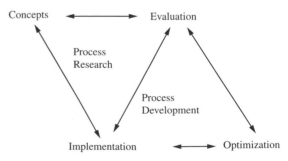

Fig. 2 Algorithm for process research and development.

Route Scouting

As the development drug candidate moves from discovery to process, a workable synthesis is available, which, however, may not be scalable. Route scouting plays a key role in identifying synthetic transformations that are safe, practical, scalable, cost effective, and environmentally friendly, thus setting the stage for eventually delivering a manufacturing synthetic process. An integral part of route scouting is to identify key intermediates that could be easily outsourced.

An example of route scouting and process improvements

Scheme 1 depicts the medicinal chemistry approach to the synthesis of BMS-180291 (Ifetroban).

A condensed schematic of the overall alternative synthesis of BMS-180291 (Ifetroban) is provided in Scheme 2.

The synthesis of the key acid ester intermediate A has been reduced dramatically from 16 to 4 steps, and the yield has been increased 10-fold from 5 to 52%. The overall synthesis of Ifetroban has been cut virtually in half (from 23 to 12 steps) and the yield (via the longest linear sequence) improved from 3 to 28%.

Process Development and Optimization

Human safety is the first priority when developing a process, followed by quality (purity, crystallinity of the product, etc.) and product yield. In addition, the process chemist takes into account the following factors:

- Hazards associated with the chemical step (human and equipment safety).
- Waste generated (disposal cost, environmental concerns).

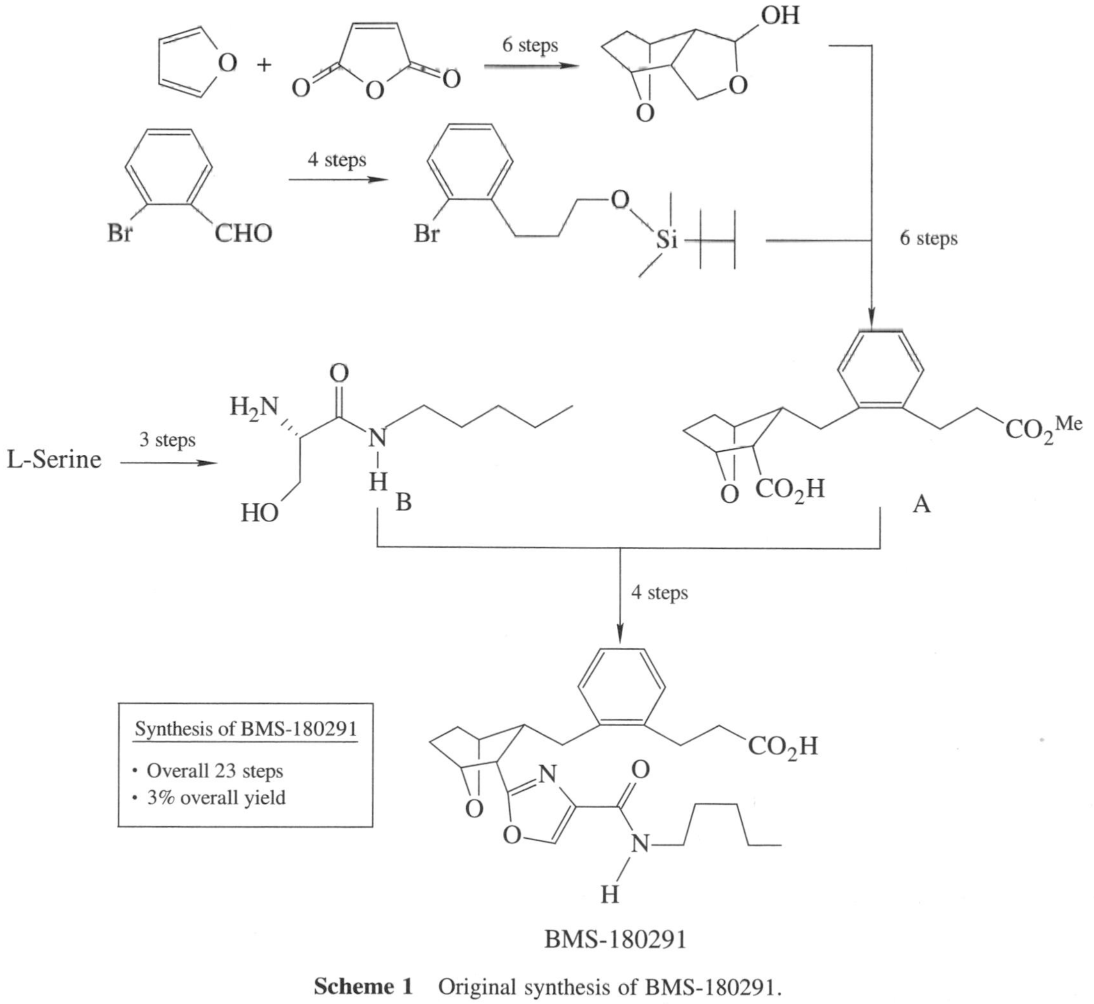

Synthesis of BMS-180291
- Overall 23 steps
- 3% overall yield

BMS-180291

Scheme 1 Original synthesis of BMS-180291.

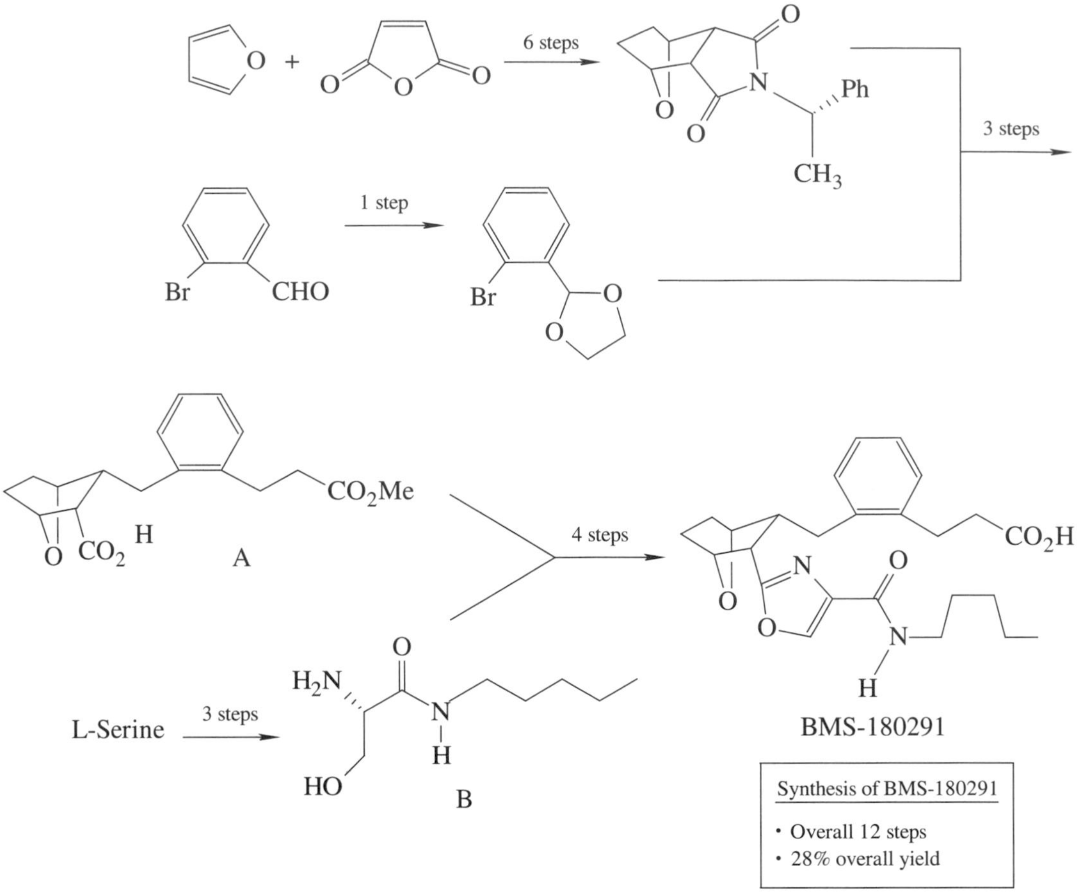

Scheme 2   Alternative synthesis of BMS-180291.

- Cost and availability of raw materials, reagents, and solvents (cost of goods, sourcing issues).
- Ease of performing the reaction on-scale (savings in capital and labor).
- Ease of product isolation (crystallization), and
- Opportunity to combine two or more chemical steps with no intermediate isolation (telescoping to increase throughput).

Once a route has been selected, the next step is to understand the effect of interactions of variables with each other on the reaction yield and quality for each and every step of the synthetic scheme and to define the limits for these process variables. This requires designing appropriate experiments including controls. This is important because as the scale of the reaction increases, every unit operation, such as addition of reagents, solvents, distillation, phase splits, etc., takes a considerably longer time. Mixing begins to play a major role as the size of the vessel increases. Due to uneven mixing, localized differences in variables such as temperature and

concentration are expected, which may have an adverse effect on the reaction.

Example 1: Process development of BMS-182205 (Scheme 3)

Issues: environmental concerns, human safety, waste management, process inefficiency.

The first step in the synthesis of the Paclitaxel® side chain has been reported in the literature by Holton (4). The drawbacks of this procedure from a process development standpoint are

1. The use of benzene and dichloromethane (human and environmental concerns).
2. No opportunity for telescoping (since the first reaction is conducted in benzene and the second in dichloromethane).
3. Low yield (68% after crystallization from ethylacetate and hexane), and
4. Brown-black product (color).

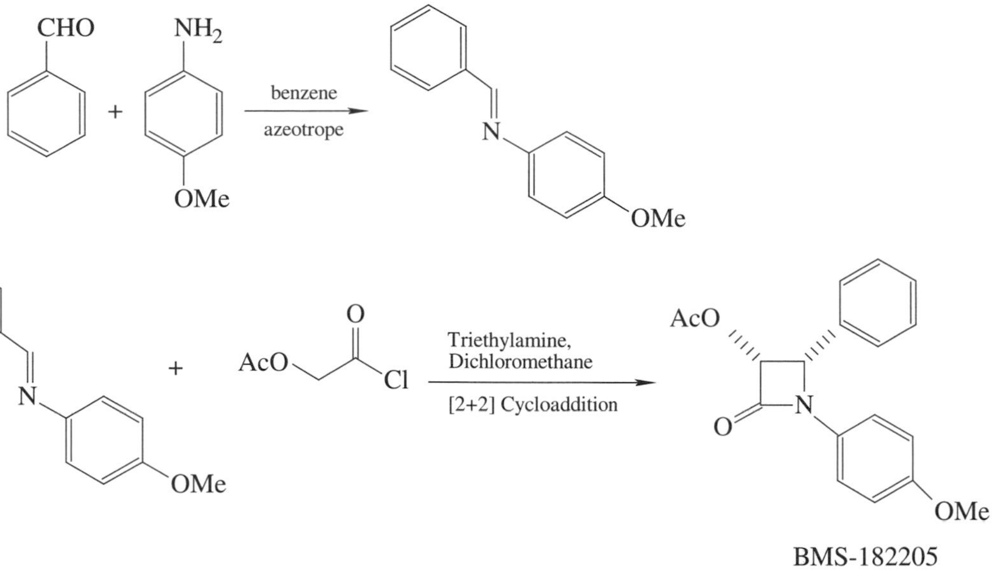

Scheme 3 Synthesis of BMS-182205.

Process improvements: *Phase I.* Benzene was replaced with a safer solvent, toluene, which was also used for the [2 + 2] cycloaddition reaction, thus facilitating the telescoping of the two reactions. However, dichloromethane was added during the work-up to prevent product precipitation. The product was crystallized from 2-propanol in 80% yield. The phase I of development eliminated the use of benzene and allowed for telescoping of the two chemical steps. However, a solvent exchange from toluene–dichloromethane to 2-propanol was still needed to crystallize the product. The color of the product after this modification was dark brown.

Phase II. Additional crystallization studies revealed that the product could be crystallized from toluene–heptane and acetone–water. The product also exhibited limited solubility in toluene. With this information at hand, both reactions were conducted in toluene as before; however, during the work-up, dichloromethane was not added. Instead, aqueous hydrochloric acid was added to neutralize excess triethylamine. Heptane was then added to precipitate the product directly from the reaction mixture. The crude wet product was crystallized from acetone–water with an overall yield of 80%. The color of the product was brown. The advantages of this modification are the elimination of several extraction and back-extraction steps and a reduction in processing time and in solvent consumption.

In an attempt to further improve the yield and address the product color issue, the following process variables were studied: the rate of addition of acetoxyacetyl chloride, the reaction temperature, and the effect of other amine bases.

The rate of addition of acetoxyacetyl chloride was optimized to be 2–3 h, at 3, 10, and 17°C. Reactions conducted at 3°C afforded the product with the highest quality. Two amines, N-methylmorpholine (NMM) and diisopropylethylamine (DIPEA), were evaluated in addition to triethylamine. In the presence of NMM, the reaction stopped after 65% conversion. In triethylamine the reaction took an additional 3 h for completion, after the addition of acetoxyacetyl chloride. However, in DIPEA, the reaction was instantaneous, the yield was further improved to 87%, and the product was free of brown-colored impurities.

Example 2: Process development of Ifetroban (Scheme 4)

Issues: environmental concerns, human safety, cost of goods (5).

In the improved synthesis of Ifetroban described previously, environmental concerns due to special handling of copper bromide waste and hazards associated with hexamethylene tetramine (HMT) on manufacturing scale led to further perfection of the synthesis. Mechanistic considerations suggested that an oxidized form of aminoamide *B* (Scheme 4) would eliminate the necessity for a late-stage copper-mediated oxidation. This was indeed accomplished. The cyclization–elimination sequence was initiated by a Lewis acid and completed by base-mediated elimination to afford the Ifetroban penultimate. In addition to eliminating the need for copper bromide and HMT, this modification helped to reduce the cost of the product by an additional 15%.

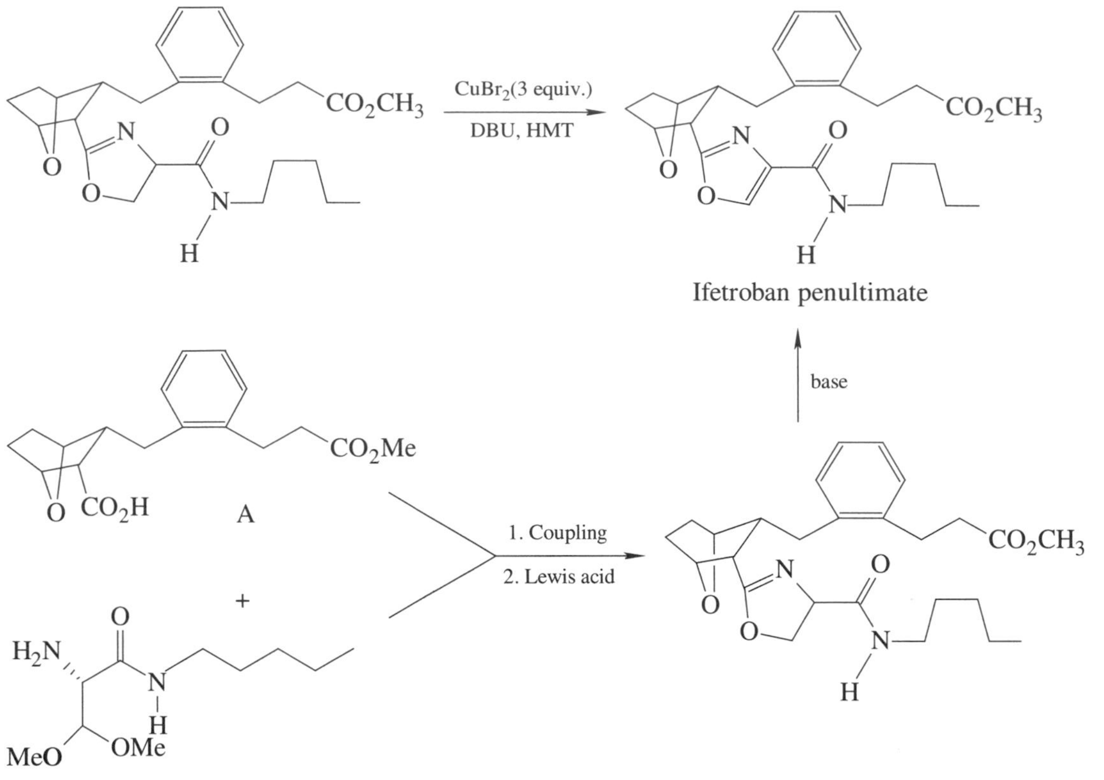

Scheme 4   Process development of Ifetroban.

Manufacturing process, route from medicinal chemistry to multi-kilos for clinical study supplies: A highly optimized and concise large-scale synthesis of a purine bronchodilator was developed by the Astra Production Chemical company from Sweden (6). Supplies for the initial biological studies were generated by the medicinal chemistry route shown in Scheme 5. The overall yield was about 14%, which was improved in the environmentally friendly manufacturing process to about 51% (Schemes 6 and 7).

Process Hazards and Safety

Process safety has become an integral part of the development of new synthetic routes, and more and more relevant information is gathered in typical process development labs (7). Many development facilities have now established special process safety departments with state-of-the-art equipment and well-trained personnel. It is important for process chemists considering alternative process routes to know the potential hazards from the main reaction and from the unwanted side reactions in each case so that the hazards of reactivity are included in the factors

reviewed in developing and selecting the final process route; three main parameters determine the design of safe chemical processes:

1. The potential energy of the chemicals involved and understanding of the inherent energy (exothermic release or endothermic absorption) during a chemical reaction.
2. The rates of reaction (energy release in the form of heat or pressure) that depend on the temperature, pressure, and concentrations. In any hazard evaluation process, the rates of reaction during normal and abnormal operations (including the worst credible case) must be considered in order to design an inherently safe process.
3. An equipment train must adequately remove any heat or pressure generated in a reaction. The effects and requirements of scale-up must be considered.

In most cases, a team of development chemists, engineers, and safety personnel evaluate and assess hazards associated with each and every step of a process, from performing a reaction to storage of waste streams in drums. The team recommends a set of safety experiments to be conducted, and data are collected for reaction

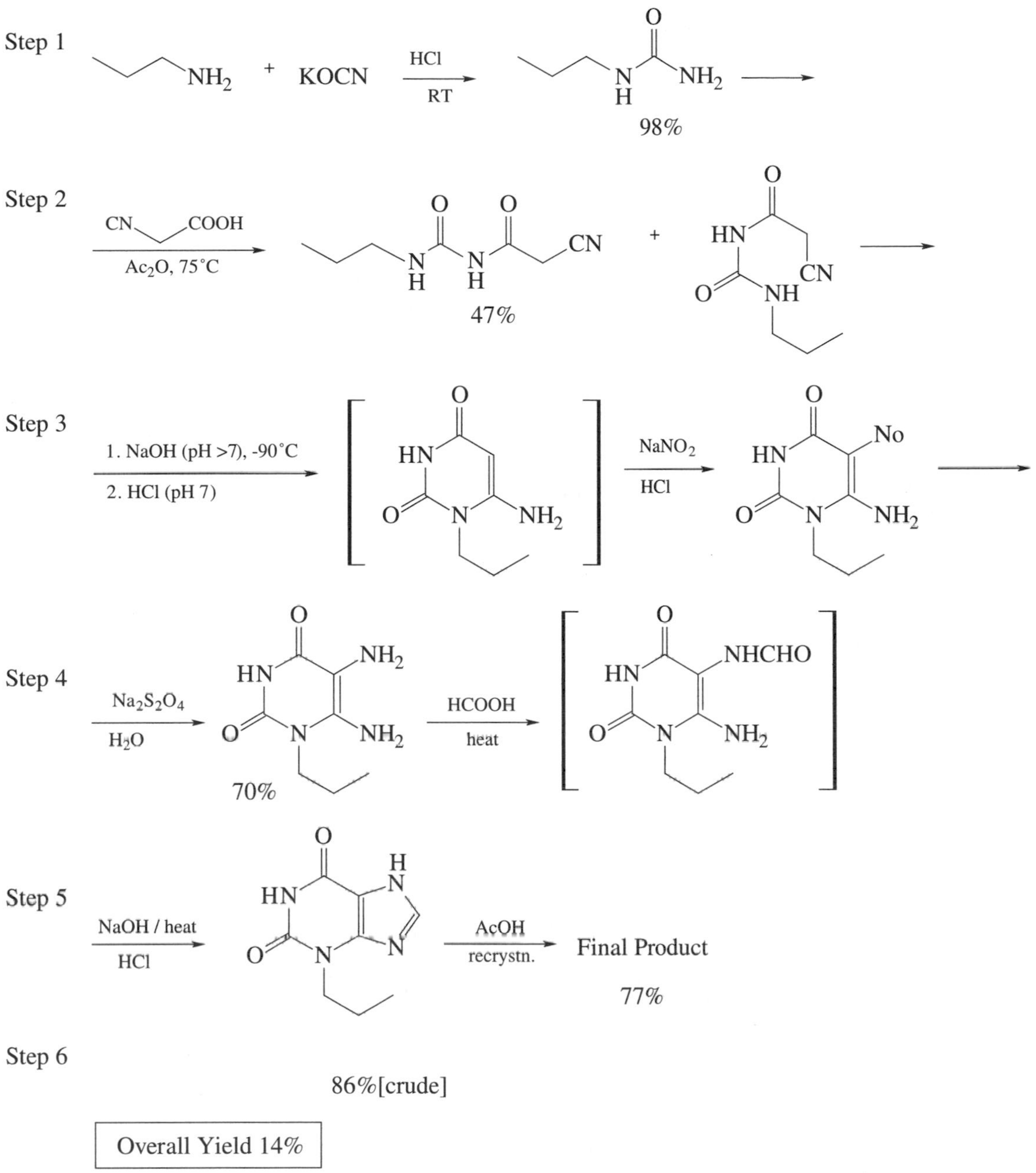

Step 1

98%

Step 2

47%

Step 3

Step 4

70%

Step 5

Final Product

77%

Step 6

86%[crude]

Overall Yield 14%

Scheme 5 Original synthesis of enprophylline by the medicinal chemistry department at Astra.

exotherms, powder explosivity, gas evolution, and compatibility of reaction mixtures or reaction waste with pilot-plant equipment and storage drums. Experiments are designed and conducted to determine the potential for initiation of a runaway reaction and the effect of decompositions that may occur on runaway. Based on the safety assessment of a process, appropriate measures are taken in the pilot plant to eliminate or minimize any hazard. During the early stages of process research (route

scouting), only small amounts of materials are available. In many cases, only theoretical information from the literature or from calculations is readily available. Screening tests can be run to identify the reaction hazards. As the route-scouting efforts enter the process development phase, additional material becomes available so that the reaction hazards can be studied more extensively to test "what-if" scenarios. During full-scale production, the chemical hazards may be reevaluated to address changed

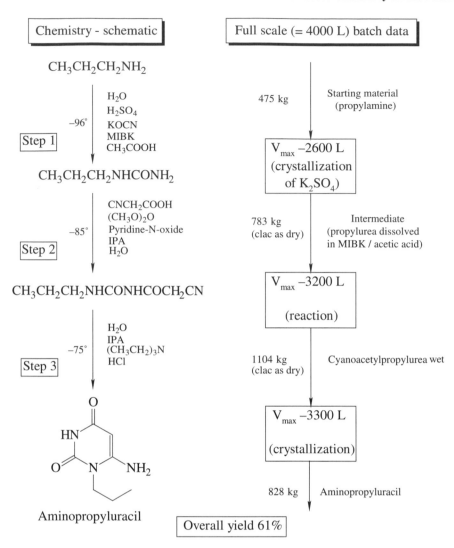

Scheme 6   Astra commercial process of 6-amino-1-propyluracil.

production requirements or other process changes such as the use of a different source of raw materials.

Numereous test methods are available using a variety of sample sizes and conditions. The tests provide qualitative or quantitative data on onset of temperature, reaction enthalpy, instantaneous heat production as a function of temperature, maximum temperature, and/or pressure excursions as a consequence of a runaway, and additional data useful for process design and operation.

"Green Chemistry": Environmental Concerns

The research that involves the end-of-process treatments to eliminate pollutants is termed "green chemistry." As Ronald Breslow (Columbia University) pointed out (8), concern for the environment is as old as the biblical injunction, "hurt not the earth, neither the sea, nor

the trees." The following example indicates approaches to the environmentally benign chemistry. The process described is high yielding with water as the by-product. Sato et al. (9) have developed an efficient, environmentally friendly method for oxidizing primary and secondary alcohols (Scheme 8). The Japanese scientists use hydrogen peroxide as an oxidant, a quaternary ammonium hydrogen sulfate as a phase-transfer agent, and tungsten as catalyst.

Enzymatic Intervention

The recent trend in pharmaceutical industries is to incorporate a microbial technology (MT) or enzymatic technology division in the process R&D and manufacturing (need basis) departments. The role of the MT division is usually to provide pharmaceutical drugs

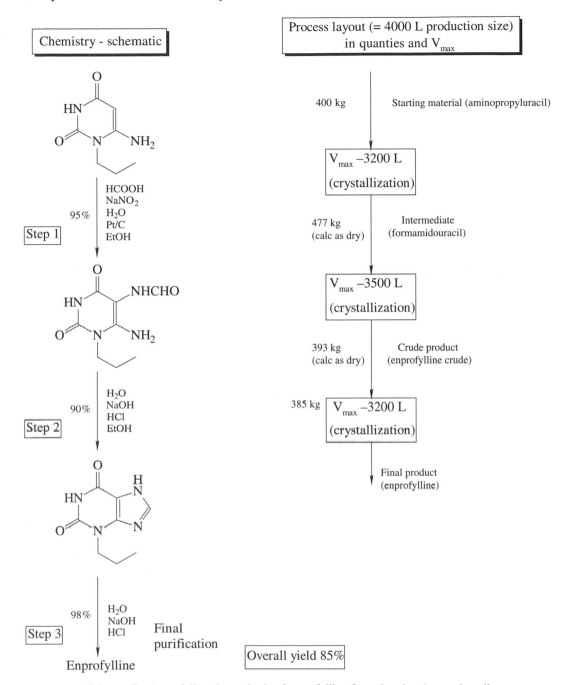

Scheme 7 Astra full-scale synthesis of enprofylline from 6-amino-1-propyluracil.

(e.g., pravastatin, β-lactam drugs, etc.), and chiral (optically pure) building blocks or synthons for the ongoing synthetic programs.

A number of cholesterol-lowering drugs (Pravachol, Zocor, and Mevacor) are prepared by enzymatic processes. Penicillin antibiotics that have been in the market for decades are produced in large quantities by the enzymatic process.

Enzymatic catalysis

The extensive use of enzymatic catalysts in organic synthesis has been documented (10–13). Enzymes represent a broad range of efficient chemical catalysts. They are classified mainly into six categories:

1. Hydrolases (hydrolysis of amides, esters, glycosides, and lactones)

2. Isomerases (C—C bond migration, E/Z isomerization, and racemization)
3. Lyases (addition to π-bonds)
4. Oxidoreductases (reversible oxidations and reductions)
5. Synthetase formation and breaking of C—C, C—N, C—O, C—S, and phosphate ester bonds
6. Transferases (transfer of acyl, glycosyl, or phosphoryl groups from one molecule to another)

Scheme 9 gives three examples.

Design of Experiments (DOE)

An understanding of how various process variables affect the chemistry is necessary for the design of a chemical process (14) that can reliably provide the product in high yield and quality. This understanding can be obtained from experimentally determined rate laws for the main and side reactions that relate temperature, concentration, pressure, solvent effects, and equivalents of each reagent to yield and impurity levels. The process chemist may take the approach of evaluating the importance of process variables by changing one variable at a time. This method can help generate chemical knowledge but is not efficient and does not easily provide the quantitative information needed to rank the importance of process variables. Furthermore, the process chemist is often faced with a task of quickly scaling up the synthesis without the benefit of completely understanding the mechanism of the chemistry involved. With the aid of statistical design approach, a great deal of

useful information can be obtained with relatively few experiments. Statistical approaches involving factorial designs are ideal for studying processes where the underlying principles are not well developed or are extremely complicated.

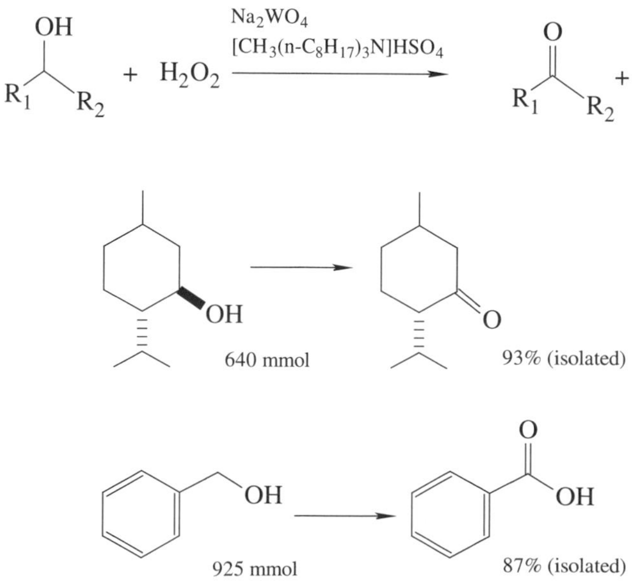

Factorial experiments consists of a systematic variation of two or more process variables at a time. For a two-level experiment, each variable is set to a high or a low value according to a standard pattern. An experimental run is conducted for each possible combination of variable settings. Selection of the low and high levels for each variable is important for obtaining meaningful results. If the levels selected are too close together, the calculated effect could be no larger than the experimental noise. Selecting widely separated levels could result in running the reaction under unrealistic conditions, for example, above the solvent boiling point, or above the decomposition temperature for reagents and reactive intermediates.

Data analysis of factorial designs involves a comparison of the experimental responses at the high and low settings of each variable. The results can be plotted in several different ways to develop an understanding of the effect of changing two or more process variables at a time with regard to reaction yield and quality of the product.

Drug Substance Crystal Form (Final Form)

The crystal form of the drug substance (15) is important for pharmaceutical industries, where products are specified not by chemical composition but by their performance. Good crystallinity, good bioavailability, satisfactory aqueous solubility and dissolution rate, and satisfactory physicochemical properties, such as stability, hygroscopicity, and flowability are required. Choosing the appropriate crystal form (final form) often involves crystallizing the drug substance from various solvent systems to search for polymorphism and screening of various salts of the drug substance (if chemically possible).

The chemical, biological, and physical characteristics of the drug substance can be manipulated and hence optimized by conversion to a salt form. Every compound that exhibits acid or base characteristics can participate in salt formation. Various salts of the same compound often behave quite differently because of the physical, chemical, and thermodynamic properties they impart to the parent compound. Table 1 lists the top 10 FDA-approved commercially marketed final drug forms, and Table 2 lists the top 10 salts that are not approved by the FDA but that are in use in other countries. Only salts of organic compounds have been considered here because most drugs are organic substances. The relative frequency with which each salt

Scheme 8 Noyori's oxidation of alcohols.

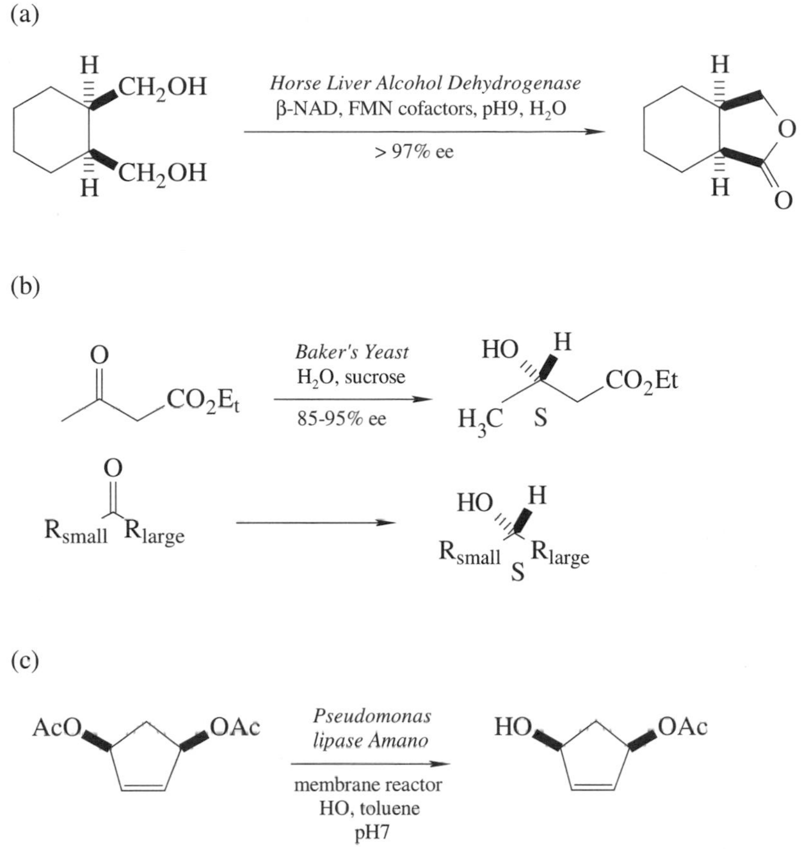

(a)

(b)

(c)

Scheme 9 Enzyme-mediated chemical transformations. (a) Enatioselective enzymatic oxidation and lactonization; (b) enzyme reduction with baker's yeast and enantioselective rule; and (c) enzymatic hydrolytic desymmetrization.

type has been used is calculated as a percentage, based on the total number of anionic or cationic salts in use.

The salt form is known to influence a number of physicochemical properties of the parent compound, such as dissolution rate, solubility, stability, and hygroscopicity. These properties, in turn, influence the absorption, distribution, metabolism, and excretion of the drug. This knowledge is essential for a complete understanding of the onset and duration of action, the relative toxicity, and the possible routes of administration. For example, certain

salts of the strong base choline have proved to be considerably less toxic than their parent compound. This observation led to the preparation of choline salicylate as an attempt to reduce the gastrointestinal (GI) disturbances associated with salicylate administration. Clinical studies indicated that choline salicylate elicited a lower incidence of GI distress, was tolerated in higher doses, and was of greater benefit to the patient than was acetylsalicylic acid (aspirin).

The chemical and physical stability of a drug can influence the choice of dosage form, the manufacturing and packaging, and the therapeutic efficacy of the final preparation. Systematic determination of the thermal stability, solution stability (at various pHs), and light sensitivity of a drug and its derivatives, both alone and in the presence of additives (excepients), provides essential information toward selecting the most suitable salt and dosage forms.

Depending on the mechanism of degradation, different salt forms impart different stability characteristics to the parent drug. Sparingly soluble salts used in the formulation

Table 1 Salts approved by the FDA

Anion	Percent	Cation	Percent
Hydrochloride	43	Sodium	62
Sulfate	7.5	Potassium	11
Bromide	5	Calcium	10.5
Chloride	4	Zinc	3
Tartarate	3.5	Meglumine	2.3

Table 2 Salts not approved by the FDA

Anion	Percent	Cation	Percent
Glycerophosphate	0.88	Piperazine	0.98
Aminosalicylate	0.25	Bismuth	0.98
Aspartate	0.25	Diethylamine	0.33
Blsulfate	0.25	Tromethamine	0.33
Hydroiodide	0.25	Barium	0.33

of suspensions reduce the amount of drug in solution and hence its degradation. Differences in hygroscopicity of several salts influence the stability of the drug in the dry state. For example, the stability of penicillin G and its salts has been widely studied because of the drug's therapeutic importance and its characteristic instability.

A solution of penicillin is not stable beyond two weeks even at refrigerator temperatures. However, the use of suspensions of sparingly soluble amine salts (procaine and hydrabamine salts) in aqueous vehicles allowed marketing of a "readymade" penicillin product.

Crystallization of the drug substance and its salt forms

In academia, a synthetic organic chemist rarely thinks about isolating a compound by crystallization, unless a single crystal structure is required. Most of the time, the chemist depends upon column chromatography to purify the compound. In contrast, in the pharmaceutical industry much depends upon crystallization. For example, crystal morphology and particle size have a direct impact on the filtration of a crystal slurry, cake compressibility, bulk stability and dissolution, bulk density, and flow characteristics. Crystallization is the preferred way of isolating the product from a reaction mixture. Knowledge of various crystallization systems from which the drug substance could be crystallized can provide information on polymorphism, thus expediting the selection of final crystal form. In polymorphism, two crystal forms with the same molecular structure are distinguished by the way in which the molecules are packed within the crystal lattice; each form has distinct physical and thermodynamic properties. In 1998, Abbott Laboratories withdrew its HIV drug, Ritonavir, because of the unexpected appearance of a new crystal form that had different dissolution and absorption characteristics than the standard product (16).

Crystallization is generally preceded by two types of nucleation. The primary nucleation occurs with the formation of clusters of molecules at the submicron level. When the concentration exceeds saturation to afford supersaturation, the clusters become nuclei. The secondary nucleation is caused by particles due to primary nucleation or seeds. There are many strategies to achieve supersaturation to initiate crystallization such as cooling, evaporation, and antisolvent addition.

Early on in the drug development program, only small amounts of material are available for crystallization studies. Parallel crystallization technique in test tubes allows for the identification of many solvent systems using small amounts of material. On a small scale, it is not easy to control the rate of cooling or the rate of evaporation to achieve supersaturation. However, the antisolvent addition strategy to achieve supersaturation in combination with seeding allows rapid identification of several crystallization systems using a minimum amount of compound.

Salts of a substrate having an acid or an amine functionality are prepared by dissolving the substrate and the counter-base (or acid) separately in appropriate solvents, mixing the two solutions in equimolar ratios, and removing the solvents under vacuum to afford a solid. This method has two distinct advantages: First, the composition of the substrate remains the same during various crystallization attempts, and second, this portion of the work can be automated with the use of liquid handling systems.

The next step is to determine the solubility of the substrate (or its salts) in different solvents. This can also be performed by an automated liquid handling system. Depending upon the solubility of the substrate in water-miscible solvents (alcohols, acetone, tetrahydrofuran, etc.) and water-immiscible solvents (ethyl acetate, methyl-*tert*-butyl ether, heptane, etc.), the process chemist can identify one or many solvent systems from which the substrate (or its salts) could be crystallized using the antisolvent addition strategy.

Another crystallization technique is used when the isolation of a highly water-soluble compound in its salt form is required from aqueous reaction mixtures. This technique takes advantage of the common-ion effect and is based on the le Chatelier's principle, which states that, "if, to a system in equilibrium, a stress is applied, the system will react so as to relieve the stress." Thus, in aqueous solutions, the solubility of the compound in salt form can be reduced by adding large amounts of a common ion that is more soluble than the salt of the compound.

Example: BMS-187745 is a potent inhibitor of squalene synthase and an efficient cholesterol-lowering agent in orally dosed animals. The final step of the synthesis involved oxidation of the penultimate in water with hydrogen peroxide and formic acid. The disodium salt was chosen as the final crystal form. Because of

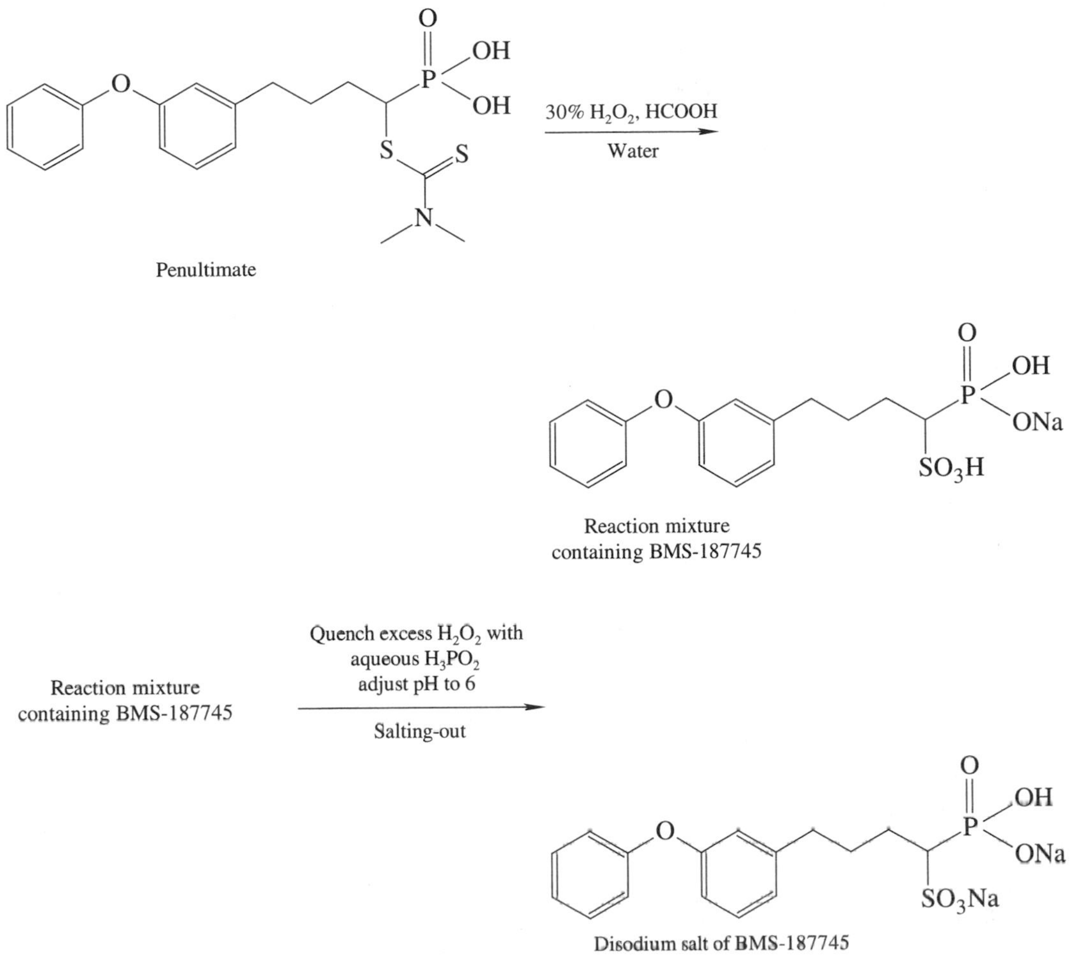

Scheme 10 BMS-187745 crystallization by salting-out.

extremely high solubility of the disodium salt in water, it cannot be extracted from water by common organic solvents. However, by employing the concept of the common-ion effect, the disodium salt can be easily crystallized from water. To accomplish this, the pH of the reaction mixture, after quench with hypophosphorous acid, is adjusted to the desired range of 6.05–6.25 (pKa of disodium salt of BMS-187745 is 6). In this pH range, sodium salts of formic, hypophosphorous, and phosphoric acids are present in high enough concentration to help lower the solubility of the disodium salt of BMS-187745 and effect crystallization (Scheme 10).

Automation in Process Chemistry Laboratories

Since the 1960s, automation has been the major tool for dramatically improving productivity (17–21). Automation techniques were introduced on the plant floor to

improve quality, increase safety, and streamline the work. Significant savings were realized initially from shorter delivery times, lower unit costs, smaller inventories, and fewer product failures. Due to an escalating cost of bringing a drug to market, companies are under immense pressure to shorten development time. The pharmaceutical industry has embraced new technologies in its discovery programs to increase throughput, generate precise data, and ensure accuracy.

Drug discovery scientists have already adopted tools such as combinatorial chemistry synthesizers; robotic systems for HTS; and software packages for computational chemistry, molecular modeling, and design of experiments to identify lead compounds ("hits"). As the number of "hits" grows, there is a potential for process R&D to become the "bottleneck." The number of compounds that can enter process development is limited by the number of process chemists available to work on these compounds. Without some type of automated process development machines to increase throughput, it will not be feasible to evaluate all the potential "hits." Created by the results from the HTS, demand for high-throughput development (HTD) tools is growing. Various companies, who in the past may have only addressed the needs of drug discovery scientists, are in the process of inventing and developing instruments that can be used by process chemists to perform many experiments in parallel. Examples of commercially available HTD tools are described below.

Parallel reactions

Charybdis Technologies: In the Calypso Reaction Block™, multi-well reaction arrays are designed for both solution and solid-phase synthesis applications. Well volumes range from 2 to 10 ml, pressures up to 207 kPa (30 psi), and temperatures from −80 to +180°C.

Quest Synthesis Technology: Quest 210 is designed for up to 20 reactions in 5- or 10-ml reaction vessels. Each of the 20 vessels can be efficiently stirred, heated, or cooled, and maintained under an inert atmosphere. Quest 205 is designed for synthesis on a large scale, with two banks of five 100-ml reaction vessels.

Argonaut Technologies: Endeavor™ allows parallel reactions under pressures up to 3.3 MPa (33 atm) and temperatures up to 200°C. Each of the eight vessels (working volume 15 ml) can be independently controlled for temperature, pressure, and gas delivery.

Surveyor™: Suitable for parallel process development and optimization with online sampling and integrated HPLC analysis, it employs 10 reaction vessels (working volume 15–45 ml), with individually controlled reaction temperatures from −40° to +150°C, with the ability to reflux. Reagent addition, reaction parameter control, sampling, and HPLC injection are controlled by built-in software.

Bohdan Automation, Inc: The process development workstation can run up to 12 independent reactions with working volumes of 25 ml. The following operations are automatically carried out: reagent preparation and addition, individual heating, cooling, and mixing, reaction sampling and quenching, and transfer to optional HPLC or FTIR modules.

Parallel purification

Isco, Inc: The CombiFlash™ Sg 100c System is suitable for purifying 10–35 g of material. It provides time- or peak-based fraction collection with on-line UV detection and a linear and/or step gradient with two solvents at a flow rate of 10–100 ml/min.
The CombiFlash Si 10x System simultaneously purifies up to 10 samples, with a linear and/or step gradient with two solvents with a total flow rate of 10–100 ml.

Automated sample handling and analysis

Bohdan Automation, Inc: The Balance Automator™ offers a cost-effective alternative to manual weighing, reduces errors and operator tedium, and processes up to 120 samples per hour. This system can accommodate various container sizes and balances with the help of interchangeable parts.

Gilson: The Gilson 215 Liquid Handler is a versatile, large-capacity, septum-piercing liquid handler for safe and efficient transfer. It helps in transferring samples to other analytical systems or inject samples directly to an on-line HPLC system.

OUTSOURCING

Outsourcing covers a broad range of services (22). It can eliminate the need for additional staff, facilities, and/or equipment. Outsourcing in drug discovery and development is expected to continue its remarkable growth over the next decade as drug synthesis becomes more complex. This dynamic growth is due to a number of factors, including the ongoing consolidation in the pharmaceutical industry and a tight labor market. As larger companies consolidate, they seek synergies resulting in release of R&D personnel. Retrospectively, companies need to get more done with fewer internal resources and this promotes outsourcing. The tight labor market has made it increasingly difficult to recruit and retain staff, and many companies are turning to outsourcing to gain access to highly trained scientists who are available. Pharmaceutical companies are also looking into long-term relationships with outsourcing partners.

FDA GUIDELINES AND REGULATORY ISSUES

The guidelines on drug preparation (GLP and cGMP compliance) regulatory issues are described in details in the Center for Drug Evaluation and Research (CDER) by the FDA (23). A complete section is dedicated to API and the GMP issues. The readers are encouraged to seek the reference for further details.

REFERENCES

1. Picano, G.P.; Wheelwright, S.C. The New Logic of High-Tech R&D. Harvard Business Review (**Sept./Oct. 1995**), 93.
2. Gadamasetti, K.G., Ed.; *Process Chemistry in the Pharmaceutical Industry*; Marcel Dekker, Inc.: New York, 1999.

3. Mueller, R.H. A Practical Synthesis of Ifetroban Sodium. *Process Chemistry in the Pharmaceutical Industry*; Gadamasetti, K.G., Ed.; Chap. 3; Marcel Dekker, Inc.: New York, 1999; 37–55.

4. Holton, R.A. Method for Preparation of Taxol. Eur. Pat. Appl. **1990**.

5. Swaminathan, S.; Singh, A.K.; et al. Tetrahedron Lett. **1998**, *39*, 4769.

6. Federsel, H.-J.; Jakupovic, E. A Highly Optimized and Concise Large Scale Synthesis of Purive Bronchodilator. *Process Chemistry in the Pharmaceutical Industry*; Gadamasetti, K.G., Ed.; Chap. 6; Marcel Dekker, Inc.: New York, 1999; 91–106.

7. *Guidelines for Chemical Reactivity Evaluation and Application to Process Design*; Center for Chemical Process Safety of the American Institute of Chemical Engineers: New York, 1995.

8. Breslow, R. The Greening Chemistry. Chem. & Eng. News **Aug., 1996**.

9. Sato, K.; Akoki, M.; Takagi, J.; Noyori, R. J. Am. Chem. Soc. **1997**, *119*, 12386.

10. Azerad, R. Bull. Soc. Chim. Fr. **1995**, *132*, 17.

11. Theil, F. Chem. Rev. **1995**, *95*, 2203.

12. Wong, C.-H.; Whitesides, G.M. *Enzymes in Synthetic Organic Chemistry*; Pergamon: Oxford, 1994.

13. Collins, A.N., Sheldrake, G.N., Crosby, J., Eds. *Chirality in Industry*; John Wiley & Sons: New York, 1992, 1997; I and II.

14. Pilipauskas, D.R. Using Factorial Experiments in the Development of Process Chemistry. *Process Chemistry in the Pharmaceutical Industry*; Gadamasetti, K.G., Ed.; Chap. 22; Marcel Dekker, Inc.: New York, 1999; 411–428.

15. Berge, S.M.; Bighley, L.D.; Monkhouse, D.C. Pharmaceutical Salts. J. Pharm. Sci. **1977**, *66* (1), 1.

16. Blagden, N.; Davey, R. Polymorphs Take Shape. Chem. in Brit. **March 1999**, 44.

17. Owen, M.; Dewitt, S. Laboratory Automation in Chemical Development. *Process Chemistry in the Pharmaceutical Industry*; Gadamasetti, K.G., Ed.; Marcel Dekker, Inc.: New York, 1999; 429–455.

18. Conner, K. The Drive to Improve the Bottom Line. Today's Chemist at Work **Nov 1999**, 29.

19. Sullivan, M. Automation Accelerates Synthesis. Today's Chemist at Work **Sept 1999**, 48.

20. Studt, T. Raising the Bar on Combinatorial Discovery. Drug Discovery Development **Jan/Feb 2000**, 24.

21. Harness, J.R. Automated Sample Handling Supports Synthesis and Screening. Drug Discovery & Development **Jan 1999**, 69.

22. Waring, J. Strategic Outsourcing Fuels Research Growth. Drug Discovery & Development **Jan/Feb 2000**, 40.

23. CDER web site: http://www.fda.gov/cder. *A Complete section is Dedicated to the Internationally Harmonised Guide for Active Pharmaceutical Ingredients (API) and Good Manufacturing Practice (GMP)*; Washington, Sept 1997.

PRODRUG DESIGN

Bernard Testa
Joachim Mayer
University of Lausanne, Lausanne, Switzerland

A CASE FOR PRODRUG DESIGN

Drug disposition and metabolism are of essential significance in pharmaceutical research because of the interdependence of pharmacokinetic and pharmacodynamic processes. Limited intestinal absorption, inadequate distribution, fast metabolism, and toxic metabolites are some of the causes of failure of drug candidates during development. To reduce the rate of attrition resulting from such pharmacokinetic defects, disposition and metabolic studies should be initiated as early as possible in the screening of lead candidates.

Avoidance of the foreseeable or proven pharmacokinetic defects thus assumes considerable significance in drug research. However, pharmacokinetic (PK) and pharmacodynamic (PD) optimization may not be compatible, meaning that efficacy at the target may be decreased or lost during PK optimization (1). A telling example of such a situation is provided by the novel drug class of neuraminidase inhibitors of therapeutic value against type A and B influenza in humans. Here, target-oriented rational design has led to highly hydrophilic, poorly absorbed agents such as Ro-64-0802, which shows very high in vitro inhibitory efficacy toward the enzyme but low oral bioavailability because of its high polarity (2). To circumvent this problem, Ro-64-0802 is marketed as Oseltamivir, its ethyl ester prodrug (Fig. 1). After intestinal absorption, the prodrug undergoes rapid enzymatic hydrolysis and produces high and sustained plasma levels of the active agent. As demonstrated by this example, the prodrug concept may thus prove to be a valuable alternative to disentangle PK and PD optimization. In other words, rather than attempting to improve lead candidates within a unitary rational design process, it may be that PK optimization can be achieved by the application of the prodrug concept to research compounds with high in vitro activity. Some of the concepts of interest in prodrug design are examined here.

OBJECTIVES AND PRINCIPLES OF PRODRUG DESIGN

Prodrugs are defined as therapeutic agents that are inactive per se but are predictably transformed into active metabolites (3, 4). As such, prodrugs must be contrasted with soft drugs, which are active per se and yield inactive metabolites.

Prodrug design aims at overcoming a number of barriers to a drug's usefulness (Table 1). The major objectives of prodrug design derive from these considerations and are also listed in Table 1.

Many successes have been recorded in prodrug design, and a large variety of such compounds have proven their therapeutic value. Several complementary viewpoints can be adopted when addressing prodrugs, namely, their chemical classification, their mechanism of activation (i.e., enzymatic and/or nonenzymatic), their tissue selectivity, the possible production of toxic metabolites, and the gain in therapeutic benefit (Table 2).

The chemical classification distinguishes between carrier-linked prodrugs (drugs linked to a carrier moiety by a labile bridge) and bioprecursors, which do not contain a carrier group and are activated by the metabolic creation of a functional group (4). In the former, the carrier moiety is often and conveniently linked to polar groups such as —OH, —NHR, and —COOH. Relevant examples of bioprecursors are provided by chemotherapeutic agents whose activation occurs by reduction in oxygen-deprived cells. Thus, the one-electron reduction of 3-amino-1,2,4-benzotriazine 1,4-dioxide to a cytotoxic nitroxide is believed to account for the antitumor activity of this bioprecursor (5). Such bioprecursors appear as a viable class of prodrugs because they avoid potential toxicity problems caused by the carrier moiety. However, attention must be given here to metabolic intermediates. A special group of carrier-linked prodrugs are the site-specific chemical delivery systems (6). Macromolecular prodrugs are synthetic conjugates of drugs covalently bound (either directly or via a spacer) to proteins, polypeptides, polysaccharides, and other biodegradable

Encyclopedia of Pharmaceutical Technology

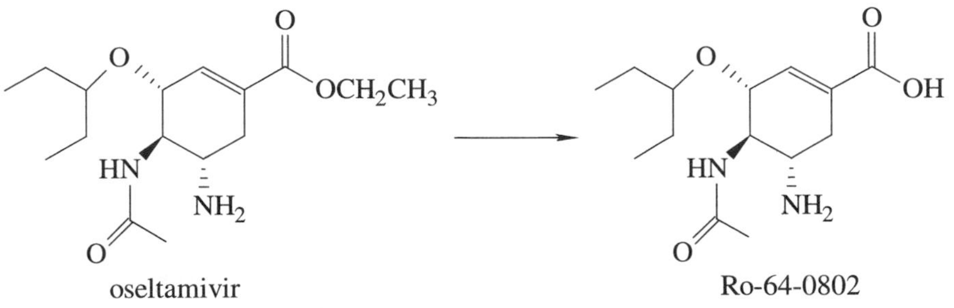

Fig. 1 The structure of the neuraminidase inhibitor Ro-64-0802 and its ethyl ester prodrug Oseltamivir.

polymers (7). A special case is provided by drugs coupled to monoclonal antibodies.

Prodrug activation occurs enzymatically, nonenzymatically, or sequentially (enzymatic step followed by nonenzymatic rearrangement). As much as possible, it is desirable to reduce biological variability, hence, the particular interest currently received by nonenzymatic reactions of intramolecular cyclization–elimination (8) presented at length below. The problem of tissue or organ targeting is another important aspect of prodrug design. Various attempts have been made to achieve organ-selective activation of prodrugs, such as dermal delivery (9) and brain penetration (6). For example, the selective presence of cysteine conjugate β-lyase in the kidney suggests that this enzyme might be exploited for delivery of sulfhydryl drugs to this organ (10).

The toxic potential of metabolic intermediates, of the carrier moiety, or of a fragment thereof must also be kept in mind. This is illustrated by formaldehyde-releasing prodrugs such as N- and O-acyloxymethyl derivatives or Mannich bases. Similarly, arylacetylenes assayed as potential bioprecursors of antiinflammatory arylacetic acids proved many years ago to be highly toxic because of the formation of an intermediate ketene. The gain in therapeutic benefit provided by prodrugs is an issue with no general conclusion. Depending on both the drug and its prodrug, the therapeutic gain may be modest, marked, or even significant. In the case of marketed drugs endowed with useful qualities but displaying some unwanted property, the expected therapeutic gain is usually modest to marked. In the case of difficult candidates showing excellent target properties but suffering from some severe physicochemical and/or pharmacokinetic drawback, a marked to significant benefit can be obtained.

CHEMICALLY ACTIVATED PRODRUGS: REACTIONS OF CYCLIZATION–ELIMINATION

So many biological factors may affect enzymatic reactions that the resulting interspecies and interindividual variability renders prodrug design unreliable and sometimes even problematic. To circumvent such difficulties, an increasing

Table 1 Barriers to drug usefulness and corresponding objectives of prodrug design

Pharmaceutical barriers	Pharmaceutical objectives
Insufficient chemical stability	Improved formulation (e.g., increased hydrosolubility)
Poor solubility	Improved chemical stability
Offensive taste or odor	Improved patient acceptance and compliance
Irritation or pain	
Pharmacokinetic barriers	Pharmacokinetic objectives
Low oral absorption	Improved bioavailability
Marked presystemic metabolism	Prolonged duration of action
Short duration of action	Improved organ selectivity
Unfavourable distribution in the body	
Pharmacodynamic barriers	Pharmacodynamic objectives
Toxicity	Decreased side effects

(From Ref. 3.)

Table 2 Complementary viewpoints in prodrug design

Chemical classification
  Bioprecursors
  Classical carrier-linked prodrugs
  Site-specific chemical delivery systems
  Macromolecular prodrugs
  Drug–antibody conjugates

Mechanisms of activation
  Enzymatic
    ⇒ biological variability
  Nonenzymatic
    ⇒ no biological variability

Mechanisms of tissue/organ selectivity
  Tissue-selective activation of classic prodrugs
  Site-specific delivery of ad hoc chemical systems

Potential toxicity
  Of a metabolic intermediate
  Of the carrier moiety or a metabolite thereof?

Gain in therapeutic benefit
  Prodrugs of marketed drugs (post hoc design); modest to
    marked benefit
  Prodrugs of difficult candidates (ad hoc design); marked to
    significant benefit

$X = O$ or NH
Nu = basic N, N^-, COO^-, OH

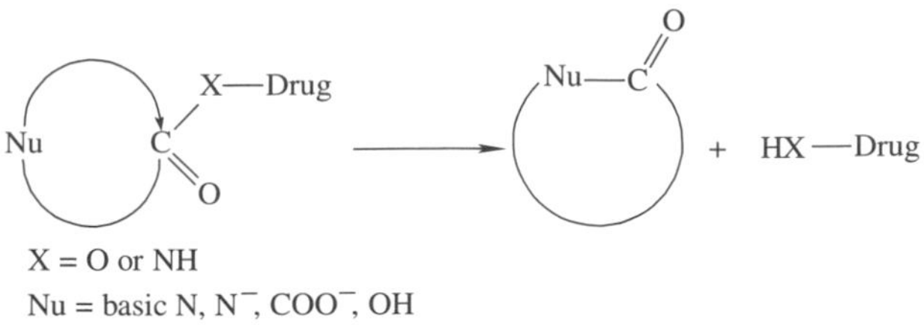

Fig. 2 General reaction scheme for the intramolecular activation of prodrugs by cyclization–elimination. (Modified from Ref. 11.)

• esters and amides undergoing intramolecular nucleophilic cyclization–elimination.

Here, we focus on prodrug activation by intramolecular cyclization–elimination (8, 11). These reactions occur in specifically designed prodrugs of phenols, alcohols, and amines. A number of design strategies exist to achieve such mechanisms, as illustrated below with selected examples. The general chemical principle of these reactions is shown in Fig. 2. In such a schematic representation, the carrier moiety is a side chain attached to the drug by a carbonyl group (i.e., by an ester or amide function) and containing a nucleophilic group symbolized by "Nu." The latter directly attacks the carbonyl in a reaction of nucleophilic substitution whose outcome is cyclization of the carrier moiety and elimination of the drug molecule.

Cyclization–Elimination Due to a Basic Amino Group

Nucleophilic attack by a basic amino group has proven to be a useful strategy to achieve and modulate cyclization–elimination. The radiation sensitizer

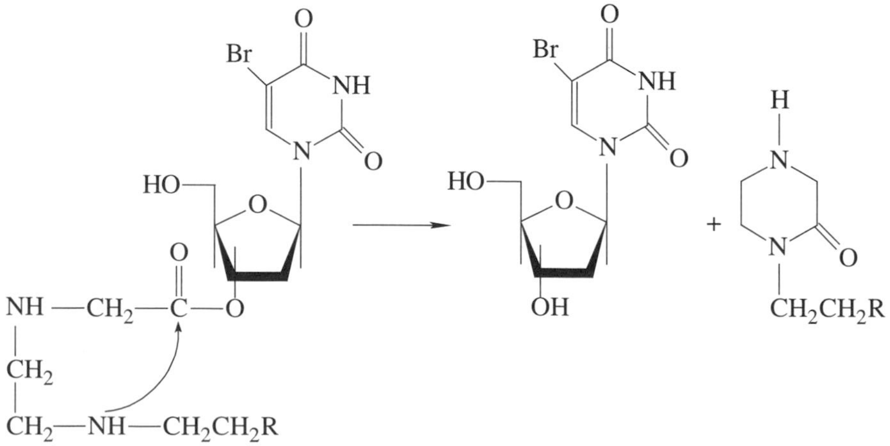

number of studies have proposed and investigated prodrugs activated by a purely or predominantly nonenzymatic mechanism. Prodrug of this type include:

• (2-oxo-1,3-dioxol-4-yl)methyl esters
• Mannich bases
• oxazolidines
• esters with a basic side chain sterically able to catalyze intramolecular hydrolysis

Fig. 3 Activation of basic ester prodrugs of 5-bromo-2′-deoxyuridine by cyclization of the promoiety. (Modified from Ref. 12.)

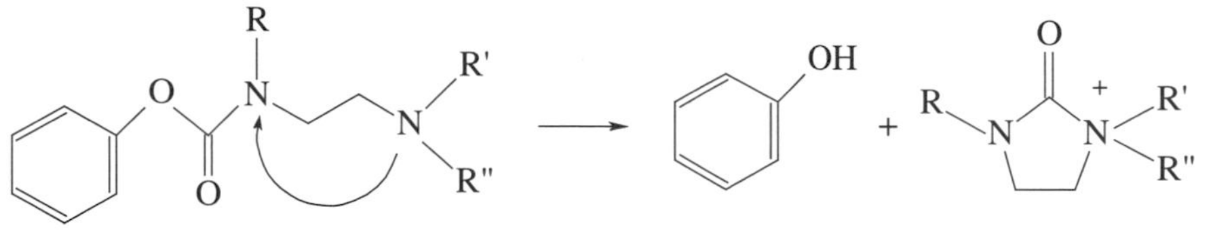

Fig. 4 Activation of basic carbamates of phenols by cyclization–elimination of the promoiety. (From Ref. 13.)

5-bromo-2′-deoxyuridine was derivatized with diamino acids to obtain the prodrugs shown in Fig. 3, with R = H or cyclohexyl (12). The reaction of cyclization proceeded cleanly to yield the drug and a piperazinone derivative without any other detectable product being formed. No hydrolysis was seen in acidic solutions. At pH 7.4 and 37°C in a buffer solution, the half-life for the two prodrugs was 23 and 30 min, respectively. In human plasma under the same conditions, the values were 70 and 47 min, respectively, suggesting protection from breakdown by binding to proteins. In rat plasma, the half-life of the first compound was 47 min, again suggesting protection, but it was 5 min for the second compound. This is an indication that enzymatic hydrolysis by rat plasma hydrolases is possible in some cases.

Thus, intramolecular activation by cyclization–elimination was modulated by steric factors. In addition, this example shows that hydrolysis may be catalyzed by enzymes depending on substrates and biological conditions.

Valuable insights can be found in an informative study on the reactivity of phenyl carbamates of ethylenediamines (Fig. 4) (13). Their half-lives of chemical activation at pH 7.4 and 37°C showed that N,N'-dimethyl and N,N',N'-trimethyl substitution gave the fastest rates of cyclization, whereas N-H, N'-H, and/or N-ethyl groups markedly decelerated the reaction. The other major interest of this study is the proof it reported that no enzymatic hydrolysis occurred. Indeed, these compounds were incubated with human plasma, pig liver homogenates, and rat liver homogenates, the half-lives of release of

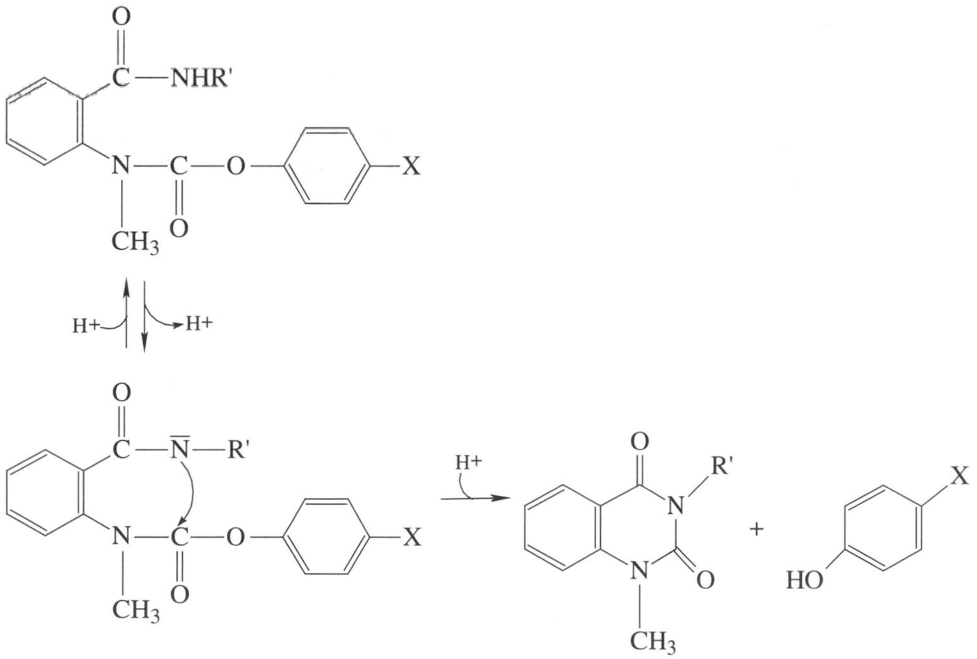

Fig. 5 Simplified reaction mechanism of intramolecular cyclization–elimination of phenyl carbamates of anthranilamides. (From Ref. 14.)

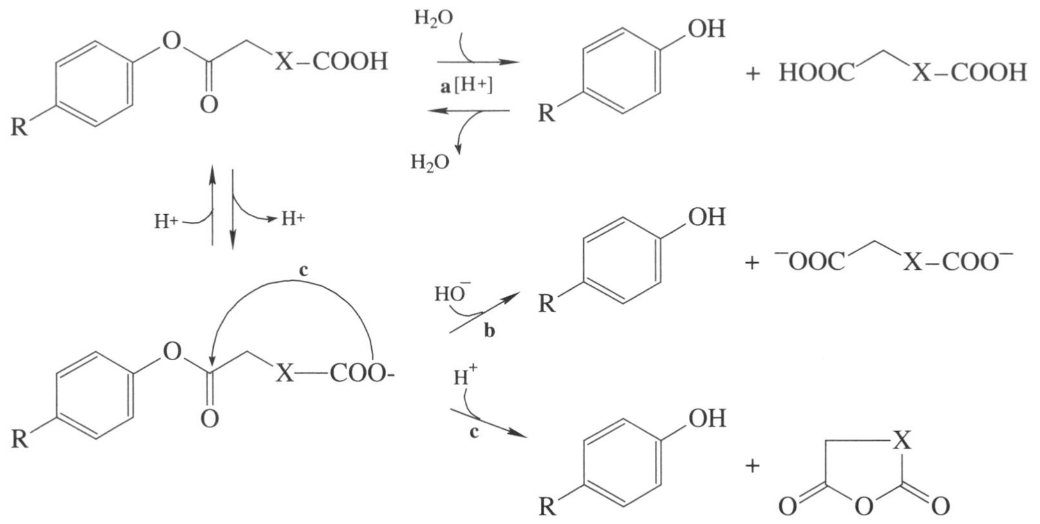

Fig. 6 Activation of hemiester prodrugs of phenols by proton-catalyzed hydrolysis (reaction a), hydroxyl-catalyzed hydrolysis (reaction b), or cyclization–elimination (reaction c). Enzymatic hydrolysis is not represented. (Adapted from Ref. 15.)

phenol being either identical to those in buffer, or slightly larger, because of protein binding.

Cyclization–Elimination Due to an Acidic Amido Group

In addition to attack by a basic nitrogen, there exists also the possibility of an intramolecular attack by an anionic nitrogen, i.e., a deprotonated amido nitrogen. This is exemplified by N-(2-carbamoylphenyl)carbamates of model phenols (Fig. 5; X = H, Cl, or OCH$_3$) (14). In such promoieties, the deprotonated carboxamido group attacks the carbamate carbonyl to form a quinazolinedione and release the phenol. The stability of a large series of N-(2-carbamoylphenyl)carbamates was explored in buffer solutions and in diluted human plasma. The rate of nonenzymatic cyclization–elimination was highly sensitive to the nature of the carboxamido substituent (R' in Fig. 5). An alkyl substituent larger than methyl strongly decreased reactivity, presumably by steric hindrance. In contrast, an electron-withdrawing

substituent increased reactivity by facilitating deprotonation. Globally, these effects were significant because the rates span four orders of magnitude.

In human plasma, two groups of compounds were seen. In most cases, the reaction in plasma (i.e., chemical plus enzymatic activation) was approximately two-fold faster than in buffer. This indicates that enzymatic hydrolysis in human plasma, if any, was modest at best. Only for the three prodrugs with an unsubstituted carboxamido group (R' = H) was the enzymatic reaction several-fold faster than was intramolecular catalysis, suggesting these compounds to be substrates of plasmatic hydrolases. Thus, the N-(2-carbamoylphenyl)carbamate promoiety allowed a highly modulatable intramolecular activation with little enzymatic activation.

Cyclization–Elimination Owing to a Carboxylate or Hydroxyl Group

Intramolecular cyclizations are not restricted to attack by a nucleophilic nitrogen (basic amino or acidic amido group).

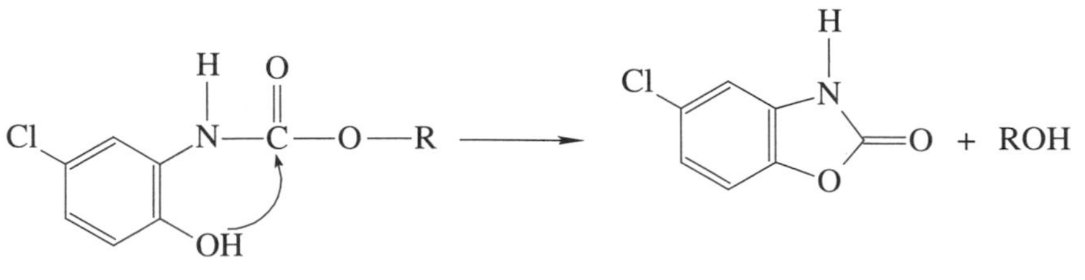

Fig. 7 Cyclization of N-2-hydroxyphenyl carbamates as potential prodrugs of benzoxazoles and phenols. (From Ref. 16.)

Table 3 Specific difficulties in prodrug design and development

Objectives	Strategy	Restrictive conditions
Minimize the number of proposed candidates	Careful prodrug design based on prediction of target phys-chem and PK properties	Available
Maximize the explored space of phys-chem and PK properties		Local quantitative models Global qualitative models (e.g., "rule of 5")Dubious
Minimize the additional synthetic work		Global quantitative models
Reach target phys-chem profile	Careful weighing of costs and benefits	Limited acceptance of additional costs and efforts
	HTP phys-chem profiling Virtual screening	Limited or dubious relevance of some HTP techniques Dubious predictive capacity of some models (see above)
Reach target PK profile	HTP PK profiling Virtual screening	Limited or dubious in vivo relevance of some HTP screens Dubious predictive capacity of some models (see above)
Reach target metabolic behavior, in particular target rate of activation	Fast in vitro metabolic assessment	Dubious extrapolation to in vivo situation
Lack of toxicity of prodrug, promoiety or fragment thereof	Knowledge-based design Toxicity screens	Incomplete knowledge Limited or dubious in vivo relevance of screens

HTP = high throughput; phys-chem = physicochemical; PK = pharmacokinetic.

They can also be catalyzed by a nucleophilic oxygen as found in a carboxylate, phenolic, or alcoholic group. Illustration of the catalytic role of a carboxylate group can be found in hemiester prodrugs of phenol (taken as model compound) or paracetamol (Fig. 6; R = H or NHCOCH$_3$, respectively) (15). In addition to enzymatic hydrolysis, three mechanisms of chemical hydrolysis were seen, namely, acid-catalyzed, base-catalyzed, and an intramolecular nucleophilic attack, resulting in cyclization–elimination (Fig. 6, reactions a, b, and c, respectively). In buffer solutions, the relative importance of these three pathways was clearly pH-dependent. At physiological pH, cyclization–elimination was the predominant reaction, with half-lives ranging from 1 to 350 min at 37°C. Reactivity at this pH was markedly influenced by the length and degree of substitution of the promoiety and by the pK$_a$ value of the phenol. Thus, succinate esters (Fig. 6; X = CH$_2$CH$_2$) were approximately 150 times more reactive than were glutarate esters (X = CH$_2$CH$_2$CH$_2$); C-methylation of the promoiety (X = CH$_2$CH(CH$_3$)CH$_2$) also increased reactivity. Esters of paracetamol (R = NHCOCH$_3$) were degraded about twice as fast as were esters of phenol (R = H).

In most cases, the hemiesters in Fig. 6 underwent no or little enzymatic degradation in human plasma, in agreement with the known inertness of hemiesters toward cholinesterase. In contrast, very rapid hydrolysis was usually seen in pig and rat liver preparations, indicating the involvement of carboxylesterases. The only inert compound was the 3,3-dimethylglutarate hemiester of paracetamol (Fig. 6; X = CH$_2$C(CH$_3$)$_2$CH$_2$). It certainly would be interesting to have data on the hydrolysis of such prodrugs by human hepatic enzymes.

The hydroxyl functionality in phenols and alcohols is also of potential interest as an intramolecular nucleophile. One example of this type is presented here (16). N-2-hydroxyphenyl carbamates (Fig. 7) undergo intramolecular cyclization with quantitative liberation of a phenol or an alcohol. The interest of this approach is that the product of cyclization is itself a drug, namely, the skeletal muscle relaxant chlorzoxazone. A large variety of phenols and alcohols were investigated in this work, most of them model compounds, but paracetamol was among them. In this case, a prodrug of this type liberates not one but two drugs and can be called a mutual prodrug.

The mechanism of activation in Fig. 7 was demonstrated to be an intramolecular nucleophilic attack by the phenolate ion on the carbonyl group. As a consequence, the rate of reaction increased linearly with pH, up to a plateau at 8–9 and beyond. The major factor influencing the rate of reaction was the acidity of the leaving ROH molecule, with $t_{1/2}$ values at pH 10 and 25°C ranging from 290 days for ROH = CH$_3$CH$_2$OH (pK$_a$ 16.0) to 3–12 s for ROH = phenols of pK$_a$ 9–10. The $t_{1/2}$ value for ROH = paracetamol was 7.1 s at pH 7.4 and 37°C (16). Some prodrugs and mutual prodrugs in Fig. 7 were also examined for their stability in human and rat plasma (16). These N-2-hydroxyphenyl carbamates showed two- to threefold increases in $t_{1/2}$ values in human and rat plasma compared with buffer. This indicates the absence of an enzymatic hydrolysis and a modest stabilization owing to binding to plasma proteins.

SOME PROBLEMS IN PRODRUG RESEARCH

The benefit brought forth by a prodrug relative to the active agent is worth considering. Schematically, it appears from innumerable data in the literature that the gain will be considerable when the development of an innovative and very promising agent is blocked by a major pharmacokinetic or pharmaceutical defect that a prodrug strategy can overcome. In contrast, the gain will be negligible when the drug defect is tolerable or barely improved by transformation to a prodrug. But what of the specific difficulties encountered in designing and developing prodrugs? Table 3 schematically presents some of these difficulties (17), to which one can add possible complications in registration.

Thus, it's no wonder so many medicinal chemists are critical of prodrugs. However, and this is our conclusion, a lucid view cannot ignore the potential benefit, in this case the mere existence of a number of successful prodrugs. Nabumetone, oseltamivir, and pivampicilline are just a few examples that come to mind. They demonstrate that in a number of cases, prodrug design may indeed allow the separate optimization of PK and PD properties.

REFERENCES

1. Testa, B.; Caldwell, J. Prodrugs Revisited—The Ad Hoc Approach as a Complement to Ligand Design. Med. Res. Rev. **1996**, *16*, 233–241.
2. Oxford, J.S.; Lambkin, R. Targeting Influenza Virus Neuraminidase—a New Strategy for Antiviral Therapy. Drug Discov. Today **1998**, *3*, 448–456.
3. Stella, V.J.; Charman, W.N.A.; Naringrekar, V.H. Prodrugs: Do They Have Advantages in Clinical Practice? Drugs **1985**, *29*, 455–473.
4. Wermuth, C.G. Designing Prodrugs and Bioprecursors. *Drug Design: Fact or Fantasy?*; Jolles, G., Woolridge, K.R.H., Eds.; Academic Press: London, 1984; 47–72.
5. Riley, R.J.; Workman, P. Enzymology of the Reduction of the Potent Benzotriazine-di-N-oxide Hypoxic Cell

Cytotoxin SR 4233 (WIN 59075) by NAD(P)H: (Quinone Acceptor) Oxidoreductase (EC 1.6.99.2) Purified from Walker 256 Rat Tumour Cells. Biochem. Pharmacol. **1992**, *43*, 167–174.

6. Bodor, N. Redox Drug Delivery Systems for Targeting Drugs to the Brain. Ann. N.Y. Acad. Sci. **1987**, *507*, 289–306.

7. Duncan, R. Drug-Polymer Conjugates: Potential for Improved Chemotherapy. Anti-Cancer Drugs **1992**, *3*, 175–210.

8. Testa, B.; Mayer, J.M. Design of Intramolecularly Activated Prodrugs. Drug Metab. Rev. **1998**, *30*, 787–807.

9. Chan, S.Y.; Li Wan, PoA. Prodrugs for Dermal Delivery. Int. J. Pharmaceut. **1989**, *55*, 1–16.

10. Hwang, I.Y.; Elfarra, A.A. Cysteine S-Conjugates May Act as Kidney-Selective Prodrugs: Formation of 6-Mercaptopurine by the Renal Metabolism of S-(6-purinyl)-L-Cysteine. J. Pharmacol. Exp. Ther. **1989**, *251*, 448–454.

11. Shan, D.; Nicolaou, M.G.; Borchardt, R.T.; Wang, B. Prodrug Strategies Based on Intramolecular Cyclization Reactions. J. Pharm. Sci. **1997**, *86*, 765–767.

12. Saari, W.S.; Schwering, J.E.; Lyle, P.A.; Smith, S.J.; Engelhardt, E.L. Cyclization-Activated Prodrugs. Basic Esters of 5-Bromo-2'-Deoxyuridine. J. Med. Chem. **1990**, *33*, 2590–2595.

13. Thomsen, K.F.; Strøm, F.; Sforzini, B.V.; Begtrup, M.; Mørk, N. Evaluation of Phenyl Carbamates of Ethyl Diamines as Cyclization-Activated Prodrug Forms for Protecting Phenols Against First-Pass Metabolism. Int. J. Pharma. **1994**, *112*, 143–152.

14. Thomsen, K.F.; Bundgaard, H. Cyclization-Activated Phenyl Carbamate Prodrug Forms for Protecting Phenols Against First-Pass Metabolism. Int. J. Pharma. **1993**, *91*, 39–49.

15. Fredholt, K.; Mørk, N.; Begtrup, M. Hemiesters of Aliphatic Dicarboxylic Acids as Cyclization-Activated Prodrug Forms for Protecting Phenols Against First-Pass Metabolism. Int. J. Pharma. **1995**, *123*, 209–216.

16. Vlgroux, A.; Bergon, M.; Zedde, C. Cyclization-Activated Prodrugs: N-(Substituted 2-Hydroxyphenyl and 2-Hydroxypropyl)Carbamates Based on Ring-Opened Derivatives of Active Benzoxazolones and Oxazolidinones as Mutual Prodrugs of Acetaminophen. J. Med. Chem. **1995**, *38*, 3983–3994.

17. Testa, B.; Mayer, J.M. Concepts in Prodrug Design to Overcome Pharmacokinetic Problems. *Pharmacokinetic Optimization in Drug Research—Biological, Physicochemical and Computational Strategies*; Testa, B., van de Waterbeemd, H., Folkers, G., Guy, R., Eds.; Wiley—VCH: Weinheim, in press.

18. Balant, L.P.; Doelker, E. Metabolic Considerations in Prodrug Design. *Burger's Medicinal Chemistry and Drug Discovery*; 5th Ed., Wolff, M.E. Ed.; Wiley: New York, 1995; 1, 949–982.

19. Borchardt, R.T., Repta, A.J., Stella, V.J., Eds. *Directed Drug Delivery—A Multidisciplinary Approach*, Humana Press: Clifton NJ, 1985.

20. Bundgaard, H., Hansen, A.B., Kofod, H., Eds. *Optimization of Drug Delivery*, Munkgaard: Copenhagen, 1982.

21. Bundgaard, H. *A Textbook of Drug Design and Development*; Krogsgaard-Larsen, P., Bundgaard, H., Eds.; Harwood: Reading, 1991; 113–191.

22. Harper, N.J. Drug Latentiation. *Progress in Drug Research*; Jucker, E., Ed.; Birkhäuser: Basel, 1962; 4, 221–294.

23. Testa, B.; Jenner, P.; *Drug Metabolism: Chemical and Biochemical Aspects*; Marcel Dekker, Inc.: New York, 1976.

24. Testa, B.; *The Metabolism of Drugs and Other Xenobiotics—Biochemistry of Redox Reactions*; Academic Press: London, 1995.

25. Testa, B. Drug Metabolism. *Burger's Medicinal Chemistry and Drug Discovery*; 5th Ed.; Wolff, M.E., Ed.; Wiley: New York, 1995; 1, 129–180..

26. Testa, B.; Mayer, J.M.; *Hydrolysis in Drug and Prodrug Metabolism—The Biochemistry and Enzymology of Hydrolases*; Wiley—Verlag Helvetica Chimica Acta: Zurich, in preparation.

27. Widder, K.J., Green, R., Eds. *Drug and Enzyme Targeting (Methods in Enzymology)*; Academic Press: Orlando, FL, 1985; 112.

PROJECT MANAGEMENT

Jerry J. Groens
Abbott Laboratories, Abbott Park, Ilinois

Cara R. Frosch
Covance Central Laboratory Services, Inc., Indianapolis, Indiana

INTRODUCTION

New products are developed and introduced in organizations primarily through the use of projects and teams. Research of new technologies and innovation is essentially accomplished through the use of projects as well. The processes for developing and introducing new products are certainly more structured and well understood when compared with research; however, the essence of each is that they are projects.

A project is a *temporary endeavor undertaken to create a unique product or service* (1). Project management provides the processes, tools, techniques, skills, and knowledge needed to manage a project such that the results meet or exceed the stakeholder needs and expectations. Stakeholders are the individuals or organizations whose interests may be positively or negatively impacted by the project.

Searching for sources of project management in the literature, an individual finds hundreds of books, articles, and cases covering the topic in all industries, environments, and situations. These sources emphasize that every project is different and that projects exist in an environment of change, uncertainty, and inconsistency. However, some of these sources then proceed to state that "project management is a science" and that the processes of project management are consistent across all industries and environments. Any successful practitioner in project management in the fields of product development and, more specifically pharmaceutical development, knows that this is not correct. Project management is more, much more of an art than a science, and the application of project management is not consistent across industries, environments, and situations.

For example, many of the elements of project management applied in the construction and telecommunications industries do not work in pharmaceutical development. This includes earned value, configuration management, and detailed representations of the work breakdown structures. These concepts actually provide too much structure when applied to pharmaceutical or any product development and could potentially have a negative impact on innovation, creativity, and effective teaming. Therefore, the creation of a development framework, based upon the principles and practices of project management, is required to address the uncertain world of pharmaceutical development. This chapter will focus on that framework.

A PROJECT MANAGEMENT FRAMEWORK

A project management framework has six elements. These are:

- Project definition,
- Project team and organization,
- Project planning, scheduling, and control,
- Problem solving and decision making using prototypes,
- Senior management review and control, and
- Proactive, real-time change management (2).

Each of these items is key to the successful management of a new product development project. For example, the project definition processes develop:

- The project scope and objectives,
- The business case and the technologies utilized,
- The project strategy or direction being pursued,
- The sponsorship and championship for the new product
- Concept, and
- The final product performance targets and deliverables.

This project management chapter will cover each of these elements of a project management framework and provide sources for further study.

PROJECT DEFINITION

This first element of a project management framework is used to define project scope and objectives. It outlines what is within and not within the project boundaries,

Encyclopedia of Pharmaceutical Technology

the business case and market need, the technologies to be used to solve that business case, and the initiation, selling, and sponsoring of the project.

The scope of the project includes not only the definition of the final product deliverable but the level of work effort required to complete this project. For example, a new pharmaceutical drug will be used to reduce long-term intractable pain, will be in an injectable form, and will use existing packaging configurations in defined concentrations and formulations. This is an initial, general definition of the product scope. The project scope, however, is much more time consuming and complex to develop and would include:

- The number, type, and cost of clinical studies or trials (including number of patients and sites) required in each phase of development to complete the project;
- The formulation, analytical chemistry, packaging and sterilization/microbiological work needed; and
- The manufacturing processes, equipment, and other resources required to produce the product.

Resource estimates (hours and dollars) for people's time, expenses, and capital are projected along with an approximation of the timing of the need for these resources. This becomes the basis for a project approval document or *charter*, which also includes the product scope, project objectives, business case, and financial evaluation.

Project objectives are also a key element of project definition and set the direction for a product development project. These objectives operate in an environment where trade-offs are necessary, and are often referred to as the *triple constraint* (see Fig. 1). Looking at these three constraints, a few questions may come to mind. For example:

- How often have you been on a project where the scope did not change? Probably never, and if you have, this is very unusual.
- How often have you been able to estimate the original resources required on a new project as closely as ±5%? Probably never, and if you have, this is very unusual.
- How often are you allowed as much time as needed to complete the project? Probably never and, in fact, cycle time reductions are the norm.

Given these experiences, and assuming that these are typical and true, a project manager recognizes the magnitude of the challenges in being successful because meeting these objectives is the measurement of success. This emphasizes the relevance of an old phrase that many project managers quote from time to time: "fast, cheap, or good; pick two." This may be a catchy phrase, but it highlights a crucial dilemma in project management. To help solve this dilemma, the project manager needs to understand the expectations of the sponsor and key stakeholders and to periodically assess them throughout the project life cycle. The project manager may identify some "give" or slack on one and possibly more of these expectations depending on the project, with its unique uncertainties and challenges. In the pain management example, most likely a specific target level of pain reduction is crucial to successfully achieve the product (product performance) requirements. This will probably represent the area where changes in project scope and direction will most likely occur. Since getting the product to market quickly is a goal (time-to-market), providing sufficient funding (resources) to support these objectives is critical. So, where is the "give" in the objectives based upon the needs of the management stakeholders? Managing the triple constraint and the expectations of management with regards to these objectives requires the development and management of the project's business case with financials.

The business case for a new product project should include the following:

- An evaluation of the market and customer needs including appropriate market research studies,
- An analysis of the competition including their potential products and strengths and weaknesses,

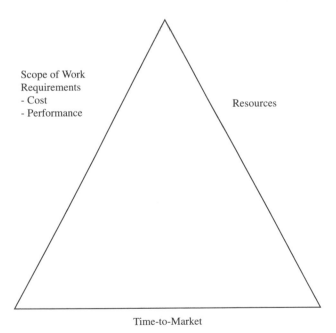

Fig. 1 New product projects objectives. (Adapted from Ref. 3.)

Scope of Work
Requirements
- Cost
- Performance

Resources

Time-to-Market

- A technical assessment of the capability of the organization as it relates to the product competing in the market,
- A statement of alignment to the organization's business strategy, and
- A preliminary evaluation of the financial opportunity of the new product, which may include use of return on
- Investment, discounted cash flow and internal rate of return, net present value, and break-even time (4).

Due to the uncertainty involved in the evaluation of new products, financial analysis tools that consider risks and opportunities are more appropriate and valuable than deterministic approaches. These new approaches to project financial evaluation that consider uncertainty include options analysis and Monte Carlo simulation. Due to their proactive handling of uncertainty, these tools can more accurately calculate the risks and opportunities of a new product concept (5). With the use of a financial analysis model, basic trade-off statements can be developed by the project manager to assist in understanding the importance of each objective. In the pain management product example, a statement emphasizing the value of time would be "a week delay in the project costs $1 million in today's money" (6).

Of course, all of this project definition process and effort, hopefully, will lead to an approved and ultimately successful new pharmaceutical product. The need for a concurrent process of project selling and support is emphasized due to the nature of new product development, the uncertainty of the projects, high cost, and limited resources. To accomplish this task, a new product project requires two types of individuals early in its life cycle:

champions and sponsors. Project champions are individuals within the organization who support the project and sell it to management. Project sponsors are senior-level executives whose support is needed to fund and provide resources for the project. Of course, the more champions that a new product has selling the concept, the greater the potential for funding and support from senior-level executives. The level of support needed and number of senior executives increases as the funding requirements of the project increase. This is probably obvious, and yet not recognizing them can result in missing a key new product concept.

Early in the life of a new product, its future is tenuous and requires an approach that not only puts it through a rigorous business, technical, and financial evaluation but allows it to nurture and grow into a development project where appropriate. An organization should have an early new product process that: 1) captures and provides an opportunity for all the valuable new concepts that an organization is researching to be evaluated on a level playing field, and 2) focuses the organization on those key few projects that allow for fast product development. This concept, called the "funnel" (Fig. 2) in some sources (2), shows the need for the following elements of successful initial project definition:

- A proactive process of mining both externally and internally for new product concepts,
- Research for these new product concepts and funding for the same to assure that the concepts are developed to an appropriate level prior to evaluation, and
- A process to evaluate new product concepts to assure that the best concepts are fully funded based upon the criteria identified above under business case.

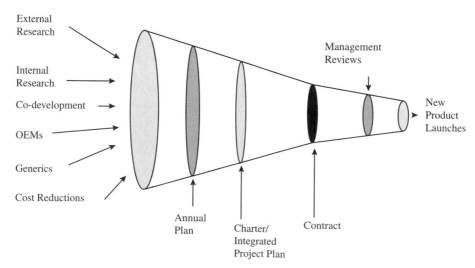

Fig. 2 New product "funnel."

The evaluation process, sometimes known as "stage gates" and "phased reviews"(7), needs to be accomplished early in the development project life and continue on throughout the life of a project as needed and defined in a *contract or integrated project plan*. The project plan will be reviewed later in this chapter along with its use in project reviews and stage gates.

PROJECT TEAM AND ORGANIZATION

A team is a small number of people with complementary skills who are committed to a common purpose, performance goals, and approach for which they hold themselves mutually accountable (8). Teams, however, are not necessarily the answer to all business endeavors, but the challenges of new pharmaceutical drug development lends itself very well to this organizational approach.

"Core" or primary team and support teams are used often to keep the number of team members small. A graphical illustration of this type of core and support team is shown in Fig. 3. Core team members represent the different functions of an organization, have significant authority and responsibility in the organization (especially for high priority projects), and have both specialist/technical and generalist/business skills. In the pain management example, the core team may include team members from:

- Program management,
- Marketing management,
- Clinical development,
- Formulation development,
- Analytical chemistry,
- Process development,
- Operations management, and
- Regulatory management.

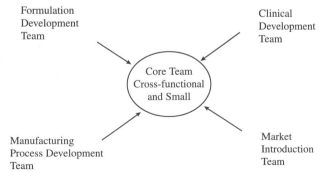

Fig. 3   Design of a project team.

This team example meets the definition criteria in that it is small in number and contains team members that have complementary skills and represent all or most of the functions in the project. Support teams and support team members would then be set up to work on the major elements of the project. In the graphical illustration shown in Fig. 3, these support teams would work on formulation development, clinical development, market introduction, and manufacturing process development.

To be small and effective, a core team should have around twelve members. For major, high-priority projects each team member must have considerable authority and responsibility within their respective functional organization. Each team member

- Ensures functional expertise on the project,
- Represents functional perspective on the project,
- Ensures functional deliverables are met, and
- Proactively raises functional issues that impact the team (2).

This "heavyweight" team member has the authority to either make the decisions and solve the problems on their own or involve the right functional support for decision making and problem solving.

Team members also represent the team. "Heavyweight" team members

- Share responsibility for team results,
- Revise project tasks and content,
- Establish project status reporting and other organizational responsibilities,
- Participate in monitoring and improving team performance,
- Share responsibility for ensuring effective team processes,
- examine issues from an executive point of view, and
- Understand, recognize, and responsibly challenge the boundaries of the project and team processes (2).

Team members must realize that they are part of a team. For the team to be most productive and effective, team members must collaborate with other team members, put aside their own personal or functional agenda, and use dialogue (10, 11) to develop a common understanding and create the best cross-functional approach for the project and the organization.

The term "heavyweight" has been used in this section to designate team members with significant authority and responsibility. Essentially, a heavyweight team is one where more decision making and problem-solving authority and responsibility reside in the team rather than in the functions. As shown in Fig. 4, teams need both a functional or specialist perspective and a project or

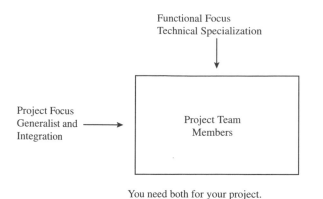

You need both for your project.
The question is which one is most important.

Fig. 4 Project organization structures.

generalist perspective to be effective. Depending on the needs of the project, either the functional or project perspective will be more important to its success. For example, a research project requires more of a technical specialization than a generalist perspective to be successful. Consequently, a functional approach would be more appropriate. Also, a small, generic drug project may not require the team clout and generalist perspective that a larger, proprietary drug would require. Consequently, a "lightweight" team, one where the functional perspective is more important and decisions are made mainly within the functions, may be more appropriate. A "heavyweight" team would have a stronger team oriented, cross-functional perspective rather than a functional perspective. A project or venture team, one where the team members are removed from their functions to report directly to the project leader, may be appropriate in some proprietary drug projects. Such a "heavyweight" team should be created in situations where a new business or market is being entered (12).

Leading a "heavyweight" team requires a project manager who has significant authority, responsibility, and skills, both technical and generalist, to be successful. A "heavyweight" project manager is one who manages, leads, and evaluates other members of the core team, champions the core concept, manages "in motion," is a multilingual translator (being fluent in different functional languages), and provides direct interpretation of market and customer needs. These individuals "earn the respect and right to carry out these roles based on prior experience, carefully developed skills, and status earned over time. A qualified leader who can play those roles as a heavyweight project manager is a prerequisite to an effective heavyweight team structure (2).

For an effective and productive team-oriented structure, organizations must support cross-functional

teams and use these teams in a way that makes them more effective. Support of teams requires teams be recognized formally as the approach for developing and introducing new pharmaceutical drugs to market. This may sound obvious, but in practice this requires new approaches to

*   Performance appraisal—including team-member and total team results with functional evaluations,
*   Promotion and pay—creating incentives based upon team results and involvement in successful new product teams, and
*   Career development—providing lateral career paths across the functions that develop heavyweight team members.

Anything less than changing the core approaches to these items will result in a team environment that is less than optimal (13).

PROJECT PLANNING, SCHEDULING, AND CONTROL

Although project management was certainly applied in practice prior to the mid-1950's, the development of the critical path method and the Project Evaluation and Review Technique (PERT) is considered to be the initiation of the modern practice of project management. The critical path method is a network analysis technique used to predict project duration by analyzing which sequence of activities or path most likely has the least amount of scheduling flexibility or the least amount of float. This critical path determines the earliest completion of the project (1). The critical path method relies on one estimate for the duration of a task, whereas PERT uses three estimates. These are most likely (i.e., the critical path method), worst case, and best case estimates. In practice, PERT becomes a very cumbersome approach to scheduling and tracking time.

Network logic determines the relationship between the tasks or team member deliverables, either sequential (finish to start) or overlapping (start to start and/or finish to finish). There are numerous software packages available at low cost to support calculation of the critical path and float. However, the real challenge of project management tools is the creation of the project network based upon historical experience and team involvement. By definition projects are unique and, in the pharmaceutical arena, each project is different. Therefore, the importance of team member involvement in the development, tracking, and adjustment of the project schedule is crucial to successful application of project management basics.

A popular approach for team members to develop a project network diagram is a concept known as the "yellow sticky" method. This method uses post-it notes, roll-paper, and markers and the team to develop a network diagram. The suggested steps of the "yellow sticky" method are as follows:

1. Identify the milestones that the project team will trackwith management along with target completion dates.
2. Identify the team member deliverables or responsibilities that need to be completed prior to the milestone dates (this provides ending linkages for deliverables).
3. Create the network diagram as follows:

   - Identify which tasks can be started today, based availability of information not upon availability of resources.
   - Identify which tasks can be started after the initial tasks are completed, which tasks can be completed after that and so forth to the end of the project or the next major milestone.

4. Obtain team member commitments to deliverables— usually best accomplished after the first planning meeting.
5. Negotiate between project milestone dates and team member deliverable dates.

Step 2 uses a very valuable tool known in project management as the work breakdown structure. The work breakdown structure is a "deliverable-oriented grouping of project elements which organizes and defines the total scope of the project" (1). In this example, recommended for pharmaceutical development use, the project is organized at the first level by the milestones that will be tracked. These are the milestones that senior management wants to see in the project. Examples are FDA submission, IND submission, product first lot to stock, first clinical supplies produced, etc. Under the milestones, each team member has deliverables, which are "any measurable, tangible, verifiable outcome, result or item that must be produced to complete a project or part of project" (1). Example of team member deliverables would be to develop the analytical method, develop the product formulation, develop the sterilization process, develop the manufacturing process, develop the specifications, produce clinical supplies, develop the clinical program, and prepare regulatory submissions. Project planning at a level of detail below this can certainly be done. However, a good rule of thumb is to plan down to the level of detail where a team member accepts primary responsibility for the deliverable and no further, unless two things happen:

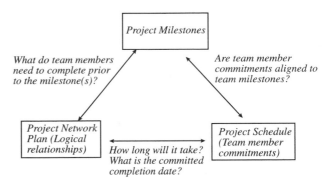

Fig. 5 Team-based project planning and scheduling approach.

- A team member does not understand the job and/or
- A team member is not motivated to do the job.

Standard operating procedures should handle the first issue and having the right team members should handle the second issue. Planning in more detail than this will result in unmotivated team members (i.e., micromanagement) and a schedule that is too cumbersome and detailed for tracking.

Steps 1–3 of this planning method are best accomplished in a core team meeting, along with support team members. Steps 4 and 5 are best accomplished after the meeting when the team members have time to evaluate their workload and commit to the deliverables. Negotiating the deliverable dates with project milestones is also best accomplished after the meeting. Project team members should be advised of the status of this process, but the project manager needs to accomplish this with individual team members, parts of the project team and management, and/or external stakeholder groups. This part of the process is graphically shown in Fig. 5. If there is a misalignment between management's expectations for completion of major milestones, there are a number of options:

- Change the milestone date,
- "Fast track" the project schedule, or
- "Crash" the project.

Changing the milestone date is straightforward. The target date is rescheduled because the original assumptions for this date were proven to be incorrect when the team came together to schedule the project. "Fast tracking" the project means to compress the project schedule by overlapping activities that would normally be done in sequence. This requires some risk taking, which needs to be clarified. "Crashing" the project means to decrease the total project duration after analyzing a number of alternatives to determine how to get the maximum duration compression for the least cost.

"Crashing" usually occurs by adding resources to reduce time. This happens when additional resources will not significantly reduce the time because the additional resources are not knowledgeable about the technology or part of the team process or a particular task requires a set period of time to complete.

The result of the project planning and scheduling process should be a planning document often called the project or integrated project plan. This serves to emphasize that it represents the integrated plan of all the team members. An integrated project plan should include the following information:

- The project scope and objectives,
- The business case and financial analysis and model of the project,
- The project risks and issues with contingency plans,
- The project plan and schedule (in milestone form for management review and in detailed team member deliverable form for the team members),
- The roles and responsibilities of the team members (best represented through a work breakdown structure tied to project milestones),
- Functional and technical strategies (e.g., regulatory strategy, plans, and challenges), and
- Performance measurements and incentives.

This is meant as an example for illustrative purposes, and the project manager and team should develop their own format and outline based upon their needs.

The Achilles' heel of project management is the time and resource estimate. In the majority of cases these are actually wrong. The only question is the level of inaccuracy in the estimate. There is no real scientific approach to better estimates and, similarly with all forecasts, it is more of an art and a "feel" to estimating than a science. Consequently, due to the uncertainty of projects

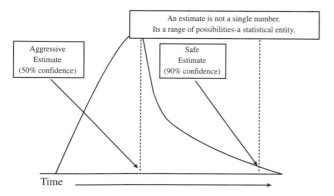

Fig. 6 Time and resource estimates: The Achilles' heel of project management.

and estimates, it is best to try to work with two numbers: the most likely and the high number (see Fig. 6). New, workable (as opposed to PERT) approaches to project management (i.e. "critical chain" project management) are available to schedule around uncertainty (14).

Once a project schedule is complete, it is used to track and review project progress towards completion. Some basic concepts on this are as follows:

- Project controls need to start with the team members.
- Team members need to take ownership for their tasks and part of this ownership is communicating status on a timely basis.
- A hierarchy of project reviews is needed in support of a pharmaceutical development project. Starting with project core and support team reviews on a weekly or more often basis, project reviews with management and other stakeholders are important to having a common understanding of project status.

Each of these elements would be part of a communication plan to be reviewed in a future section.

PROBLEM SOLVING AND DECISION MAKING USING PROTOTYPES

Pharmaceutical development projects consist of phases, technology transfer processes, milestones, and problem-solving cycles. Understanding these basic building blocks of pharmaceutical development projects in general and more specifically for your project is important towards understanding how your project will progress and how to structure that progress for status and communication purposes. For example,

- The phases of clinical development for a pharmaceutical development project: phase I, II, III, IV and post-marketing;
- The technology transfer from research to development and from development to manufacturing;
- The major milestones of a pharmaceutical project: FDA submission and first lot to stock;
- The use of different product prototyping cycles and their value towards solving problems, communicating results, and making progress.

An example of a pharmaceutical development life cycle is shown graphically in Fig. 7.

The transfer of technology from one organization to another is a key phase of the project itself. As shown in Fig. 8, there are two different approaches that can be used in the transfer of technology:

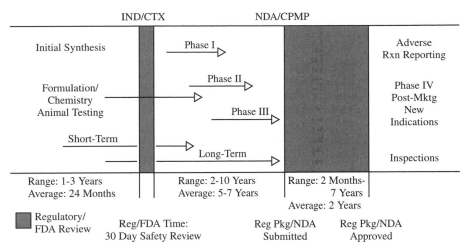

Fig. 7   Drug development phases.

- The traditional, sequential approach or
- The overlapping, concurrent approach.

The sequential approach is often known as the "throw it over the wall" approach. In this approach, the upstream group (e.g., the development team) waits until the product development effort is complete and creates specifications for the new product before communicating this information to the downstream group (e.g., the manufacturing team). Traditionally, this approach has been popular because it gives the perception of being efficient, that is, no time is wasted on incomplete designs and development work. Most often, however, this results in significant rework and inefficient use of time.

The overlapping approach is the more effective and efficient approach in practice and results in a truly integrated transfer of technology. In this approach, both the upstream and downstream groups work together to understand and solve the problems that need to be resolved to transfer the technology. Examples of these problems may include

- Development and transfer of the analytical methods.
- Development and transfer of the solution process.
- Development of product packaging, and
- Development of sterilization steps and methodology.

In an overlapping approach, team members from both the upstream and downstream groups work together to accomplish these tasks, resolve the problems, and make the necessary decisions. This requires early and intense involvement of the downstream group, even at times when it appears that progress is not occurring. This also requires early sharing of incomplete and, at times, inaccurate information by the upstream group. Sharing of this information may be considered risky due to the uncertainty of response from the downstream group. This approach requires collaboration and trust between the two groups—two basic elements to successful product development and teams (2).

Another basic building block of any product development project are design–build–test cycles. These cycles use prototypes to serve as a focal point for problem solving, testing, communication, and conflict resolution. Using these cycles provides feedback on decisions made so far and identifies issues that need to be resolved. Examples of the prototyping cycles for a clinical development project are

- Identify the bulk drug vendor,
- Determine formulation feasibility,
- Complete engineering runs,

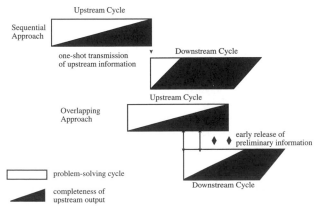

Fig. 8   Cross-functional integration requires overlapping problem solving. (Adapted from Ref. 9.)

- Produce clinical and/or stability samples,
- Ramp-up manufacturing process, and
- Produce first lot to stock product for sale.

These examples are shown to illustrate the importance of the design–build–test cycle process. Cycles will vary from project to project. Completing each of these cycles is a very effective approach to tracking and demonstrating project progress. Prototpyes can provide very focused communication about the progress to date and the remaining tasks required to complete the project (2).

SENIOR MANAGEMENT REVIEW AND CONTROL

Senior management provides the sponsorship, championship, and funding for the pharmaceutical development projects that new product teams are working on. They need to be involved and understand the importance of the project, its link to business strategy and growth, the risks and issues that the project is facing, and the status of the project. This understanding is important throughout the life of a project particularly at the start of the project. As shown in Fig. 9, the opportunity to effectively impact the project direction and scope is greater at the start of the project. However, as the project progresses, it becomes more difficult and costly to impact the project direction and scope. Typically, senior management involvement increases as the project gets closer to providing return on investment. This is usually late in the project life cycle and due primarily to an increase in project visibility as sales and marketing activities intensify.

Senior management involvement, especially at the start of the project, is key to successful project outcomes. Some

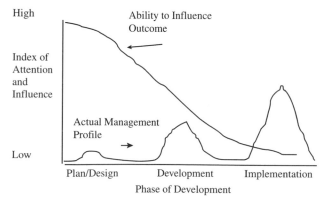

Fig. 9 Obtain senior management involvement early in setting projects direction. (Adapted from Ref. 15.)

process guidelines to assure management involvement are as follows:

1. Senior management should define strategic direction that will be used to drive new product development.
2. Senior management should define the new product project portfolio and the aggregate set of projects that will achieve their strategic objectives.
3. Senior management should be actively involved in assigning the type of project team (see earlier section) and type of project, i.e., where this project falls in the portfolio.
4. Senior management should develop and support a project review process that encourages early involvement in the project to validate the business assumptions and decrease project surprises (12).

The project manager of a pharmaceutical development project should proactively drive these process elements to assure active and early involvement of senior management in their project. The project must have the right support and visibility. Additionally, these process mechanisms assist in timely and appropriate project discontinuations.

Project reviews with senior management are a key element of the new product process. The project manager should have the ability to interface directly with senior management. As previously mentioned, a hierarchy of reviews is important to assure timely, continual communication of project status and issues. Also, stage gate reviews are a very popular process for clarifying project definition and evaluating the project's business case and technical issues. Senior management should get involved in these reviews to assure that the project continues to be on target and meet the overall goals for new product development. Senior management reviews should evaluate

- The business issues and goals of the project,
- Issues related to the customer's needs and the marketplace;
- Resource management;
- Corporate and business unit direction and product line fit;
- Sales and payback expectations;
- Project schedule;
- Timely introduction to market, and
- The availability and maturity of the technology to meet quality and cost targets;

These reviews can be scheduled to occur on a regular basis (e.g., after a phase is completed or every quarter, as stage or phase gates propose) or on an as-needed basis by senior management or the project team. The timing will be dependent upon the organization's requirements and the specifics of the project. These reviews can be mandatory (i.e., project can not proceed until this review is completed) or flexible. This is dependent upon organization's requirements and the specifics of the project. In all instances, these reviews need to be used to determine whether or not to continue with the project (e.g., make go/no go decisions) or change project direction (e.g., scope change). The concept of scope change will be the topic of the last section of this article.

PROACTIVE, REAL TIME CHANGE MANAGEMENT

As mentioned in this chapter previously, scope changes are to be expected in a pharmaceutical development project. The only question is the number and severity of these scope changes. Consequently, projects need a process for managing scope changes. Mandating the same, centralized controls for all projects, however, would probably be too constricting and result in unneeded bureaucracy—perhaps even impacting the ability for the project to be successful. The project team needs to self-regulate; manage scope changes depending on the unique needs of each project; and have the discipline to ensure appropriate process controls and management review.

Managing scope changes requires the proactive installation of a scope change process for projects that includes a method for identification and management of project risks. A suggested process for managing scope changes is the following:

1. *State the real problem*—Why is this scope change needed? It has been suggested to categorize scope changes into types to assist in determining the relative necessity and importance. Again, this may be overkill.
2. *Gather the relevant facts*—What is the impact if the scope change is implemented? What is the impact on the time to market and effect on development and final product costs? What will happen if the scope change is not implemented? These facts should be obtained from the appropriate people (i.e., the stakeholders that will be impacted one way or another by this scope change).
3. *Develop several alternative solutions*—Should nothing be done? Implement the total scope change as requested? Is there a compromise solution? Which stakeholders are interested in each solution and what are their expectations?
4. *Analyze and review impact for alternatives*—What are the impacts on time to market, investment cost, and product cost for each alternative? Financial analysis is a key element of this step because senior management

uses financials as a critical business indicator. Therefore, each alternative needs to be evaluated versus a financial model. What are the risks and trade-offs to consider for each alternative?
5. *Adopt the best alternative*—This is the connection to the senior management review process. For major scope changes, the project manager should provide an analysis of the major solutions. Based upon financial analysis and qualitative factors, the project manager should present the project team's recommendation to key stakeholders and senior management for their agreement and support.
6. *Tell everyone*—Obviously, the project team should be advised of the change in project scope because they will need to implement it. Project stakeholders also need to be advised so that they can support the scope change with the appropriate resources.
7. *Audit the outcome*—This step is undervalued. The success or failure of a project often relies on how well a scope change was or was not implemented. There are lessons to be learned from capturing the events that led to and caused scope changes and whether the change had a positive or negative impact on project success (17).

As mentioned previously, financial analysis of scope changes and the development of alternative solutions are critical steps towards the successful implementation of a scope change. Senior management needs this information to understand the financial impact on the business and the project manager must provide it. A suggested approach is illustrated graphically in Fig. 10. This approach requires that the project manager use a financial model for the project (which all projects should have) and understand

- The cost/benefit of time delays or improvements;
- The financial impact of increased or reduced product cost and/or project investment; and
- The benefit of improved product use, indications, functionality, or features.

Outlining the relationship of each of these variables to the scope change is an important first step. For example, delaying the project by one week costs approximately $5 million in division margin. A second step is to understand the specific impact of the scope change on each variable. For example, a scope change to add an additional product use and indication could delay the project three months (a 50% probability), cost an additional $5 million to implement, and result in additional division margin of $50 million over the life of the product. Is this worth the investment? Of course, the intangibles also need to be considered.

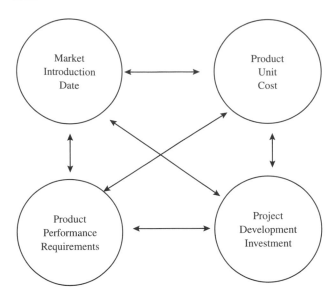

Fig. 10 Financial evaluation for justification of a scope change. (Adapted from Ref. 16.)

This "broad brush strokes" type of financial analysis is fundamental towards making informed decisions regarding trade-offs around the project objectives and scope changes (6). Given the magnitude of uncertainty of and complexity associated with pharmaceutical development, scope changes in this environment require more sophisticated analysis approaches (e.g., Monte Carlo simulation, options analysis, etc.). These tools are beyond the scope of this chapter, and the reader is asked to review the sources mentioned in the earlier sections of this chapter.

Uncertainty is reality in pharmaceutical development projects. Project uncertainty can be found in

- *The marketplace and the competitors*: What other companies will enter this market with a new drug and indication and what will be the impact?
- *The technology and its maturity*: Will our pharmaceutical and medical technology successfully solve the customer's problem or, at the least, produce better customer outcomes? Will the customer understand and use this technology?
- *The regulatory and governmental environment*: Will the regulatory bodies and government agencies modify the rules? If so, will it affect the basic assumptions of the project? Is there impact on the development, approval, or marketing of the product?
- *The suppliers of bulk, unique commodities and services*—Can the suppliers deliver on the sub-objectives of the project? Are there risks related to their technology, capabilities, or governing environment?

- *The project internal risks (e.g., funding, schedule, team components)*: Are the project team members capable of doing their tasks? Will the funding be available to support the project? Can the schedule be met?

These are general categories of risks and not meant to be all inclusive. Using these risk categories as a starting point, the project manager should expand on and flesh out specific details in order to define the most complete picture.

Risk identification is the first step of a risk management process. After risk identification, the project team needs to evaluate each risk in terms of two elements: 1) the probability of occurrence and 2) the financial impact. A popular tool in this process is a risk matrix shown graphically in Fig. 11. The matrix is used to identify the most important risks—those for which a contingency plan needs to be developed. The most important risks would fall into Quadrant IV of the matrix—those with a high probability of occurrence and high financial impact. As the example matrix indicates, the lines drawn between high and low is not quantitatively set but based upon the input of the project team. For risks in Quadrants II and III, continual monitoring is needed to determine whether the situation has changed significantly to warrant a contingency plan even though such a plan was not developed initially.

The basic concepts for risk management in a new product project environment are as follows:

1. Risk identification, quantification, and contingency planning is best accomplished with the full core team being involved.
2. Contingency plans will not be implemented for all risks that have been identified. However, when identifying risks, a common approach is to suggest a contingency plan for this risk. This can serve to encourage a proactive positive approach.

| | Probability of Occurrence | |
	Low	High
High (Financial Impact)	Quadrant II Low Probability High Impact No Contingency Plan Monitor	Quadrant IV High Probability High Impact Develop Contingency Plan
Low	Quadrant I Low Probability Low Impact No Contingency Plan	Quadrant III High Probability Low Impact No Contingency Plan Monitor

Fig. 11 Risk management plan.

3. Risk management is an ongoing process. You can't complete it and leave it. Many a project manager learned this hard way. Continual monitoring of risks, especially those in Quadrants II and III, is essential.
4. In general, risks resulting from project uncertainty are potentially the most damaging scope changes that could impact the project. It behooves the project manager and the team to proactively manage scope changes through a risk management process.

CONCLUSION

Traditional project management methodology (i.e., for the construction industry) developed 40 years ago has metamorphosed into an approach for managing new product development projects. This more flexible form of the application works well within a decentralized, team-oriented environment—an environment that is conducive to successful pharmaceutical new product development. Project management within the pharmaceutical arena plays a key role in bringing teams together, integrating solutions across functions, and providing a generalist view of projects to balance the more scientific/technical perspective. The future successful project manager will have a generalist orientation, hold team effectiveness and cross-functional integration as the top priority, and strive to overcome the barriers that would undermine these core tenets.

It is not enough to understand the concepts or utilize some of the tools of project management. For the most optimal results, organizations need to recognize the importance and fully support the role of project managers. Often organizations not fully committed to project management opt for interim or temporary solutions such as dual project leadership—a project having both a technical leader and a project manager. A similar tactic would be to have "dual hat" project managers—those who are project managers as a secondary role to their primary role as a functional or technical manager. These need to be replaced with a project manager performing solely that role and who will possess enough skills, knowledge, and clout to get the project completed. This is not an easy solution, but organizations will find that the right solutions are not often the easy ones (18).

REFERENCES

1. Project Management Institute (PMI) Standards Committee. *Project Management Body of Knowledge*; PMI, 1995.
2. Wheelwright, S.C.; Clark, K.B. *Revolutionizing Product Development*; Free Press: New York, 1992.
3. Reinertsen, D.G. *Managing the Design Factory*; Free Press: New York, 1997.
4. House, C.; Price, R. The Return Map: Tracking Product Teams. Harvard Bus. Rev. **1991**, Jan/Feb.
5. Amram, M.; Kulatilaka, N. *Real Options*; Harvard Business School Press: 1999.
6. Smith, Preston; Reinertsen, Donald. *Developing Products in Half the Time*; Van Nostrand Reinhold: New York, 1998.
7. Cooper, R.G. *Winning at New Products*; Addison-Wesley: Reading, MA, 1993.
8. Katzenbach, J.R.; Smith, D.K. *The Wisdom of Teams*; Harper Business, 1994.
9. Hayes, R.H.; Wheelwright, S.C.; Clark, K.B. *Dynamic Manufacturing*; Free Press: New York, 1988.
10. Issacs, W. *Dialogue, The Art of Thinking Together*; Currency Doubleday, 1999.
11. Senge, Peter. *The Fifth Discipline*; Currency Doubleday, 1990.
12. Wheelwright, S.C.; Clark, KimB. *Leading Product Development*; Free Press: New York, 1994.
13. Holahan, P.; Markham, S. Factors Affecting Multifunctional Team Effectiveness. *The PDMA Handbook of Product Development*; Rosenau, M.D., Jr., Ed.; John Wiley & Sons, Inc.: New York, 1996.
14. Newbold, Robert C. *Project Management in the Fast Lane*; APICS Series on Constraints Management. The St. Lucie Press, 1998.
15. Gluck, F.W.; Foster, R.N. Managing Technological Change: A Box of Cigars for Brad. Harvard Bus. Rev. **1985**, *141*, Sept–Oct.
16. Smith, P.; Reinertsen, D.G. *Developing Products in Half the Time*; VNR: New York, 1998.
17. Rosenau, M. *Successful Project Management*; John Wiley & Sons, Inc.: New York, 1998.
18. Bowen, H.K.; Clark, K.B.; Holloway, C.A.; Wheelwright, S.C. Make Projects the School for Leaders. Harvard Bus. Rev. **1994**, Sept/Oct.

PROTEIN BINDING OF DRUGS

Sylvie Laganière

Origenix Technologies, Inc., Quebec, Canada

Iain J. McGilveray

McGilveray Pharmacon, Inc., Ottawa, Ontario, Canada

INTRODUCTION

When a drug reaches the systemic circulation, either after intravenous administration or after absorption following extravascular administration, it can be distributed in the elements of blood (erythrocytes, etc.) or bind to plasma proteins. Blood transports the drug to different organs where it diffuses at different rates. The drug not bound to plasma proteins will diffuse in the extravascular compartments and tissues where it can then bind to other proteins or other tissue components.

The free drug concentrations are more closely correlated to the desirable or undesirable (toxic) pharmacological responses of a drug, because it is the unbound drug that is available to reach tissue receptors (1–3). However, it is the total (bound + unbound) drug concentration, measured in plasma or blood that is most often used in therapeutic drug monitoring to warn of ineffective or toxic levels and to adjust doses if needed. It is easier to measure total drug concentration after a simple blood draw, and usually the ratio of free to total drug concentration is constant. This chapter reviews different aspects of drug-protein binding.

METHODS FOR THE DETERMINATION OF DRUG PROTEIN BINDING

The most commonly used methods to determine drug binding to plasma proteins are equilibrium dialysis, ultrafiltration, and microdialysis. All have advantages and disadvantages, and results are method- and condition-specific.

As well as measuring the binding level of drugs in plasma, procedures can examine the number of binding sites, the affinity constants, and the nature of the protein involved (4) that allow interpretation of the impact of binding on drug pharmacokinetics and response. The general procedures involve separation of the free ligands, usually small drug molecules, from bound species attached to the protein.

Equilibrium Dialysis (ED)

Introduced in 1943 (5), ED remains the most frequently used procedure (6). A membrane separates two compartments, and at equilibrium, one compartment contains the plasma or serum with protein and bound ligand, whereas free drug is sequestered to the buffer solution compartment. The unbound fraction is determined by the ratio of drug concentration on the buffer side [D] divided by that in the plasma [D] + [DP]. Results are influenced by drug properties, proteins (content and concentration), volume of compartments, buffer strength, and ionic composition as well as by the thickness and physicochemical characteristics of the membrane (4). Time and temperature are major environmental factors, and dialysis for 4 h (or less) at 37°C has been found optimal for acidic and basic drugs (6).

In general, natural cellulose membranes are applied (7). Adsorption is low with drugs having acidic or hydrophilic characteristics. Nonspecific drug adsorption should be investigated when studying basic and lipophilic drugs (4).

In experiments, dilution or volume shifts from osmotic gradients between plasma and buffer compartments may be considerable and require correction (8). Poorly water-soluble drugs are difficult to study because use of organic solvents interferes with equilibrium distribution, and such drugs may also aggregate and adhere to membrane surfaces (7).

Ultrafiltration

Although introduced at the same time as ED (9), routine application of ultrafiltration has only recently become feasible because of improvements in membranes and equipment. Separation of the protein and bound ligand from the free drug in solution occurs using a suitable membrane that retains the proteins and is assisted either by positive pressure or more commonly by centrifugation.

Encyclopedia of Pharmaceutical Technology

The key advantage of ultrafiltration is speed (as little as 15 min), which is an important criterion for clinical monitoring situations (6) and for unstable drugs. As with ED, membrane properties and volume are important. The membranes (e.g., Amicon®) are permiselective and the cut-off can be directed at protein molecular weight sizes e.g., separation of albumin and globulins such as α1-acid glycoprotein (AAG). However, in some cases, high-molecular-weight drugs can be retained (7). Adsorption of drugs on the membrane is problematic with low concentrations, especially of lipid-soluble ligands. Saturation of the adsorbing sites with study drug or coating with silicone has been applied to overcome such problems.

Theoretically, the free ligand concentration will be constant in the ultrafiltrate and retentate (10). Nonetheless, a decrease in concentration of free drug in the retentate will result in the dissociation of bound ligand. However, provided the ultrafiltrate is not greater than 40% of the initial volume, the free ligand concentration is not affected (11). A disadvantage of both ED and ultrafiltration for low-concentration or highly bound ($\geq$90%) drugs is the need for radioisotopes to provide the sensitivity for quantitation.

Microdialysis

Microdialysis perfusion is proposed as an alternative to traditional techniques for studying drug–protein interaction. Small molecules in the sample, such as a drug, diffuse in the fiber and are transported to collection vials for analysis. The dialysis membrane excludes larger molecules such as protein and drug–protein-bound drugs. The dialysate could be analyzed using standard techniques. Microdialysis perfusion is as rapid as ultrafiltration, but the samples do not suffer from re-equilibration during separation of free drug from bound drug.

Because the technique requires more chromatographic analysis, it has a longer analytical time compared with the ultrafiltration technique. This technique could be used for in vitro determination of protein binding, also, because microdialysis probes can be implanted intravenously, binding of drug could be determined in vivo under physiological conditions after dosing (12). There has been some validation of the technique used for in vitro determination of the unbound fraction of drugs in plasma. Although there is good agreement between equilibrium dialysis and microdialysis for phenytoin and racemic aminoglutethimide, the unbound fractions are significantly higher for furosemide and disopyramide using microdialysis (13). Good correspondence was demonstrated

between ultrafiltration and microdialysis for acebutolol, acetaminophen, cephalothin, chloramphenicol, isoniazid, phenytoin, salicylic acid, theophylline, and warfarin (14). It appears that the microdialysis technique may not be suitable for all compounds because of their physicochemical properties and analytical limitations (15, 16).

Pacifici and Viani (6), commenting on comparisons among results from different methods applied to protein binding, warn that methods for drug binding need to be standardized. Currently, results depend greatly on technique and interpretation of results; thus, experimental details such as anticoagulant used, type of dialysis or filtration membrane, buffer characteristics, duration of experiment, and temperature should be taken into account.

PROTEIN BINDING PARAMETERS

Drugs bind to different proteins, such as albumin, globulins (e.g., α1-acid glycoprotein AAG and transcortin), and lipoprotein in plasma, and to tissue proteins. The reversible binding of a drug to macromolecules such as proteins is an equilibrium process. The relationship is described by the law of mass action:

$$[D] + [P] \underset{k_2}{\overset{k_1}{\rightleftharpoons}} [DP] \tag{1}$$

where [D], [P], and [DP] are the molar concentration of unbound (free) drug, unoccupied proteins, and the drug–protein complex, respectively, and k_1 and k_2 are rate constants for the reactions.

The equilibrium association constant for this reaction K_A is defined as k_1/k_2 and provides an index of the affinity between the binding sites and the ligand. The inverse of the association constant ($1/K_A$) is the equilibrium dissociation constant K_D for the drug–protein complex:

$$K_A = \frac{k_1}{K_2} = \frac{[DP]}{[D] \cdot [P]} \tag{2}$$

At equilibrium, the unbound fraction of drug (f_u) can be calculated from the following relationship:

$$f_u = \frac{[D]}{[D] + [DP]} \tag{3}$$

A protein can have several independent binding sites such that they may exhibit either the same or different affinities for the drug. The binding to one site may not affect binding to another site. The capacity constant (N_{TOT}) is the number of sites per mole of protein times the molar concentration of protein and has units of sites/L.

The concentration of bound drug can be expressed as the following:

$$[DP] = \sum_{n=1}^{n=i} \frac{N_{TOT,i}[D]}{K_{D,i} + [D]} \tag{4}$$

where i is the number of classes of binding sites, $N_{TOT,i}$ the capacity constant, [D] the unbound drug concentration, and $K_{D,i}$ the dissociation constant for the i site. Therefore, the extent to which a drug binds depends on the affinity of the drug, the number of binding sites per molecule, and the concentrations of both drug and binding proteins.

Fig. 1 shows a plot of [DP] versus [D] for a single class of binding sites. As the unbound drug concentration increases, the concentration of bound sites increases. When [D] is much larger than K_D, the equation predicts that [DP] reaches a maximum where it is equal to the maximum number of sites N_{TOT}. The dissociation constant K_D represents the concentration of unbound drug when half the sites are occupied, [DP] = $N_{TOT}/2$. The plots of Eq. 3 after linear transformations such as the Scatchard plot, the Woolf plot, and the double reciprocal plot can be used to determine the dissociation and capacity constants. The plots will be linear when there is one class of binding sites and will be curvilinear in presence of two or more classes of binding sites on the protein or if it binds to sites in more than one protein (17). For example, the Scatchard equation for a single class of binding site is:

$$\frac{[DP]/P_T}{[D]} = N \cdot K_A - \{(K_A \cdot [DP])/P_T\} \tag{5}$$

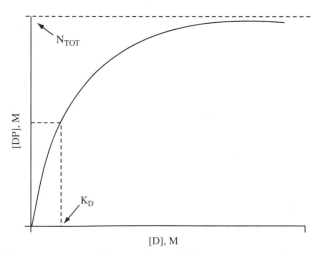

Fig. 1 A plot of bound drug [DP] versus unbound drug concentration [D] for a single class of binding sites.

where P_T is the molar concentration of total protein (occupied + unoccupied), and N the number of sites per mole of protein. A plot of ([DP]/P_T)/[D] versus [DP]/P_T gives a linear slope of $-K_A$ and a y-intercept of $N\cdot K_A$. Refined estimates of the capacity and affinity constant can be generated using a nonlinear least-squares computer program such as PCNONLIN (18).

Once the capacity and affinity constants have been obtained, the unbound plasma fraction of drug that binds to a single class of binding sites can be calculated for any value of free drug concentration:

$$f_u = \frac{[D]}{[D] + [DP]} = \frac{K_D + [D]}{N_{TOT} + [D] + K_D} \tag{6}$$

When a drug binds to two classes of binding sites such as albumin and AAG, the equation is:

$$f_u = \frac{1}{1 + \dfrac{N_{TOT1}}{K_{D1} + [D]} + \dfrac{N_{TOT2}}{K_{D2} + [D]}} \tag{7}$$

These equations indicate that the unbound fraction of the drug is dependent on the binding capacity N_{TOT}, the dissociation constant K_D, and the unbound drug concentration at equilibrium. At low free drug concentrations (i.e., [D] ≪ K_D), the unbound fraction will be independent of change in drug concentration.

DRUG BINDING PROTEINS

Human plasma contains more than 60 proteins (19). There are three main proteins associated with the binding of drugs: albumin, AAG, and lipoproteins. This article does will not review drug transport proteins of recent interest such as p-glycoproteins, organic anion transporters, and dipeptide transporters, which have been reviewed recently (20).

Albumin

zAlbumin (MW 66,300), an important binding protein present in plasma (40%) and interstitial fluid (60%) (21), which binds mostly to acidic (anionic) drugs (22) but also to cationic drugs, accounts for approximately 60% of total plasma protein (23). This water soluble protein has an isoelectric point of approximately pH 5. Therefore, at physiological pH, this protein is negatively charged, and acidic drugs bind usually to the N-terminal group. Normal serum concentrations are 38–48 g/L. Albumin is synthesized in the liver, and its half-life is approximately 19 days (23).

Two primary high-affinity drug binding sites for human albumin have been described. Binding site I, initially described for warfarin, was also shown to be involved in the binding of other drugs such as sulfonamides, phenytoin, valproic, acid and phenylbutazone. Site II (the benzodiazepine binding site) binds semisynthetic penicillins and probenecid. Naproxen, indomethacin, and tolbutamide have been shown to bind to both sites.

AAG

AAG (orosomucoid) is synthesized and metabolized by the liver with a half-life of approximately 5.5 days (24) and is an α1-globulin protein that is smaller (MW 40,000) than albumin. It is an acute phase reactant, and concentrations increase in stress situations including diseases. At least four polymorphic patterns and four genetic variants in human plasma have been reported (25, 26).

Many basic drugs (cationic) such as propranolol, lidocaine, and neutral drugs bind significantly to AAG (normal concentration 0.07–1.1 g/L) (27) and/or to lipoproteins in addition to albumin. Generally, the affinity of a drug that binds to both albumin and AAG is higher for AAG. Because the concentration of AAG in plasma in lower than that of albumin, the AAG is referred to as a low-capacity, high-affinity protein. AAG also binds to some acidic (28, 29) and neutral drugs such as carbamazepine (17) and prednisolone (30). Interpatient variability in the plasma free fraction of several drugs such as propranolol (31), carbamazepine (32), disopyramide (33), alprenolol (34), imipramine (34), lidocaine (35), and methadone (36), is related to AAG concentration in plasma.

Lipoproteins

The lipoproteins are a heterogeneous group of proteins (MW 2,500,000 for β-lipoprotein). They are classified into four groups: chylomicrons, very low-density lipoproteins (VLDL), low-density lipoproteins (LDL), and high-density lipoproteins (HDL) (37, 38). Lipoproteins can account for 95% of total probucol binding in plasma (37). Neutral and basic lipophilic drugs most commonly bind to lipoproteins; some acid drugs may bind to a lesser extent (37). Drugs that bind to lipoproteins include probucol, cyclosporin, propranolol, lidocaine, pindolol, digoxin, digitoxin and tetracycline (37, 39–41). Quinidine and some antidepressants drugs such as amitriptyline and nortriptyline exhibit saturable binding to lipoproteins. An inverse relationship was reported between the unbound fraction of drugs and concentrations of various lipoproteins

in serum for amitriptyline, imipramine, nortriptyline, and cyclosporin (37, 39, 42).

A list of some acidic, basic, and neutral drugs highly bound (>70%) to the different plasma proteins after therapeutic doses is given in Table 1 (43).

INFLUENCE OF BINDING ON DRUG DISPOSITION

Volume of Distribution

The apparent volume of distribution at steady state (V_{ss}) is influenced by plasma and tissue protein binding according to equation:

$$V_{SS} = V_P + (f_P/f_T)V_T \tag{8}$$

where f_P and f_T are the unbound fraction of drug in plasma and tissue, respectively, and V_P and V_T, are the volumes of distribution in plasma and tissue (44). The importance of binding in the plasma versus the tissue compartment is the primary determinant of the apparent volume of distribution for a drug. The distribution equilibrium of the drug in the body varies among tissues.

Tissue binding

Tissue binding can be a major determinant of pharmacokinetic characteristics of drugs, including volume of distribution and half-life. At present, no entirely satisfactory method is available for the determination of tissue binding. Sampling is invasive, and experimental animal values are difficult to validate for human correlations (45).

Examples of changes in tissue binding are the tissue displacement of digoxin by quinidine (46) and the decrease in tissue binding of digoxin in uremia (47). As a result in both cases, the volume of distribution of digoxin is decreased.

The binding of drug to tissue is usually reversible. In some cases, however, there is covalent binding, which by definition is not reversible. This applies to drug or metabolite and could be important because it could be related to toxicity (48). A good correlation has been reported in animals between the degree of covalent binding to hepatic protein and the severity of hepatic necrosis of paracetamol, isoniazid, adriamycin, and furosemide (48).

Characteristics of drugs with a large volume of distribution include weak binding to plasma proteins, high affinity to tissue protein, and high liposolubility. Increased volume of distribution can be related to an increased unbound fraction in plasma as, for example, for propranolol in chronic stable liver disease (47). Increased

Table 1 Predominant binding proteins of drugs >70% bound to plasma proteins

Albumin (% bound)	Albumin and AAG (% bound)	Albumin and lipoproteins (% bound)	Albumin, AAG, and lipoproteins (% bound)
Ceftriaxone (A)	Alprenolol (B)	Cyclosporine (N)[a]	Amitriptylline (B)
Clindamycin (A)	Carbamazepine (N)	Probucol (N)[a]	Bupivacaine (B)
Clofibrate (A)	Disopyramide (B)[b]		Chlorpromazine (B)
Dexamethasone (N)	Erythromycin (B)		Diltiazem (B)
Diazepam (B)	Lidocaine (B)		Imipramine (B)
Diazoxide (A)	Meperidine (B)		Nortriptyline (B)
Dicloxacillin (N)	Methadone (B)		Perazine (B)
Digitoxin (N)	Verapamil (B)		Propranolol (B)
Etoposide (N)			Quinidine (B)
Ibuprofen (A)			
Indomethacin (A)			
Nafcillin (A)			
Naproxen (A)			
Oxacillin (A)			
Phenylbutazone (A)			
Phenytoin (A)			
Probenecid (A)			
Salicylic acid (A)			
Sulfisoxazole (A)			
Teniposide (N)			
Thiopental (A)			
Tolbutamide (A)			
Valproic acid (A)			
Warfarin (A)			

[a]Albumin is minor binding protein.
A, indicates acid; B, base; N, neutral.
(From Ref. 43.)

volume of distribution could also result from shift of albumin-bound drug from the vascular to the interstitial space, as reported for ceftriaxone during open-heart surgery (49). For an AAG-bound drug, a decrease in volume of distribution would be related to an increase in binding in plasma because of stress-related conditions, increasing available AAG. Distribution equilibrium is achieved when unbound drug concentrations are the same in plasma and tissue.

Clearance

Hepatic clearance

The simple venous equilibrium model of organ clearance developed by Rowland (50) and Wilkinson (51) can be used to predict the effect of protein binding on hepatic plasma clearance:

$$Cl_H = \frac{Q(Cl_{l,u}f_u)}{Q + (Cl_{l,u}f_u)} \qquad (9)$$

where $Cl_{l,u}$ is the intrinsic unbound hepatic clearance, Q the hepatic plasma flow, and Cl_H the hepatic clearance.

Other models of hepatic clearance include the sinusoidal model and the dispersion model (52). All these models assume that only unbound drug can move freely through cell membranes and that the unbound fraction of a drug measured in the systemic circulation is the same as the fraction available for hepatic metabolism. The $Cl_{l,u}$ value is measured by dividing the intrinsic clearance of total drug by the measured unbound fraction.

There is, however, evidence of nonrestrictive clearance by the liver when the fraction of drug available for metabolism may not be restricted to the unbound fraction of drug (53). Drugs that bind to AAG or lipoproteins could be taken up directly by the hepatocytes by endocytosis (54, 55).

Restrictive drug clearance

A drug is said to be restrictively cleared if the extraction efficiency by an eliminating organ (E) is less than or equal to the unbound fraction of drug measured in the venous circulation. For these drugs, only the unbound fraction is available for distribution in the tissues, biotransformation, and excretion. For restrictive drugs with low extraction efficiency ($Cl_{I,u} \cdot f_u$ Q), a change in unbound fraction will affect the blood clearance as Eq. 9 simplifies to Eq. 10:

$$Cl_H = Cl_{i,u} \cdot f_u \tag{10}$$

The average steady-state drug concentration in plasma for a restrictively cleared and poorly extracted drug is determined by:

$$C_u = \frac{F D/\tau}{Cl_{l,u}} \tag{11}$$

where τ is the dosage interval. Therefore, a change in the unbound fraction will not affect the unbound concentration. It will then not be necessary to alter drug dosage after a change in binding in this situation.

It is important to note that an increase in the f_P value (fraction unbound in the plasma) caused by a displacement from drug during drug–drug interaction will cause only a transient rise in the unbound drug concentration, followed by a return to the predisplacement value when steady state has been reached (56, 57).

The influence of altered plasma or tissue binding on the elimination half-life depends on the relative influence of binding on the volume of distribution and the clearance. For a restrictively cleared and poorly extracted drug with moderate to large volume of distribution (i.e., >0.4 L/kg), the equation to reflect the half-life could be represented as:

$$t_{1/2} = 0.693 \left(V_T / Cl_{l,u} \cdot f_T \right) \tag{12}$$

and a change in plasma binding would have little influence on the half-lives of restrictively cleared drugs (e.g., diazepam, phenytoin) (56). For a drug with a small volume of distribution (<0.4 L/kg) such as warfarin, the $t_{1/2}$ value will be affected by a change in plasma or tissue binding.

Examples of significant drug interactions in which protein binding displacement is the major factor are phenytoin displacement by salicylic acid and tolbutamide and warfarin displacement by trichloroacetic acid, a metabolite of chloral hydrate (57). A change in dosage regimen is not necessary for phenytoin because, as described above, a displacement of restrictively cleared drugs from protein will decrease the total drug concentration but at steady state will not affect the average unbound concentrations. For warfarin, it might be necessary to temporarily adjust the dosage regimen because

this is a narrow therapeutic index drug with a long half-life and small volume for distribution.

Renal clearance

In the kidney, only the unbound drug is filtered. If the drug is not bound and there is absence of drug secretion and reabsorption, the renal clearance is a measure of the glomerular filtration rate (GFR). If the drug is protein-bound, the renal clearance of total drug in the plasma is less than the GFR, but the clearance of the free drug is equal to the GFR, as described by the relationship $Cl_R = f_u \cdot GFR$. For a drug that is either reabsorbed or secreted, the effect of altered protein binding is less predictable. Renal clearance expressed in terms of the renal processes is as follow:

$$Cl_R = (Cl_{RF} + Cl_{RS})(1 - FR) \tag{13}$$

where Cl_{RF} is the renal filtration clearance, Cl_{RS} the renal secretion clearance, and FR the reabsorbed fraction, and

$$Cl_{RS} = RBF f_u Cl_l / (RBF + f_u Cl_l) \tag{14}$$

where RBF is the renal blood flow. The clearance of drugs that undergo extensive tubular secretion (e.g., penicillins) is independent of plasma protein binding. The lack of reported side effects for the interaction of ceftriaxone with probenecid may be explained by the wide therapeutic index of the ceftriaxone (58).

Nonrestrictively cleared drugs

For nonrestrictively cleared drugs ($E > f_B$), which are highly cleared by an organ ($Cl_I > Q$), the unbound fraction is not rate-limiting because the clearance is determined primarily by the organ blood flow, and a change in unbound fraction will not affect the blood clearance. For example, the bioavailability of an oral dose will be independent of changes in blood or plasma protein binding. Changes in the plasma binding of nonrestrictively cleared drugs, given orally or intravenously, should not affect the average total drug concentration (56). Examples of nonrestrictively cleared drugs include morphine, meperidine, lidocaine (59), verapamil (60), and tricyclic antidepressants (61).

Drugs, that are nonrestrictively cleared by renal tubular secretion include penicillin and acetazolamide (57). Although significant displacement of penicillins by aspirin and sulfonamides occurs, as shown by an increase of up to 88% in unbound fractions of penicillins and no change in total drug concentration, this interaction is not clinically important because of the wide therapeutic index of these drugs (62). It is worth noting that although the clearance is not affected by a change in binding, a change in the f_u value may affect the drug response. The elimination half-lives of nonrestrictively cleared drugs is affected in relation to the equation:

$$t_{1/2} = \frac{0.693(V_P + (V_T \cdot f_B/f_T))}{Q} \tag{15}$$

For a drug with a large volume of distribution, such as propranolol, a smaller unbound fraction in the plasma will result in a shorter half-life, a greater fluctuation during the dosage interval, and no change in the average total drug concentration. For drugs with small volumes of distribution, such as penicillins, a change in plasma or tissue binding will have little influence on their half-lives. A change in drug binding to tissues alters the apparent volume of distribution. Therefore, an increase in tissue binding will produce an increase in volume of distribution and half-life.

Concentration Dependent Binding

The degree of binding of a drug is independent of drug concentration when the molar unbound concentration is well below the dissociation constant of the drug–protein complex. Nonlinear binding during therapeutic doses may occur when the K_D value and the therapeutic concentrations are close (see Fig. 1). For valproic acid (63), the K_D value for the high-affinity site is 5×10^{-5} M, and the therapeutic range of free concentrations is 0.7 to 2×10^{-4} M. For salicylic acid (22), the K_D value is 10^{-5} M and the therapeutic range of free concentrations is 3 to 7×10^{-5} M. Nonlinear binding is also reported for diflunisal, an anti-inflammatory drug (64), and for thiopental (65) and diazoxide (66) all of which bind predominantly to albumin. Important examples of concentration dependent binding are shown for disopyramide (2, 67) over the therapeutic concentration range and for lidocaine at the upper boundary of the therapeutic range (68, 69). The concentration-dependent binding of prednisolone, observed at very low unbound concentrations, is explained by its high-affinity binding to transcortin (70).

For a restrictively cleared drug with concentration-dependent binding, such as disopyramide, the unbound drug concentration increases proportionally with the increase in dosage regimen. Also, with the increase in the fraction unbound, the clearance also increases. Although the total concentration also increases, it is less than proportional to the increase in dosage rate. In this case, the total concentration can be misleading, and dose adjustment should be based on the unbound concentration

of disopyramide or, if unavailable, on the patient's response (2, 71).

Blood Versus Plasma Clearance

Pharmacokinetic parameters should preferably be determined from blood, but usually drug concentration is measured in plasma or serum. Although the free fraction will be different in tissue versus plasma, the unbound concentration will be the same at equilibrium as $(f_P C_P) = (f_B \cdot C_P)$.

The determination of the blood/plasma ratio will help estimate the importance of the distribution of the drug in the erythrocytes. Drug binding to erythrocytes is usually rapidly reversible.

Drugs that bind strongly to red blood cells may exhibit concentration-dependent uptake from plasma. This is reported for acetazolamide (72), chlorthalidone (73), and cyclosporine (74). The determination of the blood to plasma (B/P) ratios can be method specific. For example, the determination of the B/P ratio of cyclosporine A increases from 1.5 to 3.0 when estimated at body temperature (37°C) compared with a ratio of 2.5–10.0 at room temperature (20°C) (75). Drugs reported to bind strongly to the erythrocytes (B/P ratio > 1) are promazine, chlorpromazine, propranolol, salicylate, phenobarbital, pentazocine, and phenytoin (48).

Usually, the pharmacokinetic parameters are calculated from plasma rather than from whole blood data. The use of plasma-related parameters to measure organ extraction ratios and intrinsic clearance could, however, be misleading. When drug binding is similar in plasma and red blood cells, $C_B \approx C_P$ because $f_B \approx f_P$. However, if the binding in plasma is greater than that in red blood cells, $C_B < C_P$ and $AUC_B < AUC_P$ and use of plasma clearance will provide an underestimate of the blood clearance. Maximum errors are of the order of 40%. If the B/P ratio is >1, the clearance determined from plasma concentrations would significantly overestimate blood clearance and could exceed hepatic blood flow.

Usually, total plasma concentration of drug is measured in plasma. The total drug concentration in blood can be estimated by:

$$C_B = C_{RBC} \cdot HCT + C_P(1 - HCT) \tag{16}$$

where HCT is hematocrit, and C_{RBC} is the drug concentration in red blood cells. Although drug binding to plasma proteins is usually rapidly reversible, some studies reported the presence of irreversible binding to albumin (e.g., the acyl glucuronide metabolite of zomepirac (76) and tolmetin (77)).

Stereoselectivity

For acidic drugs, stereoselectivity was demonstrated for both albumin binding sites I and II (78). Stereoselective binding was reported for ibuprofen enantiomers, with the mean averaged unbound fraction of the R(−) enantiomer being 0.419%, significantly less than that of the S(+)-enantiomer of 0.643%. The percentage unbound of each enantiomer was concentration-dependent over the therapeutic range and was influenced by the presence of its optical antipode (79). Stereoselective binding in humans was reported for acidic drugs such as etodolac, flurbiprofen, ibuprofen, moxalactam, pentobarbital, phenprocoumon, and warfarin and for basic drugs such as chloroquine, disopyramide, methadone, propranolol, mexiletine, and verapamil. A list of human plasma protein binding of drug enantiomers was summarized by Jamali et al. (80).

Stereoselectivity in protein binding of enantiomers can also differ among species. For propranolol, a basic drug bound to AAG, the R-enantiomer binds less than the S-isomer in humans and dogs, and the reverse is observed in rat. Also, although the difference in binding is small in humans and dog, it is significant in rat (81).

Although the enantiomers of disopyramide displaced each other from AAG binding sites, resulting in a 2- to 2.6-fold change in f_u value in vitro (82), no significant enantiomer–enantiomer interaction in serum was found in vivo, presumably because of the buffering effect of serum albumin (60). The free fraction of verapamil enantiomers, determined from ex vivo volunteer samples after intravenous therapy (R-verapamil 0.06 ± 0.01, and S-verapamil 0.12 ± 0.02), was similar to that observed in vitro in the subjects' predose serum. The free fraction of both enantiomers was higher after oral drug therapy, the R- and S-isomers being 0.13 ± 0.02 and 0.23 ± 0.03, respectively. The difference in binding might be attributable to competition for serum binding sites from verapamil metabolites, which reach higher concentrations after oral administration (60).

A difference in the binding of the two isomers, quinine and quinidine, was reported (1, 2), and the f_u value of quinine and quinidine was 7.5 ± 2.2% and 12.3 ± 2.3%, respectively, in normal human plasma.

INFLUENCE AND CONSEQUENCES OF BINDING ON DRUG PHARMACODYNAMIC EFFECTS

The free fraction of drug is most likely to relate to pharmacological effect. None-the-less, because it is methodologically easier to determine total drug concentrations in blood or serum and the free/total drug concentration is usually constant, total concentrations are commonly applied in therapeutic drug monitoring. However, for some drugs the free/total ratio is variable, and disease conditions and drug interactions may alter it. In general, for monitoring of drug concentrations, the plasma or serum is used as the liquid of reference for practical reasons, but blood concentration is preferable because it reflects total drug concentration available for distribution.

Monitoring of Free Drug Concentrations

The monitoring of free drug concentrations may be necessary for drugs with concentration-dependent binding over the therapeutic range or in patients with diseases or conditions for which the unbound fraction of a drug could be significantly altered from normal (83). Compared with drugs that are mostly free in plasma, drugs that are highly bound ($f_u < 30\%$) would be candidates for monitoring because they are most likely to show significant differences in the unbound fraction under certain conditions.

Drugs for which total drug concentrations are usually measured and for which there would be advantage in monitoring free drug concentrations include carbamazepine, phenytoin, valproic acid, disopyramide, lidocaine, and quinidine (84–86). For disopyramide, monitoring of free drug concentration should be applied to the active enantiomer (87). However, monitoring of free concentration of these drugs in all patients is not recommended unless one of the following criteria is exhibited: 1) patients with disease likely to be associated with altered unbound fraction, 2) patients under treatment with a drug combination with potential protein binding interaction, and 3) patients showing unexpected drug response at a determined total drug concentration.

FACTORS AFFECTING PROTEIN BINDING AND CLINICAL CONSEQUENCES

Changes in protein binding may be related to factors affecting the concentration of proteins, to the variation in conformation of the binding protein such as for albumin, and to displacement from a protein binding site. The consequences of alteration in protein binding may be more important clinically for drugs highly bound (<90%) to plasma proteins at therapeutic concentrations and drugs with small a volume of distribution and narrow therapeutic index (88). A list of pathologic/physiologic conditions

Table 2 Pathological/physiological conditions associated with altered protein concentrations

	Albumin	AAG	Lipoproteins[a]
↓ Plasma protein concentration	Acute febrile infections Acute viral hepatitis Acute pancreatitis Advanced age[a] Analbuminemia[a] Burn injury[a] Cancer[a] Cirrhosis[a] Cystic fibrosis Hyperthyroidism Malabsorption Malnutrition Neonates/young infants Nephrotic syndrome[a] Pregnancy[a] Prolonged bedrest Protein-losing nephropathy Renal failure Rheumatoid arthritis Stress Surgery[a] Trauma injury[a]	Advanced age Cirrhosis Neonates/young infants Oral contraceptives Pregnancy Severe liver disease	Familial deficiencies[a] Hyperthyroidism Low cholesterol diet
↑ Plasma protein concentration	Dehydration Gynecological syndrome Optic neuritis/retinitis Psychosis Unspecified neuroses	Acute myocardial infarction[a] Administration of some enzyme inducers[a] Advanced age Burn injury[a] Cancer Chronic pain syndrome Inflammatory disease[a] Pneumonia Renal transplant Surgery[a] Trauma injury[a]	Alcoholism Antihypertensive drugs Biliary obstruction Diabetes mellitus Familial-hyperlipoproteinemia[a] Gout High-cholesterol diet Hypothyroidism Liver disease Nephrotic syndrome Pancreatitis Phenytoin or cyclosporine administration. Pregnancy Renal failure

[a]Conditions likely to be associated with major changes.
(From Ref. 43.)

associated with altered protein concentrations is given in Table 2.

Physiologic Conditions

Age

The plasma protein binding of drugs bound to albumin and AAG in neonates is significantly lower than that in healthy adults. AAG is low at birth and increases gradually over 12 months to reach a normal concentration (89). Factors associated with the decrease in binding are lower albumin and AAG concentrations and the presence of fetal albumin. Also, high serum concentrations of bilirubin and free fatty acids occur in the neonate, and these can compete for the albumin binding sites (90–93).

In the elderly, a small decrease in albumin concentration is associated with a small decrease in binding for salicylate (94), diazepam (95, 96), phenylbutazone (94) and valproic acid (97). Also in the elderly, an increase in concentration of AAG is associated with an increase in binding of AAG-bound drugs (98). Such an increase in AAG concentrations could be related to the greater incidence of inflammatory diseases in this population.

Pregnanoy

Significant decreases in protein binding of albumin-bound drugs are reported particularly during the third trimester of pregnancy, and are related to decreased albumin concentrations and higher, concentration of fatty acids, especially during labor. As a result, increases in the unbound fraction of salicylate (70–80%) (64–69), sulfisoxazoles (70–80%) (99), phenytoin (30%) (99–101), diazepam (40–60%) (99, 100), and valproic acid (50%) (100) occur.

For AAG-bound drugs, a 35–80% increase of the unbound fraction in the third trimester is reported for propranolol (92), lidocaine (92), and bupivicaine (102). After pregnancy, whereas albumin takes 1 month to return to normal levels, AAG and free fatty acid levels return to normal within as few days of delivery (101).

Ethnicity

Formely, much of the information obtained on drugs was acquired in Caucasian subjects. A report on inter–ethnic differences in drug response showed differences in drug protein binding between Chinese and Caucasian subjects. No difference was shown for warfarin, which is an albumin-bound drug, whereas the binding of lidocaine was significantly lower in Chinese subjects and related to lower concentrations of the binding protein AAG (103). Because lidocaine toxicity is related to free drug, this difference could have therapeutic significance. A similar reduction in

the binding of propranolol and disopyramide was also reported previously (104, 105). This ethnic difference does not seem to extend to drugs bound to albumin. Studies, that examined diazepam and salicylic acid, describe findings similar to those observed for warfarin (106).

Gender, smoking, obesity, nutritional status, surgery

The unbound concentration of diazepam is 14% greater in females than in males, whereas there are no significant differences in the binding of lidocaine (107). Although McNamara (69) reported a small increase in plasma binding of lidocaine, resulting in a decrease in free fraction from 0.31 to 0.26 in smokers, another study reported no effect of smoking on the plasma binding of lidocaine and diazepam (96).

In obese women, the AAG concentrations are doubled, and the unbound plasma fraction of propranolol is 30% lower than that in women with normal body weight (108). In the obese, the albumin concentrations, and phenytoin binding are normal, whereas diazepam binding is slightly reduced (108). In undernourished or hospitalized patients, the AAG concentrations are 30–40% higher than those in unhospitalized patients, and the propranolol free fraction is reduced by approximately, 30% (109). A marked decrease in albumin concentration has been reported in malnutrition, and it seems associated with a reduction in protein synthesis (81).

In postoperative situations, with lower albumin and increased AAG concentrations, the unbound free fractions of propranolol (101) and quinidine (111) are 30–40% reduced and 100–150% higher for the albumin-bound phenytoin (112, 113). For drugs such as quinidine, which are restrictively cleared and bound to AAG, the concentration of which would rise after surgery, no effect on unbound drug concentration should be anticipated (111). In patients undergoing open-heart surgery, the unbound free fraction of ceftriaxone is up to four-fold higher compared with that in healthy volunteers because of low plasma albumin and high free fatty acid concentrations (49, 114).

Disease States

Renal disease

The most common cause of alterations in plasma albumin concentrations is hypoalbuminemia, which is associated with a variety of physiological and pathological conditions (see Table 2). This decrease in binding capacity results in an increase in unbound concentrations in plasma. Gugler et al. (115) reported a significant inverse correlation between albumin concentration and the

Table 3   Altered plasma protein binding of drugs associated with renal dysfunction

↓ Binding			↑ Binding
Cephalosporins	Furosemide	Phenytoin	Chlorpromazine
Chloramphenicol	Midazolam	Prazosin	Lidocaine
Clofibrate	Morphine	Salicylic acid	
Diazepam	Naproxen	Sulfonamides	
Dicloxacillin	Penicillin G	Triamterene	
Diazoxide	Pentobarbital	Warfarin	
Diflunisal	Phenobarbital		
Digitoxin	Phenylbutazone		

(From Ref. 43.)

unbound plasma fraction of phenytoin in patients with nephrotic syndrome in chronic renal failure and uremia, a decrease in the binding of albumin-bound drugs was reported and related to the presence of endogenous inhibitors that accumulate (116, 117). A list of drugs associated with altered plasma protein binding in renal dysfunction is given in Table 3 (43).

Liver disease

In liver disease, the changes in drug binding may be related to a decrease in albumin and AAG concentrations attributable to either a decreased rate of synthesis or a loss of plasma proteins to the interstitial compartments. Changes may also be caused by an accumulation of endogenous inhibitors of drug binding such as bilirubin (59). For albumin-bound drugs such as diazepam and tolbutamide, the mean unbound fractions are 65–75% higher in chronic alcoholics (118) and correlate with albumin concentrations. For the AAG-bound erythromycin, the unbound fraction is two to four times higher in patients with cirrhosis compared with control subjects (119) and correlates with AAG concentrations. Increases in unbound fraction have been reported for prazosin, propranolol, morphine, diazepam, tolbutamide, phenylbutazone, phenytoin, quinidine, triamterene, theophylline, and lidocaine (48).

Pathologies associated with inflammatory conditions

AAG is a protein known as an acute phase reactant. As a result of inflammation, injury during physiological trauma, and stress (21, 39, 84, 88, 114), an increase in the binding capacity of AAG is commonly observed in patients. For a drug that is highly bound, an increase in AAG plasma levels will result in a significant decrease in unbound plasma fraction. Examples include propranolol (120), lidocaine (121), and disopyramide (34) after myocardial

infarction and propranolol and chlorpromazine (122) in Crohn's disease.

An increase in AAG concentrations after an acute myocardial infarction causes a decrease in the unbound plasma fraction of propranolol and lidocaine (nonrestrictively cleared drugs). With intravenous or oral propranolol, an increase in dosage regimen may be required (120). For lidocaine, it is recommended that normal infusion rates be used because total drug concentrations increase during long-term infusion, and the increase in binding indicates that the unbound fraction does not change significantly (121).

Cancer and burn injury

Cancer and burn injury are associated with increased concentrations of AAG and decreased concentrations of albumin in plasma. For AAG-bound drugs, a 20–30 % decrease in the unbound fractions of lidocaine (123), methadone (36), propranolol (31), and imipramine (124) is observed, whereas the unbound fractions of albumin-bound drugs increase for tolbutamide (30%) (123), diazepam (180%) (124), and phenytoin (150%) (125).

Diabetes mellitus

The decreased plasma binding of sulfisoxazole in patients with diabetes is related to in vivo glycosylation of albumin, whereas the decreased plasma binding of diazepam may be caused by high concentrations of free fatty acid displacers (126, 127).

Thyroid disease

A decrease in concentration of proteins and an increase in concentration of free fatty acids in plasma are observed in hyperthyroidism. For propranolol and warfarin, an increase of up to 20–30 % in the unbound plasma fractions has been reported (128).

Table 4   In vivo drug interactions caused by protein displacement

Drug	Displacer	Drug	Displacer
Bupivacaine	Lidocaine	Phenytoin	Salicylic acid
Carbamazepine	Valproic acid[a]		Tolbutamide
Ceftriaxone	Probenecid[a]		Phenylbutazone[a]
Diazepam	Valproic acid[a]		Valproic acid[a]
Methotrexate	Salicylic acid[a]	Valproic acid	Salicylic acid[a]
	Probenecid[a]	Warfarin	Diflunisal
	Sulfisoxazole[a]		Phenylbutazone[a]
Penicillin	Aspirin		
	Sulfamethoxy pyridazine		

[a]Drugs also known to inhibit renal tubular secretion or hepatic metabolism of displaced drugs.
(From Ref. 43.)

Cystic fibrosis

Cystic fibrosis is associated with hypoalbuminemia (129). For theophylline, the unbound fraction in plasma is 30% higher in these patients compared with control subjects (129).

Drug Interactions

A change in the binding affinity of a drug may be related to the displacement by other drugs. Competitive displacement may result in an increase in the free fraction of drug in plasma, as the apparent dissociation constant (K_{Dapp}) for the displaced drug is then expressed by:

$$K_{Dapp} = \frac{K_D(1 + [I])}{K_I} \qquad (17)$$

where [I] is the unbound concentration of the inhibitor in plasma, and K_I is the dissociation constant for the binding of the inhibitor.

There appear to be more cases of drug displacement involving drugs that are highly bound to albumin compared with drugs that bind to AAG and albumin. For example, the unbound free fraction of lidocaine can be increased significantly by therapeutic concentrations of bupivicaine of 3–4 mg/L (130, 131). No significant binding interaction has been reported for disopyramide, which binds almost exclusively to AAG (2). Other examples of in vivo displacement resulting in increased unbound fraction of drugs in plasma are listed in Table 4 (43).

In Vitro Artifacts

The use of vacutainer tubes and heparin was shown to alter the determination of protein binding. Heparin was shown

to decrease the plasma binding of certain drugs including phenytoin, propranolol, lidocaine, diazepam, quinidine, and verapamil (132–134). This is also an in vitro artifact attributable to continued ex vivo activity of the lipoprotein lipase enzyme and accumulation of fatty acids in the blood collection tube.

High unbound fraction of basic drugs was attributed to displacement from the AAG binding sites by a plasticizer in the cap stopper (135, 136). Since then, the stoppers have been reformulated. Storage containers and other anticoagulants have also been responsible for altering binding measurements. Binding inhibitors such as plasticizers in bags could be responsible for the alteration in the binding of disopyramide (2). The unbound fraction of phenytoin and meperidine is 80% higher in citrated plasma compared with serum or heparinized plasma (137).

Drug Regulatory Concerns

A New Drug Submission should provide information on the quality, safety, and efficacy of the drug product under the conditions of proposed use. Therefore, the chemical, pharmacokinetic, biopharmaceutical, pharmacological, toxicological, and clinical aspects should be investigated and reported. This includes detailed information on the protein binding, with an emphasis on populations at risk, such as with renal or hepatic insufficiency or when AAG may be altered. The ICH Common Technical Document on efficacy indicates the sections where proteins binding of a new active substance should be documented. The submission should include the preclinical and human pharmacokinetic information necessary to fully understand the biodisposition of the drug and its relation to the pharmacodynamic response and therapeutic and/or toxic effect. In addition, for drug–drug or other interactions, the clinical importance of alterations in protein binding and the mechanism of the interaction should be determined, for example, if total or free concentration is affected only under initial displacement and whether these persist during chronic dosage.

It is also essential to include clinically significant protein binding information in the product monograph. In the clinical setting, the information should help explain the inter and intrapatient variations in pharmacokinetics that would be reflected in variable pharmacodynamic effects and would certainly indicate when a dose or dosage adjustment is necessary. As noted above, changes in protein binding do not always require that adjustment in dosage regimens is needed, and there must be sufficient information for proper inferences to provide safe and effective therapy to patients.

REFERENCES

1. McDevitt, D.G.; Frisk-Holmberg, M.; Hollifield, J.W.; Shand, D.G. Clin. Pharmacol. Ther. **1976**, *20*, 152–157.
2. Lima, J.J. J. Pharmacol. Exp. Ther. **1981**, *219*, 741–747.
3. Evans, W.E.; Rodman, J.H.; Relling, M.V.; Petros, W.P.; Stewart, C.F.; Pui, C.; Rivera, G.K. J. Pharmacol. Exp. Ther. **1992**, *260*, 71–77.
4. Sebille, B. Fund. Clin. Pharmacol. **1990**, *4* (Suppl. 2), 151s–161s.
5. Davis, B.D. J. Clin. Invest. **1943**, *22*, 753.
6. Pacifici, G.M.; Viani, A. Clin Pharmacokinet. **1992**, *23*, 449–468.
7. Sebille, B.; Zini, R.; Madjar, C.; Thuaud, N.; Tillement, J.P. J. Chromatog. Biomed. **1990**, *531*, 1–77.
8. Tozer, T.; Gambertoglio, G.; Furst, D.; Avery, D.; Holford, N. J. Pharm. Sci. **1983**, *72*, 1442–1446.
9. Rehberg, P.B. Acta Physiologica Scandinavica **1943**, *5*, 115–126.
10. Bowers, W.F.; Fulton, S.; Thompson, J. Clin. Pharmacokinet. **1984**, *9* (Suppl 1), 49–60.
11. Whitlam, J.B.; Brown, K.F. J. Pharm. Sci. **1981**, *70*, 146.
12. Scott, D.O.; Bell, M.A.; Lunte, C.E. J. Chrom. **1990**, *506*, 461–469.
13. Ekblom, M.; Hammarlund-Udenaes, M.; Lundqvist, T.; Sjöberg, P. Pharm Res. **1992**, *9* (1), 155–158.
14. Herrera, A.M.; Scott, D.O.; Lunte, C.E. Pharm. Res. **1990**, *7*, 1077–1082.
15. Sjöberg, P.; Olofsson, I.M.; Lundqvist, T. Pharm. Res. **1992**, *9*, 1592–1598.
16. Wong, S.L.; Wang, Y.; Sawchuk, R.J. Pharm. Res. **1992**, *9*, 332–338.
17. MacKichan, J.J.; Zola, E.M. Br. J. Clin. Pharmacol. **1984**, *18*, 487–493.
18. Metzler, G.M. *A User's Manual for NONLIN and Associated Programs*; The Upjohn Co.: Kalamazoo, 1974.
19. Putnam, F.W. The Roster of the Plasma Proteins. *The Plasma Proteins*; Putnam, F.W., Ed.; Academic Press: New York, 1975; 57–131.
20. Sadee, W.; Gravel, R.C.; Lee, A.Y. Pharm. Biotechnol. **1999**, *12*, 29–58.
21. Tillement, J.P.; Lhoste, F.; Giudielli, J.F. Clin. Pharmacokinet. **1978**, *3*, 44–154.
22. Jusko, W.J.; Gretch, M. Drug Metab. Rev. **1983**, *14*, 427.
23. Peters, T., Jr. Serum Albumin. *The Plasma Proteins*; Putnam, F.W., Ed.; Academic Press: New York, 1975; 133–181.
24. Schmidt, K. α1-Acid Glycoprotein. *The Plasma Proteins*; Putnam, F.W., Ed.; Academic Press: New York, 1975; 183–228.
25. Lunde, P.M.K. Inflammation and α1-Acid Glycoprotein: Effect on Drug Binding. *Drug-Protein Binding*; Reidenberg, M.M., Erill, S., Eds.; Praeger Publishers: New York, 1986; 201–219.
26. Tinghely, D.; Baumann, P.; Conti, M.; Jonzier-Perey, M.; Schopf, J. Eur. J. Clin. Pharmacol. **1985**, *27*, 661–666.
27. Wagner, J.G. Protein Binding. *Pharmacokinetics for the Pharmaceutical Scientist*; Technomic Publishing Co. Inc.: Lancaster, PA, 1993; 243–258.
28. Urien, S.; Albengres, E.; Zini, R.; Tillement, J.P. Biochem. Pharmacol. **1982**, *31*, 3687–3689.
29. Urien, S.; Albengres, E.; Pinquier, J.L.; Tillement, J.P. Clin. Pharmacol Ther. **1986**, *39*, 683–689.
30. Milsap, R.L.; Jusko, W.J. J. Steroid. Biochem. **1983**, *18*, 191.
31. Abramson, F.P.; Jenkins, R.N.; Ostchega, Y. Clin. Pharmacol. Ther. **1982**, *32*, 659–663.
32. Baruzzi, A.; Contin, M.; Perucca, E.; Albani, F.; Riva, R. Eur. J. Clin. Pharmacol. **1986**, *31*, 85–89.
33. David, B.M. Br. J. Clin. Pharmacol. **1983**, *15*, 435–441.
34. Piafsky, K.M.; Borga, O. Clin. Pharmacol. Ther. **1977**, *22*, 545–549.
35. Edwards, D.J.; Lalka, D.; Cerra, F.; Slaughter, R.L. Clin. Pharmacol. Ther. **1982**, *31*, 62–67.
36. Abramson, F.P. Clin. Pharmacol. Ther. **1982**, *32*, 652–658.
37. Lemaire, M.; Urien, S.; Albengres, E. Lipoprotein Binding of Drugs. *Drug-Protein Binding*; Reidenberg, M.M., Erill, S., Eds.; Praeger Publishers: New York, 1986; 201–219.
38. Scanu, A.M.; Edelstein, C.; Keim, P. Serum Lipoproteins. *The Plasma Proteins*; Putnam, F.W., Ed.; Academic Press: New York, 1975; 317–391.
39. Piafsky, K.M. Clin. Pharmacokinet. **1980**, *5*, 246–262.
40. Lemaire, M.; Tillement, J.P. J. Pharm. Pharmacol. **1982**, *34*, 715–718.
41. Hughes, T.A.; Gaber, A.O.; Montgomery, C.E. Ther. Drug. Monit. **1991**, *13*, 289–295.
42. Lindholm, A.; Henricsson, S. Ther. Drug Monit. **1989**, *11*, 623–630.
43. MacKichan, J.J. Influence of Protein Binding and Use of Unbound Drug Concentrations. *Applied Pharmacokinetics*; Evans, W.E., Schentag, J.J., Jusko, W.J., Eds.; Applied Therapeutics Inc.: Vancouver, WA, USA, 1992; 33–37.
44. Gibaldi, M.; McNamara, P.J. Eur. J. Clin. Pharmacol. **1978**, *13*, 373–378.
45. Fichtl, B. Tissue Binding of Drugs: Methods of Determination and Pharmacokinetic Consequences. *Plasma Binding of Drugs*; Belpaire, F., Bogaert, M.,

Tillement, J.P., Verbeeck, R., Eds.; Academia Press: Gheny, 1991; 149–158.

46. D'Arcy, P.F.; McElnay, J.C. Pharmacol. Ther. **1982**, *17*, 211–220.

47. Klotz, U. Clin. Pharmacokinet. **1976**, *1*, 204.

48. Labaune, J.P. Fixation au Niveau Des Fractions Sanguines. *Pharmacocinetique*; Labaune, J.P., Ed.; Masson Publisher: Paris, 1984; 116–130.

49. Jungbluth, G.L.; Pasko, M.T.; Beam, T.R.; Jusko, W.J. Antimicrob. Agents Chemother. **1989**, *33*, 850–856.

50. Rowland, M.; Benet, L.Z.; Graham, G.G. J. Pharmacokinet. Biopharm. **1973**, *1*, 123–136.

51. Wilkinson, G.; Shand, D. Clin. Pharmacol. Ther. **1975**, *18*, 377–390.

52. Morgan, D.J.; Smallwood, R.A. Clin. Pharmacokinet. **1990**, *8*, 61–76.

53. Wilkinson, G.R. Plasma Binding and Hepatic Drug Elimination. *Drug-Protein Binding*; Reidenberg, M.M., Erill, S., Eds.; Praeger Publishers: New York, 1986; 220–232.

54. Gupta, S.K.; Benet, L.Z. Pharm. Res. **1990**, *7*, 46–48.

55. Meijer, D.K.F.; van der Sluijs, P. Pharm. Res. **1989**, *6*, 105–118.

56. MacKichan, J.J. Clin. Pharmacokinet. **1984**, *9* (Suppl 1), 32–41.

57. MacKichan, J.J. Clin. Pharmacokinet. **1989**, *16*, 65–73.

58. Stoeckel, K.; Trueb, V.; Buback, U.C.; McNamara, P.J. Eur. J. Clin. Pharmacol. **1988**, *34*, 151–156.

59. Blaschke, T.F. Clin. Pharmacokinet. **1977**, *2*, 32–44.

60. Gross, A.S.; Heuer, B.; Eichelbaum, M. Biochem. Pharmacol. **1988**, *37*, 4623–4627.

61. Tozer, T.N. Implications of Altered Plasma Protein Binding in Disease States. *Pharmacokinetic Basis for Drug Treatment*; Benet, L.Z., Ed.; Raven Press: New York, 1984; 173–93.

62. Kunin, C.M. Clin. Pharmacol. Ther. **1966**, *7*, 180–188.

63. Patel, I.H.; Levy, R.H. Epilepsia. **1979**, *20*, 85–90.

64. Lin, J.H. Clin. Pharmacokinet. **1987**, *12*, 402–432.

65. Morgan, D.J.; Blackman, G.L.; Paull, J.D.; Wolf, L.J. Anesthesiology **1981**, *54*, 468–473.

66. Pearson, R.M. Clin. Pharmacokinet. **1977**, *2*, 198–204.

67. Meffin, P.J.; Robert, E.W.; Wincle, R.A.; Harapat, S.; Peters, F.A.; Harrison, D.C. J. Pharmacokinet. Biopharm. **1979**, *7*, 29–48.

68. Tucker, G.T.; Boyes, R.N.; Bridenbaugh, P.O.; Moore, D.C. Anesthesiology **1970**, *33*, 287–314.

69. McNamara, P.J.; Slaughter, R.L.; Visco, J.P.; Elwood, C.M.; Siegel, J.H.; Lalka, D. J. Pharm. Sci. **1980**, *69*, 749–751.

70. Jusko, W.J.; Rose, J.Q. Ther. Drug Monit. **1980**, *2*, 169–176.

71. Lima, J.J. Disopyramide. *Applied Pharmacokinetics*; Evans, W.E., Ed.; Applied Therapeutics, Inc.: Spokane WA, 1986; 1210–1253.

72. Wallace, S.M.; Riegelman, S. J. Pharm. Sci. **1977**, *66*, 729–731.

73. Dieterle, W.; Wagner, J.; Faigle, W. Eur. J. Clin. Pharmacol. **1976**, *10*, 37–42.

74. MacKichan, J.J.; Zola, E.M. Br. J. Clin. Pharmacol. **1984**, *18*, 487–493.

75. Van der Berg, J.W.O.; Werhoef, M.L.; De Boer, A.S.H.; Schalm, S.W. Clin. Chem. Acta. **1985**, *147*, 291–297.

76. Smith, P.C.; McDonagh, A.F.; Benet, L.Z. J. Clin. Invest. **1986**, *77*, 934–939.

77. Hyneck, M.L.; Smith, P.C.; Munafo, A.; McDonagh, A.F.; Benet, L.Z. Clin. Pharmacol. Ther. **1988**, *44*, 107–113.

78. Simonyi, M.; Fitos, I.; Visy, J. Trends Pharmacol. Sci. **1986**, *7*, 112–116.

79. Evans, A.M.; Nation, R.T.; Sansom, L.N.; Bochner, F.; Somogyi, A.A. Eur. J. Clin. Pharmacol. **1989**, *36*, 283–290.

80. Jamali, F.; Mehvar, R.; Pasutto, F.M. J. Pharm. Sci. **1989**, *78*, 695–715.

81. Belpaire, F.M.; Vermeulen, A.M.; Bogaert, M.G. Stereoselectivity of Plasma Protein Binding and Its Pharmacokinetic Consequences. *Plasma Binding of Drugs*; Belpaire, F., Bogaert, M., Tillement, J.P., Verbeeck, R., Eds.; Academia Press: Gheny, 1991; 137–147.

82. Lima, J.J. Life Sci. **1987**, *41*, 2807–2813.

83. Levy, R.H.; Moreland, T.A. Clin. Pharmacokinet. **1984**, *9* (Suppl 1), 1–9.

84. Svensson, C.K.; Woodruff, M.; Baxter, J.; Lalka, D. Clin. Pharmacokinet. **1986**, *11*, 450–469.

85. Perucca, E. Clin. Pharmacokinet. **1984**, *9* (Suppl 1), 71–78.

86. Woosley, R.L.; Siddoway, L.A.; Thompson, K.; Cerkus, I.; Roden, D.M. Clin. Pharmacokinet. **1984**, *9* (Suppl 1), 79–83.

87. Lima, J.J.; Wenzke, S.C.; Boudoulas, H.; Schaal, S.F. Ther. Drug Monit. **1990**, *12*, 23–28.

88. Wilkinson, G.R. Drug Metab. Rev. **1983**, *14*, 427–465.

89. Bienvenu, J.; Sann, L. Clin. Chem. **1981**, *27*, 721–726.

90. Besunder, J.B.; Reed, M.D.; Blumer, J.L. Clin. Pharmacokinet. **1988**, *14*, 189–216.

91. Kurz, H.; Mauser-Ganshorn, A.; Stickel, H.H. Eur. J. Clin. Pharmacol. **1977**, *11*, 463–467.

92. Wood, M.; Wood, A.J. J. Clin. Pharmacol. Ther. **1980**, *29*, 522–526.

93. Morselli, P.L. Clin. Pharmacokinet. **1976**, *1*, 81–98.

94. Wallace, S.; Whiting, B. Br. J. Clin. Pharmacol. **1976**, *3*, 327–330.

95. Greenblatt, D.J. Clin. Pharmacol. Ther. **1980**, *27*, 301–312.

96. Davis, D.; Grossman, S.H.; Kitchell, B.B.; Shand, D.G.; Routledge, P.A. Br. J. Clin. Pharmacol. **1985**, *19*, 261–265.

97. Perucca, E.; Grimaldi, R.; Gatti, G.; Pirrachio, S.; Crema, F.; Frigo, G.M. Br. J. Clin. Pharmacol. **1984**, *17*, 665–669.

98. Kelly, J.G.; O'Malley, K. Drug-Protein Binding in Old Age. *Drug-Protein Binding*; Reidenberg, M.M., Erill, S. Eds.; Praeger Publishers: New York, 1986; 163–171.

99. Dean, M.; Stock, B.; Patterson, R.J.; Levy, G. Clin. Pharmacol. Ther. **1980**, *28*, 253–261.

100. Perucca, E. J. R. Soc. Med. **1981**, *74*, 422.

101. Bardy, A.H.; Hiilesmaa, V.K.; Teramo, K.; Neuvonen, P. J. Ther. Drug Monit. **1990**, *12*, 40–46.

102. Denson, D.D.; Coyle, D.E.; Thompson, G.A.; Santos, D.; Turner, P.A.; Myers, J.A.; Knapp, R. Clin. Pharmacol. Ther. **1984**, *35*, 702–709.

103. Feely, J.; Grimm, T. Br. J. Clin. Pharm. **1991**, *31*, 551–552.

104. Zhou, H.J.; Roshaki, R.P. New Engl. J. Med. **1989**, 565–570.
105. Zhou, H.J.; Adedoyin, A.; Wilkinson, G.R. Clin. Pharm. Ther. **1990**, *48*, 10–17.
106. Ghoneim, M.M.; Kortila, K.; Chiang, C.K.; Jacobs, L.; Schoenwald, R.; Mewaldt, S.; Kayaba, K.-O. Clin. Pharmacol. Ther. **1981**, *29*, 749–756.
107. Routledge, P.A.; Shand, D.; Barchowsky, A.; Wagner, G.; Stargel, W. Clin. Pharmacol. Ther. **1981**, *30*, 154–157.
108. Benedek, I.H.; Fiske, W.D., III; Griffen, W.O.; Bell, R.M.; Blouin, R.A.; McNamara, P.J. Br. J. Clin. Pharmacol. **1983**, *16*, 751–754.
109. Jagadeesan, V.; Krishnaswamy, K. Eur. J. Clin. Pharmacol. **1985**, *27*, 657–659.
110. Feely, J.; Forrest, M.B.; Gunn, A.; Hamilton, W.; Stevenson, I.; Crooks, J. Clin. Pharmacol. Ther. **1980**, *28*, 759–764.
111. Fremstad, D. Eur. J. Clin. Pharmacol. **1976**, *10*, 441–444.
112. Elfstrom, J. Clin. Pharmacokinet. **1979**, *4*, 16–22.
113. Elfstrom, J. Acta. Neurol. Scand. **1977**, *55*, 455.
114. Jungbluth, G.L.; Pasko, M.T.; Jusko, W.J. J. Pharm. Sci. **1989**, *78*, 807–811.
115. Gugler, R.; Azarnoff, D.L. Clin. Pharmacokinet. **1976**, *1*, 25–35.
116. Reidenberg, M.M.; Drayer, D.E. Clin. Pharmacokinet. **1984**, *9* (Suppl 1), 18–26.
117. Niwa, T.; Takeda, N.; Maeda, K.; Shibata, M.; Tatematsu, A. Clin. Chem. Acta **1988**, *173*, 127–138.
118. Thiessen, J.J.; Sellers, E.M.; Denbeigh, P.; Dolman, L. J. Clin. Pharmacol. **1976**, *16*, 345–351.
119. Barre, J.; Houin, G.; Rosenbaum, J.; Zini, R.; Dhumeaux, D.; Tillement, J.P. Br. J. Clin. Pharmacol. **1984**, *18*, 652–653.
120. Routledge, P.A.; Stargel, W.; Wagner, G.; Shand, D. Br. J. Clin. Pharmacol. **1980**, *9*, 438–439.
121. Routledge, P.A.; Stargel, W.; Kitchell, B.B.; Barchowsky, A.; Shand, D. Br. J. Clin. Pharmacol. **1981**, *11*, 245–250.
122. Piafsky, K.M.; Borga, O.; Odar-Cederlof, I.; Johansson, C.; Sjoqvist, F. New Eng. J. Med. **1978**, *299*, 1435–1439.
123. Jackson, P.R.; Tucker, G.T.; Woods, H.F. Clin. Pharmacol. Ther. **1982**, *32*, 295–302.
124. Martyn, J.A.; Abernethy, D.R.; Greenblatt, D.J. J. Clin. Pharmacol. Ther. **1984**, *5*, 535–539.
125. Bowdle, T.A.; Neal, G.D.; Levy, R.H.; Heimbach, D.M. J. Pharmacol. Exp. Ther. **1980**, *213*, 97–99.
126. Ruiz-Cabello, F.; Erill, S. Clin. Pharmacol. Ther. **1984**, *6*, 691–695.
127. Erill, S.; Calva, R. Post-Translational Changes of Albumin as a Cause of Altered Drug-Plasma Protein Binding. *Drug-Protein Binding*; Reidenberg, M.M., Erill, S., Eds.; Praeger Publishers: New York, 1986; 220–232.
128. Feely, J.; Stevenson, I.H.; Crooks, J. Clin. Pharmacokinet. **1981**, *6*, 298–305.
129. Prandota, J. Drugs **1988**, *35*, 542–578.
130. McNamara, P.J.; Slaughter, R.L.; Pieper, J.A.; Wyman, M.G.; Lalka, D. Anesth. Analg. **1981**, *60*, 395–400.
131. Goolkasian, D.L.; Slaughter, R.L.; Edwards, D.J.; Lalka, D. Eur. J. Clin. Pharmacol. **1983**, *25*, 413–417.
132. Wood, M.; Shand, D.; Wood, A.J. Clin. Pharmacol. Ther. **1979**, *25*, 103–107.
133. Brown, J.E.; Kitchell, B.B.; Bjornsson, T.D.; Shand, D.G. Clin. Pharmacol. Ther. **1981**, *30*, 636–643.
134. Dube, L.M.; Davies, R.F.; Beanlands, D.S.; Mousseau, N.; Beaudoin, N.; Chan, B.; Ho-Ngoc, A.; McGilveray, I.J. Biopharm. Drug Dispos. **1989**, *10*, 55–68.
135. Borga, O.; Piafsky, K.M.; Nilsen, O.G. Clin. Pharmacol. Ther. **1977**, *22*, 539–544.
136. Midha, K.; Loo, J.C.K.; Rowe, M. Res. Commun. Psychol, Psychiatry Behav. **1979**, *4*, 193–203.
137. Jackson, A.J.; Miller, A.K.; Narang, P.K. J. Pharm. Sci. **1981**, *70*, 1168–1169.

PYROGENS AND ENDOTOXIN DETECTION

James F. Cooper

Charles River Endosafe, Charleston, South Carolina

INTRODUCTION

A pyrogen is defined as a fever-producing agent. Pyrogens are substances that cause febrile reactions when sufficient amounts enter the circulatory system. Bacterial endotoxin is the most significant pyrogen because of its potency and ubiquity. The Bacterial Endotoxins Test has generally replaced the rabbit pyrogen test in the pharmaceutical applications.

Early Research Efforts Involving Intravenous Therapy and Pyrogens

Our awareness of pyrogens began with the advent of intravenous therapy by Sir Christopher Wren in 1656 (1). During the development of experimental medicine in the late 18th and early 19th century, many documented reports describe intravenous infusion therapy to humans that were frequently accompanied by febrile episodes. The mechanism of fever induction by infusion therapy was unknown. Since septic fever or wound fever occurred frequently when tissue from open wounds or surgical sites decomposed, physicians speculated that pyrogens might be formed in these tissues from processes such as fermentation or putrefaction. After Louis Pasteur (1822–1895) discovered that bacteria were the infectious agents that caused fermentation, there was additional thought that pyrogens were associated with bacteria. However, it was unclear whether the pyrogens were produced by bacteria or were inherently a part of bacteria. The history relevant to bacterial pyrogens in medicine has been reviewed elsewhere (2–4).

Pyrogen research beginning more than a century ago concentrated on the chemical, physiological, and pharmacological nature of bacterial pyrogens. In 1894, Centanni extracted pyrogenic substances from a large variety of bacteria, including *Escherichia coli* and typhoid (5). He also showed that these bacterial pyrogens were not proteins and that they were heat stable. Hort and Penfold's studies, published in 1912, provided the best understanding of the nature of injection fevers to that date (6–8). They used rabbits to standardize an assay for fever. By utilizing their fever assay and the staining procedure of Gram, they demonstrated that the pyrogenic bacteria were predominately gram-negative, whereas the nonpyrogenic types were gram-positive. They were usually able to correlate the pyrogenic activity of the distilled water used in their studies with its bacterial count and showed that dead Gram-negative bacteria (GNB) were also capable of inducing pyrogenicity. They concluded that the cause of all injection fevers was a filterable, heat-stable bacterial substance.

The classic investigations of Seibert during 1923–1925 established conclusively that injection fevers were caused by heat-stable, filterable components of GNB (4, 9–11). She also successfully developed a process to consistently produce infusion fluids that could pass rabbit pyrogen assays.

Advent of Large Volume Parenteral (LVP) Solutions

Seibert's methods for producing nonpyrogenic intravenous (IV) fluids enabled hospital pharmacies to produce solutions that were safe for patient therapy (10, 11). Her manufacturing methods also launched the commercial LVP solutions industry in the decade preceding World War II. Production of today's commercial LVP solutions relies on the availability of large volumes of nonpyrogenic water, known as Water for Injection (WFI), which is typically generated by distillation. Raw material ingredients are screened for the absence of pyrogen and added to WFI. After nonpyrogenic ingredients are verified, they are mixed with the WFI in depyrogenated tanks and dispensed through filling equipment into depyrogenated containers. These filled containers are immediately autoclaved to sterilize the solution and prevent the growth of any GNB, pyrogen-producing organisms that might be present in the mixture.

NATURE OF PYROGENS

The term "pyrogen" is frequently used to describe the pyrogen most significant to the pharmaceutical industry, GNB endotoxin. Since pyrogen is a general term for any substance that causes fever after IV administration or inhalation, it is important to differentiate nonmicrobial and microbial pyrogens. Nonmicrobial pyrogens include pharmacological agents like bleomycin, colchicine, and polynucleotide poly-I:C. For sensitized hosts, there can be antigens of human blood products, such as human serum albumin, penicillin drugs, or other therapeutic agents (12, 13).

Microbial pyrogens are by far the most significant problem for pharmaceutical manufacturers. Bacteria (killed and live), fungi, plasmodia (malarial parasites), and viruses (live) can all act as pyrogens. Additionally, bacterial products, including streptococcal exotoxins, staphylococcal enterotoxin and bacterial endotoxin lipopolysaccharide (LPS), as well as fungal products, can also act as pyrogens (13). Because the LPS component in the endotoxin is toxic in very small quantities, GNB endotoxin is the microbial pyrogen most significant for pharmaceutical producers, as mentioned above. The amount of USP Reference Standard Endotoxin needed to initiate pyrogenicity in humans and rabbits is about 1 ng/kg (14). Whole cells induce pyrogenicity when large numbers are phagocytized by the macrophages they encounter as they enter the bloodstream. Therefore, although it requires the administration of at least 10,000 organisms/kg of the most pyrogenic GNB bacteria to cause a pyrogenic reaction in rabbits (15), the number of gram-positive or fungal organisms required to induce the same effect is orders of magnitude higher, $10-10^8$/kg (12, 16, 17).

Mechanism of Fever Induction

Endotoxin pyrogen induces fever by an indirect process. On entry into the circulatory system, endotoxin is bound to LPS-binding protein (LPB) that transports it to receptor cells in the reticuloendothelial system. The main target cells are circulating mononuclear cells, which produce proinflammatory cytokines such as interleukin-1 (IL-1), interleukin-6 (IL-6), and tumor necrosis factor-α (TNFα) (18,19). These cytokines are involved in acute and chronic inflammation, induce fever, and modulate the host's response to bacterial infection (20).

Bacterial Endotoxin Pyrogen

Bacterial endotoxin is a high molecular weight complex that constitutes an integral component of the outer cell wall membrane of GNB. These bacteria constantly shed endotoxin into the environment as they grow and multiply, as well as when they die and disintegrate (21). Consequently, bacterial endotoxin can either exist in a cell-associated state or in a free state. Endotoxin that remains cell-associated can be removed from a solution by microporous sterilizing filters, but endotoxin in a free state easily passes through most sterilizing filters. Since bacterial endotoxin is heat stable, it is not fully destroyed by a routine autoclave process. Endotoxin is ubiquitous and can be found wherever GNBs exist. Endotoxin is found in the soil, in food, in ground waters, and on any surface touched by these substances. Since the vast majority of bacteria that grow and multiply in water systems are gram-negative, bacterial endotoxin is a normal constituent of ordinary water. For this reason, it is a common contaminant in laboratories and in wet manufacturing areas, including laboratory glassware, research equipment, and water baths. It can contaminate sampling equipment, storage containers, and any reusable materials that retain moisture.

Chemical Nature and Structure of Endotoxins

Naturally occurring bacterial endotoxins contain the lipid, carbohydrate, and protein makeup of the outer cell membrane of GNB (see Fig. 1). However, most of the commercial endotoxin preparations have been purified by various extraction procedures and are generally free of nucleic acids, proteins, phospholipids, and other bacterial cell components (21). The primary chemical configuration that remains after purification is a polysaccharide structure that is covalently bound to a lipid component called Lipid A. Based on its chemical nature, which is common to various bacterial families, this substance is referred to as lipopolysaccharide (LPS). Although the terms endotoxin and LPS are often used interchangeably, most reference "endotoxin" standards are purified preparations that are more correctly described as LPS.

The Lipid A component of LPS is embedded in the outer membrane of the bacterial cell, whereas the polysaccharide protrudes into the environment (21). The polysaccharide component is composed of two parts, the core oligosaccharide that is connected to Lipid A and a longer oligosaccharide O-specific chain that is attached to the core (Fig. 2). The O-specific chain is the most variable component of the complex. It consists of 20–40 repeating units that include up to eight sugars, and it is responsible for the specific immune reaction that each type of GNB is able to evoke in a host. The core oligosaccharide is much less variable than the O-specific chain, and its influence on the host is less profound, although it can trigger antibody production in response to mutant endotoxins that lack an O-specific chain. The core

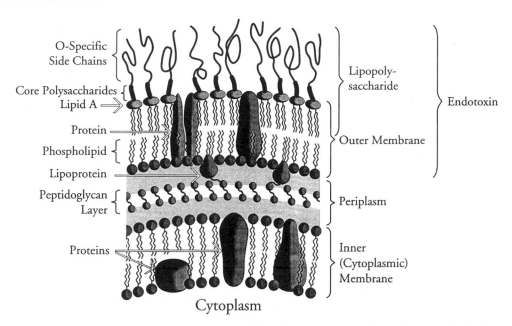

Fig. 1 Cell membrane of a gram-negative bacteria, including the lipopolysaccharide, protein, and phospholipid of the outer membrane (O-specific = oligosaccharide-specific).

is divided into the inner core that attaches to Lipid A and the outer core that links up to the O-specific chain. The inner core is the more interesting of the two segments because it bears two unusual sugars, a seven-carbon heptose and 3-deoxy-D-manno-2-octulosonic acid KDO. KDO links the polysaccharide core to Lipid A and is found in all endotoxins, but it occurs nowhere else in nature, except in certain plants and algae (22).

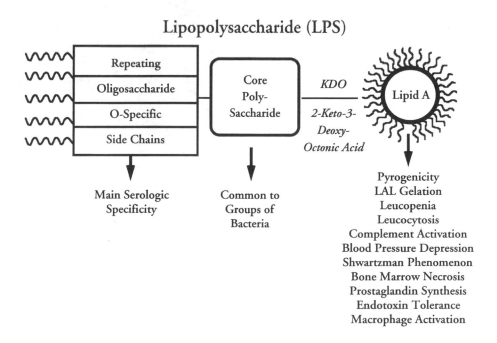

Fig. 2 The major components of lipopolysaccharide (LPS).

Lipid A is the least variable component of LPS. It consists of a disaccharide of glucosamine, which is highly substituted with amide-linked and ester-linked long-chain fatty acids, each with a backbone of about 14 carbon atoms (21). Lipid A is responsible for the vast majority of both the harmful and the beneficial biological activities that have been attributed to endotoxin. A partial list of these activities is shown in Fig. 2.

Biological Properties of Endotoxins

Bacterial endotoxins have fascinated investigators for years, in part because of their extensive and diverse biological properties and activities. Endotoxins are potent substances, which elicit a broad spectrum of the harmful physiologic responses that are produced in hosts by pathogenic GNB (21). At the extreme, they can produce profound alterations in organ function, such as hypotension and disseminated intravascular coagulation, which can lead to severe morbidity or death. On the other hand, endotoxins are also active stimulators of the mammalian defense system, which can enhance the body's capacity to cope with both microbial infections and malignant tumors. This dichotomy of biological activity continues to intrigue research scientists who are attempting to modify the Lipid A component of endotoxin in such a way that its toxic effects can be reduced or eliminated while its beneficial effects are retained (23).

Fever

Fever is one of the dramatic biological effects produced by endotoxin and one of the easiest to measure. For this reason, it is one of the most studied and best understood of the many physiological activities that are initiated by endotoxin. The current understanding of the pathogenesis of fever is shown in Fig. 3 (21). When exogenous pyrogens enter the blood stream, they are removed from circulation by phagocytosis. The host's phagocytic cells (primarily peripheral monocytes) are thereby stimulated to synthesize a family of cytokines, or endogenous pyrogens, that are released into the circulation. These endogenous pyrogens travel to the hypothalmus, the thermoregulatory center of the body, via arterial blood supply. There the endogenous pyrogens induce various cells to increase the level of arachidonic acid metabolites (primarily the cyclooxygenase-derived prostaglandins, prostacyclins, and thromboxanes). There is considerable evidence that prostaglandin E_2 (PGE_2) is the major arachidonic acid metabolite associated with increasing the hypothalamic thermostat to febrile levels. During fever, levels of PGE_2 are elevated in the cerebral spinal fluid; the ability of aspirin and other antipyretics to reduce fever is directly

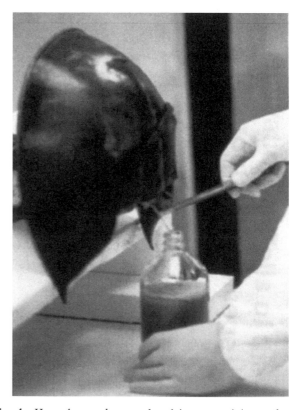

Fig. 4 Horseshoe crabs are placed in a restraining rack and passively bled for a few minutes. They are promptly returned to the sea unharmed. Amebocyte blood cells are concentrated, washed, and lysed to produce LAL reagent. (Photo provided by J. Cooper, Endosafe, Charleston, SC.)

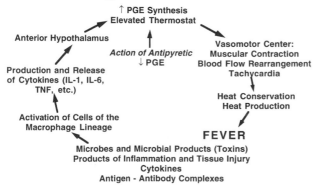

Fig. 3 The sequential events that produce fever in humans and animals.

related to their ability to block brain cyclooxygenase. The new thermostatic setting signals the nerves that stimulate peripheral blood vessels to constrict those vessels and conserve body heat. This causes the body to chill, and the discomfort that results stimulates other physiologic mechanisms within the body to generate more heat in order to return the body to a homeostatic condition. The end result is fever (18, 24).

The systemic response to threshold pyrogenic doses of endotoxin in humans is described in studies that were conducted by the National Institutes of Health. The USP Reference Standard Endotoxin (RSE), *Escherichia coli* 0113:H10:K0, was injected into healthy volunteers at dosages ranging from 2 to 4 ng/kg (25). About 1 h after administration, a monophasic rise in temperature was observed, accompanied by chills and rigors. The chills lasted for 15 to 30 min and were followed by varying degrees of myalgias, arthralgias, headache, and nausea over the next 2 h. During this period, the subjects appeared sallow and exhibited general malaise. The peak core temperature (38.5–40°C) occurred at 3 h, followed by defervescence and symptomatic improvement over the next 3–5 h.

Septic shock

As mentioned earlier, bacterial endotoxin is a concern to the pharmaceutical industry because of its ability to induce pyrogenic reactions at intravenous dosages as low as 1 ng/kg. In higher dosages, endotoxin can be lethal. In one report, a self-administered intravenous dose of 1 mg of *Salmonella minnesota* endotoxin initiated the full clinical manifestations of septic-shock syndrome in a middle-aged laboratory worker (26). Septic-shock syndrome includes a high-cardiac-output form of hypotension, disseminated intravascular coagulation, abnormalities of hepatic and renal function, and noncardiogenic pulmonary edema. This patient was diagnosed and treated promptly and survived the episode.

Beneficial biological effects of endotoxins

Tumor reduction was attributed to endotoxin (27). Other beneficial effects of endotoxins on the host defense system include enhanced immune protection, protection from lethal irradiation, enhanced nonspecific resistance to infection, and resistance to toxic doses of endotoxin (tolerance). A hypothesis has been proposed (28) to explain the seemingly contradictory findings of the toxic vs. beneficial effects of endotoxins. It suggests that they are the primary signals that animals use to detect potentially harmful GNB and that the host defense system employs many of the body's defenses to both detect and to react against the threat of bacterial infection. This hypothesis also proposes

that the body possesses feedback mechanisms that, in most cases, attempt to match the bacterial endotoxin threat with an appropriate response. Thus, the intensity of the responses to endotoxins has evolved to maximize protection while minimizing the biological cost and self-damaging effects to the host. In general, the benefits of these responses far outweigh the risks, and when harmful events do occur, they are examples of inappropriate activity of overly protective systems (28).

Physical Properties of Endotoxins

It is important to be aware of the various physical properties of endotoxins in order to understand why they change their behavior when placed into different environments. An understanding of these physical properties is also essential for designing effective processes for depyrogenation.

Heat stability

It has long been known that endotoxins are thermostable in the presence of moist heat and that they are not appreciably destroyed by routine autoclaving processes. Early research showed that boiling was not completely effective (9). However, endotoxins can be destroyed by dry heat at temperatures above 180°C. In fact, dry heat is the method of choice for depyrogenating heat-resistant materials, such as glass and equipment.

Size

The size of endotoxin is dependent on its aggregation state, which, in turn, is dependent on its surrounding environment. In an aqueous environment, LPS is arranged in a bilayer. Its hydrophilic Lipid A components are clustered in the center of the bilayer, whereas its hydrophilic components are exposed to the surrounding solution. Bacterial LPS is stabilized by divalent cations, and in the presence of magnesium and calcium, it forms bilayer sheets and vesicles with a diameter of about 100 nm (21). However, if the divalent cations are removed from the environment, the bilayer breaks down into micellular forms that are 20–70 nm long and about 3–7 nm thick. In the presence of detergents, these micelles can be even further broken down into subunits of 0.8–1.2 nm in diameter and 10–60 nm in length.

The tendency for endotoxin to aggregate into larger and larger entities in an aqueous environment is due to the attraction that the hydrophobic groups of the LPS molecules have for one another. Aggregated endotoxin vesicles of 0.1 μm in diameter have been visualized by using electron microscopes. Even in its largest aggregation state, endotoxin passes through 0.22 μm sterilizing filters. Conventional reverse-osmosis membranes that are nominally rated at pore sizes on the order of 1.0 nm are able to remove endotoxin from water (29). This process also removes any salts that may be present.

Molecular weight

In a typical aqueous environment that contains small amounts of divalent cations, endotoxin has a molecular weight of about 10^6 Da (21). If divalent cations are removed from the aqueous environment by chelators, the endotoxin bilayers break down into micelles of 300,000 to 1,000,000 molecular weight. When these micelles are further broken down in the presence of surface-active agents, their molecular weight drops again to about 10,000–20,000. However, these steps are completely reversible; if the detergents are dialyzed out, and divalent cations are added back to the endotoxin, the micelles and then the membranous structures reassemble themselves (30).

As the salt concentrations in water increase, endotoxin forms larger and larger molecular weight aggregates. The aggregation state of endotoxin affects both its solubility and biological reactivity. As the molecular weight of endotoxin increases, its solubility in water decreases. Additionally, as the molecular weight of endotoxin increases, toxicity in rats, rate of clearance from blood, interaction with complement, and affinity for cells also increase. However, endotoxin lethality in mice decreases as its molecular weight increases, as does its pyrogenicity in rabbits (31).

Electrostatic properties

At pH levels above 2, endotoxin aggregates are negatively charged and behave as anions (21). This property accounts for the attraction that endotoxin aggregates have for divalent cations in solutions. It is also the characteristic that provides the mechanism of action for endotoxin removal by cationically charged adsorbents.

PYROGEN TESTING

The development of the large volume parenteral (LVP) drug industry prompted the need for pyrogen testing to assure their safety. Pyrogen contamination is a greater problem for manufacturers of LVPs than it is for producers of small volume injectables because the initiation of patient fevers by parenteral solutions is dose dependent rather than concentration dependent. In other words, the onset and extent of injection fever depends on the total amount of pyrogen delivered to a patient and not on the concentration of pyrogen per milliliter of drug. Therefore,

an LVP must meet a more stringent standard for nonpyrogenicity than lesser volume drugs.

The heavy demand for LVP drug therapy prior to and during World War II and the need to ensure that commercial infusion fluids were free from pyrogens caused the United States Pharmacopeia (USP) to undertake the development of a compendial test for pyrogens (32). In 1941, the Committee of Revision of the USP authorized Subcommittee 3 on Biological Assays to begin the first USP collaborative study of pyrogen. Using *Pseudomonas aeruginosa filtrates*, prepared by the Division of Bacteriology of the FDA, the collaborative study was undertaken by the FDA, the NIH, and 14 pharmaceutical manufacturers (33,34). The study utilized the rabbit pyrogen test used earlier by Hort and Penfold and Seibert and her co-workers (7–9). Large numbers of rabbits were challenged with both pyrogenic material and physiologic saline solution. The results of the study, which were published in 1943, led to the inclusion of the first compendial pyrogen test in the 12th edition of the USP in 1942. Although refinements have been added from time to time, the USP rabbit pyrogen test remains relatively unchanged from the original format.

Basically, the pyrogen test involves measuring the rectal temperature of rabbits, both prior to and after the intravenous injection of a test solution in the ear veins. If the animals exhibit febrile responses that exceed established limits, the test solution is judged to be pyrogenic. Rabbits became the animal of choice because they are relatively inexpensive, are easy to handle, and have a labile thermoregulatory mechanism. Rabbits frequently produce false-positive pyrogen tests. For this reason, a negative result is more significant than a positive test, which makes the rabbit a good choice for assuring the absence of pyrogen in a test solution (32).

In 1969, Greisman and Hornick compared three purified endotoxin preparations on a dose-per-weight basis in rabbits and healthy adult males (35). Their results showed that rabbits and humans require approximately the same amount of endotoxin on a weight basis to induce threshold pyrogenic responses.

USP Rabbit Pyrogen Test

The USP <151> Pyrogen Test (36) is designed for solutions that can be tolerated by the rabbit in doses that do not exceed 10 ml/kg body weight and can be delivered within a time frame that does not exceed 10 min. Exceptions to these requirements are given in individual USP product monographs or federal regulations for biologics. Specifications for pyrogen test material handling, calibration limits for recording equipment, and requirements for housing and conditioning the rabbits are also given in the <151> test chapter.

For the initial pyrogen tests, groups of three healthy, mature rabbits are chosen. Accurate temperature-sensing devices, such as clinical thermometers or thermistor probes, are inserted into the rectum of the rabbits to record their body temperature. If these probes remain inserted throughout the test period, the rabbits must be restrained with light-fitting neck stocks that permit them to move about. During the test, food but not water is withheld from the animals.

A control temperature is determined not more than 30 min prior to injection of the test dose. This is the base for determining any temperature increase resulting from the injection. Test solutions are warmed to 37 ± 2°C prior to injection. After injection, rabbit temperatures are recorded at 30-min intervals between 1 and 3 h. Temperature decreases are considered as zero rise. If no rabbit shows an individual temperature rise of 0.5°C or more above its control temperature, the product meets the requirements for the absence of pyrogens. If any rabbit shows an individual temperature rise of 0.5°C or more, the test is continued with an additional five rabbits. If not more than three of the eight rabbits show individual temperature rises of 0.5°C or more, and if the sum of the eight individual maximum increases does not exceed 3.3°C, the material under examination meets the USP <151> requirements for the absence of pyrogens (36).

Human Cell-Based Pyrogen Test

Pyrogens induce human monocytes to release proinflammatory cytokines such as IL-1, IL-6, IL-8, and TNF-α, as previously discussed. Test methods have been designed that include incubation of a test sample with monocytes in whole blood or in cultured cell lines and analysis of a specific cytokine after a suitable time. This cell-based methodology may provide an alternative to rabbit pyrogen testing that is required for human blood products. More development is needed to determine the optimum cytokine for analysis and to assess the nature of interference conditions (37, 38).

BACTERIAL ENDOTOXINS TEST (BET)

A *Limulus* amebocyte lysate (LAL) reagent is the basis for an in vitro pyrogen test method that is specific for bacterial endotoxin pyrogen. For this reason, it is now referred to as the bacterial endotoxins test (BET), although BET and

LAL testing are used interchangeably. When it was first introduced, there was concern by the industry and regulators that its specificity would limit its application in the parenteral industry (39). However, experience gained in this industry over the past 25 years confirms that endotoxin is the principal pyrogen of concern to pharmaceutical and medical device manufacturers. The BET has steadily gained acceptance globally as a replacement for the rabbit pyrogen test.

Discovery of *Limulus* Amebocyte Lysate (LAL) Reagent

The LAL test reagent is prepared by lysing amebocyte blood cells obtained from the American horseshoe crab, *Limulus polyphemus*. The origin of LAL reagent is traced to Frederick Bang, who first recognized the association between bacterial endotoxin and *Limulus* blood coagulation in studies of marine organisms at the Marine Biological Laboratory in Woods Hole, MA. An interest in immunity and infectious disease led Bang to study how *Limulus* would respond to an injection of bacteria. He observed that gram-negative *Vibrio* bacteria and its extracted endotoxin caused death in horseshoe crabs, not from infection but from intravascular coagulation (40).

Jack Levin, who had an interest in the effects of endotoxin on platelets and human blood coagulation, joined Bang at Woods Hole, MA, for several summers to do research on endotoxin-initiated *Limulus* blood coagulation. This collaboration produced several publications that explained a simple mechanism of enzyme-mediated interaction of LAL with endotoxin (41, 42). Levin discovered a way to harvest the intracellular fluid by osmotic lysis of stabilized amebocytes. Modern-day preparation of LAL reagent still follows Levin's basic methods.

Levin's original interest in the LAL test was for its potential as a clinical diagnostic tool for endotoxemia. However, a collaboration between Levin and Cooper produced the test's most celebrated application as a pyrogen test for the parenteral industry. The advent of short-lived radioactive drugs in the late 1960s prompted a need for a pyrogen test that was quick and required only a small volume of test material. As Cooper searched for an alternative endotoxin test for these drugs, he compared LAL sensitivity with rabbit response. The threshold pyrogenic level in rabbits was determined for LPS derived from *Escherichia coli* and *Klebsiella*. An excellent correlation was found between rabbit febrile response (fever index) and LAL reactivity (gel time), which indicated that the in vitro test was indeed an indicator of a biological response (43). The LAL test yielded unmatched sensitivity and reproducibility.

Cooper and Mills set up the first commercial LAL production facility in 1971 in Chincoteague, VA, for Mallinckrodt, Inc. Production sites for LAL reagent are located on the eastern coast of the United States where horseshoe crabs are found abundantly in shallow coastal waters. The LAL test succeeded as the first "alternative to an animal test" because of amazing similarity between *Limulus* and mammalian response to endotoxin (44). The activation of human monocytes in blood by endotoxin to produce proinflammatory cytokines compares strongly to the activation of amebocytes in *Limulus* to produce clotting enzymes. As LAL reagents became commercially available, the pharmaceutical industry began to investigate the use of LAL testing as an alternative to the rabbit pyrogen test.

LAL clotting mechanism

The LAL test is based on the primitive blood-clotting defense mechanism that protects the horseshoe crab from the hostile sea of GNB that surrounds it. When a crab is wounded and invading bacteria enter its blood stream, its amebocyte blood cells respond by releasing granules that contain a coagulagen protein substance. Intracellular serine protease zymogens in the crab's blood are triggered by the presence of endotoxin to initiate a series of activations that subsequently produce a coagulin gel clot from this coagulagen protein. The sequential activation of Factor C, Factor B, and the clotting enzyme in this coagulation cascade results in an enormous amplification in sensitivity of LAL for endotoxin.

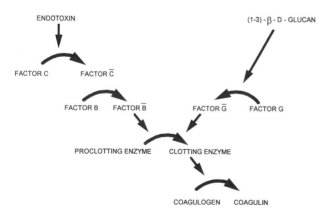

Fig. 5 Stages in the blood coagulation system of horseshoe crab amebocytes.

Figure 5 shows a coagulation scheme proposed by Nakamura (45).

The horseshoe crab is also exposed to fungus and yeast in its environment, which may explain why Factor G responds to a $(1 \rightarrow 3)$-β-D-glucan, a component from the cell well of these organisms. This pathway gives rise to a nonendotoxin activation of the LAL coagulation system (46).

Bacterial Endotoxins Test Methods

The observation of gel formation in a test tube as an endpoint for an endotoxin assay provides the means for a very simple test. The need for more objective quantitative methods has led scientists to develop a variety of automated methods for endotoxin measurement. This discussion is limited to the three methods that were accepted by the Food and Drug Administration (FDA).

Gel-clot BET

The gel-clot end point is the most commonly used endotoxin test. It is simple and requires minimal laboratory equipment and facilities. Equal volumes of test solution and LAL reagent (usually 0.1 ml each) are mixed in 10×75 mm glass test tubes. After incubation at 37°C for 1 h, the tubes are observed for clot formation after inverting them. Formation of a solid gel clot that withstands inversion of the tube constitutes a positive test. Each lot of gel-clot reagent licensed by the FDA must be labeled with its sensitivity (λ) to the reference standard endotoxin (RSE). The test can be used qualitatively to judge samples as positive or negative at the reagent's sensitivity; this method is called a Limit test. The test may be also used as a semi-quantitative assay by titrating positive samples to an endpoint and multiplying the last positive sample dilution by the labeled sensitivity.

Kinetic turbidimetric assay

During the LAL-endotoxin reaction, the solution mixture becomes increasingly turbid. The kinetic turbidimetric assay (KTA) requires an incubating microplate or tube reader driven by an endotoxin-specific software. The reaction mixtures in a KTA system are continually monitored for changes in optical density in each sample that are caused by scattering and absorption of light. Generally, the KTA method measures the onset time needed to reach a predetermined absorbance by each reaction mixture. The onset times of samples are compared with those of endotoxin standards to yield quantitative values for each sample or control that contains endotoxin.

Kinetic and endpoint chromogenic assays

Unlike previously described tests, chromogenic LAL tests do not utilize the coagulagen protein from LAL reagent to produce an endpoint. Although endotoxin activates the same enzymatic cascade from the reagent, as previously described, the clotting enzyme reacts with a synthetic substrate that has been added to the reaction mixture. The substrate consists of a colorless amino acid chain attached to a chromophore. The activated clotting enzyme cleaves the bond that holds the chromophore to the amino acid; the amount released is proportional to the concentration of endotoxin (47). The chromophore that is released changes the color of the reaction mixture, thereby increasing the optical density. In the kinetic chromogenic assay (KCA), the reaction times of assay mixtures are determined with the same methods and readers used for KTA determinations. Endpoint chromogenic reactions may be done with nonincubating readers, where LAL, substrate, and quenching agent are added sequentially. After the reaction is terminated, the absorbency is read over a one-log range. In contrast, the kinetic turbidimetric and chromogenic assays may be conducted over a 2-to-4 log range.

Compendial and Regulatory Status of the BET

As confidence grew in the capability of the LAL test, as a screening tool for endotoxin pyrogen, pharmaceutical and medical device industries began to replace the rabbit test with the new in vitro test. The USP has continually revised the BET to keep abreast of advancements in LAL methodology.

The USP <85> Bacterial Endotoxins Test

The <85> BET first appeared in 1980 as an informational chapter in the *USP XX*. Significantly, the USP adopted the FDA *E. coli 0113* endotoxin standard as its reference standard and assigned units of potency to it (48). It also included information about calibrating a control standard endotoxin (CSE) to the RSE.

The first large-scale conversion of the rabbit test to the BET occurred in Supplement 5 to *USP XXII* when the BET became the official endotoxin test for 185 USP articles. The *USP 24* has endotoxin limits for over 650 USP articles.

Endotoxin limit

Endotoxin limits were introduced by the FDA to ensure the absence of unsafe levels of endotoxin in parenteral products. Because endotoxin is ubiquitous, it was necessary to assign an allowable, safe limit that was below the threshold dose of endotoxin for pyrogenicity. In 1983, the USP officially replaced the <151> Pyrogen Test in USP monographs for 29 radiopharmaceuticals and five pharmaceutical waters. The USP subcommittee, responsible for revising the general chapters of the compendium, announced in 1987 its intent to replace the <151> Pyrogen Test with the BET for all USP articles for which the BET could be validated (48). Endotoxin limits were applied to USP articles using the K/M formula that was devised by the FDA. The endotoxin tolerance limit for humans, K, was set at 5 USP endotoxin units (EU) per kilogram of body weight (5 EU/kg), and M was defined as the maximum dose of the substance administered to an individual per kilogram per hour. The maximum dose is usually taken from the labeling of the parenteral manufacturer. The endotoxin limit for a substance is expressed in EU/mg or unit of product if it is administered on a weight basis, such as a small volume parenteral. Infusion solutions and medical device extracts have an endotoxin limit of 0.5 EU/ml. Drugs that are dosed on a volume basis also have an endotoxin limit in EU/ml.

Endotoxin limit for cerebrospinal fluid administration

Intrathecal administration applies to parenteral drugs that are infused directly into cerebral spinal fluid spaces. The tolerance limit, K, for these drugs is 0.2 EU/kg because intrathecal administration is the most toxic route for endotoxin pyrogen. An outbreak of aseptic meningitis followed intraspinal administration of nuclear imaging agents that were contaminated with endotoxin, but had passed the USP Pyrogen Test (49). One-milliliter volumes of the agents that had less than 10 EU per dose produced serious patient reactions and prompted the tighter endotoxin limit.

Harmonized BET

A harmonized text for <85> bacterial endotoxins test (BET) became effective in January of 2001 (50). It was a product of the International Conference on Harmonization (ICH). It was drafted by the Japanese Pharmacopeia and agreed on by the European Pharmacopeia and the USP. In adopting the harmonized BET, the USP chapter introduced radical changes. The text was simplified to make it easier to understand and follow. Whereas the previous version was a gel-clot test only, the new BET provides standardization for both gel-clot and photometric LAL methods. Any validated method may be used for a USP article however, the gel-clot method is the referee test in the unlikely case of a dispute.

FDA Validation Guideline for the LAL Test

The FDA was actively involved from the outset in developing the BET as an alternative to pyrogen testing. In 1972, a collaboration of Cooper with the FDA Bureau of Biologics (now Center for Biologics Evaluation and Research) established LAL methodology within the FDA. A study that compared LAL and rabbit tests on a group of biological and radiopharmaceutical drugs indicated that the LAL test was a rapid, sensitive, and reproducible way to detect pyrogen in these products (51). In 1973, the *Federal Register* announced the intention of the FDA to license LAL reagents as a biological product. That announcement also proclaimed the usefulness of the reagent for detecting endotoxin (52).

A *Federal Register* announcement in 1977 gave conditional approval for the BET as a release test for medical devices and biological products, provided that product manufacturers submitted appropriate test-validation data to each respective agency to amend their product's registration documents or license (53). The Bureau of Medical Devices established its own endotoxin standard and supported an industry collaborative study to develop an endotoxin limit and uniform test method for parenteral devices. As acceptance of LAL testing grew, the FDA decided to prepare a single guideline that would apply to all Agency-regulated products that were subject to screening for endotoxin. A FDA Task Force was formed with representatives from the Agency's various Centers to standardize test-validation criteria. A guideline for end-product testing by LAL methods was published in 1987 (54).

The FDA LAL test-validation guideline describes how to use all LAL methods and identifies three basic requirements:

1. The LAL reagent used in all validation, in-process, and end-product tests must be licensed by CBER.
2. The product manufacturer must perform an initial qualification of their laboratory personnel and facility.
3. Inhibition and enhancement tests must be conducted on test products to ensure that the products do not interfere with the detection of endotoxin.

This guideline has been the most influential document in LAL testing to date. Annual updates of the Appendix E, endotoxin limits for established parenteral products, were published by the FDA until 1994. With the upgrades in test procedures and endotoxin limits published in individual product monographs, the FDA no longer has a need to revise the 1987 guideline.

Overcoming Inhibition and Enhancement Conditions

Conditions for the LAL reaction with endotoxin require pH neutrality and optimum levels of sodium and divalent cations. A uniform temperature of 37°C optimizes the rate of reaction. Most therapeutic drug products require dilution with LAL reagent water (LRW) before testing to avoid interference, which is recognized by improper recovery of the positive product control (PPC). Inhibition is a failure to recover the PPC, whereas enhancement is high recovery of the PPC. Cooper (55) has described ways to identify the concentration of a substance, which is chemically compatible with the BET, and to validate the BET with drug products and excipients.

Inhibition mechanisms

There are three principal causes of inhibitory effects in gel-clot and kinetic LAL testing (55). One is an adverse chemical condition, such as a nonneutral pH, suboptimum levels of sodium ions and divalent cations (magnesium and calcium), or inhibition by trivalent cations such as soluble forms of aluminum and gadolinium. The LAL manufacturer can alleviate many of these problems by incorporating optimum concentrations of all necessary components into the LAL formula, in particular, significant amount of an organic buffer. The second important type of inhibition is loss of purified endotoxin used for the PPC. This invalidity is somewhat of an artifact because purified endotoxin, LPS, is more unstable in water than in native endotoxin, which has a stabilizing protein attached. This instability leads to container adsorption and molecular aggregation that makes the positive control unavailable for LAL detection, and this loss is not always overcome by vortex mixing. Optimum formulation of the CSE by the supplier is critical to the recovery of positive controls. Finally, interference results from inadequately controlled test parameters including test accessories, reagents, and analyst's proficiency.

Enhancement

The LAL reaction is specific for endotoxin with the exception of a glucose polymer from cellulose, yeast, and certain other microbial sources, known as $(1\rightarrow3)$-β-D-glucan (46). This glucan activates LAL the same as endotoxin and produces a synergistic enhancement of the PPC in kinetic LAL studies. The BET allows glucan-containing products to be tested by LAL reagents that are treated to make them specific for endotoxin and avoid a false-positive result.

Preparation of a positive product control (PPC)

The PPC, required by the FDA Guideline, is a sample of the test material that contains a concentration of endotoxin that is double the labeled sensitivity of the LAL reagent (54). The PPC must be tested with each sample in a Limits test or kinetic LAL assay to ensure that a result is valid and free of interference. The most accurate and reliable technique is the "hot spike" method that requires adding 10 μl of endotoxin standard to the reaction vessel (tube or well) before addition of LAL. The gel clot method requires the addition of 10 μl of 20λ to the reaction mixture. Kinetic methods require the addition of 10 μl of a standard, 10 times greater than the spike concentration, to the wells or tubes designated as PPCs. Only inhibition is seen in gel-clot Limits tests, whereas both inhibition and enhancement are seen in kinetic LAL methods.

Sensitivity of a BET

The results of endotoxin tests for in-process solutions, bulk materials, and finished parenteral products should be reported in the same units as those assigned to the product. Two factors determine the sensitivity of a BET. For infusion solutions and device extracts, the gel-clot sensitivity or the lowest point on the standard curve (lambda for kinetic LAL) and the amount of dilution determine test sensitivity (55). For products that have an endotoxin limit in EU/mg, the choice of lambda and the concentration of the test material determine sensitivity. The formula for product-specific sensitivity (PSS) is a convenient way to calculate the sensitivity of a BET for this type of product, where:

$$PSS = \frac{Lambda\ (EU/mL)}{Test\ concentration\ (mg/mL)}$$

DEPYROGENATION

A process that removes or destroys endotoxin in a solution or on a material is "termed"? depyrogenation. Endotoxin is difficult to eliminate because it is ubiquitous in nature, stable, and pervious to sterilizing filters. Chemical destruction requires treatment with strong base or oxidants, which is usually too corrosive for practical use. Aseptic processing of parenteral products requires that all components, excipients, and active ingredients be made endotoxin-free (depyrogenated) before filling or assembly (55, 56). The BET is the test of choice to monitor the effectiveness of depyrogenation.

Water

Municipal water systems usually contain 5-to-50 EU/mL of endotoxin. Pharmaceutical waters are treated by ultrafiltration, distillation, or reverse osmosis to separate endotoxin from water (55). The principal source of endotoxin is bacteria within a water system in the form of biofilm or colonies entrapped in resin beds, etc. A water system will be contaminated unless there is an ongoing sanitization program. The endotoxin limit for Water for Injection was set at 0.25 EU/ml because it is a critical vehicle and a major source of pyrogens.

Glassware

Dry heat sterilization is used to depyrogenate glassware and other heat-stable materials (55, 57). Temperatures in the range of 250°–325°C rapidly inactivate endotoxin by thermal incineration. The size and mass of a load influence the time required to reach equilibrium within the oven; therefore, empirical data are required to verify that desired conditions were achieved. Overkill cycles in the range of 4–6 log reduction values (LRV) are common. A heat exposure of 250°C for at least 30 min provides greater than a 3-log reduction.

Oven cycles are most accurately challenged with an endotoxin indicator that contains 1000–10,000 EU per container in a 5- to 10-ml vial. This configuration enables complete recovery of the endotoxin challenge because it is small enough to vortex mix. Indicators are placed inside a glass pack of vials or large vessels, exposed to the oven cycle, and analyzed for log reduction.

Elastomeric Closures

Closures are traditionally sterilized and depyrogenated by a combination of washing, rinsing, and steam sterilization. All three of these steps are effective in reducing endotoxin and should be considered in the validation process. Steam sterilization as a depyrogenation process is underappreciated (58). The combined steps consistently give >3-log reduction values. The recovery of endotoxin challenge levels from closures is less efficient than recovery from glass because of the porous nature of the closure and inability to apply vortex mixing efficiently. An acceptable recovery for challenge stoppers is >10% (55).

Bulk Products

Outbreaks of pyrogenic reactions underscore the need to assign endotoxin alert limits (EAL) and to screen blood and fermentation products for endotoxin. Two clusters of pyrogenic reactions were traced to a bulk producer of gentamicin (59). Patients reacted to endotoxin levels similar to the threshold pyrogenic dose of 4.1 EU/kg determined in a study of reference endotoxin in a population of healthy male volunteers (60).

An EAL for a bulk product is a fraction of the endotoxin limit (EL) for the finished product. An appropriate range for an EAL is at least four to five times less than the EL, depending on solubility and interference properties of the material. A validated method for a bulk substance should include a specific method to dissolve the drug and dilute it to a compatible concentration (55).

Biotherapeutic products

The elimination of endotoxin from a recombinant or fermentation product is challenging because the host organism often contributes enormous amounts of endotoxin to the bulk material. The product is usually separated from endotoxin and feedstream impurities by affinity columns.

Future of the BET

The trend among pharmaceutical and medical device manufacturers is to move from gel-clot to kinetic LAL methods to quantify results, enhance test efficiency, and improve management of BET data. Powerful endotoxin-specific software for kinetic methods addresses the needs for simplicity, comprehensive reporting, trend analysis, and compliance with software validation requirements. In the past 25 years, the BET has enabled the parenteral industry to greatly reduce the levels of endotoxin pyrogen in its products. Competition between bait fishermen and the LAL industry for the horseshoe crab has brought about coast-wide conservation measures to maintain *Limulus* resources. The BET will continue to be an essential tool for assuring the safety of parenteral products.

REFERENCES

1. Annen, G.I.I. An Exhibition of Books on the Growth of Our Knowledge of Blood Transfusion. Bull. N.Y. Acad. Med. **1939**, *15*, 622–632.
1b. Dudrick, S.J.; Rhoades, J.E. JAMA **1971**, *215*, 923–949.
2. Macht, S.D. Three Hundred Years of Parenteral Nutrition: The History of Intravenous Nutritional Therapy. Conn. Med. **1980**, *44* (1), 27–30.
3. Westphal, O.; Wesphal, U.; Sommer, T. The History of Pyrogen Research. Microbiology. **1977**, 221–238.
4. Seibert, F.B. Pyrogens from an Historical Viewpoint. Transfusion. **1963**, *3*, 245–249.
5. Centanni, E. Untersuchungen über Das Infektionsfieber, Das Fiebergift Der Bakterien. Deutsch. Med. Wochenschr. **1894**, *10*, 148.

6. Hort, E.; Penfold, W.J. Microorganisms and Their Relation to Fever. J. Hyg. Camb. **1912**, *12*, 361–390.
7. Hort, E.; Penfold, W.J. A Critical Study of Experimental Fever. Proc. Roy. Soc. Med., London, Ser. B. **1912**, *85*, 174–186.
8. Hort, E.; Penfold, W.J. The Reaction of Salvarsan Fever to Other Forms of Injection Fever. Proc. Roy. Soc. Med., Part III, Pathology. **1912**, *5*, 131–139.
9. Seibert, F.B. Fever-Producing Substances Found in Some Distilled Waters. Am. J. Physiol. **1923**, *67*, 90–104.
10. Seibert, F.B. The Cause of Many Febrile Reactions Following Intravenous Injections. Am. J. Physiol. **1925**, *71*, 621–651.
11. Seibert, F.B.; Mendel, L.B. Temperature Variations in Rabbits. Am. J. Physiol. **1923**, *67*, 83–89.
12. Pearson, F.C., III Pyrogens Other than Endotoxin. *Pyrogens*; Marcel Dekker, Inc.: New York, 1985; 64–76.
13. Dinarello, C.A. Production of Endogenous Pyrogen. FASEB. **1979**, *38*, 52–56.
14. Elin, R.J.; Wolff, S.M.; McAdam, K.P.W.J.; Chedid, L.; Audibert, F.; Bernard, C.; Oberling, F. Properties of Reference Escherichia Coli Endotoxin and Its Phthalylated Derivative in Humans. J. Infect. Dis. **1981**, *144*, 329–336.
15. Marcus, S.; Anselmo, C.; Luke, J. Studies on Bacterial Pyrogenicity, II. A Bacteriological Test for Pyrogens in Parenteral Solutions. J. Am. Pharm. Assoc. **1960**, *9*, 616–619.
16. Atkins, A.; Freedman, L.R. Studies in Staphylococcal Fever, I. Responses to Bacterial Cells. Yale J. Bio. Med. **1963**, *35*, 451–471.
17. Braude, A.I.; McConnell, J.; Douglas, H. Fever from Pathogenic Fungi. J. Clin. Invest. **1960**, *39*, 1266–1276.
18. Atkins, E. Pathogenesis of Fever. Physiol. Rev. **1960**, *40*, 580–605.
19. Dinarello, C.A. Interleukin-1 and Its Biologically Related Cytokines. Adv. Immuniol. **1989**, *44*, 155–205.
20. Bendtzen, K. Interleukin-1, Interleukin-6 and Tumor Necrosis Factor in Infection, Inflammation and Immunity. Immunol. Lett. **1988**, *19*, 183–192.
21. Pearson, F.C., III Endotoxin. *Pyrogens*; Marcel Dekker, Inc.: New York, 1985; 23–56.
22. Rietschel, E.T.; Brade, H. Bacterial Endotoxins. Sci. Am. **1992 (August)**, 55–61.
23. Rietschel, E.T. Foreword. Immunobiol. **1993**, *187*, 167–168.
24. Hellon, R.; Townsend, Y. Mechanisms of Fever. Pharm. Ther. **1983**, *19*, 211–244.
25. Martich, G.D.; Boujoukos, A.J.; Suffredini, A.F. Response of Man to Endotoxin. Immunobiology. **1993**, *187*, 403–416.
26. Taveira da Silva, A.M.; Kaulbach, H.C.; Chuidian, F.S.; Lambert, D.R.; Suffredini, A.F.; Danner, R.L. Brief Report: Shock and Multiple-Organ Dysfunction After Self-Administration Of *Salmonella* Endotoxin. New Eng. J. Med. **1993**, *328*, 1457–1460.
27. Naunts, H.C. Bacterial Pyrogens: Beneficial Effects on Cancer Patients. *Biomedical Thermology*; Alan R. Liss, Inc.: New York, 1982; 687–696.
28. Legrand, E.K. An Evolutionary Perspective of Endotoxin: A Signal for a Well-Adapted Defense System. Med. Hypoth. **1990**, *33*, 49–56.

29. Nelson, L. Application of Reverse Osmosis in Pyrogen Removal. *Depyrogenation, Technical Report No. 7*; Parenteral Drug Association: Philadelphia, 1985; 28–36.

30. Sweadner, K.J.; Forte, M.; Nelson, L. Filtration Removal of Endotoxin (Pyrogens) in Solution in Different States of Aggregation. Appl. Environ. Microbiol. **1977**, *34*, 382–385.

31. Galanos, C.; Freudenberg, M.A.; Luderitz, O.; Rietschel, E.T.; Westphal, O. Chemical, Physicochemical and Biological Properties of Bacterial Lipopolysaccharides. *Biomedical Applications of the Horseshoe Crab (Limulidae)*; Cohen, E., Ed.; Alan R. Liss: New York, 1979; 32–332.

32. Weary, M. The Rabbit Pyrogen Test. *Pyrogens*; Marcel Dekker, Inc.: New York, 1985; 104–118.

33. Welch, H.; Calvery, H.D.; McClosky, W.T.; Price, C.W. Method of Preparation and Test for Bacterial Pyrogens. J. Am. Pharm. Assoc. **1943**, *32*, 65–69.

34. McClosky, W.T.; Price, C.W.; Van Winkle, W.J.; Welch, H.; Calvery, H.O. Results of First USP Collaborative Study of Pyrogens. J. Am. Pharm. Assoc. **1943**, *32*, 69–73.

35. Greisman, S.E.; Hornick, R.B. Comparative Pyrogenic Reactivity of Rabbit and Man to Bacterial Endotoxin. Proc. Soc. Exp. Biol. Med. **1969**, *131*, 1154–1158.

36. <151> Pyrogen Test. *U.S. Pharmacopeia 24*; United States Pharmacopeial Convention, Inc.: Rockville, MD, 2000; 1850.

37. Taktak, Y.S.; Selkirk, S.; Bristow, A.F.; Carpenter, A.; Ball, C.; Rafferty, B.; Poole, S. Assay of Pyrogens by Interleukin-6 Release from Monocytic Cell Lines. Pharm. Pharmacol. **1991**, *43*, 578–582.

38. Dinarello, C.A.; Gatti, S.; Barfai, T. Fever: Links with an Ancient Receptor. Curr. Biol. **1999**, *9*, R147–150.

39. Pearson, F.C.; Weary, M. The Significance of Limulus Amebocyte Lysate Test Specificity on the Pyrogen Evaluation of Parenteral Drugs. J. Parenter. Drug Assoc. **1980**, *34*, 103–108.

40. Bang, F.B. A Bacterial Disease Of *Limulus Polyphemus*. Bull. Johns Hopkins Hosp. **1956**, *98* (3), 325–351.

41. Levin, J.; Bang, F.B. The Role of Endotoxin in the Extracellular Coagulation Of *Limulus* Blood. Bull. Johns Hopkins Hosp. **1964**, *115* (3), 265–274.

42. Levin, J.; Bang, F.B. Clottable Protein In *Limulus*: Its Localization and Kinetics of Its Coagulation by Endotoxin. Thromb. Diathes. Haemorrh. **1968**, *19*, 1186–1197.

43. Cooper, J.F.; Levin, J.; Wagner, H.N., Jr. Quantitative Comparison of In Vitro (*Limulus*) and In Vivo (Rabbit) Methods for the Detection of Endotoxin. J. Lab. Clin. Med. **1971**, *78*, 138–148.

44. Flint, O. A Timetable for Replacing, Reducing and Refining Animal Use with the Help of In Vitro Tests: The Limulus Amebocyte Lysate Test (LAL) as an Example. *Alternatives to Animal Testing. New Ways in Biomedical Sciences*; Reinhardt, C.A., Ed.; Weinheim: Germany, 1994; 27–43.

45. Nakamura, T.; Morita, T.; Iwanega, S. Lipopolysaccharide-Sensitive Serine-Protease Zymogen (Factor C) Found in *Limulus* Hemocytes. Eur. J. Biochem. **1986**, *153*, 511–521.

46. Cooper, J.F.; Weary, M.E.; Jordan, F.T. The Impact of Non-Endotoxin LAL-Reactive Materials on Limulus Amebocyte Lysate Analyses. PDA J. of Pharm. Sci. Technol. **1997**, *51*, 2–6.

47. Harada, T.; Morita, T.; Iwanaga, S.; Nakamura, S.; Niwa, M. A New Chromogenic Substrate Method for the Assay of Bacterial Endotoxins Using *Limulus* Hemocyte Lysate. *Biomedical Applications of the Horseshoe Crab (Limulidae)*; Cohen, E., Ed.; Alan R. Liss, Inc.: New York, 1979; 209–220.

48. Weary, M.E. Understanding and Setting Endotoxin Limits. J. Parenteral Sci. Technol. **1990**, *44*, 16–18.

49. Cooper, J.F.; Harbert, J.C. Endotoxin as a Cause of Aseptic Meningitis After Radionuclide Cisternography. J. Nucl. Med. **1975**, *16*, 809–813.

50. <85>Bacterial Endotoxins Test. *USP 24-NF 19*; The United States Pharmacopeial Convention, Inc.: Rockville, MD, 2000; 2875–2879, Supplement 2.

51. Cooper, J.F.; Hochstein, D.H.; Seligmann, E.B. The Limulus Test for Endotoxin (Pyrogen) in Radiopharmaceuticals and Biologicals. Bull. Parent. Drug Assoc. **1972**, *26*, 153–162.

52. U.S. Public Health Service. Limulus Amebocyte Lysate: Additional Standards. Fed. Reg. **1973**, *38*, 26130.

53. Dabbah, R.; Ferrry, E.; Gunther, D.A.; Hahn, R.; Mazur, P.; Neely, M.; Nicholas, P.; Pierce, J.; Slade, J.; Watson, S.W.; Weary, M. Pyrogenicity of E. Coli 055:B5 by the USP Rabbit Pyrogen Test—HIMA Collaborative Study. J. Parenter. Drug Assoc. **1980**, *34*, 212–216.

54. US Food and Drug Administration. *A Guideline on Validation of the Limulus Amebocyte Lysate Test as an End-Product Endotoxin Test for Human and Animal Parenteral Drugs, Biological Products and Medical Devices*; Food and Drug Administration: Rockville, MD, 1987.

55. Cooper, J.F. Bacterial Endotoxins Test. *Microbiology in Pharmaceutical Manufacturing*; Prince, R., Ed.; Parenteral Drug Assoc., Bethesda, Davis Horwood International Publication, Ltd.: Modalmeny, UK, 2001; p. 537–567.

56. Weary, M. Depyrogenation. *Pyrogens*; Marcel Dekker, Inc.: New York, 1985; 203–218.

57. Tsuji, K.; Harrison, S. Dry Heat Destruction of Lypopolysaccharide: Dry Heat Destruction Kinetics. Appl. Environ. Microbiol. **1978**, *36*, 710–714.

58. Bamba, R.; Matsui, R.; Watabe, I. Effect of Steam-Heat Treatment with/without Divalent Cations of the Inactivation of Lipopolysaccharides from Several Bacterial Species. PDA J. Parenter. Sci. Technol. **1996**, *50*, 129–135.

59. Fanning, M.M.; Wassel, R.; Piazza-Hepp, T. Pyrogenic Reactions Associated with Gentamicin Therapy. N. Eng. J. Med. (2000) 343, 1658-1659.

60. Hochstein, H.D.; Fitzgerald, E.A.; McMahon, F.G.; Vargas, R. Properties of US Standard Endotoxin (EC-5) in Human Male Volunteers. J. Endotoxin Research. **1994**, *1*, 52–56.

RADIOCHEMICAL METHOD OF ANALYSIS

R. Raghavan
Jose C. Joseph
Abbott Laboratories, Abbott Park, Illinois

INTRODUCTION

In nuclear medicine, drugs containing radioactive metals, metal complexes, and metal conjugates are used for diagnosis and therapy of various diseases. Radioactive materials used as pharmaceuticals are not only small organic and inorganic molecules but are also macromolecules such as monoclonal antibodies and antibody fragments that are attached to radioactive metals. Nuclear medicine has become a \$12 billion medical industry, and more than one-third of the hospitals in the United States currently use radioisotopes for such procedures. It is anticipated that diagnostic procedures in the United States are likely to exceed 20 million by the end of 2000. The successful use of radiochemicals needs a basic understanding of radiation, radioactivity, and the nature and characteristics of instruments to detect and quantitate radiation. This article addresses these applications related to radioactivity and radiochemical methods of measurement.

ATOMIC STRUCTURE, NUCLEAR STABILITY, AND RADIOACTIVITY

Atomic physics describes the structure of atoms in complex mathematical terms of quantum mechanics. However, the model of the atom as described by Niels Bohr in 1913 is very simple, pictorial, and more than adequate for a basic understanding of the phenomenon of radioactivity. Bohr's planetary model of the atom consists of a dense positively charged nucleus surrounded by negatively charged electrons (e) in orbits of well-defined energy states. The nucleus consists of positively charged protons and neutral particles called neutrons. The protons and neutrons are held together by very a strong nuclear force of attraction, effective at very close distances (approximately 10^{-13} cm). These strong forces for each nucleus are computed in terms of binding energy. The electroneutrality of the atom is maintained by the orbital electrons, which are equal in number to that of the protons. This number is called the atomic number, Z. The masses of the atoms (A) and other particles are described in terms of

atomic mass units (amu). The amu is defined as 1/12th the mass of a carbon atom with atomic mass of 12.0000. The properties of these nuclear particles known as nucleons and electron are summarized in Table 1.

Any configuration of protons and neutrons is called a nuclide. There are three nuclides of the element hydrogen with atomic number 1. Some characteristics of the nuclides are listed in Table 2.

The notation $^a_Z X$ is used to indicate the nuclide of an element. The three nuclides of hydrogen are called isotopes of hydrogen. Tritium with an N/Z ratio of two is unstable. When the N/Z ratio becomes higher, the nucleus become unstable and results in the disintegration of the nucleus so as to achieve a stable N/Z ratio and therefore a stable nucleus. This process is called radioactive decay. This radioactive process can be spontaneous in some naturally occurring nuclides; then these elements are said to be naturally radioactive. When such instability is brought about by bombarding stable nuclides with high-energy particles, it is called artificial radioactivity. Of nearly 3000 known nuclides of elements, which are either man-made or natural, 287 nuclides of 83 elements are stable; the rest are unstable to varying degrees. The unstable nuclides disintegrate to form stable nuclides with release of energy and nuclear particles. Binding energy and nuclear stability are found to be dependent on the ratio of number of neutrons to protons (N/Z or n/p ratio). To be stable, at least one proton is required. The most stable heavy nuclide is $^{209}_{83} X$, with 83 protons and 126 neutrons ($N/Z = 1.5$). In general, when the N/Z ratio is greater than 1.6, the radioactive nuclide readjusts to a stable ratio of N/Z with the release of energy and particles of matter. The three nuclides of hydrogen are called isotopes. Other members of the nuclide family are isobars and isotones. The characteristics of these nuclides are given in Table 3.

Radioactive Decay

Different radioactive species undergo disintegration at different rates. The rate of this decay or activity is characteristic of the individual nuclide and is proportional to the number of radioactive nuclides present at the beginning of this time interval. The proportionality constant

Encyclopedia of Pharmaceutical Technology

Table 1 Mass, charge, and energies of nucleons and electrons

Particle	Mass (Kg)	Mass (amu)	Charge	Energy[a] (MeV)	Comments
Electron (e)	0.9108×10^{-30}	0.000549	-1	0.511	—
Proton (p)	1.6721×10^{-27}	1.00728	$+1$	938.8	—
Neutron (n)	1.6744×10^{-27}	1.00867	0	939.9	—
Alpha (α)	6.6465×10^{-27}	4.003874	$+2$	3726.7	Binding energy of the α-Particle is 28.29 MeV
Beta (β^-)	0.9108×10^{-30}	0.000549	-1	0.511	Variable kinetic energy depending on how ejected
Positron (β^+)	0.9108×10^{-30}	0.000549	$+1$	0.511	Variable kinetic energy depending on how ejected
Neutrino (v)	0	0	0	—	—
Photon	0	0	0		Varying energy

[a]Energy is based on the rest mass of the particle.

is called the decay constant and is denoted by λ. The decay constant is a measure of the probability that a certain radioactive nucleus will disintegrate within a specified time interval. These disintegrations are characteristic of the nuclide and are unaffected by pressure, temperature, concentration, and other physical or chemical properties of the radionuclide. This rate constant is conveniently denoted in terms of $t_{\frac{1}{2}}$, or halflife. The halflife of a radionuclide is the time required for the sample activity to decrease to half its initial value. $t_{\frac{1}{2}}$ is related to rate constant (λ) as follows:

$$\lambda = 0.6932/t_{1/2}$$

In fact, less than 1% will be radioactive in seven halflives, and after 10 halflives, greater than 99.9% of the radioactive nuclide will have lost its activity. The halflife refers to that of a pure nuclide. In a sample containing mixtures of disintegrating radionuclides, the total activity is the sum of the separate activities. From a plot of relative activity against time, the individual halflives can be computed. However, in practice, this can be realized for mixtures containing 3 or <3 nuclides. Other commonly used terms in nuclear medicine and pharmacy are average (mean) halflife, biological halflife, and effective halflife. Average halflife is the mean lifetime of a nuclide, and it is equal to $1.44 \times t_{\frac{1}{2}}$. Biologic halflife, t_b, is the time required

for the body to eliminate half the administered dose by normal biological process of elimination. Effective halflife (t_{eff}) is a measure of how fast the body eliminates the radioactive material by the combination of biological elimination and radioactive decay:

$$1/t_{\text{eff}} = 1/t_b + 1/t_{1/2}$$

Unit of Activity

The fundamental SI unit of activity is the Becquerel (Bq). One Bq is equal to one disintegration per second (dps). Because this is a very small unit, it is more often expressed in kilobequerels or kBq. However, the older historical unit of activity C_i is normally used for radiopharmaceuticals. The Curie was defined in terms of the number of disintegrations per second of 1 g of ^{226}Ra and is equal to 3.7×10^{10} dps. Other commonly used units are millicurie and microcurie (mC_i and μC_i). The unit of C_i represents absolute activity (A). However, relative activity R is proportional to the efficiency of the counting device. The device reports in counts per minute.

$R = qA$; $q =$ efficiency quotient. Sometimes specific activity, in terms of radioactivity per unit mass of an element or radiolabeled compound or unit volume of solution is also specified. In these case, the mass or volume should be clearly specified.

Table 2 Configuration of nuclides of hydrogen

Nuclide	No. of protons (Z)	No. of neutrons (N)	N/Z (n/p) ratio	Notation	Nuclear stability
Hydrogen	1	0	0	$^{1}_{1}H$	Stable
Deuterium	1	1	1	$^{2}_{1}H$	Stable
Tritium	1	2	2	$^{3}_{1}H$	Unstable

Table 3 Characteristics of nuclides

Nuclide	Atomic number (Z)	Mass number	Neutron number	Chemical property	Examples
Isotopes	Same	Different	Different	Same	$^{15}_{8}O$, $^{16}_{8}O$, $^{17}_{8}O$, $^{18}_{8}O$
Isobars	Different	Same	Different	Different	$^{67}_{29}Cu$, $^{67}_{30}Zn$, $^{67}_{31}Ga$,
Isotones	Different	Different	Same	Different	$^{59}_{26}Fe$, $^{60}_{27}Co$, $^{62}_{29}Cu$, (33 neutrons each)
Isomers	Same	Same	Same	Same	$^{99m}_{43}Tc$, and $^{99}_{43}Tc$. (^{m}) meta stable isomer

Decay Processes

The radioactive decay process involves the emission of radiation, which is dependent on the mode of decay of the particular radionuclide. Radiation resulting from any decay process can be classified as alpha (α), beta (β), gamma rays (γ), and/or other emissions.

α-Particles

Alpha (α)-particles are doubly charged, highly energetic helium nucleus. α-Particles originate in the nuclei of heavier atoms. The emission involving α-Particles is the most efficient process for a radionuclide to attain stability because the nuclide loses both charge and mass. Because α-Particles are very heavy (7400 times of that of an electron) and doubly charged, they attract electrons from the surrounding medium when they pass through a medium. This results in the ionization of the medium. An α-Particle loses energy, slows down, and finally becomes a helium nucleus. In each ionization process, it loses 34 eV per event. For example, a loss of 3.4 MeV of energy causes 100,000 ionization events. These particles travel very short distances, called the range. Because they are extremely efficient in ionizing, they lose energy very rapidly. This range is approximate 4 cm in air and a few thousandths of a centimeter in biological tissues. Because of this tremendous amount of energy transfer, α-Particles can cause extensive damage to organs and tissues when they are exposed to this radiation. Generally, α-Particles arise during the natural decay of elements with a Z value greater than 83. A typical alpha decay process is represented below:

$$^{238}_{92}U \longrightarrow {}^{234}_{90}Th + {}^{4}_{2}He + Energy$$

β-Particles

A β-Particle is a high-velocity nucleon ejected out of a decaying nucleus. β-Particles have the rest mass (0.000548 amu) of an electron. If it is negatively charged, it is called a negatron and if positively charged, it is called a positron. In common usage, β-Particle emission refers to the negatron (β^-) and β^+-Emission is called positron emission. For example, the decay of $^{32}_{15}P$ to $^{32}_{15}S$ results in the emission of β^-, antineutrino, and release of energy. The difference in the masses of the two nuclides, 0.001836 amu (31.965675 for P $-$ 31.9638390 for S), results in the release of energy equivalent to 1.70 MeV. Part of this energy is used up in the ejection of particles, and the remaining is used in the release of antineutrino. Because no other energy is emitted, ^{32}P is called a pure β-Emitter. Sometimes some portion of the energy difference may be retained in the nucleus, and consequently the nuclide resides in a nuclear excited state. The excited nucleus may lose the excess energy and return to the stable ground state in the form of electromagnetic radiation (gamma-rays). β-Particles are emitted with variable energy from zero to the maximum of the difference in energy between the parent and daughter nucleus. The variability in energy arises from the distribution of energy between the β-Particle and the antineutrino.

Negatively charged β-Particles are emitted when the radionuclide has more neutrons than required by the number of protons for stability. Sometimes more than one β-Particle may be emitted. For example, ^{131}I decays with the emission of six β-Particles and 14 γ-Rays of different energies:

$$^{131}_{53}I \longrightarrow {}^{131}_{54}Xe + \beta^- + \beta^- + \gamma + antineutrino + Energy$$

Nearly 100% of all these decay processes correspond to β-Particles of energy 0.61 MeV and γ-Radiations of energy 0.364 MeV. The decay to form stable nuclides may involve the formation of many unstable intermediate radionuclides. For example, the decay of $^{127}_{50}Sn$ to $^{127}_{53}I$, shown below, involves the formation of a number of intermediate nuclides:

$$^{127}_{50}Sn \longrightarrow {}^{127}_{51}Sb \longrightarrow {}^{127}_{52}Te \longrightarrow {}^{127}_{53}I$$

In general, β^-- and β^+-Particles penetrate deep into the medium; however, they do not cause damage to tissues and organs. Radionuclides that decay by β-Particle emissions are used very extensively in nuclear medicine for diagnostic and therapeutic applications. Positron-emitting nuclides are used in nuclear medicine for diagnostic purposes. β^+-Emitting radionuclides are under active study for use in radiotherapy. An example of a decay process involving emissions of positrons follows:

$$^{15}_{8}O \longrightarrow {}^{15}_{7}N + {}^{0}_{1}\beta^+.$$

γ-Rays (γ)

During the disintegration of the nucleus, part of the energy is used in the creation of excited-state radionuclide. In the excited state, the nuclide is unstable. The release of energy while the excited nucleus returns to the ground state appears as electromagnetic radiation. These radiations are called γ-Rays. γ-Emission is common when the difference between the excited state and the lowest energy ground state nucleus is greater than 100 keV. Because γ-Emission is electromagnetic radiation, there is no change in the neutron number or mass number or atomic number. Therefore, invariably, γ-Radiation is always preceded by a nuclear decay reaction involving emission of α, β^-, β^+ particles.

γ-Rays are high-energy electromagnetic radiation such as X-Rays with no electrical charge. γ-Rays are different from X-Rays in that they differ with respect to their origin. X-Rays originate from orbital electrons, whereas γ-Rays originate from the decay of a nuclide. The γ-Rays also ionize the medium by striking orbital electrons with high energy and by knocking the electrons out of the atom. These ejected electrons cause secondary ionization referred to as indirect ionization. The degree of penetration of γ-Rays is extremely high. There are at least seven different processes by which γ-Rays can interact with matter. However, the processes associated with γ-Ray interaction or production, which are pharmaceutically relevant, are electron capture, isomeric transition, and internal conversion. These are briefly discussed below.

Electron capture is a decay process in which an orbital electron loses energy and becomes absorbed into the nucleus. As a result, outer-shell electrons jump to fill the inner-shell vacancy resulting in an electron orbit reshuffling. This process result in the release of X-Rays, and these electrons are subsequently absorbed and result in the release of weakly bound orbital electrons. These are called Auger electrons. When the decay process involves in positron emission, it is almost always followed by electron capture. As a result of nuclear reaction, an excited radionuclide (with energy >100 keV) loses energy by de-excitation:

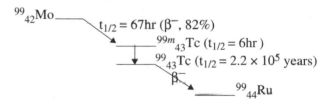

More often, these occur in multiple steps with the release of γ-Ray photons of multiple energy. Thus, the resulting γ-Ray spectrum is unique to the decaying radionuclide; this uniqueness, therefore, is used to identify the unknown nuclide. γ-Rays with no mass and charge can penetrate into matter and bring about other chemical reactions in the system. γ-Rays are widely used in nuclear medicine.

An excited radionuclide may remain in several excited states before reaching ground state. However, transitions can occur within these excited states with the emission of γ-Rays. These transitions are called isomeric transitions. When these isomeric transitions are significantly long-lived, these are called metastable states.

An example of the decay process is shown below. (↘▲— increase in Z, ↙— (left arrow) decrease in Z)

$$^{99}_{42}Mo$$
$$t_{1/2} = 67hr\ (\beta^-, 82\%)$$
$$^{99m}_{43}Tc\ (t_{1/2} = 6hr)$$
$$^{99}_{43}Tc\ (t_{1/2} = 2.2 \times 10^5\ years)$$
$$\beta^-$$
$$^{99}_{44}Ru$$

A process alternative to isomeric transition is called internal conversion (IC). In some cases, the γ-energy is absorbed by a K-shell (inner) electron. This electron is ejected out with lower energy. This ejected electron is the internal conversion electron, and the process is called internal conversion. Some diagnostic and therapeutic radionuclides with corresponding halflives are given below.

Diagnostic raidonuclides: ($t_{\frac{1}{2}}$ in units as indicated are given in parentheses.) $t_{\frac{1}{2}}$ hours: ^{67}Cu (62.0); ^{67}Ga (78.3); ^{90}Y (64.1); ^{117}In (67.9); ^{99m}Tc (6); ^{201}Tl (72) {β^--particles}-t min; ^{11}C (20.4); ^{13}N (10.1); ^{15}O (2.0); ^{18}F (1.9); ^{68}Ga (68.0); and ^{82}Rb (1.25) {β^+}.

Therapeutic radionuclides: $t_{\frac{1}{2}}$ days: D; ^{32}P(14.3); ^{47}Sc (3.4); ^{67}Cu (2.6); ^{64}Cu (0.5); ^{90}Y (2.7); ^{105}Rh (1.5); ^{111}Ag (7.5); ^{117m}Sn (13.6); ^{131}I (8.0); ^{149}Pm (2.2); ^{153}Sm (1.9); ^{166}Ho (1.1); ^{177}Lu (6.7); ^{186}Re (3.8); ^{188}Re (0.7).

RADIATION DETECTION AND MEASUREMENT

Interaction of Radiation with Matter, Ionization Chamber, and GM Counters

The detection and quantitation of nuclear radiation are based on its interaction with material contained in the detector. Ionization of the gas particles in the medium and scattering are the two most common types of interaction of radiation with matter. Radiation causes darkening of photographic emulsion, ionization of a gas or a mixture of gases, or fluorescent scintillation. In radiology, exposure and observation of the photographic film are most commonly used. When α-Particles with high kinetic energies impinge on gases enclosed in a chamber, they produce approximately 40,000 (±10,000) ion pairs per cm. The range of α-particles is short (approximately 6 cm in air and 2 μM in lead); β-Particles have longer and irregular paths and produce approximately 100–700 ion pairs per cm. A typical ionization chamber, shown in Fig. 1, consists of a sealed tube containing helium, neon, or gas–air mixtures placed in a space between two electrodes. The incoming particles create ion pairs; the ions are separated and collected at the electrodes of opposite charge. Electrons are collected at the anode. The number of such ions collected at each electrode is also a function of the applied voltage across the electrodes. If the response is measured in terms of pulse height (proportional to the number of electrons collected), a plot of this value against applied voltage will exhibit a characteristic response as given in Fig. 2. The different regions in Fig. 2 are explained below. Region I is called the recombination region. In this region, ion pairs produced increase linearly as a function of applied voltage (<100 V) as recombination is proportionately decreased. This is not a useful region for measurement. In region II (100–400 V), pulse height attains a plateau because all ions formed are collected. This region is used in ionization chambers to measure energies of γ-Rays and X-Rays. This region is also used for identification of α- and β-Particles because the height at which plateau occurs is characteristic of the nature of the particle. Dose meters and dose rate meters, which measure high-intensity radiation fields,

operate in this region. In region III (400–800 V), the number of pulses produced is proportional to the intensity of radiation. The size of the pulses counted gives a measure of the primary ionization produced. In this region, the primary electrons are accelerated with high gain in energy. This high energy causes additional secondary electrons to be generated as a result of interaction with gases in the ionization chamber. These secondary electrons cause further ionization. The net effect is pulse amplification; the size of the amplification is of the order of 100–10,000 times that of the size of the ions initially produced in the ionization chamber.

In Fig. 2, the two response plots correspond to two particles of different energy. Ionization chambers operate in this region.

Region IV (applied voltage 800–1000 V) is limited proportional region and is not important for purposes of detection. When the applied voltage is between 1000 and 1500 V, the size of the pulse is no longer proportional to the initiating event. However, each pulse corresponds to a single event. The counters that operate in this region are called Geiger–Mueller counters or GM counters. The GM counters are very sensitive. Because of the high gain involved, these are used primarily in regions where the radioactivity is of very low intensity, (e.g., radioactive contamination). The readings are given in milli-, micro-, or Roentgens/h or in counts per minute. In the GM counter, ionization produced spreads to the entire gas. Therefore, the counter may not respond to a succeeding second incoming pulse before a recovery time of approximately 100–300 μs. This dead time for recovery is unusually high compared with the dead time for the proportional counter, which is approximately 1 μs. Secondly, because a fixed amount of gas is present in the chamber, the purity of the gas in the chamber decreases. Therefore, the GM counter has to be calibrated frequently, using standard ^{226}Ra or ^{137}Cs sources

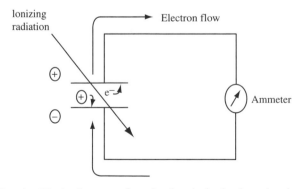

Fig. 1 Block diagram of a simple air ionization chamber. Electrons are attracted to the positive plate, and positive ions go to the negative plate.

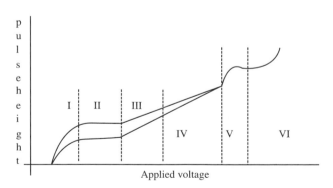

Fig. 2 Pulse height versus applied voltage response.

per Nuclear Regulatory Commission (NRC) requirements. Above an applied voltage of 1500 V, continuous discharge occurs, and this is not useful for any measurement.

Scintillation Detectors

When radiation interacts with certain substances called fluors or phosphors, it produces a flash of light called scintillation. The scintillation is then detected using a sensing element, amplified, sorted, and recorded by counting. The scintillation-detecting instruments include well counters, scanners, thyroid probes, and scintillation cameras called Auger cameras. In addition, all these instruments consist of a collimator (excluding well counters), photomultipliers, a high-voltage power supply, an amplifier, a gain control unit, a pulse height analyzer, and instruments or computers for appropriate display modes. The scintillation cameras also contain coordinate-positioning (x,y) circuits.

Solid-State Detectors

These detectors are made of semiconducting materials. In these detectors, solid-state electrodes are made from Li doped with Si or Ge. The resolution is approximately 1–2 keV for 1 MeV γ-Rays and sometimes provides a greater than 10-fold improvement over NaI (Tl) scintillation detectors, described below. These are commercially available and more often used in research-grade instruments.

A brief review of scintillation phosphors and their uses are given in Table 4.

Liquid Scintillators

The sample radionuclide is dissolved in a liquid scintillator called the scintillation cocktail. It consists of two principal components. The first is a primary solvent such as toluene, xylene, or 1,2,4-Trimethylbenzene (pseudocumene). The second component is the fluor solute, 2,5-Diphenyloxazole (PPO) that emits UV light at ~380 nm. The cocktail may also contain one or more the following:

- A secondary solvent such as dioxane to improve solubility of aqueous samples or surfactants such as sodium dodecylbenzenesulfonate as emulsifier
- A secondary scintillator to shift the wavelength of photons emitted (~380 nm) to the wavelength response of some photomultiplier tubes (PMT, ~420 nm)
- One or more adjuvants for purposes of suspending or solubilizing biological tissues.

A brief description of other components of scintillation detectors (generally applicable to liquid scintillators also) is given below.

Photomultiplier (PM) tubes

The PM tube has a light-sensitive electrode called the photocathode. It emit electrons when photons strike it. The electrons are then accelerated from the photocathode to the anode of PM tube by the application of approximately 1000 V in steps of approximately 100 V by a series of electrodes called the dynodes. In the PM tube, secondary electrons are produced, resulting in pulses of 10^5 to 10^8 electrons. Typically a phototube with 10 dynodes delivers approximately 4^{10} electrons. This gain or amplification is dependent on the dynode voltages.

Preamplifier

Even though such a large number of secondary electrons are generated, these are not adequate to generate enough current. The voltage pulse is amplifed by a factor of 4–5 by the preamplifier without loss of power. The preamplifier also provides the driving force necessary to prevent loss in the several feet of connecting cables.

Linear amplifier

The pulses received from preamplifier have wide variation in energies of the particles. The gain in the amplifier is of the order of 8000 such that a 1-mV signal is amplified to approximately 8 V while still maintaining the proportionality of the energy delivered by the particle (more often γ-Ray) to the detectors. The amplified pulse is then delivered to pulse height analyzer.

Pulse height analyzers (PHA)

The pulses that emerge from the amplifier usually have different amplitudes owing to differences in energies. These analyzers are essentially energy sorters. Single-channel PHAs count pulses of a given amplitude, whereas multichannel analyzers (MCAs) scan whole energy range and record the pulses in each channel. For example, by using an MCA, γ-Ray spectrum can be recorded and, thus, these instruments that use MCAs are called γ-Ray spectrometers. MCAs may have as many as 4000 channels.

X-Y-positioning circuits

These are unique to scintillation cameras, known as Auger cameras, used in nuclear medicine studies. Approximately 19–91 PMTs are mounted on a Na(Tl) crystal used in the camera. These crystals are typically–thick. The number of PMTs, which are optically coupled to the back of the crystal, is determined by the size and shape of the crystal. A maximum amount of light will be received by the PMT nearest to the point of interaction compared with the other PMTs, which are positioned differently. The amount of light received in these PMTs is proportional to the solid

Table 4 Scintillation phosphors and their uses

Particle detected	Phosphors used	Characteristics/comments
Alpha (α)	Thin sheet of plastic scintillator or zinc sulfide embedded in a transparent tape	Phosphors are wrapped in very thin aluminized mylar foil to exclude light. α-Particles, because of low penetrating power, lose all their energy to scintillators. β- and γ-Particles produce only smaller pulses and by adjustment of appropriate setting of the discriminator, α-Particles alone can be counted.
Beta (β)	Single crystals of anthracene, *trans*-stillbene are commonly used. Sometimes naphthalene doped with anthracene can also be used.	For β-Particle counting, especially low-energy particles from ^{14}C and tritium, liquid scintillators are commonly used (see discussion below on liquid scintillators).
Gamma (γ)	Sodium iodide doped with thallium iodide are used [NaI(Tl)]; thallium, which is present at 0.1–0.4% of sodium emits 420 nm scintillations. This phosphor is very efficient in absorbing γ radiation because of high atomic number of iodine and high density of sodium iodide.	Sodium iodide is hermetically sealed. It is normally used in well counters. A typical well counter used in laboratory and that used in cameras in nuclear medicine are show in Figs. 3 and 4.

angle subtended by the PMT. Therefore, $X-Y$-positioning of the camera has to be controlled and known so that $X-Y$-coordinate of the γ-Ray interaction can be assessed accurately. These data are stored in a computer and then processed or recorded on Polaroid or X-Ray films.

Efficiency of detection in scintillation detectors

In gas-filled as well as scintillation detectors, the observed count rate is typically less than the actual decay rate of the radionuclide. The efficiency of detection may differ from particle to particle under identical conditions using the same type of detector. The factors that affect the efficiency of detection are operating voltage, resolving time, geometry of the instrument used in relation to the position of the sample with respect to the detector, scaler, energy resolution, absorption by cells, and sometimes constituents of the sample itself. For example, the scintillation cocktail sometimes reduces counts considerably. This effect is known as quenching. For accurate measurements of radioactivity, appropriate correction for quenching is required.

Frequent calibration of the instruments with the use of appropriate standards is required to make suitable allowances for decreases in the efficiency of the instruments. Such calibration standards are available from the National Institute of Standards and Technology (NIST). Other sources traceable to NIST standards through active program of participation in comparison measurements also provide such standards. The United States Pharmacopeia (USP) also provides nuclear decay data for new calibration standard. USP 24 lists $t_{\frac{1}{2}}$, energy of photons, and number of

photons per disintegrations, for the following radionuclide standards: ^{137}Cs, ^{137m}Ba, ^{22}Na, ^{60}Co, ^{57}Co, ^{54}Mn, ^{109}Cd, ^{109}Ag, and ^{129}I.

Tomographic Imagers

Tomography is a process in which three-dimensional images are constructed using a large number of two-dimensional slices of images from an object. Computed tomography uses rigorous mathematical algorithms to reconstruct these images. When radionuclide emissions are used, it is called emission tomography. Two common techniques are now used to obtain images using emission tomography, namely, single photon emission computed tomography (SPECT) and positron emission tomography (PET). In SPECT, γ-Emitting nuclides are used, whereas in PET, positron-emitting nuclides are used. In the SPECT system, an object is photographed using many Auger cameras at a number of small angles (between 3 and 10°) around the object. The total span may be between 0 and 180° or between 0 and 360°. Because the rotating cameras provide two-dimensional digital images, these are stored as 64 × 64 matrix (for 180° span) or as 128 × 128 matrix (for 360° span) digital information. The Auger cameras use NaI (Tl) crystals in the detector heads. In PET, positron-emitting radionuclides are used. Each positron emitted from these radionuclides travels through tissues, deposits energy, and finally is annihilated by interaction with an electron. The annihilation results in the formation of two photons traveling in opposite directions (180° apart) with energy of 0.511 MeV. Two Auger cameras are placed 180°

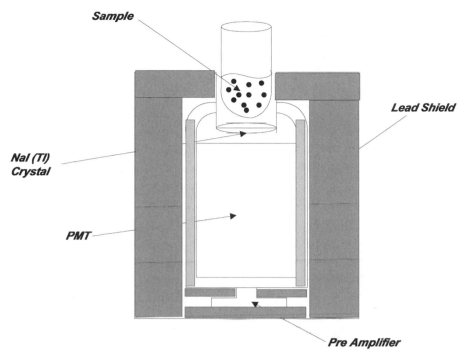

Fig. 3 A typical well counter used for measurement of gamma rays.

apart but at the same distance from the object. Each camera detects a photon at the same time. By appropriately moving cameras in pairs, the data are collected over many angles and stored in 64 × 64 or 128 × 128 matrix. Thus, this electronic collimation brought about by simultaneous detection increases sensitivity and reduces the need for use of collimators as in SPECT. Additional advantages of PET include easy availability of radionuclides with short halflives of isotopes of elements commonly found in organic molecules (such as F, N, C, and O). (See USP 24 for additional details of requirements for radiopharmaceuticals for PET.)

ANALYSIS OF RADIOCHEMICALS

Radiochemical methods of analysis are considerably more sensitive than other chemical methods. Most spectral methods can quantitate at the parts-per-million (ppm) level, whereas atomic absorption and some HPLC methods with UV, fluorescence, and electrochemical methods can quantitate at the parts-per-billion (ppb) levels. By controlling the specific activity levels, it is possible to attain quantitation levels lower than ppb levels of elements by radiochemical analyses. Radiochemical

analysis, in most cases, can be done without separation of the analyte. Radionuclides are identified based on the characteristic decay and the energy of the particles as

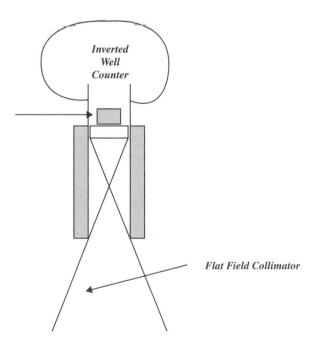

Fig. 4 A typical well counter used in nuclear medicine.

described in detection procedures presented above. Radiochemical methods of analysis include tracer methods, activation analysis, and radioimmunoassay techniques.

Tracers and Tracer Methods of Analysis

Radiochemical tracers or radiotracers are compounds labeled with radioisotopes. For tracer methods, the compound to be measured or a suitable reagent is radiolabeled. A measurement of the redistribution of tracer within such a sample–reagent reaction system provides the required quantitative analytical information. Major advantages of tracer methods are high sensitivity, simplicity, and speed. Radiotracers are more commonly used for following mechanisms of biological and/or chemical processes or if there is need to eliminate complicated separation procedures, especially in biological processes.

Isotopic dilution analysis

In isotope dilution analysis, a known amount of radiolabeled compound with known specific activity is spiked to a known amount of an unknown mixture containing the same compound made up of stable isotopes. Then, the components of the radiotracer-diluted samples are mixed thoroughly to form a homogeneous mixture. This istopically diluted mixture, with known levels of dilution, is then suitably treated to isolate a small amount of the desired constituent. The radioactive isotope content of the isolated portion is determined by measuring its specific activity. From the specific activities of the tracer before and after dilution, the concentration of the component in the mixture can then be calculated. The major advantage is that these isolation procedures need not be quantitative; however, it is necessary that the compound isolated should be pure enough for an activity determination. Isotope dilution analyses are used for determination of inorganic trace elements and for the determination of organic compounds in biological systems. If separations are required and the radioisotope concentration is not adequate to bring about separation, dilutions can be accomplished by using a nonradioactive compound (or carrier) with similar chemical behavior. For example, if radio strontium is to be precipitated and it is in low amounts such that it cannot be quantitatively precipitated, it can be coprecipitated along with a calcium salt by the addition of calcium before precipitation. An alternative procedure to isotope dilution, reverse or inverse isotope dilution, can be used to determine the quantity of radioactive compound by dilution with an inactive compound. This procedure is applicable when a system contains an unknown amount of isotopically labeled substance of known specific activity.

Radioisotope exchage

For understanding mechanisms and kinetics of organic or biological reactions, nonradioactive atoms in molecules or ions are allowed to exchange with appropriate radio-labeled compound. After chemical exchange between a labeled compound and the test sample (the chemical form of the element being different in the two solutions, e.g., iodine in CH_3I vs $^{131}I^-$ in labeled sodium iodide), the specific activity of the element becomes the same in the sample and reagent. A measured decrease in the activity of the reagent or increase in the activity of the sample can then be related to the amount of element present in the sample. Isotopic exchange methods of analysis are very sensitive, rapid, and specific. Isotopic exchange plays a very important role in pharmacokinetic studies. For example, a drug molecule may be labeled with tritium to follow the drug distribution. Exchange of tritium with an unlabeled compound or with a water molecule in the vicinity may lead to erroneous interpretation of the drug distribution if suitable precautions are not taken to avoid potential isotopic exchange reactions.

Radiotracers as radiopharmaceuticals: Methods for radiopharmaceutical analysis

When radiolabeled compounds (radiotracers) are used for diagnostic and therapeutic purposes, it is called a radiopharmaceutical. A radiopharmaceutical should be easily produced, inexpensive, readily available, have relatively short halflife, and preferably should be a γ-Emitter with an energy between 30 and 300 keV. Such a γ-Emitting nuclide should invariably decay by electron capture or isomeric transition. When positron-emitting nuclides are used, they must have specific localization in the desired organ or tissue and should not result in undue radiation exposure. Radiotracers, used as pharmaceuticals, are produced in one of two ways: either as a product of nuclear fission reactions or as a product of nuclear reactions induced by high-energy accelerator particles or neutrons. Particle accelerators are instruments that cause nuclear reactions by bombarding target nuclides with highly accelerated and energized particles such as protons, deutrons, and electrons. For production of radiopharmaceuticals, on-site accelerators called cyclotrons are used. For production of positron-emitting radionculides linear accelerators are used. Readily transportable instruments, which serve as sources for short-lived radionuclides, are called generators. Typically, in a generator, a long-lived parent nuclide is allowed to decay to a short-lived daughter radionuclide. Using differences in chemical properties, the daughter nuclide is separated from the parent. Typical pharmaceutically relevant radionuclides and their sources are summarized in Table 5.

A radiopharmaceutical is a radioactive chemical used as a pharmaceutical. Therefore, as pharmaceuticals, they should have proper ionic strength, pH, isotonicity, and osmolarity. In addition to chemical purity, radionuclide purity and radiochemical purity also have to be demonstrated. The radionuclide purity refers to the ratio of the amount of radioactivity corresponding to that of desired radionuclide to the total amount of radioactivity owing to other isotopes and other isotopic impurities. Radionuclide purity is determined by measuring halflives and other characteristics of radiation of the radionuclide. Radiochemical purity refers to the fraction of total radioactivity in the desired form. Radiochemical impurities are general chemical impurities formed by the chemical as a result of decomposition of the chemical entity, whereas all the resulting impurities may still be radioactive. Potential decomposition pathways are the same as for any other pharmaceutical. Examples include acid and base hydrolysis products, oxidized and reduced species, additional radiolysis products, and photochemical and thermal decomposition products of the chemical. For example in many ^{99m}Tc-labeled complexes, free unreacted ^{99m}TcO$_4^-$ and hydrolyzed ^{99m}Tc are radiochemical impurities. A number of analytical methods can be used to detect and determine radiochemical impurities. For example, when separating the impurities from radiochemical compound of interest using HPLC, if a radiochemical detector is used, all the radioactive impurities that are separated can be quantitated, and radiochemical purity can be ascertained. These include but are not limited to distillation, precipitation, paper, thin layer, gel chromatography, HPLC, ion exchange, solvent extraction, and other separation and purification techniques. The techniques and principles of these techniques are the same as for any other pharmaceutical. Thus, these techniques are not addressed here.

Activation Analysis

Activation analysis is a process in which a target trace element in a sample matrix is irradiated with particles in a nuclear reactor. As a result, an activated radionuclide is formed. The characteristic particles or γ-Rays emitted are used for qualitative identification and, more often, for quantitative measurement. The most common activation analysis is neutron activation analysis (NAA). In this technique, a sample containing the element is irradiated with neutrons in a reactor. After irradiation, γ-Emissions ensue from the decaying radionuclide. These are quantitated by using appropriate semiconductor radiation detectors. Detecting γ-Rays of a specific energy identifies the radionuclide. These particular energy values correspond to unique energies characteristic of the decaying radionuclides. For example, when ^{24}Na decays to ^{24}Mg, the γ-Rays released have unique energies of 1.268 and 2.754 MeV. A plot of γ-Ray counts versus energy yields a γ-Ray spectrum; the area under the curve is proportional to the radioactivity of the sample. The rate at which γ-Rays are emitted is proportional to the concentration of the radionuclide. When a large number of elements in a single sample matrix are analyzed using appropriate instruments for quantitation, without separation of the elements, it is called instrumental neutron activation analysis. When there is spectral interference in the sample matrix and if chemical separation is carried out to isolate the element, it is called radiochemical neutron activation analysis. When other charged particles are generated for analysis by activation, it is called charged particle activation analysis (CPAA). CPAA is applied to the determination of elemental concentration in surface layers.

All methods of activation analysis are very accurate and sensitive, and a precision of approximately 2% RSD is easily attainable. Detection limits in parts per per billion or lower, depending on the element and sample matrix, are

Table 5 Examples of radionuclides and their production mode

Production mode →	Reactor	Accelerator	Generator
Radionuclides Produced → (some examples)	^{99}Mo, ^{131}I, ^{137}Cs, ^{133}Xe, ^{32}P, ^{51}Cr, ^{125}I, ^{135m}Ba, ^{195m}pt.	^{123}I, ^{57}Co, ^{67}Ga, ^{201}Tl, ^{111}In, ^{127}Xe, ^{81}Rb. The following positron generating nuclides are produced on site: ^{11}C, ^{13}N, ^{15}O, ^{18}F;	^{99}Mo to ^{99m}Tc, to ^{99}Tc[a], ^{113}Sn to ^{113m}In, to ^{113}In, 87Y to ^{87m}Sr, ^{81}Rb to ^{81m}Kr, to ^{81}Kr, ^{195m}Hg to ^{195m}Au, to ^{195}Au; other elements used for generator reactions include ^{68}Ge, ^{62}Zn, ^{137}CS, and ^{82}Sr.

[a]Decay as indicated below: parent to daughter to granddaughter.

easily attainable. As many as 60 different elements that can form radionuclide can be analyzed using NAA. NAA finds wide application in a number of other fields, and these are summarized in Table 6.

Radioimmunoassay

Radioimmunoassay (RIA) is a technique based on the formation of antigen–antibody complex. This technique essentially involves the application of isotope dilution analysis. An antigen is typically a protein of molecular weight greater than 10,000 that stimulates the production of antibody in an animal body. The antigen subsequently binds with the antibody. Antigen is usually measured in the patient's sample, and the antigen becomes the analyte. To an antibody, a mixture of labeled and unlabeled antigen is added in excess such that the quantity of antibody needed to bind is allowed to be insufficient. As a result, both types of antigen compete with the limited amount of antibody in the sample. The reaction in an RIA mixture can be described as follows.

$$
\begin{array}{l}
Ag^* \\
 + Ab \xrightleftharpoons[k_2]{k_1} \quad Ag^*\text{--}Ab \quad + Ag^* \\
Ag \quad Ag\text{--}Ab \quad + Ag
\end{array}
$$

k_1 and k_2 are rate constants; equilibrium constant $K = k_1/k_2$.

To a constant amount of labeled antigen and antibody, increasing amounts of unlabeled antibody are added. The initial amount added is still in excess of the antibody needed for binding. As a result of competing reactions of the labeled and unlabeled antigen, the greater the concentration of the unlabeled antigen added, the less is the amount of bound labeled complex (Ag^*–Ab complex) and hence greater is the free (unbound) antigen. After incubation to equilibrium at a specified temperature and time, unique to the system, separation of the free labeled Ag^*, the fraction of the bound labeled antigen is determined by measuring the activity of the radioactive nuclide. By plotting the percent of bound labeled antigen versus the concentration of antigen added, the concentration of the unknown antigen can be determined. Several radionuclides such as ^{14}C, ^{3}H, ^{131}I, ^{32}P, ^{75}Se, ^{59}Fe, ^{99}Mo, and ^{57}Co have been used for RIA. However, ^{125}I is the most commonly used radionuclide for RIA. The earliest method of separation included electrophoresis and chromatography. However, today RIA kits are marketed by commercial manufacturers with detailed description of the principles of the method, methods of use, sensitivity, precision, and limitations of use for specific uses. The RIA methods are very rapid, sensitive, specific, and inexpensive, especially for large biological samples in complex sample matrices.

The RIA technique is applied in assays of hormones, steroids, peptides, aminoglycosides such as tobramycin and gentamycin, insulin, many immunoglobulins, different types of viral heptitis, plasma catecholamines, angiotension-converting enzymes, many vitamins including vitamine B_{12}, human growth hormones, many folate derivatives, and others. Many commercially available RIA kits, unique to each kit, contain series of standards with known concentrations of unlabeled antigen, a vial of suitable labeled antigen, a vial of antibody solution, and appropriate precipitants or other analytical aides.

RADIATION SAFETY

When radiation energy is absorbed by tissues, depending on the dose received, rupture of chemical bonds occurs that causes damage to cells and tissues. Such damage may not be clinically apparent even for years if the absorbed

Table 6   Application of neutron activation analysis

Field of application	Typical application
Geology	Characterization of elemental deposition or formation
Environmental science	Atmosphere, soil, and water pollution
Industrial engineering	Corrosional and frictional effects
Agriculture	Nutrient deficiency
Chemical studies	Contamination, characterization of reference standards, surface effects
Forensic science	Sample identification, correlation of samples to crime scenes

dose is small. Radiation damage is measured in terms of absorbed dose. Dose is defined as the energy imparted to a material per unit mass. The SI unit of dose is called Gray, or Gy (joules/Kg). The traditional unit is rad. One Gy = 100 rads. However, the effectiveness of all radiations is not the same. The effectiveness is dependent on the nature of the particle, the thickness of the tissue or organ, and the characteristics of the material or organ to which such a dose is administered. Thus, to account for such differences in effectiveness, another term, called dose equivalent, is used. The SI unit of dose equivalent is Sievert, which is numerically equivalent to Gy multiplied by the appropriate weighting factor corresponding to biological tissue or organ. For example, the weighting factor (W_R) for many tissues is 0.3, whereas it is 0.03 for bone surfaces. The radiation weighting factor is also dependent on the energy of the particles. For example, for neutrons with less than 10 keV, W_R, = 5, whereas it is equal to 20 for neutrons greater than 100 keV.

For purposes of administered dose of a radiopharmaceutical, the package insert contains a table that lists dosage for the "average" patient as a function of administered activity. This information may be used for calculation of radiation dose. If needed, a medical physicist will calculate administered dose based on Medical Internal Radiation Dose (MIRD) committee recommendations.

External exposure to ionizing radiation as a result of occupation is measured using dosimeters. Three different types of dose monitors are commercially available. They are pocket dosimeters, film badges, and thermoluminescent detectors (TLDs). Pocket dosimeters are GM counting-based digital dosimeters, which provide immediate reading. Film badges are the least expensive and most popular. Using appropriate filters in the film holder, accurate readings to exposure to different particles can be measured. The major disadvantage with film badges is the waiting period required for developing and processing films. In TLDs, the radiation received is stored in holders containing crystals of LiF or manganese-activated calcium fluoride. Subsequently, during measurement, the crystals are heated to required temperatures such that they emit light. When measured, the emitted light provides a measure of absorbed dose.

REGULATORY REQUIREMENTS

The regulations of various advisory groups and government organizations have to be met in handling, use, and disposal of radioactive material and radiopharmaceuticals. These include the FDA, NRC, Department of Transportation (DOT), Environmental Protection Agency (EPA), and Occupational Safety and Health Administration (OSHA). Of these, the FDA regulates safety, stability, efficacy, and toxicity of the radiopharmaceuticals; NRC regulates all reactor-produced by-products regarding use, handling, disposal, and radiation safety and protection of workers and the public using the facilities. Title 10 of the Code of Federal Regulations, 10 CFR 20, contains the regulations for radiation protection, whereas 10 CFR 35 addresses medical uses of radioactive materials. Title 49, 49 CFR, addresses packaging and transportation of radioactive materials. In addition, all USP requirements have to be met for a radiopharmaceutical. The International Committee on Radiation Protection (ICRP) and the National Committee on Radiation Protection (NCRP) provide radiation dose recommendations for adoption to other regulatory agencies. The NRC requires that licensees follow the ALARA philosophy regarding radiation exposure. ALARA is an acronym for as low as reasonably achievable. Under the ALARA concept, when radiation exposure of a worker exceeds 10% of the allowed occupational limit, an investigation is required. If it exceeds 30%, investigation and corrective action are necessary per NRC requirements.

As with any other pharmaceutical, radiotracers used as pharmaceuticals are subject to all regulatory requirements. The radiopharmaceutical manufacturer must, at a minimum, satisfy the requirements of the NRC and the FDA.

BIBLIOGRAPHY

1. Alfassi, Z.B. *Chemical Analysis by Nuclear Methods*; John Wiley & Sons: Chichester, UK, 1994.
2. Anderson, C.J.; Welch, M.J. Chem. Revs. **1999**, *99*, 2219.
3. Bernier, D.R.; Christian, P.E.; Lanagan, J.K. *Nuclear Medicine Technology and Techniques*, 4th Ed.; Mosby: St. Louis, MO, 1997.
4. Bhargava, K.; Du, J.; Raghavan, R.; Joseph, J. *Encyclopedia of Pharmaceutical Technology*, 1st Ed.; Swarbrick, J.S., Boylan, J.C., Eds.; Marcel Dekker, Inc.: New York, 1996; 13, 255–281, and References Contained Therein.
5. Britton, K.E.; Granowska, M. *Nuclear Medicine in Clinical Diagnostics and Treatment*; Murray, P.C., Ell, P.J., Eds.; Churchill Livingstone: New York, NY, 1994; 2, 779–800.
6. Chattel, J.F.; Mahe, M. *Nuclear Medicine in Clinical Diagnostics and Treatment*; Murray, P.C., Ell, P.J., Eds.; Churchill Livingstone: New York, NY, 1994; 2, 865–876.
7. Collier, B.D.; Krasnow, A.Z.; Hellmann, R.S. *Skeletal Nuclear Medicine*; Collier, B.D., Fogelmann, I., Rosenthall, L., Eds.; Mosby: St. Louis, MO, 1996.
8. Early, P.J.; Sodee, D.B. *Principles and Practice of Nuclear Medicine*; Mosby: St. Louis, MO, 1995.

9. Ehmann, W.D.; Vance, D.E. *Radiochemistry and Nuclear Methods of Analysis, Vol. 116: Chemical Analysis*; John Wiley & Sons: New York, NY, 1991.

10. Helmer, R.G. *Kirk-Othmer Encyclopedia of Chemical Technology*, 4th Ed.; Kroschwitz, J.I., Howe-Grant, M., Eds.; John Wiley & Sons Inc.: New York, NY, 1996; 20, 871–906.

11. Kist, A.A. J. Anal. Chem. **1996**, *51*, 80, (Transl. of Zh. Anal. Khim).

12. Kolesov, G.M. J. Anal. Chem. **1996**, *51*, 71, (Transl. of Zh. Anal. Khim).

13. Lazewatsky, J.L.; Crane, P.D.; Scott, Edwards, D. *Kirk-Othmer Encyclopedia of Chemical Technology*, 4th Ed.; Kroschwitz, J.I., Howe-Grant, M., Eds.; John Wiley & Sons: New York NY, 1996; 20, 930–962.

14. Marek, M.J.; Lambert, C.R.; Rhodes, B.A. *Techniques for Direct Radiolabeling of Monoclonal Antibodies*; RhoMed Incorporated: Albuquerque, NM, 1994.

15. Mettler, F.A.; Guiberteen, M.J. *Essentials of Nuclear Medicine*, 3rd Ed.; W.B. Saunders Co.: Philadelphia, PA, 1991.

16. Muller, S. *Nuclear Medicine in Clinical Diagnostics and Treatment*; Murray, P.C., Ell, P.J., Eds.; Churchill Livingstone: New York, NY, 1994; 1, 195–212.

17. Perkins, A.C. *Nuclear Medicine in Pharmaceutical Research*; Perkins, A.C., Frier Eds.; Taylor and Francis: Philadelphia, PA, 1999; 15–30.

18. Pimm, M.V. *Nuclear Medicine in Pharmaceutical Research*; Perkins and Frier Ed.; Taylor and Francis: Philadelphia, PA, 1999; 133–162.

19. Powsner, E.R.; Widman, J.C. *Tietz Textbook of Clinical Chemistry*, 3rd Ed.; Burtis, C.A., Ashwood, E.R., Eds.; W.B. Saunders Co.: Philadelphia, PA, 1999; 113–132.

20. Powsner, R.A.; Powsner, E.R. *Essentials of Nuclear Medicine Physics*; Blackwell Science Inc.: Malden, MA, 1998.

21. Saha, G.B. *Fundamentals of Nuclear Pharmacy*, 3rd Ed.; Springer-Verlag: New York, NY, 1992.

22. Skoog, D.A.; Holler, F.J.; Nieman, T.A. *Principles of Instrumental Analysis*, 5th Ed.; Harcourt Grace College Publishing: Chicago, 1988; 810–828.

23. Stroebel, H.A.; Heinemann, W.R. *Instrumental Analysis: A Systematic Approach*; John Wiley & Sons Inc.: New York, 1989.

24. Spencer, R.P. *Nuclear Medicine in Clinical Diagnostics and Treatment*; Murray, P.C., Ell, P.J. Eds.; Churchill Livingstone: New York, NY, 1994; 2, 647–665.

25. Taillefer, R.; Tamaki, N. *New Radiotracers in Cardiac Imaging, Principles and Applications*; Appleton and Lance: Stamford, CT, 1999.

26. *United States Pharmacopial Convention, United States Pharmacoepia*; 24th Revision: New York, NY, 2000, 1981–1990; USP Convention.

27. Volkart, W.A.; Hoffmann, T.J. Chem. Rev. **1999**, *99*, 2269.

28. Weber, D.A.; Eckermann, K.F.; Dillman, L.T.; Rayman, J.C. *MIRD Radionuclide Data and Decay Schemes*; New York Society of Nuclear Medicine, 1989.

29. Yalow, R.S. J. Chem. Ed. **1999**, *76*, 767.

30. Ekin, R.P. J. Chem. Ed. **1999**, *76*, 769.

31. Ullmann, E.F. J. Chem. Ed. **1999**, *76*, 781.

32. http://www.psich.,/www.lrp.hn/lrp.

33. http://www.triumf.ca/safety/rpt/html.

34. http://www.brighamrad.harvard.edu/education/online/BrainSPECT/.

35. http://www.research.atlantech.fr/Topic.

36. http://www.fz-rossendorf.de/FWB/fwbc/handzet/.

37. http://www.anl.gov./labDB/current/Ext/.

38. http://www.catcmb.cua.edu/receptor.htm.

39. http://www.tardis.jyu.fi/ECRIS/rip.

40. http://www.fkpi.com/Release_Comp/Releases/International/.

41. http://www.radio-isotopes.com/nucmed.htm.

RADIOLABELING OF PHARMACEUTICAL AEROSOLS AND γ-SCINTIGRAPHIC IMAGING FOR LUNG DEPOSITION

Hak-Kim Chan
University of Sydney, Sydney, New South Wales, Australia

OVERVIEW

Inhalation aerosols have been used successfully to deliver drugs to the lung for local and systemic therapeutic effects. In vivo evaluation of pharmaceutical inhalation products is achieved by γ-Scintigraphic imaging of the aerosol deposited in the lung. Imaging provides direct information on the amount and location of the drug deposited in the lung after inhalation (1). This local bioavailability, rather than the systemic bioavailability after absorption, is pertinent to drugs that act directly on the lung. For drugs that act systemically, deposition site will affect the rate and extent of absorption in the lung. As a result, lung deposition using γ-Scintigraphy has been proposed for bioequivalence studies of aerosol products (2). The deposition data can be linked further to the clinical response and in vitro particle size distribution, adding a new dimension to the inter-relationship between them.

To measure lung deposition by imaging, the aerosol must be first labeled or tagged with a suitable radionuclide. Radiolabeling techniques have been developed for current inhalation products including nebulizers, propellant-driven metered-dose inhalers (MDIs), and dry powder inhalers (DPIs).

Lung imaging is achieved using a γ-Camera. The camera creates an image of the γ-Rays emitted by the radionuclide in the lung (3). In the past, numerous lung deposition studies on radiolabeled aerosol products have been carried out using planar imaging by which only the anterior or posterior 2-Dimensional view of the lung is collected. However, because the lung is a 3-Dimensional object, spatial distribution of the aerosol in the lung can be best obtained using tomographic (rather than planar) imaging such as single photon emission computed tomography (SPECT). SPECT is a technique for producing cross-sectional images of radionuclide distribution in the body. This is achieved by imaging the lung at different angles (e.g., 64 or 128 images/180° or 360°) around the thorax using a rotating γ-Camera, followed by computational image reconstruction.

BACKGROUND OF RADIOLABELING PHARMACEUTICAL AEROSOLS

It is a prerequisite that the pharmaceutical aerosols can be suitably radiolabeled before any lung scintigraphic imaging can begin. Ideally, the drug can be directly radiolabeled, i.e., chemically by substitution of an atom in the drug molecule with a radioactive isotope. This can be achieved using positron emitters, e.g., C-11, N-13, and O-15 atoms. Positrons are positively charged electrons that when combined with an electron, produce two γ-Rays with equal energy (511 keV) emitted at 180° to each other. Theoretically, because C, N, and O atoms are present in all organic molecules, they can be used to label virtually any drug. In reality, the use of these atoms is limited by their short half-lives (e.g., 20, 10, and 2 min for C-11, N-13, and O-15 atoms, respectively), relative to the time taken for manipulating the drug (including organic synthesis for radiolabeling and successive processing for product characteristic assurance such as particle size distribution of the aerosol particles). Further, to produce these positron emitters, it is necessary to have a nearby cyclotron facility, which means extra cost. So far, only three antiasthmatic compounds have been successfully radiolabeled by positron emitters: ipratropium bromide (Br-77) (4), triamcinolone acetonide (C-11), and fluticasone proprionate (F-18) (5). This is indicative of the difficulties for direct radiolabeling.

Because of the forementioned limitation, γ-Emitters have been used to radiolabel the drug indirectly for γ-Scintigraphy. In this case, the radiolabel associates with the drug by physical means instead of by chemically incorporating into the drug molecule via covalent bonds. Thus, instead of being a direct chemical approach, it is an indirect radiolabeling. Technetium-99m is the most commonly used pure γ-Emitter for indirect radiolabeling of pharmaceutical aerosols. The γ-Ray of ^{99m}Tc has sufficient energy (140 keV) to penetrate body tissues without significant absorption or scattering, but when it reaches the detector of the γ-Camera, it will be absorbed and converted into light photons, thus optimal for γ-Camera imaging. The half-life of ^{99m}Tc is 6 h, which is long enough for handling and imaging but not too long as to increase the radiation dose to the subject unnecessarily. As a result, ^{99m}Tc is used for the majority of nuclear medicine imaging studies. Once inhaled into the lung, ^{99m}Tc can have a much shorter biological half-life depending on the physical form, e.g., as diethylenetriamine penta-acetic acid (DTPA) or DTPA complex, it will be absorbed rapidly from the lung into systemic circulation, followed by glomerular filtration in the kidney to the bladder where it is excreted in the urine. The whole process could take less than 2 h if the subject drinks plenty of water.

Regardless of the type of aerosol products to be radiolabeled, a fundamental requirement in the radiolabeling of aerosol products is that the radiolabel must associate with the drug such that not only the radiolabel distribution matches the drug distribution but also that the radiolabel distribution matches that of the unlabeled commercial product.

RADIOLABELING OF NEBULIZER SOLUTIONS

Radiolabeling of nebulizer solutions is by far the simplest among the aerosol products and is achieved by simply mixing the radionuclide with the drug solution. Because the radionuclide and the drug are uniformly distributed in the solution and provided that there is no precipitation of the ingredients occurred, each nebulized aerosol droplet would contain both radioactivity and drug in proportion to the droplet size. ^{99m}Tc in complexing with DTPA or human serum albumin is widely used as the radionuclide. Sodium pertechnetate is not suitable because the free anion, as with iodide, has a high affinity for the thyroid. Lung deposition of nebulized salines and drug solutions, including nedocromil sodium (6), salbutamol, fenoterol, ipratropium bromide, carbenicillin, pentamidine isethionate (7), flunisolide (8), and liposomes containing beclomethasone dipropionate (9), has been studied using this radiolabeling technique of mixing the radionuclide with the drug solution.

RADIOLABELING OF PROPELLANT-DRIVEN MDIs

Historically, there are three major approaches of radiolabeling suspension MDIs, developed by Few et al. (10), Newman et al. (11), and Kohler et al. (12). The first two methods were initially developed for polymeric

Scheme 1 MDI radiolabeling (10)

Elution of ^{99m}Tc as sodium pertechnetate from a ^{99}Mo-^{99m}Tc generator
Adjustment of pH to 7–9 with concentrated NH_4OH
Addition of a drop of 5% tetraphenylarsonium (TPA) chloride aqueous solution
Extraction of ^{99m}Tc-TPA into chloroform[a]
Separation by passing through phase-separation paper[b]
Collection of the filtrate (the $CHCl_3$ phase containing the ^{99m}Tc-TPA)
Evaporation of the $CHCl_3$ to dryness
Reconstitution in the appropriate medium containing the compound for radiolabeling

[a]For example, by mechanical shaking or sonication the solution with $CHCl_3$.

[b]For example, Whatman 1_s^P silicone-treated phase-separation filter paper.

particles but were later modified for the radiolabeling of drugs.

Early in 1970, Few et al. (10) radiolabeled polystyrene particles for a mucociliary clearance study. The radiolabeled aerosols were produced by a spinning disk generator. The radiolabeling technique involves the key steps of extracting sodium pertechnetate ($Na^{99m}TcO_4$) into chloroform as tetraphenylarsonium pertechnetate followed by evaporation of the chloroform. A solution of polystyrene is then added to the radioactive residue and dispersed (Scheme 1). This technique has subsequently been adopted by other workers for radiolabeling pharmaceutical MDIs of sodium cromoglycate (13, 14). It is important to note that in this technique, the complexing agent tetraphenylarsonium chloride is classified as poisonous (15). Although the actual amount of the compound inhaled is in the nanogram range, safety to the researchers and the subjects inhaling the aerosols has to be carefully ensured.

Another way to radiolabel the pharmaceutical MDI is to use Teflon particles with a size distribution similar to that of the drug of interest (Scheme 2). This was carried out in 1981 by Newman et al. (11) who used Teflon particles of mean size 2 ± 0.4 μm to mimic the MDI aerosols of bronchodilators. Thus, the Teflon particles were used as a surrogate for the drug. The Teflon particles were almost monodispersed and were produced using a spinning disk aerosol generator. However, this approach is limited by the physicochemical characteristics of the Teflon particles being different from those of the drug particles. Also, the aerosol particle size distribution of the Teflon may not match that of the drug. By co-administering a physical mixture of the radiolabeled Teflon particles with the drug

Scheme 2 MDI radiolabeling (11)

Elution of ^{99m}Tc as sodium pertechnetate from a ^{99}Mo-^{99m}Tc
  generator
Removal of sodium by passing the eluate through a cation
  exchange column
Collection of the filtrate
Evaporation of the filtrate to dryness
Addition of Teflon particles suspended in 40% alcohol
Generation of radiolabeled Teflon particles by spinning disc
  technique[a]
Collection of radiolabeled Teflon particles
Transfer of the radiolabeled particles to an empty canister
Addition of the content from a commercial MDI[b] into the
  canister[c] containing the radiolabeled particles, followed by
  recrimping of the MDI
Mixing by sonication

[a]For example, a spinning speed of 62,000 RPM had been used.
[b]For example, the MDI is chilled at $-60°C$ before the transfer is carried out.
[c]For example, the canister is chilled at $-60°C$ before the transfer is
carried out.

salbutamol, the lung deposition and clinical response have
been monitored simultaneously (16, 17).

The first attempt to radiolabel drug particles (instead of
polymers such as polystyrene or Teflon particles) for
pharmaceutical aerosols was carried out on fenoterol and
salbutamol by Kohler et al. (12) (Scheme 3). However, it
was later found that the method would change the particle

Scheme 3 MDI radiolabeling

Elution of ^{99m}Tc as sodium pertechnetate from a ^{99}Mo-^{99m}Tc
  generator
Extraction of ^{99m}Tc-TPA into methyl ethyl ketone (MEK).[a]
  Repeat the extraction if necessary.
Separation of the aqueous and MEK phases[b]
Collection of the MEK phase (containing the pertechnetate)
Evaporation of the MEK to dryness in a glass beaker
Addition of propellant[c] and surfactant[d] to the dry pertechnetate
Concentration by evaporating the propellant to 0.2 mL
Transfer of the propellant containing the pertechnetate and
  surfactant into an MDI canister to be radiolabelled, followed
  by recrimping of the MDI
Mixing by shaking

[a]For example, by shaking the pertechnetate solution with approximately
equal volume of MEK.
[b]For example, in a separating funnel.
[c]For example, Freon 11, 5–10 ml had been used.
[d]For example, 1% sorbitan trioleate had been used.
(From Ref. 12.)

Scheme 4 MDI radiolabeling

First 4 steps are the same as in Scheme 3.
Evaporation of the MEK (containing the pertechnetate) to
  dryness in an empty canister
Transfer of the content from a commercial MDI into the canister
  containing the pertechnetate for radiolabeling, followed by
  recrimping of the MDI
Mixing by sonication

This method is simpler than Scheme 3 as it does not involve the propellant
concentration step and the subsequent transfer of the concentrate.
(From Ref. 18)

size distribution of the labeled aerosol, resulting in a
coarser aerosol than the unlabeled product. The method,
after subsequent improvement by Summers et al. (18)
(Scheme 4), has become widely used for the radiolabeling
of MDIs. This method is preferred over other methods
because it does not involve extraction with tetraphenylarsonium chloride and chloroform.

It is worth noting that each of the radiolabeling
examples noted previously can be further modified for the
study need. For example, the drug particles can be
suspended in the organic phase containing the radiolabel
and spray-dried, followed by reconstitution in the
propellants, as carried out on salbutamol sulfate (19).

Although the radiolabeling methods have been widely
used, the mechanism of association between the radiolabel
and the drug particles has been studied only recently. The
study by Farr (20) on the MDI systems indicated that in the
CFC formulation, the radiolabel ^{99m}TcO$_4^-$, being hydrophilic, would associate with hydrophilic domains including the surface of hydrophilic drug particles and the
interior of surfactant reverse micelles. There is a need to
extend the study to other systems on hydrophobic drugs
and on non-CFC propellants. See Table 1 for methods of
radiolabeling MDIs.

RADIOLABELING OF DPIs

A method of wide application to radiolabeling of dry
powders is by adsorbing the radiolabel on the particles
in a suitable liquid (Scheme 5). This is achieved by
wetting the drug particles with a nonsolvent containing
the radiolabel, followed by evaporation of the solvent,
leaving the radiolabel on the surface of the drug particles.
The method has been applied to radiolabel terbutaline
sulfate and budesonide (32, 33). Factors affecting the
radiolabeling of dry powder formulations include the
physicochemical nature of the drug, choice of nonsolvent

Table 1   Examples of radiolabeling pharmaceutical MDIs

Drug MDI	Study objective	Reference
Salbutamol sulfate	Development of radiolabeling method[a]	19
Salbutamol	Radiolabeling method development; simultaneous measurement of lung deposition and bronchodilator response[b]	16
Salbutamol	Comparison of lung deposition and bronchodilator response among MDI, DPI and nebulizer[b]	17
Sodium cromoglycate	Development of radiolabeling method[c]	30
Sodium cromoglycate	Comparison of MDI with DPI	31
Sodium cromoglycate	Effect of spacer	13
Sodium cromoglycate	Effect of higher dose (5 mg/puff); effect of spacer	14
Nedocromil sodium	Development of radiolabeling method	18
Nedocromil sodium	Ventilator suitability	21
Terbutaline sulfate, salbutamol	Development of radiolabeling method	22
Nacystelyn	Lung deposition	23
Salbutamol and fenoterol	Development of radiolabeling method and lung deposition	24
Flunisolide and fenoterol	Lung deposition and effect of a spacer	25
Salbutamol	Development of radiolabeling method and comparison of MDI with DPI	26
Beclomethasone diproprionate in hydro fluorocarbons	Correlation of in vitro particle sizing with in vivo deposition	27
Fenoterol	Comparison of nebulizer with MDI plus a holding chamber	28
Salbutamol	Aerosol delivery by microprocessor control (SmartMist[TM])	29

[a]Drug particles were suspended in the chloroform phase and spray-dried.
[b]Radiolabeled Teflon was used (the drug itself was not radiolabeled).
[c]Spray-drying of the drug was followed by reconstitution in an MDI.

Scheme 5   DPI radiolabeling

First 4 steps are the same as in Scheme 3
Evaporation of the MEK (containing the pertechnetate) to dryness
Redissolution of the pertechnetate in a suitable liquid[a]
Addition of the pertechnetate solution to the drug powder to be radiolabeled[b]
Evaporation of the liquid[c]
Filling of the radiolabelled powder to the DPI[d]

[a]The liquid must be a nonsolvent for the drug powder to be radiolabeled; some suitable ones include water for budesonide, chlorofluorocarbon 11 for salbutamol
[b]Mixing, e.g., by sonication for 20 min, if required
[c]Freeze drying has been used for water removal.
[d]Blend with lactose carrier, if required.

for the drug, solubility of radiolabel in the nonsolvent, moisture level, electrostatic charge, and the number of processing steps (30). Unfortunately, the details still generally remain as proprietary information and are not available in the literature. For example, exactly how the spherical agglomerates of budesonide powder are to be wetted with the ^{99m}Tc solution to ensure reproducible radiolabeling has not been reported.

Alternatively, a method resembling Scheme 1 can be used, provided the drug to be radiolabeled will not dissolve in CHCl$_3$. This method involves the same first six steps as in Scheme 1. After the filtrate (the CHCl$_3$ phase containing the ^{99m}Tc-TPA) is collected, it is added to the drug powder. The CHCl$_3$ is then evaporated, e.g., at 70°C, leaving the radiolabel with the powder. The powder is ready for filling into the DPI. Bronchodilators (salbutamol, terbutaline sulfate) and prophylactics (nedocromil sodium)

Scheme 6 DPI radiolabeling

Preparation of solution of the drug to be radiolabeled[a]
Addition of sodium pertechnetate to the drug solution[b]
Spray drying of the solution[c]
Collection of dry powder
Filling of the radiolabelled powder to the DPI[d]

---

[a]For example, 6% w/w for sodium cromoglycate
[b]For example, 1 ml of pertechnetate in normal saline
[c]For example, Buchi Minispray dryer, model 190, liquid feedrate 60 ml/min, inlet air temp 180°C, air throughput 2.4 m^3/min and nozzel air pressure 800 kPa.
[d]For example, Blend with lactose carrier, if required

for asthma have been successfully labeled using this technique for lung deposition studies (31, 34).

There was also an earlier method for the radiolabeling of dry powders (primarily sodium cromoglycate) by spray-drying (35, 36). The basic principle can be considered the same as that in Scheme 1 for MDI in that radiolabeled particles were produced by evaporation of radiolabel-containing atomized droplets. The method is very straightforward (Scheme 6) but suffers the limitation that spray-dried particles may not be physicochemically the same as those in the commercial products. This is because milling rather than spray-drying is normally used for micronization of the drug particles. Spray-drying, following ^{99m}Tc adsorption to the surface of the particles, has also been used to prepare radiolabeled cromogycic acid and nedrocromil powders (37).

The exact mechanism of association between the radiolabel and the drug particles is unknown and is generally regarded as a surface-coating phenomenon. However, the surface is proportional to the square of the particle size, whereas the volume (drug mass) the cube of the particle size. It follows that to have a match between the radiolabel and drug mass in the aerosol, the radiolabeled particles must exist as agglomerates rather than as single particles. See Table 2 for examples of radiolabeling DPIs.

γ-SCINTIGRAPHIC IMAGING FOR LUNG DEPOSITION

Aerosol deposition in the lung is measured by γ-Scintigraphyroutinely used in nuclear medicine. A γ-Camera consists of a collimator located in front of a detector, behind which is an array of photomultiplier tubes (3). The collimator allows only γ-Rays with a defined angle to reach the detector. The detector, which is a scintillation crystal made of sodium iodide, converts the γ-Rays to light photons. The photomultiplier tubes then transform the light photons into an electrical signal that can be displayed in the X- and Y-position on a monitor such as a cathode-ray tube or a computer. Planar imaging, which provides 2-Dimensional anterior and/or posterior views of the lung, has been commonly used in the past to study deposition. This involves inhalation of the radiolabeled aerosols with a collimated γ-Camera placed in front of or behind the chest of the subject. The image is formed as the γ-Ray photons emitted from the radiolabeled aerosol in the lung fall on the camera detector. The primary advantage of planar imaging is that the image acquisition and data processing are less effort-demanding. Also, compared with tomographic imaging (see SPECT, below), it can utilize a lower radioactivity dose. However, a severe limitation of planar imaging is that it compresses the 3-Dimensional lung into a 2-Dimensional view, and thus it cannot provide 3-Dimensional spatial information about the aerosol distribution in the lung. This may become more critical if

Table 2 Examples of radiolabeling pharmaceutical DPIs

Drug DPI	Study objective	Reference
Terbutaline sulfate	Development of radiolabeling method for Turbuhaler in lung deposition study	33
Nedocromil sodium	Lung deposition study and comparison with an MDI	34
Budesonide	Nasal distribution study	32
Budesonide	Lung deposition in children with cystic fribrosis	38
Salbutamol	Lung deposition study using a new DPI	30
Disodium cromoglycate	Lung deposition comparison between a conventional MDI and a new DPI	34
Salbutamol sulfate	Development of radiolabeling method and comparison with an MDI	26
Cromoglycic acid and Nedocromil	Development of radiolabeling method	37

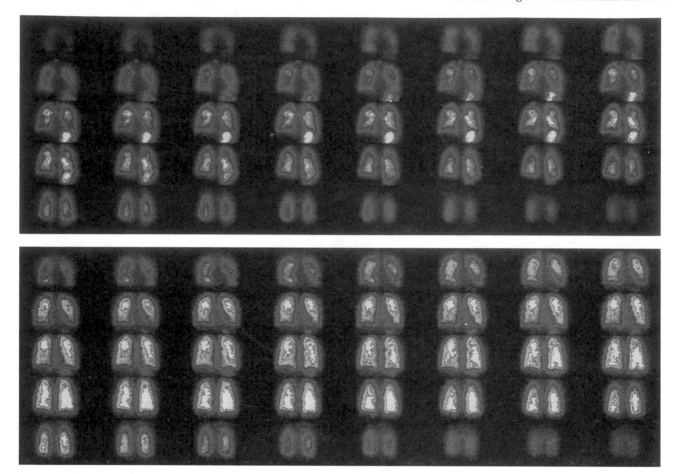

Fig. 1 Fast 1-min SPECT coronal section lung images of a healthy subject after inhalation of normal saline aerosols containing ^{99m}Tc-DTPA in large and small droplets (7 μm, top 3 μm, bottom) generated by air-jet nebulizers. The difference in deposition between the two aerosols is clearly shown in these images.

thelung deposition data are to be used for bioequivalence comparison (1,2).

Three-dimensional image data can be achieved by SPECT. SPECT has been used to measure lung deposition of aerosols in a number of studies (6, 39–44, 49). This involves imaging the lung at different angles using a SPECT camera rotating round the chest of the subject after radioaerosol inhalation. The acquired raw data are then processed by high-speed computers to reconstruct the lung images in the coronal, sagittal, or transverse section (e.g., see Fig. 1 for the coronal section images). The question remains as to whether SPECT offers any advantage over planar γ-Scintigraphy for quantitation of total (as opposed to regional) lung deposition. This can be answered by comparing the measurement of a known amount of radioactivity in a lung phantom (e.g., a perspex container with size and shape similar to the human lung) using both techniques. The results of this comparison are not yet published.

Misconceptions of SPECT

High-dose radiation has often been quoted as a disadvantage of SPECT (1). Obviously, the radioactive dose should never be administered more than required, regardless of whether SPECT or planar imaging is used. It is interesting to note that a number of planar imaging studies were carried out in the past using radiation doses comparable with those for SPECT (43). In practice, the dose consideration must be balanced by the benefits of the deposition details gained using SPECT. If planar imaging cannot provide the required deposition details, then SPECT should be considered. Otherwise, carrying out a suboptimal study using planar imaging without obtaining the deposition data required is not justified because it exposes the subjects to unwanted radiation exposure. The amount of radioactivity delivered to the lung for SPECT is approximately 60 MBq, which is equivalent to an effective whole-body dose of 0.4 mSv. In comparison, the

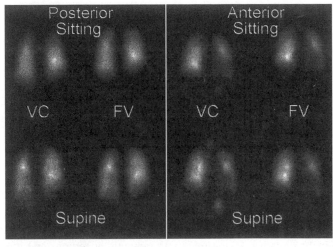
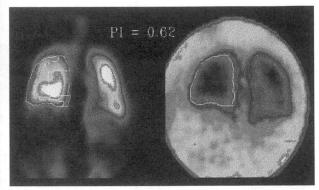

Fig. 2 Lung images of a healthy subject after inhalation of an aqueous aerosol containing ^{99m}Tc-DTPA generated by a novel aerosol inhaler, the AERx system of Aradigm Inc. (Ref. 42). *Left*: planar images from aerosols inhaled using two different breathing maneuvers [vital capacity (VC) or fixed volume (FV) of 1 L above the functional residual capacity] and two different postures as stated. *Right*: a midcoronal image acquired using SPECT. Superposition of the lung outline from the transmission SPECT image (right) on the emission SPECT image confirmed the excellent peripheral deposition of the aerosol.

average radiation dose from background radiation is approximately 2–3 mSv in a year, depending on the geographic location.

Another common misconception about SPECT is the long image-acquisition time and the associated problem of relocation of deposited aerosol particles in the lung (1). Historically, this was true when a single-head SPECT γ-Camera was used in the 1980s for lung deposition because the imaging process took approximately 15–20 min (43). During this length of time, relocation of the radiolabel occurred as confirmed by comparing lung images immediately before and after the SPECT acquisition. Radiolabel movement would create problems of inconsistent projection during image reconstruction, leading to artifacts in the reconstructed images. Despite these limitations, SPECT has been shown to be superior to planar imaging in differentiating lung deposition among aerosols (39). In a more recent study on a novel inhaler using different breathing maneuvers (42), SPECT was able to detect a subtle difference in the aerosol deposition that was not observed using planar imaging (Fig. 2). The problem of long acquisition time has recently been resolved by fast dynamic SPECT (44, 49). Using a triple-head γ-Camera, the SPECT acquisition time has been reduced to only 1 min (Fig. 1). Thus, 20–30 complete individual 1-min SPECT image acquisitions can be collected in 20–30 min, making dynamic study feasible. The technique can also be applied to study clearance of an aerosol from the lung after deposition (Fig. 3).

Attenuation and Scatter Correction

Attenuation occurs when the γ-Ray photons emitted from the radionuclide in the lung are absorbed by the body tissues before reaching the camera detector. Attenuation causes a reduction in measured radioactivity counts. Because of the heterogeneous nature of the thorax tissues (lung, muscles, bones), the attenuation cannot be assumed to be uniform and must be measured. Experimentally, the attenuation information can be obtained from a

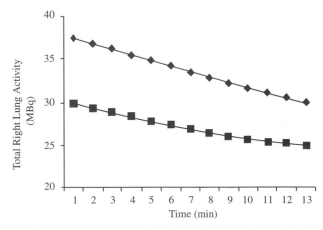

Fig. 3 The time course of activity clearance from the lung measured by fast 1-min SPECT on a healthy subject after inhalation of normal saline aerosols containing ^{99m}Tc-DTPA in large and small droplets (7 μm, ◆; 3 μm, ■). In the plot, 2-min frames are used for clearer illustration.

transmission scan that uses an external γ-Radiation source for imaging of the thorax. To avoid uncertainty in image re-alignment between studies, transmission imaging is best carried out simultaneously with the aerosol (emission) study (45). This can be achieved by attaching the radiation source to the γ-Camera during the aerosol lung image acquisition. The use of the same radionuclide for the transmission as the emission imaging would eliminate uncertainties attributable to differences in the photon energy. When simultaneous emission–transmission imaging is not feasible, the attenuation information can also be obtained from a separate transmission study before the aerosol inhalation. Alternatively, x-ray computerized tomography (CT) scanning can be carried out, but it involves a higher radiation dose to the subject. Also, the separate transmission scan would require extra time, and image re-alignment may be more difficult.

Scatter occurs when the γ-Ray photons emitted from the radionuclide in the lung encounter the thorax tissues and change the traveling direction from their original path. Therefore, scatter causes mispositioning of the detected counts, leading to a loss of image contrast and quantitative accuracy. Quantitative assessment of aerosol deposition would require both attenuation and scatter correction. The latter is also important for proper image reconstruction in SPECT. For additional reading, texts of SPECT imaging are recommended (46, 47).

Data Analysis

Image processing

Planar images can be analyzed on the anterior or posterior view. Because the lung has a thickness, the radiolabel may occur anywhere along the thickness. The effect owing to deposition at varying thicknesses can be minimized by taking the geometric mean of the anterior and posterior images.

Compared with planar images, SPECT data require more rigorous treatment involving mathematical image reconstruction algorithms. Because of simplicity and speed, the filtered back-projection algorithm has been used in clinical SPECT studies including aerosol deposition in the lung. Filtered back-projection uses summation techniques using projections (count rate profiles) of the acquired image data. Artifacts in the back-projected image are corrected by filtering (using mathematical operations) the data before or after reconstruction. Because of the nonuniform attenuation regions of the thorax, other iterative reconstruction techniques involving attenuation and scatter correction have also been used (46, 47).

Drawing of the lung region

The lung outline is obtained from the transmission image or from ventilation image using radioactive gases such as ^{81m}Kr, when available. After superimposing the lung outline on the aerosol emission image, the lung is then divided into different regions of interest, and the amount of activity in each region is measured. Regions such as apex and basal or central and middle and peripheral are most commonly used. A conventional way to analyze aerosol distribution (or deposition pattern) is to express it as the ratio of the activity in one region to another, e.g., peripheral to central, which is conventionally defined as the penetration index. However, there is no consensus on how the size and shape of each region should be drawn. For example, both rectangular regions and lung shape regions have been used for the planar images in the past, but the regions can vary from laboratory to laboratory. Thus, there is a need to standardize the methods for drawing lung regions for comparing studies among different laboratories. The rationale of drawing the lung regions is that the peripheral region should contain more small airways than the central region. In a planar image, there will inevitably be extensive overlapping of structures in the lung. In relative measurement or comparative studies using the same subject as his or her own control, the region size and shape may not be as crucial as in the absolute measurement when the aim is to assign the deposition to certain anatomical structures. The latter is a formidable task because the whole lung contains approximately 1.6 million airway branches. It has recently been attempted on SPECT images with the aid of computer modeling (48). Success will provide valuable information for interpreting the γ-Camera images in relation to the aerosol distribution in the airways.

CONCLUDING REMARKS

Radiolabeling of nebulizer solutions, propellant-driven MDIs, and DPIs is generally well documented. For some DPIs, the procedure may still be lacking in sufficient detail to ensure reproducible radiolabeling. Deposition of radiolabeled aerosols in the lung has been measured primarily by planar imaging. Tomographic imaging using SPECT can provide 3-Dimensional information about the spatial distribution of the aerosol in the lung. The recent development of fast dynamic SPECT has made it the method of choice for aerosol imaging in the new millennium.

ACKNOWLEDGMENTS

I am grateful to Karen Smith for technical assistance and to Stefan Eberl for the availability of Figs. 1, 2 and 3.

REFERENCES

1. Snell, N.J.C.; Ganderton, D. Assessing Lung Deposition of Inhaled Medications. Resp. Med. **1999**, *93*, 123–133.
2. Newman, S.P.; Wilding, I.R. Gamma Scintigraphy: An In Vivo Technique for Assessing the Equivalence of Inhaled Products. Int. J. Pharm. **1998**, *170*, 1–9.
3. Eberl, S.; Zimmerman, R.E. Nuclear Medicine Imaging Instrumentation. In *Nuclear Medicine in Clinical Diagnosis and Treatment*; Murray, I.P.C., Ell, P.J., Eds.; Churchill Livingstone: Edinburgh, 1998; 2, 1559–1570.
4. Short, M.D.; Singh, C.A.; Few, J.D.; Studdy, P.R.; Heaf, P.J.D.; Spiro, M.D. The Labelling and Monitoring of Lung Deposition of an Inhaled Synthetic Anticholinergic Bronchodilating Agent. Chest **1981**, *80 Suppl*, 918–921.
5. Berridge, M.S.; Lee, Z.; Zheng, L.; Heald, D.L. Nasal Distribution of Inhaled Drugs Determined by Positron Tomography. J. Aerosol Med. **1999**, *12*, 117.
6. Chan, H.K.; Phipps, P.R.; Gonda, I.; Cook, P.; Fulton, R.; Young, I.; Bautovich, G. Regional Deposition of Nebulised Hypodense Non-Isotonic Solutions in the Human Respiratory Tract. Eur. Resp. J. **1994**, *17*, 1483–1489.
7. Newman, S.P. Scintigraphic Assessment of Therapeutic Aerosols. Crit. Revi. Ther. Drug Carrier Sys. **1993**, *10*, 65–109.
8. Newman, S.P.; Steed, K.; Reader, S.J.; Hooper, G.; Zierenberg, B. Efficient Delivery to the Lungs of Flunisolide Aerosol from a New Portable Hand-Held Multidose Nebulizer. J. Pharm. Sci. **1996**, *85*, 960–964.
9. Vidgren, M.T.; Waldrep, J.C.; Arppe, J.; Black, M.; Rodarte, J.A.; Cole, W.; Knight, V. A Study of 99m Technetium-Labelled Beclomethasone Dipropionate Dilauroylphospatidylcholine Liposome Aerosol in Normal Volunteers. Int. J. Pharm. **1995**, *115*, 209–216.
10. Few, J.D.; Short, M.D.; Thomson, M.L. Preparation of 99m Tc Labelled Particles for Aerosol Studies Radiochem. Radioanal Lett. **1970**, *5*, 275–277.
11. Newman, S.P.; Pavia, D.; Moren, F.; Sheahan, N.F.; Clarke, S.W. Deposition of Pressurised Aerosols in the Human Respiratory Tract. Thorax **1981**, *36*, 52–55.
12. Kohler, D.; Fleischer, W.; Matthys, H. New Method for Easy Labeling of Beta-2-Agonists in the Metered Dose Inhaler with Technetium 99m. Respiration **1988**, *53*, 65–73.
13. Newman, S.P.; Clark, A.R.; Talaee, N.; Clarke, S.W. Pressurised Aerosol Deposition in the Human Lung with and without an Open Spacer Device. Thorax **1989**, *44*, 706–710.
14. Newman, S.P.; Clark, A.R.; Talaee, N.; Clarke, S.W. Lung Deposition of 5mg Intal from a Pressurised Metered Dose Inhaler Assessed by Radiotracer Technique. Int. J. Pharm. **1991**, *74*, 203–208.
15. In *The Merck Index*; Merck & Co. Whitehouse Station: NJ, 1996.
16. Zainudin, B.M.Z.; Tolfree, S.E.J.; Biddiscombe, M.; Whitaker, M.; Short, M.; Spiro, S.G. An Alternative to Direct Labelling of Pressurised Bronchodilator Aerosol. Int. J. Pharm. **1989**, *51*, 67–71.
17. Zainudin, B.M.Z.; Biddiscombe, M.; Tolfree, S.E.J.; Short, M.; Spiro, S.G. Comparison of Bronchodilator Responses and Deposition Patterns of Salbutamol Inhaled from a Pressurised Metered Dose Inhaler, as a Dry Powder, and as a Nebulised Solution. Thorax **1990**, *45*, 469–473.
18. Summer, Q.A.; Clark, A.R.; Hollingworth, A.; Fleming, J.; Holgate, S.T. The Preparation of a Radiolabelled Aerosol of Nedocromil Sodium for Administration by Metered-Dose Inhaler that Accurately Preserves Particle Size Distribution of the Drug. Drug Invest. **1990**, *2*, 90–98.
19. Arppe, J.; Vidgren, M. Practical Gamma Labelling Method for Metered-Dose Inhalers and Inhalation Powders. STP Pharm. Sci. **1994**, *4*, 19–22.
20. Farr, S.J. The Physico-Chemical Basis of Radiolabelling Metered Dose Inhalers with 99mTc. J. Aerosol. Med. **1996**, *9* (Suppl 1), S27–S36.
21. Everard, M.L.; Stammers, J.; Hardy, J.G.; Milner, A.D. New Aerosol Delivery System from Neonatal Ventilator Circuits. Arch. Dis. Child. **1992**, *67*, 826–830.
22. Aug, C.; Perry, R.J.; Smaldone, G.C. Technetium [99m] Radiolabeling of Aerosolized Drug Particles from Metered Dose Inhalers. J. Aerosol. Med. **1991**, *2*, 127–135.
23. Hardy, J.G.; Everard, M.L.; Coffiner, M.; Fossion, J. Lung Deposition of a Nacystelyn Metered Dose Inhaler Formulation. J. Aerosol. Med. **1993**, *6*, 37–44.
24. Ballinger, J.R.; Calcutt, L.E.; Hodder, R.V.; Proulx, A.; Gulenchyn, K. Improved Method to Label Beta-2 Agonists in Metered-Dose Inhalers with Technetium-99m. J. Aerosol. Med. **1993**, *24*, 787–794.
25. Hammermaier, A.; Bidlingmaier, A.; Waitzinger, J.; Stechert, R.; Wenske, H.; Jaeger, H. Radio Labelling of Drugs in a Metered Dose Inhaler (MD) and Lung Deposition in Human Subjects. J. Aerosol. Med. **1994**, *7*, 173–176.
26. Biddiscombe, M.F.; Melchor, R.; Mak, V.H.F.; Marriott, R.J.; Taylor, A.J.; Short, M.D.; Spiro, S.G. The Lung Deposition of Salbutamol, Directly Labelled with Technetium-99m, Delivered by Pressurised Metered Dose and Drug Powder Inhalers. Int. J. Pharm. **1993**, *91*, 111–121.
27. Leach, C.L.; Davidson, P.J.; Boudreau, R.J. Improved Airway Targeting with the CFC-Free HFA-Beclomethasone Metered-Dose Inhaler Compared CFC-Beclomethasone. Eur. Resp. J. **1998**, *12*, 1346–1353.
28. Fuller, H.D.; Dolovich, M.B.; Posmituck, G.; Wong, P.W.; Newhouse, M.T. Pressurised Aerosol Versus Jet Aerosol Delivery to Mechanically Ventilated Patients. Am. Rev. Resp. Dis. **1990**, *142*, 440–444.
29. Farr, S.J.; Rowe, A.M.; Rubsamen, R.; Taylor, G. Aerosol Deposition in the Human Lung Following Administration from a Microprocessor Controlled Pressurised Metered Dose Inhaler. Thorax **1995**, *50*, 639–644.
30. Pitcairn, G.R.; Newman, S.P. Radiolabelling of Dry Powder Formulations. In *Respiratory Drug Delivery VI*;

Dalby, R.N., Byron, P.R., Farr, S.J. Eds.; InterPharm Press Inc. Buffalo Grove IL, 1998, 397–399.

31. Pitcairn, G.; Lunghetti, G.; Ventura, P.; Newman, S. A Comparison of the Lung Deposition of Salbutamol Inhaled from a New Powder Inhaler at Two Inhaled Flow Rates. Int. J. Pharm. **1994**, *102*, 11–18.

32. Thorsson, L.; Newman, S.P.; Weisz, A.; Trofast, E.; Moren, F. Nasal Distribution of Budesonide Inhaled via a Powder Inhaler. Rhinology **1993**, *31*, 7–10.

33. Newman, S.P.; Moren, F.; Trofast, E.; Talaee, N.; Clarke, S.W. Deposition and Clinical Efficacy of Terbutaline Sulphate from Turbuhaler, A New Multi-Dose Powder Inhaler. Eur. Resp. J. **1989**, *2*, 247–252.

34. Pitcairn, G.; Lim, J.; Hollingworth, A.; Newman, S.P. Scintigraphic Assessment of Drug Delivery from the Ultrahaler Dry Powder Inhaler. J. Aerosol. Med. **1997**, *10*, 295–306.

35. Vidgren, M.T.; Karkkainen, A.; Karjalainen, P.; Paronen, T.P. A Novel Labelling Method for Measuring the Deposition of Drug Particles in the Respiratory Tract. Int. J. Pharm. **1987**, *37*, 239–244.

36. Vidgren, M.; Paronen, P.; Vidgren, P.; Vainio, P.; Nuutinen, J. Radiotracer Evaluation of the Deposition of Drug Particles Inhaled from a New Powder Inhaler. Int. J. Pharm. **1990**, *64*, 1–6.

37. Chan, H.-K.; Gonda, I. Preparation of Radiolabeled Materials for Studies of Deposition of Fibers in Human Respiratory Tract. J. Aerosol. Med. **1993**, *6*, 241–249.

38. Devadason, S.G.; Everard, M.L.; MacEarlan, C.; Roller, C.; Summers, Q.A.; Swift, P.; Borgstrom, L.; Le Souef, P.N. Lung Deposition from the Turbuhaler in Children with Cystic Fibrosis. Eur. Resp. J. **1997**, *10*, 2023–2028.

39. Phipps, P.R.; Gonda, I.; Bailey, D.L.; Borham, P.; Bautovich, G.; Anderson, S.D. Comparisons of Planar and Tomographic Gamma Scintigraphy to Measure the Penetration Index of Inhaled Aerosols. Am. Rev. Resp. Dis. **1989**, *139*, 1516–1523.

40. Chua, H.L.; Collis, G.G.; Newbury, A.M.; Chan, H.-K.; Bower, P.N.; Sly, P.D.; Le Souef, P. The Influence of Age on Aerosol Deposition in Children with Cystic Fibrosis. Eur. Resp. J. **1994**, *7*, 2185–2191.

41. Phipps, P.R.; Gonda, I.; Anderson, S.D.; Bailey, D.; Bautovich, G. Regional Deposition of Saline Aerosols of Different Tonicities in Normal and Asthmatic Subjects. Eur. Resp. J. **1994**, *7*, 1474–1482.

42. Chan, H.-K.; Daviskas, E.; Eberl, S.; Robinson, M.; Bautovich, G.; Young, I.H. Deposition of Aqueous Aerosol of Technetium-99m Diethylene Triamine Penta-Acetic Acid Generated and Delivered by a Novel System (AER$_x$) in Healthy Subjects. Eur. J. Nucl. Med. **1999**, *26*, 320–327.

43. Chan, H.-K. Use of Single Photon Emission Computed Tomography in Aerosol Studies. J. Aerosol. Med. **1993**, *6*, 23–36.

44. Chan, H.K.; Eberl, S.; Daviskas, E.; Constable, C.; Young, I.H. Dynamic SPECT of Aerosol Deposition and Clearance in Healthy Subjects. J. Aerosol. Med. **1999**, *12*, 135.

45. Bailey, D.L. Transmission Scanning in Emission Tomography. Eur. J. Nucl. Med. **1998**, *25*, 774–787.

46. Bailey, D.L.; Parker, F.A. Single Photon Emission Computed Tomography. In *Nuclear Medicine in Clinical Diagnosis and Treatment*; Murray, I.P.C., Ell, P.J. Eds.; Churchill Livingstone: Edinburgh, 1998; 2, 1589–1602.

47. Meikel, S.R.; Hutton, B.F.; Bailey, D.L. A Transmission-Dependent Method for Scatter Correction in SPECT. J. Nucl. Med. **1994**, *35*, 360–367.

48. Fleming, J.S.; Hashish, A.H.; Conway, J.H.; Hartley-Davies, R.; Nsaaim, M.A.; Guy, M.J.; Coupe, J.; Holgate, S.T.; Moore, E.; Bailey, A.G.; Martonen, T.B. A Technique for Simulating Radionuclide Images from the Aerosol Deposition Pattern in the Airway Tree. J. Aerosol. Med. **1997**, *10*, 199–212.

49. Eberl, S.; Chan, H.-K.; Daviskas, E.; Constable, C.; Young, I.H. Aerosol Deposition and Clearance Measurement: A Novel Technique using Dynamic SPET. Eur. J. Nucl. Med. **2001**, *28*, 1365–1372.

RECEPTORS FOR DRUGS: DISCOVERY IN THE POST-GENOMIC ERA

Jeffrey M. Herz
Applied Receptor Sciences, Mill Creek, Washington

William J. Thomsen
Arena Pharmaceuticals, San Diego, California

INTRODUCTION

A paradigm shift has occurred in receptor-based drug discovery based upon the elucidation of the complete human genome and advances in genomics research, which have revealed a plethora of potential new receptors on which to focus drug discovery efforts. Based on sequence, structural, and functional similarities of a great number of receptors, these receptor targets can be grouped into relatively few multigene superfamilies. Molecular biological approaches have also revealed that additional receptor subtypes and isoforms are generated through multiple mechanisms. The current challenge lies in the development and application of new strategies for rapidly mining the receptor genome sequences to establishing and understanding their function, which has been referred to as "functional genomics." Practical problems and approaches to assays for the characterization of the ligand binding and elucidating signaling properties of expressed orphan receptors are critically evaluated. The ensuing characterization of orphan receptors is expected to reveal therapeutically important receptor targets that will serve as a platform for much of the drug discovery enterprise. These findings will spur the discovery and development of a new generation of receptor-subtype specific drugs with enhanced therapeutic specificity.

CONCEPT AND DEFINITION OF RECEPTORS

To paraphrase Voltaire, if receptors did not exist it would be necessary for pharmacologists to invent them. In fact, this is precisely what J.N. Langley did around the turn of the century when he suggested the existence of "receptive substances" through which tissues were able to selectively recognize agonist and antagonist chemicals (i.e., ligands) and, importantly, also provide a mechanism for the translation of this recognition event into a physiological response. Thus, a basic and enduring operational definition of a receptor is that it "must recognize a distinct chemical entity and translate information from that entity into a form that the cell can read to alter its state accordingly, for example, by a change in membrane permeability, activation of a guanine nucleotide regulatory protein, or an alteration in the transcription of DNA" (1). Hence, the attributes of *ligand recognition* and *signal transduction* are both fundamentally necessary to define receptors. The transduction process may be mediated through an integral part of the receptor structure and may involve receptor interactions with additional nonreceptor proteins. A signal transduction feature of many ligand–receptor interactions is the activation of a kinase domain that initiates phosphorylation in a signal transduction pathway.

This definition has been the basis for an enormous body of scientific investigation into the function and regulation of receptors and mechanisms of drug action. However, final proof of the existence of receptors did not occur until relatively recent applications of modern biochemistry and molecular biology to purify, sequence, clone, and express pure receptor proteins. This lack of proof notwithstanding, the therapeutic basis of many modern, and not so modern, drugs resides in their specific interactions with receptor molecules located in the plasma membrane or cytosol of target cells. In fact, these specific interactions have provided the experimental basis for their discovery and development.

CRITERIA FOR RECEPTOR CLASSIFICATION

Primacy of Molecular Structure

Historically, pharmacologists classified receptors based on the concept that a single receptor mediated a pharmacological response to a single endogenous agonist and that receptor subtypes could be defined primarily by pharmacological properties. Receptor subclassification systems were dependent upon the availability of selective and potent natural substances (toxins and alkaloids) or synthetic ligands, which could selectively elicit or inhibit biochemical and physiological responses from receptors. In some cases, subtypes could be distinguished by different signal transduction mechanisms associated with each receptor subtype. While this approach led to understanding the molecular and cellular mechanisms of many drugs and to significant therapeutic advances, it did not provide evidence of the numerous and diverse subtypes that are now known to comprise all receptor families.

The enormous molecular diversity and multiplicity of receptor subtypes for a given neurotransmitter or hormone were not fully appreciated until the application of modern molecular biology techniques. The GPCRs (G-protein coupled receptor) currently comprise the single largest receptor superfamily, with estimates of over 1000 receptors in the human genome. Within each receptor family, the multiplicity of receptor subtypes has greatly exceeded the numbers that were predicted on the basis of pharmacological data alone. Now frequent cloning of many receptor genes and the study of the encoded recombinant proteins have both revolutionized the criteria necessary for classification of receptors, which otherwise could not be distinguished pharmacologically and provided fundamental insight into mechanisms of drug action at the molecular level.

Current classification criteria for receptors developed by the Committee for Receptor Nomenclature and Drug Classification of the International Union of Pharmacology (NC-IUPHAR) are based on a combination of information derived from molecular structure (structural), pharmacological characteristics of the receptor (operational or recognitory) and on signal transduction mechanisms used by the receptor (transductional) (1). Of these three essential criteria, the amino acid sequence of the receptor provides a definitive identification of a distinct protein and thus serves as an unambiguous primary basis for classification. Identification of the endogenous ligand or ligands provides a secondary means to group receptors into families. Integration of pharmacological evidence obtained from radioligand binding studies of selective agonists, antagonists, and allosterics (modulatory ligands), and their characterization in functional assays (changes in intracellular cAMP levels, calcium, or reporter gene assays) enables a comprehensive assessment for classification based upon all three essential criteria.

Receptors can be most reliably subclassified and defined on the basis of antagonist affinities, whereas data obtained with agonists are considered much less useful since intrinsic activity and potency have been found to be cell and tissue dependent. Information on receptor-effector mechanisms that reflect the molecular signaling properties of the receptor provides another tier for receptor classification, although transduction mechanisms for novel receptors may be unclear and subject to controversy.

Furthermore, the use of heterologous cellular expression systems for the study of recombinant receptors has revealed the potential for receptor subtypes to initiate signaling events not normally associated with their physiological role. These studies have also demonstrated that the ultimate response to receptor activation is cell-type specific. Hence, the potential ambiguity that may arise in defining receptor transductional characteristics has led to the recognition that this characteristic has more limited value among classification criteria. The question of how to integrate receptor structural information, pharmacological characteristics, and transductional properties into a rational scheme of receptor classification and nomenclature is a subject of continuing discussion among pharmacologists (2).

Receptor Superfamilies, Families, and Subtypes

From the vast number of amino acid sequences deduced from fully sequenced genomes and from cloned receptor proteins, primary amino acid and structural similarities have been identified that are common to numerous receptor types that possess distinct pharmacology. Putative receptor genes usually contain recognizable sequence motifs to suggest a superfamily of receptor they might encode. This homology method has been widely used to find common sequence motifs that typically occur in the extracellular ligand binding domains, transmembrane domains, or within intracellular domains of receptors. This has enabled receptor classification into superfamilies based on sequence similarities that encompass many receptor proteins that differ pharmacologically but are structurally and functionally similar since they share a single molecular signal transductional mechanism. The "common structure–common function" concept is not unique to receptors but originates from the observation that families of proteins are derived from a common ancestral gene. Receptor subtypes within a superfamily are generally considered to have arisen through evolutionary mechanisms of gene duplication and genetic drift leading to divergence from a common progenitor receptor gene rather than reconstruction of new genes de novo. Indeed, members of a family are often clustered in a relatively small region of the human chromosome, and the genomic organization of highly homologous receptors (and receptor subunits) often reveals identical structures consisting of the same number of protein-encoding exons. For many members of the GPCRs superfamily, the entire protein is encoded by only a single exon.

Despite the enormous multiplicity of receptor subtypes, a limited number of basic superfamilies have been recognized that currently suffice to accommodate all of the signal transducing receptors. As an example, in the GPCRs superfamily, the signature motif of these single subunit receptors is seven distinct hydrophobic domains of 20–30 amino acids, which are linked by hydrophilic amino acid sequences of varying length. As shown in Fig. 1, the aligned amino acid sequences of the five subtypes of human somatostatin receptors are shown, using the single-letter amino acid code. The seven transmembrane regions are indicated, which show the highest level of sequence identity from the overall receptor sequences. Biophysical and biochemical studies have shown that these sequences

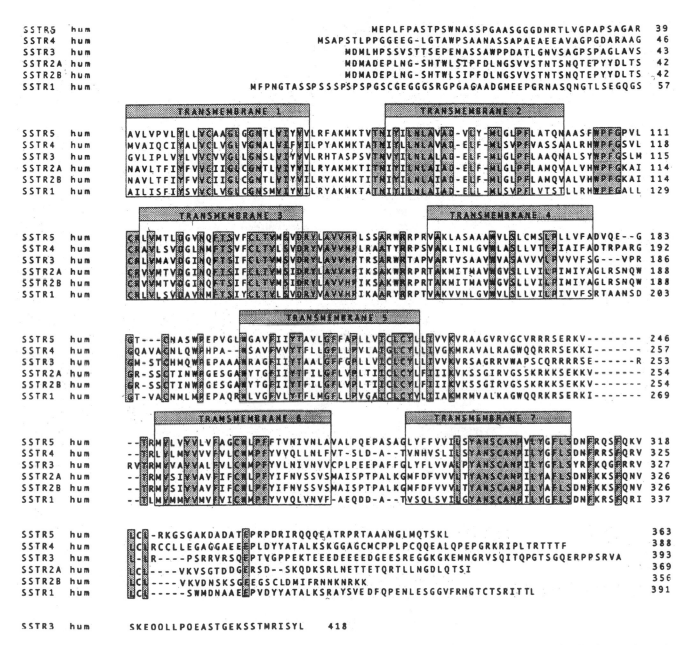

Fig. 1 Primary amino acid sequence comparison between five members of the human somatostatin receptor family. The amino acid sequences are aligned, using the single-letter amino acid code. Gaps introduced in the sequences to optimize the alignments are represented with dashes (−). The boxes indicate amino acids that are identical in all five receptor subtypes. The highest level of homology occurs within the seven canonical transmembrane domains of the human SST receptors (indicated above the sequences) and these domains have been derived by a combination of hydropathy analysis and comparison with the transmembrane domains of the other G-protein coupled receptors. The high level of homology among the members of the SST receptor family in the seven membrane spanning domains is shared by other G-protein coupled receptors that are coupled to inhibition of adenylyl cyclase.

form a bundle of transmembrane α-helices in the plasma membrane and that the amino terminus is present on the extracellular surface and the carboxyl terminus is present on the cytoplasmic surface of the membrane. Other smaller structural motifs act as functional microdomains in GPCRs. These domains have been mapped by site-directed and deletion mutagenesis studies, generation of receptor chimeras, and through the use of antibodies and include sequences critical for ligand binding, coupling to G-proteins and phosphorylation (Fig. 2). Functionally, all agonist-activated GPCRs signal through interaction with heterotrimeric G proteins, triggering a diverse array of cellular responses. Other major recognized superfamilies include the ligand gated-ion channel receptor (LGCR), receptor tyrosine kinase (RTK), receptor protein tyrosine phosphatase, tumor-necrosis factor (TNF)/nerve growth factor (NGF) receptor, TGF-β serine/threonine kinase receptor, and nuclear receptor superfamilies. Undoubtedly, as many novel sequences of receptors become known that cannot be accommodated within the existing superfamily framework, and their signal transduction properties are defined, new superfamilies of receptors will be proposed. Receptors are further subclassified into receptor families and subfamily groups on the basis of relative

sequence homologies, operational and signal transduction mechanisms. The nomenclature system frequently employed has been to name families with reference to their endogenous ligands, for example, glutamate, serotonergic (5-HT), dopaminergic, epidermal growth factor. Each family typically consists of multiple receptors subtypes that share similarities in their molecular biological, pharmacological, biochemical, and physiological properties. Within a receptor family, members of one subfamily are more closely structurally homologous to one another (on average between 50 and 80%) than to members of other subfamilies (in the range of 25%). However, the current nomenclature system carries forward several notable idiosyncrasies with regard to ligand–receptor systems in which a single endogenous ligand serves as the neurotransmitter for receptors belonging to two distinct superfamilies. Hence, acetylcholine is the transmitter for muscarinic acetylcholine receptors that are GPCRs with seven transmembrane domains (3) and the unrelated nicotinic acetylcholine receptors that are multisubunit ligand-gated ion channel receptors (LGCRs) (4). Similarly, several neurotransmitters interact with receptors that belong to these two different superfamilies. Glutamate receptors are divided into metabotropic (GPCRs) and the

GPCR Domains

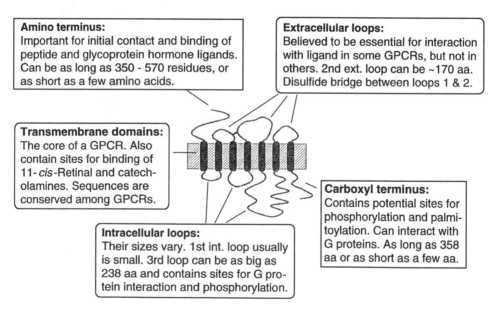

Amino terminus:
Important for initial contact and binding of peptide and glycoprotein hormone ligands. Can be as long as 350 - 570 residues, or as short as a few amino acids.

Extracellular loops:
Believed to be essential for interaction with ligand in some GPCRs, but not in others. 2nd ext. loop can be ~170 aa. Disulfide bridge between loops 1 & 2.

Transmembrane domains:
The core of a GPCR. Also contain sites for binding of 11-*cis*-Retinal and catecholamines. Sequences are conserved among GPCRs.

Carboxyl terminus:
Contains potential sites for phosphorylation and palmitoylation. Can interact with G proteins. As long as 358 aa or as short as a few aa.

Intracellular loops:
Their sizes vary. 1st int. loop usually is small. 3rd loop can be as big as 238 aa and contains sites for G protein interaction and phosphorylation.

Fig. 2 Seven transmembrane spanning model of the a typical G-protein coupled receptor showing functional domains. The core of about 175 amino acid residues that forms the transmembrane domains (defined by hydrophobicity analysis) are highly conserved among superfamily members. The extra- and intracellular loop regions and C-terminus are much more divergent, even among closely related receptors. Sites for glycosylation are found on the amino terminus and a palmitolylation of a Cys in the C-terminal domain are shown. Intracellular residues involved in G-protein coupling and interaction with receptor-specific kinases that mediate desensitization occur on the intracellular loops.

ionotropic, which include the NMDA, AMPA, and kainate families (LGCRs). GABA receptors are classified as GABA$_B$ (GPCRs) and GABA$_A$ (LGCRs), and purinergic P2 (P2X and P2Y) receptors also have subtypes in both superfamilies. All serotonergic receptors (5HT$_1$–5HT$_7$) belong to the GPCR superfamily with the exception of the 5HT$_3$ receptor, which is a LGCR 5,6).

Multiligand/Multireceptor Families

It is well recognized that all superfamilies contain examples of receptor subtypes that interact with more than one species of endogenous ligand. Receptor binding and tissue-culture experiments have shown that a structurally related family of ligands may bind and activate a single receptor. The existence of families of endogenous ligands that activate either one or more closely related receptor subtypes presents a significant challenge of "receptor promiscuity" to both receptor classification and drug–receptor design. The newly recognized prevalence of such multi-ligand receptor families present among diverse receptor superfamilies suggests that the classical pharmacological dictum of one ligand per one receptor is no longer tenable.

Within the GPCR superfamily, the individual subtypes of CC-chemokine receptors bind and are activated by multiple CC-chemokine ligands. Determining chemokine structure and function is extremely difficult especially when cells contain an ensemble of receptors on their membrane. For example, most chemokine receptors have more than one high-affinity endogenous agonist, and most chemokines bind to more than one receptor subtype. Within the 11 member CC-chemokine receptor family, there are at least five subtypes of chemokine receptors involved in binding the CC-chemokines (also known as β-chemokines): MCP-1, MIP-1α, and RANTES. Based on studies to date, one receptor (CCR-1) binds all three ligands, another (CCR2) binds only MCP-1, and RANTES binds to CCR1, CCR3, and CCR5. Similar observations of complex ligand–receptor promiscuity are seen with the CXC- or α-chemokine family and five receptor subtypes. Two closely related neutrophil-derived CXC (IL-8) receptors, CXCR-1(IL8R$_A$) and CXCR-2 (IL8$_B$), have been cloned whose binding characteristics account for the binding observed with neutrophils. CXCR-1 receptors interact with three ligands (IL-8, GCP-2, and NAP-2) that are also known to bind CXCR-2 receptors.

A second example of multiligand/multireceptor interactions is illustrated by the bone morphogenetic proteins (BMPs), which are members of the TGF-β superfamily. The BMP family of protein ligands has diverse functional roles, including bone and cartilage formation, cell proliferation, apoptosis, differentiation, and morphogenesis. A number of BMPs have been discovered and, based upon sequence homology, most of the GDFs (growth/differentiation factors) have been added to the BMP family, bringing the number of ligands in this family to around 25. TGF-β, BMP-2, and BMP-7 interact with at least six receptor subtypes of the potentially multimeric Type 1 and Type II receptors in the TGF-β receptor serine/threonine kinase superfamily. The complexities in devising a uniform, rational nomenclature scheme that incorporates endogenous multiligand/-multireceptor interactions and also is consistent with instances in which a cell surface receptor can simultaneously function as both a ligand for a receptor on another cell and as an independent receptor entity are substantial.

Receptor Subtypes Composed of Combinatorial Subunits

The central tenet of the current classification system is to define a unique receptor subtype for each receptor that is composed of only single polypeptide encoded by distinct gene. As an example, the dopamine receptor family is known to contain at least five distinct subtypes, dopamine D$_1$–D$_5$ receptors, each receptor consisting of one subunit encoded by separate genes. A more complex system arises in the case of multisubunit oligomeric receptors, as in the case of the LGCR superfamily. These multisubunit receptors are known to exist as hetero-oligomers with many subunit combinations that comprise distinct subtypes. For several families, homologous genes encoding highly related receptor subunits have been designated by a combination of greek letters and numbers. Molecular cloning studies of GABA$_A$ receptors have identified five different subunit types named α, β, γ, δ, and ρ, which share significant amino acid sequence identity with each other (30–40%) and with other members of the ligand-gated ion channel superfamily. Nearly all of these subunits also have a number of different isoforms (α1–6, β1–4, γ1–3, δ, and ρ1–2) and all sequences within each isoform family are highly homologous (70–80% identity). Individual GABA$_A$ receptor subtypes are thus defined by the distinct combination of subunits and stoichiometry that compose the oligomeric complexes, such as α2α3β3γ2, α1α3β2γ2, and α1α3β2γ2. However, subunits of the NMDA, AMPA, and kainate receptor-ion channel complexes have been classified using an alternate system; NMDA1 and NMDA2A-D, and glu1-7 and ka1-2. The combinatorial mechanism of receptor assembly has the potential for producing a large number of receptor subtypes and is a common feature of the multigene families that comprise the LGCR superfamily.

Molecular Mechanisms Producing a Diversity of Receptor Isoforms

Additional variation in receptor sequences occurs through naturally arising mutations, naturally occurring allelic variants, RNA splicing, and RNA editing. For example, the human dopamine D_4 receptor subtype contains a direct repeat of a 16 amino acid segment in the putative third intracellular loop of the receptor. Naturally occurring allelic variants of this receptor subtype contain variable numbers of direct repeat units (e.g., 2, 4, 7 repeats; dopamine $D_{4.2}$, $D_{4.4}$, $D_{4.7}$) producing a substantial number of receptor variants in the human with different primary amino acid sequence but as yet indistinguishable receptor binding and signal transduction pharmacology for a wide range of ligands (7). Other subtype variants occur at the level of RNA splicing giving rise to length variants of the receptor subtype. For example, differential splicing results in the long and short isoforms of the dopamine D_2 receptor, D_{2L} (D_{2A}) and D_{2S} (D_{2B}) 7), and produces two proteins differing by 29 amino acids. RNA editing is yet another mechanism producing sequence and functional diversity and has been found to produce seven different edited forms of the kainate GluR6 subunit, all encoded by only one gene. While many receptors are subject to posttranslational modifications, such as phosphorylation, which modulate receptor properties, these differences are not considered to define a receptor subtype.

Species homologs of the same receptor subtype display a high degree of amino acid sequence homology, typically showing 85–95% sequence identity between species. This is a greater sequence similarity than is usually found between distinct receptor subtypes in the same species. The introduction of cloning has enabled identification of species homologs of receptors that otherwise might be defined as distinct receptor subtypes due to their species-specific pharmacology, as was found in the case of the rat 5-HT$_{1B}$ and human 5-HT$_{1B}$ (5HT$_{1D\beta}$) receptors (8). Since a change in as little as a single amino acid within the binding site domain can markedly alter ligand affinity, some receptor species homologs exhibit distinctive pharmacology. A notable example is the comparative binding of the nonpeptide antagonist ligands, CP96345 and RP67580, to the human and rat neurokinin NK$_1$ receptors. While CP96345 binds with nanomolar affinity to the human NK$_1$ receptor, it exhibits two orders of magnitude lower affinity for the rat receptor, whereas RP67580 shows selectivity for the rat receptor. The magnitude of the selectivity difference is noteworthy given that the rat and human receptors are 95% identical. Construction of single residue substitutions in recombinant NK$_1$ receptors demonstrated that an exchange of two residues was sufficient to reverse the species selectivity of the two ligands. Due to the number of cases in which species homologs differ from human receptor pharmacology, the use of cloned human receptors for drug discovery screening programs is increasingly favored.

Orphan Receptors

Putative receptors identified by gene cloning that exhibit homology to known receptors in the existing superfamilies but for which no known ligands have been identified are referred to as *orphan receptors*. Initially, these novel receptors may be classified based upon the level of sequence homology. When the endogenous ligand for an orphan receptor remains unknown, the receptor may be provisionally named based on the binding of a synthetic ligand to the receptor until the endogenous ligand is identified. As the functions of an orphan receptor are uncovered, these novel receptors frequently become targets for the development of new therapeutics.

LIGAND–RECEPTOR INTERACTIONS DEPEND UPON RECEPTOR CONFORMATIONAL STATES

Resting, Activated, and Densensitized Receptor States Differ in Ligand Affinity

One of the major criteria in receptor subtype classification is the pharmacological selectivity profile as defined by ligand affinities (equilibrium dissociation constant, K_d) and activation constants. Since binding data overcome many of the limitations inherent in studies of biological responses, ligand affinities have provided a practical method to define and classify related subtypes. Nevertheless, accurate comparisons of agonist affinities of cloned receptors with binding affinities characteristic of the native cell type or tissue may be difficult to obtain. Agonist affinities determined for recombinant receptors expressed in distinct heterologous cell types have been found to vary substantially and differ from value characteristic of the native cell type (9). These findings underscore the need to compare ligand affinities and function of an expressed recombinant receptor in several host cell lines and for related receptor subtypes to be expressed in a common host cell line in order to allow accurate pharmacological comparisons (10). Receptor classification schemes will need to take into account the host cell environment when evaluating ligand affinity and functional data.

In contrast to traditional receptor theory, it is now evident from molecular pharmacological analysis that transitions between receptor states can be induced by interaction of a receptor with a full spectrum of ligands that have very different capacities to activate the receptor. Ligand-induced changes in the population distribution of receptor molecules between these states govern the binding and functional properties of the receptor. As discussed in detail ahead, measurements in vitro and in situ have revealed the importance of temporal responses in characterizing multiphasic ligand–receptor interactions for the ligand-gated ion channel and GPCRs superfamilies.

An agonist, by virtue of the molecular "information" it contains (e.g., size, 3D configuration, charge distribution, hydrogen- or ionic-bonding residues, chirality), selectively binds to a complementary 3D surface or binding site domain formed by amino acid residues of a receptor protein and initiates a cellular response. Drugs classified as full agonists elicit the maximal response while compounds that only elicit a fractional response are referred to as partial agonists. Regardless of whether the agonist is an endogenous physiological ligand, a natural product, or a synthetic compound, agonist binding is coupled to conformational changes in the receptor protein that involve a molecular transition to a common, active receptor state. As an example, binding of either full, strong, or weak partial agonists to the nicotinic acetylcholine receptor induced a transition to a open channel state that is characterized by the same unitary conductance. Although the frequency and duration of the receptor open state differ, this is indicative of a single, active conformation of the receptor. The simplest schemes for receptor activation take into account that occupation of a receptor (R) by an agonist (L) results in a conformational change in the receptor to create an agonist-activated state (LR^*), which can bring about an effect or response, and can be represented as:

$$L + R \underset{K_d}{\rightleftharpoons} LR \underset{E}{\rightleftharpoons} LR^* \rightarrow Response$$

where L is the agonist, R represents the unoccupied (inactive) receptor, R^* is the active state of the receptor, K_d is the dissociation constant for agonist-receptor binding, and E is the constant describing the equilibrium between the LR and the LR^* states of the receptor.

Contemporary models of receptor activation attempt to incorporate increasingly detailed knowledge of multiple conformational states, including desensitized receptor states. A fundamental component of these molecular activation schemes for receptors is that receptors exist in a dynamic equilibrium between three states, an inactive (R), an active conformation (R^*) and a desensitized state (R'), and that the biological response to a given ligand is governed by its ability to change the equilibrium (or its relative preference for binding) between the three receptor

states. Continued exposure of LGCRs to agonists promotes a multiphasic conversion to desensitized receptor states that develop on time scales ranging from milliseconds to minutes. Generally, GPCR activation is also followed rapidly by a loss of responsiveness, also termed desensitization, which is then followed by a period of recovery or resensitization. These changes in signaling are tightly regulated, primarily via mechanisms that involve rapid GPCR phosphorylation, internalization of receptors that remove them from the cell surface, and either degradation or recycling back to membrane surface (11).

Many receptors that function as ligand-gated ion channels can be described by a two-state cyclic scheme for receptor desensitization (including only one desensitized state), which was initially deduced from extensive studies of the kinetics of nicotinic acetylcholine receptor (AChR) state transitions induced by ligand binding (12). This model was expanded to a general coupled-equilibria model that described the molecular species and influence of agonists and noncompetitive inhibitors (noncompetitive antagonists) on receptor states (13). As shown in Fig. 3, the model incorporated the fact that the AChR contains two interacting agonist binding sites and a topographically distinct binding site for an allosteric, noncompetitive inhibitors.

For many receptors, the agonist binding site of the receptor protein can interconvert between high and low affinity binding states or receptor conformations. Moreover, differences in affinity of the agonists for the same site in different receptor states may be dramatic. In the case of LGCRs, the desensitized states display higher agonist binding affinity and no receptor-mediated ion permeability. It is the preference for ligand binding to the desensitized receptor that is the driving force underlying conversion to the desensitized state. The binding affinity (K_d) of acetylcholine to the muscle subtype of the nicotinic acetylcholine receptor measured at equilibrium is about 10 nM (desensitized state), 4–5 orders of magnitude below the apparent dissociation constant for the permeability response (activatable state) mediated through the same binding site (14).

Multiple agonist-affinity receptor states have also been described for many GPCR receptor families. GPCRs may adopt either a high-affinity or low-affinity state for agonists (K_H and K_L), which may differ by 1000-fold when characterized in native membranes purified from either brain tissue or derived from cell lines. Low-affinity agonist states for receptors, which typically cannot be determined by direct binding of a radiolabeled agonist, have been measured by employing radiolabeled antagonists and examining the pattern of competition over a wide range of agonist concentrations. For recombinant GPCRs, agonistinduced changes in affinity depend upon efficient coupling of the expressed recombinant receptor to endogenous G-proteins present in the host cell line, and coupling is highly dependent on the combination of receptor and clonal cell line. For example, agonist-stimulated D_3 dopamine receptor-mediated effects were lacking, and an inability to demonstrate significant affinity shifts for agonist ligands was found in the presence of guanine nucleotides in COS or CHO cells 14). However, receptor coupling to inhibition of adenylyl cyclase was readily obtained for closely related subtypes in the D_2 receptor subfamily, recombinant D_2 and D_4 receptors, expressed in a variety of cell lines (CHO-K1, HEK-293, C6-glioma, Ltk$^-$) (15,16).

Antagonist Modulation of Receptor Conformational States

According to classical models for drug–receptor interaction, full competitive antagonists and agonists share the ability to bind to a common site on the receptor molecule but differ in that antagonists are devoid of intrinsic activity. While a competitive antagonist occupies the binding site of the receptor, it does not promote conversion of the receptor to the active conformation. Indeed, at the biochemical level, nicotinic acetylcholine receptor agonists and antagonists that differ in size and structure (acetylcholine, tubocurarine, and snake venom α-toxins) have been mapped to the same molecular site on the receptor α-subunit and their binding is mutually exclusive. However, recent data suggest that no overlap in the binding site for competitive ligands is required if they bind in a mutually exclusive manner to different binding sites that are present only in different receptor conformations. Competitive antagonists may be subclassified into at least two categories: 1) neutral antagonists that do not exhibit a preference for an inactive or active receptor conformation and have no effect on basal receptor

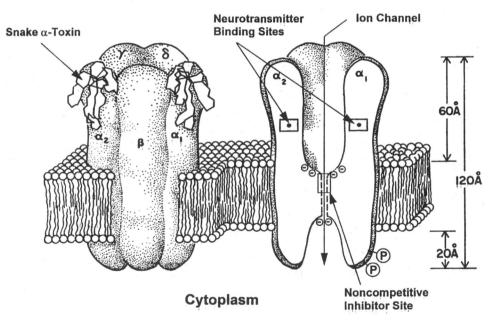

Fig. 3 Structure and ligand binding sites of the muscle subtype of the nicotinic acetylcholine receptor. The structure is derived from electron microscopy of two-dimensional crystals of receptors in *Torpedo* membranes. The five subunits together form a cylindrical shape approximately 120 Å long with a 70 Å diameter, which spans the membrane. The receptor on the right shows a section along the axis of the receptor and the cation conducting pathway in profile. A 60 Å diameter central hydrophilic tube is present on the synaptic side which is the entrance to the transmembrane ion channel which narrows at the level of the membrane. Current resolution of the receptor cannot resolve dimensions of the ion channel within the membrane bilayer which permeability studies have defined as an aqueous pore of about 7 Å diameter. Locations of the ligand binding sites have been mapped within the receptor structure by fluorescence energy transfer techniques. The two agonist binding sites, one on each α-subunit, are 20–30 Å from the membrane surface and the single allosterically-coupled noncompetitive inhibitor site is located in the channel. Positions of two snake venom α-toxin molecules (peptides of 7500 kD, peptide backbone shown) bound to the synaptic surfaces of the α-subunits are shown for the receptor on the left.

activity and 2) negative antagonists, also termed inverse agonists, which exhibit the defining property of inhibiting agonist-independent receptor activity and possess negative intrinsic activity. Furthermore, negative antagonists stabilize a different receptor conformation (state) than neutral antagonists.

For both LGCRs and GPCRs, whose activity is governed by distributions between inactive and active states, negative antagonists promote conversion of the receptor to an inactive conformation and stabilize a conformation of the receptor that is distinct from the unliganded receptor (resting state). For G-protein coupled receptors, studies of receptors expressed at high levels, using the baculovirus expression system in Sf9 cells or of receptors that have been rendered constitutively active by site-directed mutagenesis, have provided an experimental system in which agonist-independent, spontaneous adenylyl cyclase activity can be measured. This phenomenon has been best characterized for the β_2-adrenergic receptor but has also been observed for the bradykinin, dopamine D_1, and 5-HT_{2C} receptors, suggesting it is likely to be a general feature of the superfamily. A group of well-characterized β_2-adrenergic receptor antagonists were found to inhibit, to varying degrees, receptor dependent spontaneous activity (17). Negative antagonists have been shown to promote the dissociation of spontaneously occurring receptor–G-protein interactions, using constitutively active mutant receptors. As an example, the ligand ICI118551 has been shown to inhibit the basal signaling activity of the β_2-adrenergic receptor, thus acting as a negative antagonist (18).

Inverse agonist drugs may also span a range of activities, and thus current ligand and drug classification schemes recognize full agonists, partial agonists, neutral antagonists, and partial and full inverse agonists. For the ligand-gated ion channels, pharmacological studies of the interaction of the nicotinic acetylcholine receptor with a series of N-substituted analogs of decamethonium identified several compounds as antagonists but unique in their capacity to antagonize receptors that had been previously exposed to agonists. Through an extensive series of equilibrium and kinetic binding experiments, it was shown that these antagonists preferentially bound to the desensitized receptor state and had the ability to promote the conversion of the nicotinic acetylcholine receptor to this inactive state. In contrast, classical antagonists, such as tubocurarine, demonstrated the same affinity for both resting and desensitized receptor states. Antagonists that demonstrated enhanced affinity for the desensitized receptor state were termed metaphilic antagonists.

Noncompetitive Antagonists

Noncompetitive antagonists interact with a spatially distinct site (NCI site), which may be allosterically regulated by the agonist binding site(s) and block receptor function through an allosteric mechanism. In the absence of agonist, the allosteric constant, M, is increased by binding of these inhibitors, and in the presence of agonist, the rate of agonist-elicited conversion to the desensitized state is accelerated. For the LGCRs, the allosterically coupled NCI site is fundamentally different from the agonist site in its pharmacology. A study of the interaction of a phenylphenanthridium ligand, ethidium, with the high-affinity NCI site of the nicotinic acetylcholine receptor determined that it bound with extremely high selectivity to the desensitized state relative to a state stabilized by interaction with snake α-toxin at equilibrium, showing a ratio greater than 2800 13). Conversely, ethidium binding at the NCI site and its occupation converted the receptor to a state of higher agonist affinity. Similarly, association rates for the binding of radiolabeled phencyclidine (PCP) to the NCI site increased by a factor of 1000–10,000 for the transient open-channel state relative to the toxin stabilized receptor state (19). Potential explanations for these findings are that the binding site location within the transmembrane ion channel is sterically inaccessible in a toxin-stabilized receptor conformation (Fig. 3) and that binding occurs only to selected conformational states, such as the open channel state (20). Numerous ligands act through allosteric mechanisms to regulate receptors in the LGCR superfamily. As in the case of the AChR, drugs such as MK-801 and PCP bind within the ion channel domain of NMDA receptors, blocking agonist-dependent activation. $GABA_A$ receptor function is also regulated by the binding of benzodiazepines, barbiturates, and steroids at distinct allosteric sites on the receptor.

Methods to Study Drug–Receptor Interactions in Real Time

Drug–receptor interactions may quantitatively differ among rapidly converting multiple receptor states that are induced by agonist binding. While most studies commonly focus on analysis of ligand–receptor interactions and cellular responses under presumed steady-state conditions, experimental techniques available for the quantitative analysis of drug–receptor interactions with transient receptor conformational states are more limited. Since the actions of many receptors regulate rapid (within seconds) and transient changes in intracellular calcium and protein kinase activity, the magnitude and the duration of the response to either transient or sustained agonist stimulation will determine the integrated cellular response. Thus, the effects of drugs on the temporal integration of individual receptor responses are critical in determining the response of a cell to extracellular stimuli.

Molecular pharmacological techniques have been applied to study rapid, real-time analysis of ligand–receptor conformational states and cellular signaling. A variety of rapid mixing techniques have provided sensitive and rapid measurements capable of defining receptor conformational transitions induced by agonist or drug binding to membrane-bound receptors. The earliest ligand–receptor kinetic studies measured radioligand binding of agonists and functional responses, using rapid filtration, but were technically limited in kinetic resolution. Direct spectroscopic measurements extending into the millisecond time domain have been made of conformational transitions for the nicotinic acetylcholine receptor (LGCR) and the formyl peptide (fMLP, GPCR) receptor because the affinity of fluorescent agonist ligands is greatly altered by interaction with their respective receptors (21). Real-time analysis of fluorescent formyl peptide ligand binding to intact human neutrophils by both spectrofluorometric and flow cytometric methods has led to a model of signal transduction dynamics and ligand–receptor–G-protein ternary complex interactions (22). Extrinsic fluorescence labeling of receptors by covalent modification of the receptors with reporter groups has also provided evidence for conformational changes in LGCRs and GPCRs. Spectroscopic signals originating from incorporation of an environmentally sensitive fluorescent probe into the purified, human β2-adrenergic receptor provided kinetic information indicative of both agonist and negative antagonist-mediated receptor conformational changes (23).

Electrophysiological analysis of drug interactions with single receptor ligand-gated ion channels and voltage-dependent channels has provided another invaluable approach to analyze the activated open-channel states and closed states of LGCRs and voltage-activated ion channels with time resolution unmatched by other techniques. Using the methods of patch clamping, these high-resistance seals (gigaohm) attached to membrane patches or intact cells have recorded changes in conductance arising from the opening of individual transmembrane channels. Studies of this nature have been crucial in defining functional characteristics of many subtypes of receptor-ion channels and allowed the investigation of the mechanism of interactions of drugs with open channel states of these receptors, which are otherwise not amenable to study. In a classic study, the channel blocking mechanism of the local anesthetic QX-222 with the nicotinic acetylcholine receptor was defined (24). Rapid and repeating flickering changes in conductance of one channel were observed as single drug molecules stochastically entered, blocked, and left the receptor ion channel. Kinetic constants derived from such measurements can define state-dependent blockade of receptor channels.

Flow cytometry has been utilized as a powerful approach to collect multiparameter kinetic data to evaluate multiple activation parameters simultaneously in individual cells and to correlate these parameters with the ligand occupancy of each cell. Cellular functional parameters that can be measured employing this technique include intracellular calcium, magnesium, pH, and membrane potential. Choices of functional parameters depend only upon the availability and utilization of a wide range of specific fluorescent probes that can act as reporters of the desired cellular parameter. Now a common procedure is to employ a fluorescent probe for calcium to measure continuous changes in intracellular calcium in populations of cells in suspension or in cellular monolayers of immobilized cells, using conventional spectrofluorometers. Utilized in combination with fluorescence digital imaging microscopy, spatial gradients reflecting changes in ion concentrations within individual living cells in the millisecond time domain have been visualized. New instrumentation has enabled adaption of this technique to a high-density plate format that is suitable for high-throughput screening in drug discovery programs.

Progress in defining the spatial and temporal cellular location of receptors in living cells during signal transduction has advanced through the use of confocal fluorescence microscopy coupled with the development of receptor-specific fluorescent probes. Receptor fluorescent probes, in particular, green fluorescent protein (GFP), have become a popular reporter molecule that has allowed measurements agonist mediated events in real time. Tagging of GPCRs with the GFP has enabled the direct visualization of real-time trafficking of GPCRs in living cells (11). The approach utilized has been to generate expression constructs that contains GFP fused to the carboxyl terminus of the receptor. Synthesis and expression of over 20 different GPCR–GFP chimeric fusion receptors has shown rapid changes in GPCR receptor cellular distribution in the membrane and the subsequent internalization of ligand and receptor. Such analyses have provided crucial insight into the mechanisms involved in controlling GPCR function and enable the studies of the actions of GPCR drug agonists. While basic receptor studies employing fluorescent ligands are still few, this nascent area is expanding as additional specific fluorescent ligands, recombinant receptors, and instrumentation become widely available. These studies have also established fluorescence-based detection methods as the preferred format for ultrahigh throughput screening in drug discovery programs.

FUNCTIONAL ROLES FOR A MULTIPLICITY OF RECEPTOR SUBTYPES

The approach of molecular cloning has greatly expanded our knowledge of many receptor subtypes and has revealed an impressive heterogeneity of receptors not previously envisioned. The discovery of multiple receptor subtypes that are highly homologous has provoked examination of key questions related to their physiological functional significance and their importance as individual drug discovery targets. Substantial efforts have been made to define specific physiological roles and advantages conferred to the organism by expression of multiple receptor subtypes that have apparently identical endogenous ligand binding and signal transduction properties. Despite examples of receptor subtypes that exhibit indistinguishable binding and functional coupling properties, these closely related subtypes and isoforms may exhibit differences in properties that include the time course of activation, ionic selectivity, desensitization, regulation, and efficacy in coupling to distinct second messenger systems. Furthermore, homologous receptor subtypes within a family often display differentially regulated expression in particular cell types and tissues in response to specific stimuli.

Molecular Mechanisms Generating Diversity

Small differences in receptor structure (one to several amino acids) have been found to endow important pharmacological and functional differences to receptor subtypes and species homologs. Within the GPCR superfamily, a change in a single amino acid residue was found to underlie the major pharmacological differences between the rat 5-HT_{1B} and the $5\text{HT}_{1D\beta}$ receptors (25). Similarly, a change of one residue (Asn351Asp) in the dopamine D_5 receptor results in a 10-fold decrease in dopamine binding affinity while mutations in the D_2 receptor lead to differences in binding affinities for typical and atypical neuroleptic drugs used in the treatment of psychotic disorders. Essential differences in coupling of splice variants of the dopamine D_2 receptor, mglu1 receptor, somatostatin sst_2 receptor, and prostaglandin EP_3 receptor have been observed. Within the ligand-gated ion

channel superfamily, it has been found that the charge and size of a single amino acid residue in a critical channel site (the Q/R site of the GluR-B subunit) determines the particular ionic selectivity and permeability properties that characterize subtypes of AMPA-kainate-activated channels (26). For the muscle subtype of the nicotinic acetylcholine receptor, the functional properties of the receptor (channel conductance and open time) are altered during development by substitution of one of the subunits in the pentameric complex; from $(\alpha 1)_2 \beta 1 \gamma \delta$ in embryonic muscle to $(\alpha 1)_2 \beta 1 \varepsilon \delta$ in the adult muscle. Thus, the highly signficant changes in receptor structure and function that can result from subtle variations in the genetic sequence encoding receptors can affect target identification, characterization, and validation in the drug discovery process.

Cellular and tissue expression patterns for related receptor subtypes may overlap but are often highly specific and tightly regulated. For example, there are striking differences in the cellular distribution of CXCR1 (IL-8R1) and CXCR2 (IL-8R2) receptors (77% sequence identity overall). CXCR1 expression is restricted to neutrophils, monocytes, and a few myeloid cell lines, whereas CXCR2 is widely distributed in myeloid cell lines but also in lymphocytes, melanoma cells, melanocytes, and fibroblasts (27). These specific cellular distributions suggest that the main function of the CXCR1 receptor is neutrophil activation and mobilization of phagocytes in host defense while the CXCR2 receptor serves to mediate migration and growth of cells not involved in defense. In situ hybridization studies of mRNAs encoding subunits of the neuronal nicotinic acetylcholine receptor gene family (LGCRs) and subtypes of GPCRs have documented that transcripts corresponding to homologous receptor subunits and subtypes within a receptor family exhibit distinct anatomical distributions in the mammalian brain (28). Among the family of human dopamine receptor subtypes, D_2 receptors are most highly expressed in the striatum, D_3 and D_5 receptors exhibit a preferential localization in the limbic area of the brain and low expression in motor areas such as the basal ganglia, while D_1 and D_4 receptors are both abundant in the cerebral cortex. Thus, the operative paradigm is that functional diversification and heterogeneity in expression patterns for receptor subtypes allows each subtype and isoform to perform a unique physiological role.

Defining Receptor Subtype Function

The process of defining receptor subtypes associated with cloned sequences and their associated physiological and pharmacological properties remains a major challenge, particularly for the ligand-gated ion channel superfamily. The molecular diversity of subunits that comprise the nicotinic acetylcholine, GABA$_A$, and glutamate LGCRs families allows for a plethora of subtypes composed of unique heteromeric subunit combinations. Many of the subunits do not directly bind ligands but nevertheless dictate binding properties for the receptor complex. Expression of distinct combinations of subunits is required to understand the individual roles each subunit plays in creating pharmacologically distinct receptor subtypes when expressed in heterologous cells. Such expression studies have shown that recombinant GABA$_A$ receptors composed of different α-subunit isoforms in combination with invariant β and γ subunits display distinct benzodiazepine pharmacology, GABA−benzodiazepine interactions, and steroid modulation. The existence of multiple receptor subtypes with unique pharmacological characteristics and differential subanatomical localization provides the rationale for their use as molecular targets in the development of novel subtype-selective drugs that are targeted to specific tissues and are hopefully devoid of the side effects associated with existing nonselective drugs.

CLONED HUMAN RECEPTORS AS DRUG DISCOVERY TARGETS

An important application of recombinant DNA technology has been the capability to provide human, cloned receptor subtypes as expressed functional proteins for drug discovery efforts. Prior to the availability of the cloned receptor targets, screening programs relied upon utilization of receptors obtained from animal tissue homogenates that had the inherent disadvantages of receptor heterogeneity, nonhuman pharmacology, and low receptor expression levels. The development and utilization of stable cell lines that express high levels of a single human receptor subtype for drug screening allow for a more accurate and selective pharmacological screening method compared with conventional methods and have enabled the discovery of highly selective drugs that discriminate between various receptor subtypes. Furthermore, cell lines have been engineered to express a recombinant receptor linked to a second messenger or other downstream biochemical response so that the functional consequences of receptor occupancy can be detected. Thus, not only can drug binding affinity of novel lead compounds be quantitatively defined, but the use of such recombinant cell lines permits rapid characterization of agonist or antagonist activity and measurements of compound efficacy at the cellular level.

Many human recombinant receptor subtypes expressed in a wide variety of human and other mammalian host cell backgrounds (e.g., CHO, HeLa, L-cells) have been found to exhibit ligand binding properties indistinguishable from their nonrecombinant "native" receptor counterpart. However, the use of recombinant receptor systems for receptor classification and pharmacological characterization can generate misleading data if heterologous host cell-specific properties have been imposed on the receptor. Ligand binding and signal transduction properties of many GPCRs have been found to depend upon the host cell as well as the expression level of the receptor, and thus agonist affinities and coupling mechanisms determined in different recombinant expression systems may not be identical. In the case of the expression of the human 5HT$_{1A}$ in HeLa cell lines, certain compounds acted as agonists in a cell line with a high receptor density but acted as pure antagonists in a cell line with only a sixfold lower density of receptors. Similarly, data for other GPCRs have been obtained showing the dependence of agonist efficacy and pharmacological properties on receptor density.

The question of analyzing receptor function must be viewed within the context of the functional level for analysis as to whether the molecular entity is the single receptor, a signal transduction pathway, or an integrated cellular response. For example, activation of a specific signal transduction pathway is often viewed as a constituting a receptor response. Insight into the complexities of analyzing the responses of recombinant receptors in heterologous cells is provided by studies of the signal transduction properties resulting from the activation of the D$_2$ dopamine receptor stably expressed in two different cell lines. Activation of D$_2$ receptors in either GH$_4$C$_1$ rat pituitary cells or mouse Ltk$^-$ fibroblasts produced inhibition of adenylyl cyclase activity (29). However, while D$_2$ receptor activation caused a rapid stimulation of phosphatidylinositol (PI) hydrolysis and an increase in intracellular calcium in Ltk$^-$ cells, it failed to effect PI hydrolysis and induced a decrease in intracellular calcium in GH$_4$C$_1$ cells. Similarly, activation of the 5HT$_{1A}$ receptor expressed in Ltk$^-$ cells was coupled to an increase in intracellular calcium but resulted in a decrease in calcium influx when expressed in GH$_4$C$_1$ cells. Since the cell-specific differences in the signaling pathways for the D$_2$ and 5HT$_{1A}$ receptors were the same, these effects may most likely be attributed to the complement of G-proteins present in each host cell type. Thus, the effector systems and responses of a transfected receptor depend not only on the receptor but upon the particular cell type in which it is expressed.

The high level of membrane expression for recombinant GPCRs in insect cells (1−40 pmol/mg in Sf9 or Sf21 cells) using the baculovirus system has demonstrated appropriate receptor pharmacology for antagonist ligands (affinities and rank order potencies), whereas anomalous agonist binding properties and lack of functional coupling have been observed for some receptors. The GPCRs expressed using baculovirus typically show only a single, low-affinity binding state for agonists, whereas the same receptors demonstrate high- (coupled) and low-affinity (uncoupled) agonist binding states in mammalian cells. Similarly, the pharmacological properties of GPCRs expressed in yeast (M_1 muscarinic and D_2 dopamine receptors) were not comparable with mammalian cells since only a single low-affinity agonist binding state was detected, indicating that the recombinant receptors do not to couple to the endogenous G-proteins present in these cells (30, 31).

Cellular engineering to coexpress recombinant GPCRs and the appropriate G-protein has been found to provide an approach to overcome such limitations. Toward this end, it was recently found that heterologous coexpression of the G protein α-subunit $G\alpha_{16}$ with a variety of GPCRs in mammalian cells enabled coupling to PLCβ activity and increases in intracellular calcium. In yeast, functional coupling was only achieved using a mutant strain lacking one yeast G-protein α-subunit and including a cDNA encoding an appropriate G-protein (31).

The integration of molecular biological approaches into receptor pharmacology has been useful in elucidating receptor structure–function relationships. Construction of chimeric receptors (hybrid polypeptides composed of adjacent portions of two related receptor subtypes) has helped to identify functional domains of many individual receptors. Such studies have successfully identified ligand-binding domains and cytoplasmic domains mediating signal transduction of many receptors. Using in vitro mutagenesis to change single amino acids to create point-mutated receptors has defined critical residues involved in receptor–ligand interactions, conformational transitions, ion channel selectivity, signal transduction, and sites of receptor phosphorylation. Due to the lack of high-resolution structural data for most membrane receptors, this approach often requires making the assumption that overall receptor conformation and the equilibrium distribution between receptor states (resting, active, and desensitized) have not been altered in the mutated receptor. Nevertheless, this experimental approach has been the basis for a large body of molecular modeling aimed at understanding the specific functional groups on receptors that interact with drug ligands. The combination of such molecular pharmacological and modeling approaches can be expected to reveal the structural determinants of drug binding and novel allosteric sites on

the receptor protein for drug interaction. Ultimately, the ability to produce large amounts of purified receptor protein from recombinant expression systems will enable the use of physical methods (NMR, electron microscopy,

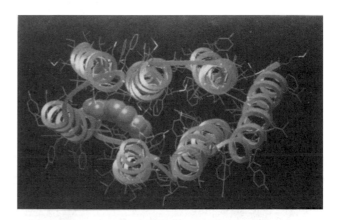

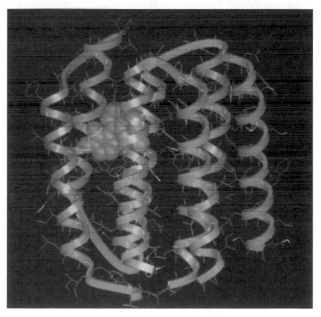

Fig. 4 A molecular model of the dopamine D2 receptor with a ligand docked in the binding site. The model of the D2 receptor transmembrane helices was constructed from the coordinates of the bacteriorhodopsin structure derived from two-dimensional electron diffraction experiments and is consistent with the projection structure for rhodopsin. The transmembrane helices are represented by a solid ribbon and the drug, apomorphine, is a space filling representation. The top view looking down the helical axis of the receptor clearly delineates the seven transmembrane helices that are the key structural motif for the GPCR superfamily. Some of the helices are inclined relative to the perpendicular to the membrane plane. The bottom view is in the plane of the membrane with the extracellular space at the top of the figure. (Adapted from Ref. 57.)

X-ray crystallography) to obtain high-resolution receptor structural data that will delineate ligand-binding sites and precisely define drug–receptor interactions. The recent elucidation of the high-resolution structure of rhodopsin is a major step towards the detailed understanding of the 3D structures of the GPCR superfamily, as shown in Fig. 4 for the dopamine D_2 receptor.

Drug Discovery Using Adopted Orphan Receptors

There are now numerous examples of orphan receptors that have been identified as novel types or subtypes of existing receptor families for which functional roles have been characterized as proven therapeutic drug targets. Many of these orphan receptors are of immediate interest as potential drug discovery targets since they represent novel receptor subtypes that extend existing receptor families that have members that are therapeutically important drug receptor targets. The close structural relatedness that is the molecular basis for organization of the receptor superfamilies has allowed a rational-based search for new members of the ligand-gated ion channel, G-protein coupled, receptor tyrosine-kinase, and nuclear receptor superfamilies. In general, discovery of new receptors (or subunits) has been accomplished by screening cDNA libraries, using sequences conserved among the receptor family at low stringency (homology screening). An alternative method has been to employ PCR amplification of human genomic DNA with degenerate oligonucleotides encoding conserved receptor domains.

Initial efforts to identify orphan receptors exploited PCR methodology to clone several novel orphan receptors belonging to the GPCR superfamily (32). These orphan receptors were subsequently shown to include the adenosine A_1 and A_{2a} receptors (33), a 5-HT$_{1D}$ receptor (34, 5), and a central cannabinoid receptor (CB$_1$). PCR using degenerate primers was subsequently used to identify cDNAs encoding the NK$_1$, NK$_2$, dopamine D_1 and D_5 (36), histamine H$_3$, adenosine A_3(37), olfactory receptors, and numerous other GPCRs. The application of these approaches has been highly successful and has led to the cloning of a series of orphan receptors (or novel subunits) in each superfamily for which functions have not yet been assigned. To date, more than 40 additional members of the nuclear receptor superfamily have been cloned for which ligands have not been identified. In addition, the ligands for the many orphan members of the receptor–protein tyrosine phosphatase superfamily have also not yet been established. Numerous orphan receptor–tyrosine kinases belonging to the EPH family have been identified that likely function by transducing signals initiated by direct cell–cell interaction (38). Many of the EPH receptors are specifically expressed in the nervous system (39), and these receptors have been implicated in the control of axon guidance, in regulating cell migration, and in defining compartments in the developing embryo.

Strategies for Ligand Identification for Orphan GPCR Receptors

Since GPCRs constitute the largest superfamily of receptors in man and these receptors also represent important drug targets that have been subject to intense biochemical and pharmacological studies, the following discussion will focus on the orphan receptors that belong to the GPCR superfamily. An explosion of the number of orphan GPCRs has been primarily due to advances in both cloning and sequencing technologies. Specifically, directed studies employing a combination of low stringency hybridization, polymerase chain reaction, an increasing database of ESTs (expressed sequence and tagged cDNA) and high throughput sequencing technologies have led to an exponential increase in the number of orphan GPCRs that await ligand identification.

The new paradigm for orphan receptor-based drug discovery is shown diagrammatically (Fig. 5). A first step toward ligand identification for a given orphan GPCR is to generate a full-length clone if the cDNA sequence is incomplete. To accomplish this, a specific tissue is identified that contains the orphan receptor gene and a full-length cDNA clone is typically generated using RT-PCR. Next, the cDNA is fully sequenced, and the sequence is compared with the sequence of known GPCRs through the use of genomic databases. If the identity of an orphan GPCR approaches 45% with a known receptor, it is likely that the orphan receptor and the highly homologous GPCR will share the same ligand (40). Successful application of this approach led to the identification of the ligand for the human 5-HT$_{1D}$(41), C3a (42), and CGRP (43) receptors. However, there are subfamilies of GPCRs that do not show this degree of similarity. Furthermore, many orphan GPCRs may reveal no significant identity with known GPCRs but will demonstate high homology to other orphan receptors, leading to the identification of new GPCR families, as typified by the important discovery of the edg family of lysophopholipid receptors (44).

Most orphan receptors share a low degree of overall sequence homology, which may be in the range of 20–30% overall amino acid identity. In these cases, a useful step in ligand identification is to evaluate the both the tissue and cell type distribution of the orphan receptor mRNA through Northern blot analysis or RT-PCR. A very

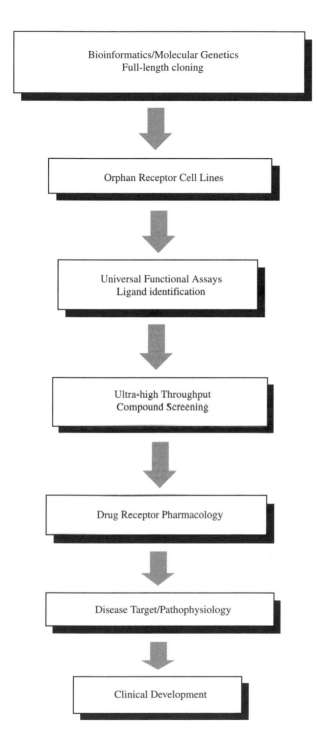

Fig. 5 Strategy for using orphan receptors as targets for drug discovery. The flow diagram illustrates the paradigm shift in receptor-based drug discovery, which is based upon a reverse molecular pharmacological strategy. The starting material for drug discovery is a sequence corresponding to an orphan receptor of unknown function.

restricted distribution pattern for an orphan GPCR may help provide clues concerning the physiological function of the receptor. Differential expression between normal and diseased tissue may indicate a role in the pathophysiology and suggest a potential therapeutic relevance for drugs targeted to the orphan receptor. Knowledge of the distribution of an orphan GPCR can also guide selection of cells or tissues to be used as sources of the endogenous cognate ligand for reverse pharmacology or ligand fishing studies. With the advent of chip technology, potentially thousands of orphan receptor cDNAs can be attached to a chip, thereby enabling the simultaneous evaluation of the expression levels under diverse pathological conditions.

Ligand Fishing for Orphan Receptors

Orphan receptors of interest may exhibit no significant homology with known GPCRs, and distribution studies may not provide any clues to the identity of the endogenous ligand. In this case, reverse pharmacology or ligand fishing studies are pursued (Fig. 5), especially for peptide receptors that often exhibit high affinity for their endogenous ligand. In this approach, the orphan receptor is used as bait to isolate the endogenous ligand from cell or tissue extracts suspected to contain the ligand (40, 44, 45). This approach has led to the discovery of novel endogenous peptide ligands orphanin FQ/nociceptin (46), orexin (47), prolactin-releasing peptide (48), melanin concentrating hormone (49), and APJ (50) as the cognate ligands for their respective orphan receptors. The specific high-affinity interaction of the endogenous ligand contained in extracts with the expressed orphan GPCR is measured in an appropriate functional second messenger assay. Once the active extract is identified, it can be fractionated, purified by HPLC, and the identity of the active component may be determined by analytical methods that may include peptide sequencing, mass spectroscopy, and NMR.

Expression of Orphan GPCRs

A critical step in ligand fishing for an orphan GPCR is to express the receptor in an appropriate cellular expression system. As previously discussed, choices may include mammalian cells, insect cells, bacteria, oocytes, or yeast. Initial considerations for choosing an expression system may focus on the type of functional assay to employ in screening procedures. A basic requirement for any given functional assay is the presence of the appropriate signal transductionmachinery in the expression system. While it is often not possible to predict specific coupling mechanims and signal transduction pathways activated by an orphan receptor, several mammalian cells have been confirmed as suitable for human orphan receptor expression, including CHO and HEK 293 cells. All of these contain a full repertoire of signal transduction components required for measurement of most GPCR-mediated changes in second messenger systems (44). Another factor to be weighed in selecting an appropriate expression system is the potential interference of endogenous receptors present in the host cell line. This factor can be experimentally addressed through parallel screening of the parental cell line. Additionally, it is important to establish that the orphan receptor is expressed at sufficient densities and present on the membrane surface. Expression levels have been evaluated by epitope tagging of the receptor and measurement of receptor on the membrane surface by fluorescence activated cell sorting (FACS) or, alternatively, by Western blot analysis.

Functional Assays Used for Orphan Receptor Ligand Identification

For the full value of the receptor gene sequence to be realized, the function of the expressed orphan receptor, as well as its regulation and expression need to be elucidated. In many cases, exemplified by the nociceptin receptor, the orphan receptor will be activated by an as yet unknown endogenous ligand (transmitter, peptide, or hormone) or the endogenous ligand may be identified as a previously characterized molecule whose function has not been assigned. Strategies for identification of either the endogenous or surrogate ligands for an orphan receptor are frequently based upon utilization of high and ultrahigh throughput "agonist screening" assays in which ligand binding is coupled to a cellular functional response.

Functional assays based upon measurements of common cellular signal transduction pathways (i.e., mobilization of intracellular calcium, cAMP, transcription response elements) have been employed. Since many types of receptors (LGCRs, GPCRs, and RTKs) mediate cellular responses through elevations in intracellular calcium, real-time measurements of intracellular calcium, using fluorescent probes, have provided a rapid, generic assay for receptor activation. In addition, cell-based transcriptional activation assays represent a functional screening method that requires engineering of stable cell line(s) expressing the recombinant orphan linked to a luminescent or fluorescent-based reporter gene (i.e., luciferase or green fluorescent protein) under the transcriptional control of a promoter element (i.e., cAMP response element (CRE), NFAT, or STAT binding elements). The advantages inherent in these one-step screening approaches include high detection sensitivity, compatibility with automation, and high throughput.

The first consideration for developing a functional assay for screening extracts or compounds to identify endogenous ligands or surrogate agonists for orphan GPCRs is to determine which G-protein(s) mediate coupling to the receptor. Certainly, this is difficult to determine unless the orphan receptor of interest contains a high level of homology to other known GPCRs activating well-characterized signal transduction pathways. In some cases, evaluation of extracts or compounds in both G_s, G_i and G_q-associated functional assays is necessary. Once the type of assay endpoint is chosen, there is a variety of high throughput and robust functional assays that can be utilized in ligand fishing. Advances in commercially available technology have enabled the development of ultrahigh throughput screening methods and systems that have led to the miniaturization of assays from 96-well plate formats to 1536-well formats that require only microliter volumes of reagents. Functional assays based upon one of several fluorescence detection techniques, including fluorescence resonance energy transfer, polarization, time-resolved fluorescence, and luminescence, now allow receptor-activated signaling events in live cells to be rapidly measured.

Reporter gene assays

Reporter gene assays have been widely used as high-throughput, cell-based functional assays for numerous GPCRs. In these assays, gene transcription is activated by a receptor-associated transduction event, such as increases in cellular cAMP or intracellular calcium. Reporter genes typically consist of a specific responsive element placed upstream of a minimal promoter, which together control the expression of the reporter gene, such as β-galactosidase luciferase. Commonly used response elements include the cAMP response element that is suitable for either G_s- and G_i-coupled receptors or a calcium-sensitive response element suitable for G_q-coupled receptors (51).

Another cell-based functional gene transcription assay has been developed by Tsien and co-workers that permits real-time receptor activation of gene expression to be measured in live cells. For this assay, mammalian cells are transfected with receptor and the gene for β-lactamase that acts as a reporter by hydrolyzing an exogenous substrate that is loaded intracellularly. The highly sensitive fluorescence assay permits clonal selection of single cells by flow cytometry and forms the basis for a high-throughput screen.

A bioluminescent reporter assay for G_q-coupled receptors has been described in which the receptor of interest is cotransfected with the calcium-sensitive protein aequorin. Agonist activation of receptor-mediated increases in intracellular calcium lead to activation of aequorin and subsequent luminescent responses (52). Due to the considerable amplification occurring after agonist activation of the GPCR, this assay can be significantly minaturized and run in 96-, 384-, and 1536-well formats. Transient expression of apoaequorin in CHO cells and reconstitution with the co-factor coelenterazine resulted in a large, concentration-dependent agonist-mediated luminescent response following cotransfection with the endothelin ET_A, angiotensin AT_2, thyrotropin-releasing hormone (TRH), and neurokinin NK_1 receptors, all of which interact predominantly with the $G_{\alpha q}$-like phosphoinositidase-linked G-proteins. To generate a system amenable for the study of agonist activity at virtually any G-protein-coupled receptor, the α-subunit of the receptor promiscuous G-protein $G_{\alpha 16}$ was either transiently or stably expressed in CHO cells together with apoaequorin. In cells expressing $G_{\alpha 16}$, but not in its absence, agonists at a series of receptors that normally interact with either $G_{\alpha s}$ or $G_{\alpha i}$ were now able to cause a luminescent response from mitochondrially targeted apoaequorin. In the case of the A_1 adenosine receptor, this response was clearly a result of activation of $G_{\alpha 16}$ and not a consequence of the release of the $G_{\alpha i}$-associated β/γ complex, as the luminescent response was unaffected by pertussis toxin treatment of the cells, whereas agonist-mediated inhibition of adenylyl cyclase activity was attenuated. These studies describe the use of coexpressed apoaequorin as a reporter for G-protein-coupled receptor-mediated calcium signaling. Furthermore, coexpression of $G_{\alpha 16}$ and apoaequorin provides a basis for a generic mammalian cell microplate assay for the assessment of agonist action at virtually any GPCR, including orphan receptors for which the physiological signal transduction mechanism may be unknown.

Use of Engineered Cells for Developing Cell-Based Functional Assays

Advances in molecular engineering have facilitated the design of recombinant cells that can be used to design universal assays for orphan receptors. As a tool to analyze the function of newly discovered orphan receptor genes, "promiscuous" G-proteins have been utilized to develop screens for orphan GPCRs that can be used to search for compounds that activate such receptors. For example, coexpression of the "universal adapter" $G_{\alpha 16}$ G-protein with an orphan GPCR of interest allows the activated

receptor to couple to increases in intracellular calcium, although the receptor may not couple to G_q in nonengineered cells. Another common approach to designing a universal functional ligand-screening system for any GPCRs is to construct and coexpress chimeric G-proteins with an orphan GPCR (53). Chimeric G-protein α-subunits have been constructed in which the backbone of either G_s, G_i, or G_q, is combined with small peptidic sequences corresponding to the C-terminus of G_s, G_i, and G_q. The C-terminal end of the chimera dictates receptor coupling and the G-protein backbone determines which effector system is activated. For example, short C-terminal portions of G_s or G_i can be combined with the backbone of G_q, resulting in an engineered G-protein chimera that can universally signal through increases in intracellular calcium or activate calcium sensitive reporter assays (53, 54). Conversely, chimeras can be constructed with the backbone of the G_s-α-subunit and the C-terminus of G_q to develop an assay system in which cAMP is measured. The design of universal assay systems for orphan GPCRs can greatly facilitate throughput for analysis of large numbers of candidate receptors.

Recently, a number of GPCRs have been reported to activate second messenger responses, even in the absence of their natural ligands or surrogate agonists. GPCRs that possess this ligand-independent activity are referred to as constitutively active GPCRs. Three different methods have been employed to produce constitutively activated receptors and include: 1) overexpression of the native receptor in heterologous expression systems, 2) overexpression of the appropriate G-protein that couples to the receptor, or 3) mutation of specific aminoacid residues of the receptor, typically in transmembrane regions or in intracellular loops of the receptor. A number of pharmaceutical companies are now utilizing constitutively activated orphan GPCRs for identification of either inverse agonists or agonists from small molecule libraries using functional ligand-independant screens. Thus, drug discovery for orphan GPCRs doesnot now require previous identification of the endogeneous ligand or a surrogate agonist to develop a functional screen for drug discovery. Molecules discovered in these screens can be used not only as potential therapeutics but also as tools to furhter evaluate the physiological functions of the orphan GPCRs and their potential therapeutic relevance.

Screening for Endogenous and Surrogate Ligands

After a reliable and robust functional assay is developed for an expressed orphan receptor, screening can ensue.

Several approaches can be taken. First, cell and tissue extracts or biological fluids can be evaluated for activation of the orphan receptor. If an active extract is identified, it is further fractionated and then subjected to HPLC followed by further testing of fractions in the functional assay. After substantial purification, the identity of the active component can be elucidated by numerous analytical methods including mass spectroscopy and NMR. Another approach is to screen a collection of compounds with known pharmacological actions and biological compounds for which the mechanism of action is unknown. A third approach is to screen peptide or small molecule libraries. This can easily be accomplished rapidly due to advances in high-throughput screening and laboratory automation. Once the surrogate ligand is identified, clues as to the physiological function of the orphan receptor and possibly the endogenous ligand can be often obtained.

The identification of gene sequences is only the beginning of the process for the development of the useful small molecule therapeutic agent. Analysis of a stretch of only 10–25 amino acids from an orphan receptor sequence may be sufficient to identify whether the orphan of interest is homologous to either a known protein or a recognizable motif that corresponds to a ligand recognition or functional domain characteristic of a receptor superfamily. Based upon the level of observed sequence homology with known receptors, it may be possible to either deduce the class of ligand bound by the orphan receptor and/or postulate a mechanism of signal transduction. The systematic search for natural cognate ligands of orphan receptors is more difficult when the properties of such receptors are not well predicted by sequence comparisons to known receptors and/or the orphan receptors exhibit novel pharmacology.

As an example of the first strategy, the process leading to the characterization of the orphan ORL1 (Opioid Receptor-Like I) receptor, which has become known as the orphanin or nociceptin receptor (46), is of interest since it represents one model that can be readily adapted to other orphan receptors. The ORL1 receptor is a novel G-protein coupled receptor that is most closely related to the opioid receptors. Based upon substantial sequence identity of the ORL1 receptor with opioid receptors (50% overall, 65% within transmembrane domains), it was reasonable to hypothesize that the related orphan receptor would share signal transduction properties in common with the μ-, δ-, and κ-opioid receptor subtypes. Since opioid receptors are all negatively coupled to adenylyl cyclase, a stable recombinant CHO cell line expressing ORL1 was constructed for use in a functional screen, using untransfected CHO cells as a control. A survey of opiate ligands identified etorphine, a nonselective opiate agonist, as mediating inhibition of forskolin-induced accumulation

of cAMP, although its potency was found to be about three orders of magnitude less compared with other opioid receptors. However, additional efforts to characterize the pharmacology of the ORL1 receptor by analysis of agonist effects induced by endogenous opioid peptides (endorphins, enkephalins, and dynorphins) or other synthetic opioid ligands were not successful.

Based upon the structural homology of ORL1 with opioid receptors, in particular, the acidic extracellular loop 2 of the κ-opioid receptor, it was hypothesized that the endogenous ligand might be a peptide that resembled dynorphin. A biochemical fractionation procedure was used to isolate a pituitary peptide whose structure was identified as a 17 amino acid neuropeptide that shares many features in common with other opioid peptides and is now known as nociceptin. Isolation of the endogenous ligand was achieved through a functional assay on the basis of its ability to inhibit adenylyl cyclase in a stable recombinant cell line. The identity of nociceptin was confirmed through synthesis of a radiolabeled derivative that was found to bind in a saturable manner with high affinity and to be a potent and specific activator of the ORL1 receptor. In vivo activity of nociceptin induced hyperalgesia when administered intracerebroventricularly to mice, indicating the agonist of the ORL1 receptor appears to possess pronociceptive properties. The unique pharmacology, physiology, and brain distribution of this novel receptor make it an important target for drug discovery.

An alternative approach may be to employ an immobilized orphan receptor to capture the cognate ligand from biological extracts, fractions, and other combinatorial chemistry libraries. Orphan receptor screening efforts will be able to take advantage of large-scale synthetically produced random peptide, peptidomimetic, and combinatorial chemical libraries, as well as phage display libraries that are available as novel sources of chemical and structural diversity for discovery of potent and selective chemical entities for each of the receptors. Finding new natural product-based lead compounds by screening fermentation broths and extracts from plant and marine organisms may yield ligands with novel structures, as was found in the case of the subtype-selective endothelin receptor peptidic antagonists.

Among the GPCR superfamily, the discovery and characterization of the large number of novel receptor subtypes belonging to the chemokine, dopaminergic, serotoninergic, somatostatin, and opioid receptor families provide examples of the tremendous impact of gene cloning. As a consequence of the original cloning of the orphan receptor sequence corresponding to the 5-HT$_{1D}$ receptor in 1989 (55), the human receptor sites involved in the action of acute antimigraine drugs were subsequently identified. Studies of these receptors have led to significant insights into the pathophysiology of migraine and the development of new antimigraine drugs, such as naratriptan and zolmitriptan, which were selected for development based upon their high affinity and selectivity for the human recombinant 5-HT$_{1D}$ receptors. Clearly, the value inherent in orphan receptor characterization for drug discovery has been proven and will continue to lead to the discovery of substantial numbers of novel, human receptors designated as "orphans" that will provide novel targets for drug development.

Human Genome Sequencing—New Orphan Receptors and Subtypes

The most intensive research project in biomedicine is under way—the immense task of sequencing the human genome and identifying all of the expressed human genes. This effort is driving a paradigm shift in the fundamental approach to drug discovery as genomic data becomes the initiation point for the drug discovery process. Considerable progress has been made by the Human Genome Project as advances in cloning, mapping, and sequencing technologies have jointly contributed to an explosion in the volume of human sequence data. The rapidly approaching completion of the human genome sequence will lead to structure of all of the roughly 25,000–35,000 different human genes. To integrate and analyze the vast database of genomic data, the field of bioinformatics is providing powerful computational algorithms and methods for searching databases and complex data sets to allow molecular classification and extrapolate receptor structure and function from numerous new sequences. The impact of this effort will be an exponential increase in the number of novel orphan receptors requiring further study to define their potential role as targets for drug discovery. At the conclusion of this project, the identification and sequence of all receptor genes in the human genome will be available for study. Based upon estimates that 2–3% of the genome is likely to consist of receptors, this would suggest that the total number of receptors to be identified will be approximately 600–900. Yet another benefit of these genomic efforts will be the identification single disease-causing genes that are responsible for common or inherited diseases. Numerous examples exist for disease states that are associated with either deficient receptor responses, unregulated signaling function, or enhanced responses to neurotransmitter or hormonal signaling, indicating the biomedical importance for identifying the molecular etiology of a disease state and gaining access to disease-relevant receptor targets. The recent cloning of a Karposi's sarcoma-associated herpevirus (KSHV, or

human herpesvirus 8) genome fragment revealed an open reading frame encoding a putative GPCR that was homologous to human CXCR1 and CXCR2 receptors (56). Expression studies showed that it was indeed a bona fide signaling receptor that exhibited binding characteristics of a chemokine receptor, with affinity for a range of chemokines in the CXC and CC families. The receptor demonstrated constitutive (agonist-independent) activity in COS cells and stimulated cellular proliferation, making it a candidate viral oncogene.

Technological extensions based upon the human genome sequencing platform that enhance receptor-based drug discovery include development and construction of biochips containing DNA microarrays of gene sequences. These biochips enable high-throughput screening using fluorescent hybridization of total cDNA or mRNA libraries from particular cell types or rare tissues and permit quantitative examination of large numbers of specific receptor sequences expressed in normal and disease samples. The large-scale quantitative examination of large numbers of specific receptor sequences expressed in normal and disease samples is called expression profiling. Such differential gene expression studies can detect different levels and patterns of a receptor gene expression in different tissue states and can be used as a tool to decipher receptor gene function and potentially define a relationship to a particular disease state.

In summary, the application of molecular genetics to large-scale sequencing, analysis of DNA sequence information, and new experimental approaches for rapid functional analysis of receptor molecules from these sequences can be expected to lead to the identification of an abundance of novel receptors that will become molecular targets for the development of highly selective drugs. Indeed, gene-based discoveries are already providing an entirely new approach to the development of a novel drug pharmaceuticals. The parallel utilization of all receptor subtypes that comprise a family of human receptors in high-throughput primary screening programs has demonstrated the value of this approach for the identification of receptor-subtype specific drugs. This development in the field of drug discovery holds great promise since drugs with therapeutic activity that emerge from such screening programs should possess high molecular specificity.

The current challenge in receptor functional genomics will be to develop successful experimental strategies and new technologies for the identification of ligands that can activate orphan receptors or inhibit these receptors, should they exhibit constitutive, basal activity. Although progress has been made, the continued application of molecular biological approaches to receptor pharmacology coupled with advances in biophysical methods should serve as tools that will enable a precise delineation of receptor binding sites and drug–receptor interactions at the molecular level. A more complete understanding the molecular events that transduce ligand binding into receptor activation will ultimately aid in the in the discovery of more selective agents for specific conformational states of existing receptor subtypes. Furthermore, the rapid elucidation of receptor–protein interaction partners and mapping intracellular signal transduction pathways associated with receptor signaling will accelerate understanding of novel receptor function. Finally, methods to localize and image the expression of receptor genes in living cells and animals can be expected to provide a foundation for novel pharmacological interventions targeted to specific cell types and tissues.

The application of many new technologies is synergistically accelerating the process of moving from novel receptor gene sequences to validated drug discovery receptor targets and ultimately, new drugs. The ongoing sequencing of the human genome and ensuing characterization of orphan receptors coupled with the precise molecular analysis of receptor structure, function, expression, and role of these receptors in disease processes will continue to reveal new drug receptor targets that will serve as a platform for much of the drug discovery enterprise.

REFERENCES

1. Kenakin, T.P.; Bond, R.A.; Bonner, T.I. Definition of Pharmacological Receptors. Pharmacol. Rev. **1992**, *44*, 351–362.
2. Alexander, S.; Peters, J. TIPS Receptor and Ion Channel Nomenclature Supplement. Trans. Pharmacol. Sci. Elsevier.
3. Hulme, E.C.; Birdsall, N.J.; Buckley, N.J. Muscarinic Receptor Subtypes. Annu. Rev. Pharmacol. Toxicol. **1990**, *30*, 633–673.
4. Changeux, J.P.; Devillers-Thiery, A.; Chemouilli, P. Acetylcholine Receptor: An Allosteric Protein. Science **1984**, *225*, 1335–1345.
5. Bowery, N.G. GABA$_B$ Receptor Pharmacology. Annu. Rev. Pharmacol. Toxicol. **1993**, *33*, 109–147.
6. Burt, D.R.; Kamatchi, G.L. GABA$_A$ Receptor Subtypes: from Pharmacology to Molecular Biology. FASEB J. **1991**, *5*, 2916–2923.
7. Seeman, P.; Van Tol, H.H. Dopamine Receptor Pharmacology. Trends Pharmacol. Sci. **1994**, *15*, 264–270.
8. Hamblin, M.W.; Metcalf, M.A. Primary Structure and Functional Characterization of a Human 5-HT1D-Type Serotonin Receptor. Mol. Pharmacol. **1991**, *40*, 143–148.
9. Adham, N.; Ellerbrock, B.; Hartig, P.; Weinshank, R.L.; Branchek, T. Receptor Reserve Masks Partial Agonist Activity of Drugs in a Cloned Rat 5-Hydroxytryptamine 1B Receptor Expression System. Mol. Pharmacol. **1993**, *43*, 427–433.
10. Hill, P.; Hnilo, J.; Karla, M.; Bounds, S.; Herz, J.M. Cloning, Expression and Comparison of the Binding Characteistics of the Known Human Dopamine Receptors. Adv. Neurolo. **1996**, *69*, 41–52.
11. Kallal, L.; Benovic, J.L. Using Green Fluorescent Proteins to Study G-Protein-Coupled Receptor Localization and Trafficking. Trends Pharmacol. Sci. **2000**, *21*, 175–180.
12. Sine, S.M.; Taylor, P. The Relationship Between Agonist Occupation and the Permeability Response of the Cholinergic Receptor Revealed by Bound Cobra Alpha-Toxin. J. Biol. Chem. **1980**, *225*, 10144–10156.
13. Herz, J.M.; Johnson, D.A.; Taylor, P. Interaction of Noncompetitive Inhibitors with the Acetylcholine Receptor. The Site Specificity and Spectroscopic Properties of Ethidium Binding. J. Biol. Chem. **1987**, *262*, 7238–7247.
14. Sokoloff, P.; Andrieux, M.; Besancon, R. et al. Pharmacology of Human Dopamine D3 Receptor Expressed in a Mammalian Cell Line: Comparison with D2 Receptor. Eur. J. Pharmacol. **1992**, *225*, 331–337.
15. Chio, C.L.; Drong, R.F.; Riley, D.T.; Gill, G.S.; Slightom, J.L.; Huff, R.M. D4 Dopamine Receptor-Mediated Signaling Events Determined in Transfected Chinese Hamster Ovary Cells. J. Biol. Chem. **1994**, *269*, 11813–11819.
16. Lahti, R.A.; Evans, D.L.; Stratman, N.C.; Figur, L.M. Dopamine D4 Versus D2 Receptor Selectivity of Dopamine Receptor Antagonists: Possible Therapeutic Implications. Eur. J. Pharmacol. **1993**, *236*, 483–486.
17. Chidiac, P.; Hebert, T.E.; Valiquette, M.; Dennis, M.; Bouvier, M. Inverse Agonist Activity of Beta-Adrenergic Antagonists. Mol. Pharmacol. **1994**, *45*, 490–499.
18. Samama, P.; Pei, G.; Costa, T.; Cotecchia, S.; Lefkowitz, R.J. Negative Antagonists Promote an Inactive Conformation of the Beta 2-Adrenergic Receptor. Mol. Pharmacol. **1994**, *45*, 390–394.
19. Oswald, R.E.; Bamberger, M.J.; McLaughlin, J.T. Mechanism of Phencyclidine Binding to the Acetylcholine Receptor from Torpedo Electroplaque. Mol. Pharmacol. **1984**, *25*, 360–368.
20. Herz, J.M.; Atherton, S.J. Steric Factors Limit Access to the Noncompetitive Inhibitor Site of the Nicotinic Acetylcholine Receptor. Fluorescence Studies. Biophys. J. **1992**, *62*, 74–76.
21. Neubig, R.R.; Sklar, L.A. Subsecond Modulation of Formyl Peptide-linked Guanine Nucleotide-Binding Proteins by Guanosine 5′-O-(3-Thio)Triphosphate in Permeabilized Neutrophils. Mol. Pharmacol. **1993**, *43*, 734–740.
22. Posner, R.G.; Fay, S.P.; Domalewski, M.D.; Sklar, L.A. Continuous Spectrofluorometric Analysis of Formyl Peptide Receptor Ternary Complex Interactions. Mol. Pharmacol. **1994**, *45*, 65–72.
23. Gether, U.; Lin, S.; Kobilka, B.K. Fluorescent Labeling of Purified β2-Adrenergic Receptor. Evidence for Ligand-specific Conformational Changes. J. Biol. Chem. **1995**, *270*, 28268–28275.
24. Neher, E.; Steinbach, J.H. Local Anaesthetics Transiently Block Currents Through Single Acetylcholine-Receptor Channels. J. Physiol. **1978**, *227*, 153–176.
25. Oksenberg, D.; Marsters, S.A.; O'Dowd, B.F.; et al. A Single Amino-acid Difference Confers Major Pharmacological Variation Between Human and Rodent 5-HT1B Receptors. Nature **1992**, *360*, 161–163.

26. Burnashev, N.; Villarel, A.; Sakmann, B.; Jingami, H. Dimensions and Ion Selectivity of Recombination AMPA Kainate Receptor Channels and Their Dependence on Q/R Site Residues. J. Physiol. **1996**, *496*, 165–173.

27. Moser, B.; Barella, L.; Mattei, S. et al. Expression of Transcripts for Two Interleukin 8 Receptors in Human Phagocytes, Lymphocytes and Melanoma Cells. Biochem. J. **1993**, *294*, 285–292.

28. Goldman, D.; Deneris, E.; Luyten, W.; Kochhar, A.; Patrick, J.; Heinemann, S. Members of a Nicotinic Acetylcholine Receptor Gene Family are Expressed in Different Regions of the Mammalian Central Nervous System. Cell **1987**, *48*, 965–973.

29. Vallar, L.; Muca, C.; Magni, M.; et al. Differential Coupling of Dopaminergic D2 Receptors Expressed in Different Cell Types. Stimulation of Phosphatidylinositol 4,5-Bisphosphate Hydrolysis in LtK-fibroblasts, Hyperpolarization, and Cytosolic-Free Ca^{2+} Concentration Decrease in GH4C1 Cells. J. Biol. Chem. **1990**, *265*, 10320–10326.

30. Payette, P.; Gossard, F.; Whiteway, M. Dennis M. Expression and Pharmacological Characterization of the Human M1 Muscarinic Receptor in Saccharomyces Cerevisiae. FEBS Lett. **1990**, *266*, 21–25.

31. King, K.; Dohlman, H.G.; Thorner, J.; Caron, M.G.; Lefkowitz, R.J. Control of Yeast Mating Signal Transduction by a Mammalian β2-Adrenergic Receptor and Gs Alpha Subunit. Science **1990**, *250*, 121–123.

32. Libert, F.; Vassart, G.; Parmentier, M. Current Developments in G-Protein-Coupled Receptors. Curr. Opin. Cell Biol. **1991**, *3*, 218–223.

33. Libert, F.; Schiffmann, S.N.; Lefort, A. et al. The Orphan Receptor CDNA RDC7 Encodes an A1 Adenosine Receptor. EMBO J. **1991**, *10*, 1677–1682.

34. Hamblin, M.W.; Metcalf, M.A. Primary Structure and Functional Characterization of a Human 5-HT1D-Type Serotonin Receptor. Mol. Pharmacol. **1991**, *40*, 143–148.

35. Zgombick, J.M.; Weinshank, R.L.; Macchi, M.; Schechter, L.E.; Branchek, T.A.; Hartig, P.R. Expression and Pharmacological Characterization of a Canine 5-Hydroxytryptamine 1D Receptor Subtype. Mol. Pharmacol. **1991**, *40*, 1036–1042.

36. Zhou, Q.Y.; Grandy, D.K.; Thambi, L. et al. Cloning and Expression of Human and Rat D1 Dopamine Receptors. Nature **1990**, *347*, 76–80.

37. Zhou, Q.Y.; Li, C.; Olah, M.E.; Johnson, R.A.; Stiles, G.L.; Civelli, O. Molecular Cloning and Characterization of an Adenosine Receptor: The A3 Adenosine Receptor. Proc. Natl. Acad. Sci. U.S.A. **1992**, *89*, 7432–7436.

38. Lindberg, R.A.; Hunter, T. cDNA Cloning and Characterization of ECK, an Epithelial Cell Receptor Protein-Tyrosine Kinase in the EPH/ELK Family of Protein Kinases. Mol. Cell. Biol. **1990**, *10*, 6316–6324.

39. Bartley, T.D.; Hunt, R.W.; Welcher, A.A. et al. B61 is a Ligand for the ECK Receptor Protein-Tyrosine Kinase. Nature **1994**, *368*, 558–560.

40. Marchese, A.; Sawzdargo, M.; Nguyen, T. et al. Discovery of Three Novel Orphan G-Protein-Coupled Receptors. Genomics **1999**, *56*, 12–21.

41. Maenhaut, C.; Van Sande, J.; Massart, C. et al. The Orphan Receptor CDNA RDC4 Encodes a 5-HT1D Serotonin Receptor. Biochem. Biophys. Res. Commun. **1991**, *180*, 1460–1468.

42. Ames, R.S.; Li, Y.; Sarau, H.M. et al. Molecular Cloning and Characterization of the Human Anaphylatoxin C3a Receptor. J. Biol. Chem. **1996**, *271*, 20231–20234.

43. Kapas, S.; Clark, A.J. Identification of an Orphan Receptor Gene as a Type 1 Calcitonin Gene-Related Peptide Receptor. Biochem. Biophys. Res. Commun. **1995**, *217*, 832–838.

44. Wilson, S.; Bergsma, D.J.; Chambers, J.K. et al. Orphan G-Protein-Coupled Receptors: The Next Generation of Drug Targets? Br. J. Pharmacol. **1998**, *125*, 1387–1392.

45. Civelli, O. Functional Genomics: The Search for Novel Neuro-transmitters and Neuropeptides. FEBS Lett. **1998**, *430*, 55–58.

46. Meunier, J.C.; Mollereau, C.; Toll, L. et al. Isolation and Structure of the Endogenous Agonist of Opioid Receptor-like ORL1 Receptor. Nature **1995**, *377*, 532–535.

47. Sakurai, T.; Amemiya, A.; Ishii, M. et al. Orexins and Orexin Receptors: A Family of Hypothalamic Neuropeptides and G-Protein-Coupled Receptors that Regulate Feeding Behavior. Cell **1998**, *92*, 573–585.

48. Hinuma, S.; Habata, Y.; Fujii, R. et al. A Prolactin-Releasing Peptide in the Brain. Nature **1998**, *393*, 272–276.

49. Chambers, J.; Ames, R.S.; Bergsma, D. et al. Melanin-Concentrating Hormone is the Cognate Ligand for the Orphan G-Protein-Coupled Receptor SLC-1. Nature **1999**, *400*, 261–265.

50. Tatemoto, K.; Hosoya, M.; Habata, Y. et al. Isolation and Characterization of a Novel Endogenous Peptide Ligand for the Human APJ Receptor. Biochem. Biophys. Res. Commun. **1998**, *251*, 471–476.

51. Colquhoun, D.; Hawkes, A.G. A Note on Correlations in Single Ion Channel Records. Proc. R. Soc. London, Ser. B. Biol. Sci. **1987**, *230*, 15–52.

52. Stables, J.; Green, A.; Marshall, F. et al. A Bioluminescent Assay for Agonist Activity At Potentially Any G-Protein-Coupled Receptor. Anal. Biochem. **1997**, *252*, 115–126.

53. Milligan, G.; Rees, S. Chimaeric G Alpha Proteins: Their Potential Use in Drug Discovery. Trends Pharmacol. Sci. **1999**, *20*, 118–124.

54. Conklin, B.R.; Herzmark, P.; Ishida, S. et al. Carboxyl-Terminal Mutations of Gq Alpha and Gs Alpha that Alter the Fidelity of Receptor Activation. Mol. Pharmacol. **1996**, *50*, 885–890.

55. Maenhaut, C.; Van Sande, J.; Massart, C. et al. The Orphan Receptor CDNA RDC4 Encodes a 5-HT1D Serotonin Receptor. Biochem. Biophys. Res. Commun. **1991**, *180*, 1460–1468.

56. Arvanitakis, L.; Geras-Raaka, E.; Varma, A.; Gershengorn, M.C.; Cesarman, E. Human Herpesvirus KSHV Encodes a Constitutively Active G-Protein-Coupled Receptor Linked to Cell Proliferation. Nature **1997**, *385*, 347–350.

57. Teeter, M.; Fromanitz, M.; Stec, B.; Du Ravid, J. Homology Modelling of the Dopamine D2 Receptor and Its Testing by Docking of Agonist and T Ricyclic Antagonists. J. Mod. Chem. **1994**, *37*, 2874–2878.

SCALE-UP AND POSTAPPROVAL CHANGES (SUPAC)

Jerome P. Skelly
Consultant, Alexandria, Virginia

OVERVIEW

In the process of developing a new drug product, the batch sizes used in the earliest human studies are small. As one proceeds through Phase 1 testing (i.e., the first introduction of a new chemical entity to humans), Phase 2 (discovering an indication for use), and Phase 3 (determining dose, side-effect profile, etc.), the size of the batches is gradually increased. When a New Drug Application (NDA) is approved by the Food and Drug Administration (FDA), the drug product is scaled up to a significantly larger batch size to meet the demands of the anticipated market. Similarly, in the development of a generic version of an already approved marketed product, a small batch is produced and tested for, among other things, bioequivalence to the FDA reference listed drug product. When the generic product meets FDA approval criteria, the Abbreviated New Drug Application (ANDA) or generic antibiotic application (AADA) is approved for marketing. It, too, is then scaled up to meet the demands of its anticipated market.

Whether a new chemical entity being brought to market for the first time or an approved generic version of previously marketed product, the size of the batch is almost inevitably scaled up to a significantly larger batch. In the process of scaling up, certain changes in the formula (composition) and/or in the manufacturing process and/or in the equipment may be necessary. In addition, the site at which the product will be manufactured may differ from where the smaller (pilot) batches were manufactured. The scale-up process and the changes made after approval in the composition, manufacturing process, manufacturing equipment, and change of site have become known as Scale-Up and Postapproval Changes, or SUPAC. The FDA has issued various guidances for SUPAC changes designated SUPAC-IR (1) (for immediate-release solid oral dosage forms), SUPAC-MR (2) (for modified-release solid oral dosage forms), and SUPAC-SS (3) (for non-sterile semisolid dosage forms including creams, ointments, gels, and lotions).

Although scale-up may occur at any point in the lifetime of a product, it most often occurs after the firm has been notified that the drug product is approvable, i.e., it meets all the conditions required by the FDA for marketing. With the submittal of Final Printed Labeling, a showing that the marketed product will meet the conditions for marketing as approved by the FDA (and in the case of generics, production of three consecutive scaled-up batches), and satisfactory completion of a preapproval inspection by the local FDA district office, the product is formally approved to be manufactured and sold in the United States. At this point, SUPAC begins to exert its effect.

Although SUPAC is a means of decreasing regulatory burden by empowering industry to make regulatory decisions, it does not affect any compliance or inspection requirement. It also is limited to scale-up and postapproval changes, even though the underlying science applies to preapproval changes as well. The major affect of SUPAC is a significant decrease in the time required to implement changes.

BACKGROUND

For years, the FDA had approved generic drug applications (ANDAs), using bioequivalence as a surrogate for clinical effectiveness. Aware that changes in the scale of the batch or the manufacturing equipment could affect a product's bioavilability, the FDA required that batches used in the ANDA-submitted bioequivalence studies be "production-sized batches made on production equipment." The FDA failed to verify the truthfulness of this statement, which had been submitted in virtually every ANDA and AADA. At one point, however, FDA inspectors noted that one firm, having obtained approval of a generic version of an approved marketed drug, had great difficulty scaling up that product to market-size batches. On investigation, the FDA discovered that the production-size batch made on production equipment consisted only of a few hundred dosage units produced on laboratory equipment. Although the samples from this very small batch when tested were bioequivalent to the innovator product, the firm could not scale up to the million plus units per batch they wished to market.

The FDA immediately promulgated rule 22–90, requiring that the minimum batch size for bioequivalence studies would henceforth be 100,000 units or 10% of

Encyclopedia of Pharmaceutical Technology

the anticipated market batch size, whichever is greater. Although this rule solved an immediate problem, it was not based on science. To address the question, the FDA used a method previously used to address quite controversial issues involving controlled-release dosage forms (4, 5) and bioanalytical methods (6). With the American Association of Pharmaceutical Scientists, it held three public workshops, bringing together outstanding industrial, academic, and FDA scientists to openly discuss the scientific and regulatory issues. The discussions were followed by the publication of consensus White Papers (7–9).

SUPAC

The premise of the consensus White Papers was that if: 1) the source of the drug substance for the smaller and larger batches was the same; 2) the drug substance particle size (both mean and distribution) was the same; 3) the excipients were the same; 4) the excipient particle size (both mean and distribution) was the same; 5) the order of addition was the same; 6) the equipment was the same; 7) the processing was the same; and, most important, 8) a surrogate test for bioequivalence testing (dissolution) was the same, the two batches were indeed the same. Over the previous 20 years the FDA Biopharmaceutics Program had established that within definable limits, dissolution was predictive of in vivo bioequivalence, for the same formulation, processed under the same conditions, on the same equipment. These criteria became the fundamental principle of the SUPAC initiative. (The percutaneous diffusion test is similarly used as a surrogate bioequivalence test for nonsterile, semisolid formulations.)

To establish the validity of the approach recommended by the three consensus papers, the FDA contracted the College of Pharmacy of the University of Maryland to study several drug products chosen on the basis of their solubility and permeability. The data revealed that the workshop recommendations were conservative and could be safely implemented. In fact, the studies showed that even broad differences in in vitro dissolution that resulted from major compositional changes failed to translate into bioavailability differences. Subsequently, the FDA published its *SUPAC Guidance for Immediate Release Solid Oral Dosage Forms* and followed with guidances for modified-release (controlled-release) and nonsterile semisolid dosage forms. In November 1999 (modified slightly in December 1999), the FDA extended the SUPAC concept to address changes in analytical methodology, packaging, and labeling and sterile semisolid dosage forms (10). This last guidance also updated the previously published guidances on immediate-release, modified-release, and nonsterile, semisolid dosage forms. In particular, the issue of multiple postapproval changes (which had been addressed differently in the previously published guidences) were now the same. The FDA now allowed multiple postapproval changes for every solid oral dosage form, using the same requirements as its SUPAC Semisolid Guidance.

The SUPAC Guidances published by the FDA define various levels of change and for each level of change specifies the 1) recommended chemistry, manufacturing, and control tests; 2) in vitro dissolution testing and/or in vivo bioequivalence tests; and 3) documentation that the FDA requires to be filed in the NDA, ANDA, or AADA to support the change. These guidances do not affect other compliance or inspection documentation required by the FDA Center for Drug Evaluation and Research Office of Compliance (CDER-OC) or the FDA field investigation units.

DOCUMENTATION

An annual report must be filed for every active application pending at the FDA. This report, which must be filed annually, updates all activity covered by the various FDA regulations affecting drug products under development or approved for marketing in the United States. Any change to an FDA-approved product must be submitted in a Supplemental New Drug Application, which requires review and approval. Until SUPAC, all supplements were Prior Approval Supplements (PAS). However, with SUPAC, the Agency allowed the use of a new Changes Being Effected (CBE) supplement, which allows industry to implement certain moderate changes on the very day the supplement is sent to the FDA. This eliminated the previously required and often lengthly FDA prereview and comment period. On the other hand, the Agency, after its review, reserves the right to require a PAS rather than a CBE if it disagrees with the industry decision. When the FDA published its new and updated guidance in December 1999, it provided for a new supplemental application called Changes Being Effective in 30 days (CBE-30). This procedure primarily applies to sterile dosage forms for which the Agency, obviously, requires a more exacting level of review.

LEVELS OF CHANGE

SUPAC lists three levels of change (Fig. 1) including: 1) minor changes, which are unlikely to have any

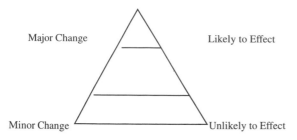

Fig. 1 Levels of change to FDA-approved products.

detectable effect on formulation quality and/or performance; 2) moderate changes, which could have a significant effect on formulation quality and/or performance; and 3) major changes, which are quite likely to have a significant effect on formulation quality and/or performance of the dosage form.

For a minor change, the chemical testing required and submitted to the FDA is routine. For example, accelerated stability testing and a commitment to perform long-term stability testing, plus those tests contained in the compendia and/or in the NDA/ANDA/AADA, would have to be performed. The data must be filed in the next annual report. On the other hand, a major change could involve dissolution-testing profiles to be determined in several media, an in vivo bioequivalence study, and a requirement for all data to be submitted in a supplemental filing to the application, which would require FDA preauthorization before implementation.

CHEMICAL, MANUFACTURING, AND CONTROLS TESTS

The FDA chemical testing for immediate-release, solid oral dosage forms (including the surrogate dissolution test) takes into consideration whether the drug has a narrow therapeutic index. The chemical, manufacturing, and control testing (including dissolution) is more onerous for narrow therapeutic index drug products than for other immediate-release, solid oral dosage forms.

In addition, although the testing criteria for changes in the composition of nonrelease-controlling excipients in delayed release (i.e., enteric-coated) dosage forms and controlled-release (i.e., extended) dosage forms are very similar to those for immediate-release, solid oral dosage forms, the criteria for those excipients affecting the release rate are, understandably, more onerous.

On the other hand, the comparability of the drug substance and excipients with those of the innovators product listed by the FDA as the "Reference Listed Drug"

(RLD), assumes (under the FDA's SUPAC guidelines) considerably greater importance for sterile and nonsterile semisolid formulations than, for solid oral dosage forms. With the semisolid dosage forms, the FDA uses various types of diffusion analyses in lieu of dissolution as a surrogate for in vivo bioequivalence.

In general, semisolid dosage forms are complex formulations having complex structural elements. Often, they are composed of two phases (oil and water), one of which is a continuous (external) phase and the other of which is a dispersed (internal) phase. The active ingredient is often dissolved in one phase, although occasionally the drug is not fully soluble in the system and is dispersed in one or both phases, creating a three-phase system. The physical properties of the dosage form depend on various factors including the size of the dispersed particles, the interfacial tension between phases, the partition coefficient of the active ingredient between phases, and the product rheology. These factors combine to determine the release characteristics of the drug as well as other characteristics such as viscosity.

Although for a true solution, the order in which solutes are added to the solvent is usually unimportant, this is not true for dispersed formulations. Because dispersed matter can distribute differently depending on the phase to which a particulate substance is added, the order of addition for these formulations is of critical importance. Any change in the order of addition, therefore, is a major change.

Over a period of years, the FDA, monitoring the performance of a variety of physical and chemical tests commonly performed on semisolid products and their components (e.g., solubility, particle size, and crystalline form of the active component; viscosity; and homogeneity of the product), has determined that these tests provide evidence of consistent performance. Although the evidence available at this time is less convincing than in vitro dissolution as a surrogate for in vivo bioequivalence in the case of solid oral dosage forms, the FDA is using diffusion testing (i.e., in vitro release-rate testing) to assess product "sameness" to allow certain SUPAC for semisolid products.

STABILITY

In addition, the FDA requires that every marketed product be stable, meeting its approved specifications throughout its marketed shelf-life. Generally, for minor changes, in addition to the application or compendial chemistry and manufacturing control requirements

(CMC), long-term stability data from one batch must be filed when available in the annual report. For moderate changes, the general requirement is for accelerated (3-month) stability data from one batch filed in either a CBE supplement or a PAS, plus long-term stability data from one batch filed in an appropriate annual report. For major changes, in addition to the long-term stability data for one batch filed in an annual report, 3-month accelerated stability data must be submitted in a PAS for either one or three batches, depending on how long that particular product has been in the marketplace. For new chemical entities, the period is 5 years, whereas for a new dosage form of an approved chemical entity, the period is 3 years. If the product meets this market criterion, a "substantive body of information" is said to exist, and data from one batch are required to be submitted. If a product does not meet this marketing criterion, a "significant body of information" is said not to exist, and data from three batches are required to be submitted. In any case, the data must be filed in a supplement requiring FDA preapproval (i.e., PAS).

SURROGATE MEASURES OF EFFICACY

For 30 years, the FDA has satisfactorily used in vivo bioequivalence as a surrogate of clinical efficacy for the development of new dosage forms and strengths of innovative products and for approval of generic versions of approved marketed drugs. It additionally requires human in vivo bioequivalence studies for most major postapproval changes, as well as for moderate post-approval changes for narrow therapeutic index drugs. In those cases where an in vivo/in vitro correlation has been established for a particular product, it may be used in lieu of in vivo bioequivalence.

However, the FDA uses in vitro dissolution as a surrogate for in vivo bioequivalence testing for most minor and moderate postapproval changes. For implementation of minor changes, the dissolution requirement is usually the same as that required by the FDA for the release of an approved product into the marketplace. On the other hand, for moderate changes, the FDA usually requires additional in vitro dissolution testing. The type of dissolution study required for solid oral dosage forms varies depending on several drug variables, e.g., solubility, permeability, therapeutic index, and dosage form.

Minor changes may be implemented for drugs that are both soluble (at the largest strength marketed) and permeable (bioavailability >90%) if the product meets

the SUPAC single-point dissolution criteria of 85% in 15 minutes. Those that fail this test must meet a more onerous multipoint dissolution test in which samples are taken every 15 min until either 85% is dissolved or an asymptote is reached, thus establishing a dissolution rate profile. Modified-release preparations must additionally meet the profile criterion in water and buffered aqueous solutions. The dissolution profiles comparing product manufactured after the change with that manufactured before the change must be comparable. The FDA accepts comparability if the profiles meet the FDA "F-2" similarity test criterion (11). Failure to establish comparable dissolution profiles would normally necessitate human in vivo bioequivalence studies or use of an in vivo/in vitro correlation. In addition delayed-release solid oral dosage forms must pass the compendial 2-h acid-dissolution test.

In the case of semisolid dosage forms, the FDA uses a standard open-chamber diffusion cell fitted with a synthetic membrane as the in vitro release test to be used as a surrogate for in vivo bioequivalence studies. It uses this test for semisolid dosage form SUPAC changes, just as it used dissolution in the case of solid oral dosage forms. The FDA guidance recommends using the test on all creams, ointments, and gels. In this test, a plot of the amount of drug released per unit area of membrane ($\mu g/cm^2$) versus the square root of time should yield a straight line. The regression (slope of the line) represents the drug release rate. Comparisons of the release rate before and after making the change are required. In the case in which the change is not similar, in vivo bioequivalence data would be required to implement the change.

POSTSCRIPT

SUPAC is a revolutionary change in drug regulation. For nearly all of the 20th century, congressional action increased industry's regulatory burden in response to what was perceived as industry's irresponsible actions. This was accompanied by an ever-increasing cost to develop and market new drugs and a concomitant increase in the time required to obtain marketing approval from the FDA. In the last 2 decades, many perceived that the United States was falling behind in the drug development process and that, as a result, Americans were not able to obtain new state-of-the-art treatments for serious diseases in timely manner. With the passage of the Food and Drug Administration Modernization Act (FADAMA), Congress allowed the FDA to employ additional scientists while at the same time mandated management efficiencies in the drug review process. SUPAC is a reversal of the ever-increasing authority of the U.S. drug regulatory body. It empowers the industry to take responsibility for its actions, while simultaneously allowing adequate overview of the drug development and marketing process by the FDA.

Because of FADAMA, the SUPAC process has been extended by the FDA to include sterile dosage forms, analytical methods, product labeling, and product packaging postapproval changes.

Two important updates of previously published SUPAC guidances include the change in multiple SUPAC changes and the redefinition of "site of manufacturer". For all SUPAC guidances, multiple postapproval changes are now permitted. The requirements that must be fulfilled default to those for the most restrictive change proposed. For example, three level-one changes and one level-two change would have to meet the more restrictive level-two criteria.

In addition, although the definition of "same site/different site" will remain the same for foreign manufacturers until a May 14, 1999, proposed regulation requiring registration of foreign manufacturers who want to market drugs in the United States is published in final form, the definition for domestic manufacturers has been changed. In the latter case, Same Site is defined as the site in which the new and old buildings are included under the same drug establishment registration number, and the operations in both are inspected by the same FDA district office. Different site is defined as the site where the new and old buildings have different drug establishment registration numbers or when the operations are inspected by different FDA district offices.

REFERENCES

1. *Immediate Release Solid Oral Dosage Forms: Scale-Up and Post Approval Changes*, Center for Drug Evaluation and Research (CDER): March 1995; FDA Guidance for Industry.

2. *SUPAC-MR—Modified Release Solid Oral Dosage Forms: Scale-Up and Post Approval Changes*, Center for Drug Evaluation and Research (CDER): Sept 1997; FDA Guidance for Industry.

3. *Non-Sterile Semisolid Dosage Forms: Scale-Up and Post Approval Changes*, Center for Drug Evaluation and Research (CDER): May 1997; FDA Guidance for Industry.

4. Skelly, J.P.; Barr, W.; Benet, L.; Doluisio, J.; Goldberg, A.; Levy, G.; Lowenthal, D.; Robinson, J.; Shah, V.; Temple, R.; Yacobi, A. Report of a Workshop on Controlled Release Dosage Forms: Issues and Controversies. Pharm. Res. **1987**, *4* (1), 75–77.

5. Skelly, J.P.; Amidon, G.L.; Barr, W.; Benet, L.; Carter, J.R.; Robinson, J.; Shah, V.; Yacobi, A. In Vitro and In Vivo Testing and Correlation for Oral Controlled/Modified Release Forms. J. Pharm. Sci. **1990**, *79* , 849–854.

6. Shah, V.; Midha, K.K.; Dighe, S.; Skelly, J.P.; Layloff, T.; McGilveray, I.J.; Viswanathan, C.T.; Yacobi, A. Analytical Method Validation: Bioavailability, Bioequivalence, and Pharmacokinetics Studies. Pharm. Res. **1992**, *9*, 588–590.

7. Skelly, J.P.; Van Buskirk, G.; Savello, D.R.; Amidon, G.L.; Arbit, H.M.; Dighe, S.; Fawzi, M.B.; Gonzalez, M.; Malick, A.W.; Malinowski, H.; Nedich, R.; Pearce, D.M.; Peck, G.E.; Schwartz, J.B.; Shah, V.P.; Shangraw, R.F.; Truelove, J.P. Scale-Up of Solid Oral Immediate Release Dosage Forms. J. Pharm. Res. **1993**, *10*, 313–316.

8. Skelly, J.P.; Van Buskirk, G.A.; Savello, D.; Augsburger, L.; Theeuves, F.; Leeson, L.; Lesko, L.; Barr, W.H.; Amidon, G.; Gonzalez, M.; Malinowski, H.; Berge, S.; Fox, D.; Wheatly, T.; Nixon, P.; Porter, S.; Clevenger, J.; Dighe, S.; Arbit, H.; Pearce, D.M.; Peck, G.E.; Jerussi, R.; Hoiberg, C.; Schwartz, J.; Shah, V.P.; Robinson, J.; Shangraw, R. Scale-Up of Oral Extended Release Dosage Forms. Pharm. Res. **1993**, *10*, 1800–1805.

9. Van Buskirk, G.A.; Shah, V.; Adair, D.; Arbit, H.M.; Dighe, S.; Fawzi, M.; Feldman, T.; Flynn, G.L.; Gonzalez, M.; Gray, V.; Guy, R.; Herd, A.K.; Hem, S.L.; Hoiberg, C.; Jerussi, R.; Kaplan, A.S.; Lesko, J.; Malinowski, H.; Meltzer, N.; Nedich, R.; Pearce, D.; Peck, G.E.; Rudman, A.; Savello, D.; Schwartz, J.B.; Skelly, J.P.; Vanderlaan, R.K.; Wang, J.C.; Weiner, N.; Winkel, D.; Zatz, J.L. Workshop III Report: Scale-Up of Liquid and Semisolid Disperse Systems. Pharm. Res. **1994**, *11* (8), 1216–1220.

10. *Changes to an Approved NDA or ANDA*, US, DHHS, FDA, Center for Drug Evaluation and Research (CDER), Nov 1999; FDA Guidance for Industry.

11. *Dissolution Testing of Immediate Release Solid Oral Dosage Forms* US, DHHS, FDA, Center for Drug Evaluation and Research (CDER), Aug 1997; FDA Guidance for Industry.

SECONDARY ELECTRON MICROSCOPY IN PHARMACEUTICAL TECHNOLOGY

Peter C. Schmidt
University of Tübingen, Tübingen, Germany

BASIC PRINCIPLES OF ELECTRON MICROSCOPY

Introduction

Basic principles of imaging

The principle of an electron microscope is based on the light microscope except that electrons are used instead of light. The resolving power of any microscope is given by Abbe's equation:

$$d_0 = \frac{0.61 \cdot \lambda}{n \sin \alpha} [\text{nm}] \tag{1}$$

where d_0 = minimum resolvable separation distance; λ = wavelength of the light; n = refractive index of the medium between the object and the objective lens; and α = half-angle subtended by the objective at the object.

The lower the minimum resolvable distance the higher the resolution of the instrument. Therefore, the resolution is enhanced by a short wavelength of the light, a high refractive index of the medium between the objective lens and the object, and a small distance between the object and the lens. The product $n \sin \alpha$ is called the numerical aperture of the objective lens. Since α can never exceed 90°, an objective in air can never resolve distances smaller than 0.61 λ. The limits of a light microscope are given in Table 1.

De Broglie (2) showed that an electron has a dual character. It can be regarded either as a moving charged single particle or as a radiation with a distinct wavelength. The relation between the two is given by Eq. 2:

$$\lambda = \frac{h}{m v} [\text{nm}] \tag{2}$$

where λ = wavelength; h = Planck's constant; m = mass of the electron; and v = velocity of the electron.

The velocity of the electron depends on the voltage applied and can be used to calculate the wavelength, λ, and the minimum resolvable distance, d_0, as shown in Table 2.

The advantage of the use of electrons as a light source compared with visible light is obvious.

Types of electrons in electronic imaging

When an electron beam is interacting with a specimen surface, different reactions can occur. The various signals arising from the specimen's surface on incidence of the primary electron beam are shown in Fig. 1.

Secondary electrons (SEs): A collison of electrons from the primary electron beam with the surface of the specimen results in a detachment of the so-called SEs. The number of SEs depends on the surface topography, the accelerating voltage, and the atomic number of the surface elements. They create the SE current, which is collected for imaging.

Backscattered electrons (BSEs): These are primary electrons that have been reflected from the specimen surface in a way that they return back out of the specimen again. Depending on the individual collision, they have energies ranging from the full primary energy of the electron beam down to the level of secondary electrons. Their intensity increases with increasing atomic number. They give information on the topography of the sample and the atomic number of the sample elements.

X-ray photons (X): Photons of X-radiation are emitted from the specimen under electron bombardment. They are characteristic for elements and could be used to determine the element distribution on the surface of the sample under investigation.

Transmitted electrons (TEs): TEs are those penetrating through a thin specimen that are focussed into images on a phosphor luminescence screen or on a photosensitive material.

Absorbed electrons (AEs): Some of the primary electrons are absorbed by the specimen and are grounded as a current. If there is no ground connection, the specimen will charge up.

Cathodoluminescence (CL): This is a light emission of the specimen under electron bombardment. The light could be visible or invisible.

In secondary electron microscopy (SEM), in most cases, SEs are used for imaging. BSE detectors are closely connected with element analysis of the specimen. Other types are more or less seldom used in electron microscopy.

Table 1 Minimum resolvable distance, d_0, of a light microscope depending on the wavelength λ, the refractive index n, and the angle α

Wavelength λ (nm)	Angle α (°)	Refractive index n	Minimum resolving distance d_0 (nm)
800	15	1.000[a]	1885
400	15	1.000[a]	942
800	30	1.000[a]	976
400	30	1.000[a]	488
800	60	1.000[a]	563
400	60	1.000[a]	281
800	60	1.516[b]	371
400	60	1.516[b]	185

[a]Air.
[b]Oil.
(Adapted from Ref. 1.)

Table 2 Variation of electron velocity, wavelength, and minimum resolvable distance with accelerating voltage for an electron microscope

Acceleration voltage (kV)	Velocity (km/h)	λ (nm)	d_0[a] (nm)
1	18, 370	0.03876	0.0169
10	58, 460	0.01220	0.0053
100	164, 400	0.00370	0.0016

[a]According to Eq. 1, assuming that $n \cdot \sin \alpha = 1.4$.
(Adapted from Ref. 3.)

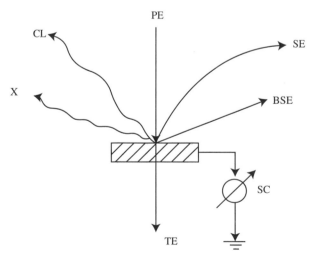

Fig. 1 Signals arising from the specimen's surface on incidence of the primary electronic beam (4), where PE = primary electronic beam; SE = secondary electrons; BSE = backscattered electrons; X = X-ray photons; TE = transmitted electrons; SC = absorbed electrons; and CL = cathodoluminescence.

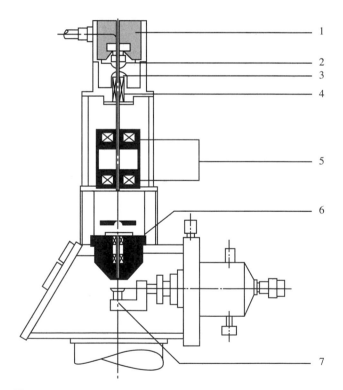

Fig. 2 The design of a secondary electron microscope (4), where 1 = electronic gun; 2 = Wehnelt cylinder; 3 = anode; 4 = beam alignment coils; 5 = condensor lenses; 6 = objective lens; and 7 = specimen holder.

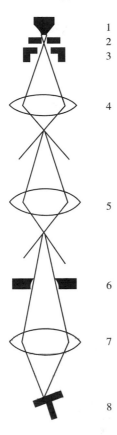

Fig. 3 The electronic beam arrangement modified from (4), where 1 = cathode; 2 = Wehnelt cylinder; 3 = anode; 4 + 5 = electromagnetic condensor lenses; 6 = aperture; 7 = objective lens; and 8 = specimen surface.

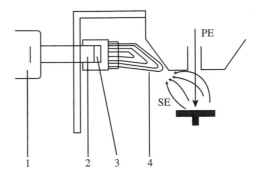

Fig. 5 The secondary electron detector (4), where 1 = photomultiplier; 2 = light guide; 3 = scintillator; 4 = collector; PE = primary electron beam; and SE = secondary electron beam.

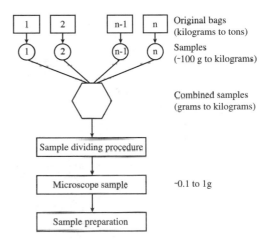

Fig. 6 Sampling procedure to create a small sample ready for microscopic examination.

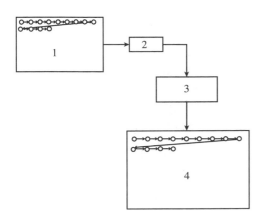

Fig. 4 Principle of the scanning mode of a secondary electron microscope (4), where 1 = specimen surface; 2 = detector; 3 = video processing; and 4 = monitor screen.

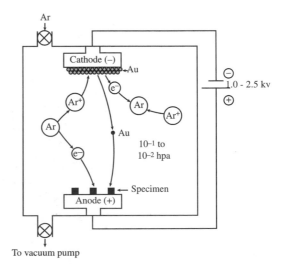

Fig. 7 Principle of the cathodic sputtering process.

In transmission electron microscopy (TEM), transmitted electrons will be processed to give an image.

Secondary Electron Microscope

Among the different types of electron microscopes such as the secondary electron microscope (SEM), the transmission electron microscope (TEM), the scanning transmission electron microscope (STEM), and the field emission scanning transmission electron microsope (FESTEM), the SEM finds greater application in the field of pharmaceutical technology, followed by the TEM. This article will focus only on the principle of the SEM.

The design of a SEM is shown in Fig. 2.

It consists of the electronic gun (**1**), the Wehnelt cylinder (**2**), the anode (**3**), and beam alignment coils (**4**) on the top of the instrument. The condensor lenses (**5**), the aperture, and the objective lens (**6**) focus the beam onto the specimen that is mounted on the specimen holder (**7**). The latter one could be moved in X-, Y-, and Z-direction within the specimen chamber. In addition, the sample could be moved by rotation. The arrangement to create the electronic beam is shown in Fig. 3.

The electrons are emitted by the cathode (**1**) from a filament, normally a heated tungsten wire. The emitted electron current is controlled by a Wehnelt cylinder (**2**) having a negative polarity against the cathode. The electrons are picked up by the anode (**3**) after being

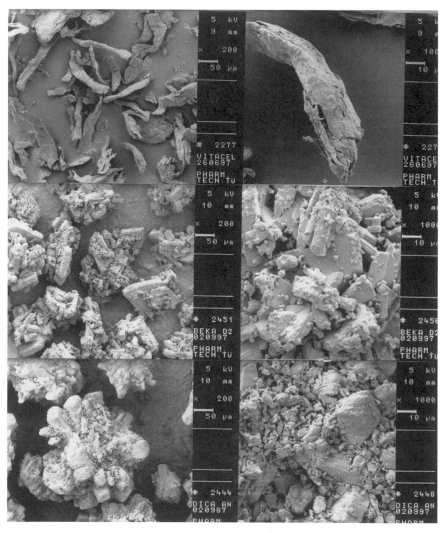

Fig. 8 Microcrystalline cellulose (Vitacel) (top), dicalcium phosphate dihydrate (Bekapress D2) (middle), and dicalcium phosphate anhydrous (Dicaphos AN) (bottom).

accelerated by the accelerating voltage of approximately 1–25 kV. The cathode assembly and the anode are arranged so as to produce a crossover of the electron beam between the components. Through the bore hole of the anode the electron beam enters two electromagnetic condensor lenses (**4** and **5**), which reduce the crossover. After passing the aperture (**6**), the electron beam is focussed by the objective lens (**7**) so that the focal spot is imaged on the specimen surface (**8**).

The specimen is scanned point by point by the electron beam as shown in Fig. 4. Secondary electrons that are emitted from the specimen's surface (**1**) are collected by the detector (**2**) and undergo a video processing (**3**) leading to the image formed on the video screen (**4**).

The electron beam is moved on the surface of the specimen by an electromagnetic deflection system that is integrated in the objective lens moving the beam in a raster over the specimen as mentioned above. The deflection system consits of two sets of crossed saddle coils for deflection in X and in Y direction. The saddle coils produce distortion-free images at lowest magnifications and permit large deflection angles.

The secondary electron detector (Fig. 5) (**4**) is mounted to the side of the microscope chamber. Primary electrons (PEs) liberate secondary ones (SEs) from the specimen's surface, which are caught by the collector (**4**) having a positive potential for the detection of SE. The electrons pass through the grid and move toward the scintillator (**3**). This is biased to +10 kV and accelerates the low-energy SEs to a higher energy level. These electrons strike the scintillator, where they generate photons, which are guided out of the detector chamber through a light guide (**2**) to the photomultiplier (**1**). The photomultiplier converts the light current by amplification again into an electron current that presents the video signal at the output of the subsequent preamplifier. If the collector is at a negative potential, only backscattered electrons (BSE) can strike the scintillator and a BSE image is produced in this mode.

Electrons move over long distances only under vacuum. The whole system, therefore, has to be operated under a vacuum of 10^{-5} to 10^{-7} hPa. The vacuum system consists of a rotary pump giving a vacuum up to 10^{-3} hPa combined with a water-cooled turbomolecular pump leading to the desired high vacuum. In some instruments, an oil-diffusion pump is used instead of a turbomolecular pump. An automatic control ensures that the system cannot be run without water cooling and at a low vacuum level.

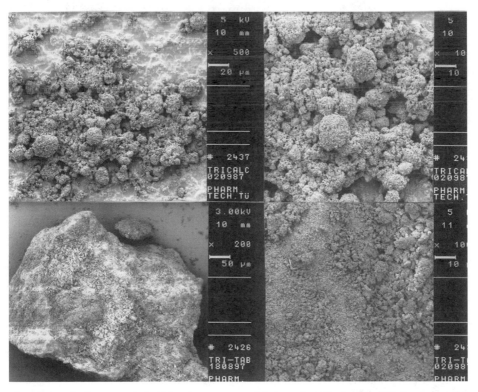

Fig. 9 Tricalcium phosphates (hydroxyapatite). Tricaphos, a spray-dried product (top), and Tritab, prepared by roller compaction (bottom).

SAMPLE PREPARATION IN SCANNING ELECTRON MICROSCOPY

Introduction

Most of the samples being investigated by SEM in the field of pharmaceutical technology are powders prepared by different methods, granules, pellets, tablets, and films from coated tablets. The sample preparation of bulk materials includes the following steps:

1. choosing a representative sample from the bulk material;
2. mounting the sample on a suitable sample holder (specimen); and

3. preparing the specimen for observation by coating, if it is not self-conducting.

In pharmaceutical technology, materials are handled quite often as a bulk. Due to the fact that electron microscopic imaging is based on very small samples, the sampling procedure itself and the preparation of the final sample become very important. An overview for sampling procedures is given by Sommer (5). A scheme for powder sampling is given in Fig. 6.

The initial samples from the original bags are normally taken by hand. Depending on the size of the bag they have to be taken from different places. They are then combined by mixing before undergoing the sampling procedure.

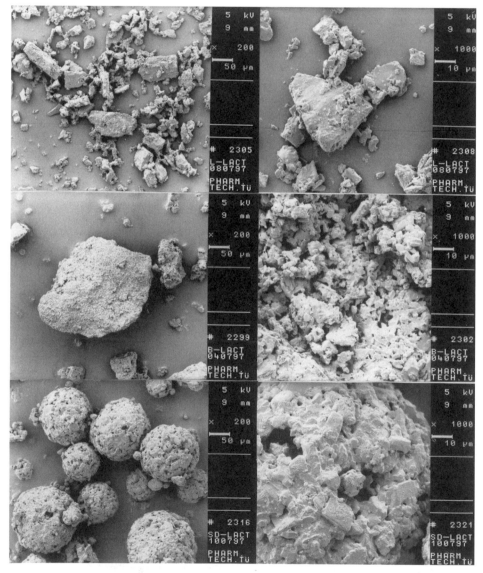

Fig. 10 Lactoses. α-lactose monohydrate (top), β-lactose (middle), and spray-dried lactose (bottom).

Today, these procedures are carried out by sampling machines like a rotary sample divider.

Depending on the size of the combined sample, the procedure has to be done in several steps if necessary. At the end a sample size directly applicable to the microscopic sample preparation must be achieved.

Specimen Preparation for Secondary Electron Microscopy

In pharmaceutical technology, most of the samples that are examined by an SEM are powders. After the sampling procedure, the final sample has to be distributed uniformly onto a stub and later on—if it is not self-conducting—covered by a layer of a conducting material. The stubs are either pin-type mushroom or cylinders normally made from aluminum. In most of our work, simply metal rivets were used instead of the expensive aluminum stubs offered by the suppliers of SEM accessories. The stubs have to be cleaned carefully by a surfactant solution followed by distilled water and acetone in an ultrasonic bath. Finally, the traces of acetone should be removed by a warm air stream. The surface of the stubs is then covered by a double-adhesive tape. Conductivity of the tape is ensured by a small droplet of conducting silver fluid, which is placed between one end of the tape and the stub. Coarse powders

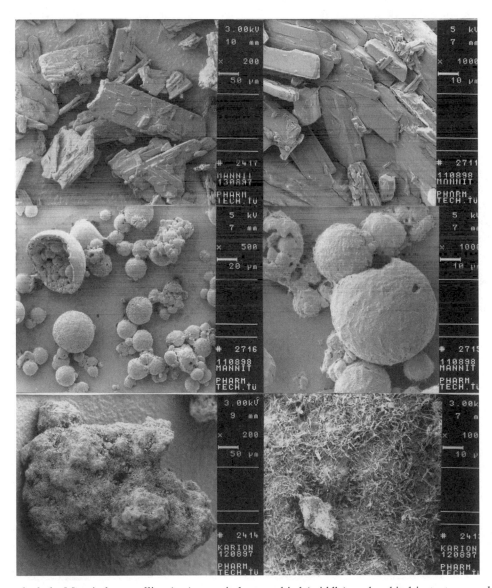

Fig. 11 Sugar alcohols. Mannitol, crystalline (top), mannitol, spray dried (middle), and sorbitol-instant, spray dried (bottom).

are directly sprinkled onto the so-prepared stubs, and fine ones have to be desagglomerated. Depending on the degree of agglomeration this could be done either by blowing the material onto the stub by an air stream or by sucking it through a pipe by vacuum. Also, the "Rhodos" dry powder desaggregation unit of the Sympatec-Helos Particle Sizer (6) could be used to blow the powder onto a stub. Other samples like tablets, coated tablets, pellets, packaging materials, and needles of syringes can be directly mounted to the stub by the use of colloidal silver paste, bonding the sample to the stub mechanically and electrically. For other preparation methods the reader is recommended to refer to a special literature (7).

A part of the primary electron beam, amounting 10^{-12} to 10^{-6} A, is emitted as secondary or backscattered electron current. The difference between the two currents must be allowed to leak away to earth via the stub, otherwise the specimen will charge up. If a sample is not self-conducting it has to be provided with a thin conducting coat. Only at a low accelerating voltage in

the range of 1 kV, a sample does not need to be conductive. The coating is performed under vacuum either by evaporating carbon, gold/palladium, or platinum or by d.c. sputtering. The latter is the most popular and easy technique to apply conductive coatings to a sample. The principle of sputtering is shown in Fig. 7.

The apparatus consists of an evacuated chamber, a cathode, and an anode. The air within the chamber is replaced by an inert gas, preferably argon, and the voltage applied to the system is in the range of 1.0–2.5 kV. Under these conditions a glow discharge is set up between cathode and anode. Neutral gas atoms are ionized to positively charged argon ions and electrons. The ions are attracted by the cathode, where they cause an emission of a gold atom and an electron from the cathode material. The electron neutralizes an argon ion, the Au atom is moving toward the anode. On the way there are a lot of collisions with gas atoms and as a result the Au atoms arrive at the anode from different directions where they settle onto the specimen's surface. Free electrons are accelerated in

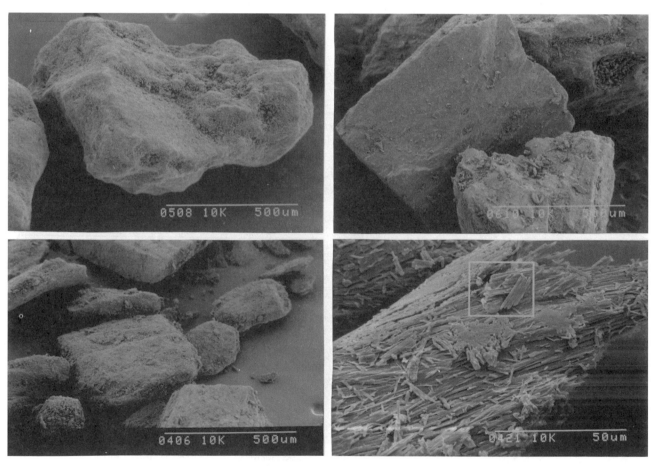

Fig. 12 Different types of sorbitol.

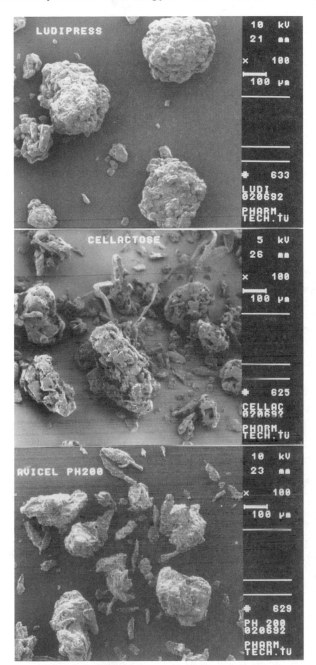

Fig. 13 Ludipress (93% α-lactose monohydrate, 3.5% soluble povidone, 3.5% cross-linked povidone) (top), Cellactose (75% α-lactose monohydrate, 25% powdered cellulose) (middle), and Avicel PH 200 (agglomerated microcrystalline cellulose) (bottom).

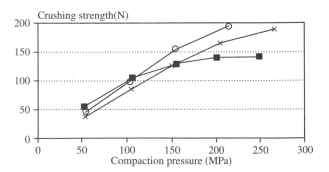

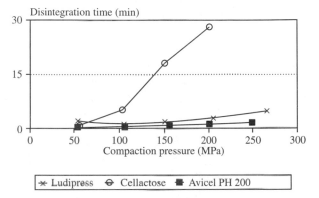

Fig. 14 Compressional pressure/hardness-profile and compressional pressure/disintegration profile of the coprocessed materials, Ludipress, Cellactose, and Avicel PH 200.

the direction of the anode, and when reaching the anode, create heat in the specimen.

The process itself and the deposition of metal atoms onto the specimen's surface depends on the target material, the type and pressure of the inert gas within the chamber, the cathode potential, the current, the time of sputtering, and the distance between the target, and the sample. The preferred gas is argon, having the lowest price of all inert gases. Air could not be used because it causes oxidation of metals, e.g., gold. A black coating indicates the presence of air during the sputtering process. With argon the sputtering rate of gold and silver is high compared with carbon. The coating thickness is determined by the sputtering rate, the distance between the target and the sample, and the time. There is a linear correlation between the thickness of the gold layer and the sputtering time at constant conditions.

The quality of the coat has to be judged by the homogeneity of the thickness, adhesion onto the surface of the sample, and its mechanical stability. Plain surfaces result in a uniform coating thickness. At rough surfaces, a uniform coating can only be achieved when the metal atoms settle diffuse from all directions. This could be predetermined by the vacuum applied. The optimum coating thickness is a compromise between the conductivity of the coated sample and the resolution of fine surface structures. If the conductivity is not high enough, a charge up of the specimen is observed. For routine imaging a coating thickness of 1 to 2.0 nm is sufficient.

APPLICATION OF SECONDARY ELECTRON MICROSCOPY IN PHARMACEUTICAL TECHNOLOGY

The application of SEM in the field of pharmaceutical technology is widespread. Solid starting materials for any kind of formulation can be visualized as well as powder mixtures, granulations, pellets, tablets, coatings, spray- and freeze-dried products, microparticles, liposomes, and packaging materials. Although there are articles dealing with SEM investigations of raw materials (8–10) and some other materials, a general review on the applications of SEM in pharmaceutical technology is not available. Thus, this section attempts to fill the gap in the literature. The following examples were taken from our own experience over 13 years. They do not cover the whole field, but they have been selected to demonstrate that a lot of problems can be solved by the view through a microscope.

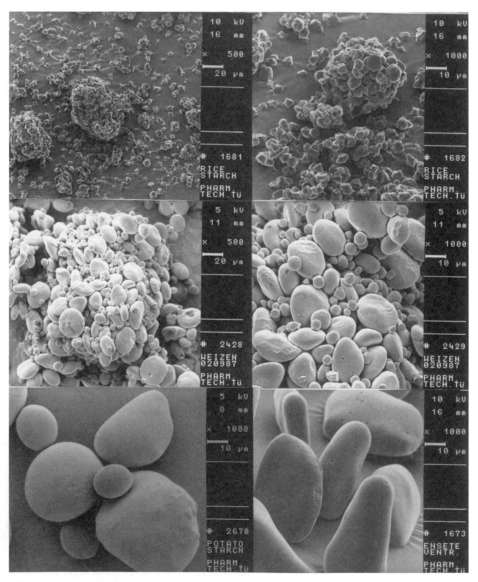

Fig. 15 Starches used in pharmacy. Rice starch (top), wheat starch (middle), potato starch (bottom left), and enset starch (false banana) (bottom right).

Starting Materials

Filler/binders

Filler/binders are used in direct compression of tablets. The requirements they have to fulfill are summarized by Khan and Rhodes (11). An important factor in the evaluation of filler/binders is their so-called "dilution potential," i.e., giving an amount of active ingredient that can be taken up by the filler/binder to produce a tablet according to previously fixed specifications.

Filler/binders belong to the following classes of substances: microcrystalline and powdered celluloses, lactoses, phosphates, particularly calcium phosphates, sugar alcohols, and the so-called "co-processed materials,"

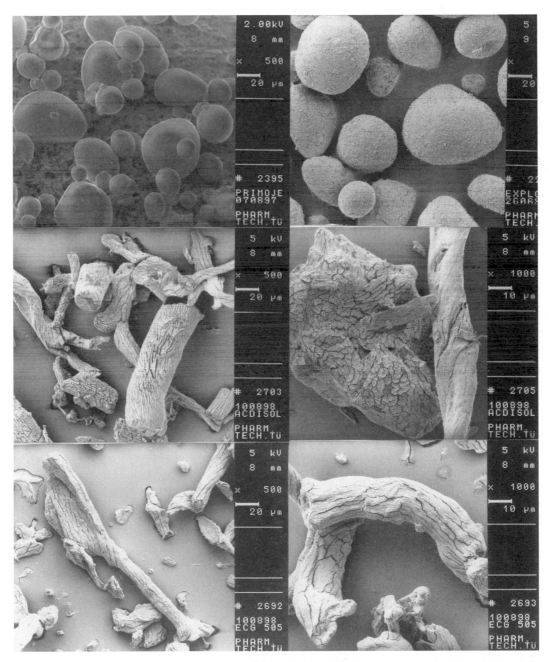

Fig. 16 Disintegrants. Primojel (top left), Explotab, both sodium starch glycolates (top right), cross-linked carboxymethyl cellulose (middle), and calcium carboxymethyl cellulose (bottom).

which are especially designed combinations for-direct compression (12). The following figures (Figs. 8–13) show filler/binders at differant magnifications. Figure 8 (top) depicts microcrystalline cellulose (Vitacel). The fibrous structure is typical for all products of this type and differs significantly from the calcium phosphates shown below. The dicalcium phosphate dihydrate (Bekapress D2) in the middle is composed of small agglomerates, whereas

the anhydrous type (Dicaphos AN) is agglomerated to a higher extent. In Fig. 9 two types of tricalcium phosphates are presented. Crystallographically both are hydroxyapatites. Tricaphos (top) is a spray-dried product showing typically rounded particles built from very small crystallites, whereas Tritab is a granulation prepared by roller compaction (bottom). For detailed description of calcium phosphates see the relevant literature (13–16).

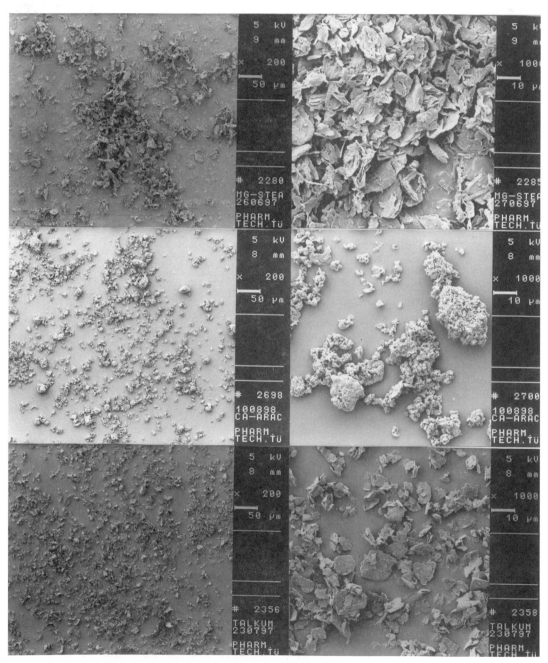

Fig. 17 Lubricants. Magnesium stearate (top), calcium arachinate (middle), and talc (bottom).

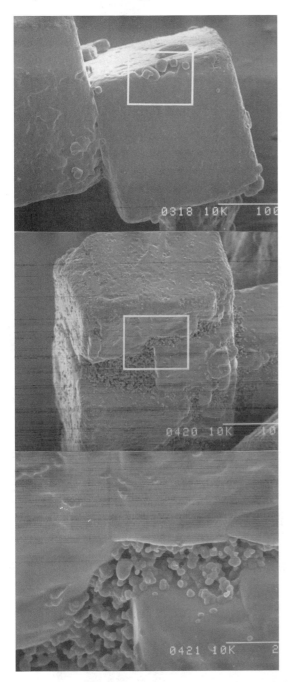

Fig. 18 Partially interactive powder mixture between sodium chloride (top) and micronized etilefrine HCl. The bottom picture is an extension of the middle. Etilefrine HCl settle at crystal irregularities of the cubic sodium chloride.

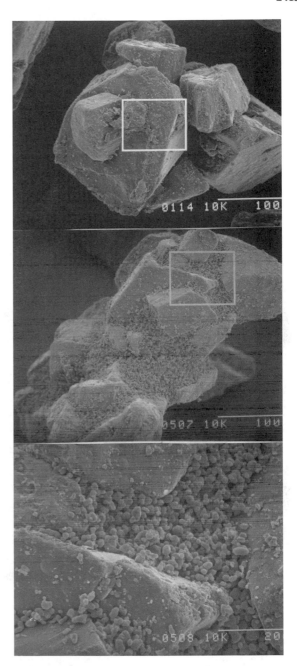

Fig. 19 Interactive mixture between lactose (top) and micronized etilefrine HCl. The bottom picture is an extension from the middle. Due to more crystal irregularities, there is a higher adherence of the etilefrine HCl onto the carrier.

Figure 10 presents three different types of lactoses. The typically wedge-shaped α-lactose monohydrate (top) differs significantly from the roller dried β-lactose (middle), and the ball-shaped, spray-dried lactose (bottom), which shows the highest compactability due to

its agglomerated form and its content of 8–15% of amorphous lactose (17).

The sugar alcohols, mannitol and sorbitol are quite often used in the preparation of buccal and sublingual tablets as well as lozenges. Fig. 11 shows the morphological differences between a crystallized (top) and a spray-dried mannitol (middle). Sorbitol, of which the γ-polymorph is used in direct compression, has to be regarded as the "chameleon" of tablet excipients. The spray-dried instant product (Fig. 11, bottom) is of irregular shape and shows fine needles on higher magnification. A product obtained from a melt (Fig. 12, top left) has a more regular surface as well as products that have been produced by crystallization (top right and bottom left). At higher magnifications the latter product exhibits a completely different structure compared to spray-dried sorbitol (18–20).

Figure 13 depicts the SEM pictures of three different co-processed materials (21). Ludipress, being mostly α-lactose monohydrate, shows fairly round agglomerates,

Cellactose, containing 25% of a powdered cellulose, is composed of lactose agglomerates from which the incorporated cellulose fibers protrude like tentacles. Avicel PH 200, a pure microcrystalline cellulose is an agglomerated irregular-shaped product (22).

The compressional properties of these materials with respect to hardness are similar, whereas the disintegration time shows for Cellactose a tremendous increase at compressional pressures above 100 MPa as shown in Fig. 14 (23).

Disintegrants

Starches are used as disintegrants in tablets, as binders after gelatinization in granulations, as carriers in spray drying, and as fillers and moisture absorbers in external

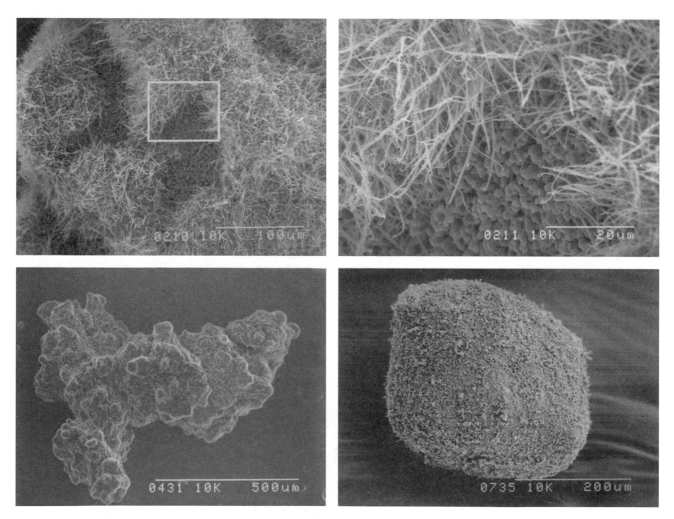

Fig. 20 Interactive mixtures with sorbitol as a carrier. Sorbitol plus 16% micronized etilefrine HCl, part of the granule (top left), sectional view from left showing the fine sorbitol needles and the micronized particles of etilefrine (top right). Pure sorbitol instant (bottom left), sorbitol plus 16% propranolol (bottom right).

powders. As disintegrants they are used in quite high concentrations ranging from 10 to 15% of a tablet formulation. Figure 15 presents rice (top) and wheat (middle) starches in two different magnifications. On the bottom left potato starch (one of the most commonly used starches) is shown together with starch from an Ethiopian plant called Enset false banana (*Ensete ventricosum*) showing particles of a very distinctive shape having a similar size as potato starch (24).

Besides starches, starch derivatives like sodium starch glycolate (Primojel, Explotab) are used as disintegrants as they exhibit enhanced disintegrating power. Although both products (Primojel and Explotab) are chemically identical, their microscopic behavior is different (Fig. 16, top). Primojel has a smooth surface and Explotab has a rough surface, resulting from their preparation methods that attribute to the differences in their disintegrating action (25).

Derivatives of celluloses like Ac-di-Sol and E.C.G. 505 act as the so-called "super disintegrants" (26, 27). Their microscopic pictures are similar to cellulose fibers. The

materials, however, could not be distinguished by microscopic examination.

Lubricants

Among lubricants, magnesium stearate is the most widely used one. It appears in different crystal forms, shows different particle size and shape, and occurs in several hydrate forms (28, 29). Its lubricating effectiveness was described by Delacourte et al. (30). The platelet form (Fig. 17) seems to have some advantages. Magnesium stearate is capable of forming films on other tablet excipients during prolonged mixing, leading to a prolonged drug liberation time (31), a decrease in hardness, and an increase in disintegration time (32, 33). For comparison reasons, calcium arachinate and talc are presented in Fig. 17. Calcium arachinate differs from the others by showing a microparticle structure instead of platelets.

The lubricating ability of talc is less compared with magnesium stearate, although both substances are microscopically similar (34).

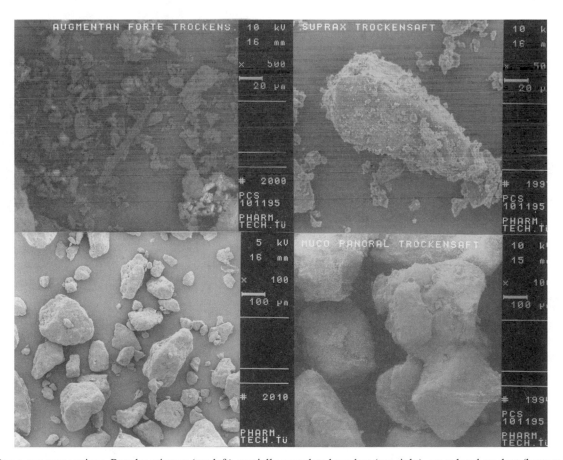

Fig. 21 Dry syrup preparations. Powder mixture (top left), partially granulated product (top right), granulated product (bottom left), and coated crystals, partially agglomerated (bottom right).

Powder Mixtures

Powder mixtures could be random (35–39) or "ordered" mixtures (40). The latter were later on called "interactive" mixtures (41) due to the fact that they are not of a higher degree of order. The mixing homogeneity of an interactive mixture is not better compared with a random one, but it leads to an interaction between a fine component and a coarse carrier and then to a higher stability of the system. Pharmaceutical powder mixtures are quite often between a random and an interactive mixture, and hence they are partially interactive. The degree of interaction depends on the following parameters:

1. particle size of the "adherent" fine powder;
2. particle size and surface structure of the coarse carrier;
3. cohesion forces between the "fines";
4. adhesion forces between the "fines" and the coarse carrier particles; and
5. relation between the amount of "fines" and coarse particles.

The following examples deal with interactive powder mixtures (42, 43). Figure 18 shows on top a sodium chloride crystal. When mixing the sodium chloride with 16% of a micronized etilefrine HCl, a partially interactive powder mixture results (Fig. 18, middle and bottom). The micronized active ingredient is preferentially adhered onto crystal irregularities. In these regions multilayers of etilefrine HCl are obtained. When choosing lactose as a carrier instead of sodium chloride, the situation changes (Fig. 19). Due to the more irregular crystals, there is a higher degree of visible adhering particles (middle). The extension of this figure (bottom) shows again the concentration of fines at crystal irregularities. Special effects could be achieved when using sorbitol instant as a carrier. Sorbitol instant is produced by spray drying and subsequent instantization. Fig. 20 presents such a particle showing an irregular shape and a rough surface. Mixing this product with 16% of etilefrine HCL (top left) results in an adherence tendency to the "valleys" of the sorbitol particle. The extension (top right) shows the fibrous structure of the spray-dried sorbitol and the micronized particles. When using 16% of micronized propranolol HCl instead of etilefrine as the active ingredient being mixed, a total coverage of the sorbitol particle is obtained. Since propranolol has a higher adhesion and cohesion tendency, after filling up the sorbitol "valleys" it covers the whole surface.

Dry Syrup Preparations

Dry syrup preparations are powdered or granular formulations prepared for reconstitution. They are filled up to volume by a liquid, normally water, just before use. During production and storage they are solids and during administration they are either solutions or suspensions. The main reason for the development of dry syrups is the instability of the active ingredient in the liquid state. They

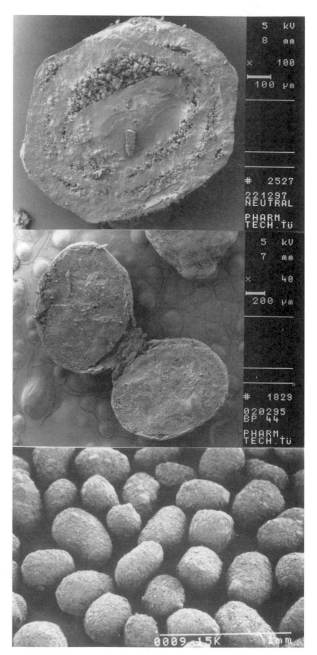

Fig. 22 Pellets prepared by different methods. Cross-sectional view of a pellet prepared by powder layering (top), cross-sectional view of a pellet prepared by extrusion/spheronization (middle), and size and shape of pellets prepared by extrusion/spheronization (bottom).

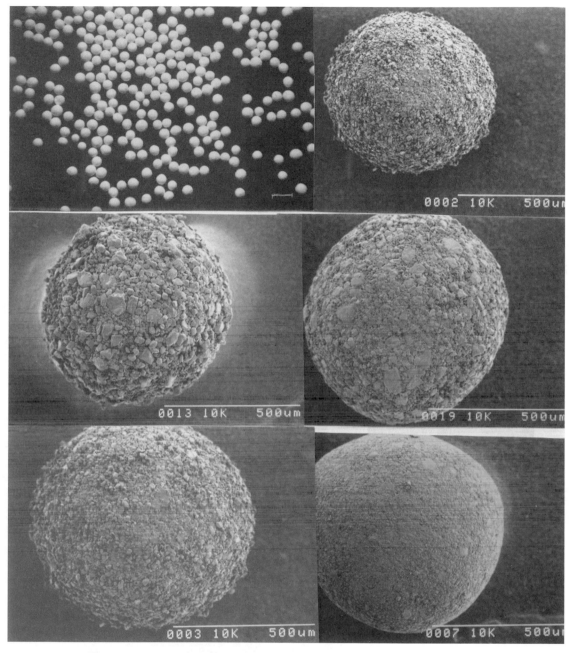

Fig. 23 Pellets prepared by spherical agglomeration. Overview about ascorbic acid pellets prepared from powder of a mean particle diameter of 8.8 μm. The bar is 1 mm (top left). SEM picture from left (top right). Ascorbic acid pellet prepared from powder of a mean diameter of 8.8 μm without the addition of povidone (middle left). Pellet from left prepared with the addition of 2% PVP (middle right). Ascorbic acid pellet prepared from powder of a mean particle diameter of 3.0 μm without the addition of povidone (bottom left). Pellet from left with the addition of 2.0% povidone (bottom right).

have to be used within a limited period of time after conversion into a suspension or solution. Most of the medicaments formulated as dry syrups belong to the group of antibiotics. It was shown that the bioavailability of a dry syrup could be superior compared with an oily suspension (44). In addition to the active ingredient, the formulations (45) contain carriers like saccharose, sorbitol, and xylitol, acting also as sweeteners, microcrystalline cellulose and starch, viscosity enhancers, mainly xanthan gum, artificial sweeteners, preservatives,

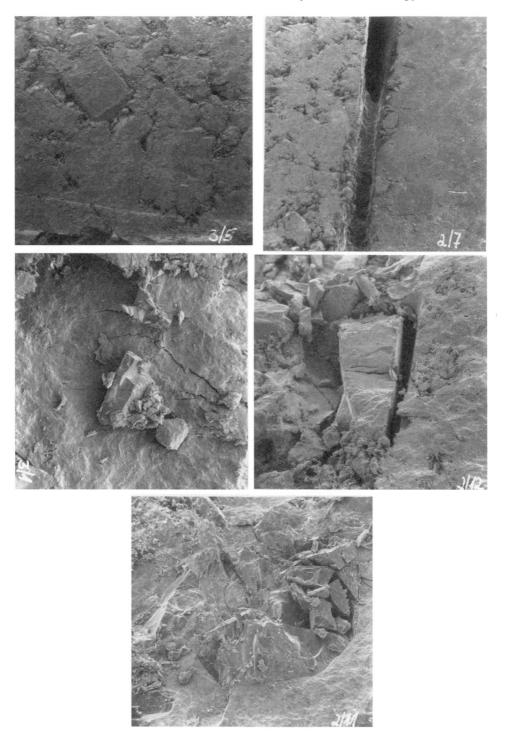

Fig. 24 Differences in the deformation behavior of substances during tableting demonstrated by sorbitol instant as an example for a plastically deforming substance and ascorbic acid as a more brittle one. Tablet compressed at 5 kN (10 mm in diameter) (top left) and 30 kN on top right. Inner part of a broken tablet showing an ascorbic acid crystal being totally embedded into plastically deformed sorbitol (middle left) and a crystal being partially removed from the sorbitol matrix through the break down of the tablet (middle right). A cracked ascorbic acid crystal in a sorbitol matrix (bottom).

wetting and complexing agents, and buffer substances. They could be prepared as powder mixtures, completely or partially granulated products, and as coated coarse carriers. Fig. 21 (top left) shows as an example for a powder mix, amoxicilline trihydrate, and clavunlinic acid containing preparation. A lot of small particles of different size and shape indicate a mixture. A partially granulated product containing cefixim trihydrate is shown on top right. Besides small size particles granules are visible. A granulated dry syrup prepared from acetylcysteine is presented on bottom left, while coated carriers that are partially agglomerated containing bromhexine hydrochloride and cefaclor monohydrate are shown on bottom right. In three of the four formulations

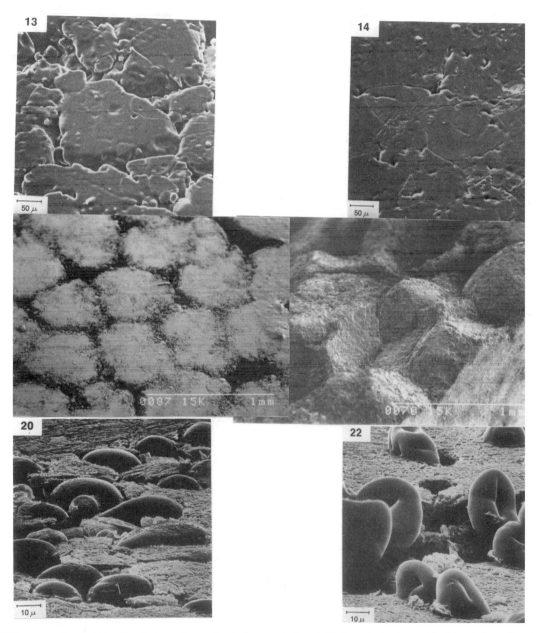

Fig. 25 Differences observed in the deformation of substances during tableting. Potassium chloride at low (top left) and high compressional forces (top right), pellets prepared by spherical agglomeration in a tablet surface (middle left) and in the inner part of a broken tablet (middle right), surface of an ASA tablet containing 10% sodium carboxymethyl starch (bottom left) and the same surface after moistening with a finger (bottom right) (54).

mentioned above xanthan gum is used as viscosity enhancing agent.

Pellets

Pellets are mainly prepared by four different methods: powder layering, rotating fluidized bed, extrusion/-spheronization, and the agglomeration method. The oldest one is the so-called, "powder layering method" (46), where seed crystals in a drum are moistened by a binder solution and subsequently dusted by a fine powder. After a drying phase, the next moistening step is carried out followed by a powder application and so on. These types of pellets are characterized by

a core corresponding to the seed crystal, surrounded by fine particles. Figure 22 (top) represents such a pellet.

Pellets prepared by extrusion/spheronization (47) have uniform cross-sectional area (Fig. 22, middle) but differ slightly in shape and size, which is based on the spheronization process following extrusion (Fig. 22, bottom). They are harder compared with pellets produced by powder layering. Their appearance is similar to pellets obtained by fluidized-bed granulation using the so-called "rotating fluidized-bed" (48). Due to the fact that ideally round pellets are desired, several attempts were made to quantify their roundness (49, 50). The spherical agglomeration is a completely different method that is

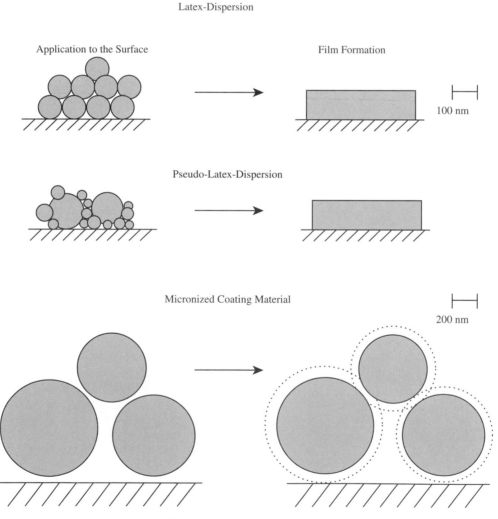

Fig. 26 Differences observed in the mechanism of film formation from latex and pseudolatex dispersions-and from micronized coating materials.

employed to develop pellets that are round and uniform in size. In this, particles are agglomerated in suspension (51, 52).

The resulting pellets are round and uniform in size (Fig. 23, top left); the shape of an ascorbic acid pellet prepared from a fine powder having a mean diameter of 3.0 μm is shown in Fig. 23 top right. Increasing the particle size of the starting material to a mean diameter of 8.8 μm, the surface of the pellets becomes more rough (middle left). The addition of 2% of povidone during pellet preparation smoothes the surface (middle right). A finer starting material of 3 μm leads to a smoother surface (bottom left) that could become very smooth by the addition of 2% of povidone (bottom right). This example clearly demonstrates that by spherical agglomeration, it is possible to adapt the surface of the pellets being produced by a proper choice of the particle size of the starting material as well as by the addition of a polymer (53).

Tablets

SEM was widely used to investigate the structure of tablets. An excellent review is presented by Hess (54). Imaging of tablets is a useful tool to demonstrate differences in compression behavior of substances. Figure 24 shows an example where the plastically deforming spray-dried sorbitol instant was compressed together with the more brittle ascorbic acid in one tablet. At low compressional force of 5 kN for a 10 mm tablet, the rectangular ascorbic acid crystals as well as the partially deformed sorbitol particles are visible (top left). On top right the surfaces of two tablets compressed at 5 kN (left) and 30 kN (right) are compared. At higher compressional forces, a uniform, flat, and smooth tablet surface is formed, but within this surface a single unchanged ascorbic acid crystal could be detected. Observation of a broken tablet (Fig. 24, middle), which was prepared at a high compressional force of 30 kN, reveals that the ascorbic

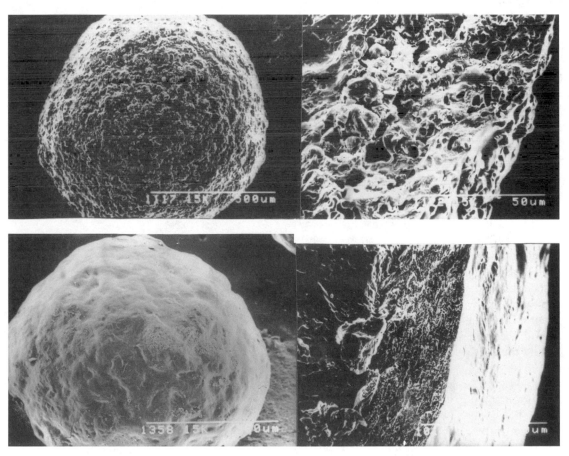

Fig. 27 Influence of the type of polymer application on film properties (top and side view). HP55 (HPMCP)-coated pellet, prepared from a micronized film dispersion (top). HP55 (HPMCP)-coated pellet, prepared from an organic solution (bottom).

acid crystal is totally fixed within a matrix of plastically deformed sorbitol. Even when the crystal was partially removed from the sorbitol matrix, during the break down of the tablet, the sorbitol matrix is still intact (middle right). This is supported by the bottom picture, where an ascorbic acid crystal was cracked during the breaking of the tablet, but it is still surrounded by plastically deformed sorbitol. These findings are similar to investigations of Hess (54), who used the plastically deforming potassium chloride (Fig. 25, top). On the top right, after compressing at low compressional forces, the single potassium chloride particles are separated by dips between them, while after compressing at high forces—although the original particles are still detectable—there are no visible dips.

When compressing pellets into tablets, their deformation depends on their hardness (55). When hard pellets produced by spherical agglomeration are compressed (Fig. 25, middle), the single pellets are still visible at the surface (left) and are only partially deformed in the inner part of the tablet [right, (53)]. This is of high importance, when pellets having an enteric or a sustained-release coat are compressed with the aim not to damage the coating.

The bottom pictures of Fig. 25 show differences in the elastic recovery of substances after compression. The left picture depicts the surface of an ASA-tablet containing 10% of sodium carboxylmethyl starch as a disintegrant. The plastically deforming ASA remains plain after compression, whereas the starch derivative shows elastic recovery. After moistening the surface with finger the starch derivative particles start swelling moving out of the tablet surface (54).

Coatings

Coatings are applied to solid dosage forms for several reasons: taste masking, moisture prevention, gastric resistancy, and sustained-release action being the most common ones (56). They could be handled as a solution, a latex or pseudolatex dispersion, or as a suspension containing a micronized polymer powder as the film-forming agent. The film formation is easiest from a polymer solution because single polymer molecules can interact to build the coating. Using latex or pseudo latex dispersions or even micronized polymers the situation is different as demonstrated in Fig. 26. The size of true latex particles is uniform and it is in the range of 100–200 nm. A pseudolatex shows a broader particle size distribution although the mean particle diameter could be in the same range. In contrast, the particle size of a micronized particle of a film forming agent is 10 to 30 times higher compared to a latex, which is in the range of 1 to 3 or even more

micrometers. For a complete film formation, the plasticizer has to penetrate uniformly into the polymer. This is easily achieved when a latex dispersion is used. With a pseudolatex dispersion, however, the larger particles would not be plasticized completely. With a micronized polymer, on the other hand, only the outer part of the particles will be penetrated by the plasticizer. The resulting differences are presented in Fig. 27. On top, the rough surface and cross-sectional area of a pellet coated with the micronized polymer hydroxypropyl methylcellulose (HPMCP, HP55) are shown. The cross-sectional view

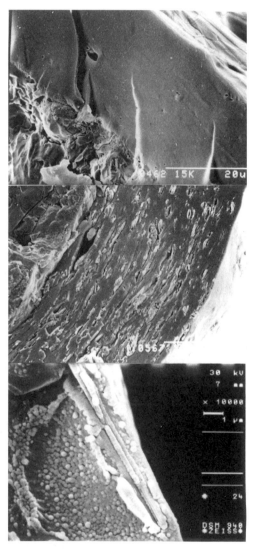

Fig. 28 Cross-sectional areas of different films. Eudragit L 30 D without pigments, film thickness approx. 25 μm (top), Eudragit L 30 D film containing 50% of magnesium stearate, film thickness approx. 25 μm (middle), incomplete film formation at higher magnification, showing individual latex particles from an Eudragit L 30 D dispersion in the film (bottom).

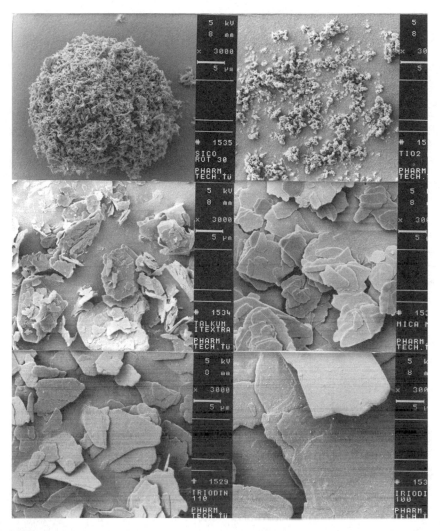

Fig. 29 Comparison of differences in size of pigments at the same magnification. Red iron oxide (top left), titanium dioxide (top right), talc (middle left), mica (middle right), and two pearl luster pigments Iriodin 110 (bottom left) and Iriodin 100 (bottom right).

hardly allows distinction between the coat and the inner part of the particle. The thickness of the film is approximately 25 μm. The pellet shown on the bottom was coated using an organic solution of HP55 showing a smooth surface and a more uniform cross-sectional view of the film. A more detailed structure of films is depicted in Fig. 28, where the influence of composition and conditions of preparation is apparent. The top picture represents a film that is produced without pigments. The addition of 50% of magnesium stearate results in a more structured layer (middle). On the bottom of Fig. 28 the cross-sectional view of an incomplete film at a higher magnification is presented. A pigment platelet is located near the surface. The latex particles around the platelet form a film, whereas those that one in the inner part of the coat still exist as latex

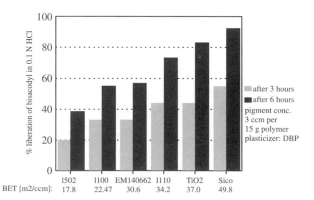

Fig. 30 Liberation of theophylline from aquacoat ECD 30 coated pellets with different pigments in relation to the BET surface of the pigments.

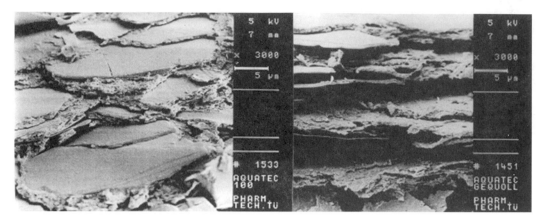

Fig. 31   Cross-section of films from Aquacoat ECD 30 pigmented with 20% (V/V) of the pearl luster pigment Iriodin 100.

particles in the range of 100–200 nm. Obviously the minimum film-forming temperature was not reached in this region. The pictures clearly demonstrate the differences between the various application forms of film-forming agents.

Pigments could influence the mechanical properties of a film as well as the dissolution behavior of a drug substance from coated tablets or pellets. According to Rowe (57) different pigments should be compared on the bases of the pigment volume concentration, which takes density differences into account (Eq. 3),

$$\text{PVC} = \frac{V_\text{P}}{V_\text{P} + V_\text{B}} \tag{3}$$

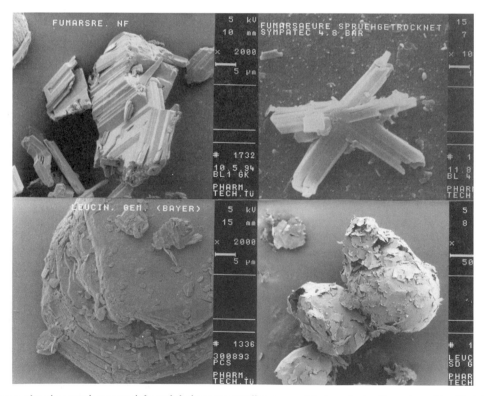

Fig. 32   SEM picture showing starting materials and their corresponding spray-dried products. Fumaric acid milled (top left) and spray dried (top right), L-leucine milled (bottom left) and spray dried (bottom right). Before spray drying both substances show a layered crystal structure but differ significantly after the spray-drying process.

where PVC = pigment volume concentration; V_P = pigment volume; and V_B = polymer volume.

Pigments exhibit different shape and size. Figure 29 clearly demonstrates that for red iron oxide (top left) and titanium dioxide (top right) on one hand, and talc, mica (middle), and two pearl luster pigments (bottom) on the other. The primary particle size of the two metal oxide crystallites is below 1 μm. The red iron oxide is more agglomerated compared with titanium dioxide. Talc (middle left) and mica (middle right) show platelet structure with a broader particle size distribution of talc. The two pearl luster pigments, both based on mica, coated with metal oxides also show the typical platelet structure and higher particle sizes. For titanium dioxide (58) and talc (59) the influence of the amount of pigment added to the film-coating formulation on the drug dissolution was shown. Up to the critical pigment volume concentration, the permeability of the films is decreased and therefore the sustained release effect is prolonged. Above the critical concentration the permeability of the films increases due to defects in the uniform film layer caused by the pigments (60).

With pearl luster pigments, depending on their particle size and/or BET-surface, respectively, this effect could be used to control drug liberation of sustained-release preparations. Figure 30 compares the in vitro dissolution of theophylline in water after 3 and 6 h from pellets that were coated with an Aquacoat ECD 30 dispersion pigmented with 20% of different pigments based on the amount of polymer used. Sicopharm (red iron oxide) and titanium dioxide, both fine crystallites, show the highest release rates. The others having a more or less pronounced platelet structure show a decrease in drug liberation that is directly correlated to the BET-surface of the pigments (60). The reason for the reduced film permeability lies in the special structure of films containing platelet-shaped pigments. Figure 31 (left) shows a section of such a film under an angle of approximately 45°. The roof-like structure of the coating is obvious. Therefore, substances penetrating the film have to permeate around the solid platelets, which prolongs the diffusion. Path consequently, the drug liberation is delayed. During the dissolution process, the film swells due to the swelling properties of the polymer. At the end of the process a picture shown in Fig. 31 (right) is obtained. The cross-sectional area of the swollen film in this case was observed under an angle of 90°. The pigment platelets are still in their original overlapping position. The degree of swelling depends on the type of polymer used. Aquacoat ECD 30 shows only a slight effect compared with Eudragit RL 30 D and RS 30 D.

Spray-Dried Products

Spray drying is used to convert solutions, emulsions, or suspensions into powders (61). The applications in pharmaceutical technology are numerous. Raw materials are spray dried, for instance, to enhance the compressional properties of substances such as lactose (62) and tricalcium phosphate (13), to distribute a minor component like digoxin more uniformly in a matrix, and to enhance

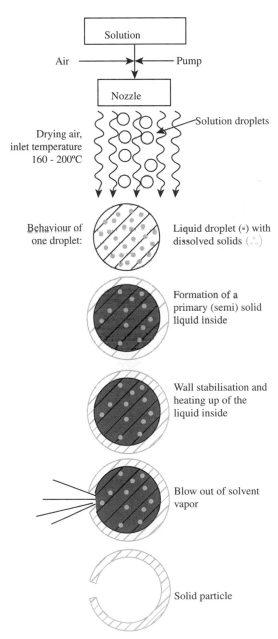

Fig. 33 Spray-drying process of extracts with respect to the behavior of a single droplet.

their dissolution rate as described for digoxin in combination with a hydrophilic polymer (63).

Normally one would expect round- to nearly ball-shaped particles from a spray-drying process when starting from a solution or an emulsion. When using a suspension, the resulting particles could also be more or less irregular agglomerates as shown earlier for spray-dried lactose and some of the so-called "multi-purpose excipients." But even when starting from a solution round particles may not be obtained. This is demonstrated in Fig. 32. Fumaric acid and L-leucine in their original state are both crystals compasing of thin lamellae. After spray-drying fumaric acid forms small star-like agglomerates (Fig. 32, top right), whereas L-leucine forms hollow spheres built from small and very thin platelets (Fig. 32, bottom right). These spheres have advantages as lubricants in effervescent tablets compared with a milled product because the spheres are broken during compression, forming a thin

film of small L-leucine platelets on the punches and die of a tablet press. Thus, an amount of 3.75% of spray dried L-leucine in an effervescent tablet formulation was more effective compared with 5% of the milled product (64). Spray drying of extracts is quite often used to prepare readily soluble tea preparations (65). The advantages are a quicker solubility, a uniform distribution of active ingredients, and a free-flowing, dust-free powder. The drying process of a single droplet can be schematically described as shown in Fig. 33.

In the first step, liquid droplets are formed by the nozzle of the spray dryer with the aid of a pump and compressed air or by an airless system. Due to the high temperature of the drying air, the solvent evaporates first from the outer surface of the droplet and a solid "skin" is formed around the liquid that acts as a barrier for further evaporation. As a result, the pressure within the droplet increases until the wall breaks and the solvent is blown out of the droplet. At

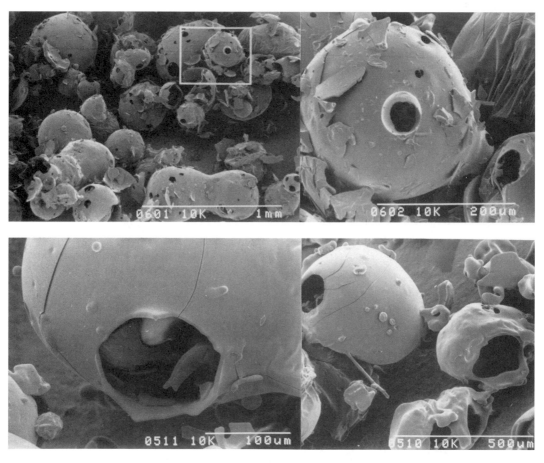

Fig. 34 Spray-dried plant extract solutions used to prepare readily soluble tea preparations. Spray-dried product from an airless high-pressure system leading to a coarse particle size distribution (top left) and a magnification thereof (top right), detailed view of one particle showing fragments inside (bottom left), and the product from above after a wrong sample preparation (bottom right).

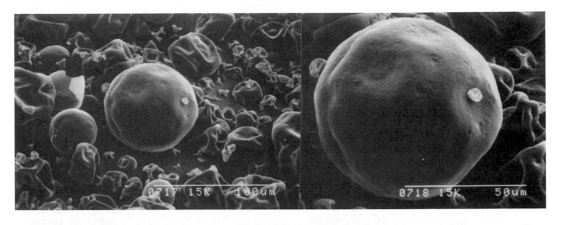

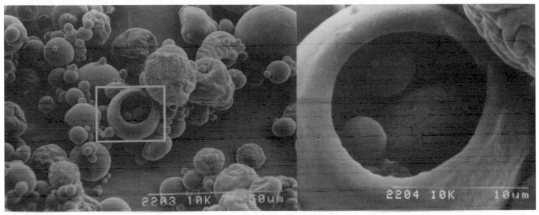

Fig. 35 Spray-dried extracts and pantothenate solution. Spray dried calcium pantothenate: overview (top left) and detail (top right), showing mainly particles that were damaged during preparation of the SEM sample either by the high vacuum of the SEM or by the heat created during the sputter coating process. Spray dried *Tussilago farfara* extract prepared by a system using atomizing air to form droplets and leading to small particle sizes (bottom left) and a magnification thereof (bottom right).

the end, a hollow solid particle results showing small holes, where the liquid was blown out. Depending on the excipients in the formulation particles could more or less break down during the process. The fragments then adhere to other fragments and to the spheres. This behavior is demonstrated by Fig. 34 (top left). The extract particles on

Table 3 Manufacturing data of porous ceramic pellets of β-Tricalcium Phosphate and hydroxyapatite, respectively

Type (see Fig. 44)	Compaction pressure (MPa)	Firing temperature (°C)	Size (d/h; mm)[a]	Density[b] (%)
a[c]	48	1075	4.4/4.0	64.9
b[c]	48	1125	4.1/3.7	78.4
c[c]	168	1075	4.4/4.0	79.8
d[d]	111	1150	4.4/4.0	63

[a] d = Diameter; h = Height.
[b] Percent density based on the true density of the starting materials.
[c] β-Tricalcium phosphate.
[d] Hydroxyapatite.

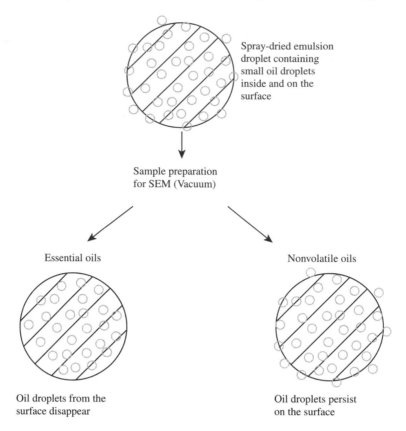

Fig. 36 Differences between spray-dried emulsions containing essential oils and nonvolatile oils during sample preparation. The oil droplets of the volatile essential oils disappear during sample preparation under vacuum, while nonvolatile oil droplets stay permanently.

that figure originating from an airless spraying system result in particle size ranges from approximately 100 to 500 μm. Fragments adhering to other particles are present as well as agglomerates of two or three spheres. The higher magnification of one of the particles (Fig. 34, top right) shows the "blow out hole" and also adhering fragments. A higher magnification of one of the "blow out holes" (bottom left of Fig. 34) demonstrates the presence of fragments and smaller spheres within a bigger particle. In the picture, at bottom right, some of the particles show irregular surfaces. These are artifacts, which are formed during sample preparation. They are built as a result of overheating during the sputter process with gold. A similar case is demonstrated in Fig. 35 (top). Most of the spray-dried calcium pantothenate particles are collapsed due to instability of the previously formed thin walled spheres under the high vacuum of the SEM. From time to time one can observe the collapsing of the particles under the SEM.

The bottom pictures of Fig. 35 demonstrate the difference to particles mentioned before when using an air-driven nozzle instead of an airless one. The particle size range of the *Tussilago farfara* extract shown in the figure is now in the range from 1 to 20 μm. Some of them are damaged by heat during sputtering (bottom left).

At higher magnification (bottom right) one single particle of roughly 20 μm in diameter is shown containing smaller ones inside. The wall thickness is in the range of 1 μm or below. In some cases emulsions containing oil in the inner phase are submitted to spray drying. The spray-dried particles contain the small oil droplets inside as well as on the surface as schematically drawn in Fig. 36. During the sputtering process of the samples under vacuum essential oil droplets are evaporated from the surface of the spray-dried particles, whereas nonvolatile oil droplets stay on the surface and are coated by gold. The different situations are demonstrated in Fig. 37 by SEM pictures. On top, an azulene containing spray-dried particle to which smaller ones are adhered is shown. Here, no oil droplets on the surface are visible due to the fact that azulene belongs to the group of essential oils. In the middle, the surface of a 50% vitamin E acetate containing spray-dried particle is depicted. The surface is rough and higher magnification of the same (bottom of Fig. 37) clearly demonstrates the presence of small oil droplets on the surface of the spray-dried particle.

Freeze-Dried Products

Freeze drying was first carried out in 1890 by Altman (66) but became well known through the industrial development of the process. The process is used in the food industry e.g., for the production of instant coffee, tea, and other products. In the field of pharmaceutical technology, it was for a long time restricted to only few formulations for injection containing the active ingredient in the freeze-dried state in an ampoule to be dissolved just before application. With the increasing interest in protein and peptide formulations, freeze-dried products became more important. These are discussed under "microparticles for injection" in the following section.

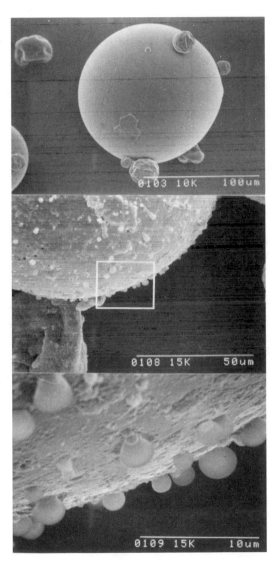

Fig. 37 Spray-dried emulsions. Particle from an emulsion containing a volatile essential oil (azulene) (top). Particle from an emulsion containing a nonvolatile oil (vitamin E acetate) (middle and bottom).

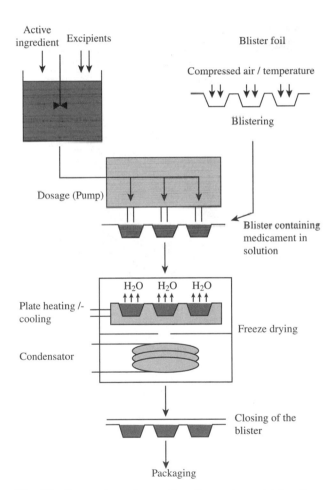

Fig. 38 Preparation scheme of medicaments containing-freeze dried platelets.

Instantenously soluble freeze-dried platelets (67) became known during the last few years. They were mainly developed for people having problems of swallowing a tablet. Their production scheme is presented in Fig. 38. A solution containing the active ingredient together with excipients like mannitol and if necessary polymers, sweeteners, colors, and flavors is dosed by a pump into preformed blisters of PVC or a combination of PVC and PVDC. The blisters containing the solution are freeze dried and an aluminum foil covering the blister is applied at the end of the process. The platelets have the size of tablets as shown on top of Fig. 39 and they adapt to the form of the blister through the freeze-drying process. The surface shows small holes from channels where water was evaporating during drying. These channels form a percolating system within the tablet (Fig. 39, middle). Their microstructure is shown on bottom of Fig. 39 indicating the loose structure of the platelets having a high internal surface. Through the channels, water is penetrating quickly into the platelet leading to a very fast dissolution.

Microparticles for Injection

During the last decade, peptides and proteins became more and more important as medicaments. Most of them are unstable in an acidic environment and in the

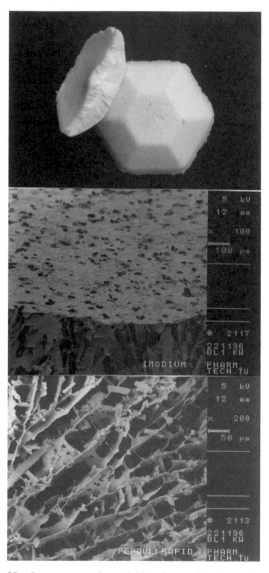

Fig. 39 Instantaneously soluble freeze-dried medicament platelets/tablets. Cross-sectional side view and top view (top), border line between the surface (upper part), and the cross-section (lower part of the picture) (middle), inner part of the platelet (bottom).

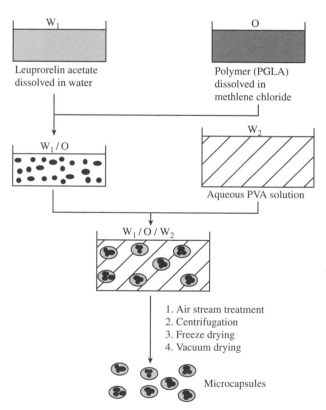

Fig. 40 Preparation of leuprorelin acetate containing microcapsules according to the "in-water-drying" process.

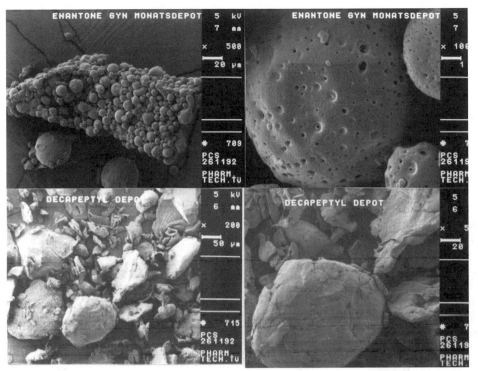

Fig. 41 Microparticles for injection prepared by the "in-water-drying" process (top) and by freeze drying (bottom) for two LH-RH super agonists.

presence of enzymes. Therefore, they could not be administered or applied via the peroral route (68). Since the development and registration of poly-lactide-glycolides as biodegradable polymers for injectable

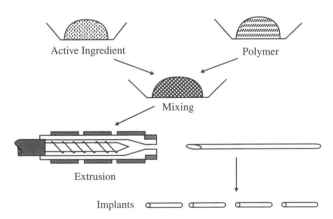

Fig. 42 Preparation of sterile injectable implants by extrusion of a mixture of d,l-poly(lactide-glycolide) and an active ingredient.

sustained release preparations (69), methods of preparation of injectable microparticles became very interesting. As preparation methods, spray and freeze drying and the so-called "in-water-drying" process are in use (70). The latter is demonstrated in Fig. 40. Leuprorelin acetate dissolved in water and a polylactide-glycolide solution in methylene chloride are mixed forming a W/O-Emulsion, where the methylene chloride solution is the outer phase of the emulsion. By the addition of an aqueous polyvinyl alcohol (PVA) solution, a water/oil/water multiple emulsion is formed with PVA solution in the outer phase. The main part of the methylene chloride is evaporated by an air treatment leading to a precipitation of polylactide-glycolide. The resulting particles are centrifuged, freeze dried, and dried under vacuum to remove traces of methylene chloride (71). Fig. 41 shows (top) the resulting round particles as a bulk before redispersion for injection (left) and single particles at higher magnification (right). The single particle exhibit pores with small holes where the methylene chloride has evaporated. For comparison reasons, a freeze-dried product is shown on the bottom of Fig. 41.

Implants

Implants can be biogradable or nonbiogradable ones. In earlier times tablets were implanted by a small surgery and removed after a certain time period. Modern implants consist of biogradable organic or inorganic materials. The most commonly used organic material since the introduction of Zoladex® is *d*,l-poly(lactide-glycolide) (71). The implants are cylindrical in shape and have a diameter enabling the application by syringes and injection needles. A scheme of the preparation of this type of implants is presented in Fig. 42.

The active ingredient and the polymer are mixed, extruded to a cylindrical rod, and cut into pieces of approximately 1 cm in length. These pieces are introduced into syringes and applied to the patient as an implant through a needle. Fig. 43 presents one end of the cylindrical implant at two magnifications. The higher magnification shows small irregularities at the end of the rod that could be responsible for the pain sometimes reported during the application of the systems.

A second type of implant that is used for the local antibiotic treatment of bone infections is based on β-tricalcium phosphate ceramic pellets (72). The pellets are prepared by granulation and subsequent thermal treatment between 975 and 1300°C. They are loaded with antibiotic drugs like gentamycin. The drug liberation is affected by the pore volume of the pellets leading to a sustained release of the antibiotic. Fig. 44 presents a SEM picture of some materials, showing the influence of the thermal treatment and compaction pressure of the green pellets on the structure of the material. The manufacturing data are given in Table 3.

An increase in firing temperature from 1075 to 1125°C leads to a smaller pellet and a higher density corresponding to a lower porosity. Similar compacts can be obtained at the lower firing temperature by the application of a higher compaction pressure. Hydroxyapatite shows differences compared with β-tricalcium phosphate leading to low densities at high thermal treatment. A prolonged drug liberation up to 14 days was achieved by this method.

SUMMARY

The application of secondary electron microscopy (SEM) has become widespread in pharmaceutical technology. Besides other techniques like particle size analysis, surface measurements, X-ray diffraction, and differential scanning calorimetry, it is a useful tool to characterize raw materials. Intermediates like powder mixtures, granules, and other bulk materials could be visualized by SEM. For interactive powder mixtures it is the only method making the interaction visible. Pellets could be investigated with respect to size and shape as well as for surface characteristics and properties of coatings being applied to them. Tablets show their internal structure in SEM. Spray-dried and freeze-dried products are further interesting examples for the application of SEM. In general one could state that more than 50% of all problems could be solved by the view through a microscope.

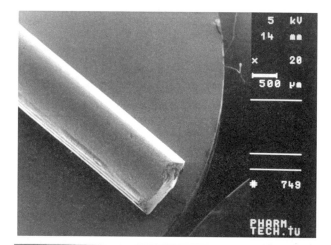

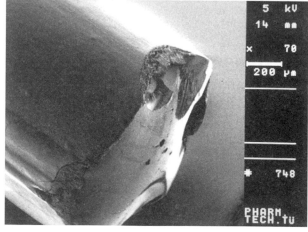

Fig. 43 SEM picture of a Zoladex® cylindrical implant. The stripes at the lower surface result from small irregularities of the extrusion nozzle (top). One end of a Zoladex® implant at a higher magnification. The cross-sectional area shows irregularities resulting from the cut off of single cylinders (bottom).

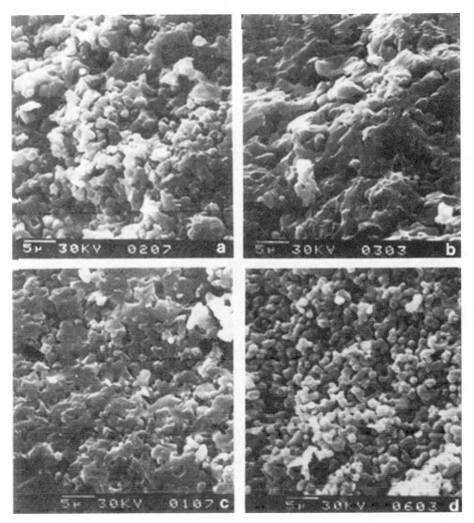

Fig. 44 Scanning electron micrographs of the structure cross-section of porous ceramic pellets of β-tricalcium phosphate (a–c) and hydroxyapatite (d).

ACKNOWLEDGMENTS

This chapter was written on the basis of a 13 years experience with SEM in pharmaceutical technology. The author would like to thank Mr. Klaus Weyhing for his permanent involvement in the practical work with the SEM and for his graphical support as well as Mrs. Renate Beer for typing and editing this work. Thanks should also be given to Professor Dr. Tsige Gebre-Mariam, University of Addis Ababa, for correction of the manuscript.

REFERENCES

1. Watt, I.M. Microscopy with Light and Electrons. *The Principle and Practice of Electron Microscopy*, 2nd Ed.; Cambridge University Press: New York, Melbourne, 1997; 8–10.

2. de Broglie, L.A. Tentative Theory of Light Quanta. Phil. Mag. **1924**, *47*, 446.

3. Watt, I.M. Microscopy with Light and Electrons. *The Principle and Practice of Electron Microscopy*, 2nd Ed.; Cambridge University Press: New York, Melbourne, 1997; 14.

4. DSM 940. A-Design of Instrument. *Operation Manual*; Zeiss: Oberkochen, 1990; 4–5.

5. Sommer, K. Sampling Procedures. *Sampling of Powders and Bulk Material*; Springer-Verlag: Berlin, New York, Tokyo, 1986; 80–124.

6. Sympatec Rhodos 12SR Rhodos Operationg Instructions. *Operation Manual*; Sympatec GmbH: Clausthal-Zellerfeld, 1985; 3.1–3.52.

7. Watt, I.M. Specimen Preparation for Electron Microscopy. *The Principle and Practice of Electron Microscopy*, 2nd Ed.; Cambridge University Press: New York, Melbourne, 1997; 136–187.

8. Shangraw, R.F.; Wallace, J.W.; Bowers, F.M. Morphology and Functionality in Tablet Excipients for Direct Compression. Part I. Pharm. Technol. **1981**, *5*, 69–78.

9. Doelker, E.; Massuelle, D.; Veuillez, F.; Humbert-Droz, P. Morphological, Packing, Flow, and Tableting Properties of New Avicel Types. Drug Dev. Ind. Pharm. **1995**, *21*, 643–661.

10. Larhrib, H.; Wells, M.H.; Rubinstein, M.H.; Ricart, G. Characterization of PEGs using Matrix-Assisted Laser Desorption/Ionisation Mass Spectrometry and Other Related Techniques. Int. J. Pharm. **1997**, *14*, 187–198.

11. Khan, K.A.; Rhodes, C.T. The Production of Tablets by Direct Compression. Can. J. Pharm. Sci. **1973**, *8*, 1–5.

12. Shangraw, R.F. The Design and Evaluation of Coprocessed Tablet Excipients and Direct Compression Active Ingredients. FMC **1981**, *1*, 1–20.

13. Schmidt, P.C.; Herzog, R. Calcium Phosphates in Pharmaceutical Tableting. Part I: General Properties, Pharm. World Sci. **1993**, *15*, 105–115.

14. Schmidt, P.C.; Herzog, R. Calcium Phosphates in Pharmaceutical Tableting. Part II: Comparison of Tableting Properties. Pharm. World Sci. **1993**, *15*, 116–122.

15. Carstensen, J.T.; Ertell, L. Physical and Chemical Properties of Calcium Phosphates for Solid-State Pharmaceutical Formulations. Congr. Int. Technol. Pharm., 5th, Ass. Pharm. Gal. Ind. **1989**.

16. Hou, X.P.; Carstensen, J.T. Compression Characteristics of Basic Tricalcium Phosphate ($Ca_3(PO_4)_2$,$Ca(OH)_2$). Int. J. Pharm. **1985**, *25*, 207–215.

17. Lerk, C.F. Physikalisch-Pharmazeutische Eigenschaften Von Lactose. Pharm. Unserer Zeit **1987**, *16*, 39–46.

18. Schmidt, P.C.; Vortisch, W. Einfluß Der Herstellungsart von Füll- und Bindemitteln auf Ihre Tablettierfähigkeit: Vergleich von Acht Marktüblichen Sorbit-Typen. Pharm. Ind. **1987**, *49*, 495–503.

19. Schmidt, P.C. Tableting Characteristics of Sorbitol. Pharm. Technol. **1983**, *7*(11), 65–74.

20. DuRoss, J.W. Modification of the Crystalline Structure of Sorbitol and Its Effects on Tableting Characteristics. Pharm. Technol. **1984**, *8*, 42–53.

21. Schmidt, P.C.; Rubensdörfer, C. Evaluation of Ludipress as a "Multi-Purpose Excipient" for Direct Compression. Part I: Powder Characteristics and Tabletting, Drug Dev. Ind. Pharm. **1994**, *20*, 2899–2925.

22. Pesonen, T.; Paronen, P.; Puurunen, T. Evaluation of a Novel Cellulose Powder as a Filler-Binder for Direct Compression of Tablets. Pharm. Weekbl. Sci. Ed. **1989**, *11*, 13–19.

23. Schmidt, P.C.; Rubensdörfer, C. Evaluation of Ludipress as a "Multi-Purpose Excipient" for Direct Compression. Part II: Interactive Blending and Tabletting with Micronized Glibenclamide Drug, Dev. Ind. Pharm. **1994**, *20*, 2927–2952.

24. Gebre-Mariam, T.; Schmidt, P.C. Isolation and Physico-Chemical Properties of Enset Starch. Starch/Stärke **1996**, *48*, 208–214.

25. Bolhuis, G.K.; van Kamp, H.V.; Lerk, C.F. On the Similarity of Sodium Starch Glycolate from Different Sources. Drug Dev. Ind. Pharm. **1986**, *12*, 621–630.

26. Ferrero, C.; Munoz, N.; Velasco, M.V.; Munoz-Ruiz, A.; Jiménez-Castellanos, R. Disintegrating Efficiency of Croscarmellose Sodium in a Direct Compression Formulation. Int. J. Pharm. **1997**, *147*, 11–21.

27. Bertoni, M.; Ferrari, F.; Bonferoni, M.C.; Rossi, S.; Caramella, C. Functionality Tests for Tablet Disintegrants: The Case of Sodium Carboxymethylcelluloses. Pharm. Technol. Eur. **1995**, *7*, 17–24.

28. Ertel, K.D.; Carstensen, J.T. Chemical, Physical, and Lubricant Properties of Magnesium Stearate. J. Pharm. Sci. **1988**, *77*, 625–629.

29. Steffens K.-J. Koglin J. The Magnesium Stearate Problem III, International Conference on Pharmaceutical Ingredients and Intermediates 1992; 118–125

30. Delacourte, A.; Guyot, J.C.; Colombo, P.; Catellani, P.L. Effectiveness of Lubricants and Lubrication Mechanism in Tablet Technology. Drug Dev. Ind. Pharm. **1995**, *21*, 2187–2199.

31. Frömming, K.-H.; Gröbler, S. Einfluß Von Füllmitteln Und Von Magnesiumstearat Auf Die Wirkstofffreisetzung Aus Hartgelatinekapseln. Pharm. Ztg. **1983**, *128*, 786–793.

32. Roblot, L.; Puisieux, F.; Duchêne, D. A Study on Lubrication by Magnesium Stearate. The Influence of the Proportion of Lubricant and the Mixing Process on the Tablet Characteristics. Labo. Pharma. Probl. Tech. **1983**, *31*, 843–847.

33. Jarosz, P.J.; Parrott, E.L. Effect of Lubricants on Tensile Strengths of Tablets. Drug Dev. Ind. Pharm. **1984**, *10*, 259–273.

34. Williams, R.O., III; McGinity, J.W. A Study of the Influence of Magnesium Stearate or Talc on the Compaction Properties of Direct Compression Excipients using Tableting Indices. Pharm. Tech. Tabl. Tech. **1987**, *1*, 157–165.

35. Stange, K. Beurteilung Von Mischgeräten Mit Hilfe Statistischer Verfahren. Chem. Ing. Tech. **1954**, *26*, 150–155.

36. Stange, K. Die Mischgüte Einer Zufallsmischung Als Grundlage Zur Beurteilung Von Mischversuchen. Chem. Ing. Tech. **1954**, *26*, 331–337.

37. Egermann, H.; Frank, P. Novel Approach to Estimate Quality of Binary Random Powder Mixtures: Samples of Constant Volume. I: Derivation of Equation. J. Pharm. Sci. **1992**, *81*, 551–555.

38. Egermann, H.; Frank, P. Novel Approach to Estimate Quality of Binary Random Powder Mixtures: Samples of Constant Volume. II: Applications of Equation to Optimize Tableting Conditions. J. Pharm. Sci. **1992**, *81*, 667–669.

39. Egermann, H.; Krumphuber, A.; Frank, P. Novel Approach to Estimate Quality of Binary Random Powder Mixtures: Samples of Constant Volume. III: Range of Validity of Equation. J. Pharm. Sci. **1992**, *81*, 773–776.

40. Hersey, J.A. Ordered Mixing: A New Concept in Powder Mixing Practice. Powder Technol. **1975**, *11*, 41–44.

41. Egermann, H.; Orr, N.A. Ordered Mixtures—Interactive Mixtures. Powder Technol. **1983**, *36*, 117–118.

42. Schmidt, P.C.; Ben, E.S. Vereinfachung Der Kapselrezeptur Durch Bildung Inaktiver Mischungen. Pharm. Ztg. **1987**, *132*, 2550–2557.

43. Schmidt, P.C.; Walter, R. Investigation of the Cohesion Behavior of Powders and Their Adhesion to a Carrier by an Electronic Tensiometer. Pharmazie **1994**, *49*(2,3), 183–187.

44. Sievert, M.; Blume, H.; Stenzhorn, G.; Lenhard, G.; Kieferndorf, U. Zur Qualitätsbeurteilung Von Phenoxymethylpenicillinhaltigen Fertigarzneimitteln 2. Mitteilung:

Vergleich Der Bioverfögbarkeiten Eines Trockensaftes Und Einer Üligen Suspension. Pharm. Ztg. Wiss. **1990**, *135*, 103–107.

45. Ryder, J. The Formulation of Dry Syrup Preparations. Int. J. Pharm. Technol. Prod. Manuf. **1979**, *1*, 14–25.

46. Rothgang, G. APV-Info. **1974**, *20*, 39.

47. Vervaet, C.; Baert, L.; Remon, J.P. Extrusion-Spheronisation—A Literature Review. Int. J. Pharm. **1995**, *116*, 131–146.

48. Schmidt, W.G.; Mehnert, W.; Frömming, K.-H. Controlled Release from Spherical Matrices Prepared in a Laboratory Scale Rotor-Granulator—Release Mechanism Interpretation using Individual Pellet Data. Eur. J. Pharm. Biopharm. **1996**, *42*, 348–350.

49. Eriksson, M.; Alderborn, G.; Nyström, C.; Podczeck, F.; Newton, J.M. Comparison between and Evaluation of Some Methods for the Assessment of the Sphericity of Pellets. Int. J. Pharm. **1997**, *148*, 149–154.

50. Lindner, H.; Kleinebudde, P. Anwendung Der Automatischen Bildanalyse Zur Charakterisierung Von Pellets. Pharm. Ind. **1993**, *55*, 694–701.

51. Kawashima, Y. An Experimental Study of the Kinetics of Spherical Agglomeration in a Stirred Vessel. Powder Technol. **1974**, *10*, 85–92.

52. Kawashima, Y. Spherical Crystallization as a Novel Particle Design Technique for the Development of Pharmaceutical Preparations. Kona. **1987**, *5*, 75.

53. Wolf, J. Untersuchung Der Hergestellten Agglomerate. *Herstellung, Charakterisierung und Tablettiereigenschaften Von Sphärischen Arzneistoffagglomeraten*; Thesis University of Tübingen: Tübingen, 1990; 59–61.

54. Hess, H. Tablets Under the Microscope. Pharm. Technol. Int. **1978**, *1*, 18–43.

55. Beckert, T.E.; Lehmann, K.; Schmidt, P.C. Compression of Enteric-Coated Pellets to Disintegrating Tablets. Int. J. Pharm. **1996**, *143*, 13–23.

56. McGinnity, J.W. *Aqueous Polymeric Coatings for Pharmaceutical Dosage Forms*; Marcel Dekker, Inc.: New York, 1997.

57. Rowe, R.C. The Effect of Pigment Type and Concentration on the Incidence of Edge Splitting on Film-Coated Tablets. Pharm. Acta. Helv. **1982**, *57*, 221–225.

58. Thomas, N.L. The Barrier Properties of Paint Coatings. Prog. Org. Coat. **1991**, *19*, 102–121.

59. Asbeck, W.K.; Van Loo, M. Critical Pigment Volume Relationships. Ind. Eng. Chem. **1949**, *41*, 1470–1475.

60. Maul, K.A.; Schmidt, P.C. Influence of Different-Shaped Pigments and Plasticizers on Theophylline Release from Eudragit RS30D and Aquacoat ECD30 Coated Pellets. S. T. P. Pharm. Sci. **1997**, *7*, 498–506.

61. Herbener, R. Staubarme Pulver Durch Sprühtrocknen—Erfahrungen Mit Neueren Techniken. Chem. Ing. Tech. **1987**, *59*, 112–117.

62. Vromans, H.; Bolhuis, G.K.; Lerk, C.F.; van de Biggelaar, H.; Bosch, H. Studies on Tableting Properties of Lactose. VII. The Effect of Variations in Primary Particle Size and Percentage of Amorphous Lactose in Spray-Dried Lactose Products. Int. J. Pharm. **1987**, *35*, 29–37.

63. Nürnberg, E.; Dölle, B. Darstellung Von Digoxin-Sprüheinbettungen Aus wäβrigen Systemen: Eigenschaften Dieser Produkte. Pharm. Ind. **1980**, *42*, 1019–1026.

64. Röscheisen, G.; Schmidt, P.C. Preparation and Optimization of L-Leucine as Lubricant for Effervescent Tablet Formulations. Acta Pharm. Helv. **1995**, *70*, 133–139.

65. Rinkel, R. Sprühtrocknung Pharmazeutischer Produkte. APV-Info. **1970**, *15*, 170–180.

66. Oetjen, G.-W. *Gefriertrocknen*; VCH-Verlagsgesellschaft mbH: Weinheim, 1997; 3.

67. Corveleyn, S.; Remon, J.P. Formulation and Production of Rapidly Disintegrating Tablets by Lyophilisation using Hydrochlorothiazide as a Model Drug. Int. J. Pharm. **1997**, *152*, 215–225.

68. Chen, T. Formulation Concerns of Protein Drugs. Drug Dev. Ind. Pharm. **1992**, *18*, 1311–1354.

69. Brannon-Peppas, L. Recent Advances on the Use of Biodegradable Microparticles and Nanoparticles in Controlled Drug Delivery. Int. J. Pharm. **1995**, *116*, 1–9.

70. Lill, N. Injizierbare Arzneiformen Auf Basis Biodegradabler Polymere. Pharm. Ztg. Prisma **1995**, *2*, 269–278.

71. Schmidt, P.C.; Maul, K.A. Moderne Arzneiformen für Urogenitalerkrankungen. Dtsch. Pharm. Ztg. **1993**, *138*, 837–842.

72. Thoma, K.; Alex, R.; Fensch-Kleemann, E. Biodegradable Controlled Release Implants Based on β-Tricalcium Phosphate Ceramic. I. Preparation and Characterization of Porous β-Tricalcium Phosphate Ceramic Pellets. Eur. J. Pharm. Biopharm. **1992**, *38*, 101–106.

FURTHER READING

Alexander, H. *Physikalische Grundlagen der Elektronenmikroskopie*; Teubner Studienbücher: Stuttgart, 1997.

Flegler, S.L.; Heckman, J.W.; Klomparens, K.L. *Elektronenmikroskopie: Grundlagen, methoden, Anwendungen*; Spektrum: Heidelberg, 1995.

Watt, I.M. *The Principles and Practice of Electron Microscopy*, 2nd Ed.; Cambridge University Press: Cambridge, 1997.

SEMISOLID PREPARATIONS

Guru Betageri
Sunil Prabhu
Western University of Health Sciences, Pomona, California

INTRODUCTION

Pharmaceutical semisolid preparations may be defined as topical products intended for application on the skin or accessible mucous membranes to provide localized and sometimes systemic effects at the site of application. In general, semisolid dosage forms are complex formulations having complex structural elements (1). They are often composed of two phases (oil and water), one of which is a continuous (external) phase and the other a dispersed (internal) phase. The active ingredient is often dissolved in one or both phases, thus creating a three-phase system. The physical properties of the dosage form depend on various factors, including the size of the dispersed particles, the interfacial tension between the phases, the partition coefficient of the active ingredient between the phases, and the product rheology. These factors combine to determine the release characteristics of the drug as well as other characteristics such as viscosity. Although a majority of semisolid preparations contain medicinal agents for therapeutic effect, some nonmedicated semisolid preparations are used for their physical effects as protectants and lubricants. The design of a semisolid preparation is based on its ability to adhere to the surface of application for a reasonable duration before they are washed or worn off. The adhesion is brought about by a plastic rheologic behavior that allows the semisolids to retain shape and cling as a film until acted on by an outside force, whereupon they deform and flow. One can assess this behavior by thrusting a finger through the semisolid mass, which leaves a track that does not fill up when the finger is withdrawn (2, 3). Semisolids are characterized by a three-dimensional structure that is sufficient to impart solid-like character to the undisturbed system but that is easily broken down and realigned under an applied force. In broad terms, semisolid preparations may be classified as ointments, creams, pastes, and gels.

Ointments are composed mostly of fluid hydrocarbons meshed in a matrix of higher melting solid hydrocarbons. Common examples of ointment bases include mineral oil, petrolatum, and polyethylene glycol. Creams are semisolid emulsion systems with an opaque appearance. Their consistency and rheologic properties are based on whether the emulsion is o/w or w/o and on the nature of the solid in the internal phase. Pastes are basically ointments into which a high percentage of insoluble solids has been added. Powders such as zinc oxide, titanium dioxide, starch, and kaolin are incorporated in high concentrations into a preferably lipophilic greasy vehicle to form a paste-like mass. Gels are semisolid systems in which a liquid phase is constrained within a three-dimensional polymeric matrix in which a high degree of physical cross-linking has been introduced. Most of the semisolid preparations are applied to the skin for topical relief of dermatologic conditions, whereas a lesser portion of these preparations are applied to mucous membranes such as rectal and buccal tissue, vaginal mucosa, urethral membrane, external ear lining, nasal mucosa, and cornea. Whereas normal skin permeation is limited to localized effects, the mucous membranes permit more ready access to systemic circulation. Overall, even though the nature of the underlying structures differ remarkably across all the different semisolid systems, they all share the property that their structures are easily broken down, rearranged, and reformed.

OINTMENTS AND CREAMS

Ointments utilize certain bases that act as vehicles to deliver the drug and to impart emollient and lubricant properties to the preparation. Usually, but not always, they contain medicinal substances (4). Properties of ointments may vary from product to product depending on their specific use, ease, and extent of application. In general, ointment bases may be classified into four general groups: hydrocarbon, absorption, water-removable, and water-soluble bases.

Hydrocarbon Bases

Also known as oleaginous bases, the hydrocarbon bases are essentially water-free, incorporating aqueous preparations only in small amounts and with considerable difficulty. The primary features of this type of base include its emollient effect, retention on the skin for prolonged periods, prevention of escape of moisture from the skin to the atmosphere, and difficulty in washing off. They act as occlusive dressings, thus increasing skin hydration by reducing the rate of loss of surface water. Also, they do not dry out or change noticeably on aging. Hydrocarbon-based semisolids comprise fluid hydrocarbons C_{16} to C_{30} straight chain and branched, entrapped in a fine crystalline matrix of yet higher-molecular-weight solid hydrocarbons. The high-molecular-weight fraction precipitates out substantially above room temperature, forming interlocking crystallites (5). The extent and specific nature of this structure determine the stiffness of the ointment. In general, hydrocarbon-based ointments liquefy on heating because the crystallites melt. Moreover, when cooled very slowly, they assume fluidity much greater than when rapidly cooled because slow cooling leads to fewer and larger crystallites and, therefore, less total structure.

Common examples of these bases include:

1. *Petrolatum, USP*—a mixture of semisolid hydrocarbons obtained from petroleum. It is an unctuous mass, varying in color from yellowish to light amber. It melts at temperatures between 38 and 60°C and may be used alone or in combination with other agents as an ointment base. Petrolatum of varying melting ranges and consistencies are commercially available as given in Table 1.

2. *White petrolatum, USP*—a petrolatum that has been decolorized, either partially or wholly. It is used for the same purpose as petrolatum but is more esthetically acceptable to a patient than petrolatum because of its lighter color. White petrolatum is particularly useful to treat diaper rash (impervious to urine and protects the baby's skin) and dry skin (helps the skin retain moisture). Example 1 illustrates an ointment preparation that incorporates 95% white petrolatum resulting in an ointment base with firm consistency.

3. *Yellow ointment, USP*—the purified wax obtained from the honeycomb of the bee. It contains 5% yellow wax and 95% petrolatum in the formulation.

4. *Mineral oil*—a mixture of liquid hydrocarbons obtained from petroleum. These are useful as levigating agents to wet and incorporate solid substances (e.g., salicylic acid, zinc oxide) into the preparation of ointments that consist of oleaginous bases as their vehicle. There are two types of mineral oils listed in the *U.S. Pharmacopeia/National Formulary* (USP/NF). Mineral oil USP is also called heavy mineral oil with a specific gravity between 0.845 and 0.905 and a viscosity of not less 34.5 cSt (cSt = mm²/s) at 40°C. Light mineral oil, NF has a specific gravity between 0.818 and 0.880 and a viscosity of not more than 33.5 cSt. Table 2 lists the commercially available mineral oil fractions.

Blending of increasing quantities of mineral oil with petrolatum can produce ointments of various consistencies as desired. For example, blending 10% w/w mineral oil with 90% w/w white petrolatum base can produce an ointment with less drag or resistance to spreading, making it ideal for application to burns or other painful areas. As illustrated in Example 2, melting the petrolatum and mineral oil together and allowing them to cool forms a soft base or vehicle. By increasing the quantity of the mineral oil in the mixture, a base is

Table 1 Specifications of a range of petrolatum[a]

	Melting point °F (°C)	USP or ASTM consistency	Sabolt viscosity at 210°F	Typical congealing point °F (°C)
White petrolatum, USP	122/135 (50–57)	175/205	64/75	125 (51.6)
	118/130 (47–54)	210/240	57/70	120 (48.8)
	130/140 (54–60)	155/190	60/70	130 (54.4)
Yellow petrolatum, USP	118/130 (47–54)	210/240	57/70	118 (47.7)
	122/135 (50–57)	175/205	57/70	123 (50.5)

[a]Witco Chemical Corporation, Greenwich, CT.

Table 2 Specifications of a range of mineral oils[a]

Type	Viscosity, cSt at 40°C	Specific gravity at 60°C
Mineral oil, USP	65.8/71.0	0.870/0.887
	72.0/79.5	0.864/0.878
	60.0/63.3	0.863/0.883
	38.4/41.5	0.859/0.882
	34.9/37.3	0.858/0.882
Light mineral oil, NF	28.1/30.3	0.856/0.882
	24.2/26.3	0.854/0.873
	17.7/20.2	0.842/0.870
	14.2/17.0	0.845/0.860
	7.6/8.7	0.831/0.842

[a]Penzoil Products Company, Karns City, PA.

obtained that has a gel-like consistency indicating a more viscous preparation (Example 3). Hydrocarbon vehicles have several advantages, such as stability and emolliency; however, they suffer from one major disadvantage—greasiness—which may stain clothing and is usually difficult to remove (6).

Ophthalmic Ointments

Ophthalmic ointments differ from conventional ointments in that they must be sterile. Although the USP does not specify any particular base in the ophthalmic drug monographs, it states that the ingredients used must be sterilized under rigid aseptic conditions and again in its final container (7). In choosing an ointment base for an ophthalmic preparation, it must meet several qualities such as having the ability to diffuse the medication throughout the secretions bathing the eye, being nonirritating to the eye, and having the ability to diffuse the medication throughout the secretions bathing the eye. It must also have a softening point close to body temperature, both for patient comfort and for drug release. To avoid the risk of damage to the eye, it is imperative that the ointment be free of large particles and any metal particles. Mixtures of mineral oil and white petrolatum are commonly used as the base in medicated and nonmedicated (lubricating) ophthalmic ointments. Usually, the medicinal agents are added to an ointment base either as a solution or as a finely micronized powder and are subjected to fine milling to render the preparation uniform and smooth. The ophthalmic ointments also must meet the USP sterility tests and the test for metal particles in ophthalmic ointments. Rendering an ophthalmic ointment sterile requires special

Example 1 White ointment, USP

White petrolatum	95 (% w/w)
White wax	5

Procedure: Melt the white wax and add the petrolatum; continue heating until a liquid melt is formed. Congeal with stirring. Heating should be gentle to avoid charring (steam is preferred), and air incorporation by too vigorous stirring is to be avoided.

Example 2 Soft petrolatum base

White petrolatum, USP	90.0 (% w/w)
Mineral oil, NF	10.0

Procedure: Melt the white petrolatum and mineral oil together and allow to cool.

Example 3 Gelled petrolatum base

White petrolatum, USP	75.0 (% w/w)
Mineral oil, NF	25.0 (% w/w)

Procedure: Melt the white petrolatum and mineral oil together and allow to cool.

aseptic techniques and processing. Each drug, along with other components, is rendered sterile separately, aseptically weighed, and incorporated in preparing a final product that meets the sterility requirement (8). This is done because of difficulty in terminal product sterilization, such as lack of penetration of steam into the ointment base and instability of components owing to high dry heating. Antimicrobial preservatives such as methylparaben (0.05%) and propylparaben (0.01%) and its combinations phenylmercuric acetate (0.0008%), chlorobutanol (0.5%), and benzalkonium chloride (0.008%) are used as needed.

Absorption Bases

Absorption bases, as such, are hydrophilic, anhydrous materials (w/o emulsions) or hydrous bases (w/o emulsions that have the ability to absorb additional water). Addition of lanolin, lanolin isolates, cholesterol, lanosterol, or acetylated sterols renders the hydrocarbon base hydrophilic. Such hydrophilic mixtures have been known as absorption bases; however, the word absorption is a misnomer. Although the bases do eventually absorb aqueous solutions to be considered w/o emulsions, they do not absorb water on contact, but after sufficient agitation only. They are conventional ointments that contain w/o emulsifiers in appreciable quantity. A w/o emulsion is formed when an aqueous medium, perhaps containing the drug in solution, is worked into the base. Thus, these bases can be classified as: 1) those that permit the incorporation of aqueous solutions, resulting in the formation of w/o emulsions (e.g., hydrophilic petrolatum), and 2) those that are already w/o emulsions (emulsion bases) that permit the incorporation of small, additional quantities of aqueous solutions (e.g., cold cream). These bases are useful as emollients, although they do not provide the degree of occlusion as oleaginous bases. They are also used pharmaceutically to incorporate aqueous solutions of drugs (e.g., sodium sulfacetamide solution) into oleaginous bases. A typical example of an anhydrous absorption base is hydrophilic petrolatum, USP (Example 4). Here, cholesterol confers the w/o emulsion property, whereas inclusion of stearyl alcohol and white wax enhances firmness and heat stability. Diverse additives including cholesterol, lanolin (which contains cholesterol, cholesterol esters, and other emulsifiers), semisynthetic lanolin derivatives, and assorted ionic and nonionic surfactants are used to emulsify water into these systems, singularly or in combination. Lanolin is probably the best known substance for the emulsification of water in an anhydrous base. Anhydrous lanolin, USP is capable of absorbing up to 30% of its weight of water to form an emulsion. Its water-absorbing capacity is improved to 50% by the addition of cholesterol. Among the absorption bases, lanolin is the oldest and best known. However, because of its tackiness and viscous nature and reports of allergic reactions, the use of lanolin is very limited. Advents in technology have successfully produced a number of emulsifiers for w/o emulsions. Used in specific formulations, emulsifiers such as polyglyceryl esters form w/o emulsions (Example 5). Absorption bases impart excellent emolliency and a degree of occlusiveness on application. However, they are also greasy when applied and are difficult to remove. The anhydrous types of absorption

Example 5   Water-in-oil emulsion formulation

Mineral oil	40.0 (% w/w)
White wax	6.0 (% w/w)
Polyglyceryl 5 trioleate	8.0 (% w/w)
Isopropyl palmitate	3.0 (% w/w)
Sorbitol monostearate	3.5 (% w/w)
Polysorbate 60	2.5 (% w/w)
Propylene glycol	4.0 (% w/w)
Water	33.0 (% w/w)
Preservative, q.s.	

bases can be used when the presence of water causes stability problems with specific drug substances such as antibiotics. Commercially available absorption bases include Aquaphor (Beiersdorf, Hamburg, Germany) and Polysorb (Fougera, Melville, NY). Absorption bases, either hydrous or anhydrous, are seldom used as vehicles for commercial drug products because the w/o emulsion is more difficult to handle than the more conventional o/w system, and also there is reduced patient acceptance because of greasiness.

A new group of w/o emulsifiers based on the linkage of polymethoxysiloxane chains with alkyl side chains and polyol groups has been constituted (9). These emulsifiers, known as organosilicone polymers, have the capability of producing w/o emulsions with a high water content. Although the polymethylsiloxane chains possess both hydrophilic and lipophilic properties, the alkyl side chains supply the necessary lipophilic and polyol groups to provide the hydrophilic characteristics of the emulsifier. Other examples of w/o emulsifiers include cetyl dimethicone copolymer (10), polyethylene glycol-20-com glycerides (11), and a series of caprylic–capryl stearates (12).

Water-Removable Bases (Water-Washable Creams)

These are the most commonly used o/w emulsion bases that are capable of being washed from skin or clothing with water. They may contain water-soluble and -insoluble components. From a therapeutic viewpoint, they have the ability to absorb serous discharges in dermatologic conditions. The water-removable bases form a semipermeable film on the site of application after the evaporation of water. As such, the base consists of three component parts: the oil phase, the emulsifier, and the aqueous phase. The oil phase, also called the internal phase, is typically made up of the petrolatum

Example 4   Hydrophilic petrolatum, USP (anhydrous absorption base)

White petrolatum	86.0 (% w/w)
Cholesterol	3.0 (% w/w)
Stearyl alcohol	3.0 (% w/w)
White wax	8.0 (% w/w)

Procedure: Melt the stearyl alcohol and white wax together on a steam bath, then add the cholesterol and stir until it completely dissolves. Add the white petrolatum and mix. Remove from the bath and stir until mixture congeals.

and/or liquid petrolatum. Other ingredients such as cetyl and stearyl alcohol may be added to make up the oil phase. A typical water-removable emulsion base is hydrophilic ointment, USP, as shown in Example 6. The stearyl alcohol serves as an adjuvant emulsifier. Petrolatum in the oil phase contributes to the water-holding ability of the overall formulation. The aqueous phase contains preservative materials, emulsifier, and humectant. Humectants are added to minimize water loss in the finished composition and to add to the overall physical product acceptability. Common examples of humectants used include glycerin, propylene glycol, and a polyethylene glycol. The aqueous phase also contains the water-soluble components of the emulsion system, together with any additional stabilizers, antioxidants, buffers, etc., that may be necessary for stability, pH control, and other considerations associated with aqueous systems. Another example of an o/w emulsion base is illustrated in Example 7 (vanishing cream). The vanishing creams are so called because on application and rubbing into the skin, there is little or no visible evidence of their presence. The addition of an emulsifying agent is critical to formulating an emulsion. Emulsifiers must meet the following criteria before incorporation:

1. be a surfactant to reduce surface tension;
2. be able to prevent coalescence by being absorbed quickly around the dispersed droplets;
3. facilitate mutual repulsion between particles by imparting an adequate electrical potential to the droplets;
4. be able to increase viscosity to ensure a semisolid system; and
5. be effective at low concentrations.Emulsifiers used in cream formulations may be classified into three different categories: anionic, cationic, and nonionic emulsifiers.

Anionic emulsifiers

The active portion of this class of emulsifiers is the anion. In general, these emulsifiers are more acid-stable and permit adjustment of the emulsion pH level to the desirable range of 4.5 and 6.5. Common examples include sodium lauryl sulfate and soaps such as triethanolamine stearate. Triethanolamine stearate is one of the most popular emulsifiers for creams and lotions in use today. It is usually prepared in situ during manufacture from stearic acid in the hot oil phase and from triethanolamine in the hot aqueous phase. The amount of triethanolamine controls the pH level of the resulting product.

Example 6 Hydrophilic ointment, USP

Stearyl alcohol	25.0 (% w/w)
White petrolatum	25.0 (% w/w)
Methylparaben	0.025 (% w/w)
Propylparaben	0.015 (% w/w)
Sodium lauryl sulfate	1.0 (% w/w)
Propylene glycol	12.0 (% w/w)
Purified water	37.0 (% w/w)

Procedure: Melt the stearyl alcohol and white petrolatum in a steam bath and warm to 75°C. Add the other ingredients previously dissolved in water and warmed to 75°C, and stir mixture until it congeals.

Example 7 Vanishing cream (cream base o/w)

Oleaginous phase	
Stearic acid	13.0 (% w/v)
Stearyl alcohol	1.0
Cetyl alcohol	1.0
Aqueous phase	
Glycerin	10.0
Methylparaben	0.1
Propylparaben	0.05
Potassium hydroxide	0.9
Purified water, q.s.	100

Procedure: Heat the oil phase and water phase to approximately 65°C. Add the oil phase slowly to the aqueous phase with stirring to form a crude emulsion. Cool to approximately 50°C and homogenize. Cool with agitation until congealed.

Cationic emulsifiers

Cationic compounds are highly surface-active but are used less frequently as emulsifiers. The cation portion of the molecule is usually a quaternary ammonium salt including a fatty acid derivative such as dilauryldimethylammonium chloride. These emulsifiers are irritating to the skin and eyes and have a considerable range of incompatibilities, including anionic materials.

Nonionic emulsifiers

This class of emulsifiers shows excellent pH and electrolyte compatibility in emulsions, owing to the fact that they do not ionize in solution. Although nonionic emulsifiers range from lipophilic to hydrophilic members, a typical emulsifier system may include a mixture of both a lipophilic and a hydrophilic member to produce a hydrophilic–lipophilic balance (HLB). As devised by Griffin (13), an HLB scale can be used to establish a range of optimum efficiency for a suitable emulsifier for a certain activity such as wetting agent,

Table 3 Activity and HLB value of emulsifiers

Activity	Assigned HLB
Antifoaming	1–3
Emulsifiers (w/o)	3–6
Wetting agents	7–9
Emulsifiers (o/w)	8–18
Solubilizers	15–20
Detergents	13–15

Example 9 Water-in-oil cream formulation HLB 12

Part A	
Mineral oil	50.0 (% w/w)
White wax	15.0 (% w/w)
Sorbitan monostearate	2.0 (% w/w)
Part B	
POE[a] sorbitan monostearate	3.0 (% w/w)
Water, q.s.	30.0 (% w/w)

Procedure: Same as in Example 8.
[a]Polyoxyethylene

antifoaming agent, detergent, etc. Although the numbers have been assigned up to 40, the usual range is between 1 and 20. Materials that are highly polar or hydrophilic are assigned higher numbers than materials that are less polar and more lipophilic. Generally, those emulsifiers with an assigned value between 3 and 6 are greatly lipophilic and produce w/o emulsions, whereas those in the range between 8 and 18 are hydrophilic and produce o/w emulsions. By using this scale, it is possible to relate various emulsifiers to suitable applications. Table 3 illustrates the relationship between HLB numbers and the type of activity expected from emulsifiers. Emulsions containing nonionic emulsifiers are prepared by dissolving or dispersing the lipophilic component in the oil phase and the hydrophilic component in the aqueous phase. The two phases are heated separately and combined. Emulsions containing nonionic emulsifiers are generally low in irritation potential, stable, and have excellent compatibility characteristics. Examples 8 and 9 illustrate the use of these emulsifiers in the formulation of creams.

The Cosmetic, Toiletry and Fragrance Association's *International Cosmetic Ingredient Dictionary* (14)

provides an exhaustive listing of the variety of emulsion-base components, particularly the oil phase components. Over 6000 ingredients, cross-referenced to more than 25,000 trade names and synonyms, are presented. These include emulsifiers, coemulsifiers, surfactants, and stabilizers. Another source is The *McCutcheons Detergents and Emulsifiers* (15), which also lists thousands of emulsifiers and surfactants. These lists are important sources of information and help formulators in the pharmaceutical and cosmetic industry. Commonly used oils and surfactants in formulating semisolid emulsions are shown in Tables 4 and 5.

Microemulsions

Microemulsions are fluid, transparent, thermodynamically stable oil and water systems, stabilized by a surfactant usually in conjunction with a cosurfactant that may be a short-chain alcohol, amine, or other weakly amphiphilic molecule (16, 17). An interesting characteristic of microemulsions is that the diameter of the droplets is in the range of 100–1000 Å, whereas the diameter of droplets in a kinetically stable macroemulsion is 5000 Å. The small droplet size allows the microemulsion to act as carriers for drugs that are poorly soluble in water. The suggested method of preparation of microemulsions is as follows: the surfactant, oil, and water are mixed to form a milky emulsion and titrated with a fourth component, the cosurfactant, until the mixture becomes clear (18). If more oil is added to a w/o system, the system becomes cloudy, but the addition of more cosurfactant again gives a clean transparent emulsion. As illustrated in Example 10, the formulation results in clear, transparent "ringing gels" with good stability. Microemulsions are optically clear because the diameter of the particles in the colloidal system is less than one-quarter of the wavelength of incident light. Because of this effect, the particles do not scatter light and result in a transparent system (19, 20). Microemulsions, once made, must be packaged while hot

Example 8 Oil-in-water cream formulation HLB 13

Part A	
Stearic acid	10.0 (% w/w)
Mineral oil	8.0 (% w/w)
White petrolatum	6.0 (% w/w)
Sorbitan monostearate	2.0 (% w/w)
Part B	
POE[a] sorbitan monostearate	1.0 (% w/w)
Water	73.0 (% w/w)
Preservative, q.s.	

Procedure: Part A is heated at 70°C until completely melted. Part B is added at 70°C and the mixture is cooled to room temperature.
[a]Polyoxyethylene.

Table 4 Oil phase emulsion components

Type	Composition	Physical state
Hydrocarbon	Mineral oils	Liquid
Hydrocarbon	Petrolatum	Semisolid
Hydrocarbon	Polyethylene polymers	Solid
Hydrocarbon	Synthetic waxes	Solid
Esters	Vegetable oils	Liquid
Ester	Lanolin	Liquid
Esters	Synthetics (e.g., butyl stearate)	Liquid or solid
Alcohols	Long chain	Liquid or solid
Fatty acids	Long chain	Liquid or solid
Ethers	Polyoxyethylene	Liquid or solid
	Polyoxypropylene	Liquid or solid
Silicones	Polymers	Liquid or solid
Natural products	Plant and animal waxes	Solid

and in the liquid form. After they are cooled, they cannot be reheated and melted because they will lose transparency because of coalescence of the oil globules to a size where they reflect light.

Water-Soluble Bases

These bases contain only water-soluble components. Water-soluble bases are also referred to as greaseless because of a lack of oleaginous materials. Incorporation of aqueous solutions is difficult because they soften greatly with the addition of water. They are better used for nonaqueous or solid substances. Polyethylene glycols (PEG) make up the majority of components of the water-soluble base. PEGs may exist as liquids or waxy solids, identified by numbers that are an approximate indication of their molecular weight. The lowest number signifies a liquid state, which transitions to a waxy solid state as the numbers increase. For example, PEG 400 is a liquid, whereas PEG 4000 is a waxy solid. Polyethylene glycol is a polymer of ethylene oxide and water represented by the formula $OHCH_2$ (CH_2OCH_2) CH_2OH. They are nonvolatile, water-soluble, or water-miscible compounds and chemically inert. PEGs of interest as vehicles include the 1500, 1600, 4000, and 6000 products, ranging from soft, waxy solids to hard waxes. PEG, particularly 1500, can be used as a vehicle by itself, but better results are often obtained using blends of high- and low-molecular-weight glycols as in polyethylene glycol ointment, NF (Example 11). PEGs also serve as excellent bases for suppository insert dosage forms. Various combinations of PEGs may be used to achieve a suppository base of desired

Table 5 Emulsifiers for semisolid emulsions

Anionic	Cationic	Nonionic
Alkyl sulfates	Quaternary ammonium compounds	Polyoxyethylene alkyl–aryl ethers
Soaps	Alkoxyalkylamines	Polyoxypropylene alkyl–aryl ethers
Dodecyl benzenesulfonates		Polyoxyethylene fatty acid esters
Lactylates		Polyoxyethylene sorbitan esters
Sulfosuccinates		Polyoxyethylene-polyoxypropylene block polymers
Monoglyceride sulfates		
Phosphate esters		Sorbitan fatty acid esters
Silicones		Glyceryl fatty acid esters
Sarcosinates		
Taurates		

Example 10 Microemulsion

Mineral oil, NF	16.0 (% w/w)
Sucrose distearate	5.0 (% w/w)
Sucrose stearate	5.0 (% w/w)
Diethylamine oleylether—10 phosphate	2.0 (% w/w)
Diethylamine oleylether—3 phosphate	5.0 (% w/w)
1,3-Ethylhexane diol	2.5 (% w/w)
Propylene glycol	5.0 (% w/w)
Water	59.5 (% w/w)

Example 12 Zinc oxide paste, USP

Zinc oxide	25.0%
Starch	25.0%
Calamine	5.0%
White petrolatum, q.s.	100%

Procedure: Titrate the calamine with the zinc oxide and starch and incorporate uniformly in the petrolatum by levigation in a mortar or on a glass slab with a spatula. Mineral oil should not be used as a levigating agent, because it would soften the product. A portion of petrolatum can be melted and used as a levigating agent if so desired.

consistency and characteristics. For example, PEG 1000 blended with PEG 4000 results in a higher melting product, whereas blending with a liquid polyethylene glycol lowers the melting point. Some drugs lower the melting points of PEG and, therefore, each ingredient must be considered in selecting a base. The advantage of PEG suppositories is that they may be designed to prevent melting at body temperature but rather to dissolve slowly in the body fluids. Thus, they can be prepared at temperatures higher than that of the body. They also can be stored without the need for refrigeration and do not tend to leak from the orifice on insertion because of higher melting temperatures.

PASTES

Pastes maybe defined as ointments incorporating a high percentage of insoluble particulate solids, sometimes as much as or more than 50% (2). The use of this high amount of insoluble particulate matter renders a stiffness to the system as a result of direct interactions between the dispersed particulates and by absorption of the liquid hydrocarbons from the vehicles onto the surface of the particles. Because of the stiffness, they remain in place after application and are used effectively to absorb serous secretions. Pastes as such are not suited for application to hairy parts of the body. Examples of insoluble ingredients serving as the dispersed phase include starch, zinc oxide, and calcium carbonate. Pastes

Example 11 Polyethylene glycol ointment, NF

Polyethylene glycol 3350	40 (% w/w)
Polyethylene glycol 400	60 (% w/w)

Procedure: Heat the two ingredients in a water bath to 65°C. Allow to cool and stir until congealed.

make good protective barriers for the following reasons. In addition to forming an unbroken film, pastes also absorb and neutralize certain harmful chemicals before they reach the skin surface. This last feature is attributed to the presence of insoluble particulate matter within the paste formulations. For example, for the treatment of diaper rash, when spread over the baby's bottom, the pastes absorb irritants formed by bacterial action on urine. Pastes also provide a protective layer over skin lesions and, when covered with suitable dressings, prevent excoriation of the patient's skin by scratching. Pastes afford emollient action as do ointments. In addition, the water-impermeable film formed on application is opaque and thus can often serve as a sunblock. Pastes are less greasy than ointments because of the absorption of the fluid hydrocarbon fraction to the insoluble particles. A clinically distinctive feature, which is generally attributed to pastes, is the ability to absorb exudates by nature of the powder or other absorptive components (21). Among the few pastes in use today is zinc oxide paste (Lassar's Plain Zinc Paste) (Example 12), which is prepared by levigating and then mixing 25% each of zinc oxide and starch with white petrolatum. The product is very firm and is better able to protect the skin and absorb secretions than is zinc oxide ointment.

GELS

Gels are defined as semisolid preparations consisting of dispersions of small or large molecules in an aqueous liquid vehicle rendered jelly-like through the addition of a geling agent (22). Gels are an intermediate state of matter, containing both solid and liquid components. The solid component comprises a three-dimensional network of interconnected molecules or aggregates that immobilizes the liquid in the continuous phase (23). Gels may be

Example 13 Carbomer 941 gel

Carbomer 941	0.5 (% w/w)
Glycerine	10.0 (% w/w)
Triethanolamine	0.5 (% w/w)
Water	89.0 (% w/w)
Preservative q.s.	

Procedure: Water, glycerine, and preservative are mixed and the carbomer added by sprinkling on the surface while constantly mixing at high speed. Triethanolamine is added with slow agitation until a clear viscous gel forms.

classified into two primary types: hydrogels, which have an aqueous continuous phase, and organogels, which have an organic solvent as the liquid continuous medium. Gels may also be classified based on the nature of the bonds involved in the three-dimensional solid network: chemical gels form when strong covalent bonds hold the network together, and physical gels form when hydrogen bonds and electrostatic and van der Waals interactions maintain the gel network (24). Gelling agents commonly used are synthetic macromolecules (e.g., carbomer 934), cellulose derivatives (e.g., carboxymethylcellulose and hydroxypropylmethylcellulose), and natural gums (e.g., tragacanth). Carbomers in particular are high-molecular-weight water-soluble polymers of acrylic acid cross-linked with allyl ethers of sucrose and/or pentaerythritol. The NF contains monographs for six such polymers: carbomers 910, 934, 934P, 940, 941, and 1342. They are used as gelling agents at concentrations of 0.5–2.0% in water. Carbomer 940 yields the highest viscosity: between 40,000 and 60,000 CP as a 0.5% aqueous dispersion. Depending on their polymeric composition, different viscosities result. Gels may be classified as two-phase or single-phase systems. A two-phase gel system consists of floccules of small distinct particles rather than large molecules, thus called

Example 14 Carbomer 934 alcoholic gel

Carbomer 934 resin	3.0 (% w/w)
Glycerine	10.0 (% w/w)
Ethanol	40.0 (% w/w)
2-Ethylhexylamine	2.5 (% w/w)
Water	44.5 (% w/w)

Procedure: The carbomer is dispersed in the glycerine and water, and a solution of the 2-Ethylhexylamine in ethanol is added to the water solution with mixing until a clear transparent gel is formed.

a two-phase system often referred to as a magma. Milk of magnesia (or magnesia magma), which comprises a gelatinous precipitate of magnesium hydroxide, is an example of such a system. The gel structure in the two-phase systems is not always stable and thus may thicken on standing, forming a thixotrope, and must be shaken before use to liquefy the gel and enable pouring. Single-phase systems are gels in which the macromolecules are uniformly distributed throughout a liquid with no apparent boundaries between the dispersed macromolecules and the liquid. Examples of such gels include tragacanth and carboxymethylcellulose. A typical gel formulation may contain, apart from the gelling agent and water, a drug substance, cosolvents such as alcohol and/or propylene glycol, antimicrobial preservatives such as methylparaben and propylparaben or chlorhexidine gluconate, and stabilizers such as edetate disodium. Medicated gels may be prepared for administration by various routes including topically to the skin or eye, nasally, vaginally, and rectally. Some simple gel formulations are shown in Examples 13 and 14. Example 15 gives the formulation for a firm, rigid gel.

MANUFACTURING METHODS

Ointments

There are two primary methods of manufacturing ointment dosage forms: incorporation and fusion. Each may be used on a small scale (laboratory) or large scale (industry) for the manufacture of semisolid dosage forms.

Incorporation (laboratory scale)

On a small scale, as in a pharmacy, small quantities of ointments may be prepared using a mortar and pestle or

Example 15 Solubilized mineral oil gel

Polyethylene glycol 3 oleyl ether phosphate	6.8 (% w/w)
Polyethylene glycol 3 oleyl ether	4.0 (% w/w)
Polyethylene glycol 5 oleyl ether	2.7 (% w/w)
Mineral oil 220 SUS	13.6 (% w/w)
2-Ethyl-1,3-Hexanediol	13.4 (% w/w)
Propylene glycol	1.4 (% w/w)
Water	68.1 (% w/w)

Procedure: All components except water are heated to 75°C. The water is added at 75°C to the oil with mixing to form a soft gel, which on stirring and cooling sets at approximately 35°C.

an ointment slab (porcelain or glass) and spatula. The finely divided drug material is dispersed into an appropriate vehicle by mixing the components or rubbing the ingredients together to form an ointment. Sometimes, nonabsorbent parchment paper may be used to cover the working surface, which is then subsequently disposed of, thus eliminating the time to clean the ointment slabs.

When incorporating solids by the method of spatulation, the ointment base is placed on one side of the slab, and the finely divided drug powder components are placed on the other side. A small portion of the powder is mixed with a small portion of the base and worked in together to form a uniform mass. The procedure is repeated with the remaining base and powdered materials until all of the components are uniformly combined and blended. A broad blade spatula, made of metal or hard plastic, may be used for this task. Hard plastic spatulas are used when a component (e.g., phenol) of the mixture sometimes reacts with the metal.

Often it is desirable to keep the particle size of powder components in an ointment to a minimum to avoid roughness or grittiness of the preparation. Methods of particle size reduction include use of the mortar and pestle and the process of levigation. In this, the finely divided powdered material is levigated thoroughly with a small quantity of ointment base to form a concentrate. Sometimes, levigating agents such as mineral oil (for oleaginous bases) and glycerin (for aqueous bases) can also be used to form smooth dispersions. The levigating agent should be physically and chemically compatible with the drug and base. The concentrate is then diluted geometrically with the remainder of the base until a uniform mix is achieved. The process of levigation is usually carried out using a mortar and pestle to reduce particle size as well as to disperse the powdered material into the concentrate. After levigation, the dispersion may either be transferred onto an ointment slab or mixed further using the mortar and pestle with the remainder of the ointment base. If the drug substance is soluble in solvents such as alcohol or water, the powdered materials are first dissolved in the solvent of choice and then incorporated with the remainder of the base using a mortar and pestle. Spatulation is inconvenient because the water- or alcohol-dissolved components are free-flowing.

When incorporating liquids or solutions of drugs into ointment bases, care must be taken to select the appropriate ointment base with regard to its capacity to accept the volume of drug in solution. To incorporate liquids into hydrophobic bases such as oleaginous bases,

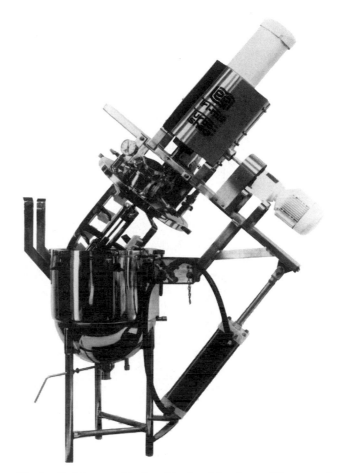

Fig. 1 Stainless steel jacketed kettle with agitator. (Courtesy of Lee Industries, Inc., Philipsburg, Pennsylvania.)

the liquid solution must first be incorporated in a minimum amount of hydrophilic base and subsequently added to the hydrophobic base. Care must be taken not to exceed the liquid-retaining capacity of the bases beyond which they become too soft or semiliquid in state.

Incorporation (industrial scale)

Mechanical mixers are used to prepare ointments in large quantities, especially in the Pharmaceutical industry. Stainless steel kettle mixers may be used to manufacture hydrocarbon and water-soluble base ointments (Fig. 1). The stainless steel kettle is jacketed for heating and cooling and is equipped with a mixing device. The kettle configuration is especially well-suited for the melting and mixing of oils and waxes and for complete bottom-emptying. Depending on the formulation to be processed, the mixer may be either a propeller or an anchor–agitator design. If the formulation is primarily liquid, a propeller

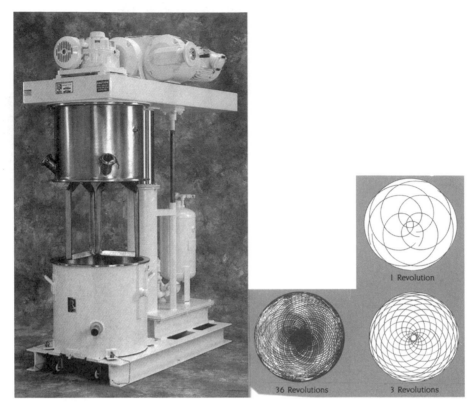

Fig. 2 Double planetary mixer showing mixing patterns at different stirring speeds. (Courtesy of Charles Ross & Son Co., Hauppauge, New York.)

mixer is more suitable. If the formulation consists of solid waxes, lanolin, petrolatum, and similar components, a kettle with a removable agitator, as shown in Fig. 1, is indicated.

Planetary mixers (Fig. 2) may also be used for large-scale preparations of the ointments. Here, the finely divided powdered materials are added slowly or sifted into the vehicle (ointment base) previously placed inside the rotating mixer. On achieving a uniform consistency, the ointment preparation may be processed through the roller mill to ensure complete dispersion and reduce the size of aggregates that may have formed during processing. The roller mills force the coarsely formed ointments through stainless steel rollers to produce ointments that are uniform in composition and smooth in texture.

Fusion Process

The process of fusion uses heat to melt all or some of the components of the ointment; the mixture is then allowed to cool with constant stirring until congealed. Additional components of the ointment preparation that were not subject to the initial melting process are added to the congealing mixture as it is being cooled and stirred. Heat-labile substances are added to the preparation after careful observation that the temperature of the mixture is sufficiently low so as not to cause decomposition or volatilization of the components.

Substances may also be added by levigating a portion of the base with the milled drug to form a concentrate. The concentrate is then added to or dispersed in the remainder of the vehicle using a mixer such as porcelain dish or glass beaker (on a small scale) or a steam-jacketed vessel (on a large scale) and allowed to cool and congeal as noted earlier. Once congealed, the mixture is rubbed with a spatula or mortar and pestle (on a small scale) or allowed to pass through an ointment roller mill (on a large scale) to ensure a uniform and smooth texture. Some common examples of components that are subjected to the fusion process include beeswax, paraffin, stearyl alcohol, and high-molecular-weight polyethylene glycols (PEG). The order of addition of components in the process of fusion plays a role in the manufacture of ointments. In general, one way to mix all components together is to choose the component with

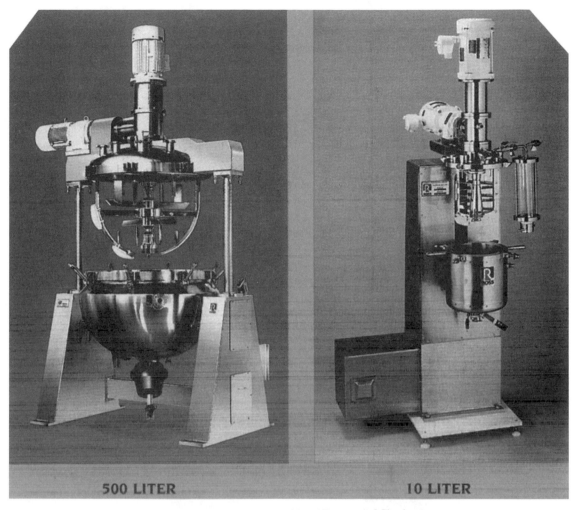

Fig. 3 High-turbulence mixers (turboemulsifiers) of varying capacities. (Courtesy of Charles Ross & Son Co., Hauppauge, New York.)

the highest melting point and use the minimum amount of heat to melt it. Subsequently, all the other components may be added with constant stirring and cooling of the melt until the mixture is congealed. Alternatively, the component with the lowest melting point may be added first. With increasing temperature, the remaining materials may be added to melt the entire mixture and then the process of cooling and congealing followed as before.

Emulsion Products

Emulsions are prepared by means of a two-phase heat system. In the first phase, the oil phase ingredients are combined in a jacketed tank and heated between 70 and 75°C to melt or liquefy all the ingredients to a uniform state. In a separate tank, the second phase, aqueous phase

ingredients are heated together to slightly above 75°C. The aqueous phase is then slowly added to the oil phase through constant agitation. The mixture is cooled slowly with continuing agitation as the emulsion is formed. The medicinal ingredients may be added when the emulsion is in the cooling stage. Usually, these ingredients are added as concentrated slurry that has been previously milled to a finely divided state. At times, when the aqueous phase of the emulsion system is larger, a large kettle may be required with a more complex mixer. As the oil phase is heated in a kettle, the aqueous phase is prepared in a kettle almost twice the size of the oil phase kettle. This size difference accommodates the volume of the final emulsion. Both phases may be heated between 70 and 80°C. For convenience and efficiency, the oil phase kettle should be mounted directly above the aqueous phase so as to introduce the oil phase mixture into the lower emulsifying

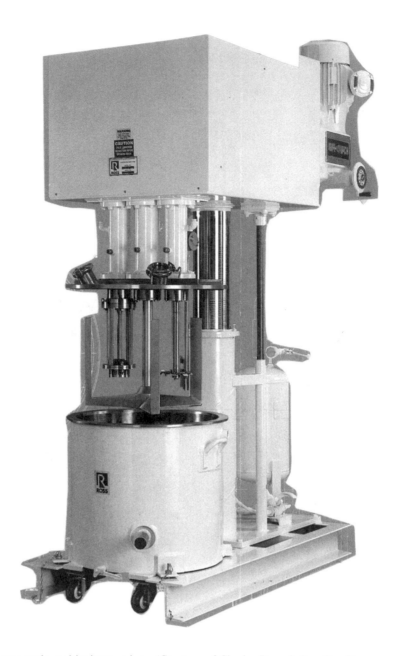

Fig. 4 Large-scale multiagitator mixer. (Courtesy of Charles Ross & Son Co., Hauppauge, New York.)

unit. The oil phase is introduced into the aqueous phase kettle in a relatively small stream to allow rapid dispersion and emulsification by an appropriately sized agitator. For capacities of 200 gallons or less, a single high-turbulence agitator may be used in most cases. Figure 3 shows two models of a high-turbulence emulsifier consisting of three top-entering coaxial agitators including an anchor–agitator and self-adjusting Teflon scrapers for thorough mixing of the preparation. For larger batches of up to 1000 gallons, a large-scale

multiagitator mixer may be used (as shown in Fig. 4) that involves a mixer–emulsifier (for high degree of shear), a high-speed disperser (to disperse solids into viscous liquids), and an anchor–agitator (to provide maximum movement of product under low shear conditions in the mix vessel). Another design for large batches uses a double-motion, counterrotating agitation combined with a homogenizing action that allows for versatility in mixing applications (Fig. 5). After the addition of the phases, the rate of cooling is generally slow to allow for adequate

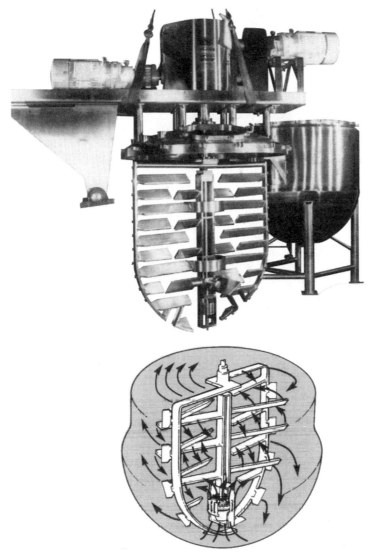

Fig. 5 Large-scale manufacturing unit (Tri-mix Turboshear) with counter-rotating mixing bars. (Courtesy of Lee Industries, Inc., Philipsburg, Pennsylvania.)

mixing while the emulsion is still in liquid form. Cooling should be at a rate consistent with the mixing of the emulsion and scraping of the kettle walls to prevent formation of congealed masses of ointment or cream, especially when the semisolid contains a large amount of high-melting substances. If drugs are introduced during the manufacture of the product, oil-soluble drugs should be dissolved in the oil phase and water-soluble drugs in the aqueous phase. All emulsions are susceptible to bacterial contamination, thus, preservative agents should be added while the emulsion is still hot to effect complete solution. To improve the stability of the oil phase, colloid mills may be used to disperse the oil phase further once the emulsion is formed. As shown in Fig. 6, a colloid mill can be a portable unit that can be lowered into the kettle and operated as the mixing of phases continues. It operates by a shearing action of a high-speed rotor against a stationary stator with a clearance of a few thousandths of an inch. The colloid mill may also be located outside of the kettle and the emulsion pumped through it to the filling equipment or holding tank (Fig. 7). Sometimes, a homogenizer may be used to reduce the size of the oil globules by exerting a smearing action in which the emulsion is forced through a small orifice under high pressure. It is located between the emulsifying kettle and the filling line or holding tank. The advantage of the homogenizer over the colloid mill is that it does not incorporate air into the emulsion. However, the throughput

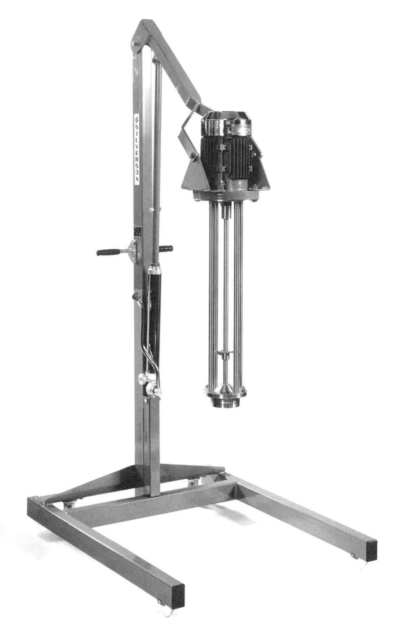

Fig. 6 Portable batch mixer on mobile hydraulic floor stand (Courtesy of Silverson Machines, Inc., East Long Meadow, Massachusetts).

of the homogenizer is 10–100 times lower than that of the colloid mill. When the emulsion is pumped from one vessel to another, an in-line colloid mill may be installed. Instead of producing an emulsion in a kettle or other vessel, several phases may be introduced into the pipeline in their proper proportions using metering pumps and emulsified en route by the action of the in-line colloid mill (Fig. 8).

Another in-line method of emulsification is the ultrasonic process, which uses a sonolator and the principle of the Pohlman whistle (25). This process uses a very high-intensity mixing device that mechanically generates ultrasonic acoustic energy to produce emulsions and dispersions. Liquid to be processed is pumped through a special orifice, forming a flat, high-pressure stream. This jet impinges on the edge of a flat blade enclosed in a tube, causing it to vibrate at ultrasonic frequencies. Cavitation produces violent local pressure changes that act on the liquid, causing instantaneous and intense dispersion of any immiscible liquids or insoluble particles. Water-in-oil

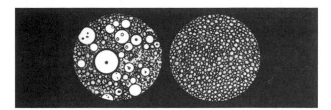

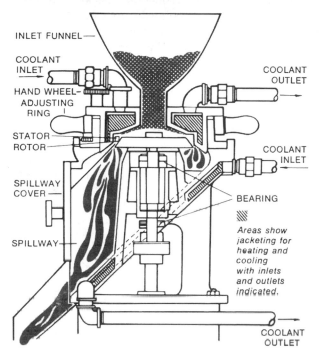

Fig. 7 Schematic representation of colloid mill and microphotographs showing emulsion globule size before and after milling. (Courtesy of Premier Mill Corp., Reading, Pennsylvania.)

emulsions are manufactured in the same equipment as o/w emulsions except that the phases are reversed in the equipment.

Miscellaneous Preparations

Heating, melting, and cooling in a single kettle in the same manner as with ointment preparations may be used to process the water-soluble bases composed of polyethylene glycols, ranging from liquids to waxy solids. They may be allowed to cool and solidify and to be stored until needed. Then they are remelted and packaged. Gels can be processed similarly in a single mixing kettle with slow agitation to avoid air entrapment, which may occur if mixed rapidly. This is especially important because all gels appear to be transparent or translucent, and air bubbles appear as a visible contamination.

PRESERVATIVES

Semisolid dosage forms must meet acceptable standards for microbial content, and preparations that are prone to microbial growth must contain antimicrobial preservatives. Antimicrobial preservative substances are included in ointment formulations to maintain the potency and integrity of product forms and to protect the health and safety of the consumer. The USP addresses this subject inits monograph *Microbiological Attributes of Non-SterilePharmaceutical Products*. An ideal preservative system should have attributes such as effectiveness at lowconcentrations against a host of microorganisms, solubility, nontoxicity, nonsensitizing, compatibility with other components, absence of odor, stability, and inexpensive. In addition, they must have the appropriate oil/water partition coefficient and be effective at the pH level of the products.

Several sources of contamination include water, raw materials, and poor sanitation conditions during manufacture, storage, and use. As such, preparations that contain water tend to support microbial growth to a greater extent than do preparations that are water-free. In the case of emulsion manufacture, the process of heating between 70 and 80°C usually kills most of the microorganisms. However, contamination may still occur as a result of unclean transfer lines and from improperly cleaned, sanitized, and protected filling equipment. It is not unusual to use a combination of preservatives to broaden their spectrum of activity because use of a single antimicrobial compound is generally insufficient for adequate preservation.

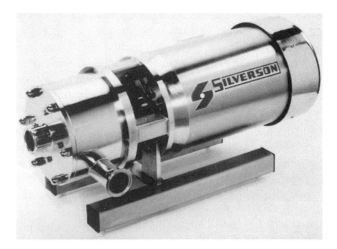

Fig. 8 Ultra-hygienic in-line mixer. (Courtesy of Silverson Machines, Inc., East Long Meadow, Massachusetts.)

Two categories of microorganisms are cause for concern in preservation of topical semisolid products. They are those liable to cause pathogenic symptoms and include staphylococci and hemolytic streptococci, *Pseudomonas aeruginosa* and *cepacia*, and *Escherichia coli*, and microorganisms liable to cause spoilage, which include water and airborne molds and yeasts. The following section describes the properties of some commonly used preservatives (26).

Parabens

The two most widely used agents are methylparaben and propylparaben. They are effective against molds and yeasts, but less effective against bacteria. They are more effective against Gram-positive than against Gram-negative bacteria. Parabens are most active at acidic pH levels less so in alkaline media. They are usually combined; an effective combination is 0.20% methylparaben and 0.05% propylparaben.

Dowcill 200 (Dow Chemical Co., Midland, MI) is a water-soluble, broad-spectrum antimicrobial and antifungal compound. It is not inactivated by nonionic, cationic, or anionic formulations, and it is particularly effective against *Pseudomonas*. Its activity is independent of pH; effective concentration is 0.02–0.30%.

Glydant (MDMH) (Lonza, Inc. Fairlawn, NJ): dimethylol-5,5,dimethylhydantoin is a water-soluble, highly active, broad-spectrum preservative. It functions over a wide range of temperatures and pH levels. It is noncorrosive, toxicologically acceptable, and biodegradable; effective concentration is 0.005–0.10%.

Germall 115 (Sutton Laboratories, Chatham, NJ): imidazolidinyl urea is a hygroscopic water-soluble white powder compatible with essentially all cosmetic ingredients including surfactants, proteins, and other special ingredients. Germall 115 acts synergistically with all other preservatives. It is effective against Gram-negative bacteria including *Pseudomonas*. Combined with parabens, it provides a broad spectrum of activity against yeasts and molds. It is recommended in the combination of Germall 115, 0.30%; methylparaben, 0.20%; and propylparaben, 0.01%.

Germall II (Sutton Laboratories, Chatham, NJ): diazolidinyl urea is a water-soluble, hygroscopic powder effective against Gram-positive and Gram-negative species including *Pseudomonas*. It is synergistic with other preservatives including the parabens. It is not inactivated by surfactants, proteins, or emulsifiers and is effective at all usual pH levels. It is recommended in the combination of Germall II, 0.20%; methylparaben, 0.20%; and propylparaben, 0.10%.

Germaben II-E (Sutton Laboratories, Chatham, NJ) is a clear liquid preservative system, readily soluble at a concentration of 1.0% in both w/o and o/w emulsions, but not in water alone. It has the composition of Germall II, 20%; methylparaben, 10%; propylparaben, 10%; and propylene glycol, 60%.

Suttocide A (Sutton Laboratories, Chatham, NJ) is a 50% aqueous solution of sodium hydroxymethylglycinate. It is a broad-spectrum antimicrobial preservative active against Gram-positive and Gram-negative bacteria and against yeast and mold. It remains active at alkaline pH levels.

LiquaPar Oil (Sutton Laboratories, Chatham, NJ) is a 100% clear, active, stable liquid blend of isopropyl, isobutyl, and *n*-Butyl esters of *p*-Hydroxybenzoic acid. This combination of parabens is a very effective preservative even at low concentrations against Gram-positive and Gram-negative bacteria, yeasts, and molds. The higher alkyl esters are more active and more stable and resistant to hydrolysis than are the lower alkyl esters; effective concentration is 0.1–0.4%

Busan 1504 (CTFA) (Buckman Laboratories, Memphis, TN): dimethylhydroxy-methylpyrazole is a water-soluble, broad-spectrum bactericide and fungicide compatible with anionic, cationic, and nonionic ingredients. It is stable over a broad pH range and compatible with proteins; effective concentration is not given.

Ethylenediaminetetraacetic acid (EDTA) is a chelating agent that binds certain metals, especially iron and copper, which are essential to the nutrition of certain microorganisms. In this manner, it is a strong booster or enhancer of the activity of preservatives (27, 28) especially the parabens. Alone, it has the ability to increase the permeability of the bacterial cell wall and can kill *Pseudomonas aeruginosa* and *E. coli* by this activity; effective concentration is 0.05–0.10%.

Several factors may influence the success or failure of a preservative to protect a formulation against microbial contamination. These factors include the interaction of the preservative with surfactants, active substances, other components of the vehicle, sorption by the polymeric packaging materials, and product storage temperature. Although hundreds of chemicals can function as germicides, only a few substances have made it to the marketplace. The small list is not based as much on a compound's effectiveness as an antimicrobial agent as on the compound's safety and effectiveness in the final product.

The packaging of semisolid products, usually in jarsand tubes, represents the best and worst conditions for microbial contamination. When using jars, the risk of contamination is higher every time a jar is opened or each time fingers touch the product. For these reasons, semisolid products in jars require a highly effective, long-acting preservative system to remain active throughout the life of the product. With tubes, the risk of microbial contamination is significantly reduced because they expose only a very small area each time a cap is removed. Tubes also provide control of dose by an amount expressed with minimum exposure to the environment or human contact. Therefore, because products packaged in tubes are less likely to become contaminated, the use of preservative is also reduced. Thus, products packaged in tubes are less likely to cause skin irritation or sensitization.

PACKAGING

Topical dermatologic products are packaged in jars or tubes, whereas ophthalmic, nasal, vaginal, and rectal semisolid products are almost always packaged in tubes. Regardless of the container a semisolid product is eventually placed in, it must meet with the guidelines of the FDA (29) for drug products, as follows:

> Containers, closures and other component parts of drug packages, to be suitable for their intended use, must not be reactive, additive or absorptive to the extent that the identity, strength, quality or purity of the drug will be affected. All drug product containers and closures must be approved by stability testing of the product in the final container in which it is marketed. The stability test includes testing filled containers at room temperature (e.g., 70°F) as well as under accelerated conditions (e.g., 105 and 120°F).

Because it is chemically inert, impermeable, strong, and rigid, glass has FDA clearance and is the ideal container for most drug products. With the proper closure system, it provides an excellent barrier to practically every element except light. Opaque jars are used to protect light-sensitive products and are available as porcelain white or dark green or amber in color. Commercially available empty ointment jars vary in size from 0.5 ounce to 1 pound.

Plastic containers are increasing in popularity over glass and metal (aluminum). This is because of qualities such as light weight, less breakage-prone, lower shipping costs, and the convenience of silk screen and plastic heat-transferred labeling. However, the disadvantage of plastics is the risk of permeation in two directions: from the product through the plastic from the inside out and from the ambient environment through the plastic from the outside into the product.

Plastic containers used for emulsion systems must be thoroughly evaluated for physical and chemical changes in the emulsion as well as for physical changes in the container. Product–plastic interactions maybe divided into five categories: permeation, leaching, sorption, chemical reaction, and alteration in the physical properties of the plastics or products (30, 31). For adequate protection of the product, container evaluation during the development stage of the product is imperative The protocols and standard for tests to demonstrate resin equivalence are found in the USP/NF and include three categories of tests for chemical and spectral characteristics and moisture barrier (7). Some examples of plastics include high- or low-density polyethylene (HDPE or LDPE) or a blend of each, polypropylene (PP), polyethylene terephthalate (PET), and various plastic/foil/paper laminates, sometimes 10 layers thick (32). Each of these plastics has its own characteristics and advantages that make it conducive to packaging of semisolid products. For example, LDPE is soft and resilient and provides a good moisture barrier. HDPE provides a superior moisture barrier but is less resilient. PP has a high level of heat resistance, and PET offers transparency and a high degree of product chemical compatibility. Thus, plastics and plastic laminates are generally preferred over metal tubes for packaging of pharmaceutical and cosmetic products.

QUALITY CONTROL

The purpose of undertaking quality control measures is to ensure a quality product to the consumer. Quality control encompasses a broad range of responsibilities including component and final product testing as well as in-process testing and controls. Compliance with current Good Manufacturing Practices (cGMP) regulations, process validation, and good management of operations such as design, production, packaging, testing, and distribution are all integral parts in the total quality assurance effort. Quality control provides critical support in the testing and decision making required for process validation, and the activities and responsibilities of the quality control unit cover a broad range of testing and other activities (33). The goal of quality control is to ensure that different lots of a product are essentially the same by confirming that all lots meet specifications. The parameters used to determine the quality assurance of semisolid preparations include raw material specifications, in-process controls,

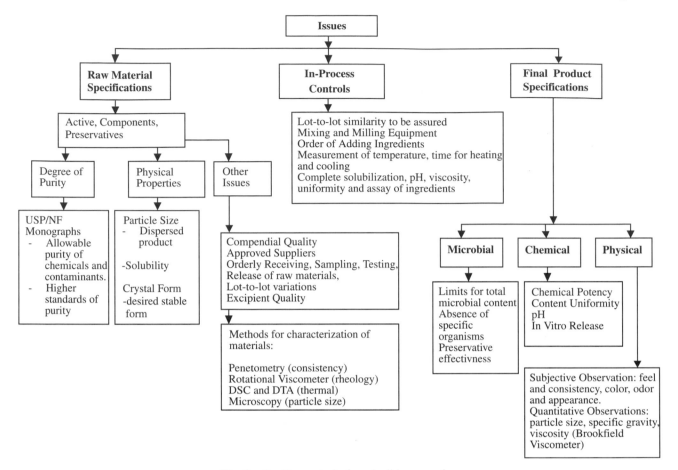

Fig. 9 Quality control of semisolid preparations.

and finished product specifications. The key parameter for any drug product is its efficacy as demonstrated in controlled clinical trials. However, the time and expense associated with such trials make them unsuitable as routine quality control methods. Therefore, in vitro surrogate tests are often used to ensure that product quality and performance are maintained over time and in the presence of change. As illustrated in the flow sheet (Fig. 9), a variety of physical and chemical tests commonly performed on products and their components (e.g., solubility, particle size and crystalline form of the active component, viscosity and homogeneity of the product) have historically provided reasonable evidence of consistent performance. More recently, in vitro release testing has shown promise as a means to comprehensively ensure consistent delivery of the active components from semisolid preparations (34). An in vitro release rate can reflect the combined effect of several physical and chemical parameters, including solubility and particle size of the active ingredient and rheological properties of the dosage form. In most cases, in vitro release rate is a useful

test to assess product sameness between prechange and postchange products. Recently, an in vitro test developed for a peptide containing gel formulation demonstrated that the release test can be modified to ensure product sameness after scale up and postapproval change (SUPAC) (35). However, with any test, the metrices and statistical approaches to documentation of sameness in quality attributes should be considered. Bioequivalence to previous lots may be considered as an additional parameter for some pharmaceutical products (36).

STABILITY

Stability testing is a routine procedure performed on drug substances and products. It is involved at various stages of product development. In early stages, accelerated stability testing (at relatively high temperatures and/or humidities) can be used to determine the types of degradation products that may be found after long-term storage. Testing under more gentle conditions (those recommended for long-term shelf storage) and slightly elevated temperatures can be used to determine product shelf life and expiration dates.

According to the FDA draft guidelines to the industry (1), semisolid preparations should be evaluated for appearance, clarity, color, homogeneity, odor, pH, consistency, viscosity, particle size distribution (when feasible), assay, degradation products, preservative and antioxidant content (if present), microbial limits/sterility, and weight loss (when appropriate). Additionally, samples from production lots of approved products are retained for stability testing in case of product failure in the field. Retained samples can be tested along with returned samples to ascertain if the problem was manufacturing- or storage-related. Appropriate stability data should be provided for products supplied in closed-end tubes to support the maximum anticipated use period, during patient use, and after the seal is punctured allowing product content with the cap/cap liner. Ointments, pastes, gels, and creams in large containers including tubes should be assayed by sampling at the surface, top, middle, and bottom of the container. In addition, tubes should be sampled near the crimp.

For a product to be considered stable, it must retain the same properties and characteristics, within specific limits, that it possessed at the time of manufacture (7). A product must remain stable when it is stored for a period of time after the date of manufacture. When a product is subjected to stability testing, the objective is to determine whether the product has adequate shelf life under market and use conditions, when manufactured and packaged on a commercial scale. The FDA requires stability data on at least three lots of the same formulation and packaging—these data should appear on the product made by the commercial or any other equivalent process (in terms of critical parameters) to the proposed commercial process. To establish a stability profile, product stability storage tests must be carefully planned and initiated.

The commonly used predictive method of accelerated and stress testing depends on storage of products under conditions of rigidly controlled environment. Studies under accelerated conditions provide useful data for establishing expiration date and product stability information for future product development (e.g., preliminary assessment of proposed manufacturing changes such as change in formulation and scale up). These studies also assist in validation of analytical methods for the stability program and generate information that may help elucidate the degradation profile of the drug substance or product. Studies under stress conditions may be useful in

determining whether accidental exposures to conditions other than those proposed (e.g., during transportation) are deleterious to the product and also for evaluating which specific test parameters may be the best indicators of product stability.

A stability program typically involves aging the product under accelerated conditions of temperature, humidity, and light. Other types of accelerated or stress testing include centrifugation, shipping tests, and some form of product use test. The purpose of the product use test is primarily to evaluate preservative efficacy and ensure that the physical properties of the product remain stable under the conditions of use and are suitable for the intended application. Another useful test is to subject the product to low-intensity shaking for a period of hours or days. The key parameters of a stability program include the selection of specific accelerated storage conditions, how stability samples are stored at the test conditions (or stability stations), testing intervals, and testing the stability samples. A representative stability program may be illustrated as follows:

Samples: Each sample is one unit placed inverted in the storage chamber. An equal number of units are placed upright as control samples. The sample may also include units placed sideways. Additional samples should be placed at each stability station to make provision for samples for further investigations if this becomes necessary.

Stability Stations and Sampling Periods: Three 24-h freeze–thaw cycles are used: 1, 2, and 3 months at 50°C; 1, 3, 6, and 12 months at 40°C; and 1, 6, 12, 18, 24, and 36 months at 25°C (room temperature). At the end of each period, the sample is evaluated for chemical and physical properties as applicable (as noted earlier). The sample should also be examined to evaluate product–package compatibility. Microscopic examination of the sample can provide a very useful evaluation of changes in particle size and crystal structure. Tests for evaluating the compatibility of the product with the container include weight loss and moisture loss (if applicable). Reduction in the concentration of critical ingredients would indicate loss owing to binding with the container material or permeation through the container walls. The container should also be examined to evaluate interaction of the product with the container surface. The purpose of a stability program is to measure the changes observed in samples subjected to various stress conditions. The most difficult aspect of stability testing is to apply this information to determine the stability profile of the product and to project an expected shelf life under market conditions. This is particularly difficult with semisolid preparations because the accelerated environmental and other stress tests used for stability testing are likely to cause substantial changes in critical properties of formulation ingredients. Higher storage temperatures can cause changes in the solubility and partitioning profile of drug and preservatives and alteration of the rheological profile of a product system. There may also be changes in the interfacial properties of ingredients that help stabilize emulsion systems. Therefore, results of stability testing can be misleading if the stress conditions used for stability evaluation do not reflect realistic product exposure conditions. It is generally recognized that application of stress testing to develop the stability profile of a product is useful. However, subjecting the product to unrealistic stress conditions is not useful for predicting shelf life under normal market and use conditions (37). Therefore, it is important to recognize the specific properties that are affected by the stress conditions of the stability test and whether the sample will return to normal after stress is removed. For this assessment, the pharmaceutical scientist must depend on the knowledge developed by appropriate studies to characterize the physical and chemical properties of the system.

REFERENCES

1. Shah, V.P. FDA Guidance for Industry Document. *Nonsterile Semisolid Dosage Forms*; Center for Drug Evaluation and Research: Rockville, MD, 1997; 1–40.
2. Flynn, G.L. Cutaneous and Transdermal Delivery: Processes and Systems of Delivery. *Modern Pharmaceutics*, 3rd Ed.; Banker, G.S., Rhodes, C.T., Eds.; Marcel Dekker, Inc.: New York, 1995; 272–298.
3. Idson, B.; Lazarus, L. Semisolids. *Theory and Practice of Industrial Pharmacy*, 3rd Ed.; Williams and Williams: Baltimore, MD, 1986; 534–563.
4. Block, L.H. Medicated Applications. *Remington: The Science and Practice of Pharmacy*, 17th Ed.; Gennaro, A.R. Ed.; Mack Publishing Co. Easton, PA, 1995; 1577–1597.
5. Erdi, N.Z.; Cruz, M.M.; Battista, O.A. Rheological Characteristics of Polymeric Gels. J. Colloid Interface Sci. **1968**, *28*, 36.
6. Franks, A.J. Hydrocarbon Bases for Ointments and Creams. Soap, Perfumes and Cosmetics **1964**, *37*, 221–319.
7. Ophthalmic Ointments. In *United States Pharmacopoeia*, 23rd Ed.; The Pharmacopoeial Convention, Inc.: Rockville, MD, 1995; 1812.
8. Lee, J.Y. Sterilization Control and Validation for Topical Ointments. Pharm. Tech. **1992**, *16*, 104–110.

9. Hameyer, P. Novel Emulsifiers for w/o Emulsion Preparations. Household Profess. Prod. Indust. **1993**, *4*, 27–31.
10. Information About Cosmetic Ingredients. *Dow Corning Bulletin*; Midland, MI, 1988.
11. Surface Active Agents. *Croda Formulary Update*; Croda, Inc.: New Jersey, 1999; 11–15.
12. In *Creanova Product Literature*; Degussa-Huls America, Inc.: Piscataway, NJ, 2000.
13. Griffin, W.C. Hydrophilic-Lipophilic Balance. J. Soc. Cosmet. Chem. **1949**, *1*, 311.
14. *International Cosmetic Ingredients Dictionary*; The Cosmetic, Toiletries and Fragrance Association: Washington, DC, 2000; 1250–1261.
15. *McCutcheons Surfactants and Emulsifiers*; McCutcheon Directories: Princeton, WI, 2000; 150–166.
16. Paul, B.K.; Moulik, S.P. Microemulsions. Overview. J. Disper. Sci. Tech. **1997**, *18*, 301–367.
17. Lawrence, M.J. Surfactant Systems: Microemulsions and Vesicles as Vehicles for Delivery. Eur. J. Drug Metab. Pharm. **1994**, *3*, 257–269.
18. Bhargava, H.N.; Narurkab, A.; Lieb, L.M. Using Micro-Emulsions for Drug Delivery. Pharm. Tech. **1987**, *11*, 46.
19. Prince, L.M. Microemulsions. *Theory and Practice*; Academic Press: New York, 1977; 511–531.
20. Friberg, S.E.; Venable, R. Microemulsions. *Encyclopedia of Emulsion Technology*; Becher, P., Ed.; Marcel Dekker, Inc.: New York, 1983; 1, 128–185.
21. Juch, R.D.; Rufli, Th.; Surber, C. Pastes: What Do They Contain? How Do They Work? Dermatology **1994**, *189*, 373–377.
22. Ansel, H.C.; Allen, L.V., Jr.; Popovich, N.G. Ointments, Creams and Gels. *Pharmaceutical Dosage Forms and Drug Delivery Systems*, 7th Ed.; Lippincott, Williams and Wilkins: Philadelphia, 1999; 244–262.
23. Murdan, S.; Gregoriadis, G.; Florence, A.T. Novel Sorbitan Monostearate Organogels. J. Pharm. Sci. **1999**, *6*, 608–614.
24. Hermans, P.H. *Colloid Science*; Kruyt, H.R., Ed.; Elsevier: Amsterdam, 1969; 11, 483–651.
25. Gennaro, A.R. *Remington's Pharmaceutical Sciences* 18th Ed.; Mack Publishing Co., 3rd Ed.; Easton PA, 1990; 1640.
26. Bandelin, F.J.; Sheth, B.B. Semisolid Preparations. *Encyclopedia of Pharmaceutical Technology*, 1st Ed.; Swarbrick, J., Boylan, J.C., Eds.; Marcel Dekker, Inc.: New York, 1989; 31–61.
27. Kabara, J.J. GRAS Antimicrobial Agents for Cosmetic Products. J. Soc. Cos. Chem. **1980**, *31*, 1–10.
28. Kabara, J.J. Structure-Function Relationships of Surfactants as Antimicrobial Agents. J. Soc. Cos. Chem. **1978**, *29*, 733–741.
29. *FDA Good Manufacturing Practices Regulations*; Fed. Register, 1974; 9.
30. *Modern Plastics Encyclopedia*; McGraw-Hill Inc.: New York, 1992; 49.
31. Varsona, J.; Gilbert, S.G. *Proceedings of the Plastic Packaging Institute*; Grosset and Dunlap: New York, 1991; 122–131.
32. Forcinio, H. Tubes the Ideal Package for Semisolids. Pharm. Tech. **1998**, *22* (1), 32–36.
33. Hanna, S.A. Quality Assurance. *Pharmaceutical Dosage Forms: Disperse Systems*; Lieberman, H.A., Rieger, M.M.,

Banker, G.S., Eds.; Marcel Dekker, Inc.: New York, 1989; 2, 631–680.

34. Shah, V.P.; Elkins, J.S.; Williams, R.L. Evaluation of the Test System Used for In Vitro Release of Drugs for Topical Dermatological Drug Products. Pharm. Dev. Tech. **1999**, *4* (3), 377–385.

35. Badkar, A.; Talluri, K.; Tenjarla, S.; Jaynes, J.; Banga, A.K. In Vitro Release Testing of a Peptide. Gel. Pharm. Tech. **2000**, *1*, 44–52.

36. Van Buskirk, G.A.; Shah, V.P.; Adair, D.; Arbit, H.M.; Dighe, S.V.; Fawzi, M.; Feldman, T.; Flynn, G.L.; Gonzalez, M.A.; Gray, V.A.; Guy, R.H.; Herd, A.K.; Hem, S.L.; Hoiberg, C.; Jerussi, R.; Kaplan, A.S.; Lesko, L.J.; Malinowski, H.J.; Meltzer, N.M.; Nedich, R.L.; Pearce, D.M.; Peck, G.; Rudman, A.; Savello, D.; Schwartz, J.B.; Schwartz, P.; Skelly, J.P.; Vanderlaan, R.K.; Wang, J.C.T.; Weiner, N.; Winkel, D.R.; Zatz, J.L. Workshop III Report: Scale Up of Liquid and Semisolid Disperse Systems. Pharm. Res. **1994**, *11* (8), 1216–1220.

37. Rieger, M.M. Skin Care: New Concepts vs. Established Practices. Cosm. Toiletr. **1991**, *106*, 59–69.

SOLUBILIZATION OF DRUGS IN AQUEOUS MEDIA

Paul B. Myrdal
Samuel H. Yalkowsky
The University of Arizona, Tucson, Arizona

INTRODUCTION

Therapeutic drugs are often given systemically. Once given systemically, a drug will distribute throughout the body. By distributing in the body, the drug is essentially diluted out from its original concentration in the formulation/dosage form. Hence, the formulation is really a drug concentrate. For solid dosage forms, the dose to be delivered is not normally a physical problem. However, dose can become a significant formulation challenge for parenteral preparations, due to limitations in aqueous solubility and volume. Therefore, in order to obtain a solution formulation for drugs with poor solubility, it is necessary to alter the formulation to facilitate solubilization.

The choice of solubilization method will depend upon how efficiently the drug can be solubilized, stability in the system, and upon the biocompatibility of the vehicle for a given delivery route. For solid dosage forms, it may be possible to alter the solid phase to enhance dissolution. For parenterals, the four most commonly used techniques for solubilization are: pH adjustment; cosolvent addition; micelle inclusion through surfactant addition and complexation. The following chapter is designed to summarize the theoretical as well as practical use of each of the above techniques. More extensive discussion on techniques for drug solubilization can be found in books dedicated to the subject (1, 2).

SOLUBILITY

Before attempting random laboratory experimentation, it is prudent to understand what physicochemical properties are making a given drug poorly soluble. There are two key components that govern the solubility of an organic solute in water, namely the crystal structure (melting point and enthalpy of fusion) and the molecular structure (activity coefficient). The aqueous solubility, X_w, of an organic nonelectrolyte is simply described by the addition of these two terms, i.e.,

$$\log X_w = \log X_i^c - \log \gamma^w \tag{1}$$

where X_i^c is the ideal solubility and γ^w is the activity coefficient of the compound in water.

Ideal Solubility

The ideal solubility pertains to the effect of the crystalline structure on solubility. A solute molecule must first dissociate from this crystal lattice before it can go into solution. This dissociation from the crystalline lattice is accompanied by a free energy change. The more energy it takes to free a solute molecule from its crystal (i.e., the higher the melting point), the lower the solubility.

It is possible to quantitate the molar free energy necessary to produce a hypothetical supercooled liquid at a given temperature T, through the use of an enthalpy–temperature thermodynamic cycle (3). Rigorously, it is necessary to sum the corresponding enthalpy and entropy changes that it takes to heat the crystal to the melting point, melt the crystal, then cool the liquid back to the reference temperature. For this discussion it is convenient to omit any change in enthalpy with temperature (heat capacity). This allows for the simplified mathematical expression

$$\log X_i^c = \frac{\Delta S_m (T_m - T)}{2.303 RT} \tag{2}$$

where X_i^c is the ideal solubility (mole fraction), R is the universal gas constant (1.98 cal/deg mol), ΔS_m is the entropy of melting and T_m is the melting point of the compound in Kelvin.

If the entropy of melting, ΔS_m, is not known experimentally, an approximation for rigid organic molecules of 13.5 cal/degmol can be made (4). If the temperature of interest is 298 K then Eq. 2 becomes

$$\log X_i^c = -0.01(T_m - 298) \tag{3}$$

or

$$\log X_i^c = -0.01(MP - 25) \tag{4}$$

where MP is the melting point of the compound in Celsius. If the melting point is less than 25°C (i.e., liquid at room temperature) then there is no crystal limitation on solubility and Eq. 4 is equal to zero.

Encyclopedia of Pharmaceutical Technology

For those compounds that are crystalline, it is important to emphasize that the ideal solubility is strictly a function of the pure crystal, and as a result, is solvent independent. Eq. 4 also assumes that the solvent does not effect the solid phase in any way to change the free energy.

Table 1 demonstrates the effect of melting point on solubility as described by Eq. 4. It can be seen that for every 100 degree difference in melting point, there is a corresponding change in solubility of 10 times. Thus, for a hypothetical compound that melts at 325°C, the crystal structure would be responsible for approximately a 3-fold (1000 times) decrease in solubility, relative to it as a liquid at room temperature.

Activity Coefficient

The aqueous activity coefficient of a compound describes the effect of molecular structure on aqueous solubility. If a compound mixes with water and forms an ideal solution, then the activity coefficient would be taken as unity and the last term in Eq. 1 would become zero. In such a case, then the solid phase, if any, would be the sole physical property inhibiting solubility. Most drugs are relatively nonpolar and do not form ideal solutions with water. Therefore in order to understand the extent by which the inherent molecular structure is limiting solubility, it is helpful to obtain an estimate for the aqueous activity coefficient.

Numerous methods have been developed to estimate the aqueous activity coefficient (3, 5–13). A convenient method that has been successfully applied within the pharmaceutical industry utilizes the octanol/water partition coefficient. Yalkowsky and Valvani (14) have shown that the molar activity coefficient can be directly related to the octanol/water partition coefficient, $K_{o/w}$, by the following molar relationship;

$$\log \gamma^w = -\log K_{o/w} + 0.80 \qquad (5)$$

Table 1   Comparison of different hypothetical melting points and the resulting effect on solubility as described by Eq. 4

Hypothetical melting point (°C)	Log X_i^c (Eq. 4)	Decrease in solubility
0	0	No effect (reference)
25	0	No effect (reference)
125	−1	10×
225	−2	100×
325	−3	1000×

There are numerous methods by which to estimate octanol/water partition coefficients. One of the most widely recognized is the group contribution method CLOGP (15).

Equation (5) enables a convenient tool for assessing the effect of structure on aqueous solubility. Table 2 demonstrates the decrease in solubility as partition coefficient increases. As $K_{o/w}$ increases by a factor of 10 ($\log K_{o/w} = 1$), the decrease in solubility is also a factor of 10. Thus, a compound with a partition coefficient of 1000 (log $K_{o/w} = 3$) will have a solubility that is approximately 3-fold (1000 times) less than a reference compound that has a $K_{o/w}$ of 1 (log $K_{o/w} = 0$).

Estimating Solubility

With the knowledge or estimate of the octanol/water partition coefficient and melting point, solubility can be estimated, by incorporating Eqs. 4 and 5 into Eq. 1. This gives

$$\log S_{est} = -0.01(MP - 25) - \log K_{o/w} + 0.80 \qquad (6)$$

where S_{est} is the estimated molar solubility, MP is the melting point (°C) and $K_{o/w}$ is the octanol/water partition coefficient. For drugs that are liquid at room temperature, the melting point term is zero, giving simply

$$\log S_{est} = -\log K_{o/w} + 0.80 \qquad (7)$$

While Eqs. 6 and 7 are simplified equations for estimating aqueous solubility, they can also be used to facilitate the understanding of why a drug is poorly soluble. The equations yield quantitative descriptions of which physicochemical properties are limiting solubility. If a compound has a low, or no melting point at room temperature, however and a high $\log K_{o/w}$, then molecular structure is limiting solubility and the aqueous media must be modified to facilitate solubilization. If the melting point is very high, and the $\log K_{o/w}$ is low, then modification of the aqueous media may not significantly increase solubility and manipulation of the solid phase may be necessary. If a compound has a high melting point and a high $\log K_{o/w}$, it can be appreciated that a formulator will have a significant challenge in drug solubilization.

Table 2   Comparision of different hypothetical log $K_{o/w}$s and the resulting effect on solubility as described by Eq. 5

$K_{o/w}$	log γ^w [Eq. 5]	Decrease in solubility
1	−0.8	Reference
10	−1.8	10×
100	−2.8	100×
1000	−3.8	1000×

SOLID PHASE

As discussed above, the solid phase for a solute molecule is a fundamental component of a compound's solubility. Consequently, understanding and characterizing the solid phase of a drug, in a given system, is of vital importance from a formulation standpoint. A comprehensive review on the theoretical and practical aspects of solid state chemistry and the significance to the pharmaceutical industry has been given by Byrn et al. (16).

It is important to always consider, that for any raw drug substance or formulation, only one solid phase is thermodynamically stable for a given set of environmental conditions. The most stable solid will have the lowest free energy and correspondingly the lowest solubility. The unknowing use of a metastable crystal can lead to formulation stability problems with respect to solubility. In light of this, it would seem as though little can be done in regards to increasing solubility through the use of crystal modification. It is clear that the most stable crystal is the most prudent choice for suspensions. The kinetics for solvent mediated transformation are generally too rapid or too uncontrollable for a stable product. However for solid dosage forms, it may be possible to utilize a less stable solid phase due to the decreased molecular mobility in the dry state. The key determinant for success will be if the metastable form has an intrinsically high energy barrier to reconversion and is well defined from a kinetic standpoint. To facilitate stability, it may be necessary to add excipients or impose packaging constraints to eliminate or slow down conversion.

Apparent Solubility and Dissolution Rate

The crystal form with the higher free energy may exhibit an apparent solubility that is higher than the true equilibrium solubility for the system. An apparent solubility increase can occur anytime the starting solid material is not the most stable for the given system. However, a metastable crystal will produce only a transient increase in solubility. The most stable crystal will eventually precipitate and the apparent solubility gain will diminish until the thermodynamic equilibrium solubility is reached. The degree of supersaturation and duration will depend on the characteristics of the starting material and on the nucleation rate and growth kinetics of the stable form. Consequently, an inherent difficulty in working with metastable systems is that the kinetics of conversion often cannot be predicted or controlled.

By virtue of having a higher apparent solubility, a metastable crystal will have an increased dissolution rate over the more stable form. The change in mass, M, as a function of time, t, for a solute is directly proportional to its apparent solubility, S_{app}, and is given by

$$dM/dt = K \times A(S_{app} - C) \tag{8}$$

where A is the solvent accesscible surface area, C is the concentration of the solute in solution, and K is a constant that includes the diffusion coefficient of the solute and other hydrodynamic properties of the system (17). Hence, the larger the apparent solubility of a metastable form, the greater the dissolution rate that it leads to. Hamlin et al. (18) have illustrated the dependency of dissolution rate upon solubility for a large number of pharmaceutical compounds. Yoshihashi et al. (19) have correlated initial dissolution rates for terfenadine based on heats of fusion of the starting material. In addition, since the crystal contribution to solubility is independent of the solvent, this general relationship is applicable to virtually any solvent system. Nicklasson and Brodin (20) have successfully correlated dissolution rate with solubility for ethanol cosolvent systems.

Surface area is also directly proportional to the dissolution rate of a solute. Particle size reduction is another common and often efficient means by which to achieve higher levels of drug in solution at earlier time points (21–28). As particle size decreases, the surface area per unit volume of solute increases and consequently more drug is exposed to the solvent. Also, as particle size decreases the surface molecules are of higher free energy which increases dissolution. And finally, the processing of solid material can often lead to crystal defects within a particle or surface area where crystallinity is lost (amorphous), both of which can increase the apparent solubility. Mosharraf et al. have demonstrated the effect of crystal structure disorder on solubility and dissolution rate (29).

The significance of solubility and dissolution is one to be highlighted. Insufficient oral bioavailability can be the result of a compound's low intestinal solubility and/or slow dissolution rate. It may be practical at times to use a solid material that gives a higher apparent solubility and/or an increase in dissolution rate in order to enhance bioavailability. Aguiar et al. (30, 31) were able to show that polymorph B of chloramphenicol palmitate, which can produce solubility that is roughly two times that of polymorph A, gives greater blood levels in vivo. They were able to show that as the percentage of polymorph B increases in the dosage form, there is a linear increase in blood concentration of chloramphenicol palmitate. Several other investigators (32–34) have also found that with the proper choice of the solid-state form, biological activity can be enhanced due to increased solubility or dissolution rate.

Apparent Solubility Enhancement from Different Solid Phases

In order to assess the relative increase in solubility of a metastable solid phase with respect to another, a simple solubility ratio can be defined. Here the solubility ratio is defined as the value for the higher solubility phase divided by the lower. Table 3 contains a selected list of solubility ratios for different solid phases of a selected list of example drugs.

From Table 3, it can be seen that a solubility ratio greater than one can be obtained, however there are cases in which there is no apparent increase in solubility between phases. For the data given, the transient solubility increase for solvates is similar to that of polymorphs, having solubility ratios that often range between 1 and 3.

Table 3 Examples of different drugs and their observed solubility ratios for different solid phases[a]

Drug (temp. in °C)	More soluble phase/less soluble phase	Solubility ratio	Reference
Acetohexamide (37)	II/I	1.2	35
Benzoxoprofen (25)	I/II	1.5	36
Glibenclamide (37)	II/I	1.6	37
Mebendazole	C/A	3.6	38
Mebendazole	B/A	7.4	38
Meprobamate (25)	II/I	1.9	39
Oxyclozamide (25)	II/I	2.6	40
Oxyclozamide (25)	III/I	3.9	40
Ampicillin (not cited)	Anhydrate/trihydrate	1.3	41
Ampicillin (20)	Anhydrate/hydrate	2.2	42
Ampicillin (30)	Anhydrate/hydrate	1.5	42
Calcium gluceptate (37)	Anhydrate/3.5 hydrate	18.6	43
Erythromycin (30)	Anhydrate/dihydrate	2.2	44
Lamivudine (25)	Anhydrate/0.2 hydrate	1.2	45
Paroxetine HCl (20)	Anhydrate/hemihydrate	1.7	46
Phenobarbital (20)	Anhydrate/hydrate	1.1	47
Phenobarbital (25)	Anhydrate/hydrate	1.4	47
Phenobarbital (35)	Anhydrate/hydrate	1.0	47
Piroxicam (25)	Anhydrate/monohydrate	1.0	48
Sulfamethoxazole (25)	Anhydrate/monohydrate	1.2	49
Theophylline (25)	Anhydrate/monohydrate	2.0	50
Uric acid (25)	Hydrate/anhydrate	1.6	51
Uric acid (37)	Hydrate/anhydrate	1.9	51
DMHP (25)	Formate solvate/anhydrate	8.2	52
Furosemide (37)	Dioxane solvate/anhydrate	1.3	53
Furosemide (37)	DMF solvate/anhydrate	1.2	53
Glibenclamide (37)	Pentanol solvate/anhydrate	31.8	37
Glibenclamide (37)	Toluene solvate/anhydrate	2.4	37
Caffeine (25)	Amorphous/crystalline	6.5	54
Diacetylmorphine (25)	Amorphous/crystalline	16	54
Theophylline (17)	Amorphous/crystalline	58	54
Theobromine (16)	Amorphous/crystalline	50	54
Morphine (20)	Amorphous/crystalline	268	54
Hydrochlorothiazide (37)	Amorphous/crystalline	1.1	55
Bendrofluazide (37)	Amorphous/crystalline	2.8	55
Cyclothiazide (37)	Amorphous/crystalline	6.2	55
Cyclopenthiazide (37)	Amorphous/crystalline	8.3	55
Polythiazide (37)	Amorphous/crystalline	9.8	55

[a]The different solid phases used as well as the temperature of the experiment study are also given.

While most compounds produce increases that are less than a factor of ten, calcium gluceptate and glibenclamide exhibited significant increases of nearly 20 and 30, respectively (37, 43).

Consideration of Eq. 4, would suggest that the largest gain in solubility should be realized for those solid fractions that are actually not crystalline, i.e., amorphous. For a purely amorphous material, there would be no crystal contribution to the solubility and the compound could be treated as a liquid. Since it is difficult to produce a purely amorphous material, there is often some degree of crystallinity to a "amorphous" material. Nonetheless, amorphous materials clearly have the highest free energy, relative to any crystalline solid fraction. As a result, amorphous materials can potentially give some of the largest solubility ratios. Toffoli et al. (54) and Corrigan et al. (55) have investigated the use of amorphous materials and have found a wide range of apparent solubility ratios. Some of their data is listed in Table 2, and clearly shows that the use of an amorphous material has the greatest potential for solubility enhancement. Other investigators have also observed significant solubility differenceswith amorphous compounds (56–58). Some investigators have seen practical in vivo benefits by using amorphous materials (59, 60). However, due to the high free energy of these systems their use if often not practical. Giron (61) has noted a few compounds that have relatively stable amorphous forms.

Through alteration of the solid-state form it is possible to increase the dissolution rate, or apparent solubility of a drug. These increases can potentially increase the bioavailability of a poorly water soluble drug. However, the practical use of a higher energy solid form is limited due to physical and chemical stability issues. Significant investigation must be made in order to assure that a dosage form using a metastable crystal will maintain integrity throughout the product life.

pH CONTROL

Solid-state manipulation is often not advantageous or practical, as a result, it is then necessary to alter the solvent. For organic solutes that are ionizable, changing the pH of the system may be the simplest and most effective means of increasing aqueous solubility.

For a weak monoprotic acidic drug, $HA_{(solid/liquid)}$, in water:

$$HA_{(solid/liquid)} \Leftrightarrow HA_{(solution)} \tag{9}$$

$$HA_{(solution)} + H_2O \overset{K_a}{\Leftrightarrow} H_3O^+ + A^- \tag{10}$$

where $HA_{(solution)}$ represents the free acid (unionized form) in solution and A^- is the ionized acid in solution. The total concentration of drug in solution (S_T) is equal to $[HA_{(solution)}] + [A^-]$, where $HA_{(solution)}$ is the intrinsic solubility of the drug (S_W). From Eq. 10, the ionized concentration of drug is

$$[A^-] = \frac{K_a[HA]}{[H^+]} \tag{11}$$

giving

$$S_T = S_w + \frac{K_a[HA]}{[H^+]} \tag{12}$$

Since $[HA] = S_w$, $\log K_a = pK_a$ and $\log H^+ = pH$, Eq. 12 can be simplified to,

$$S_T = S_w(1 + 10^{(pH-pK_a)}) \tag{13}$$

which relates the total solubility to the intrinsic solubility and pK_a of the weak monoprotic acid and the pH of the system.

For a weak base in an aqueous solution,

$$B_{(solid/liquid)} \Leftrightarrow B_{(solution)} \tag{14}$$

$$B_{(solution)} + H_2O \overset{K_b}{\Leftrightarrow} OH^- + HA^+ \tag{15}$$

By analogy to the weak acid the total solubility is described by

$$S_T = S_w(1 + 10^{(pK_a-pH)}) \tag{16}$$

where the pK_a refers to HA^+. Fig. 4 illustrates the general pH-solubility profiles for three solutes having the same intrinsic solubility but different pK_as.

Fig. 1 illustrates that solubilization by ionization can be very efficient for a mono acidic or basic drug. The linear solubilization slope corresponds to a 10-fold increase in solubility for a one-unit change in pH. Zwitterionic compounds, which have both acidic and basic functional groups, will have a pH solubility plot that will be a combination of those given in the top and bottom portions of Fig. 1. These compounds have a minimum solubility at a pH that is equal to the average of the pK_as 62–65). The solubilization of divalent acids and bases is similar to their monoprotic counterparts. However, upon the ionization of the second functional group, the solubilization slope is 2 instead of 1, which corresponds to a 100-fold increase in solubility for a one-unit change in pH. A complete mathematical description for the solubilization of a dibasic compound has been given by Garren and Pyter (66).

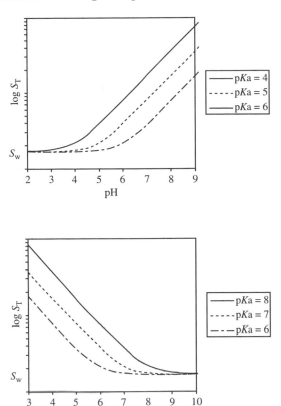

Fig. 1 (Top) Log solubility, logS_T vs. pH for typical weak acids having pK_as of 4, 5, and 6 and the same intrinsic solubility, logS_w. (Bottom) Log solubility, logS_T, vs. pH for typical weak bases (HA$^+$) having pK_as of 8, 7, and 6 and the same intrinsic solubility.

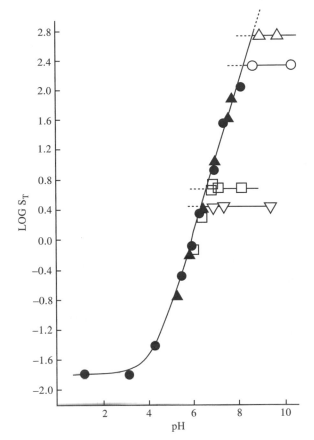

Fig. 2 Solubility-pH profiles, S_T of naproxen and four salts: $\triangle$, potassium salt; $\bigcirc$, sodium salt; $\square$, magnesium salt; and $\triangledown$, calcium salt. (From Ref. 67.)

Salt Formation

Eqs. 13 and 16 assume that the ionized species of a solute has infinite solubility. However, an ionized solute can form salts with appropriate counterions. The formation of a salt is governed by the solubility product, K_{sp}, of the salt complex. For example, the thermodynamic equilibrium for a chloride salt, BH$^+$Cl$^-$, is

$$\text{BH}^+\text{Cl}^-{}_{\text{(Solid)}} \overset{K_{SP}}{\Leftrightarrow} [\text{BH}^+] + [\text{Cl}^-] \qquad (17)$$

where BH$^+$Cl$^-_{\text{(Solid)}}$ represents the solid chloride salt, BH$^+$ is the ionized base and Cl$^-$ is the chloride counterion. As a result, the concentration of the ionized species will be limited by the solubility of the salt. Some organic salts are very soluble in aqueous systems, others are not and can significantly limit the solubility of a solute. Chowhan (67) demonstrated the effect of four different salts on the pH-solubility profile of naproxen. As shown in Fig. 2, all four salts behave identically between the pH values of 1 and 6, and can be described by Eq. 13. However, depending on

the given salt, the solubility of naproxen is limited at pH values greater then 6.5. The solubilities of the corresponding salts are indicated by plateaus, with the potassium salt having nearly 200 times the solubility of then calcium salt. Hence, at a given plateau the salt is the solid fraction that is in equilibrium with the system, which once again emphasizes the importance of characterizing the solid phase in order to understand what factors are influencing solubility.

Kramer and Flynn (68) have also previously investigated the effect of salt formation on solubility. A graph from their work is given in Fig. 3 and shows the pH-solubility profile for an organic hydrochloride. As can be seen from the data, there is a exponential increase in solubility as would be expected from Eq. 16. The solubility diverges from the expected line and roughly plateaus at pH levels under about 7.2. As pH decreases further, so does solubility, due to the disappearance of the free base from solution after the hydrochloride is formed. Kramer and Flynn illustrated how Eq. 16 can be modified to take into account salt

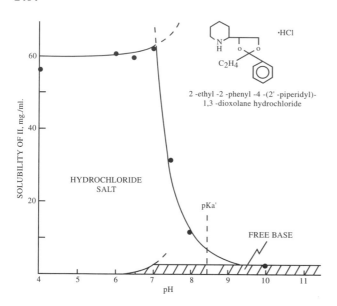

2-ethyl -2 -phenyl -4 -(2' -piperidyl)-
1,3 -dioxolane hydrochloride

Fig. 3 Solubility–pH profile of a substituted piperidyl-dioxolane (II) in 0.05 M succinate buffer at 30°C. Lines represent theoretical curves. (From Ref. 68.)

formation. Additional mathematical expressions have been developed more recently to characterize pH solubility profiles with the appreciation of counterion affects (69–71).

In addition to overall solubility, salts can have a significant impact on the dissolution rate of a solute. Hence, solubility considerations are important factors to be assessed when trying to make a rational choice of an appropriate pharmaceutical salt (72–77).

Buffers

One practical use of a buffer is to simply maintain the pH of the system over time. For pH solubilized drugs, another practical use of a buffer is to reduce or eliminate the potential for precipitation of the drug upon dilution. It has been shown that drug precipitation upon intravenous injection has been linked to phlebitis (78–82). As shown through the previous discussion, the solubility of a drug can be increased exponentially with pH alteration. However, it also then follows that the solubility can decrease exponentially with pH alteration. If a pH solubilized formulation is diluted with a medium by one half, then the drug concentration will decrease by one half. At the same time the pH of the new mixture may change. If it changes by one pH unit, in a direction that decreases ionization of the drug, then the solubility of that drug will decrease 10-fold. The drug can precipitate if the concentration in the solution exceeds the new solubility.

The degree and extent of precipitation will depend on the ability of a formulation to resist pH change when diluted. The pH change on dilution of one solution by another will depend on the initial pHs and buffer capacities of both solutions. Surakitbanharn et al. (83) illustrated the affect of initial pH and phosphate buffer concentration on pH change when diluted with Sorensen's Phosphate Buffer. Myrdal et al. (82) used the computational model of Surakitbanharn et al. as a means of selecting buffer concentration and initial pH to eliminate the precipitation potential of a weakly basic drug, levemopamil–HCl. Myrdal et al. showed that the unbuffered formulation precipitated upon dilution and resulted in phlebitis in vivo, whereas the buffered formulations did not precipitate and did not elicit any phlebitis in vivo.

Solubilization through the Use of pH Control

Under the proper conditions, the solubility of an ionizable drug can increase exponentially by adjusting the pH of the solution. From a structural point of view, a drug that can be efficiently solubilized by pH control should be either a weak acid with a low pK_a or a weak base with a high pK_a. Note that the effect of pH on solubilization is independent of the value of the solubility of the unionized form of the drug. In other words the solubility of an unionized acid with a pK_a of 4.2 and a solubility of 1.0 mg/ml and one with the same pK_a and a solubility of 0.001 mg/ml will both be increased by a factor of 1001 at pH 7.4.

Although the use of a buffer will aid in reducing the risk of precipitation upon dilution, there are pH, concentration and buffer type limitations. Physiological compatibility will depend on factors such as the route of administration, tonicity, and contact time. Other factors such as chemical stability as a function of pH must also be considered. Table 4 lists some marketed parenteral products and associated buffers, concentrations and pH values.

COSOLVENTS

A common and effective way by which to increase the solubility of a non polar drug is through the use of cosolvents. A cosolvent system is one in which a water miscible or partially miscible organic solvent is mixed with water to form a modified aqueous solution. Cosolvents have some degree of hydrogen bond donating and or hydrogen bond accepting ability as well as small hydrocarbon regions. The resulting solution will have physical properties that are intermediate to that of the pure

Table 4 Selected list of marketed products that contain buffers

Drug (product)	Route of administration	Buffer, concentration (% w/v) and pH
Methohexital sodium	IV/IV infusion reconstituted	Sodium carbonate pH 9–11
Chlorpromazine–HCl (Thorazine)	IM/IV after dilution	Ascorbic acid 0.2% pH 3.0–5.0
Amikacin sulfate	IM/IV infusion after dilution	Sodium citrate 2.8% pH 3.5–5.5
Biperidan lactate (Akineton)	IV/IM	Sodium lactate 1.4%
Thiopental sodium (Pentothal sodium)	IV infusion reconstitued	Sodium carbonate pH 10–11
Epinepherine–HCL (SusPhrine)	SC	Ascorbic acid 1.0%
Etidocaine HCl (Duranest)	Infiltration	Citric acid pH 3–5
Etoposide (VePesid)	IV infusion	Citric acid 0.2% pH 3–4
Methoxamine HCl (Vasoxyl)	IV/IM	Citric acid 0.3% pH 3–5
Methyldopate HCl (Aldomet ester HCl)	IV infusion after dilution	Sodium citrate 0.3% Citric acid 0.5% pH 3.5–4.2
Nalbuphine HCl (Nubain)	IV/IM/SC	"Citrates" 2% pH 3.5
Perphenazine (Trilafon)	IM/IV/SC	Citric acid pH 4–5.5
Chlordiazepoxide–HCL (Librium)	IM/IV	Maleic acid 1.6% pH 3
Topotecan (Hycamtin)	IV infusion	Tartaric acid 2% pH 2.5–3.5
Diazepam (Valium)	IM/IV	Sodium benzoate/benzoic acid 5.0% pH 6–7
Midazolam–HCL	IM/IV	pH 3
Octreotide acetate 84-(Sandostatin)	SC/IM/IV after dilution	Lactic acid 0.34% pH 4.2
Prochlorperzine edislate (Compazine)	IM/IV/IV infusion after dilution	Sodium biphosphate 0.5% Sodium tartrate 1.2% pH 4–6
Phenytoin sodium (Dilantin)	IM/IV	Sodium hydroxide pH 10–12.3

(From Refs. 84–86.)

organic solvent and water through the reduction of water–water interactions. This affords a system that is more favorable for nonpolar solutes.

Table 5 gives some physical properties of commonly used pharmaceutical cosolvents in water. Note that n-octanol is added in the table as a reference, since compounds that have large octanol/water partition coefficients have poor aqueous solubility. The use of cosolvent systems that have physical properties that are more similar to those of n-octanol would be expected to have greater success in solubilizing a nonpolar drug. In the following section it will be demonstrated that aqueous solubilization via colsovency is dependent on both the solute and cosolvent physical properties.

Mathematical Description for Cosolvency

Numerous methods have been proposed to predict or describe the effect of a particular cosolvent system (86–102) on drug solubility. A practical cosolvent model was developed by Yalkowsky and coworkers (103–106) by assuming the mixed solvent system is a linear

Table 5 Physical properties of some common cosolvents and their reference to water and n-octanol

Solvent	$\log K_{o/w}$	Solubility parameter	Surface tension	Dielectric constant
Water	−4.00	23.4	72.0	81.0
Glycerin	−1.96	16.5	64.9	42.5
Propylene glycol	−0.92	12.6	37.1	32.0
PEG-400	−0.88	11.3	46.0	13.6
Dimethyl sulfoxide	−1.09	12.0	38.0	46.7
Dimethyl acetamide	−0.66	10.8	35.7	37.8
Ethanol	−0.31	12.7	22.2	24.3
n-Octanol	2.94	10.3	20.5	10.3

combination of the pure components. They found that this approach yields the log-linear relationship

$$\log S_{\text{mix}} = \log S_{\text{w}} + \sigma f_{\text{c}} \tag{18}$$

where the logarithm of the solubility of a nonpolar solute S_{mix} will increase with the cosolvent fraction (f_{c}), having a slope of σ, and an intercept of log S_{w}. On a linear scale, an exponential increase in solubility is observed with an increase in cosolvent composition. Figure 4 illustrates the linear and exponential solubilization profiles.

For solid solutes, the melting point contributes only to the intercept of the solubilization profile. The independence of the intrinsic solubility and the solubilization slope can be demonstrated by the isomers benzo(a)pyrene and perylene. Figure 5 (top) shows the solubilization of benzo(a)pyrene and perylene in ethanol/water systems.

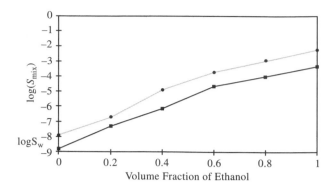

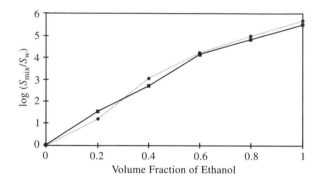

Fig. 5 (Top) Solubilization profile of ◆, benzo(a)pyrene and ■, perylene in ethanol–water mixtures. (Bottom) Relative solubilization (log($S_{\text{mix}}/S_{\text{w}}$)) of ◆, benzo($a$)pyrene and ■, perylene in ethanol–water mixtures.

The log$K_{\text{o/w}}$'s (or aqueous activity coefficients) can be considered to be equal for these two compounds, however, their melting points are different. Benzo(a)pyrene has a melting point of 179°C, while perylene has a melting point of 273°C, and as a result, the latter has a lower intrinsic solubility. Yet both compounds have solubilization slopes (σ) which are nearly identical. This is because σ is soley a function of the activity coefficients (log $K_{\text{o/w}}$).

Since the intrinsic solubility does not directly affect the solubilization slope, it is convenient to arrange Eq. 18 to

$$\log(S_{\text{mix}}/S_{\text{w}}) = \sigma f_{\text{c}} \tag{19}$$

By plotting $\log(S_{\text{mix}}/S_{\text{w}})$ versus f_{c}, solubilization lines are normalized with respect to the intrinsic solubility and pass through the origin on a semi log plot. This facilitates comparisons among different drugs as well as different cosolvents. Fig. 5 (bottom) shows the solubilization plots of benzo(a)pyrene and perylene using the expression of Eq. 19.

The ability of a cosolvent to solubilize a given solute can be related to the properties of both the solute and cosolvent. The solubilization slope, σ, for a given cosolvent system is dependent upon the polarity of

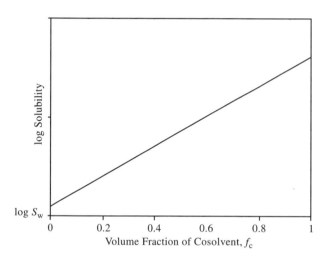

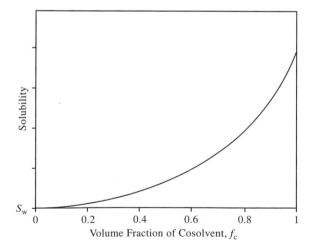

Fig. 4 Typical cosolvent solubilization curves for a nonpolar drug. (Top) Log-linear scale. (Bottom) Linear scale.

the drug and the polarity of the cosolvent and can be related by,

$$\sigma = s \log K_{o/w} + t \qquad (20)$$

where polarity of the drug is indicated by $\log K_{o/w}$ and the polarity and physical properties of the cosolvent are represented through the parameters s and t.

Dependence of Solubilization on Solute Properties

As illustrated in Fig. 5, isomeric compounds or compounds that have almost identical aqueous activity coefficients (i.e, similar $\log K_{o/w}$s) will have very similar solubilization slopes for a given cosolvent system. Differences in overall solubility are once again attributed to differences in the crystal contribution to solubility.

For nonpolar solutes, or those solutes that are more nonpolar than the cosolvent of choice, solubilization generally follows the log-linear model of Eq. 18. The degree of solubilization is directly related to the polarity of the solute. From Eq. 20 it has been shown that the solubilization slope, σ, can be related directly to the logarithm of the octanol–water partition coefficient ($\log K_{o/w}$). Fig. 6 shows data for a series of hydrocortisones in propylene glycol. As $\log K_{o/w}$ increases it follows that the solubilization slopes increase. Li and Yalkowsky (107) have also illustrated this relationship for nonpolar solutes in ethanol–water systems. Once again the trend maintains that as $\log K_{o/w}$ increases, solubilization is increased for a given cosolvent system (i.e, s and t are constant). For the

most nonpolar compounds (largest $\log K_{o/w}$'s) solubilization approaches several orders of magnitude.

As $\log K_{o/w}$ decreases so does the ability of an organic cosolvent to solubilize the solute. For solutes that are semipolar and polar (polarities that are between water and a given cosolvent) little gain in solubility, if any, can be expected with the addition of an organic cosolvent. Semipolar solutes will have a maximal solubility at some mixed composition at a polarity that matches the solute. After a maximum solubility the slope becomes negative, and any additional cosolvent will decrease the solubility of the solute. The overall gain in solubility for semipolar solutes is generally less than a factor of five, which is significantly less than that of nonpolar solutes.

The solubility of polar solutes decreases with the addition of an organic cosolvent to water. Although it is obvious that cosolvents would not be used for solubilizing polar solutes, it is important to understand that for formulations that have other components or excipients, the use of a cosolvent for a nonpolar drug may cause solubility problems for polar excipients. If it is a polar drug that is insoluble, a reflection to Eq. 6 will aid in understanding that it is likely the crystal contribution that is limiting the solubility. This is generally the case since polar compounds have significant polar functionalities such as hydrogen bonding moieties that generate a strong crystal structure. If any of the functional groups are acidic or basic, the choice of pH may be the most efficient means by which to solubilize these compounds. Once again the trend maintains that as incremental hydrocarbon groups are added to a base structure, solubilization is increased for a given cosolvent system (i.e, s and t are constant). For the most nonpolar compounds (largest $\log K_{o/w}$) solubilization approaches 5–6 orders of magnitude.

Dependence of Solubilization on Cosolvent Properties

The reduction of intermolecular hydrogen bonding interactions of water when an organic cosolvent is mixed with water creates a solvent system that favors the dissolution of a nonpolar solute. The more nonpolar the cosolvent, the more nonpolar the cosolvent/water system will become and the greater the solublization of a nonpolar drug. In addition to polarity considerations, it is also useful to take into account hydrogen bond donating and accepting capabilities when evaluating cosolvent systems (108). As can be seen from solubilization of benzocaine with different cosolvent systems in Fig. 7, there is a clear dependence between cosolvent polarity and solubilization. The more nonpolar the cosolvent the greater the solubilization slope.

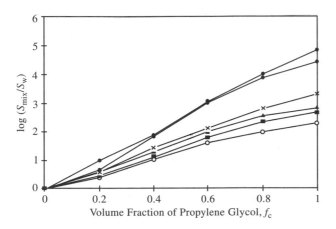

Fig. 6 Solubilization of different hydrocortisones in propylene glycol–water mixtures; ●, hydrocortisone acetate, ◆, hydrocortisone propionate, ✕, hydrocortisone butyrate, ▲, hydrocortisone pentanoate, ■, hydrocortisone hexanoate, ○, hydrocortisone heptanoate.

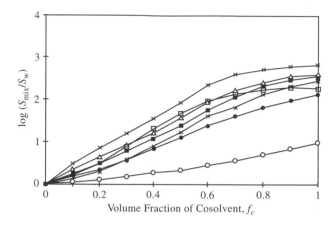

Fig. 7 Solubilization of benzocaine by *, dimethylacetamide, △, PEG-400, ■, PEG-200, □, ethanol, ×, methanol, ◆, propylene glycol; and ○, glycerin.

Relationship between Solubilization Slope, σ, and Solute Polarity

It is important to recognize that cosolvent solubilization does not rigorously follow a log-linear relationship. In fact a slight negative deviation is observed at low cosolvent compositions and a downward curving positive deviation is often observed at higher cosolvent compositions. Several investigators have attempted to explain or predict this type of behavior (89–102), however, the simplest and most useful remains the log-linear model. Another advantage of the log-linear model is that only two data points are needed to estimate the solubility of a solute in any ethanol–water composition.

With appreciation of the curvature observed for the cosolvent systems given above, a good correlation can still be obtained from simply looking at the terminal slope, σ, of a cosolvent system. That is, by using the log-linear approach (Fig. 4), the slope is simply the difference between the solubility of a solute in the pure cosolvent and in water. The general applicability of this has been demonstrated by Morris et al. (109) and Li and Yalkowsky

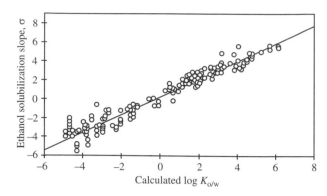

Fig. 8 Relationship between solubilization slope, σ and calculated log $K_{o/w}$ (via C log P) for a variety of different solutes in ethanol cosolvent systems. (From Ref. 107.)

(107). Figure 8 illustrates the relationship between solubilization slope, σ, and log$K_{o/w}$. The gain in solubilization potential (increase in σ) is directly related to an increase in the calculated log$K_{o/w}$.

Millard and Yalkowsky (110) have recently evaluated several cosolvent systems using log$K_{o/w}$'s calculated by CLOGP (15). They found reasonable correlations between the solubilization slope and log$K_{o/w}$ for ethanol, propylene glycol, polyethylene glycol 400, and glycerol cosolvent systems. A summary of their work is given in Table 6.

From Table 6 it is clear that cosolvent solubilization effectiveness (σ) is directly related to log$K_{o/w}$. The least polar cosolvent, EtOH, produces the highest σ value, and the most polar cosolvent, glycerol, produces the lowest σ value.

Multiple Cosolvents

The use of multiple cosolvents can be a valuable method for solubilizing a poorly water soluble drug when a dosage form necessitates limits on the amount and type of cosolvent that can be utilized. The effects of multiple cosolvents on solubility can be reasonably approximated

Table 6 Regression analysis of solubilization slope, σ, and log $K_{o/w}$ (Eq. 20) for different cosolvent systems

Cosolvent	Cosolvent log$K_{o/w}$	σ	t	n	r^2	SE
Ethanol	−0.31	0.93	0.38	120	0.96	0.53
Propylene glycol	−0.92	0.76	0.57	93	0.93	0.48
Polyethylene glycol 400	−0.88	0.73	1.19	25	0.77	0.62
Glycerol	−1.96	0.34	0.29	26	0.81	0.34

Given are the slope, σ, intercept, t, number of compounds used in the regression, n, and the regression correlation values, r^2, and standard errors, SE.

by simply expanding Eq. 18 to include a liner addition of cosolvents, i.e,

$$\log S_{mix} = \log S_w + \sigma_1 f_{c1} + \sigma_2 f_{c2} + \sigma_3 f_{c3} + \cdots \quad (21)$$

where the subscripts 1, 2, and 3 represent the slope and fraction of cosolvents 1, 2, 3, etc. Chien and Lambert (111) found that Eq. 21 adequately represented the solubility of a steroid in mixed solvent systems. Similarly, Pramar and Das Gupta (112) found that the solubility of spironolactone (Fig. 9) in multiple cosolvent systems followed a log-linear relationship. Data from Pramer and Das Gupta are presented in Fig. 10, showing the solubility of spironolactone for some ternary systems. Figure 10 demonstrates a nearly linear increase in solubility of spironolactone as the amount of propylene glycol or glycerin is added to a given PEG-400 concentration. All of the systems include 10% ethanol, giving a ternary system. Further investigation of the data, reveal that propylene glycol is a more efficient solubilizing agent than glycerol. In fact, the slope for propylene glycol is nearly twice that of glycerol, which is very similar to the findings above for the single cosolvent systems (Table 8).

Eq. 21 assumes that each cosolvent interacts independently. Of course this is not always the case. In fact the data of Pramar and Das Gupta (112) show a synergistic affect for the solubilization of the nonpolar solute, spironolactone. In addition, the use of one cosolvent can be used to increase the solubility of a partially miscible cosolvent in water. The facilitated cosolvency effect of multiple species in water has been shown by Gupta et al. (113) and Riley (114).

Solubilization through the Use of Cosolvents

Cosolvents can be a powerful tool by which to solubilize drugs. For a given cosolvent selected, it is clear that the degree of solubilization attained for any solute is directly proportional to the octanol/water partition coefficient of

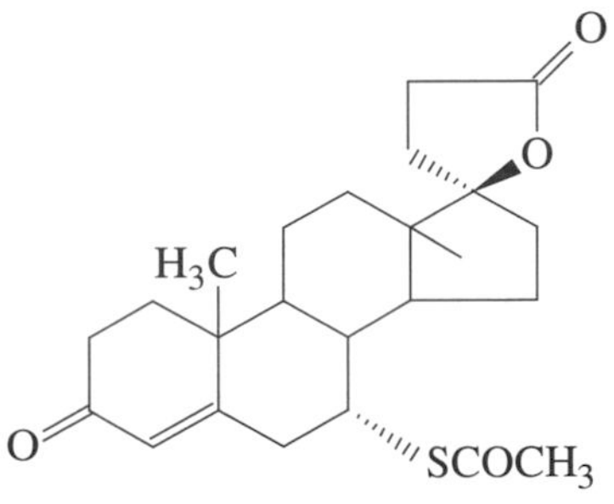

Fig. 9 Structure of spironolactone.

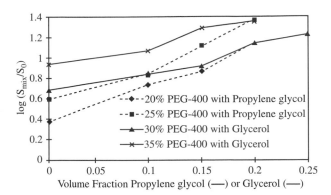

Fig. 10 Ternary cosolvent systems and resulting solubilization of spironolactone. S_o represents the solubility of spironolactone in a 10% ethanol/water system. Given in the figure are different concentrations of PEG-400 with varied propylene glycol or glycerin volume fractions. (From Ref. 112.)

that solute. However, as with pH solubilization, solubilization through cosolvents is logarithmic, and as a result there is the potential for precipitation upon dilution.

A potential limitation to the use of cosolvents may be the choice and amount of cosolvent needed. For pharmaceuticals there are relatively few organic cosolvents that are generally regarded as safe. Rubino (115) has discussed the biological effects of many of the commonly utilized cosolvents such as ethanol, propylene glycol, glycerol, polyethylene glycols, and dimethylacetamide (DMA). The permissible amount of a given cosolvent will be dependent upon the dosage form. Table 7 gives some examples of products that contain cosolvents. The introduction of new, safe cosolvents would greatly enhance the technique of using cosolvents for solubilization. However, even with the limited number of acceptable cosolvents, cosolvancy is clearly a valuable methods by which to solubilize poorly water soluble drugs.

SURFACTANTS

Surfactants are molecules with distinct polar and nonpolar regions. Most surfactants consist of a hydrocarbon segment (usually in the form of a long aliphatic chain segment) connected to a polar group. The polar group can be anionic (such as a carboxylate, sulfate, or sulfonate), cationic such as ammonium, trialkylammonium, or pyridinium), zwitterionic (such as glycine or carnitine) or nonionic such as polyethylene glycol, glycerol, or sugar. An illustration of the general structure of classical surfactants, as well as different pictorial representations, are illustrated in Fig. 11. Selected structures of non-classical surfactants are illustrated in Fig. 12. Although

Table 7 Examples of some parenteral products that contain cosolvents

Drug (product)	Route of administration	Cosolvent composition (% w/v)
Busulfan (Busulfex)	IV infusion after dilution	67% PEG 400 33% + *N,N* DMA
Chlordiazepoxide (Librium)	IV after dilution	20% Propylene glycol
Diazepam (Valium)	IM/IV	10% Ethanol 40% Propylene glycol
Digoxin (Lanoxin)	IM/IV	10% Ethanol 40% Propylene glycol
Dihydroergotamine mesylate (D.H.E.)	IM/IV	6.1% Ethanol 15% Glycerin
Esmolol–HCl (Brevibloc)	IV after dilution	25% Ethanol 25% Propylene glycol
Etoposide (VePesid)	IV infusion after dilution	30 % Ethanol 60% PEG 300
Fenoldopam (Corlopam)	IV after dilution	50% Propylene glycol
Lorazepam (Ativan)	IM/IV after dilution	18% Polyethylene glycol 400 80% Propylene glycol
Melphalan–HCl (Alkeran)	IV infusion after dilution	5% Ethanol 60% Propylene glycol
Nitroglycerin (Nitro-Bid)	IV infusion after dilution	70% Ethanol 4.5% Propylene glycol
Pentobarbital Sodium (Nembutal sodium)	IV/IM after dilution	10% Ethanol 40% Propylene glycol
Paricalcitol (Zemplar)	IV	20% Ethanol 30% Propylene glycol
Phenytoin Sodium (Dilantin)	IM/IV	10% Ethanol 40% Propylene glycol
Epinephrine (Sus-Phrine)	SC	32.5% Glycerin
Methocarbamil (Robaxin)	IM/IV after dilution	50% Polyethylene glycol 300
Oxytetracycline (Terramycin)	IM	67–75% Propylene glycol
Teniposide (Vumon)	IV infusion after dilution	42% Ethanol + 6% DMA

(From Refs. 84–86.)

these structures do not contain a single aliphatic chain and a simple polar head group, they do contain distinct polar and nonpolar regions.

Due to the differences in properties of the polar and nonpolar regions, surfactants tend to accumulate and orient at interfaces so that each region of the surfactant interacts with a separate phase. The polar portion of the surfactant will associate with the more polar phase (especially if it is water) and the nonpolar portion of the surfactant will remain in the more nonpolar solvent. In water, as the concentration of surfactant increases above a critical value, its molecules self associate into soluble structures called micelles. The concentration at which they begin to form is called the critical micelle concentration (or the CMC).

These micelles are normally spherical with the nonpolar regions of the surfactant molecules gathered in the center (core) and surrounded by a mantel of the polar regions which are in contact with the water as illustrated in Fig. 13. A nonpolar drug, which is squeezed out of water, can locate within the micelle core. A semipolar drug can locate between or partially within the core and the mantel. Since the micelles are soluble in water any drug that is incorporated into the micelle will also be soluble in the aqueous system.

The general solubilization curve for surfactants is given in Fig. 14. If the monomers of surfactant in solution do not affect the solubility of the solute, then the solute concentration will remain constant (at the intrinsic solubility, S_w) until the CMC. After the CMC the solute concentration will increase linearly with increasing surfactant (micelle) concentration. A simple mathematical

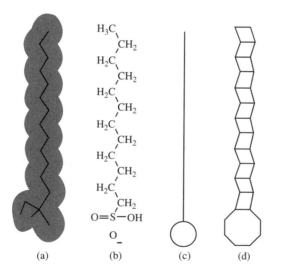

Fig. 11 Representation of classical surfactant structures: (a) Space-filling model; (b) chemical structure diagram; (c) simple line "stick" figure; (d) hybrid of diagrams a-c. (From Ref. 1.)

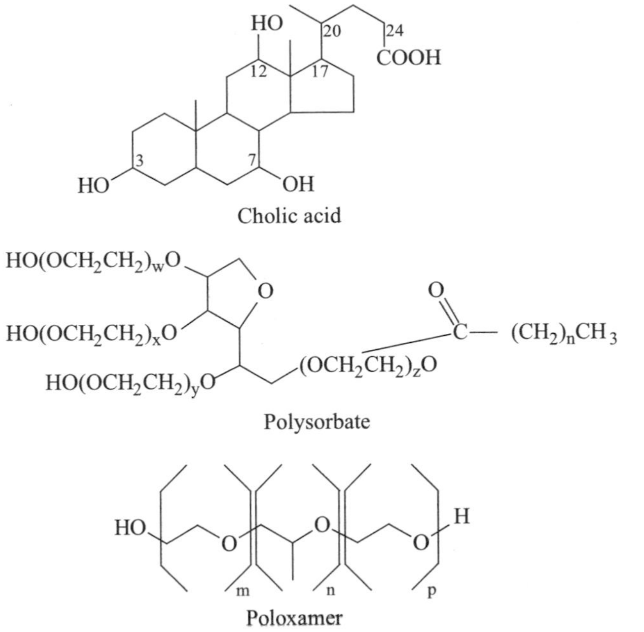

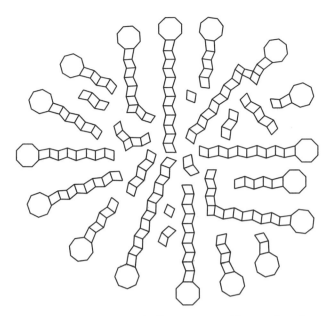

Cholic acid

Polysorbate

Poloxamer

Fig. 12 Structure for the nonclassical surfactants cholic acid and generic structural features for polysorbates and polaxamers.

representation for a solute's total solubility, S_T, in a surfactant system is

$$S_T = S_w + \kappa(C_{surf} - CMC) \qquad (22)$$

where C_{surf} is the total concentration of the surfactant and κ is the solubilization capacity. The quantity in parenthesis in Eq. 22 represents the micelle concentration. The solubilization capacity reflects the number of surfactant molecules that are required to solubilize a single solute molecule. Deviations from Eq. 22 are usually the result of changes in micelle shape or size that occur as the concentration of surfactant increases.

A micelle is a dynamic aggregation of any number of individual surfactant molecules, or monomers. Although the molecules are intertwined, they are in constant motion like those of a liquid. Thus, the interior of a micelle can be thought of as a separate phase and a micellar solution can be thought of as a microdispersion of that phase in water. If the micelle is considered to be a separate phase, it is then convenient to evaluate the solubilization capacity (κ), in terms of the partition between the micelle and water. The micellar partition coefficient, K_m, is defined as the ratio of the solute concentration in the micelle, C_m, to that of water, C_w:

$$K_m = C_m/C_w \qquad (23)$$

The micelle/water partition coefficient for many solutes have been shown to correlate to the octanol/water partition

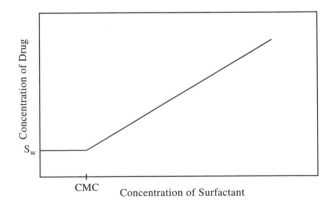

Fig. 13 Illustration of a micellar structure with nonpolar solutes in the core of the micelle.

coefficient (116–121). Data in Table 8, from Azaz and Donbrow (116), show that the micellar partition coefficients of the methylphenols increase with the number of methyl groups. Collett and Tobin (119) showed that the micellar partition coefficients of several benzoic acid derivatives are proportional to their octanol–water partition coefficient for poloxamers (Table 9). Tomida et al. (119) also illustrated that most of the 34 monosubstituted benzoic acids with Brij 35 have micellar partition coefficients that are inversely proportional to their aqueous solubilities and proportional to their octanol–water partition coefficients. The data of Tomida et al. (121) for some steroid hormones (Table 10), further illustrate the parallelism between octanol–water and micelle–water partition coefficients.

Fig. 14 General curve for solubilization with surfactants.

Table 8 Micellar partition coefficients of methylphenols by cetomacrogol

Solute	logS_w	K_M	logK_M	CLOGP
Phenol	—	42.00	1.62	1.49
2-Methylphenol	−0.62	79.50	1.90	1.95
3-Methylphenol	−0.70	76.40	1.88	1.96
4-Methylphenol	−0.85	85.10	1.93	1.94
2,3-Dimethylphenol	−1.43	169.00	2.23	2.42
2,4-Dimethylphenol	−1.29	125.00	2.10	2.30
2,5-Dimethylphenol	−1.54	197.00	2.29	2.33
2,6-Dimethylphenol	−1.31	114.00	2.06	2.36
3,4-Dimethylphenol	−1.41	151.00	2.18	2.23
3,5-Dimethylphenol	−1.40	132.00	2.12	2.35

(From Ref. 116.)

Semipolar solutes are generally solubilized by the polar regions of nonionic surfactants. The solute is absorbed into the polyoxyethylene mantle rather than the hydrocarbon core. The micellar partition coefficients of the semipolar solutes is also dependent upon their octanol–water partition coefficient. However, since these solutes are solubilized primarily in the mantle, the surfactant property that is most important is the number of polyoxyethylene units, and the alkyl chain length of the surfactant plays only a minor role in determining the micellar partition coefficient of a semipolar solute.

Materials that are solubilized in polyethylene glycol can be solubilized in the polyoxyethylene chains on the surface of a nonionic micelle. Ismail et al. (122) found that the micellar partition coefficients of barbiturates in polysorbates 20, 40, 60, and 80 is a function of the solute substituents and is proportional to the octanol–water partition coefficient of the barbiturate. Similarly, Ikeda

Table 10 Micellar partition coefficients of some steroids in Brij 35

Solute	log S_w	log K_M	CLOGP
Hydrocortisone	−2.97	1.99	1.55
Corticosterone	−3.24	2.27	1.94
Deoxycorticosterone	−3.45	2.60	2.90
Cortisone	−3.27	1.82	1.42
Hydrocortisone acetate	−4.34	2.36	2.19
Cortisone acetate	−4.21	2.31	2.10
Deoxycorticosterone	−4.63	2.86	3.08
11-Hydroxyprogesterone	−3.82	2.43	2.36
Progesterone	−4.42	3.12	3.87
Testosterone	−4.08	2.80	3.29
Prednisolone	−3.18	2.04	1.61
Prednisolone acetate	−4.37	2.45	2.40
Triamcinolone	−3.68	1.98	1.03
Betamethasone	−3.77	2.45	1.94
Dexamethasone acetate	−4.90	2.99	2.91
Betamethasone-17-valerate	−4.71	3.25	3.48

(Based on Ref. 121.)

et al. (123) showed that the solubilization of alkyl barbiturates by polyoxyethylene lauryl ether is not dependent upon the number of carbons in the substituents. Since the different polysorbates contain different aliphatic groups, the rather small dependence of solubilization upon polysorbate number (i.e., upon alkyl chain length) suggests that the barbiturates are not solubilized primarily in the hydrocarbon portion of the micelle. Gouda et al. (124) showed that the solubilization of barbiturates in polyoxyethylene stearates is proportional to the number of polyoxyethylene units in the surfactant.

Jafvert et al. (125) developed the following equation for predicting the molar solubilization capacity of organic

Table 9 Micellar partition coefficients of some benzoic acid derivatives by poloxamer L64 at 37°C

Solute	logS_w	K_M	log K_M	CLOGP
Benzoic acid	−1.52	43.50	1.64	1.81
2-Hydroxybenzoic acid	−1.76	83.00	1.92	2.38
3-Hydroxybenzoic acid	−1.21	28.50	1.45	1.50
4-Hydroxybenzoic acid	−1.23	30.80	1.49	1.58
4-Chlorobenzoic acid	−3.31	277.00	2.44	2.65
4-Bromobenzoic acid	−3.54	445.00	2.65	2.86
4-Iodobenzoic acid	−3.95	678.00	2.83	3.02
4-Nitrobenzoic acid	−2.66	92.70	1.97	1.89
4-Methoxybenzoic acid	−0.63	66.50	1.82	1.96

(From Ref. 119.)

compounds in nonionic surfactants on the basis of surfactant structure as well as solute structure.

$$K_M = K_{o/w}(0.030{\sim}L_1 - 0.0058{\sim}L_2 \\ -0.0056{\sim}L_3 + 0.0319{\sim}L_4) \quad (24)$$

where:

L_1 = number of straight chain aliphatic carbons in the hydrophobic tail

L_2 = number of repeating ethoxy groups

L_3 = number of carbons in a sorbitan group

L_4 = number of total carbons in alkylbenzene groups

This equation relates the micellar partition coefficient to the octanol–water partition coefficient. It also accounts for both the polar and nonpolar surfactant moieties.

Alvarez-Nunez and Yalkowsky (126) showed that the molar micellar partition coefficient is related to the octanol–water partition coefficient for a structurally diverse set of pharmaceutically important compounds through the relationship

$$K_M = a \log K_{o/w} + b \quad (25)$$

Which for posysorbate 80 is equal to

$$K_M = 0.92 \log K_{o/w} - 0.07 \quad (26)$$

Eq. 26 is then used to estimate total solubility by the equation

$$S_{tot} = S_w[1 + C_{polysorbate}{\sim} \times 10^{(0.92 \log K_{o/w} - 0.07)}] \quad (27)$$

where $C_{polysorbate\ 80}$ is the concentration of polysorbate 80.

While both Eqs. 24 and 26 are quite useful, they must be employed with caution, especially for solutes that have some degree of amphiphilic character. Solutes that have surface-active physicochemical properties themselves (i.e., they have separate polar and nonpolar regions) tend to be more soluble than expected because they can accumulate at the core/mantle interface or the core/water

interface. In essence, weakly amphiphilic solutes can act as cosurfactants and form mixed micelles with nonionic surfactants as well as with ionic surfactants. This can alter both the CMC and the size of the micelle. In most cases this leads to a higher degree of solubilization than would be predicted on the basis of either molecular size or partition coefficient.

In summary, micellar solubilization for both nonpolar and semipolar surfactants can be obtained. Due to the limitation on surfactant quantity that can be practically used, due to biological constraints, micellar solubilization is typically more advantageous for low dose formulations. In addition, although a large number of anionic, cationic and nonionic surfactants are available for use as solubilizing agents (128–131), only polysorbate-80 and cremephor EL have been used to any significant extent in parenteral products. Table 11 lists some parenteral formulations that contain surfactants. It should be noted that adverse clinical events have been observed for patients receiving cremophor EL.

COMPLEXATION

Complexation is the association between two or more molecules to form a nonbonded entity with a well-defined stoichiometry. The two types of complexation that are most useful for increasing the solubility of drugs in aqueous media are stacking and inclusion. Stacking complexes are formed by the overlap of the planar regions of aromatic molecules, while inclusion complexes are formed by the insertion of the nonpolar region of one molecule into the cavity of another molecule (or group of molecules).

The mathematical description for the equilibrium constant of a 1:1 complex, $K_{1:1}$, is defined by

$$K_{1:1} = [SL]/[S][L] \quad (28)$$

Table 11 Examples of some products that contain surfactants

Drug (Product)	Route of administration	Surfactant composition (% w/v)
Taxol (Paclitaxel)	IV infusion after dilution	51% Cremophor EL
Valrubicin (Valstar)	IV infusion after dilution	50% Cremophor EL
Chlordiazepoxide HCl (Librium)	IM/IV (diluent)	4% Polysorbate 80
Cyclosporin (Sandimmune)	IV infusion after dilution	65% Cremophor EL
Etoposide (VePesid)	IV infusion after dilution	8% Polysorbate 80
Amiodarone (Cordarone)	IV infusion after dilution	10% Polysorbate 80

(From Refs. 84–86.)

where S is the concentration of the free solute, L is the concentration of the free ligand, and [SL] is the concentration of the solute/ligand complex. The equilibrium constant is also commonly referred to as the stability constant or the complexation constant. If it takes two ligand molecules to complex with a solute molecule the complexation constant is defined by

$$K_{1:2} = [SL_2]/[S][L]^2 \qquad (29)$$

The total solubility of the solute, S_T, for a solute that forms a 1:1 complex is

$$S_T = S_w + [SL] \qquad (30)$$

where S_w is the intrinsic solubility of the solute in water. Similarly the total concentration of ligand, $[L^{tot}]$, in the system is

$$[L^{tot}] = [L] + [SL] \qquad (31)$$

Combining Eqs. 28, 30, and 31, gives the general equation for solubilization by 1:1 complexation,

$$S_T = S_w + [K_{1:1}S_w/(1 + K_{1:1}S_w)]L^{tot} \qquad (32)$$

where the intercept is the aqueous solubility of the solute. Eq. 32 represents a linear increase in the solubility of the solute with increasing ligand concentration, with a slope, $\sigma_{complex}$, of

$$\sigma_{complex} = [K_{1:1}S_w/(1 + K_{1:1}S_w)] \qquad (33)$$

and the stability constant is

$$K_{1:1} = \sigma_{complex}/[S_w(1 - \sigma_{complex})]. \qquad (34)$$

From the above it can be seen that, as the stability constant of a 1:1 complex increases, the slope will increase until the value converges to unity for a strong complex in which one ligand molecule solubilizes one solute molecule. The initial segment of the curve in Fig. 15 illustrates this. This linear region will continue until the solubility of the complex itself is reached, at which point the total solubility of the solute remains constant, as indicated by the central segment of the curve. A plateau is analogous to the maximum solubility of a salt as described previously. Further addition of the complexing agent can result in a reduction in of the concentration of the free solute and a leveling off of the curve at the solubility of the pure complex as illustrated by the final segment of the curve in Fig. 15.

The solubilization curve for a solute molecule that complexes with two ligand molecules is more complicated than those shown in Fig. 15. If the complexation constant for a second ligand is significantly lower than the first, a 1:1 complex will be formed at lower ligand concentration.

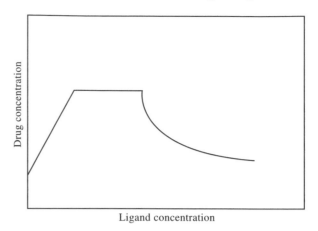

Fig. 15 General solubilization profile for complexation.

It will then combine with a second ligand to produce a 2:1 complex. Assuming that the latter is more soluble than the 1:1 complex, the solubilization curve will have two distinct slopes. If each ligand is equally capable of complexing with the solute, they will complex simultaneously to produce a convex up solubilization curve.

According to Eq. 32, the factors that determine the degree of solubilization of the solute are the complexation constant and the solubilities of the solute, the ligand, and the complex. As a result, the most useful ligands for solubilization in aqueous media are highly water soluble, and produce soluble complexes.

Self-Association and Stacking Complexation

Nonpolar moieties tend to be squeezed out of water by the strong hydrogen bonding interactions of the water. This causes some molecules to minimize the contact with water by aggregation of their hydrocarbon moities. This aggregation is favored by large planar nonpolar regions in the molecule. Just as micelles can be pure or mixed, stacked complexes can be homogenous or mixed. The former is known as self-association and the latter as complexation. Some examples of substances that interact in an aqueous media by stacking are shown in Fig. 16.

Higuchi and Kristiansen (132) found that complexes formed between compounds containing aromatic acids or amides and compounds with aromatic nitrogens, such as those depicted in the second and third row of Fig. 16, consistently had higher stability constants than complexes made of a single compound. There have been a number of attempts to quantitatively relate or classify the chemical structures of the solute and ligand with their ability to complex (132–137).

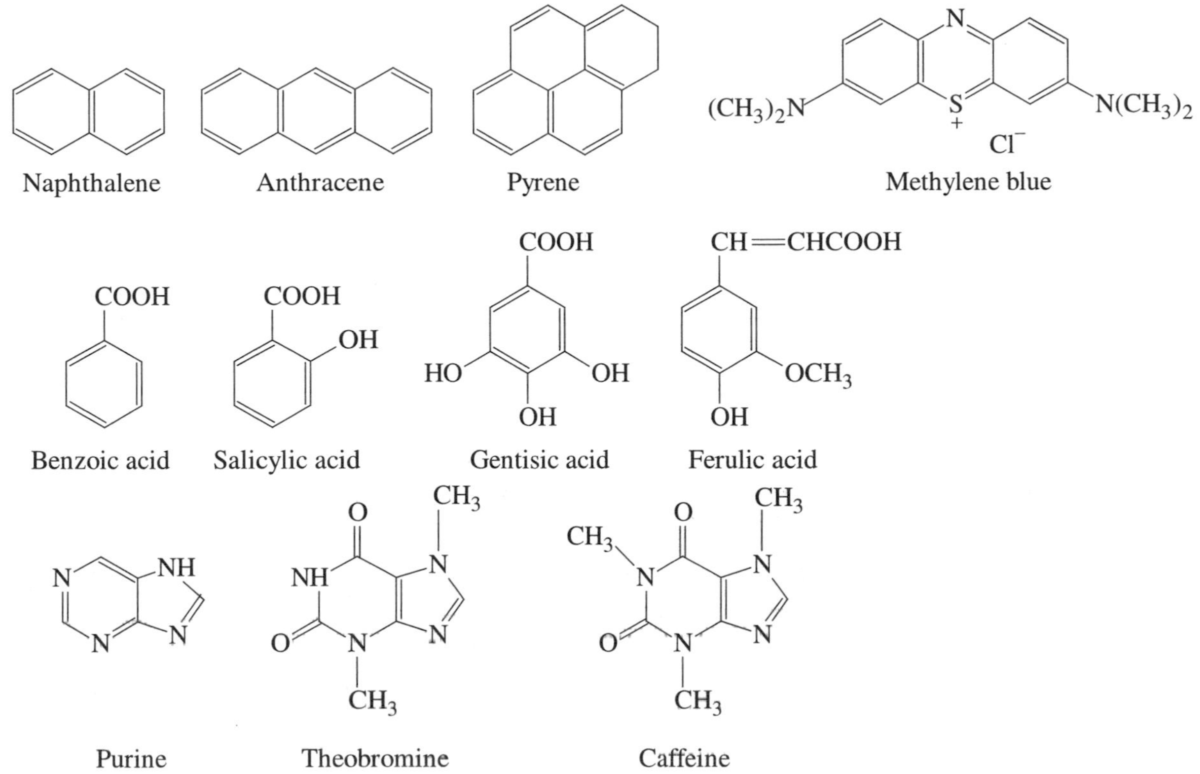

Naphthalene   Anthracene   Pyrene   Methylene blue

Benzoic acid   Salicylic acid   Gentisic acid   Ferulic acid

Purine   Theobromine   Caffeine

Fig. 16 Some compounds that are known to form stacking complexes.

Inclusion Complexes

An inclusion complex is produced by the inclusion of a nonpolar molecule or the nonpolar region of a molecule (known as the guest) into the nonpolar cavity of another molecule or group of molecules (known as the host). When the guest molecule enters the host molecule the contact between water and the nonpolar regions of both is reduced. Thus, inclusion phenomena are the result of the same driving force that produces micellization, self-association, and stacking; namely the squeezing out from water of nonpolar moities.

The major structural requirement for inclusion complexation is a snug fit of the guest into the host cavity. The host cavity must be large enough to accommodate the guest and small enough to eliminate water so that the total contact between water and the nonpolar regions of the host and the guest is reduced.

The most commonly used host molecules are the cyclodextrins. These cyclic oligomers of glucose are relatively soluble in water and have cavities large enough to accept nonpolar portions of common drug molecules. The naturally occurring cyclodextrins contain 6, 7, and 8 glucopyranose units and are termed α, β, and γ,

respectively. These are represented in Fig. 17 where "G" represents a glucopyranose unit. Modified cyclodextrins have one or more of the hydroxy groups of one or more of the glucopyranose units modified. Some of the more common modifications are with alkyl or hydroxyalky groups, or with anionic or cationic functionalities. Many of these modified cyclodextrins are more soluble than their naturally occurring precursors (138–140).

The size of the cavity in the cyclodextrin is the major factor in determining which guest solutes will be most acceptable for complexation. In general, alkyl groups will

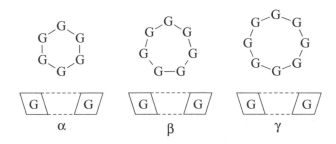

Fig. 17 Schematic representation of two views of the naturally occurring α, β, γ cyclodextrins.

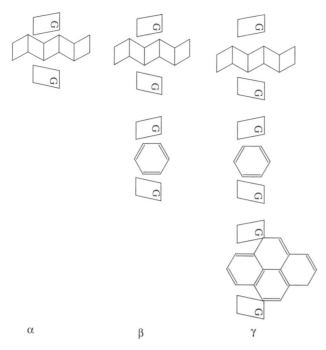

Fig. 18 Representation of the incorporation of pentane, benzene, and pyrene into α, β, and γ cyclodextrins.

fit well into the cavity of the α-cyclodextrins. The β-cyclodextrins are most well suited for accepting single aromatic rings, and the γ-cyclodextrins have large enough cavities to accommodate larger hydrocarbons such as pyrene. Fig. 18 illustrates these as well as other representative inclusion complexes.

The degree to which a solute molecule will be solubilized by a cyclodextrin molecule will depend on several properties. First the solute molecule must have a significant nonpolar portion in order to be squeezed out of the water and into the cyclodextrin cavity. Since the interior dimensions of a given cyclodextrin are fixed, a significant part of the molecule (or whole molecule) must then fit inside the cyclodextrin. Once presented to the interior cavity, it will be the fit, as well as the intermolecular interactions between the two molecules that will determine the strength of the complex. The stability constants for some compounds are given in Table 12. Note that the compounds in the upper third of the table contain aliphatic chains and are preferentially solubilized by α-cyclodextrin, while those in the middle contain aromatic rings and are best solubilized by β-cyclodextrin. The bottom third of the table contains fused ring compounds that are best solubilized by the larger γ-cyclodextrin.

Seo et al. (141) have shown the dependence of stability constant and overall solubility upon cyclodextrin ring size for spironolactone. From the data given in Fig. 19, it can be

Table 12 Apparent stability constants for complexes of α-, β-, and γ-cyclodextrins

Solute	α	β	γ
1-Butanol	89	16	
1-Octanol	6309	1479	
Carmofur	1200	670	180
Prostaglandin E1	1430	1700	530
Nonyl-*p*-hydroxybenzoate	4558	4327	
Decyl-*p*-hydroxybenzoate	4236	3306	
Octyl-*p*-hydroxybenzoate	3747	3920	
Ethyl-*p*-aminobenzoate	290	500	
Methyl-*p*-hydroxybenzoate	218	870	
Ethyl-*p*-hydroxybenzoate	178	1055	
Phenobarbital	30	1400	110
Phenytoin	90	1120	120
Anthracene	75	2000	220
Phenanthrene	16	1500	770
Benzo(*a*)anthracene	88	3225	605
Pyrene	148	543	1125
Benzo(*a*)pyrene	173	2219	63245
Triamcinolone	121	2370	9920
Triamcinolone acetonide	256	3230	26100
Triamcinolone diacetate	300	3530	12100
Dexamethasone	169	4660	26600
Dexamethasone acetate	316	9560	37300
Digitoxigenin	1700	130000	640000
Digitoxin	350	37000	78000

(Based upon Ref. 1.)

seen that for the relatively large spironolactone molecule (Fig. 9) the stability constant increases with size of the host cavity that is reflected through an increase in the linear slopes. The lowest maximum solubility was obtained with the β-cyclodextrin, which has the lowest solubility of the three cyclodextrins (142).

As discussed earlier and shown in Fig. 19, a significant limitation to the naturally occurring cyclodextrins is their limited solubility. Based on this and other physical property limitations, numerous derivatives have been prepared from the base cyclodextrins (143–147). Among the most studied of these is that of the hydroxypropyl-β-cyclodextrin, HP-β-CD and the sulfobutylethers of β-cyclodextrin, SBE-β-CD. These compounds are very soluble in water and can be used in high concentrations. Pitha et al. (148) investigated the use of high concentrations of HP-β-CD for a variety of compounds and found a wide range of solubility enhancement. The data from Pitha et al. is given in Table 13. SBE-β-CDs, have also shown good complexation characteristics. Table 14 shows the solubility enhancement for some selected compounds in a solution of Sulfobutylether

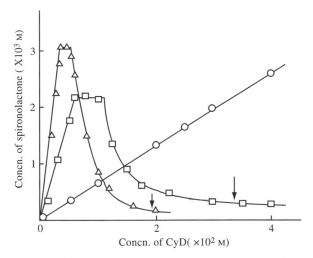

Fig. 19 Solubility of spironolactone as a function of cyclodextrin and concentration. ○, α-cyclodextrin, □, β-cyclodextrin, and, △, γ-cyclodextrin. (From Ref. 14.)

β-cyclodextrin IV. The selected data given in Tables 13 and 14 provide a good illustration of the practical range of solubilization that can be achieved by complexation.

Combination of pH and Complexation

The effect of pH on solubilization by complexation will depend entirely on the given solute and ligand. Tinwalla et al. (150) found that the combined use of ionization and complexation can be a powerful method for solubilization. They were able to significantly increase the solubility for a

Table 13 Solubility enhancement through the use of high concentrations of HP-β-CD

Solute	% HP-β-CD	Solubility enhancement
Estriol	50	13666
Estradiol	40	7000
Progesterone	40	2266
Spironolactone	40	1400
Testosterone	40	1461
Digoxin	50	971
Dexamethasone	50	240
Chlorthalidone	50	87.5
Diphenylhydantoin	50	57
Furosamide	50	24
Nitroglycerin	40	8.3
Acetamidopen	50	6
Apomorphine	50	5.8
Theophylline	50	1.3

(From Ref. 148.)

Table 14 Solubility enhancement through the use of 0.1 M SBE-β-CD (IV)

Solute	Solubility enhancement
Testosterone	2020
Prednisolone acetate	426
Dexamethasone	208
Dapsone	189
Prednisolone	106
Methylprednisolone	88
Hydrocortisone	87
Menadione	69
Benzyl guanine	68
Chloramphenicol	8

(From Ref. 149.)

thiazolobenzimidazole derivative, TBI (shown in Fig. 20), through the use of both pH and complexation via HP-β-CD.

Li et al. (151, 152) derived a mathematical expression to explain the combined effect of pH and complexation on solubilization. If either the ligand or solute ionizes with pH, the stability constant will typically decrease. However, even with a decrease in the stability constant the solubility can sometimes increase. Although the

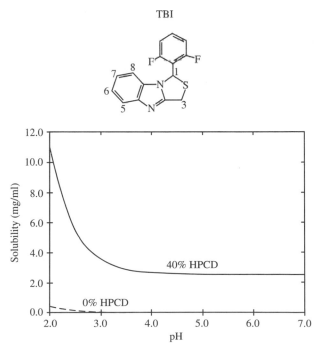

Fig. 20 Solubility of TBI (structure top, $pK_a = 3.55$), as a function of pH for 0 and 40% HP-β-CD solutions. (From Ref. 150.)

Table 15 Examples of some parenteral products that contain complexation agents

Drug (Product)	Route of administration	Surfactant composition (% w/v)
Alprostadil (Edex)	Intracavernosal (reconstituted)	α-Cyclodextrin
Itraconazole (Sporanox)	IV Infusion after dilution	40% Hydroxypropyl-β-cyclodextrin
Ziprasidone mesylate(Phase III)	IM/SC	Sulfobutylether-β-cyclodextrin
Prednisolone phosphate sodium (Hydeltrasol)	IV Infusion after dilution	2.5% Niacinamide

(From Refs. 84–86.)

stability complex for the protonated form of TBI was nearly 13-fold less than that of the neutral complex, they were still able to attain a 3-fold increase in solubility.

Solubilization through Complexation

With the general characterization for stacking complexes being planar, the list of possible candidates is extensive. Of course, not all possible ligands can be considered acceptable. Some of the planar molecules that form stacking complexes (such as those given in Fig. 16) are pharacologically active. Others like the parabens or benzyl alcohol can be used as antimicrobial agents. Furthermore, the addition of these organic compounds can also facilitate solubilization through cosolvency. Inclusion complexation has been proven to be useful for compounds with isolated hydrocarbon regions. Solutes with large or multiple hydrocarbon regions are most efficiently solubilized by complexation, however a shape requirement must be met in order for inclusion complexation to occur. An abbreviated list of excipients used in some parenteral products is given in Table 15.

REFERENCES

1. Yalkowsky, S.H. *Solubility and Solubilization in Aqueous Media*; Oxford University Press: New York, 1999.
2. Liu, R. *Water-Insoluble Drug Formulations*; Interpharm Press: Englewood, CO, 2000.
3. Prausnitz, J.M.; Lichtenthaler, R.N.; Gomes de Azevedo, E. *Molecular Thermodynamics of Fluid-Phase Equilibria*, 2nd Ed., Prentice-Hall: New Jersey, 1986.
4. Yalkowsky, S.H. Ind. Eng. Chem. Fundam. **1979**, *18*, 108–111.
5. Myrdal, P.B.; Ward, G.H.; Dannenfelser, R-M.; Mishra, D.; Yalkowsky, S.H. Chemosphere **1992**, *24*, 1047–1061.
6. Myrdal, P.B.; Ward, G.H.; Simamora, P.; Yalkowsky, S.H. SAR and QSAR in Environ. Res. **1993**, *1*, 53–61.
7. Myrdal, P.B.; Manka, A.M.; Yalkowsky, S.H. Chemosphere **1995**, *30*, 1619–1637.
8. Lee, Y-C.; Myrdal, P.B.; Yalkowsky, S.H. Chemosphere **1996**, *33*, 2129–2144.
9. Pinsuwan, S.; Myrdal, P.B.; Lee, Y-C.; Yalkowsky, S.H. Chemosphere **1997**, *35*, 2503–2513.
10. Slusher, J.T. Fluid Phase Equilib. **1988**, *153*, 45–61.
11. Ruelle, P. J. Org. Chem. **1999**, *12*, 769–786.
12. Abraham, M.H.; Le, J. J. Pharm. Sci. **1999**, *88*, 868–880.
13. Lin, S-T.; Sandler, S.I. AIChE J. **1999**, *45*, 2606–2618.
14. Yalkowsky, S.H.; Valvani, S.C. J. Pharm. Sci. **1980**, *69*, 912–922.
15. *ClogP*®, version 2.2.02b, Bio-Byte Corporation: 1997.
16. Byrn, S.R.; Pfeiffer, R.R.; Stowell, J.G. *Solid State Chemistry of Drugs*, 2nd Ed.; SSCI, Inc.: West Lafayette, IN, 1999.
17. Noyes, A.A.; Whitney, W.R. J. Am. Chem. Soc. **1897**, *19*, 930–934.
18. Hamlin, W.E.; Northam, J.I.; Wagner, J.G. J. Pharm. Sci. **1965**, *54*, 1651–1653.
19. Yoshihashi, Y.; Kitano, H.; Etsuo, Y.; Terada, K. Int. J. Pharm. Sci. **2000**, *204*, 1–6.
20. Nicklasson, M.; Brodin, A. Int. J. Pharm. Sci. **1984**, *18*, 149–156.
21. Allen, D.J.; Kwan, K.C. J. Pharm. Sci. **1969**, *58*, 1190–1193.
22. Goldberg, A.H.; Gibaldi, M.; Kanig, J.L. J. Pharm. Sci. **1966**, *55*, 487–472.
23. Kaneniwa, N.; Watari, N. Chem. Pharm. Bull. **1977**, *25*, 867–875.
24. Florence, A.T.; Salole, E.G. J. Pharm. Pharmac. **1976**, *28*, 637–642.
25. Florence, A.T.; Salole, E.G.; Stanlake, J.B. J. Pharm. Phamac. **1974**, *26*, 479–480.
26. Ikekawa, A.; Hayakawa, S. Bull. Chem. Soc. Jpn. **1981**, *54*, 2587–2591.
27. Picolo, T.; Sakr, A. Pharm. Ind. **1984**, *46*, 1277–1279.
28. Pereira De Almeida, L.; Simoes, S.; Brito, P.; Portugal, A.; Figueiredo, M. J. Pharm. Sci. **1997**, *86*, 726–731.
29. Mosharraf, M.; Sebhatu, T.; Nystrom, C. Int. J. Pharm. **1999**, *177*, 29–51.
30. Aguiar, A.J.; Krc, J.; Kinkel, A.W.; Samyn, J.C. J. Pharm. Sci. **1967**, *56*, 847–853.
31. Aguiar, A.J.; Zelmer, J.E. J. Pharm. Sci. **1969**, *58*, 983–987.
32. Kato, Y.; Kohetsu, M. Chem. Pharm. Bull. **1981**, *29*, 268–272.
33. Yokoyama, T.; Umeda, T.; Kuroda, K.; Kuroda, T.; Asada, S. Chem. Pharm. Bull. **1981**, *29*, 194–199.

S

34. Kokubu, H.; Morimoto, K.; Ishida, T.; Inoue, M.; Morisaka, K. Int. J. Pharm. **1987**, *35*, 181–183.

35. Kuroda, K.; Yokoyama, T.; Umeda, T.; Takagishi, Y. Chem. Pharm. Bull. **1978**, *26*, 2565–2568.

36. Umeda, T.; Matsuzawa, A.; Ohnishi, N.; Kuroda, T. Chem. Pharm. Bull. **1984**, *32*, 1637–1640.

37. Suleiman, M.S.; Najib, N.M. Int. J. Pharm. **1989**, *50*, 103–109.

38. Himmelreich, M.; Rawson, B.J.; Watson, T.R. Austrail. J. Pharm. Sci. **1977**, *6*, 123–125.

39. Clements, J.A.; Popli, S.D. Can. J. Pharm. Sci. **1973**, *8*, 88–92.

40. Pearson, J.T.; Varney, G. J. Pharm. Pharmacol. **1973**, *25*, 62–70.

41. Wells, J.I. Pharmaceutical Preformulation. *The Physico-chemical Properties of Drug Substances*; Ellis Horwood, Ltd.: United Kingdom, 1988; 94–95.

42. Poole, J.W.; Bahal, C.K. J. Pharm. Sci. **1968**, *57*, 1945–1948.

43. Suryanarayanan, R.; Mitchell, A.G. Int. J. Pharm. **1985**, *24*, 1–17.

44. Fukumori, Y.; Fukuda, T.; Yamamoto, Y.; Shigitani, Y.; Hanyu, Y.; Takeuchi, Y.; Sato, N. Chem. Pharm. Bull. **1983**, *31*, 4029–4039.

45. Jozwiakowski, M.J.; Nguyen, N.-A.T.; Sisco, J.M.; Spancake, C.E. J. Pharm. Sci. **1996**, *85*, 193–199.

46. Buxton, P.C.; Lynch, I.R.; Roe, J.M. Int. J. Pharm. **1988**, *42*, 135–143.

47. Sekiguchi, K.; Kanke, M.; Nakamura, N.; Tsuda, Y. Chem. Pharm. Bull. **1973**, *21*, 1592–1600.

48. Kozje, F.; Golic, L.; Zupet, P.; Palka, E.; Vodopivec, P.; Japelj, M. Acta Pharm. Jugosl. **1985**, *35*, 275–281.

49. Abdallah, O.; El-Fattah, S.A. Pharm. Ind. **1984**, *46*, 970–971.

50. Rodriguez-Hornedo, N.; Lechuga-Ballesteros, D.; Wu, H.-J. Int. J. Pharm. **1992**, *85*, 149–162.

51. Mentasti, E.; Rinaudo, C.; Boistelle, R. J. Chem. Engin. Data **1983**, *28*, 247–251.

52. Ghosh, S.; Grant, D.J.W. Int. J. Pharm. **1995**, *114*, 185–196.

53. Matsuda, Y.; Tatsumi, E. J. Pharmacobio-Dyn. **1989**, *12*, 38.

54. Toffoli, F.; Avico, U.; Signoretti, CiranniE.; Di Francesco, R.; Di Palumbo, V.S. Ann. Chem. **1973**, *63*, 1–4.

55. Corrigan, O.I.; Holohan, E.M.; Sabra, K. Int. J. Pharm. **1984**, *18*, 195–200.

56. Otsuka, M.; Kaneniwa, N. Chem. Pharm. Bull. **1983**, *31*, 230–236.

57. Higuchi, W.I.; Lau, P.K.; Higuchi, T.; Shell, J.W. J. Pharm. Sci. **1963**, *52*, 150–153.

58. Doherty, C.; York, P. Drug Dev. Ind. Pharm. **1989**, *15*, 1969–1987.

59. Mullins, J.D.; Macek, T.J. J. Pharm. Sci. **1960**, *49*, 245–248.

60. Fukuoka, E.; Makita, M.; Yamamura, S. Chem. Pharm. Bull. **1987**, *35*, 2943–2948.

61. Giron, D. Thermochim. Acta. **1995**, *248*, 1–59.

62. Cohn, E.J.; McMeekin, T.L.; Edsall, J.T.; Weare, J.H. J. Am. Chem. Soc. **1934**, *56*, 2270–2282.

63. Tsuji, A.; Nakashima, E.; Hamano, S.; Yamana, T. J. Pharm. Sci. **1978**, *67*, 1059–1066.

64. Tsuji, A.; Nakashima, E.; Yamana, T. J. Pharm. Sci. **1979**, *68*, 308–315.

65. Tsuji, A.; Nakashima, E.; Nishide, K.; Deguchi, Y.; Hamano, S.; Yamana, T. Chem. Pharm. Bull. **1983**, *31*, 4057–4069.

66. Garren, K.W.; Pyter, R.A. Int. J. Pharm. **1990**, *63*, 167–172.

67. Chowhan, Z.T. J. Pharm. Sci. **1978**, *67*, 1257–1260.

68. Kramer, S.F.; Flynn, G.L. J. Pharm. Sci. **1972**, *61*, 1896–1904.

69. Avdeef, A. Pharm. Pharmacol. Commun. **1998**, *4*, 165–178.

70. Streng, W.H.; Hsi, S.K.; Helms, P.E.; Tan, H.G.H. J. Pharm. Sci. **1984**, *73*, 1679–1684.

71. Streng, W.H. Int. J. Pharm. Sci. **1999**, *186*, 137–140.

72. Berge, S.M.; Bighley, L.D.; Monkhouse, D.C. J. Pharm. Sci. **1977**, *66*, 1–19.

73. Bighley, L.D.; Berge, S.M.; Monkhouse, D.C. Salt Forms of Drugs and Absorption. *Encyclopedia of Pharmaceutical Technology*, 1st Ed.; Swarbrick, J., Boylan, J.C., Eds.; Marcel Dekker, Inc.: New York, 1996; 13, 453–499.

74. Agharkar, S.; Lindenbaum, S.; Higuchi, T. J. Pharm. Sci. **1976**, *65*, 747–749.

75. Gould, P.L. Int. J. Pharm. **1986**, *33*, 201–217.

76. Morris, K.R.; Fakes, M.G.; Thakur, A.B.; Newman, A.W.; Singh, A.K.; Venit, J.J.; Spagnuolo, C.J.; Serajuddin, A.T.M. Int. J. Pharm. **1994**, *105*, 209–217.

77. Spurlock, C.H. J. Parent. Sci., Tech. **1986**, *40*, 70–72.

78. Jusko, W.J.; Gretch, M.; Gassett, R. J. Am. Med. Assoc. **1973**, *225*, 176.

79. Yalkowsky, S.H.; Valvani, S.C.; Johnson, B.W. J. Pharm. Sci. **1983**, *72*, 1014–1017.

80. Ward, G.H.; Yalkowsky, S.H. J. Parent. Sci. Tech. **1993**, *47*, 161–165.

81. Jamerson, B.D.; Dukes, G.E.; Brouwer, K.L.R.; Donn, K.H.; Massenheimer, J.A.; Powel, J.R. Pharmacotherapy **1994**, *14*, 47–52.

82. Myrdal, P.B.; Simamora, P.; Surakitbanharn, Y.; Yalkowsky, S.H. J. Pharm. Sci. **1995**, *84*, 849–852.

83. Surakitbanharn, Y.; Simamora, P.; Ward, G.H.; Yalkowsky, S.H. Int. J. Pharm. **1994**, *109*, 27–33.

84. Strickley, R.G. PDA J. Pharm. Sci. Technol. **1999**, *53*, 324–349.

85. Strickley, R.G. PDA J. Pharm. Sci. Technol. **2000**, *54*, 69–96.

86. Strickley, R.G. PDA J. Pharm. Sci. Technol. **2000**, *54*, 152–169.

87. Paruta, A.N.; Sciarrone, B.J.; Lordi, N.G. J. Pharm. Sci. **1965**, *54*, 1325–1333.

88. Sorby, D.L.; Liu, G.; Horowitz, K.N. J. Pharm. Sci. **1965**, *54*, 1811–1813.

89. Martin, A.; Newburger, J.; Adjei, A. J. Pharm. Sci. **1980**, *69*, 487–490.

90. Martin, A.; Paruta, A.N.; Adjei, A. J. Pharm. Sci. **1981**, *70*, 1115–1120.

91. Williams, A.; Amidon, G.L. J. Pharm. Sci. **1984**, *73*, 9–13.

92. Williams, A.; Amidon, G.L. J. Pharm. Sci. **1984**, *73*, 14–17.

93. Williams, A.; Amidon, G.L. J. Pharm. Sci. **1984**, *73*, 18–23.

94. Ochsner, A.B.; Belloto, R.J., Jr.; Sokoloski, T.D. J. Pharm. Sci. **1985**, *74*, 277–282.

95. Acree, W.E., Jr.; McCargar, J.W.; Zvaigzne, A.E.; Teng, I.L. Phys. Chem. Liq. **1991**, *23*, 27–35.

96. Escalera, J.B.; Bustamante, P.; Martin, A. J. Pharm. Pharmacol. **1994**, *46*, 172–176.

97. Barzegar-Jalali, M.; Hanaee, J. Int. J. Pharm. **1994**, *109*, 291–295.

98. Li., A.; Andren, A.W. Env. Sci. Tech. **1995**, *29*, 3001–3006.

99. Barzegar-Jalali, M.; Jouyban-Gharamaleki, A. Int. J. Pharm. **1997**, *152*, 247–250.

100. Jouyban-Gharamaleki, A.; Barzegar-Jalali, M.; Acree, W.E., Jr. Int. J. Pharm. **1998**, *166*, 205–209.

101. Jouyban-Gharamaleki, A.; Acree, W.E., Jr. Int. J. Pharm. **1998**, *167*, 177–182.

102. Jouyban-Gharamaleki, A.; Valaee, L.; Barzegar-Jalali, M.; Clark, B.J.; Acree, W.E., Jr. Int. J. Pharm. **1999**, *177*, 93–101.

103. Yalkowsky, S.H.; Amidon, G.L.; Zografi, G.; Flynn, G.L. J. Pharm. Sci. **1972**, *64*, 48–52.

104. Yalkowsky, S.H.; Valvani, S.C.; Amidon, G.L. J. Pharm. Sci. **1976**, *65*, 1488–1495.

105. Yalkowsky, S.H.; Roseman, J.T. Solubilization of Drugs. *Techniques of Solubilization of Drugs*; Yalkowsky, S.H., Ed.; Ch. 3 Marcel Dekker, Inc.: New York, 1981.

106. Yalkowsky, S.H.; Rubino, J.T. J. Pharm. Sci. **1985**, *74*, 416–421.

107. Li., A.; Yalkowsky, S. J. Pharm. Sci. **1994**, *83*, 1735–1740.

108. Rubino, J.T.; Yalkowsky, S.H. Pharm. Res. **1987**, *4*, 220–230.

109. Morris, K.R.; Abramowitz, R.; Pinal, R.; Davis, P.; Yalkowsky, S.H. Chemosphere **1988**, *17*, 285–298.

110. Millard, J.W.; Alvarez-Nunez, F.A.; Yalkowsky, S.H. submitted. J. Pharm. Sci. **2001**.

111. Chein, Y.W.; Lambert, H.J. Chem. Pharm. Bull. **1975**, *23*, 1085–190.

112. Pramar, Y.V.; Das, GuptaV. Pharmazie **1994**, *49*, 661–665.

113. Gupta, B.; Mishra, D.S.; Cheng, C-H.; Yalkowsky, S.H. Tox. Environ. Chem. **1991**, *33*, 7–21.

114. Riley, C.M. *Solubilization of Some Poorly Soluble Drugs by Cosolvents*; M.S. Thesis University of Arizona: Tucson, AZ, 1990.

115. Rubino, J.T. Cosolvents and Cosolvency. *The Encyclopedia of Pharmaceutical Technology*; Marcel Dekker, Inc. 1990; 3, 375–398.

116. Azaz, E.; Donbrow, M. J. Colloid and Interface Sci. **1976**, *57*, 11–15.

117. Fashelelbom, K.M.S.; Timoney, R.S.; Corrigan, O.I. Pharm. Res. **1993**, *10*, 631–634.

118. Collet, J.H.; Koo, L. J. Pharm. Sci. **1975**, *64*, 1253–1255.

119. Collet, J.H.; Tobin, E.A. J. Pharm. Pharmacol. **1979**, *31*, 174–177.

120. Tomida, H.; Yotsuyanagi, T.; Ikeda, K. Chem. Pharm. Bull. **1978**, *26*, 2824–2831.

121. Tomida, H.; Yotsuyanagi, T.; Ikeda, K. Chem. Pharm. Bull. **1978**, *26*, 2832–2837.

122. Ismail, A.A.; Gouda, M.W.; Motawi, M.M. J. Pharm. Sci. **1970**, *59*, 220–224.

123. Ikeda, J.; Kato, K.; Tukamoto, T. Chem. Pharm. Bull. **1971**, *19*, 2510–2517.

124. Gouda, M.W.; Ismail, A.A.; Motawi, M.M. J. Pharm. Sci. **1970**, *59*, 1402–1405.

125. Jafvert, C.T.; Van Hoof, P.L.; Heath, J.K. Water Res. **1994**, *28*, 1009–1017.

126. Alvarez-Nunez, F.A.; Yalkowsky, S.H. Int. J. Pharm. **2000**, *200*, 217–222.

127. Nakagawa, T.; Tori, K. Koll. Z. **1960**, *168*, 132–139.

128. Elworthy, P.H.; Florence, A.T.; Macfarlane, C.B. *Solubilization by Surface-Active Agents*; Chapman Hall: New York, 1968.

129. Attwood, D.; Florence, A.T. *Surfactant Systems*; Chapman Hall: New York, 1983.

130. Rosen, M. *Surfactants and Interfacial Phenomena*; Second Ed. John Wiley & Sons: New York, 1989.

131. Christian, S.D.; Scamehorn, J.F. *Solubilization in Surfactant Aggregates*; Marcel Dekker, Inc.: New York, 1994.

132. Higuchi, T.; Kristiansen, H. J. Pharm. Sci. **1970**, *59*, 1601–1608.

133. Kakemi, K.; Sezaki, T.; Mitsunaga, T.; Nakano, M. J. Pharm. Sci. **1970**, *59*, 1579–1601.

134. Kenley, R.A.; Jackson, S.E.; Winterle, J.S.; Shunko, Y.; Visor, G.C. J. Pharm. Sci. **1986**, *75*, 648–653.

135. Fawzi, M.B.; Davison, E.; Tute, M.S. J. Pharm. Sci. **1980**, *69*, 104–106.

136. Boje, K.M.; Sak, M.; Fung, H-L. Pharm. Res. **1988**, *5*, 655–659.

137. Connors, K.A. *Binding Constants*; Wiley-Interscience Publication: New York, 1987; 1–101.

138. Yoshida, A.; Arima, H.; Uekama, K.; Pitha, J. Int. J. Pharm. **1988**, *46*, 217–222.

139. Muller, B.W.; Brauns, U. Int. J. Pharm. **1985**, *26*, 77–85.

140. Okada, Y.; Kubota, Y.; Koizumi, K.; Hizukuri, S.; Ohfuji, T.; Ogata, K. Chem. Pharm. Bull. **1988**, *36*, 2176–2185.

141. Seo, H.; Tsuruoka, M.; Hashimoto, T.; Fujinaga, T.; Otagiri, M.; Uekama, K. Chem. Pharm. Bull. **1983**, *31*, 286–291.

142. Jozwiakowski, M.J.; Connors, K.A. Carbohyd. Res. **1985**, *143*, 51–59.

143. Muller, B.W.; Brauns, U. Int. J. Pharm. **1985**, *26*, 77–88.

144. Duchene, D.; Wouessidjewe, D. Pharm. Tech. **1990**, *14*, 26–34.

145. Szejtli, J. Pharm. Tech. **1991**, *15*, 36–44.

146. Szejtli, J. J. Inclus. Phenom. **1992**, *14*, 25–36.

147. Irie, T.; Uekama, K. J. Pharm. Sci. **1997**, *86*, 147–162.

148. Pitha, J.; Milecki, H.; Fales, H.; Pannell, L.; Uekama, K. Int. J. Pharm. **1986**, *29*, 73–82.

149. Data from CyDex, L. C., Overland Park, Kansas, 66212.

150. Tinwalla, A.Y.; Hoesterey, B.L.; Xiang, T.; Lim, K.; Anderson, B.D. Pharm. Res. **1993**, *10*, 1136–1143.

151. Li, P.; Tabibi, S.E.; Yalkowsky, S.H. J. Pharm. Sci. **1998**, *87*, 1535–1537.

152. Li, P.; Zhao, L.; Yalkowsky, S.H. J. Pharm. Sci. **1998**, *88*, 1107–1111.

SPECTROSCOPIC METHODS OF ANALYSIS—ATOMIC ABSORPTION AND EMISSION SPECTROPHOTOMETRY

John P. Oberdier
Abbott Laboratories, Abbott Park, Illinois

INTRODUCTION

Often it is necessary to measure the metal content of different kinds of samples in the pharmaceutical industry. These samples can be actual products that have metals, such as calcium or magnesium added for their therapeutic value or biological samples, such as blood, urine, and tissue. More recently, work has been done on the role of metals in biological processes. In addition, products can be monitored for trace metal contamination, that can lead to unexpected degradation of product. A number of techniques are available for metal analyses. Some of the more common techniques are colorimetry, titrimetry, atomic absorption spectrophotometry (AA), fluorescence spectrophotometry, and emission spectrophotometry. The most common form of emission spectrophotometry is inductively coupled plasma (ICP). Thus, the analyst must choose the best approach for the sample being analyzed. The purpose of this article is to give a general overview of the strengths and limitations of atomic absorption spectrophotometry and ICP so that the best technique can be selected for the problem to be solved.

PRINCIPLE OF OPERATION FOR ATOMIC ABSORPTION SPECTROPHOTOMETRY (1)

The basis of atomic absorption spectrophotometry is the absorbance of light by the free, ground-state atoms of the element of interest. The ground state of an atom is the electronic state in which all the electrons are in their most stable configuration or orbitals. When light is absorbed by an atom, one or more of the electrons is excited to a higher energy orbital. The word free refers to the lack of any effects that would alter the amount of energy or the wavelength of the energy that is needed to cause the electrons in the atoms to shift from the ground state to an excited state(s).

Because each element absorbs at very discrete wavelengths, the lamp used for analysis of a particular metal emits light only at the desired wavelengths and is specific for that element. The two kinds of lamps used in atomic absorption spectrophotometry are the hollow cathode lamp (HCL) and the electrodeless discharge lamp (EDL). These lamps contain a deposit of the metal of interest in an inert gas atmosphere and then use either a charged anode/cathode or a radio frequency to excite the metal atoms. As the excited atoms relax, they emit the absorbed energy as light energy at the characteristic wavelength(s) for that particular metal. This light energy is focused through the sample chamber onto the monochromator and detector as shown in Fig. 1.

The concentration of the analyte in the sample chamber is proportional to the amount of light absorbed and, under the proper experimental conditions, follows Beer's law. This relationship is defined as $A=abc$, where A is the absorbance, a is the absorption coefficient of the analyte, b is the cell path length, and c is the concentration of the analyte. The concentration of unknown samples can be readily determined by comparing the absorbance of a sample of known concentration(s) with the absorbance of the test sample.

SAMPLE INTRODUCTION TECHNIQUES AVAILABLE FOR ATOMIC ABSORPTION SPECTROPHOTOMETRY

One limitation of atomic absorption spectrophotometry is that the samples generally have to be in solution, preferably aqueous. Thus, either the sample must be directly soluble in a suitable solvent or some type of pretreatment, such as acid digestion, is necessary. One exception is that some instruments using a graphite furnace can be modified for direct injection of solids. Another limitation is that only one metal can be analyzed at a time. There are four primary methods of accomplishing this:

1. flame (aspiration of sample solution);
2. cold vapor (or chemical vaporization);
3. hydride generation (or chemical vaporization); and
4. Graphite furnace (or electrothermal atomization).

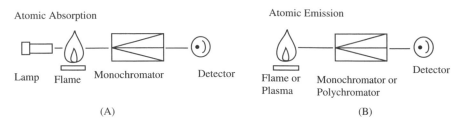

Fig. 1 Comparison of major components of atomic absorption and (A) emission spectrophotometers (B). (Courtesy of Perkin-Elmer Instruments).

All these methods have one common goal; to get the analyte atoms into the light path as free, ground-state atoms. Thus, there must be a balance of supplying enough energy so that the analyte atoms are free from association with other atoms (or molecules) in the sample matrix, versus not having excess energy, there by allowing the electrons of the analyte atoms to remain in the ground state.

The technique of flame atomic absorption spectrophotometry accomplishes this by aspirating the sample solution into a burner chamber, where it is mixed with a fuel gas and an oxidant gas. The mixture is then burned in a specially designed burner head (Fig. 2). The light beam is directed lengthway down the burner, and the absorption of the analyte atoms in the flame is measured. The most commonly used gas mixtures are air with acetylene and nitrous oxide with acetylene. Experimental conditions are

well-defined in the literature, and "cookbook" conditions are available from most instrument manufacturers. In addition, many instruments are computer-controlled, and typical conditions are available directly on the operating screen. Figure 3 shows the type of information usually available. These conditions provide excellent starting points for new methods, and in many cases the manufacturers provide information on possible interferences and the linear range for each element.

Table 1 shows the detection limits of atomic absorption spectrophotometry for various metals. In general, flame atomic absorption spectrophotometry is quantitative in the lower parts-per-million levels and is readily automated for routine, high-volume samples. The other three techniques are used primarily for trace analysis and are quantitative to the lower parts-per-million levels for many elements.

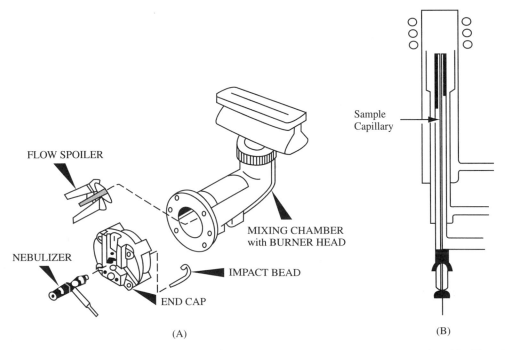

Fig. 2 Comparison of atomic absorption burner (A) and ICP argon plasma torch (B). (Courtesy of Perkin-Elmer Instruments.)

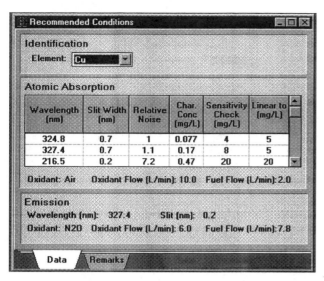

Fig. 3 Typical operation screen for copper using flame atomic absorption spectrophotometry (Courtesy of Perkin-Elmer Instruments.)

The cold vapor technique is used for mercury. This technique involves reducing the mercury to the zero valence state with either sodium borohydride or stannous chloride. The mercury is then swept into a gas cell aligned in the light path of the spectrophotometer, using a stream of nitrogen or air. Fig. 4 shows a diagram of a typical unit.

A broad peak is obtained on the graph. Either the peak height or the integrated peak area is measured and compared with that obtained for a specific volume of a known concentration. Note that this technique measures the total mercury present in the sample aliquot. Thus, both the mercury concentration and the sample volume analyzed are important in determining the sensitivity of the assay. Generally, the sample volume is less than 50 ml; however, volumes up to 100 ml have been used. One potential problem with this technique is that the mercury must be in a form that is easily reduced. If there are complexing agents or organo mercury compounds that do not yield Hg atoms, these compounds must be treated before analysis. Frequently, acid digestion of the sample before analysis brings the sample to the desired state for analysis.

The technique of hydride generation is very similar to the cold vapor technique addressed previously. Seven metals (arsenic, bismuth, germanium, antimony, selenium, tin, tellurium) can be analyzed using this method. First, the volatile hydrides are formed by reacting the sample with sodium borohydride. The metal hydride is then swept into a heated gas cell using a stream of argon. Anything in the sample matrix that prevents the metal hydride from forming easily causes an interference. However, this technique is applicable to many complicated samples that

are very difficult or impossible to analyze using other techniques.

The final technique described for atomic absorption apectrophotometry is the graphite furnace. In this technique, a tubular, high-temperature furnace is placed in the light path of the spectrophotometer so that the light is focused down the center of the sample tube. The sample tube is a hollow cylindrical tube made of compressed graphite, with or without a pyrolytic graphite coating. The tube may also be equipped with a L'vov platform. One of the primary advances of this technique have been in furnace and sample tube design to improve the uniformity of heating. Uneven heating causes reproducibility problems and spattering or loss of sample. An atmosphere of inert gas is maintained in the sample chamber to prevent oxidation of the graphite tube during the subsequent heating steps. Typically $5-50\,\mu$l of the sample are deposited on the bottom side of the tube or on the L'vov platform, and the tube is electrically heated to evaporate the sample solvent ($100-200°C$). If the sample contains organic material, the sample is usually ashed ($600-1000°C$). After this step, the inert gas flow is interrupted, and the metal is volatilized ($1500-3000°C$) and then measured. Matrix modifiers may be added to the sample to prevent loss of the analyte, before the volatilization step. All of these parameters are set up and optimized during initial method development. The preliminary settings are readily available in the literature and from most instrument manufacturers. Once the conditions have been chosen, the entire sequence can be automated, including use of an autosampler. An autosampler is especially recommended for this technique because one of the primary causes of irreproducibility is improper or inconsistent placement of the sample in the sample tube. Many autosamplers will add matrix modifiers and/or known amounts of standards to samples for standard addition-recovery experiments.

One of the inherent problems in the graphite furnace technique is background correction. When the metal atoms are volatilized, there may be absorption or loss of light that is not related to the metal atom concentration. For example, there may be small amounts of partially carbonized material that also volatilizes and causes light scattering. There are at least two methods available to correct for background effects: continuum correction and Zeeman correction. Continuum background correction assumes that absorption or loss of light, caused by effects other than atomic absorption, are constant over the entire spectral range. Thus, the sample signal is corrected by electronically subtracting the background absorption at a wavelength where the metal being measured does not absorb. This technique works well for background effects

Table 1 Typical detection limits (mg/L)

Element	Flame AA	Hg/Hydride	GFAA	ICP emission	ICP-MS	Element	Flame AA	Hg/Hydride	GFAA	ICP emission	ICP-MS
Ag	1.5		0.02	0.9	0.003	Mo	45		0.08	3	0.003
Al	45		0.1	3	0.006	Na	0.3		0.02	3	0.003[a]
As	150	0.03	0.2	50	0.006	Nb	1500			10	0.0009
Au	9		0.15	8	0.001	Nd	1500		0.3	2	0.002
B	1000		20	0.8	0.09	Ni	6			5	0.005
Ba	15		0.35	0.09	0.002	Os	120			6	
Be	1.5		0.008	0.08	0.03	P	75000		130	30	0.3
Bi	30	0.03	0.25	30	0.0005	Pb	15		0.06	10	0.001
Br					0.2	Pd	30		0.8	3	0.003
C				75	150	Pr	7500			2	<0.0005
Ca	1.5		0.01	0.02	0.05[a]	Pt	60		2.0	10	0.002
Cd	0.8		0.008	1	0.003	Rb	3		0.03	30	0.003
Ce				5	0.0004	Re	750			5	0.0006
Cl					10	Rh	6			5	0.0008
Co	9		0.15	1	0.0009	Ru	100		1.0	6	0.002
Cr	3		0.03	2	0.02	S				30	70
Cs	15				0.0005	Sb	45	0.15	0.15	10	0.001
Cu	1.5		0.1	0.4	0.003	Sc	30			0.2	0.02
Dy	50			2	0.001	Se	100	0.03	0.3	50	0.06
Er	60			1	0.0008	Si	90		1.0	3	0.7
Eu	30			0.2	0.0007	Sm	3000			2	0.001
F					10000	Sn	150		0.2	60	0.002
Fe	5		0.1	2	0.005[a]	Sr	3		0.025	0.03	0.0008
Ga	75			4	0.001	Ta	1500			10	0.0006
Gd	1800			0.9	0.002	Tb	900			2	<0.0005
Ge	300			20	0.003	Te	30	0.03	0.4	10	0.01

(Continued)

Table 1 Typical detection limits (mg/L) (*Continued*)

Element	Flame AA	Hg/Hydride	GFAA	ICP emission	ICP-MS
Hf	300			4	0.0006
Hg	300	0.009	0.6	1	0.004
Ho	60			0.4	<0.0005
I					0.008
In	30				9
Ir	900		3.0	5	0.0006
K	3		0.008	20	0.015[a]
La	3000			1	0.0005
Li	0.8		0.06	0.3	0.0001[a]
Lu	1000			0.2	<0.0005
Mg	0.15		0.004	0.07	0.007
Mn	1.5		0.035	0.4	0.002
Th					<0.0005
Ti	75		0.35	0.4	0.006
Tl	15		0.15	30	0.0005
Tm	15			0.6	<0.0005
U	15000			15	<0.0005
V	60		0.1	0.5	0.002
W	1500			8	0.001
Y	75			0.3	0.0009
Yb	8			0.3	0.001
Zn	1.5		0.1	1	0.003
Zr	450			0.7	0.004

[a] Denotes that the ICP-MS detection limit was measured under cold plasma conditions.

All detection limits are given in micrograms per liter and were determined using elemental standards in dilute aqueous solution. All detection limits are based on a 98% confidence level (3 S.D.). All atomic absorption (Model 5100) detection limits were determined using instrumental parameters optimized for the individual element, including the use of system 2 electrodeless discharge lamps where available. ICP emission (Optima 3000) detection limits were obtained under simultaneous multielement conditions with a radial plasma. Detection limits using an axial plasma (Optima 3000 XL) are typically improved by 5–10 times.

Cold vapor mercury detection limits were determined with a FIAS™-100 or FIAS-400 flow-injection system with amalgamation accessory. The detection limit without an amalgamation accessory is 0.2 µg/L with a hollow cathode lamp, 0.05 µg/L with a System 2 electrodeless discharge lamp. (The Hg detection limit with the dedicated FIMS™-100 or FIMS-400 mercury analyzers is <0.010 µg/L without an amalgamation accessory and <0.001 µg/L with an amalgamation accessory.) Hydride detection limits shown were determined using an MHS-10 Mercury/Hydride system. Graphite furnace AA detection limits were determined using 50-µl sample volumes, a L'vov platform, and full STPF conditions (Model 5100 PC with 5100 ZL Zeeman Furnace Module or Model 4110 ZL). SIMAA 6000 detection limits are similar in its multisource and are typically two to five times better in its single-source mode. Graphite furnace detection limits can be enhanced further by the use of replicate injections.

ICP-MS detection limits were determined using a 3-S integration.

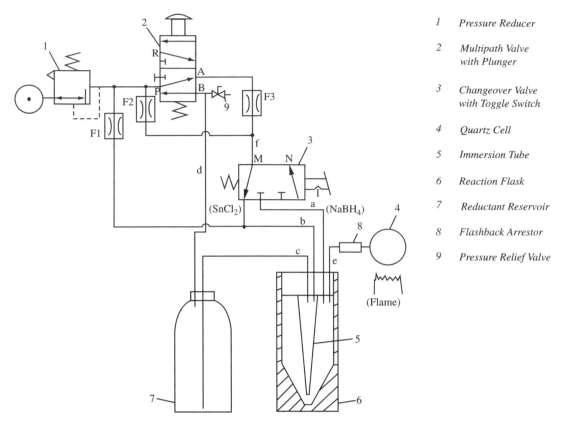

Fig. 4   Diagram of a typical unit for vapor or hydride generation technique. (Courtesy of Perkin-Elmer Instruments.)

such as light scattering that are fairly continuous over the entire spectral range. However, many background effects are not continuous, and the analyte signal is either under- or overcorrected. Zeeman background correction relies on the Zeeman effect. In simplest terms, Professor Zeeman discovered in 1896 that when an atomic line spectrum was subjected to a magnetic field, the lines were split into multiple components. Thus, the corrected sample signal can be obtained by electronically subtracting the sample absorbance in the presence and absence of a magnetic field. Because the background is actually being measured at the analyte wavelength, the measurement is generally less susceptible to error.

COMMON SOURCES OF ANALYTICAL ERROR IN ATOMIC ABSORPTION SPECTROPHOTOMETRY

The two common sources of analytical error are interference during the analytical measurement and contamination during sample preparation. During the analytical measurement, potential interferences include, matrix effects: chemical interferences, ionization interferences, and spectral interferences.

Matrix effects usually involve physical parameters, which differ between samples and standards. For example, in flame atomic absorption spectrophotometry, if the viscosity of the sample and standard solutions is significantly different, the solutions are aspirated into the burner chamber at different rates and the responses are different. Viscosity effects can often be eliminated by adding 1–2% of a metallic salt to the analyte solutions. Chemical interference can include both complexes and organically bound metals. When these type of interference are encountered, the samples often have to be digested with acid to destroy the organic material. For chemical complexes, adding a large excess of a competing ion is an alternative to acid digestion. Ionization interference is very common for sodium, potassium, and lithium. To overcome this problem, a large excess of one of the other elements is added. For example, 1–2% lithium might be added to a sample being analyzed for potassium. Ionized potassium atoms can collide with the large excess of lithium atoms, resulting in the loss of energy for the potassium atoms. These atoms will return to the ground state and be measured. Finally, there may be spectroscopic interference such as molecular or atomic absorption at the analyte wavelength. In practice, this interference can normally be overcome, and very complex samples can be analyzed rapidly and accurately, provided the analyst recognizes the potential interference and takes appropriate steps to minimize it.

Contamination during sample preparation is probably the single major source of error in this technique and is especially important when analyzing for metals at the parts-per-million level. Contamination can occur because of improperly cleaned containers or the wrong type of container (such as glass versus plastic). In addition, contamination can come from reagents used to prepare the sample. Special grade acids or matrix modifiers are usually necessary for trace metal analysis. Another source of contamination is the general environment. For example, even a dust particle can cause errors of 10-fold or more in the analysis of aluminum. In summary, serious thought must be given to every material and reagent the sample will contact during the entire sample-handling process. A series of review articles (2–6) are listed in the references for additional reading on atomic absorption spectrophotometry.

PRINCIPLE OF OPERATION AND TECHNIQUES USED IN EMISSION SPECTROPHOTOMETRY (7)

Emission Spectrophotometry is a complementary technique to atomic absorption. In this technique, the electrons in the atoms are excited by electrical or thermal energy to an unstable energy state. When the atom returns to a more stable state or the ground state, energy as light is emitted. This emitted light is detected and quantitated in emission spectrophotometry. The wavelength(s) of the emitted light is specific to the element(s) that are present. Figure 1 compares the major components of atomic absorption and emission spectrophotometry.

This emission of light from elements was reported as early as the mid-1700s and was later the basis of discovering four elements by Kirchoff and Bunsen in the mid-1800s. However, it was not until the 20th century that the technique really became a useful analytical tool. The first analytical instruments used a spark discharge to provide the energy to excite the atoms so that they would emit light. This approach gave valuable qualitative and semiquantitative information but did not have the accuracy and precision needed for many applications. The one exception was the analysis of alkali earth metals, which require very little energy to raise the electrons to an excited state. A simple propane flame is sufficient. This led to the development of a clinical analyzer for sodium and potassium in blood and urine samples that is still used routinely in clinical laboratories. It was not until the argon plasma flame was developed that a reliable source of high energy was available to excite a wide variety of atoms so that they would emit light. This led to the development of the technique commonly referred to as inductively coupled plasma (ICP) spectrophotometry.

As noted previously, the argon plasma flame provided the reliable energy source needed for ICP to become a reality. The plasma is created by passing argon gas between two concentric quartz tubes while applying an RF field (Fig. 5). This plasma flame reaches temperatures up to 10,000°K, with the sample reaching temperatures of 5500–8000°K. The shape of the flame confines the sample emission to an optically thin source resulting in a wide dynamic range for ICP. The sample is aspirated into the argon plasma flame, where it is believed to go through several steps: desolvation, varporization, atomization, and finally excitation or ionization. As the different atoms relax to a lower energy state, the emitted light strikes a monochromator or polychromator, and the intensity of the line spectra for each element is measured at the appropriate wavelength(s) for that element.

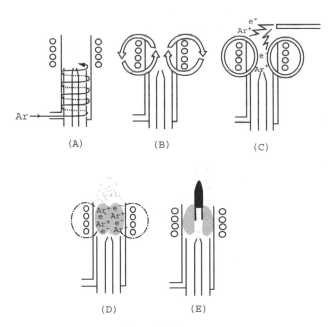

Fig. 5 Cross section of an ICP torch and load coil depicting an ignition sequence. (A) Argon gas is swirled through the torch; (B) RF power is applied to the load coil; (C) a spark produces some free electrons in the argon; (D) the free electrons are accelerated by the RF fields, causing further ionization and forming a plasma; (E) the sample aerosol-carrying nebulizer flow punches a hole in the plasma. (Courtesy of Perkin-Elmer Instruments.)

The most commonly used technique of sample introduction is aspiration of the solution into the argon plasma flame. Because of the high temperatures in the flame, many of the problems associated with atomic absorption are eliminated. However, matrix effects such as significant differences in viscosity between sample and standard solutions can still have an effect. When needed, most of the techniques of sample introduction used in atomic absorption spectrophotometry can also be used for sample introduction in emission spectrophotometry [see the review articles (8–13) listed in the references].

HOW TO CHOOSE AMONG THE TECHNIQUES

The major advantage of ICP is that multiple elements can be analyzed at the same time. The rule of thumb is if one typically assays less than four to six metals in a sample, atomic absorption is the better route. However, for more than six metals, ICP is clearly the choice. However, other factors such as sensitivity and interferences also have to be considered. One other variation of ICP that is becoming important is the hyphenated technique of ICP–MS (mass spectrophotometry). This combination gives excellent sensitivity and can even differentiate ionic species or isotopes if needed. Table 1 summarizes the sensitivities of the various techniques. As noted previously, all these techniques are complimentary, and the various strengths and weaknesses must be understood to choose the best technique.

THE FUTURE

The instrumentation for atomic absorption spectrophotometry is very well-defined and can range from a relatively simple manually operated instrument to a completely automated system that is on line to a central database. In addition, accurate results can be obtained on a wide range of samples. The future lies in using this technique to solve problems rather than to further develop instrumentation. For example, the FDA published new guidelines for the aluminum content of products used in total parenteral nutrition.

The role of ICP in the future will continue to expand, especially with the development of ICP–MS. The role of metals in biological processes and disease states is just beginning to be understood, with numerous studies being published. For multivalent metals, the exact species of metal involved in the biological process can be determined with ICP–MS. Understanding this type of detail will hopefully lead to important breakthroughs in the future. See the References (14–17) for additional information on future applications.

REFERENCES

1. Beaty, R.D.; Kerber, J.D. *Concepts, Instrumentation, and Techniques in Atomic Absorption Spectrophotometry*; Perkin Elmer: Minneapolis, KS, 1993.
2. Komaromy-Hiller, G. Flame, Flameless, and Plasma Spectroscopy. Anal. Chem. **1999**, *71* (12), 338R–342R.
3. Lagalante, A.F. Atomic Absorption Spectroscopy. A Tutorial Review. Appl. Spectrosc. Rev. **1999**, *34* (3), 173–189.
4. Hill, S.J.; Dawson, J.B.; Price, W.J.; Shuttler, I.L.; Smith, C.M.M.; Tyson, J.F. Advances in Atomic Absorption and Fluorescence Spectrometry and Related Techniques. J. Anal. At. Spectrom. **1999**, *14* (8), 1245–1285.
5. Sturgeon, R.E. Graphite Furnace Atomic Absorption Spectrometry and Environmental Challenges at the Ultratrace Level—A Review Spectrochim. Acta, Part B **1997**, *52B* (9, 10), 1451–1457.
6. Harnly, J.M. The Future of Atomic Absorption Spectrometry: A Continuum Source with a Charge Coupled Array Detector. J. Anal. At. Spectrom. **1999**, *14* (2), 137–146.
7. Boss, C.B.; Fredeen, K.J. *Concepts, Instrumentation, and Techniques in Inductively Coupled Plasma Optical Emission Spectrometry*, 2nd Ed.; Perkin Elmer: New York, 1999.
8. Suzuki, K.T. Hyphenated Techniques as Tools for Speciating Biological Metals: Metallothionein and Metal-binding Proteins. Analusis **1998**, *26* (6), M57–M61.
9. Sutton, K.L.; Caruso, J.A. Liquid Chromatography-Inductively Coupled Plasma Mass Spectrometry. Chromatogr., A **1999**, *856*, 243–258.
10. Horlick, G.; Montaser, A. Analytical Characteristics of ICPMS Induct. Coupled Plasma Mass Spectrom. **1998**, 503–613.
11. Taylor, A.; Branch, S.; Halls, D.J.; Owen, L.M.W.; White, M. Atomic Spectrometry Update: Clinical and Biological Materials, Foods and Beverages. J. Anal. At. Spectrom. **1999**, *14* (4), 717–781.
12. Pruszkowski, E.; Neubauer, K.; Thomas, R. An Overview of Clinical Applications by Inductively Coupled Plasma Mass Spectrometry. At. Spectrosc. **1998**, *19* (4), 111–115.
13. Lobinski, R.; Potin-Gautier, M. Metals and Biomolecules–Bioinorganic Analytical Chemistry. Analysis **1998**, *26* (6), M21–M24.
14. Taylor, H.E.; Huff, R.A.; Montaser, A. Novel Applications of ICPMS Induct. Coupled Plasma Mass Spectrom. **1998**, 681–807.
15. Welz, B. Speciation Analysis. The Future of Atomic Absorption Spectrometry. J. Anal. At. Spectrom. **1998**, *13* (5), 413–417.
16. Vanhaecke, F.; Moens, L. Recent Trends in Trace Element Determination and Speciation Using Inductively Coupled Plasma Mass Spectrometry. J. Anal. Chem. **1999**, *364* (5), 440–451.
17. Durrant, S.F. Laser Ablation Inductively Coupled Plasma Mass Spectrometry: Achievements, Problems, Prospects. J. Anal. At. Spectrom. **1999**, *14* (9), 1385–1403.

SPECTROSCOPIC METHODS OF ANALYSIS—DIFFUSE REFLECTANCE SPECTROSCOPY

Herbert Michael Heise

Institute of Spectrochemistry and Applied Spectroscopy, Dortmund, Germany

INTRODUCTION

In the field of molecular spectroscopy, absorption measurements with electromagnetic radiation covering the wavelengths between 200 nm and 20 µm can be used for analytical applications. By convention, tags such as ultraviolet (UV), visible (VIS), and infrared (IR) were given to special intervals of the spectrum, each yielding different specific information on organic and inorganic substances. The energy for electronic transitions between outer molecular orbitals corresponds to radiation of the first two spectral regions noted, whereas vibrational spectroscopy is connected to the infrared. Here, it can be further distinguished between near- and mid-infrared spectral subregions, which are important for routine analytical work.

In the classic spectroscopy experiment, transmission measurements are performed to analyze the radiation absorption of samples. Today, an additional powerful measurement technique is diffuse reflectance spectroscopy, which can be applied advantageously to scattering samples such as powders and other dispersed systems. It often requires less sample preparation than for a spectrum recorded in transmission. After sample penetration, the radiation is diffusely scattered and partially absorbed before part emerges back at the surface, from where it is detected using various optics and detectors. Beside identification of compounds, quantitative assays for active ingredients and fillers and in general formulation testing are available that often require special chemometric tools. Trace analysis and the study of adsorbed chemicals are additional fields. The combination with separation techniques, e.g., thin-layer chromatography, has been established, where diffuse reflectance measurement techniques are involved.

INSTRUMENTAL ASPECTS OF THE MEASUREMENT TECHNIQUE

Molecular spectroscopy plays an important role in the characterization of pharmaceutical substances (1). For chemical quality and process control, near-infrared spectroscopy has received much attention in the last years. The pharmaceutical industry was forced to develop fast measurement equipment and techniques for the identification of raw materials on receipt as well as to verify composition of pharmaceutical formulations before the products leave the premises. Some techniques are suited for process analysis because of their speed and lack of sample preparation. Further applications are concerned with the analysis in the laboratory during synthesis of compounds, identification of constituents of competitive products, and determination of additives and coatings. Additional cases can be discussed for which low detection limits are required. For best performance and high precision, instrumentation and sample preparation must be adapted to meet such demanding applications.

Instruments and Accessories

The spectral ranges noted above usually cannot be covered by a single instrument. Spectrometers with a grating monochromator are versatile instruments for recording UV/VIS and near-infrared spectra, which are equipped, depending on the spectral range to be measured, on different detectors [commonly used are silicon detectors: 200–1100 nm, indium gallium arsenide (InGaAs): 800–1700 nm (extended wavelength options are available), and lead sulfide: 1100–2500 nm]. Beside scanning instruments, also diode array spectrometers exist to measure the whole spectrum simultaneously. Other measurement technology uses a set of optical filters; such instruments are widespread in assays of food and agricultural products. A special technology that has been implemented in fast near-infrared spectrometers are acousto-optical tunable filters. Radiation sources such as tungsten halogen lamps, which provide a broad emission spectrum of electromagnetic radiation, may be replaced by light-emitting diodes or tunable lasers, broadening the applicability of future spectrometer systems.

The infrared spectral range is usually served by Fourier transform spectrometers, which contain an interferometer for wavelength dispersion. Today, the spectra are immediately calculated by using Fourier transformation of the measured interferograms. Such instrumentation can provide better spectral quality in shorter time than monochromator based systems. For the mid-infrared, thermal detectors such as those from deuterated triglycine sulfate (DTGS) or, for fast and sensitive measurements, liquid nitrogen cooled photodetectors such as those from mercury cadmium telluride (MCT) are used, whereas for the near-infrared InGaAs, germanium or indium antimonide (InSb) photodetectors are used. An overview on recent instrumentation is given by Coates (2). It is usual practice to display the infrared spectra with wavenumbers as abscissa (the transformation from wavelength λ, for example in micrometers, to wavenumbers $\tilde{\nu}$, in cm^{-1}, is given by $\tilde{\nu} = 10,000/\lambda$).

Various accessories were designed for recording diffuse reflectance spectra. Apart from special devices developed by different groups and described in the literature, several commercially available types must be noted. A few accessories are shown schematically in Fig. 1, which are representative of the diversity of optics. For a long time, integrating spheres have been in use, in particular for UV/VIS and near-infrared spectroscopy, although a few applications with sensitive MCT detectors also can be found within the mid-infrared (3). Usually, a baffle is placed within the sphere to prevent "first strike" radiation from immediately hitting the detector, which measures the scatter over all angles [hemispherical collection; see Fig. 1(a)].

As an alternative, reflection optics based on ellipsoidal mirrors or segments of such type became widespread. Several commercially available types can be noted, one is typified by Spectra-Tech's Collector [Fig. 1(b)]. To reduce the specular reflection, a blocker can be applied, which is placed vertically on the sample surface, perpendicular to the optical axis. Another accessory is Harrick's so-called praying mantis (the name was coined after its appearance), which uses an out-of-plane optical geometry to avoid the Fresnel reflection from the sample surface. The device shown in Fig. 1(c) was designed by us to improve the collection of diffusely back-reflected photons, observing the figures of merit for the case that irradiation and detection optics were to be optimized for optical throughput. Another positive feature of such a design is that small spots on large samples can be studied; for applications, see Heise (4). A critical evaluation of different types of diffuse reflectance accessories, especially for discrimination of specular and diffusely reflected radiation, has been given by Yang et al. (5). For a critical test using a high-absorbing inorganic sample-within an inert low-absorbing matrix of KCl powder, it was found that the specular component within the measured

spectrum was primarily sample rather than accessory-dependent.

Additional accessories are constructed from optical fibers. One affordable material suited for the UV/VIS and near-infrared is quartz, whereby a special quality of low-OH grade quartz provides better transmission, especially at longer wavelengths. Compared with mirror-based systems, the acceptance cone for radiation-gathering is reduced owing to the core/cladding configuration of the fiber light-guides [see Fig. 1(d)]. Bifurcated fiber bundles are often used as accessories, whereby the radiation-delivering fibers are mixed at random with the second fiber bundle, by which the reflected radiation is guided to the detector. The flexibility of such fiber optic probes is enormous and also allows measurements from powdered samples, for example, in opened casks.

The diffuse reflectance of a sample is usually measured against a nearly 100%-reflecting material, analogously to a transmittance measurement [a splendid coverage of standards for reflectance measurements is provided by Springsteen (6)]. Traditionally, freshly prepared MgO or BaSO$_4$ was used for coating the inner surface of an integrating sphere. For the spectral range of 200–2500 nm Spectralon^{TM} (Labsphere, North Sutton, NH) is now the preferred material because it is inert and easy to handle and process. It is a white thermoplastic resin that exhibits a reflectance larger than 0.99 over the spectral range of 400–1500 nm and larger than 0.95 for wavelengths up to 2500 nm. For the mid-infrared, powdered potassium bromide is usually available or gold-coated sandpaper of different grades, which we preferred. A commercially available standard material, obtainable from the same company as above, is InfraGold, which is a multilayer metallic on a mechanically roughened substrate. It exhibits a reflectance between 0.94 and 0.96 through the spectral ranges, with wavelengths between 1 and 25 μm. For dilution of samples, additional materials others than alkali halides have been proposed, which is presented below.

THEORETICAL CONSIDERATIONS

For spectroscopic studies, different measurement techniques are available. Radiation interacting with the sample may be absorbed, transmitted, or reflected. Usually, Lambert–Beer's law can be applied for absorbing samples showing no scattering. Reflection at a sample surface can be specular, in particular for a plane geometry as obtained for polished surfaces (also called Fresnel reflection), or diffuse, especially for rough surfaces as found in powders.

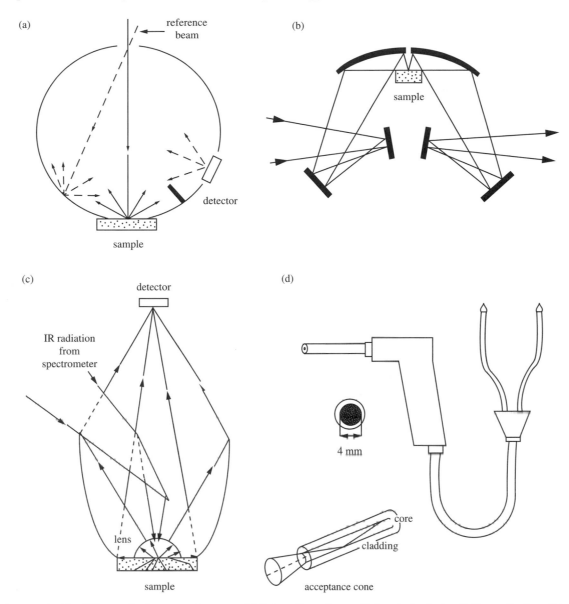

Fig. 1   Accessories for diffuse reflectance spectroscopy: (a) Integrating sphere with hemispherical radiation collection; (b) Accessory based on ellipsoidal mirrors, used within the sample compartment of the spectrometer; (c) Rotational ellipsoidal mirror device with dedicated detector; (d) Bifurcated fiber optic-based accessory (also shown is the random mixture of fibers for illumination and detection; compared with devices based on reflection optics the acceptance cone for radiation delivery and collection is limited and depends on the refractive indices of the core and cladding material).

Many reflections are a combination of both diffuse and specular components. Whereas specular reflectance can be rigorously treated using the Fresnel equations, more complex processes are reponsible for the diffuse reflection inside a scattering system. With dispersed systems, further phenomena of interaction between radiation and materials must be addressed. When radiation penetrates into a dispersed sample, the impinging radiation is partly absorbed and partly scattered by the particles so that

radiation is also reflected in a diffuse manner. This diffusely reflected radiation is useful for analytical applications and, with special functions for linearization of the diffuse reflectance signal, quantitative relations between transformed signal and concentration can be found.

As several researchers have shown empirically, the use of $-\log(\text{reflectance})$ can provide, analogous to a transmittance measurement, a linear relationship between the transformed reflectance and concentration, if the matrix is not strongly absorbing as can be found for many samples studied by near-infrared spectroscopy (7). This issue is presented in detail below. A different approach based on a physical model was considered for UV/VIS measurements and later also applied within the mid-infrared. A theory was derived by Kubelka and Munk (8) for a simple, one-dimensional, two-flux model, although it must be noted that Arthur Schuster (1905) had already come up with a reflectance function for isotropic scattering. A detailed description of theoretical and practical aspects was given by Kortüm (9). The optical absorption and scattering characteristics are described by its absorption and scattering coefficients k and s, respectively. For diffuse reflectance spectra, the transformation of the reflectance by the so-called Kubelka–Munk (K–M) function can provide a linear relationship for absorption band intensities versus concentrations (the units are often referred to as K–M units):

$$F(R) = (1 - R_\infty)^2 (2R_\infty) = k/s$$

R_∞ is the reflectance of an infinitely thick sample (in the near-infrared, this means an approximate 5-mm thickness and more). The theory was recently revisited by Loyalka and Riggs (10), who reinvestigated the accuracy of the Kubelka–Munk equations. They found that the coefficient k must be replaced by $k = 2a$ with the absorption coefficient $a = \ln(10)\ \varepsilon c$, as derivable from Beer's law; for the latter equation: $\ln(10) = 2.303$, ε the molar absorptivity, and c the molar concentration. Such a dependency for k was stated earlier by other researchers when comparing more refined radiation transport theories for biomedical applications, e.g., Ref. (11).

It must be kept in mind that the K–M theory does little more than provide an empirical model useful for quantitative work. To derive at the above equation, several assumptions were necessary such as infinite lateral extension and optical thickness, isotropy of the sample, and diffuse illumination, of which in particular the last is not met in practice when a directional sample illumination is prevailing. For isotropically scattering samples, a so-called three-flux approximation to the near-infrared radiative transfer within pharmaceutical powders and mixtures was presented recently for the derivation of scattering and absorption coefficients (12). Earlier, Hecht had studied different approaches and compared modeling results with measurements primarily in the visible (13). When the scattering inside the medium shows anisotropy as, for example, with forward scattering, more sophisticated modeling of the radiation transport inside the scattering medium is required. One tool applied recently

for spectrum prediction is Monte Carlo simulations, by which statistical averages are obtained for a large population of photons using probability functions for the scattering events. In particular, such an approach is often used for biomedical studies to analyze the photon distribution in tissues after irradiation.

Most spectroscopic software can convert spectra to K–M units on demand. With a constant scattering coefficient, at least within a limited spectral range, the transformed spectra resemble those obtained by conventional transmission spectroscopy. The relative error for K–M unit-based intensities is minimal for reflectance values between 0.2 and 0.7, which is a similar statement as obtainable for absorbance values derived from transmittance measurements and their error estimate. Studies with concern of a varying change in the reflectance of the reference material and its influence on the sample K–M units were carried out by Krivácsy and Hlavay (14).

PRACTICAL ASPECTS

The measurement of diffuse reflectance spectra from powdered samples requires less sample preparation than for the recording of transmittance spectra from solids, for which the embedding of such samples in a transparent medium is usually carried out. For mid-infrared measurements the KBr pellet technique is routinely used in the laboratory, which requires the application of high pressures to get a transparent tablet. The limitations are that the inertness of this embedding material is sometimes not given with the result of unwanted reactions. Scattering within the pellet can still exist, which is evident from evolving baseline shifts. The absorptivities of vibrational combination and overtone bands in the near-infrared are weaker than those of related bands in the mid-infrared, where many intensive bands can be assigned to fundamental vibrations. This leads to the consequence that the amount of substances required for achieving significant absorbances is much larger than for KBr pellet measurements in the mid-infrared.

In Fig. 2, a comparison of two spectra of anhydrous glucose is shown. The upper trace was recorded in transmission. For this, the pellet was placed in front of the spectrometer's detector to reduce the attenuation effects by scattering from inhomogeneities inside the pellet, because placing the pellet into the conventional sample compartment did not allow a satisfactory spectral signal-to-noise ratio. The lower spectrum was obtained using the diffuse reflectance technique on the powder, which was placed in a cup and slightly compressed by a spatulum,

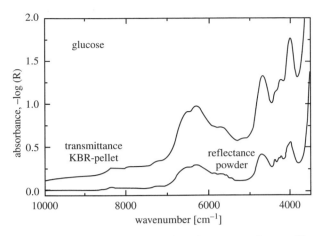

Fig. 2 Comparison of near-infrared spectra of crystalline anhydrous glucose. Spectrum measured in transmittance using the KBr pellet technique [spectral resolution 64 cm^{-1}; intensity data in absorbance (top trace) and diffuse reflectance spectrum using a spectral resolution of 32 cm^{-1} and intensity data transformed to $-\log(R)$ (bottom trace)].

illustrating the ease of sample preparation. Slight differences in the spectroscopic features arise only from the reduced spectral resolution, as used for the transmittance spectrum shown here.

The high-information density of mid-infrared spectra is well-known. In comparison, the discrimination power of near-infrared spectroscopy is illustrated in Fig. 3(a) for different monosaccharides, for which diffuse reflectance spectra were recorded. Fig. 3(b) shows the near-IR spectra of two pharmaceutical substances. In Fig. 4, the influence of finer particles, obtained by grinding the crystal material from the supplier pack on the spectrum is presented. With coarser particles, the band absorbance intensities are enlarged owing to a decrease in scattering, which means that radiation can penetrate deeper into the sample. In addition, a nearly constant attenuation can be observed, which leads just to a positive offset in the $-\log(R)$ spectrum. However, there are more severe distortions in a K–M transformed spectrum owing to baseline shifts, as pointed out by Griffiths (7).

The spectra of undiluted substances are influenced by effects from Fresnel reflection owing to strong absorption bands found within the mid-infrared spectral range. Additionally, the contrast between band intensities of strong and weak absorption bands is dramatically reduced. An example is provided in Fig. 5, which compares a KBr pellet spectrum of caffeine with that obtained from a powdered undiluted sample by using the diffuse reflectance technique. Two different representations were chosen, one with a transformation into K–M units and a

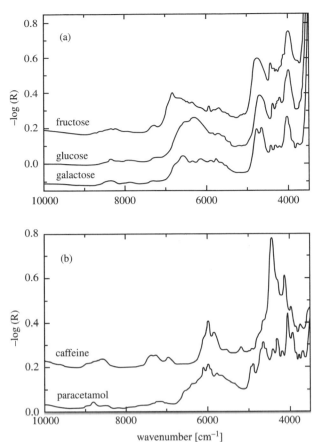

Fig. 3 Diffuse reflectance near-infrared spectra of several pharmaceutical compounds: (a) Comparison of the spectra of three different monosaccharides measured as crystalline powders; (for clarity, the spectra of fructose and galactose are offset; spectral resolution 32 cm^{-1}); (b) Comparison of spectra of pure caffeine and paracetamol (offset, spectral resolution 32 cm^{-1}).

second with $-\log(R)$. The latter shows uniquely that by using the reflectance technique, a tremendous amplification of weak absorption bands can be achieved. The distribution of intensity ratios is closer to that of the transmittance spectrum, when a dilution of the caffeine by KBr powder, for example, by a factor of 100, is used. A close-up of the mid-infrared fingerprint region in Fig. 6 provides us with the clues as to why a dilution by embedding the compound into the KBr powder must be recommended to obtain a spectrum by diffuse reflectance, which is comparable with the KBr pellet absorbance spectrum.

For strong absorption bands, a large Fresnel component shows up within the diffuse reflectance spectrum, leading to severe band distortions, which are also unmodeled by the K–M theory; the undiluted substance spectrum, in this

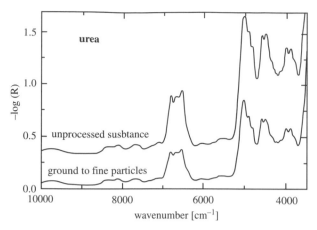

Fig. 4 Diffuse reflectance spectra of crystalline urea illustrating the effect of particle size (for the top trace, the crystalline material was unprocessed from the supplier's container), whereas for the bottom spectrum, the substance was ground to finer particles.

example of pure caffeine, shows significant shifts and band shape changes that cause certainly difficulties when comparing such a spectrum with those from spectral libraries, built from absorptivity data that were obtained from standard transmission or similar attenuated total reflection measurements. With a high-absorption index κ, which is related to the absorption coefficient by $a = \ln(10) (4\pi/\lambda)\kappa$, with λ the wavelength of the impinging radiation, the Fresnel reflection can reach unity. In this case, the band is also called the Reststrahlen band. There are applications to use the effect, e.g., for narrow optical reflection band pass filters.

Similar cases with high absorptivities can be found in the UV/VIS region, in which fundamental electronic absorptions exist. When particle size increases, the proportion caused by specular reflectance may become stronger and readily evident in the diffuse reflectance spectrum. A discussion of previous UV/VIS work is given by Wendlandt and Hecht (15).

In the past, extensive investigations were made to obtain better insight into the limitations of the diffuse reflectance measurement technique. Studies demonstrated that sample properties such as particle size and packing affect, in addition to the optical constants, the diffuse reflectance spectrum (9, 15). The characteristics of the diffuse and specular components were studied for different particle sizes and dilution within a nonabsorbing inert matrix. It was found that specularly and diffusely reflected radiation coexist in the measured diffuse reflectance spectrum, even in KCl-diluted samples. In addition, the specular component, which is certainly sample-dependent, is not necessarily the same as from the front-surface

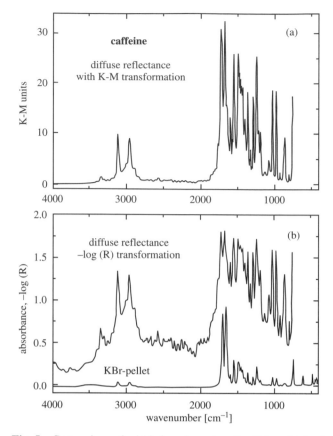

Fig. 5 Comparison of mid-infrared spectra of caffeine obtained by diffuse reflectance and transmission spectroscopy. (a) Diffuse reflectance spectrum of the pure powdered substance with transformed intensity data in K–M units. (b) Same diffuse reflectance spectrum, but using $-\log(R)$ transformation (top trace), the lower spectral range was limited by the cut-off of the MCT detector used; the bottom trace shows a transmission spectrum using the conventional KBr pellet technique transformed into absorbance, i.e., $-\log$(transmittance).

reflection (16). To prove this, a top layer of pure KCl powder was repeatedly put on top the sample to prevent front-surface reflectance. Another study to be noted is by Brimmer et al. (17) who also discussed the effect of Fresnel reflection with accessories of different optical geometries on the diffuse reflectance spectra.

The penetration depth of the probing IR-radiation is determined by both the scattering and the absorbing characteristics of the sample. Theoretical calculations were carried out by Fraser and Griffiths (18), showing that for strong and medium absorptivities, the criterion of an infinitely thick sample layer is valid for 1 mm, whereas for weaker bands, approximately about 5 mm of sample thickness was claimed. For pure KCl, under the conditions of a defined particle size distribution for the powder and the application of a certain pressure to obtain a

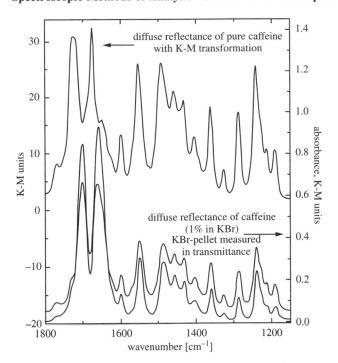

Fig. 6 Spectral differences in mid-infrared spectra of caffeine measured under different conditions. Diffuse reflectance spectrum of the pure crystalline powder (top trace), diffuse reflectance spectrum of 1% of caffeine in KBr-powder (middle trace, intensity data for both spectra in K–M units), and absorbance spectrum as recorded using the KBr pellet technique (bottom trace).

reproducible compression of the disperse sample, a depth of 2 mm was found to reach the K–M requirements of an "infinite" sample thickness, i.e., a further increase in depth causes no change in the measured reflectance (14). The packaging density of the sample, as just noted above, is another parameter that affects the spectrum. The effect of pressure applied to powders for reproducible measurements was studied also by several other spectroscopists [see, for example, Ref. (19)].

Many other materials were studied as matrix materials for diffuse reflectance spectroscopy. Beside the previously noted alkali halides, other examples are silver halides, diamond, germanium, silicon, and chalcogenide glass, preferably of small particle diameters. For an extensive survey on different matrices, see Ref. (20).

A study of the precision and accuracy limiting factors of quantitative assays using diffuse reflectance was carried out by Krivácsy and Hlavay (21), comparing these against transmission measurements. Beside a reproducible sample preparation, the effect of using an underestimated reflectance value of the reference standard ($R_{\infty,r} < 1$) in the K–M transformation approach for the quantitative evaluation of the spectra leads to a negative intercept for the calibration curves and a slightly reduced linear regression coefficient. Another prerequisite is that scattering stays constant, which is achieved by embedding the sample in a non-absorbing matrix, e.g., of KBr powder with a defined particle size distribution.

The linearity of the K–M function has been investigated for several different conditions. For caffeine, as diluted in KCl powder and reaching up to 100% of weight, maxima of weak and strong absorption bands were tested for this important analytical parameter. It was found that under the conditions given, the use of an accessory with off-axis optical geometry and with application of crossed polarizers before and after the sample, reduced contributions from specular Fresnel reflection from particles on the upper sample surface. As a result, the linear region of the absorbance–concentration dependencies was extended (22). For near-infrared spectra, an alternative linearization function for the measured diffuse reflectance based on $-\log(R)$ is noted above. An intensive investigation on the effect of an absorbing matrix was carried out by Olinger and Griffiths (23), who stated that the concentration range over which linearity holds depends on particle size and matrix absorption strength. The effects of nonlinearity are even more pronounced for mid-infrared spectra (24). Such consequences have to be taken into account when analyzing the *in situ* spectra of adsorbates on substrates, such as from thin-layer-chromatography plates. The combination of spectroscopy with separation techniques is presented below in greater detail.

An interesting study for the interpretation of diffuse reflectance spectra of powders and bulk materials was carried out by Chaffin and Griffiths (25) for the extended near-infrared spectral range, reaching from 10,000 to 2500 cm^{-1} as defined by the authors. The effects of absorption saturation and Fresnel reflection for different amounts of sample scattering are presented. Reducing the scattering inside the studied material, e.g., by application of a transparent liquid for matching the matrix refractive index, a tremendous enhancement of the absorption could be demonstrated, as predicted by the K–M theory.

Because a diffuse reflectance spectrum is scatter-dependent, information on mean particle sizes is also obtainable, which is a parameter of great importance in powder technology. An approach using near-infrared spectrometry combined with multivariate calibration has been presented by Ilary et al. (26). Included was a spectrum standardization by multiplicative scatter correction (see later).

A nonconventional approach for the qualitative analysis of difficult solid samples is to use silicon carbide abrasive paper. The sample is rubbed against the rough surface, and a small amount sticks to the substrate. A diffuse reflectance accessory is used for recording the spectrum, obtained from a "sample loaded" substrate measurement that is ratioed against that of a clean spot. Recently, metal-coated substrates were found to be even better suited, because the signal-to-noise ratio could be improved owing to much higher reflectivity, compared with the results from using uncoated abrasive paper (recommended grit size, 400). For extremely hard materials, a diamond-in-metal sampling device was used successfully (27).

For qualitative and quantitative mid-infrared studies, a dilution of a sample by a scattering, but transparent matrix is highly recommended. The diffuse reflection technique can be used for low concentrations because of enhancement effects for weak absorptions, which do not exist for transmission measurements. On the other hand, the dilution by KBr powder can add spectral impurities, and the grinding process itself carried out in a humid atmosphere could lead to an increase in water absorption band intensities owing to the hygroscopic nature of the KBr powder. Therefore, great care has to be taken when working with such a material, which should be kept dry in a desiccator or dried again in an oven. In Fig. 7 an example of a diffuse reflectance spectrum of a KBr powder is shown, for which the reference measurement was carried

out using a gold-coated diffusely reflecting substrate. As evident from the baseline offset in the spectrum, the reflectance of the KBr powder is lower than that of the gold-coated standard. The intensification of absorption bands from impurities, either inherent to the KBr used or from a polluted atmosphere, is again to be stressed when using the diffuse-reflectance technique. In this context, suprapure KBr batches and a clean bench are prerequisites for improving assay limits (28).

Diffuse reflectance has also been used extensively for trace analysis. In such a case, the sample to be studied is dissolved using a volatile solvent and transferred to KBr powder, preferably in microcups. The solvent is evaporated, and the sample has coated the KBr particles. With microsampling techniques, sample loadings lower than 100 ng can give satisfactory spectra. If strict rules for avoiding impurities and contamination are observed, detection limits even at the low nanogram level can be reached. Examples from the literature are the identification of different pharmaceuticals (28) and of chlorodibenzo-dioxins isomers (29).

When coupling separation techniques such as thin-layer chromatography (TLC) and liquid chromatography (LC) with infrared spectroscopy for component identification and, less successfully, for quantification, the diffuse reflectance technique has often been applied. Lowest detection limits were usually obtained when the analyte was isolated from its matrix, i.e., the TLC substrate or the eluent in the case of LC–IR coupling. The dissolved compound is usually transferred to a transparent powder, from which it is detected after solvent elimination [see, for example, Ref. (28)]. In situ measurements on TLC plates were also carried out by this and other groups (30). However, because of the strong and broad background absorptions from the stationary phase, such as cellulose, Al_2O_3, silica gel, and others, analyte detection limits deteriorate significantly compared with the case of a transparent matrix. In addition, substrate interactions with the separated component can often be noticed, which may cause drastic spectrum changes and certainly lead to difficulties with library searching if only normal solid-phase spectra are implemented for reference. Liquid chromatography with polar eluents, as used in reversed-phase LC, complicate the solvent elimination step, although interfaces have been constructed to enable an on-line analysis of effluents from reverse-phase high-performance liquid chromatography (RP–HPLC) (31). A review of analyte deposition-based concepts for such separation techniques is given by Somsen et al. (32). The incorporation of HPLC/FT-IR into pharmaceutical research programs and its automation are discussed by Pivonka and Kirkland (33).

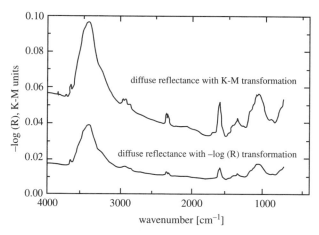

Fig. 7 Diffuse reflectance spectrum of KBr powder measured against a gold-coated diffuse reflective substrate transformed to either $-\log(R)$ or K–M units. The spectral reflectance of KBr powder is lower than that of the gold-coated standard. Furthermore, various absorption bands are noticeable: the broad band approximately at 3500 cm^{-1} and that at 1640 cm^{-1} is from adsorbed water. The doublet at 2350 cm^{-1} is from uncompensated atmospheric CO_2 within the spectrometer and accessory; bands between 1500 and 1000 cm^{-1} arise from inorganic impurities, and bands below 3000 cm^{-1} are from compounds containing aliphatic groups.

CHEMOMETRICS

Quality control, pharmaceutical product identity checks, and quantification are important fields in the broad application of the different spectroscopic methods. There are many spectroscopic aspects, e.g., concerning sample preparation, influences from different accessories, and possibly spectrometer effects, which certainly influences quantitative measurements. The latter problems could be solved using calibration transfer between different spectrometer types, for example, a scanning and an FT-near-IR spectrometer (34).

For qualitative spectrum interpretation, the conventional method for routine identification of chemical species is a library-search, based on spectral mapping algorithms. Before library-searching spectral preprocessing, i.e., elimination of baseline effects and noise, standardization, etc., is performed on the sample spectrum. Comparison of such a processed spectrum with a candidate library spectrum can be based on different principles such as correlation of spectra, similarity and distance measures, and logical operations. For an overview see Ref. (35). For the mid-infrared spectral range, many libraries are available, although only a limited number of spectra might have been recorded with the diffuse reflectance technique. On the other hand, industrial activities are on the way for near-IR libraries, in particular, recorded using the diffuse reflectance technique. For the UV/VIS range, only limited digitized information is available, whereas most spectra are from solution work. A more difficult situation is found for mixtures aiming at component identification. For a discussion and applied strategies, see Ref. (36). Procedures for classifying and interpreting spectra can be based on chemometric tools such as factor analysis, pattern recognition, cluster analysis, and artificial intelligence algorithms (37). Spectral deviations can sometimes be traced back to differences in chemical purity (e.g., water content), particle size, and size distribution or polymorphism (38). Recently, pattern recognition methods were applied for near-infrared detection of polymorphic forms and their conversion. The methods were robust enough when applied to different spectrometers to avoid the need for multivariate instrument standardization (39).

Quantification is another important field in which fast results are needed for process analysis and quality control. Multivariate techniques play an important role in quantitative assays, for which different strategies and algorithms are in use for calibration. Individual wavelength and full-spectrum methods are in use: multiple linear regression (MLR) is an example of the first category, whereas partial least-squares (PLS) and principal component regression (PCR) usually make use of broad spectral interval information. For more details, see Refs. (40, 41). Apart from so-called full-spectrum methods, spectral variable selection is a playground of chemometricians for achieving improved and more robust calibration models. A recent study also provides a review on the activities in this field (42).

It must be mentioned again that quantification based on diffuse reflectance spectra requires a reproducible sample preparation, because the reflectance depends on particle size and shape, packing density, and the texture of the sample surface. Therefore, sample preparation must be controlled (using same grinding time when using a ball and mill grinder and pressurizing the sample reproducibly). A recent example was provided by Blanco et al., who tested multivariate calibrations for active compounds in pharmaceutical mixtures based on partial least-squares regression in combination with different spectral-preprocessing methods (43). Often, baseline effects are eliminated by taking first or second derivatives of the spectral data, and, in particular, multiple scatter correction is an important preprocessing method used for the standardization of diffuse reflectance spectra (44).

PHARMACEUTICAL APPLICATIONS

The number of applications of diffuse reflectance spectroscopy for pharmaceutical analysis has increased tremendously in recent years. An overview to the activities up to 1986 is found in the first edition of the *Encyclopedia of Pharmaceutical Technology* (45). The on-line identification of pharmaceutical raw materials has been noted above because of the requirements of Good Manufacturing Practice (GMP), which is most often performed now using near-infrared spectroscopy. On the other hand, mid-infrared spectroscopy can provide more information owing to the fact that more vibrational bands from all possible molecular substructures show up within this spectral range, whereas the near-infrared comprises primarily bands corresponding to overtones and combination bands, just involving vibrations with C—H, O—H, and N–H molecular bonds. The superiority of mid-infrared spectroscopy compared with measurements in the near-infrared was shown when a special formulation type and the quantification of the active ingredients were required (46). Other applications are concerned with the development of rapid, reliable, and noninvasive testing assays for whole tablets or intact capsules. Lodder et al. described analyzing several kinds of inorganic compounds through a gelatin wall; their aim was the detection of capsule-tampering using a special clustering algorithm, which was based on near-infrared reflectance analysis (47). Another direct control of the active ingredient included in tablets without extraction or pulverization by near-infrared spectrometry was possible, as shown by other scientists (48).

Near-infrared spectroscopy was proposed as an alternative to several compendial test methods. As an example, ampicillin trihydrate was used to demonstrate that in total, eight quality criteria could be checked and its "conformity index" calculated (38). Additional chemometrics for quality control were developed by the same group (49). Their strategy was used to distinguish differences in mean particle size of various lactose samples and to study the effectiveness of a blending process for homogenous mixture preparation.

Another task often required is the determination of the water content. Quantification of moisture in hard gelantin capsules was described by Berntsson et al. who discussed its importance in monitoring for at-line process control (50). A sparse MLR calibration model with three optimized near-infrared wavelengths yielded an absolute prediction error of 0.1% over a range of 5.6–18% water content. For monitoring the production process, Han and Faulkner (51) analyzed the spectral range of 1100–2500 nm. Second derivative spectra were used for PLS calibration of moisture. Single-wavelength analysis was applied for coating thickness. Furthermore, identification of tablets inside blister packaging was also possible.

A fiber optic probe was used by Blanco et al. (52) for analysis of spasmoctyl samples with the active compound otilonium bromide and cellulose, maize starch, sodium starch glycolate, and glyceryl palmitostearate as excipients. Another study from this group covered the identification, qualification of the substance, and the quantification of the active component. A library search with a comparison to the near-infrared spectra of 163 pharmaceuticals was involved (53). An on-line monitoring for the determination of the endpoint of polymorph conversions in pharmaceutical processes was recently described (54); further investigations into this field were published and are noted previously (39).

An interesting application is the nondestructive identification of pharmaceutical tablets directly through a blister packing using a fiber optic probe (55). Three different pattern recognition methods based on full near-infrared spectra and subset wavelength ranges were tested to discriminate between film-coated and nonfilm-coated tablets as well as between active and placebo tablets. Dreassi et al. (56) used near-infrared FT spectroscopy for the quality control of solid pharmaceutical formulations. Quantitative assays were developed for solid drug preparations, for pills containing ibuprofen and tablets with paracetamol, and for powders containing benzydamine hydrochloride and tricetol. Additional work for qualitative and quantitative analysis aimed at all stages of the production, including determination of moisture, was also described by Dreassi et al. (57). Another study was concerned with the characterization of several pharmaceuticals on the basis of their physical properties, i.e., crystalline states and densities (58).

In conclusion, it can be stated that spectroscopic techniques will further dominate the analytical tools of the future with respect to qualitative and quantitative assays. This is because of their speed and the enormous information content of the spectra, especially in the infrared, and the fact that reagent-free multicomponent methodologies are available. The widespread diffuse reflection technique certainly has to compete with others in the laboratory and at the production site. However, for the study of bulk and dispersed systems, it will often be the method of choice. There are additional developments concerned with dedicated instruments and user-friendly interfaces, in which chemometrics play an important role. It is hoped that the sophisticated algorithms presented in the literature will be available soon within expert systems, allowing adaptations to special applications and broadening the general acceptance of these spectroscopic methods presented above.

ACKNOWLEDGMENTS

I am indebted to Mrs. M. Hillig for support in preparing the diagrams. Financial support from the Ministerium für Schule, Wissenschaft und Forschung des Landes Nordrhein-Westfalen, and the Bundesministerium für Bildung und Forschung is gratefully acknowledged.

REFERENCES

1. Bugay, D.E.; Williams, A.C.; Brittain, H.G., Eds.; *Physical Characterization of Pharmaceutical Solids*; Marcel Dekker, Inc.: New York, 1995.
2. Coates, J. Vibrational Spectroscopy: Instrumentation for Infrared and Raman Spectroscopy. Appl. Spectrosc. Rev. **1998**, *33*, 267–425.
3. Workman, J. Jr.; Springsteen, A. *Applied Spectroscopy—A Compact Reference for Practitioners*; Academic Press: San Diego, 1998.
4. Heise, H.M. Clinical Applications of Mid- and Near-Infrared Spectroscopy. *Infrared and Raman Spectroscopy of Biological Materials*; Gremlich, H.-U., Yan, B., Eds.; Marcel Dekker, Inc.: New York, 2001; 259–322.

5. Yang, P.W.; Mantsch, H.H.; Baudais, F. A Critical Evaluation of Three Types of Diffuse Reflectance Infrared Accessories. Appl. Spectrosc. **1986**, *40*, 974–978.

6. Springsteen, A. Standards for Reflectance Measurements. *Applied Spectroscopy—A Compact Reference for Practitioners*; Workman, J., Jr., Springsteen, A., Eds.; Academic Press: San Diego, 1998; 247–267.

7. Griffiths, P.R. Letter: Practical Consequences of Math Pre-Treatment of Near Infrared Reflectance Data: Log(1\/R) vs F(R). J. Near Infrared Spectrosc. **1995**, *3*, 60–62.

8. Kubelka, P.; Munk, F. Ein Beitrag Zur Optik Der Farbanstriche. Z. Techn. Phys. **1931**, *12*, 593–601.

9. Kortüm, G. *Reflectance Spectroscopy*; Springer-Verlag: New York, 1969.

10. Loyolka, S.K.; Riggs, C.A. Inverse Problem in Diffuse Reflectance Spectroscopy: Accuracy of the Kubelka–Munk Equations. Appl. Spectrosc. **1995**, *49*, 1107–1110.

11. van Gemert, M.J.C.; Star, W.M. Relations Between the Kubelka–Munk and the Transport Equation Models for Anisotropic Scattering. Lasers Life Sci. **1987**, *1*, 287–298.

12. Burger, T.; Fricke, J.; Kuhn, J. NIR Radiative Transfer Investigations to Characterise Pharmaceutical Powders and Their Mixtures. J. Near Infrared Spectrosc. **1998**, *6*, 33–40.

13. Hecht, H.G. A Comparison of the Kubelka–Munk, Rozenberg, and Pitts–Giovanelli Methods of Analysis of Diffuse Reflectance for Several Model Systems. Appl. Spectrosc. **1983**, *37*, 348–354.

14. Krivácsy, Z.; Hlavay, J. Effect of Sample Packing on the Scattering Properties of the Reference Material in Diffuse Reflectance Infrared Spectrometry. Talanta **1994**, *41*, 1143–1149.

15. Wendlandt, W.; Hecht, H.G. *Reflectance Spectroscopy*; Interscience Publishers: New York, 1966.

16. Yang, P.W.; Mantsch, H.H. Diffuse Reflectance Infrared Spectrometry: Characteristics of the Diffuse and Specular Components. Appl. Optics **1987**, *26*, 326–330.

17. Brimmer, P.J.; Griffiths, P.R.; Harrick, N.J. Angular Dependence of Diffuse Reflectance Infrared Spectra. I. FT-IR Spectrogoniophotometer. Appl. Spectrosc. **1986**, *40*, 258–265.

18. Fraser, D.J.J.; Griffiths, P.R. Effect of Scattering Coefficient on Diffuse Reflectance Infrared Spectra. Appl. Spectrosc. **1990**, *44*, 193–199.

19. Yeboah, S.A.; Wang, S.H.; Griffiths, P.R. Effect of Pressure in DRIFT Spectra of Compressed Powders. Appl. Spectrosc. **1984**, *38*, 259–264.

20. TeVrucht, M.L.E.; Griffiths, P.R. Quantitative Investigation of Matrices for Diffuse Reflectance Infrared Fourier Transform Spectrometry. Talanta **1991**, *38*, 839–849.

21. Krivácsy, Z.; Hlavay, J. Method for the Reliable Quantitative Analysis by Diffuse Reflectance Infrared Spectroscopy. J. Mol. Struct. **1995**, *349*, 289–292.

22. Brimmer, P.J.; Griffiths, P.R. Angular Dependence of Diffuse Reflectance Infrared Spectra. III. Linearity of Kubelka–Munk Plots. Appl. Spectrosc. **1988**, *42*, 242–247.

23. Olinger, J.M.; Griffiths, P.R. Quantitative Effects of an Absorbing Matrix on Near-Infrared Diffuse Reflectance Spectra. Anal. Chem. **1988**, *60*, 2427–2435.

24. Brimmer, P.J.; Griffiths, P.R. Effect of Absorbing Matrices on Diffuse Reflectance Infrared Spectra. Anal. Chem. **1986**, *58*, 2179–2184.

25. Chaffin, N.C.; Griffiths, P.R. Role of Scattering Coefficients in Extended Near-Infrared Diffuse Reflection Spectrometry. Appl. Spectrosc. **1998**, *52*, 218–221.

26. Ilari, J.L.; Martens, H.; Isaksson, T. Determination of Particle Size in Powders by Scatter Correction in Diffuse Near-Infrared Reflectance. Appl. Spectrosc. **1988**, *42*, 722–728.

27. Hoult, R.A.; Spragg, R.A. Abrasive Sampling for Diffuse Reflectance Using Reflective Substrates, Itoh, K., Tasumi, M., Eds.; Fourier Transform Spectroscopy, 12th International Conference, Waseda University Press: Tokyo, 1999; 506–507.

28. Otto, A.; Bode, U.; Heise, H.M. Experiences with Infrared Microsampling for Thin-Layer and High-Performance Liquid Chromatography. Fresenius Z. Anal. Chem. **1988**, *331*, 376–382.

29. Gurka, D.F.; Billets, S.; Brasch, J.W.; Riggle, C.J. Tetrachlorodibenzodioxin Isomer Differentiation by Micro Diffuse Reflectance Fourier Transform Infrared Spectrometry At the Low Nanogram Level. Anal. Chem. **1985**, *57*, 1975–1979.

30. Glauninger, G.; Kovar, K.-A.; Hoffmann, V. Possibilities and Limits of an On-Line Coupling of Thin-Layer Chromatography and FTIR-Spectroscopy. Fresenius. J. Anal. Chem. **1990**, *338*, 710–716.

31. Castles, M.A.; Azarraga, L.V.; Carreira, L.A. Continuous On-Line Interface for Reversed-Phase Microbore High Performance Liquid Chromatography/Diffuse Reflectance Infrared Fourier Transform Analysis. Appl. Spectrosc. **1986**, *40*, 673–680.

32. Somsen, G.W.; Gooijer, C.; Brinkman, U.A. Th. Analyte-Deposition-Based Detection in Column Liquid Chromatography: Concept and Examples. Trends Anal. Chem. **1998**, *17*, 129–140.

33. Pivonka, D.E.; Kirkland, K.M. Research Strategy for the HPLC/FT-IR Analysis of Drug Metabolites. Appl. Spectrosc. **1997**, *51*, 866–873.

34. Lin, J.; Lo, S.-C.; Brown, C.W. Calibration Transfer from a Scanning Near-IR Spectrophotometer to a FT-near-IR Spectrophotometer. Anal. Chim. Acta **1997**, *349*, 263–269.

35. Luinge, H.J. Automated Interpretation of Vibrational Spectra. Vibr. Spectrosc. **1990**, *1*, 3–18.

36. Chen, C.-S.; Li, Y.; Brown, C.W. Searching a Mid-Infrared Spectral Library of Solids and Liquids with Spectra of Mixtures. Vibr. Spectrosc. **1997**, *8*, 9–17.

37. Luinge, H.J. Multivariate Methods for Automated Spectrum Interpretation. *Computing Applications in Molecular Spectroscopy*; George, W.O., Steele, D., Eds.; Royal Society of Chemistry: Cambridge, 1995; 87–103.

38. Plugge, C.; van der Vlies, C. The Use of Near Infrared Spectroscopy in the Quality Control Laboratory of the Pharmaceutical Industry. J. Pharm. Biom. Anal. **1992**, *10*, 797–803.

39. Aldridge, P.K.; Evans, C.L.; Ward, H.W., II; Colgan, S.T.; Boyer, T.; Gemperline, P.J. Near-Infrared Detection of Polymorphism and Process-Related Substances. Anal. Chem. **1996**, *68*, 997–1002.

40. Martens, H.; Naes, T. *Multivariate Calibration*; John Wiley: Chichester, 1989.

41. Marbach, R.; Heise, H.M. On the Efficiency of Algorithms for Multivariate Linear Calibration Used in Analytical Spectroscopy. Trends Anal. Chem. **1992**, *11*, 270–275.

42. Norgaard, L.; Saudland, A.; Wagner, J.; Nielsen, J.P.; Munck, L.; Engelsen, S.B. Interval Partial Least-Squares Regression (IPLS): A Comparative Chemometric Study with an Example from Near-Infrared Spectroscopy. Appl. Spectrosc. **2000**, *54*, 413–419.

43. Blanco, M.; Coello, J.; Iturriaga, H.; Maspoch, S.; de la Pezuela, C. Effect of Data Preprocessing Methods in Near-Infrared Diffuse Reflectance Spectroscopy for the Determination of the Active Compounds in a Pharmaceutical Preparation. Appl. Spectrosc. **1997**, *51*, 240–246.

44. Isaksson, T.; Næs, T. The Effect of Multiplicative Scatter Correction (MSC) and Linearity Improvement in NIR Spectroscopy. Appl. Spectrosc. **1988**, *42*, 1273–1284.

45. Bornstein, M. Diffuse Reflectance Spectroscopy. *Encyclopedia of Pharmaceutical Technology*; Swarbrick, J., Boylan, J.C., Eds.; Vol. 4, Marcel Dekker, Inc.: New York, 1991; 23–35.

46. Ryan, J.A.; Compton, S.V.; Brooks, M.A.; Compton, D.A.C. Rapid Verification of Identity and Content of Drug Formulations Using Mid-Infrared Spectroscopy. J. Pharm. Biomed. Anal. **1991**, *9*, 303–310.

47. Lodder, R.A.; Selby, M.; Hieftje, G.M. Detection of Capsule Tampering by Near-Infrared Reflectance Analysis. Anal. Chem. **1987**, *59*, 1921–1930.

48. Jensen, R.; Peuchant, E.; Castagne, I.; Boirac, A.M.; Roux, G. One-Step Quantification of Active Ingredient in Pharmaceutical Tablets Using Near-Infrared Spectroscopy. Spectrosc. Int. J. **1988**, *6*, 63–72.

49. Plugge, W.; van der Vlies, C. Near Infrared Spectroscopy as a Tool to Improve Quality. J. Pharm. Biomed. Anal. **1996**, *14*, 891–898.

50. Berntsson, O.; Zackrisson, G.; Oestling, G. Determination of Moisture in Hard Gelatin Capsules Using Near-Infrared Spectroscopy: Applications to At-Line Process Control of Pharmaceutics. J. Pharm. Biomed. Anal. **1997**, *15*, 895–900.

51. Han, S.M.; Faulkner, P.G. Determination of SB 216469-S during Tablet Production Using Near-Infrared Reflectance Spectroscopy. J. Pharm. Biomed. Anal. **1996**, *14*, 1681–1689.

52. Blanco, M.; Coello, J.; Iturriaga, H.; Maspoch, S.; de la Pezuela, C. Quantitation of the Active Compound and Major Excipients in a Pharmaceutical Formulation by Near Infrared Diffuse Reflectance Spectroscopy with Fiber Optical Probe. Anal. Chim. Acta **1996**, *333*, 147–156.

53. Blanco, M.; Coello, J.; Iturriaga, H.; Maspoch, S.; de la Pezuela, C.; Russo, E. Control Analysis of a Pharmaceutical Preparation by Near Infrared Reflectance Spectroscopy. A Comparative Study of a Spinning Module and a Fiber Optic Probe. Anal. Chim. Acta **1994**, *298*, 83–191.

54. Norris, T.; Aldridge, P.K.; Sekulic, S.S. Determination of End-Points for Polymorph Conversions of Crystalline Organic Compounds Using On-Line Near Infrared Spectroscopy. Analyst **1997**, *122*, 549–552.

55. Dempster, M.A.; MacDonald, B.F.; Gemperline, P.J.; Boyer, N.R. A Near Infrared Reflectance Analysis Method for the Non-Invasive Identification of Film-Coated and Nonfilm-Coated, Blister-Packed Tablets. Anal. Chim. Acta **1995**, *310*, 43–51.

56. Dreassi, E.; Ceramelli, G.; Corti, P.; Massacesi, M.; Perruccio, P.L. Quantitative Fourier Transform Near-Infrared Spectroscopy in the Quality Control of Solid Formulations. Analyst **1995**, *120*, 2361–2365.

57. Dreassi, E.; Ceramelli, G.; Corti, P.; Perruccio, P.L.; Lonardi, S. Application of Near-Infrared Reflectance Spectrometry to the Analytical Control of Pharmaceuticals: Ranitidine Hydrochloride Tablet Production. Analyst **1996**, *121*, 219–222.

58. Dreassi, E.; Ceramelli, G.; Corti, P.; Lonardi, S.; Perruccio, P.L. Near-Infrared Reflectance Spectrometry in the Determination of the Physical State of Primary Materials in Pharmaceutical Production. Analyst **1995**, *120*, 1005–1008.

FURTHER READING

Adams, M.J. *Chemometrics in Analytical Spectroscopy*; Royal Soc. Chem.: Cambridge, 1995.

Knowles, A.; Burgess, C., Eds.; Practical Absorption Spectrometry. *Techniques in Visible and Ultraviolet Spectrometry*; Chapman & Hall: London, 1984; 3.

Korte, E.-H.; Röseler, A. Foundations and Features of Infrared Reflection Techniques. *Infrared and Raman Spectroscopy*; Schrader, B. Ed.; Wiley-VCH Weinheim 1995; 572–602.

Kramer, R. *Chemometric Techniques for Quantitative Analysis*; Marcel Dekker, Inc.: New York, 1998.

Mirabella, F.M. *Modern Techniques in Applied Molecular Spectroscopy*; John Wiley & Sons: New York, 1998.

Workman, J.J., Jr. Review of Process and Non-Invasive Near-Infrared and Infrared Spectroscopy: 1993–1999. Appl. Spectrosc. Rev. **1999**, *34*, 1–89.

SPECTROSCOPIC METHODS OF ANALYSIS— FLUORESCENCE SPECTROSCOPY

Stephen G. Schulman
Jeffrey A. Hughes
University of Florida, Gainesville, Florida

INTRODUCTION

Luminescence processes in molecules can be classified according to the source from which the excitation energy is derived. In photoluminescence, which encompasses fluorescence and phosphorescence, excitation is achieved by the absorption of light by the potentially luminescent molecule. In chemiluminescence, excitation occurs as the result of an energetic chemical reaction. Fluorescent analytical methods make up the great majority of the ultrasensitive assays carried out by light emission spectroscopy in the pharmaceutical sciences. Although they are more complicated, there has been some interest in phosphorescence and more in chemiluminescence. Accordingly, these phenomena are also briefly treated here.

MOLECULAR ENERGY LEVELS AND ELECTRONIC PROCESSES

Light absorption by an organic molecule results in the promotion of a single electron to a higher energy molecular orbital. The excited state of the molecule thus formed then has two electrons in singly occupied orbitals. The promoted electron and the one it left behind in the orbital it originally occupied can have spins that are opposite (as in the ground state), or they may have the same spin. If the electrons have opposite spins, the molecule is said to be in an excited singlet state. If, on the other hand, they acquire the same spin, the excited molecule is said to be in a triplet state. For each excited singlet state, there is a triplet state that, owing to lower electrostatic repulsion in the latter, has a somewhat lower energy than the corresponding singlet state. Luminescence originating from the electronic transition of a molecule in passing from an excited singlet state back to the ground state is called fluorescence. That originating from the transition from an excited triplet state to the ground state is called phosphorescence.

Transition may occur from the ground singlet state to a number of excited singlet states and to any of a number of vibrational levels within each of these excited singlet states as a result of scanning the sample of interest with the range of wavelengths (energies) of light that lie in the visible and near-ultraviolet regions of the electromagnetic spectrum. These electronic transitions produce the electronic absorption spectrum of the compound of interest. The "vibrational breadth" of each upper electronic state results in the broad-banded appearance of the absorption spectra of molecules, which is unlike the line-like appearance of the absorption spectra of atoms.

Subsequent to excitation, excess energy is rapidly lost by the excited molecules in collisions with the solvent. Each collisional loss of energy causes vibrational and sometimes even electronic changes in the excited molecule, which are radiationless (i.e., no light is emitted). These changes are called vibrational relaxation in the case of vibrational change and internal conversion in the case of radiationless electronic transition. In unconjugated molecules where there is great vibrational freedom, these processes may carry the excited molecule back to the ground electronic state. However, in highly conjugated molecules, especially aromatic molecules, vibrational motion may be restricted, and vibrational relaxation and internal conversion may carry the excited molecule only back to the lowest vibrational level of the lowest excited singlet state. From this state, which is about 10^6 times longer-lived than the upper vibrational and electronic states, the molecule may return to the ground electronic state by light emission (fluorescence), or it may undergo photochemical reaction or a change in spin of one of its electrons. When the latter process occurs, the molecule is said to undergo intersystem crossing, a process that results in the creation of the lowest triplet state. If light emission occurs in the demotion of the molecule from the triplet state back to the ground singlet state, it is called phosphorescence. Phosphorescence entails a change in angular momentum of the emitting molecule and is classically forbidden. This is manifested in the long decay-time of phosphorescence ($10^{-4}-10$ s). Fluorescence decay-times (reciprocal probability of decay) are typically 10^{-11}–10^{-7} s. Both forms of light emission are analytically useful, but fluorescence occurs under a much wider variety of circumstances and has been used for analytical purposes far more than has phosphorescence.

Because fluorescence and phosphorescence originate exclusively from the lowest vibrational level of the lowest excited singlet and triplet states, respectively, and terminate in any of a number of vibrational levels of the ground electronic state, there will be only one possible fluorescence band and one possible phosphorescence band observable from a single chemical species capable of fluorescing and/or phosphorescing. More than one of either is indicative of extraneous luminescing species, either impurities or products of photochemical reaction.

CHARACTERISTICS OF LUMINESCENCE SPECTRA

Fluorescence

Fluorescence is characterized by two spectra corresponding to excitation and emission. In solutions, both spectra usually appear as broad bands that may or may not show vibrational fine structure. The excitation and the absorption spectra of a compound should be the same, but with ordinary fluorescence spectrophotometers, a distorted version of the true absorption spectrum is obtained. The degree of distortion depends on the light output of the spectral excitation source and the responses of the monochromators and detector as functions of the wavelengths of exciting light. The excitation spectrum can be useful in the qualitative and quantitative analysis of mixtures. For example, the excitation spectrum of one component of a mixture can be isolated by setting the emission monochromator at the proper wavelength, provided the absorbance spectra of compounds present in the mixture differ sufficiently.

The difference in energy between the longest wavelength absorption band and the fluorescence band of an analyte is called a Stokes' shift and is usually no more than 100 nm. If the fluorescence band shows an unusually large Stokes' shift, then either the solute exhibits some form of photochemical behavior such as isomerism or prototropic dissociation in the excited state, or more than one fluorescent species is present.

The shape of the fluorescence spectrum is independent of the wavelength of light used to excite it because the fluorescence always takes place from the same level, no matter to what level the molecule was originally excited.

Quantum yield and decay-time of fluorescence

Because of the other processes that compete with fluorescence for deactivation of molecules in the lowest excited singlet state, only a fraction of the excited molecules will return to the ground state by fluorescence. This fraction is called the quantum yield of fluorescence (Φ_f) or fluorescence efficiency. Under given conditions of temperature and environment, Φ_f is a physical constant of the excited molecular species. Φ_f usually decreases with increasing temperature. The actual mean time the molecule spends in the excited state before fluorescing is referred to as the lifetime of the lowest excited singlet state (or fluorescence decay-time) and is represented by the symbol τ_R^0. The time it would spend in the lowest excited singlet state if there were no other processes competing with flourescence is called the natural life time, τ_R. The quantum yield of fluorescence, then, may be expressed as being equal to τ^0/τ_R^0. Because it is a fraction (never greater than unity), τ_R^0 is always greater than or equal to τ^0. The intensity of fluorescent light emitted depends on the concentration and molar absorptivity of the absorbing (ground state) species and the quantum yield fluorescence of the fluorescing (excited state) species.

Phosphorescence

Phosphorescence is also characterized by an excitation and an emission spectrum. Because the lowest triplet state invariably lies lower in energy than the lowest excited singlet state of the same molecule, phosphorescence will occur at wavelengths longer than those of fluorescence and, therefore, at wavelengths much longer than those of the excitation spectrum. As in the case of fluorescence, the phosphorescence spectrum and the phosphorescence excitation spectrum are distorted by the instrumental components and therefore do not represent "true" spectra.

Because of the long radiative lifetime of the lowest triplet state, most phosphorescence in fluid solutions is obviated by collisional quenching, especially by dissolved molecular oxygen. Phosphorescence, when it occurs, is usually observed at low temperatures (e.g., that of liquid nitrogen) in rigid matrices where it may demonstrate high quantum yields. In the past three decades, much interest has been focused on phosphorescence at room temperature (RTP), which sometimes can be observed in samples adsorbed on solid substrates such as filter paper. Unfortunately, the quantum yields observed in room temperature phosphorescence are low, leading to poor analytical sensitivity, and the method has not enjoyed wide popularity. Phosphorescent measurements at low temperatures require special handling techniques and are difficult to reproduce. Consequently, although low-temperature phosphorimetry is inherently a very sensitive analytical method, it too has yet to attract a substantial group of users. However, there are a substantial number of molecules of pharmaceutical interest that phosphoresce but do not fluoresce (e.g., metronidazole) or fluoresce weakly and phosphoresce intensely (e.g., warfarin), and it is probably worthwhile to pursue phosphorimetry as a valuable aspect of molecular luminescence spectroscopy.

Chemical Structural Aspects of Fluorescence Spectra

Fluorescence spectra of analytical and pharmaceutical interest arise from functionally substituted aromatic molecules, particularly those derived from benzene, naphthalene, and anthracene or their heteroaromatic analogs pyridine, quinoline, isoquinoline, and acridine.

The intensity of fluorescence observable from a given molecular species depends primarily on the quantum yield of fluorescence, which may affect the intensity of fluorescence over about four orders of magnitude and may determine whether fluorescence is observable at all. The quantum yield of fluorescence is dependent on the rates of processes competing with fluorescence for the deactivation of the lowest excited singlet state. These, in turn, depend on molecular structure.

Aromatic molecules, containing lengthy aliphatic side chains, generally tend to fluoresce less intensely than those without the side chains. This is brought about by the introduction of a large number of vibrational degrees of freedom by the aliphatic moieties, providing an efficient pathway for internal conversion. In the unsubstituted aromatic molecules, the rigidity of the aromatic ring results in wide separation of the ground and lowest excited singlet states. In general, molecular rigidity and high quantum yield of fluorescence are closely related.

The fluorescence efficiencies of aromatic molecules are reduced by heavy atom substituents such as bromine and iodine and by certain other groups such as aldehyde and keto as well as nitro groups. However, in many cases the substituents that decrease the intensity of fluorescence enhance the intensity of phosphorescence. Consequently, aromatic nitro compounds, bromo- and iodo-derivatives, aldehydes, ketones, and some N-heterocyclics tend to fluoresce very weakly or not at all. However, most of them phosphoresce quite intensely. On the other hand, many substituents that are electron donors such as amino, hydroxy, and methoxy often tend to increase the quantum yields of fluorescence of molecules to which they are attached.

The energies of the ground and lowest excited singlet states of fluorescing molecules are affected by such features of molecular structure as the presence of substituents and the molecular geometry. This is reflected in the position (energy) of the fluorescence band maximum in the spectrum. The greater the separation between the ground and lowest excited singlet states, the greater will be the frequency and the shorter will be the wavelength of fluorescence. This separation depends on the energy difference between the highest occupied and lowest unoccupied molecular orbitals and the repulsion energy between the electronic configurations corresponding to the ground and lowest excited singlet states. For aromatic molecules, the greater the extension of the conjugated system, the smaller the energy separation between the highest occupied (π) and lowest unoccupied (π^*) orbitals. Thus, the wavelengths of fluorescence (λ_f) increase with increasing extension of conjugation in the series benzene ($\lambda_f = 262$ nm), naphthalene ($\lambda_f = 314$ nm), and anthracene ($\lambda_f = 379$ nm).

The fluorescence maxima of aromatic compounds with substituents differ from those of the parent hydrocarbons. Groups such as $-NH_2$, $-OH$, and $-SH$ have unshared electron pairs of energy higher than that of the π-electrons of aromatic molecules. These can be transferred into vacant π-orbitals belonging to the aromatic ring. Thus, the energy gap between the highest occupied and lowest unoccupied orbitals of the substituted molecule is considerably smaller than that between the highest occupied and lowest unoccupied orbitals of the unsubstituted (parent) molecule, and the wavelengths of fluorescence in the former are somewhat longer. For example, 1-naphthylamine fluoresces at 372 nm in hexane whereas naphthalene fluoresces at 314 nm in the same solvent.

Groups such as carboxyl and nitrile, which are electron-withdrawing, have localized, vacant, low-energy π-orbitals in the ground state of the substituted molecule. This type of substituent introduces a vacant orbital between the highest occupied and lowest unoccupied π-orbitals of the unsubstituted molecule. The energy gap between the highest occupied and lowest unoccupied orbitals of the substituted molecule is therefore smaller than the gap between the highest occupied and lowest unoccupied orbitals of the unsubstituted molecule. Fluorescence thus appears at longer wavelengths in the substituted molecule than in the unsubstituted molecule. For example, the fluorescence of 2-naphthoic acid lies at 344 nm in hexane, 30 nm longer in wavelength than the fluorescence of naphthalene.

When an electron-withdrawing group and an electron-donating group are attached to the same aromatic ring, fluorescence may be viewed as involving transition between the lone-pair orbital of the donor group and the vacant π-orbital of the acceptor group. In this case, the energy of the transition is lower and, thus, the fluorescence wavelength is longer than when either group alone is attached to the ring. When two donor groups or two acceptor groups are attached to the aromatic ring, the position of the fluorescence band is usually determined by the donor group with the highest energy lone pair or the acceptor group with the lowest energy vacant orbital.

Solvent Effects

The solvents in which fluorescence spectra are observed play a major role in determining the spectral positions and intensities with which fluorescence bands occur. In some cases, the solvent may determine whether fluorescence is to be observed at all.

Solvent interactions with solute molecules are predominately electrostatic in nature and may be classified as dipolar or hydrogen-bonding. The position of the fluorescence band maximum in one solvent, relative to that in another, depends on the relative separations between ground and excited state in either solvent and, therefore, the relative strengths of ground- and excited-state solvent stabilization.

If the excited state of a polar molecule has a higher dipole moment than its ground state (most molecules are in this class), the excited state will be more stabilized by interaction with a polar solvent than will the ground state. As a result, upon going from a less polar to a more polar solvent, the fluorescence spectrum will shift to longer wavelengths. In a few cases, the ground state of a solute is more polar than the excited state. In this case, going to a more polar solvent stabilizes the ground state more than the excited state, causing a shift to shorter wavelengths with increasing solvent polarity.

Hydrogen-bonding solvents having positively polarized hydrogen atoms are said to be protic solvents. They interact with the nonbonded and lone electron pairs of solute molecules. Hydrogen-bonding solvents having atoms with lone or nonbonded electron pairs are called hydrogen-bond acceptor solvents. They interact with positively polarized hydrogen atoms on electronegative atoms belonging to the solute molecules (e.g., in $-COOH$, $-NH_2$, $-OH$, $-SH$). Because most hydrogen-bonding solvents are also polar, hydrogen-bonding and nonspecific dipolar interaction are usually both present as modes of solvation of functional molecules. Accordingly, the spectral shifts actually observed on going from one solvent to another are a composite of dipolar and hydrogen bonding effects that may be constructively or destructively additive.

Protic solvents interacting with functional groups that are electron-withdrawing in the excited state (e.g., carbonyl) enhance charge transfer by introducing a partial positive charge into the electron acceptor group. This stabilizes the excited state relative to the ground state so that the fluorescence spectra shift to longer wavelengths, and often the quantum yield of fluorescence increases with increasing hydrogen-bond donor capacity of the solvent. Increasing protic nature of the solvent produces shifts to shorter wavelengths and usually lower fluorescence efficiencies when interacting with lone pairs on functional groups, which are electron donors in the excited state (e.g., $-OH$, $-NH_2$). Hydrogen-bond acceptor solvents produce shifts to longer wavelengths and higher fluorescence efficiencies by solvating hydrogen atoms on functional groups that are electron donors in the excited state (e.g., $-OH$, $-NH_2$). This is a result of partial withdrawal of the positively charged proton from the functional group that facilitates transfer of electronic charge away from the functional group. Finally, solvation of hydrogen atoms on functional groups that are charge transfer acceptors in the excited state (e.g., carboxyl) inhibits charge transfer by leaving a residual negative charge on the functional group. This results in shifting of the fluorescence spectrum to higher frequency and gives rise to lower quantum yields of fluorescence.

The same considerations are applicable to the influence of the solvent on the phosphorescence wavelength, but the shifts are much smaller than in the case of fluorescence.

pH Effects

The effects of solution acidity and basicity on luminescence spectra result from the dissociation of acidic functional groups or protonation of basic functional groups associated with the aromatic portions of fluorescing and phosphorescing molecules. Protonation or dissociation can alter the natures and rates of nonradiative processes competing with luminescence and, thereby, affect the quantum yields of emission. For example, the antimalarial mefloquine fluoresces very weakly but phosphoresces well in neutral aqueous media. However, at pH < 1, its protonated form fluoresces intensely, and its phosphorescence is very weak.

Protonation and dissociation alter the relative separations of the ground and excited states of the reacting molecules and thereby cause shifting of the luminescence spectra. The shifts tend to be greater in fluorescence spectra than in phosphorescence spectra and are attributable to the electrostatic stabilization or destabilization of the excited state, relative to the ground state, produced by protonation and dissociation. The protonation of electron-withdrawing groups such as carboxyl, carbonyl, and pyridinic nitrogen causes shifts of the luminescence spectra to longer wavelengths, whereas the protonation of electron-donating groups such as the amino group produces spectral shifts to shorter wavelengths. The protolytic dissociation of electron-donating groups such as hydroxyl or sulfhydryl produces spectral shifts to longer wavelengths, whereas the dissociation of electron-withdrawing groups such as carboxyl produces shifting of the photoluminescence spectra to shorter wavelengths.

One of the interesting aspects of acid-base reactions of fluorescent molecules in fluid solutions is derived from the occurrence of protonation and dissociation during the lifetime of the excited state. This phenomenon affects the dependence of fluorescence on pH and must be considered in the development of a fluorometric analysis in aqueous solutions.

The lifetimes of molecules in the lowest excited singlet state are typically of the order of 10^{-11}–10^{-7} s. Typical rates of prototropic reactions are 10^{11} dm^3 mol^{-1} s^{-1} or lower. Consequently, excited-state proton-transfer reactions may be competitive with radiative deactivation of the excited molecules.

In the event that excited-state proton transfer and radiative deactivation are temporally competitive, the quantum yield of fluorescence will demonstrate a complex dependence on the pH level of the solution. Because the electronic distribution of a molecule is usually much different in an excited state than in the ground electronic state, the variation in fluorescence intensity caused by the pH dependence of the quantum yield of fluorescence will occur in a pH region different from the pH region in which the fluorescence intensity depends on the absorbance of the analyte. This means that in an arylammonium ion, for example, which becomes more acidic in the lowest excited singlet state, one might observe fluorescence from the conjugate base at a pH level of zero, even though the pK_a level might be as high as 5.

Quenching

The emission of light by photoexcited luminescent molecules may be decreased or even eliminated by interactions with other chemical species. This phenomenon is called quenching of luminescence.

Two kinds of quenching are distinguished. In static quenching, complexation between the potentially luminescent molecule and the quencher takes place in the ground state. The complex, when excited, fails to luminesce. The efficiency of quenching is governed by the formation constant of the complex as well as by the

concentration of the quencher. The quenching of the fluorescence of doxorubicin by Fe(III) is an example.

In dynamic quenching, the quenching species and the potentially luminescent molecule react subsequent to photoexcitation of the latter and during the lifetime of its excited state. Dynamic quenching is also called diffusional quenching, and its efficiency depends on the viscosity of the solution, the lifetime of the excited state (τ^o) of the luminescent species, and the concentration of the quencher (Q). This is summarized in the Stern–Volmer equation (Eq. 1):

$$\Phi/\Phi_f^o = \frac{1}{1 + K_Q \tau^o [Q]} \tag{1}$$

where k_Q is the rate constant for encounters between quencher and potentially luminescing species, and Φ_f^o and Φ_f are the quantum yields of luminescence in the absence and presence of concentration of the quencher (Q), respectively.

Dynamic quenching is also characterized by the dependence of the actual lifetime of the excited state on (Q). In static quenching, the lifetime of the excited state is invariant with respect to (Q).

Concentration Effects

As the concentration of a potentially luminescent solute is increased, the frequency of encounters between solute molecules is increased. This often results in the formation of solute complexes at the expense of monomeric solute molecules. Obviously, such interactions will affect the fluorescence expected from a given solution based strictly on the formal concentration of monomers and can seriously affect the results of a fluorimetric analysis.

In solutions of moderate concentration, there are two types of excited state solute–solute interaction, which are common. An excited polymer, or excimer, may form through the aggregation of excited solute molecules with ground-state molecules of the same type. Fluorescence quenching and/or a spectral red shift may result. Also, a heteropolymeric excited-state complex may form between two different solute molecules. Such a complex is referred to as an exciplex.

The transfer of electronic excitation energy from one molecule to another is another phenomenon that is related to the concentration of potentially luminescent molecules. Energy transfer occurs quite frequently in nature, either by direct collision or even over distances as great as 50 Å or more by a radiationless mechanism by which the excitation energy is transmitted from the molecules that are originally excited (donors) to the recipient molecules (acceptors). The efficiency with which an excited donor will transfer its excitation energy to an acceptor molecule (rather than fluoresce) is a function of the lifetime of the excited state of the donor, the orientations of the donor and acceptor molecules with respect to one another, and the inverse sixth power of the distance between the donor and acceptor. The energy-transfer process quenches the fluorescence of the donor and often sensitizes the fluorescence of the acceptor.

Temperature Effects

At low temperature, the efficiency of luminescence is usually increased, and the spectra often become sharper. Both effects result from the increase in solution viscosity and thus a decrease in collisional deactivation. In addition to changes in intensity, wavelength shifts also occur when the temperature of a medium is changed. At very low temperature, fluorescence originates from an excited state that is locked into the ground-state equilibrium geometry and solvent cage. At room temperature, in fluid solutions, fluorescence occurs only after the molecular geometry and solvent cage of the fluoresce have adapted to the new electronic distribution characteristic of the excited state. The emitting excited state under fluid conditions is lower in energy than under rigid conditions and, therefore, the fluorescence under the latter circumstance will be at higher energy (shorter wavelength) than in the former.

QUANTITATIVE ANALYSIS

Luminescence spectroscopy is used more often in quantitative analysis than in any other application. The quantitative relationship between fluorescence intensity F and analyte concentration C is derived from the Beer–Lambert law:

$$I = I_0 10^{-\varepsilon Cl} \tag{2}$$

where I and I_0 are the intensities of exciting light transmitted through and incident on the sample, l is the length of the light path through the sample, and ε is the molar absorptivity of the molecular species of interest at the nominal wavelength of excitation. The intensity of light absorbed I_a is then:

$$I_a = I_0 - I_0 10^{-\varepsilon Cl} \tag{3}$$

If all molecules absorbing light fluoresced, then I_a would be the intensity of fluorescence. However, only the

fraction Φ_f fluoresces. The remaining fraction $1-\Phi_f$ returns to the ground state by nonradiative means. Thus:

$$F = \phi_f I_a = \phi_f I_0 (1 - 10^{-\varepsilon Cl}) \tag{4}$$

If the absorbance (εCl) of the sample is less than 0.02, then to within an approximately 2% error, Eq. 4 becomes:

$$F = 2.3 \phi_f I_0 \varepsilon Cl \tag{5}$$

in which F is linear with respect to C. It then remains only to prepare a standard solution of concentration C_S and having fluorescence intensity F_S to be compared with the unknown solution of concentration C_U and fluorescence intensity F_U according to:

$$C_u = \frac{F_u}{F_s} C_s \tag{6}$$

It should be noted that the conditions for Eq. 5 to obtain can be met by either working with very dilute solutions or by exciting in a region of the absorption spectrum where ε is small.

Of course, it is always prudent to prepare a calibration curve for several standard solutions to check the linearity of the F versus C plot before attempting the simple relative fluorimetry expressed in Eq. 6 for a large number of samples.

In the case of phosphorescence, the intensity P is related to the concentration of analyte, following similar lines of reasoning applied to fluorescence, according to:

$$P = \phi_{ST}\phi_P I_0(1 - 10^{-\varepsilon Cl}) \tag{7}$$

where Φ_{ST} and Φ_P are the quantum yields of intersystem crossing (the fraction of excited molecules converted from the lowest excited singlet state to the lowest triplet state) and phosphorescence (the fraction of molecules arriving in the lowest triplet state that are deactivated by phosphorescence), respectively. As is the case for fluorescence, Eq. 7 can be expanded and for weakly absorbing solutions can be made analogous to Eq. 6, according to:

$$C_u = \frac{P_u C_s}{P_s} \tag{8}$$

where P_u and P_s are the phosphorescence intensities of the unknown and standard samples, respectively. Eq. 8 is, therefore, the basis of simple quantitative phosphorimetry.

INSTRUMENTATION

The basic components of luminescence instrumentation are generally arranged as shown in Fig. 1. The sample is placed in a sample cell and excited by either ultraviolet or

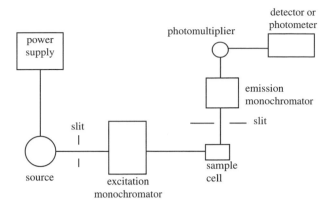

Fig. 1 General layout of luminescence instrumentation.

visible light from a source. A filter or monochromator may select a particular excitation wavelength region. The sample emits luminescence radiation in all directions, but only a portion is observed by the detection system that is usually set at 90° from the source of excitation to minimize the possibility of detecting stray light from the source. Another filter or monochromator may select the emission wavelength region, and a detector would convert the luminescence radiant flux into an electrical signal. An amplifier-readout system amplifies and processes the signal and displays it in the required form.

Sources

Sources of radiant energy are generally classified according to the spectral distribution of the radiation emitted. Continuum sources have a broad spectral distribution covering a large wavelength range. Line sources have spectra consisting of a number of sharp lines or bands. Lasers have allowed the use of extremely narrow bandwidths.

Continuum sources

Incandescent lamps are the simplest type of light source. They usually consist of a heated rod or filament of tungsten in an inert gas such as nitrogen or argon at a pressure of approximately 1 atm.

Radiation emitted by the lamp is caused by the temperature achieved by its filament, which in turn depends on the power input on the lamp. The radiation spectral distribution is a function of the temperature of the source and the wavelength, and this relationship is defined by the Planck black body equation:

$$B = \frac{2hc^2}{\lambda^5} \frac{1}{e^{hc/kT} - 1} \tag{9}$$

where B = spectral radiance in J/s m^2 nm sr; h = Planck's constant, 6.6262×10^{-34} J/s; c = velocity of light in a vacuum, 2.99792×10^8 m/s; λ = wavelength in nanometers; k = Boltzmann's constant, 1.38066×10^{-23} J/K; and T = absolute temperature in Kelvin.

A typical 500 W tungsten lamp operates at 3000 K with an emissivity of 0.4. If the spectral radiance is plotted against wavelength, the spectral radiance will have a maximum at approximately 1000 nm and swiftly drops at approximately 300 and 5000 nm, so that the tungsten lamp is most useful in the visible and near-infrared range.

Incandescent lamps are not sufficiently intense to be useful in luminescence spectrometry, although their stability cannot be matched by gas discharge and arc lamps.

Discharge lamps involve the application of voltage across two electrodes in a gas or metal vapor consisting of neutral atoms and/or molecules. If free electrons are introduced (through a high-voltage spark), then electrons are accelerated and excited, producing light emission. Gas discharge lamps use hydrogen, nitrogen, and the inert gases. Metal vapor discharge lamps use the more volatile metals such as mercury, cadmium, zinc, gallium, indium, and thallium.

With an increased voltage across the gap, higher states of excitation occur, and radiation at shorter wavelengths is emitted. When the voltage exceeds the ionization potential, the gas will be ionized by collisions resulting in increased current such that protons are accelerated to the cathode and electrons to the anode. The reformation of protonated gas atoms or molecules is very improbable at low pressures and currents because secondary electrons generated as ions may strike the cathode, neutralizing the protonated gas atom or molecule. When the secondary electrons are sufficient to maintain the discharge current, a glow discharge occurs. When the current is further increased, the cross-sectional area of the discharge increases proportionally, and the voltage becomes constant. To increase the current further, the voltage must be increased, resulting in increased brightness with a change to an arc discharge where a voltage drop occurs. A contraction in discharge into a smaller area on the cathode may also follow.

Depending on the pressure in the lamp, both line and continuum emission may be observed. Low-pressure lamps operated at low current densities and temperatures produce sharp atomic lines with little or no continuous background. Increasing pressure and temperature cause the lines to broaden and increase the intensity of the background continuum.

High-pressure xenon, mercury, or mercury–xenon arc lamps are the most common excitation sources because of their relatively high intensity, wide spectral range, and low cost. Commercially available xenon lamps are available in a wide range of power ratings and are usually operated on DC for greatest stability and longest life. Below 300 nm, the light output of the xenon lamp falls off sharply, such that the long wavelength peaks of the excitation spectrum are exaggerated and appear different from those in the absorption spectrum. Mercury–xenon lamps produce very intense light corresponding to the line emission spectrum of mercury (principal lines are at 254, 313, and 365 nm), and generally the light produced is more intense than that produced at any given wavelength by a xenon lamp of comparable power rating. However, these lamps emit very little light at other wavelengths, limiting the choice of excitation wavelength that may be used. However, because many substances have absorption spectra that overlap the mercury emission lines, they may be excited using the mercury–xenon lamp.

Pulsed discharge lamp (flash lamps) are used when high-intensity, short-lived pulses of exciting light are needed. A high-voltage capacitor is discharged across the gap, causing a short, high-current pulse to the lamp, and producing a very intense pulse of light.

The energy input to the lamp per flash is characteristic of lamp manufacture and is related to the capacitance and the voltage across the lamp:

$$Q = CV^2 \tag{10}$$

where Q = energy input in joules; C = capacitance in farads; and V = operating potential in volts.

The duration of the light flash is approximately equal to the duration of the current pulse through the lamp:

$$t_f = {}^1\!/_2 R_a C \tag{11}$$

where t_f = flash duration in seconds, and R_a = effective arc resistance in ohms.

The effective arc resistance is proportional to the arc gap length and is inversely related to the 2/3 power of the operating voltage. This implies that the shortest, most intense pulses are obtained from lamps with very short gap tubes that are operated under high voltage and low capacitance. The value of R_a for a particular lamp is given by the manufacturer and is specific for a set of conditions.

The peak input power per flash in watts is given by:

$$P_i = Q/t_f \tag{12}$$

and the peak light output per flash in watts is:

$$P_0 = \varepsilon P_i \tag{13}$$

where ε = efficiency of conversion (usually 0.25–0.5 for xenon lamps).

The average input electrical power in watts is:

$$\overline{P}_i = Qf \tag{14}$$

where f = repetition rate in hertz.

The manufacturer generally recommends the maximum P_i, value; higher-powered types may need to be forced air-cooled.

The average current drawn from the power supply is given by:

$$\overline{i} = VCf \tag{15}$$

The value of f should not exceed approximately 0.1 t_f^{-1} to prevent continuous ionization of the lamp.

The charging resistance R_c is selected so that its power rating is greater than the average input electrical power.

$$R_c = \frac{1}{5RC} \tag{16}$$

Xenon, nitrogen, and hydrogen flash lamps are available. The nature and pressure of the fill-gas affect the spectral distribution of the flash lamp.

The arc may appear narrow and filamentary when a xenon flash tube is operated below its maximum input power per flash because not all of the gas is ionized. The position of the arc tends to shift from flash to flash, causing erratic light output. It is generally not advisable to operate a flash tube very far below its maximum input.

Line sources

Glow discharge lamps (hollow cathode lamps) producing line spectra are quite similar to those propagating

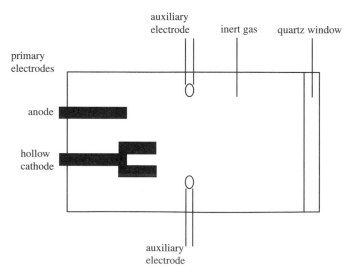

Fig. 2   Schematic diagram of a hollow cathode lamp.

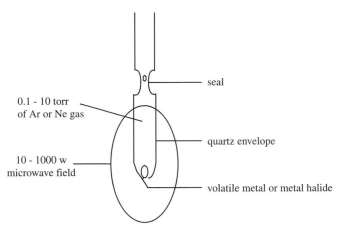

Fig. 3 Schematic diagram of an electrodeless discharge lamp.

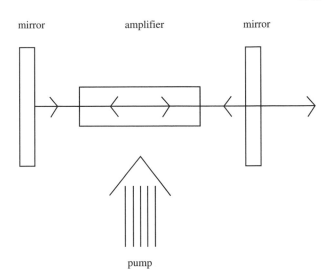

Fig. 4 Laser with conventional two-mirror cavity.

continuous spectra presented above. Accelerated electrons generate positive ions on collision with atoms of a carrier gas (Fig. 2). The ions gain energy in an electric field and collide with the cathode. Atoms of the cathode are released and are excited by inelastic collisions with the electrons. The excited metal atoms then emit light.

The lamps are usually sealed and may have auxiliary electrodes to excite atomic vapor. They are operated at DC but may be modulated and pulsed. If the primary current i_p introduced is too high, the lines emitted are self-reversed. However, this may be avoided by keeping i_p low and i_a (auxiliary current) high.

Electrodeless discharge lamps, or EDLs (Fig. 3), are easy to make, but the results obtained are not always reproducible owing to chemical effects with the walls of the lamp, poor outgassing, poor seal-off, etc. A tesla coil starter produces a few free electrons that are accelerated by a high-frequency electric field (through the use of radio- or microwaves). The electrons acquire enough energy to excite and ionize atoms produced by the thermal heating. The actual discharge is confined to a "skin effect," wherein the outer surface of the envelope minimizes self-reversal. Low pressures (0.1–1 torr) of argon or neon gas are used; helium is usually not used because it diffuses out of the quartz envelope and is not very stable in intensity.

The lamps may be operated as continuous wave sources or be modulated or pulsed. EDLs have a poor stability or poor shelf life in some cases, but they have high intensities, produce narrow spectral lines, and are relatively inexpensive.

Lasers

Modern tunable dye lasers have any of several advantages over conventional sources, including 1) extremely narrow linewidths, 2) high intensity, 3) collimation and excellent focusing abilities, 4) continuous tunability over certain wavelength regions, and 5) extremely short pulse duration. The primary disadvantages are their expense, relative complexity, and the difficulty to obtain wavelength-tunable laser output at wavelengths below 320 nm (nonlinear frequency mixing techniques may be used).

Lasers have three primary components (Fig. 4): 1) an active medium that amplifies incident electromotive waves, 2) an energy pump that selectively pumps energy into the active medium to populate selected levels and to achieve population inversion, and 3) an optical resonator, or cavity, composed of two opposite mirrors a set distance apart that store part of induced emission concentrated in a few resonator modes. A population inversion must be produced in the laser medium, deviating from the Boltzman distribution; thus, the induced emission rate exceeds the absorption rate, and an electromotive wave passing through the active medium is amplified rather than attenuated. The optical resonator causes selective feedback of radiation emitted from the excited species in the active medium. Above a pump threshold, feedback converts the laser ampler to an oscillator, resulting in emission in several modes.

The wavelength range over which the laser would operate depends on the spectral range over which the active medium and cavity have a net gain. Wavelength selection devices such as gratings, prisms, and etalons are placed in the cavity when restricting the lasing wavelength is desired; these reduce the gain of the cavity below lasing threshold for all the desired wavelengths.

The active medium in tunable dye lasers is a dye solution. The dyes are organic compounds with conjugated double bonds and have delocalized π electrons that can produce large absorption cross-sections. Because of the large dipole moments that can be generated, the spontaneous lifetime is short (<10 ns), and the quantum yield of fluorescence is large. Dye lasers are pumped by flashlamps, N_2 lasers, Cu vapor lasers, Nd-YAG, excimer, or Argon ion lasers. They oscillate within a broad band. Therefore, short pulses can be obtained.

Semiconductor lasers (laser diodes) have recently appeared as luminescence excitation sources. They have several outstanding advantages over gas and dye lasers and arc lamps as excitation sources. They are more powerful and more coherent light sources than arc lamps. They also have the advantage of producing a polarized beam that can be useful for certain applications. They are smaller, more compact, and much less expensive than other kinds of lasers, and the fact that most semiconductor lasers emit in the far-red or infrared means that less energy can be deposited in the sample so that considerably less thermal decomposition can occur than with conventional ion, excimer, and dye lasers. That until recently, emission from semiconductor lasers has been generally confined to the far-red and infrared has been a mixed blessing. On the one hand, the fact that so few substances demonstrate electronic absorption in that region of the electronic spectrum means that excitation with semiconductor laser light will be very selective. For example, the interfering luminescences of tryptophan and bilirubin from serum samples will not be problematic with semiconductor laser excitation because these substances are not excited by red light. On the other hand, because so few substances absorb red light, a new generation of fluorescent probes and labels is required for the labeling of analytes to be detected subsequent to chromatographic or immunochemical analysis.

Several of the polymethine dyes absorb in the red, far-red, and near-infrared and fluoresce efficiently as well in this spectroscopic region. Functional derivatives of these may provide excellent fluorescent labels for semiconductor laser excitation. Several research groups are currently actively involved in the synthesis and development of large polyunsaturated dye molecules that are excited and show luminescence in the red and near-infrared. This promises to be one of the most exciting areas of luminescence spectroscopy for the foreseeable future.

Wavelength Selection

The choice of limited spectral wavelength bands for excitation and emission is necessary to prevent the possibility of excitation and detection of emission from extraneous species and to spurious stray light. Mono-chromators and filters are used to select the wavelength areas of interest.

Filters

Filters are absorption type, made of tinted glass, gelatin-containing organic dyes lacquered or sandwiched between glass, or a solution of absorbing substances, or are interference filters.

Absorption filters selectively absorb portions of incident polychromatic light and allow the transmission of light of preferred wavelengths. There are three general classifications: 1) neutral tint, 2) cut-off filters, and 3) bandpass filters. Neutral tint or neutral-density filters have a nearly constant transmission over a range of wavelengths; they are used with strongly fluorescing compounds and decrease light intensity uniformly. Cut-off filters have a sharp cut-off in their transmittance characteristics; beyond a certain wavelength there is little or no transmittance. These are especially useful in preventing stray or unwanted light from falling on the detector. Bandpass filters either transmit or refuse a set wavelength band and are usually made from a series of cut-off filters.

An interference filter consists of two highly reflective but partially transmitting films of silver separated by a spacer film of completely transparent material (e.g., MgF_2). Light of wavelength corresponding to the optical separation of the silver films ($\pm 5-9$ nm), and integral multiples of this principal wavelength, are transmitted, whereas other wavelengths are eliminated by destructive interference. These filters are suited for intense sources because they absorb very little energy and rarely need to be cooled.

Monochromators

Monochromators are usually diffraction gratings with slit arrangements. Prisms were once used as monochromators but are now almost obsolete because gratings are much less expensive and less cumbersome. Polychromatic light is dispersed by the grating into its component wavelengths through constructive and destructive interference. Two types of gratings are available: transmission and reflection gratings.

A large number of parallel transparent and opaque lines are arranged alternately on a transmission grating; when a source is incident on one side of the grating, each transparent line acts as an independent line source of the original radiation. Interference will occur among the monochromatic light waves transmitted by the closely spaced transparent lines, causing an augmentation in light intensity at certain points and elimination at others.

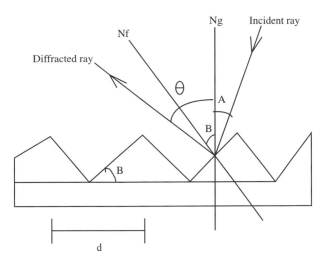

Fig. 5 Diffraction grating. Ng = normal to the grating; Nf = normal to the face of the grating; A = angle of incidence; Θ = angle of diffraction; d = grating spacing; and B = blaze angle.

A reflection grating is similar to a transmission grating except that it uses a large number of grooves on a reflective surface to cause the interference.

Fig. 5 shows a parallel light beam incident onto two adjacent grooves of a diffraction grating. At a wavelength and an angle of incidence A normal to the grating surface, constructive interference for an angle B is obtained:

$$m\lambda = d(\sin A \pm \sin B) \tag{17}$$

where m = order of interference.

The plus sign is taken if A and B are on the same side of the grating normal and the minus sign if they are not. If the light is reflected back into the direction of the incident light, the equation reduces to:

$$m\lambda = 2\,d\,\sin B \tag{18}$$

When $m = 0$, the angle of the incident radiation is equal to the angle of diffraction, and this corresponds to specular reflection of the incident radiation. When $m = 1$, the diffraction is said to be first-order and is the primary image of the spectrum. When $m = 2$, the diffraction is second-order and is the second image of the spectrum with a dispersion twice that of the first-order, and so forth for higher orders. This may cause interference. Therefore, a filter is used to eliminate higher-order spectra.

Two important factors in selecting a grating are its blaze angle and resolving power. The blaze angle e is dependent on the blaze wavelength. The output of a grating at a particular wavelength is compared with that of an aluminum mirror, and the blaze corresponds to the wavelength of maximum efficiency:

$$\Theta = \frac{A - B}{2} \tag{19}$$

A is fixed by the construction of the instrument, whereas B varies with A according to Eq. (17). The resolving power R depends on the number of grooves in the grating N and the order of interference:

$$R = mN \tag{20}$$

R is relatively independent of wavelength. A grating with a high resolution would produce better separation of the polychromatic light to its component wavelengths.

The excitation grating is on a turntable that when rotated allows light of different wavelengths to be focused through a slit and onto the sample. The sample would fluoresce, and the light would be channeled by the emission grating, which is also on a turntable, and is focused through another slit onto the detector.

Slits

Slits help focus light onto the monochromators and the detector; they regulate the wavelength range that excites and is emitted by the sample. Smaller slit widths are more selective, producing a narrower range of spectral bandpass (bandwidth at half the peak transmittance), but a decrease in transmitted light is noted and, therefore, there is a decrease in sensitivity. There are two types of slits: fixed and variable.

Fixed slits are cut in an opaque material. A series of these are found in instruments using fixed slits; the desired slit width is obtained by using any one in the group, and the results so obtained are reproducible.

Variable slits are used more commonly than fixed slits. There are two types available: unilateral or bilateral. Both involve the use of beveled blades attached to micrometers that allow the blades to shift a specified distance, although unilateral slits have only one movable blade; the other is fixed. Bilateral slits are preferred over unilateral slits because a constant center line is maintained with the former whereas that using the latter continuously changes as the slit width changes. Variable slits are more expensive but are more convenient for routine analysis. With constant use, the micrometer mechanism and blade edges become worn, resulting in a decrease in sensitivity and reproducibility. This is not considered a major problem in analytical work unless a precise knowledge of the slit widths is imperative.

Cell Compartments and Cells

Cell compartments are usually painted flat black to minimize stray light and are covered when the fluorimeter is in use to eliminate the entrance of external light. They are usually set such that the fluorescence emitted by the sample would be at a 90° angle to the line of entry of the exciting light. This arrangement decreases the interference of stray exciting light. If the sample has strong absorption at the excitation wavelength or is a solid, concentration quenching may occur, especially if the sample has a low quantum yield. Using a front-surface configuration, with the fluorescence emitted at 30° to the line of entry of the exciting light, may solve this problem. Solid sample holders with glass, quartz, or silica windows are also available.

Fluorescence cells are made of quartz, silica, or special optical glass. Glass cells are cheaper and are suitable for use with excitation wavelengths above 330 nm. For shorter wavelengths, quartz or silica cells have to be used. If analysis is to be performed at low temperatures, cryorefrigerators or Dewar flasks (Fig. 6) are used.

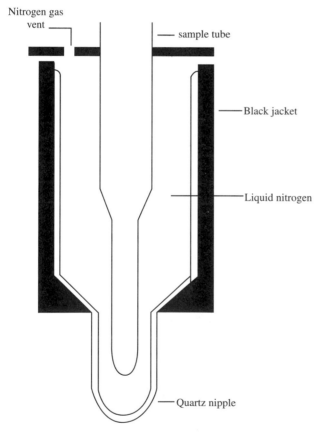

Fig. 6 Dewar flask.

At low temperatures, both fluorescence and phosphorescence may be detected when the sample in the Dewar flask is illuminated. If only phosphorescence is emitted by the sample, this setup may be used to measure phosphorescence. To isolate phosphorescence when both types of luminescence are present, a mechanical chopper with openings 180° apart is mounted in the sample compartment and rotated at a speed of several thousand revolutions per minute. This effectively cuts off the fluorescence because its lifetime is 10^{-11}–10^{-7} s, and the emitted light would have vanished completely in one quarter of a revolution. Phosphorescence has a longer lifetime (10^{-4} to several seconds) and will be registered by the detector.

Detectors

Photomultipliers

Photomultipliers are the most widely used photodetectors in fluorescence spectroscopy. They detect very low levels of light using secondary emission from a dynode chain (Fig. 7). A photomultiplier is made up of an evacuated glass or quartz tube containing a photocathode, a series of dynodes made of electron emissive material, and an anode. Fluorescence emitted by the sample strikes the photocathode, which in turn emits photoelectrons. These electrons are accelerated toward the first dynode, and more electrons are produced, hitting the second dynode and producing even more electrons, and so forth, until the last dynode, when electrons coming from the last dynode strike the anode. The anode current flows through the lead resistor, generating the signal voltage.

The amplification factor of the photomultiplier G depends on the electron gain per dynode g and the number of dynodes x:

$$G = g^x \tag{21}$$

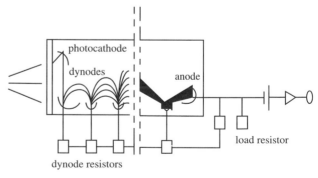

Fig. 7 Photomultiplier.

The amplification and gain per dynode of an ampler rely on the operating voltage. Thus, photomultipliers need a very stable high-voltage power supply. The spectral response depends on the cathode type and envelope material and is not affected by the electron multiplication process.

At room temperature, the noise in photomultipliers is predominantly shot noise, which is because of the fundamentally quantized nature of light energy and electrical current. Photons arrive at the cathode randomly, even though the overall intensity of light is constant. Photoelectrons emitted from the cathode arriving at the anode would thus do so randomly, even though the long-term rate of photoelectron pulses is constant and parallel to the light intensity:

$$i_s = \sqrt{2eBG\Delta f i_a} \tag{22}$$

where $B = 1 + g^{-1} + g^{-2} + \ldots + g^{-Z} = \sum_{y=0}^{z} g^{-y}$ and $f =$ electrical noise bandwidth in hertz.

The equation for shot noise current i_s owing to the total anodic current (photocurrent plus thermionic current) i_a a takes into consideration the gain of the tube G. Shot noise may often be reduced by increasing the measurement time because this would increase the signal-to-noise ratio. The thermionic component of the noise may be reduced by cooling the tube. There is a minimum temperature to which the tube may be cooled. Exposure of the tube to high light levels may cause changes in the sensitivity of the tube, and photomultipliers must never be exposed to room light or irreversible damage may result. A fatigued tube may often be restored by operating it in the dark for some time at the normal operating voltage. The cathode or anode currents must not exceed the ratings specified by the manufacturer. Photomultipliers usually have a response time of less than 10^{-8} s, which is rapid enough to detect most fluorescence decay-times.

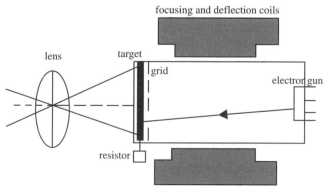

Fig. 8 Photoconductive target vidicon.

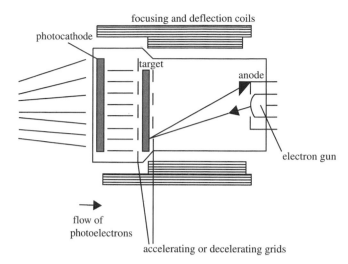

Fig. 9 Return beam vidicon.

Image detectors

Vidicons are of two types: the photoconductive target vidicon (1) and the image orthicon, or return beam vidicon (2). In the former (Fig. 8), light incident on a target previously biased by an electron beam would cause a charge separation in the photosensitive material. The carriers of the charge discharge the bias proportionate to the amount of light striking each local area, or pixel. When the raster-scanned beam returns to this region, it replaces the bias, and a signal is detected as the voltage across the load resistor is detected. The illuminated pixels cause an increase in the signal.

The return beam vidicon (Fig. 9) uses a photocathode to detect the light image. The photoelectrons are formed on a target composed of a secondary electron emitter similar to the dynodes in a photomultiplier, and secondary electrons produced are collected by a mesh, leaving the target with an image stored in the form of positively charged areas corresponding to the lit parts of the photocathode image. A low-velocity electron beam scans the target surface, and electrons are absorbed from the beam where the target is charged; the beam is scattered only in areas of little or no charge. An anode finally collects the scattered electrons. Unlike the photoconductive target vidicon, illuminated areas in the image orthicon cause a decrease in signal current.

Intensified vidicons (Fig. 10) detect photoelectrons instead of photons. There are two groups: in SEC vidicons, the target is a secondary electron conductor such as MgO, KCl, MgF, and Ag, whereas silicon-intensified target (SIT) vidicons have silicon diode arrays as their targets. SEC vidicons are approximately 10 times more sensitive

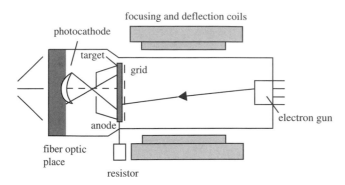

Fig. 10 Intensified target vidicon.

than ordinary vidicons, and SIT vidicons are up to 500 times more sensitive: they are capable of single-photon detection (3). The use of the latter is limited by its high noise level; however, cooling the tube and shutting the readout beam off can lower the noise by increasing the integration time (4).

Charge-coupled devices (CCD)

CCD sensors provide a higher sensitivity to light than do common detectors and photographic film, allowing for the acquisition of weaker signals. This technology has revolutionized the use of fluorescent microscopes in the biomedical sciences and has begun to have an impact on fluorescent-based analytical systems.

A CCD chip is an array of light-sensitive elements that are in fact small electronic capacitors. These capacitors are charged by the electrons generated by the emitted light. In fact, each photon that reaches the CCD array's atoms displaces some electrons that are providing a current source. These current sources are localized in small, delimited areas (the capacitors) called pixels.

Common CCD chips are composed of several pixels, for example, 192 × 165, 512 × 512, 1024 × 1024, or more. It is easy to understand that it is physically impossible to individually access each pixel. In fact, a CCD sensor provides only one serial output, through which each capacitor can be discharged (each pixel can be read). The capacitors are disposed in lines, and there are some control gates that allow the transfer of one pixel line into the next. The last line of the array can be transferred into a horizontal shift register. This shift register allows the transfer of one pixel to the next, and the last pixel of this horizontal register is connected to the output gate.

The CCD chip has one clock entry for the vertical transfer, one for the transfer gate, and one for the shift register. Thus, read out the signal, one must first transfer the last line into the shift register by providing a clock pulse on the transfer gate control pin. Then one has to provide one clock pulse on the shift register control pin for the reading of each point of this line. Finally, one must provide one clock pulse on the vertical transfer. The high number of pixels allows increases sensitivity and spatial resolution.

If a CCD array is used in a warm environment (20°C), the photosensitive area atoms produce a current, which produces noise. To reduce this noise, the CCD array atoms should be cooled so that their thermal excitation is reduced. The CCD is cooled by two primary processes: 1) electrical and 2) chemical.

Cooling a CCD by use of liquified gas is most efficient but is still reserved for the highest sensitivity purposes. This is primarily owing to the equipment needed to store and use such liquids. Thus, the most commonly used process is the use of a thermoelectric cooler, also known as a Peltier cell. It is a device working as a heat pump. The heat contained in one face of the cells is transferred to the other. These cells should be powered by direct current. Efficiency improvement of such a cell can be performed by cooling its hot face. To provide substantial cooling of the CCD, it is possible to use two Peltier cells in addition to a water- or glycol-cooling system. The first cell cools down the CCD, the second cools the first, and the liquid circuit evacuates the heat provided by the second Peltier cell.

Signal Processing

These systems amplify and process the electrical signal from the detector and show it in a read-out form. The electrical noise bandwidth is usually determined by the system, which in turn influences the amount of noise of the signal and determines the response time of the system.

DC amplifiers

DC amplifiers are the simplest and least expensive of the electronic measurement systems. They are most commonly found in commercially available fluorimeters. Ideally, the amplifier stage of a circuit contributes little or no noise to the system; the photomultiplier should produce only the noise associated with perfect performance of the photocathode and the electron multiplication process described above. However, the anode dark current of the photomultiplier adds to the noise in the signal, and the amplifier makes its own contribution to the total noise. It is therefore imperative to select the proper photomultiplier tube with low dark current so as to have a higher signal-to-noise ratio.

Photon counting

The current pulse from a single photon event would be noted at the anode as an approximate million electrons and a pulse width in nanoseconds. The amplifier changes the anode current pulse into a pair of voltage signals with sufficient gain and output impedance to couple it to the discriminator, which then shapes the pulse and rejects those below a set minimum threshold. The maximum count rate of less than 10^{7} pulses/s determined by the pulse pair resolution of the amplifier-discriminator limits pulse counting, but methods to increase the upper limit by multilevel discrimination (5) and DC switching at high light levels (6) have been described.

Correction of Spectra

Excitation and emission spectra obtained from most instruments are dependent on the wavelength-sensitive components of the particular system. To compensate for these and the different amounts of light loss per instrument, corrections for instrumental characteristics are necessary to obtain the true spectra. The results allow intrainstrument spectral comparisons to be made. Although self-correcting instruments are commercially available, these are generally too complicated and expensive for routine analytical work.

Excitation spectra may be corrected using a constant response thermopile, a chemical actinometer, a standardized phototube, or a reference compound. The latter two methods also may be used for correcting emission spectra. By reporting fluorescence intensities in relation to reference compounds, one guards against the source and photomultiplier aging characteristics of a given instrument. Any stable fluorescent compound with broad excitation and emission bands is suitable for this purpose.

SPECIAL TOPICS

The following spectroscopic topics are viewed as current areas of analytical interest. Many review articles give a more thorough discussion of these subjects, and these are cited accordingly.

Chemiluminescence

Fluorescence initiated by chemical reactions is called chemiluminescence. It is a common phenomenon in flames in which free radicals are oxidized by molecular oxygen but occurs rarely in solution because many of the reactive species necessary for the generation of chemiluminescence have very short lifetimes in solution. Phosphorescence as a form of chemiluminescence does not exist in solution because of quenching of the triplet state in the liquid phase.

A number of chemiluminescent reactions are known. The oxidation of 3-aminophthalhydrazide (luminol) has been studied extensively (7–14). The emission resulting from the reaction of certain oxalic acid derivatives is another outstanding example (15). When chemiluminescence occurs in living organisms, it is called bioluminescence. The best known example is observed in the firefly *Photinus pyralis*. Many review articles have been written about different aspects of bioluminescence; for overviews one should consult those by Gundermann and McCapra (16) and by Campbell (17).

Because chemiluminescence does not require photo-excitation, a lamp and excitation monochromator are unnecessary. Conventional fluorometric spectrophotometers may be used to measure chemiluminescence except that the excitation optics are not used.

Fiber Optic Sensors

The fiber optic fluorometer is a recent development that shows great promise for in situ fluorometry. In this device, the sample compound and cell are replaced by a fiber optic cable. Light from a source travels along an optically conducting fiber to its end where absorption, reflection, or scattering of light or fluorescence occurs. Fluorescence sensors comprise the largest group of fiber optic sensors; fluorescence sensors based on principles of direct fluorescence measurement, both single- and dual-wavelength (18, 19), fluorescence quenching (20, 21), or competitive binding (22) are available. Owing to the paucity of directly fluorescent analytes, most fluorescent optical sensors (FLOPS) are based on quenching by the analyte of the sensor fluorophore.

Instrumentation essentially consists of a light source, optical filters (if necessary), the fiber optic, a sensing zone (to which a fluorescent probe is usually covalently bound), and a detector. Lasers; xenon lamps; hydrogen-, deuterium-, mercury-, and halogen lamps; and light-emitting diodes (LEDs) have been used as excitation sources. Lasers provide high-intensity excitation with a narrow bandwidth and are especially suited for remote sensing where light losses are large. However, they are quite expensive and require a heavy power supply. The most promising light sources are the LEDs; these run at a low voltage and current, are small, have long life spans, and do not generate heat. However, they do have the disadvantage of working only from the IR region down to the blue. Fiber optic fluorescence spectrometers may be operated in a continuous or pulsed excitation mode. The latter allows for the application of time-resolved fluorometry. The material of the optical fiber would determine the wavelength used. Fused silica, glass, and plastic fibers have all been used. Silica can be used from the ultraviolet range down to 220 nm, but the fibers are expensive. Glass is suitable for use in the visible region and is reasonably priced. Plastic fibers are the lowest in cost but are limited to use above 450 nm. Measurements may be processed directly using analog and digital circuits or a microprocessor. Photomultipliers, photodiodes, photoconductor cells, photovoltaic light detectors, and CCDs have all been used as detectors.

Fiber optic sensors are less expensive, more rugged, and smaller than electrodes, which currently dominate in sensor-based analysis. In the future, we may see the former replacing the latter in various areas of analytical and clinical chemistry. Fields of application include groundwater and pollution monitoring; process control; remote spectroscopy in high-risk areas with radioactive, explosive, biological, or other hazards; titrimetry; and biosensing. Different aspects of optical sensing have been the subject of several studies (23–25). The field of FLOPS is currently one of the most active in analytical spectroscopy.

Luminescence Detection in Separation Methods

A limitation of the application of luminescence spectroscopy to the analysis of real samples is its lack of specificity owing to similarities in spectral bandshapes and spectral positions of the luminescence spectra of many compounds. An obvious solution to this problem is the separation of the analytical sample's interfering constituents from each other before quantitation by fluorescence. High-performance liquid chromatography (HPLC) and related separation methods can be coupled to fluorescence spectroscopy to take advantage of the sensitivity of the spectroscopic method and the specificity of the separation method.

Luminescence affords a very sensitive means of detection in flowing systems such as HPLC, electrophoresis, flow injection, and flow cytometry. HPLC fluorescence detectors are similar in operation to conventional fluorimeters. Most fluorescence detectors use filters for crude monochromation. Filters pass light in a wider band than do monochromators. This favors spectral sensitivity because more light excites the sample and is collected by the detector. Grating monochromators, on the other hand,

favor selectivity. The fluorimetric detector is susceptible to the usual interferences that hinder fluorescence measurements, namely, background fluorescence and quenching.

In the operation of a fluorimetric HPLC detector, the light from a UV or visible source is monochromated to some degree and focused on the cell that is on line with and receiving the effluent of the separatory column. Fluorescence is emitted by the sample in all directions so that the emitted light can be measured with the detector at right angles to the path of the exciting light and the direction of fluid flow. Stray or scattered excitation light is then blocked from the detector by a filter, and the emitted energy is then measured using a suitable detector. It is important to recognize that the solvent has a strong effect on the intensity of fluorescence. The solvent also scatters light owing to the Raman effect. This light is of slightly lower energy than the exciting light. For this reason, the emission wavelength is selected to be longer than that of the scattered Raman light. Flow cells have been designed that can be used for both fluorescence and absorption measurements. Quantitation can be considerably improved by simultaneously monitoring the absorbance and fluorescence signals that extend the linear dynamic range for fluorescent samples. At high sample concentrations in which the absorbance at the excitaiton wavelength is greater than 0.02, fluorescence intensity becomes nonlinear with concentration. At these higher concentrations, however, the light absorbance of the sample is often measurable and linear with concentration. Fluorescence, however, is often detectable at concentrations from 10^3 to 10^9 times lower than those in which absorbance is detectable.

The laser as an excitation source for luminescence detection in chromatography has become popular because of its high excitation power and its highly focused beam. The high degree of collimation of the laser beam has made it an excellent excitation source with the microbore cells, and tubing used is capillary zone electrophoresis. A typical laser beam can be focused into a spot a few microns in diameter. With laser excitation and fluorescence detected, capillary zone electrophoresis analyte concentrations below 1 attomole (at nanomole concentrations) have been measured. The advantages offered by the power and high degree of collimation of the laser as an excitation source can be exploited to measure the properties of a variety of particles including cells, algae, bacteria, larvae, etc., that either show native fluorexcence or can form fluorescent adducts. A well-defined flow of isolated particles is achieved by using hydrodynamic focusing. The particle flux is interrogated by a laser beam, which excited one particle at a time. Single-cell passage is guaranteed by adjusting the two flows; thus, collision between two cells (particles) is avoided. The method allows high-speed analysis of the cells and is called flow cytometry or fluorescent cell-sorting.

Time and Phase-Resolved Fluorimetry

The spectroscopy described thus far is based on the measurement of the intensity of fluorescence produced under steady-state conditions of excitation. Steady-state fluorimetry is derived from the excitation of the sample with a continuous beam of exciting radiation. The lamps and the power supplies used in conventional fluorimeters are sources of continuous radiation. After a short period of initial excitation of the sample, a steady state is established in which the rate of excitation of the analyte is equal to the sum of the rates of all processed, deactivating the lowest excited singlet state including fluorescence. When the steady state is established, the observed fluorescence intensity becomes time-invariant and produces the temporally constant signal that is measured by the photodetector. With the development of modern electro-optical components, it has become possible to excite a potentially fluorescent sample with a pulsed flash lamp that emits its radiation in bursts of 2–10 ns in duration with approximately 0.2 ms between pulses. Pulsed lasers generate even shorter duration pulses (typically down to 1 ps). A fluorescent sample excited by a single pulse will decay exponentially until the next pulse again excites the sample. The fluorescence from the sample excited by the pulsed source can be represented, after detection, as a function of time on a fast sampling oscilloscope used in conjunction with a multichannel pulse analyzer. The former approach is called pulse fluorimetry and the latter time-correlated single-photon counting. In either case, fluorescences with decay-times much longer than the lamp-pulse characteristics can be analyzed from a semilogarithmic plot of fluorescence intensity against time, which will yield a straight line (or a series of overlapping lines if several fluorophores have comparable but not identical decay-times) whose slope is proportional to the decay-time and whose vertical axis intercept can be compared with that of a standard solution of the fluorophore for quantitative analysis. If, however, the lamp pulse-time and the decay-time of the fluorophore are comparable, the lamp characteristics must be subtracted from the observed signal to obtain the fluorophore's decay characteristics. This is usually accomplished by using a computer to deconvolute the composite temporal characteristics of the lamp and the fluorophore output.

The pulsed source (time-resolved) method then distinguishes between the emissions of several fluorescing species by using their decay-times rather than their fluorescence intensities. This means that several strongly overlapping fluorescences such as those of catecholamines can be quantitated simultaneously without chemical or mechanical separation.

Time-resolved fluorimetry is also useful for the elimination of interferences from stray light caused by Rayleigh and Raman scatter. The latter phenomena occur on a time scale of 10^{-14}–10^{-13} because they have a much shorter duration than lamp or laser pulses. This light associated with them can be eliminated from the signal that ultimately reaches the detector. Data taken on one time-resolved fluorometer can be directly compared with that from another. This is not possible in steady-state fluorometry unless correcting wavelength variable instrumental response has been affected.

Phase fluorimetry is another useful fluorimetric technique for the determination of substances with overlapping fluorescence spectra. In phase fluorometry, the phase angle between the lamp pulse and the emission of fluorescent light allows for discrimination between fluorescences of different origin. For additional reading on this subject, see the excellent review by Demas (26).

With the introduction of powerful computers and advanced programs, traditional fluorescent devices are pushing the fringes of detection. It is now possible to observe events at a single molecule level. Information from these studies is refining our understanding of biochemistry and cell trafficking of molecules (28).

REFERENCES

1. Lubszynski, H.G. Review of TV Camera Tubes and Electron Optics. Adv. Electron. Electron. Phys. **1979**, *52*, 11.
2. Redington, R.W. *Photoelectronic Imaging Devices*; Biberman, L.M., Nudelman, S., Eds.; Plenum Press: New York, 1971; 2, 193–202.
3. Milch, J. Slow Scan Sit Detector for X-Ray-Diffraction Studies using Synchrotron Radiation. IEEE Trans. Nucl. Sci. **1979**, NS-*26*, 338.
4. Gruner, S.M.; Milch, J.R.; Reynolds, G.T. Evaluation of Area Photon Detectors by a Method Based on Detective Quantum Efficiency (DQE). IEEE Trans. Nucl. Sci. **1978**, NS-*25*, 562–565.
5. Gustafson, T.L.; Lytle, F.E.; Tobias, R.S. Sampled Photon Counting with Multilevel Discrimination. Rev. Sci. Instrum. **1978**, *49*, 1549–1550.
6. Marino, D.F.; Ingle, J.D., Jr. Microprocessor-Based Data Acquisition System for Chemiluminescence Measurements. Anal. Chem. **1981**, *53*, 1175–1179.
7. Gundermann, K.D. Chemiluminescence in Organic Compounds. Agnew. Chem. Int. Ed. Engl. **1965**, *4*, 566–572.

8. McCapra, F.Q. Chemiluminescence of Organic Compounds. Rev. Chem. Soc. **1996**, *20*, 485–572.
9. Haas, J.W., Jr. Chemiluminescent Reactions in Solutions. J. Chem. Educ. **1967**, *44*, 396–402.
10. White, E.H.; Roswell, D.F. The Chemiluminescence of Organic Hydrazides. Acc. Chem. Res. **1970**, *3*, 54–62.
11. Cormier, M.J., Hercules, D.M., Lee, J., Eds.; *Chemiluminescence and Bioluminescence*; Plenum Press: New York, 1973.
12. Gundermann, K.D. Recent Advances in Research on the Chemiluminescence of Organic Compounds. Top. Curr. Chem. **1974**, *46*, 61–65.
13. Roswell, D.F.; White, E.H. *Methods of Enzymology*; DeLuca, M.A., Ed.; Academic Press: New York, 1978; 57, 409.
14. Rauhut, M.M. *Encyclopedia of Chemical Technology,* 3rd Ed.; John Wiley & Sons: New York, 1979; 5, 416.
15. De Jong, G.J.; Kwakman, P.J.M. Chemiluminescence Detection for High Performance Liquid-Chromatography of Biomedical Samples. J. Chromatogr.-Biomed. **1989**, *492*, 319–343.
16. Decker, K.A.; Hinkkanen, A. Luminometric Determination of Flavin Adeninindinucleotide. Methods Enzymol. **1986**, *122*, 185–192.
17. Kricka, L.J. Chemiluminescence and Bioluminescence. Anal. Chem. **1999**, *71*, 305R–308R.
18. Saari, L.A.; Seitz, W.R. Immobilized Morin as Fluorescence Sensor for Determination of Aluminum (III). Anal. Chem. **1983**, *55*, 667–670.
19. Zhujun, Z.; Seitz, W.R. Optical Sensor for Oxygen Based on Immobilized Hemoglobin. Anal. Chem. **1986**, *58*, 220–222.
20. Lubbers, D.W. Opitz, N. Proceedings of the International Meeting on Chemical Sensors Fukuoka Japan. Elsevier: Amsterdam, 1983; 609–619.
21. Soper, S.A.; Warner, I.M.; McGown, L.B. Molecular Fluorescence, Phosphorescence, and Chemiluminescence Spectrometry. Anal. Chem. **1998**, *70*, 477R–494R.
22. Schultz, J.S. Affinity Sensor-A New Technique for Developing Implantable Sensors for Glucose and Other Metabolites. Diabetes Care **1982**, *5*, 245–253.
23. Seitz, W.R. Chemical Sensors Based on Fiber Optics. Anal. Chem. **1984**, *56*, 16A–34A.
24. Peterson, J.I.; Vurek, G.G. Fiber-Optic Sensors for Biomedical Applications. Science **1984**, *224*, 123–127.
25. Seitz, W.R. Optical Sensors for Clinical Applications. J. Clin. Lab. Anal. **1987**, *1*, 313–316.
26. Demas, J.N., Schulman, S.G., Eds.; *Molecular Luminescence Spectroscopy: Methods and Applications*; Part 2 Wiley-Interscience: New York, 1988; Chap. 2.
27. Weiss, S. Fluorescence Spectroscopy of Single Biomolecules. Science **1999**, *283*, 1676–1683.
28. Pederson, T. Movement and Localization of RNA in the cell nucleus. FASEB J. **1999**, *13*, S238–S242.
29. Hercules, D.M. *Fluorescence and Phosphorescence Analysis*; Wiley: New York, 1966.
30. Guilbault, G.G. *Fluorescence*; Marcel Dekker, Inc.: New York, 1968.
31. Parker, C.A. *Photoluminescence of Solutions*; Elsevier: Amsterdam, 1968.
32. Udenfriend, S. *Fluorescence Assay in Biology and Medicine*; Academic Press: New York, 1962,1968; 1, 2.
33. Becker, R. *Theory and Interpretation of Fluorescence and Phosphorescence*; Wiley: New York, 1970.
34. Pesce, A.; Rosen, G.; Pasby, T. *Fluorescence Spectroscopy*; Marcel Dekker, Inc.: New York, 1971.
35. White, C.; Argauer, R. *Fluorescence Spectrometry: A Practical Approach*; Marcel Dekker, Inc.: New York, 1971.
36. Winefordner, J.D.; Schulman, S.G.; O'Haver, T.C. *Luminescence Spectrometry in Analytical Chemistry*; Wiley: New York, 1972.
37. Zander, M. *Phosphorimetry*; Academic Press: New York, 1968.
38. Guilbault, G. *Practical Fluorescence*; Marcel Dekker, Inc.: New York, 1973.
39. Schenk, G. *Absorption of Light and Ultraviolet Radiation: Fluorescence and Phosphorescence Emission*; Allyn and Bacon: Boston, 1973.
40. Schulman, S.G. *Fluorescence and Phosphorescence Spectroscopy: Physicochemical Principles and Practice*; Pergamon: Oxford, 1977.
41. Wehry, E.L., Ed. *Modern Fluorescence Spectroscopy*; Plenum: New York, 1976,1981; 1–2, 3–4.
42. Lakowicz, J.R. *Principles of Fluorescence Spectroscopy,* 2nd Ed.; Plenum: New York, 1983,1999.
43. Schulman, S.G., Ed. *Molecular Luminescence Spectroscopy: Methods and Applications*; Part 1, Part 2, Part 3 Wiley-Interscience: New York, 1985, 1988, 1993.
44. Sharma, A.; Schulman, S.G. *Introduction to Fluorescence Spectroscopy*; Wiley-Interscience: New York, 1999.
45. Ichinose, N.; Schwedt, G.; Schnepel, F.M.; Adachi, K. *Fluorescence Analysis in Biomedical Sciences*; Wiley Interscience: New York, 1991.

SPECTROSCOPIC METHODS OF ANALYSIS—INFRARED SPECTROSCOPY

Marilyn D. Duerst
University of Wisconsin-River Falls, River Falls, Wisconsin

INTRODUCTION

Infrared (IR) spectroscopy refers broadly to the study of the interaction between matter and infrared radiation. Infrared radiation falls in the region between the visible and microwave parts of the electromagnetic spectrum, with wavelengths from 0.7 to 500 μm. Infrared spectroscopists often express this region of the spectrum in units of wavenumbers (symbol cm^{-1}) which refers to the number of waves per centimeter. This region (14,000 to 20 cm^{-1}) is usually subdivided into three regions: from 14,000 to 4000 cm^{-1} is called "near-infrared," from 4000 to 400 cm^{-1} the "mid-infrared," and from 400 to 20 cm^{-1} the "far-infrared." The mid-infrared region is widely used in the analysis of drugs and pesticides, and will be the focus of discussion here.

Chemical compounds absorb infrared radiation when there is a dipole moment change (in direction and/or magnitude) during a molecular vibration, molecular rotation, or molecular rotation-vibration. Absorptions are also observed with combinations, differences or overtones of molecular vibrations. A specific type of molecule is limited in the number of vibrations and rotations it is allowed to undergo. Therefore, each chemical compound has its own specific set of absorption frequencies and thus exhibits its own characteristic IR spectrum. This unique property of a compound allows the organic chemist to identify and quantify an unknown sample. (A special infrared technique called vibrational circular dichroism (VCD) is required to distinguish optical isomers).

Certain functional groups in a molecule (e.g., hydroxyl, carbonyl, and amine) absorb IR radiation and exhibit absorption bands at characteristic frequencies regions regardless of the structure of the rest of the molecule. These bands are termed "group frequencies." They are predictable and allow the analyst to deduce important structural information about an unknown molecule. An IR spectrum can be rapidly recorded for any phase, i.e. solid, liquid, or vapor. By coupling IR spectroscopy with other analytical techniques such as nuclear magnetic resonance (NMR) spectroscopy and mass spectrometry, the organic chemist can determine the structure of an unknown compound.

The introduction of the Fourier transform infrared (FTIR) spectrometer has revolutionized the entire field of IR spectroscopy. The typical FTIR spectrometer has a number of advantages over the conventional dispersive IR spectrometer in terms of the resolution of bands in the spectrum and the speed of acquiring the spectrum. Because of continuous improvements in sampling techniques, analysis software, and instrumentation hardware, the FTIR spectrometer has become increasingly more valuable in many areas from fundamental research to quality control to on-line process control. Recently, much interest has been focused on coupling the FTIR spectroscopic technique with chromatographic and other analytical techniques such as gas chromatography (GC–FTIR), GC-mass spectrometry (GC–MS–FTIR), high-performance liquid chromatography (HPLC–FTIR), supercritical fluid chromatography (SFC–FTIR), thin-layer chromatography (TLC–FTIR), and thermogravimetric analysis (TGA–FTIR). These methods, often termed "hyphenated techniques," employ IR spectroscopy as a means of detection to identify an unknown substance in a chromatographic eluent. Used in conjunction with a proper interfacing and sampling techniques, the limit of detection in some studies can also be in the picogram range, especially with the FTIR microscope.

This general approach will discuss the fundamental principles, instrumentation, and current applications of IR spectroscopy. Numerous reference materials, covering all aspects of infrared spectroscopy, have been published over the years (1–3). For a more in-depth understanding of the theory and instrumentation, readers can refer to the bibliography and references listed at the end of this article.

THEORY

The electromagnetic spectrum includes radiation from cosmic rays to radio waves, with wavelengths ranging from 10^{-9} nm to longer than 1000 km. In progression from short to long wavelengths, the types of radiation included in the spectrum are gamma rays, X-rays, far-, middle-, and near-ultraviolet rays, visible light, infrared rays, and microwaves.

Electromagnetic radiation may be conceptualized as a wave traveling at the speed of light (c) in a vacuum, where c is approximately 3.0×10^8 m/s. The frequency (v) is related to the wavelength by Eq. 1.

$$c = v\lambda \tag{1}$$

The wavelength, in units of cm or μm, is defined as the distance between peaks or troughs of the wave. The frequency of the wave is the number of peaks passing a fixed point per unit of time. The unit of frequency is the Hertz, i.e., the cycles or waves per second.

In infrared spectroscopy, the wavenumber, v, is often used instead of frequency, and is related to wavelength according to Eq. 2.

$$v = 1/\lambda \tag{2}$$

The wavenumber, in units of cm^{-1}, is the number of waves per centimeter. It is directly proportional to the frequency, but is not the same as frequency, as shown in Eq. 3.

$$c = v\lambda, \quad \text{thus} \quad v = v/c \tag{3}$$

The relationship between wavenumber (in cm^{-1}) and wavelength (in μm) is given by Eq. 4.

$$\underline{v} = 10^4/\lambda \tag{4}$$

INFRARED SPECTROSCOPY

Electromagnetic radiation may also be considered as photons traveling at the speed of light. The energy of a photon (E) is related to the wavelength (λ), frequency (v), and velocity of light (c) by Eq. 5, where h is Planck's constant ($h = 6.626 \ 10^{-34}$ J/s).

$$E = hv = hc/\lambda \tag{5}$$

In all spectroscopic techniques, the interaction of radiation with the molecule results in the transfer of energy to the molecule. The energy absorbed by the molecule is quantized, that is, the absorption is specific to the frequency of the radiation. Depending on the energy of the photons, the effect of an increase in energy in the molecule could cause reorientation of nuclear or electron spin states (if the molecule were in a magnetic field), changes in the energy of the valence electrons, changes in the vibrational-rotational energy, ejection of inner electrons from the molecule, or changes in the nucleus.

The absorption of IR radiation changes the rotational and/or vibrational energy states of the molecules. The IR absorption spectrum of a molecule may appear as a set of broad bands rather than discrete lines because each vibrational energy change is accompanied by a number of rotational energy changes. Three main types of absorption involving vibrations include the fundamental vibration, overtones, and combinations. The fundamental vibrational absorption bands usually appear in the mid-infrared region. It is important to realize that a molecule absorbs incident infrared radiation only when the molecular vibrational frequency is the same as the frequency of the incident radiation, and if the vibration of the atoms results in a change in the dipole moment. A symmetrical vibration does not result in a change of dipole moment; therefore, no infrared absorption will occur.

Two main types of fundamental vibrations are stretching and bending. Stretching vibrations usually appear at higher frequencies than bending vibrations. A stretching vibration consists of the movement of the atom along the bond axis, which results in changes in bond length. A bending vibration consists of a change in bond angles between bonds with a common atom. Fig. 1 shows the typical stretching and bending vibrational modes of a —CH$_2$— group within a molecule.

The intensity of vibrational absorption is proportional to the square of the magnitude of the dipole moment change. For a small dipole-moment change, the absorption band is weak, whereas a large, permanent dipole moment, such as that in a carbonyl group, exhibits strong absorption in the infrared when the carbon-oxygen distance is changed.

The stretching frequency is affected by the masses of the atoms and the strength of the bonds (i.e., the "stiffness" of the chemical bond) connecting them. Their relationship can be approximated by Eq. 6.

$$v = (1/2\pi c)(f/u)^{1/2} \tag{6}$$

where $\underline{v}$ is the the vibrational frequency (cm^{-1}), c the velocity of light (cm/s), f the force constant of the bond (mN/m or dyn/cm), u the reduced mass of the two atoms, m_1 and m_2, or $u = (m_1 m_2)/(m_1 + m_2)$.

The spatial orientation of atoms with respect to each other also affects their vibrational frequency. For example, the coupling or interaction of two fundamental vibration groups of similar frequencies in close proximity within a molecule and the inter- or intramolecular hydrogen bonding affect the vibrational frequencies of the molecule.

In general, the vibrational frequency is higher for atoms with a smaller reduced mass and a larger force constant. Vibrations of groups where one atom is hydrogen have a higher frequency than those with other, heavier atoms.

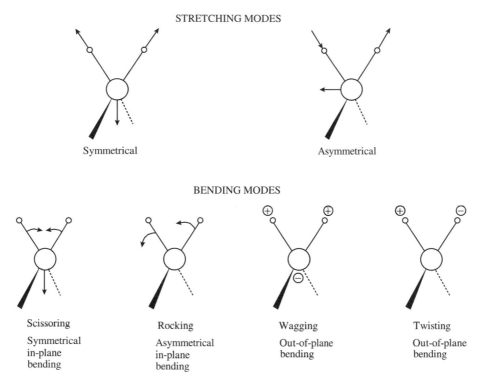

Fig. 1 Stretching and bending vibrations of a —CH$_2$— group.

For example, if the hydrogen atom in the C—H group is replaced by a deuterium atom, the vibrational frequency of C—D is lower than the vibrational frequency of C—H by a factor of about 1.414. The force constant is proportional to the bond strength (and thus to the bond order) between atoms. Therefore, for groups with atoms of the same mass, the vibrational frequency for triple-bond groups is about three times higher than that for double-bond groups. The vibrational frequency for the double-bond group is twice as high as that for the single-bond group.

Absorption bands that are attributed to overtone and combination vibrations are also observed in the IR spectrum of polyatomic molecules. Overtone vibrations occur at frequencies of approximately integral multiples of the fundamental frequencies. Combination vibrations appear at frequencies that are the sum or the difference of the frequencies of two or more fundamental vibrations. Overtone and combination bands are much less intense than fundamental bands.

Fermi resonance, which is the interaction between fundamental vibrations and overtone or combination vibrations, is also common in IR spectra. The result of Fermi resonance is the formation of two new vibration modes with one frequency higher and the other one lower than that observed when the interaction is absent. The unique quality of an IR absorption spectrum for a molecule

is partly attributed to overtone bands, combination bands, and Fermi resonance bands.

INSTRUMENTATION

Two main classes of infrared instrumentation are dispersive and nondispersive. A dispersive instrument uses a prism or grating to separate light into its frequencies. An IR spectrum generated by a dispersive instrument is normally a plot of wavenumber (cm^{-1}) or wavelength (μm) versus percent transmittance. In a nondispersive instrument, the IR radiation does not pass through a prism or grating, but through an interference filter or an interferometer, as in a Fourier transform infrared spectrometer, and is then collectively sent through the sample. An interference pattern generated by absorption within the sample is called an interferogram. It can be converted into a conventional IR spectrum by application of a mathematical operation (the Fourier transform) to the data. Using modern computer technology, this mathematical manipulation can be completed in a matter of seconds.

A typical IR spectrometer consists of the following components: radiation source, sampling area, monochromator (in a dispersive instrument), an interference filter or interferometer (in a nondispersive instrument), a detector, and a recorder or data-handling system. The instrumentation requirements for the mid-infrared, the far-infrared, and the near-infrared regions are different. Most commercial dispersive infrared spectrometers are designed to operate in the mid-infrared region (4000–400 cm^{-1}). An FTIR spectrometer with proper radiation sources and detectors can cover the entire IR region. In this section, the types of radiation sources, optical systems, and detectors used in the IR spectrometer are discussed.

RADIATION SOURCES

Infrared radiation is generated by electrically heating a source to a certain temperature. Several radiation sources (sometimes called "black body" sources) are commonly used for mid-infrared spectrometry. Table 1 summarizes the properties of each source, including the sources used for the near-IR and far-IR regions. Most sources have a maximum energy output at a certain wavelength range when heated at their optimum temperature. The energy of the radiation decreases gradually at longer wavelengths. In a dispersive instrument, however, widening the slit to allow more radiation to reach the detector can sometimes compensate for this effect.

Monochromator

A monochromator, mainly used in a dispersive instrument, is an optical device capable of separating infrared radiation into its constituent wavelengths. The monochromator normally consists of several components, including mirrors for collimating, focusing, or changing the direction of the radiation beam, and filters for attenuating the radiation and reducing stray radiation or eliminating unwanted grating orders. The most important component is the prism or the diffraction grating. By rotating the prism or grating, different wavelengths pass across a fixed slit, thereby allowing the entire wavelength range to be scanned. In most cases, the grating is preferable to the prism because the prism has several disadvantages, including lower dispersion (resulting in lower resolving power) and the introduction of unwanted reflection off its front and back surfaces.

Interferometer

The interferometer used in a nondispersive instrument is a device that divides the beam of radiation into two paths and recombines the two beams after a path difference has or has not been introduced. The basic concept of the interferometer was introduced by Michelson almost a century ago (Fig. 2). It consists of a stationary mirror, a moving mirror, and a beam splitter. The radiation from the infrared source is divided at the beam splitter; half the beam is passed to a fixed mirror and the other half is reflected to the moving mirror. The two beams are later recombined at the beam splitter and passed through the sample to the detector. For any particular wavelength, the two beams interfere constructively or destructively, depending on the difference between the optical paths of the beams in the two arms of the interferometer. The sample placed in the beam path absorbs radiation of a certain wavelength. The recorded interferogram is the sum

Table 1 Radiation sources for infrared spectrometers

Source	Composition	Operating temperature (°C)	Infrared range	Remarks
Nichrome coil	Nichrome	1100	Mid-IR	Air cooled, reliable, inexpensive, low temperature, less intense than other sources
Globar	Silicon carbide	1300	Mid-IR or Far-IR to 2000 cm^{-1}	Cooled by water, emission can be down to 80 cm^{-1}
Nernst glower	Oxides of zirconium, thorium, and yttrium	1500	Mid-IR 10,000–500 cm^{-1}	Poor emission at high wavenumbers, brittle, preheating required
High-pressure mercury arc	Mercury		Far-IR	Best for range between 200 and 10 cm^{-1}
Tungsten lamp	Tungsten		Near-IR	Best for between 33,000 and 400 cm^{-1}

of all waves except those absorbed by the sample. By a Fourier transformation of the interferogram, a conventional IR spectrum is obtained.

Detector

The detector converts infrared radiation into an electrical signal. The two main classes of detectors are thermal and quantum detectors. The heating caused by impinging infrared radiation changes some physical properties of the thermal detector itself. In quantum detectors, the quantum nature of infrared radiation changes the detector's electrical properties.

The responsivity (E) or specific detectivity (D^*) and the noise equivalent power NEP (W_n), are often used to measure the sensitivity of a detector. The responsivity depends on the wavelength of the radiation and the temperature of the detector. The NEP, also called minimum detectable power, is the quotient of detector noise (N) divided by voltage responsivity (E). The D^* is the reciprocal of NEP, thus $W_n = N/E$ and $D^* = 1/W_n$. A more sensitive detector has a smaller NEP and larger D^*, which results in less noise and a faster response time.

Thermal Detectors

Thermal detectors absorb infrared radiation and convert it to heat, resulting in a temperature change; a temperature-dependent detector property is then measured. The properties of the detector affected by the infrared radiation, depending upon the type of detector, include the expansion of a liquid, solid, or gas, electrical resistance, voltage, and electric polarization. Thermal detectors respond to radiation over a wide range of wavelengths. Since the response depends upon a change in temperature, such detectors are usually slow, typically responding in about 0.01–0.1 s. Table 2 summarizes the characteristics of various types of thermal detectors.

Quantum Detectors

Quantum detectors are usually made of semiconductor materials or mixtures. Some commonly used quantum detectors are made of lead sulfide (PbS), lead selenide (PbSe), indium antimony (InSb), or mercury cadmium telluride (MCT, HgTe–CdTe). The absorption of infrared radiation in quantum detectors excites electrons from a non-conducting state into a conducting state, resulting in a change in the current or voltage. Since the excitation of the electrons to a higher energy state is quantized, the detector exhibits a sharp cutoff frequency toward the far-infrared. Cooling is generally required to avoid thermal agitation, which produces internal electrical noise. The temperature to which the detector must be cooled depends on its sensitivity; for example, an MCT detector is usually cooled to liquid nitrogen temperature (77 K), whereas PbS and PbSe can be operated at a temperature just below ambient. Quantum detectors have much higher sensitivity and faster response times than thermal detectors; they thus are most often used in high-performance FTIR spectrometers. The response time for quantum detectors is measured in microseconds rather than in milliseconds. The sensitivity of quantum detectors is strongly dependent upon the composition of the semiconductors.

DISPERSIVE INFRARED SPECTROMETERS

Dispersive IR spectrometers can be either single-beam or double-beam; usually they are double-beam instruments. The use of a double-beam instrument significantly reduces the problem of possible interference from carbon dioxide and water vapor in the atmosphere during analysis. The absorption due to a solvent may also be nearly cancelled by placing an equivalent pathlength solvent cell in the reference beam.

A typical double-beam spectrometer is shown in Fig. 3. Radiation from the source is split into the reference beam and the sample beam. Each beam passes through a comb-shaped attenuator that regulates the beam intensity. The two beams are alternately sent through the slit into the

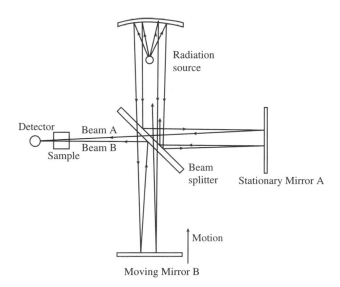

Fig. 2 Diagram of an interferometer. (Adapted from Ref. 23.)

Table 2 Thermal detectors for infrared spectrometers

Detector	Composition	Physical property affected	Remarks
Thermocouple and thermopile	Bismuth and antimony	Voltage at the junction of the two metals	Simplest and most direct measurement; slow response (30 ms)
Thermistor or thermistor bolometer	Oxides of Mn, Co, and Ni	Resistance changes	Slow response
Golay pneumatic detector	Xenon gas	Gas expansion, combined with the moving of a diaphragm, changes the illumination of a photocell	Extends to far-IR region with proper window; 15 ms response time; sensitive to intense light; microphonic disturbances; diaphragm wears out easily
Pyroelectric detector	Polarized pyroelectric materials[a] at temperatures below its Curie point	Electric polarization produces voltage changes	Low noise and fast response; used for fast-scan FTIR

[a]Such as triglycine sulfate (TGS), deuterated triglycine sulfate (DTGS), $LiTaO_3$, $LiNbO_3$.

monochromator by the chopper motor, which typically rotates at a frequency of 11 or 13 Hz. After the radiation has been dispersed into its constituent wavelengths by the monochromator, the beam is passed through the other slit and then onto the detector. The detection in a double-beam spectrometer is based on the "optical null" principle. In the absence of a sample, the two beams reach the detector with equal intensity and the recording pen is at 100% transmittance. When the sample is present, the beams are not of equal intensity. The difference in the intensity is amplified by an amplifier, which controls the pen motor. The attenuator comb in the reference beam is driven by the pen motor to adjust the intensity of the reference beam and make it equal to the sample beam. A pen moves up and down a chart to record the percent transmittance of the sample beam, and thus monitors the extent to which the attenuator must be driven. The scan motor rotates the prism or grating in the monochromator to scan the spectrum, simultaneously moving the chart under the pen. The chart records the percent transmittance versus the wavenumber (or wavelength). An alternative to the comb is to plot the difference in voltage between the reference and sample beams.

NONDISPERSIVE INFRARED SPECTROMETERS

One type of nondispersive spectrometer employs filters to isolate the wavelength desired; the other type uses an interferometer, i.e., the Fourier transform infrared (FTIR) spectrometer. Infrared analyzers utilizing simple filters to select the desired wavelength range for analysis are very useful in industrial on-line process control for monitoring a gas or liquid stream. This type of IR analyzer has high sensitivity and selectivity. A more sophisticated model (with microprocessor) can perform multicomponent analyses, calibration, and data reduction; it can also generate reports. The instrumental design of infrared analyzers is beyond the scope of this article.

Fourier transform infrared spectrometers can be single- or double-beam. Most commercial FTIR spectrometers are of single-beam design (Fig. 4). Double-beam FTIR spectrometers (Fig. 5) are less common and only a few are commercially available, and are mostly used for research purposes rather than routine tasks. A double-beam instrument is designed to compensate for atmospheric interference. In most modern IR spectrometers the optical components are manufactured in a sealed and desiccated compartment with the goal of reducing water and carbon dioxide interferences. A laser beam generates a reference signal to monitor the sampling rate and the velocity of the moving mirror, resulting in very accurate wavelengths in the spectra.

The FTIR technique has several advantages over the conventional dispersive technique. It provides a higher accuracy in wavenumber values, a better resolution, a better signal-to-noise ratio in a shorter time, and faster response time, making it useful for in-process or on-line monitoring. Dispersion or filtering of the radiation is not required.

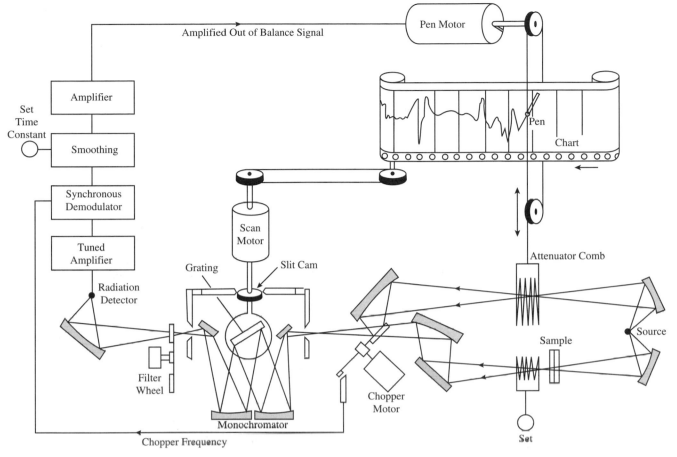

Fig. 3 Schematic of a typical double-beam spectrometer.

Data-Handling System

Most modern infrared spectrometers are equipped with a computer or microprocessor. The computer can record and store spectra, plot either absorbance or transmittance, overlay spectra for comparison, subtract one spectrum from another (to determine the difference or to remove the solvent or impurity spectrum from the sample spectrum), smooth and/or correct base lines, perform multiple scans to increase the signal-to-noise ratio and improve sensitivity, plus many other functions. A computer facilitates the Fourier transform process as well as the solving of complex mathematical matrices for multiple-component analyses.

SAMPLE HANDLING

Infrared spectra may be obtained for gases, liquids, or solids. For transmittance infrared spectroscopy, the sampling techniques may involve a solution, a film, a mull, or a pellet, depending on the type of sample. Reflectance spectroscopy differs from transmittance spectroscopy in that infrared radiation reflected from the surface of a material is studied. With a proper sampling accessory (obtainable from commercial sources), the materials analyzed by reflectance techniques normally require little or no sample preparation. The method is nondestructive, noninvasive, and very useful for analyzing materials that are too thick or have too much absorbance to be analyzed by transmittance spectroscopy.

Transmittance Spectroscopy

Obtaining the spectrum by transmittance spectroscopy normally requires sample cells with "window" materials that must be:

- Transparent in the wavelength area where the spectrum will be measured
- Chemically stable (nonreactive with the sample or the environment)

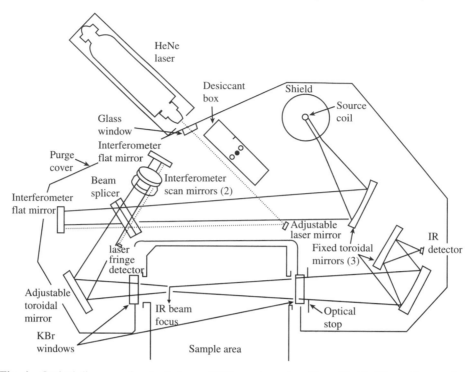

Fig. 4 Optical diagram of a single-beam FTIR spectrometer. (From Perkin-Elmer Corporation.)

- Easy to shape, grind, and polish to optical quality
- Stiff enough to retain their shape.

The most widely used window materials (Table 3) are alkali halides, particularly sodium chloride and potassium bromide.

Gases and Low-Boiling Liquids

For routine infrared analysis of gaseous samples, the type of cell normally used has a fixed path length of 10 cm. For trace level analysis, such as air monitoring, a cell with a longer path length is necessary to increase the sensitivity. A variable path cell (Fig. 6) can provide path lengths (in steps of 1.5 m) for 20-, 40-, and 120 m cells with the same volume of sample. A normal sample compartment in an infrared spectrometer does not hold a cell 120 m long. The long-path gas cell therefore utilizes a folded-path design in which the entering radiation is reflected back and forth several times before leaving the cell. Changing the angular adjustment of an internal pair of mirrors with a dial located outside the cell can vary the number of passes through the cell. Increasing the sample pressure to 10 atm in a gas cell is another way of improving the sensitivity.

Liquids and Solutions

For the analysis of liquid samples, the concentration and path lengths are selected in such a way that the transmittance lies between 15 and 75%. For neat liquids, a very thin layer (0.001–0.05 mm) is sufficient. For 0.05–10% (w/w) solutions, a cell length between 0.1 and 1 mm is normally used. For solution analysis, a compensating cell containing pure solvent is placed in the reference beam of dispersive instruments (a disadvantage for single beam FT instruments). In general, the solvent selected should not interact strongly with the solute. Several solvents are usually required to cover the entire spectrum. For example, carbon tetrachloride, transparent for the region between 4000 and 1333 cm^{-1}, and carbon disulfide, transparent for the region between 1333 and 650 cm^{-1}, may be used together. Some commonly used solvents are deuterated chloroform, methylene chloride, acetonitrile, and acetone. Information regarding the transparent regions for these solvents can be found in (1). A dilute solution in a nonpolar solvent usually gives the best spectrum.

Three types of sample cells are used in liquid analysis: sealed, demountable, and variable thickness cells (fixed and rotating windows). Fig. 7 shows a circular demountable cell and a circular sealed cell, both designed by Perkin–Elmer. A sample cell with rectangular shaped

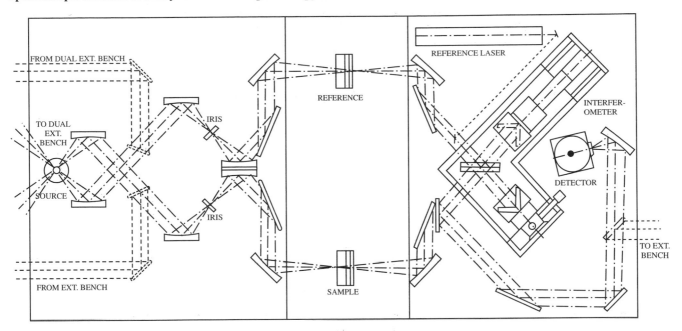

Fig. 5 Schematic of a double-beam FTIR spectrometer.

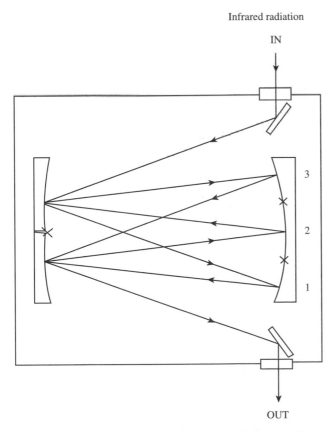

Fig. 6 A variable-path gas cell. (Adapted from Ref. 30.)

windows is also commercially available. The sealed cells are designed for quantitative analysis. The demountable cells are easily cleaned and suitable for routine sample analysis. The path length of a demountable cell can be changed with a suitable spacer. The path length of a variable-path cell in some cases can be varied continuously from 0.025 to 6 mm. This type is useful for determining extinction coefficients in liquid studies and for compensating for solvent absorption in dispersive double-beam spectrometers. Flow-through cells are available for continuous analysis of liquids such as the column effluent when an infrared spectrometer is coupled to a chromatographic system.

Solids

Solids may be examined as a deposited film, a mull, or a pressed disk, or by infrared microscopy.

Films

The deposited-film technique is particularly useful for polymers, resins, and amorphous solids. The samples are dissolved in a reasonably volatile solvent, the solution poured onto a suitable window, and the solvent evaporated by gentle heating or vacuum treatment. One disadvantage of films is that they may cause excessive light-scattering in transmittance spectrometry. This shortcoming can be

Table 3 Properties of infrared-transmitting materials

Material	Transmission range wavenumber (cm^{-1})	Refractive index^{a,b}, at 1000 cm^{-1}	Solubility g/100 g water at 20°C
Sodium chloride, NaCl	40,000–625	1.49	36.0
Potassium bromide, KBr	40,000–385	1.52	65.2
Potassium chloride, KCl	40,000–500	1.46	34.7
Cesium bromide, CsBr	10,000–270	1.67 (5000 cm^{-1})	124.3
Cesium iodide, CsI	33,000–200	1.74	160.0 (61°C)
Fused silica, SiO$_2$	50,000–2,500	1.42 (3333 cm^{-1})	Insoluble
Calcium fluoride, CaF$_2$	50,000–1,100	1.39 (2000 cm^{-1})	1.51×10^{-3}
Barium fluoride, BaF$_2$	50,000–770	1.42	0.12 (25°C)
Thallium bromide-iodide, KRS-5	16,600–250	2.37	$<4.76 \times 10^{-2}$
Silver bromide, AgBr	20,000–285	2.20	12×10^{-6}
Silver chloride, AgCl	25,000–435	2.00 (5000 cm^{-1})	Insoluble
Zinc sulfide, ZnS (Irtran-2)^a	10,000–715	2.20	Insoluble
Zinc selenide, ZnSe (Irtran-4)^a	10,000–515	2.41	Insoluble
Polyethylene (high density)	625–33	1.54 (5000 cm^{-1})	Insoluble
Germanium, Ge^a	20,000–600	4.0 (5000 cm^{-1})	Insoluble
Silicone, Si	8,300–1,500 and 360–70	3.4	Insoluble
Sapphire^a, Al$_2$O$_3$	50,000–1,780	1.74	Insoluble
Magnesium oxide, MgO (Irtran-5)	25,600–1,060	1.71 (5000 cm^{-1})	Insoluble

^{a}For attenuated total-reflectance spectrometry.
^{b}Unless otherwise indicated.

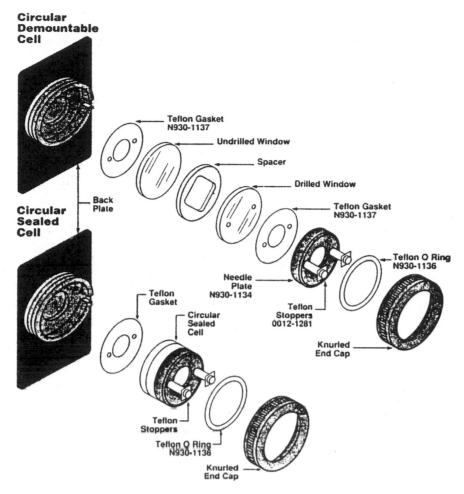

Fig. 7 Diagram of a circular demountable cell and a circular sealed cell for liquid samples. (From Perkin-Elmer Corporation.)

overcome by using attenuated total-reflection or internal-reflection sampling techniques.

Mulls

Grinding 2–5 mg of sample in a smooth agate mortar, adding a drop or two of mulling oil to the sample, and continuing the grinding forms a mull of a solid sample. The sample should be ground until the particle size is below 2 μm to avoid excessive radiation scattering. The mull is placed on the mull plates and the film thickness is adjusted so that the transmittance is between 10 and 90%T. Commonly used mulling agents are Nujol (a high-boiling mineral oil), hexachlorobutadiene, perfluorokerosene, and chlorofluorocarbon greases (fluorolubes).

Pressed disks

A pressed disk is prepared by grinding a mixture of 0.5–1.0 mg of sample and 100 mg of dry, powdered potassium bromide in a mortar or Wig-l-bug to reduce the particle size to less than 2 μm. The resulting mixture is pressed into a disk under a pressure of 68.9–103.4 MPa (10,000–15,000 psi). A simple-to-operate minipress is also available. Moisture bands near 3448 and 1639 cm^{-1} appear frequently in spectra obtained by this technique.

REFLECTANCE SPECTROMETRY

A problem that may be encountered when analyzing a solid sample by transmittance spectroscopy is radiation scattering. Employing reflectance spectroscopy can sometimes reduce this problem. With this technique, the infrared spectra of most solid materials are easily obtained with little or no sample preparation. Spectra of a wide range of solid samples can be characterized with this technique, such as coatings on beverage containers and silicon wafers, polymer films, or other intractable samples.

The reflectance technique, however, is less sensitive than the transmittance technique since about 80% of the infrared radiation is lost after being reflected off the sample surface.

Different types of reflectance spectroscopy depend upon the reflecting behavior of the radiation on the solid. Fig. 8 illustrates various categories used to distinguish techniques for reflecting radiation off solids. Specular reflection spectroscopy is used to measure the reflectance spectrum of a smooth, glossy surface. In reflection-absorption spectroscopy, the radiation passes through a thin surface film on a reflective (typically metallic) surface twice. The thickness of the surface film is normally between 0.2 and 20 μm. This technique is often used in studying the coatings on beverage containers and on silicon wafers of semiconductor devices. Diffuse-reflectance spectroscopy is applied to samples with a coarse, grainy texture such as powders, fibers, and rough surfaces.

Attenuated total-reflectance (ATR) spectroscopy is a widely used sampling technique, in which a sample is placed in contact with a reflecting medium (a plate or prism shaped material called an internal reflectance element). A beam of radiation entering the prism is reflected internally if the angle of incidence at the interface between sample and prism is greater than the critical angle (a function of the refractive index of the sample and the prism).

The sample absorbs the radiation during this process and an absorption spectrum characteristic of the sample is thus obtained. The spectrum of a sample acquired by the ATR technique is generally comparable to the transmission spectrum, but band shifts have been observed. The ATR technique has been used for materials that are too thick or absorb too strongly to be analyzed by transmission spectroscopy. Aqueous solutions can be analyzed by the liquid ATR technique, which was previously very difficult, using transmission spectroscopy.

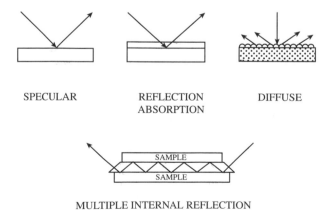

SPECULAR   REFLECTION ABSORPTION   DIFFUSE

MULTIPLE INTERNAL REFLECTION

Fig. 8 Main forms of reflective behavior.

Most reflectance spectroscopy is carried out utilizing an accessory that can be easily inserted into and removed from the sampling compartment of a conventional spectrometer. These accessories are designed for each application and usually consist of mirrors or prisms for reflecting or focusing the radiation. Most of the sampling accessories for the FTIR spectrometers and the FTIR microscopes are available commercially.

QUALITATIVE ANALYSIS

Applications of IR spectroscopy to qualitative analysis are mainly for the identification of unknown compounds. For a pure substance, an exact match of the IR spectrum of the compound with that of the reference standard is positive identification. It is important that both spectra are measured under the same conditions. A solid substance might have various crystalline forms. Therefore, the IR spectra of standard and sample in a solid state might not be identical. In such cases, equal portions of the test sample and the standard should be dissolved in equal volumes of a suitable solvent. The solutions are evaporated to dryness in similar containers under identical conditions and the test is repeated on the residues. The compound can also be recrystallized from the same solvent and the determination repeated.

INTERPRETATION OF INFRARED SPECTRA

For an unknown compound without a reference standard, important structural information can be obtained from the IR spectrum. Fig. 9 is a simplified illustration of the correlation between the absorption frequency in cm^{-1} and the functional groups [A more comprehensive description of this type of correlation chart is given in (4).] By observing the presence or absence of certain "group frequencies", related to common functional groups such as —OH, —NH$_2$, —CH$_3$, —C=O, —CN, —C—O—C, —COOH, etc., the gross structural features of an unknown compound can be quickly determined.

The IR spectrum in the mid-IR region is divided into the functional-group region, 4000–1300 cm^{-1} and the fingerprint region, 1300–400 cm^{-1}. To interpret an IR spectrum, the hydrogen-stretching vibrations, which appear between 4000 and 2500 cm^{-1}, are investigated first to determine whether the compound is aromatic or aliphatic. A sharp band at 3300 cm^{-1} suggests the presence of —C=C—H, a terminal acetylene moiety, and/or an —NH group. Aromatic and unsaturated

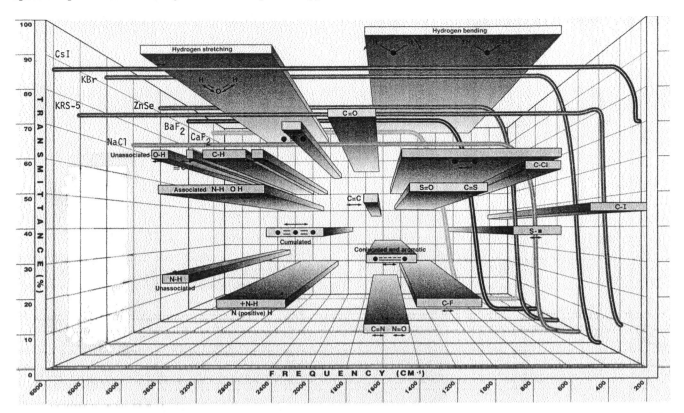

Fig. 9 Structure and infrared absorption bands correlation chart. Transmission ranges for infrared window materials CsI, KBr, ZnSe, KRS-5, Baf₂, CaF₂, and NaCl are also indicated on the chart. (From Perkin-Elmer Corporation.)

compounds appear at 3100–3000 cm⁻¹ and aliphatic compounds appear at 3000–2800 cm⁻¹. Unsaturation may also be suggested by C=C and C=C stretches between 2500–1540 cm⁻¹. Next, the group frequency is examined to establish the presence or absence of certain functional groups such as —OH, —NH, and C=O. The stretching vibration of carbonyl groups occurs in the 1850–1540 cm⁻¹ range. The fingerprint region, 1300–909 cm⁻¹, is characteristic of each molecule and, when examined in reference to the other regions, provides positive identification of certain functional groups. The lack of strong absorption bands in the 909–650 cm⁻¹ region usually indicates a nonaromatic structure. The group frequency might vary when the molecular environment changes; thus, the shift in frequency provides further structural information for an unknown substance. Some typical examples are the effects of inter- or intramolecular hydrogen bonding, the dimerization of a carboxylic acid, and ring strain within the molecule.

After the IR spectrum has been interpreted, the structural characteristics of the unknown can be narrowed down to a few compounds in a specific category. For positive identification of an unknown, information on the physical state, melting or boiling point, solubility, and the history of the compound should be obtained. The flame test should be done, and the NMR and mass spectra should be determined. Once the structure of the unknown has been deduced, the IR spectrum of the unknown can be compared with available IR reference spectra (5, 6). With FTIR spectrometers, a large collection of IR spectra can be stored in the computer's library. When the IR spectrum of the unknown is obtained, the instrument can do a library search and find the spectrum that offers the best match to the unknown.

If the unknown substance is not pure or is mixed with other components, separation of the compound from the matrix may be required. However, in many cases mixtures may be characterized. The compound can be purified by recrystallization, distillation, solvent-partitioning, pH manipulation, or chromatographic separation. Once the appropriate separation procedures have been completed, the purified unknown can undergo the structural characterization steps described above.

QUANTITATIVE ANALYSIS

The amount of infrared radiation absorbed by the sample is proportional to the concentration of the sample and the cell path length. The Beer–Lambert law, shown in Eq. 7, illustrates the mathematical relationship:

$$A = abc = \varepsilon b(c\,\mathrm{mol.\ wt.}) A = \log_{10}(I_0/I)$$
$$= \log(1/T) \tag{7}$$

The absorbance A is the logarithm (to the base 10) of the reciprocal of the transmittance (T), which in turn is the ratio of the intensity of the transmitted radiation I to the intensity of the incident radiation I_0. The absorptivity, a, is the quotient of the absorbance (A) divided by the product of concentration c in grams per liter of the substance and the absorption path length b in cm. The more commonly used molar absorptivity ε is used when the concentration is in mol/L rather than g/L.

At a constant cell path length, Beer's law shows that the absorbance of radiation through a medium is proportional to the concentration of the solute. Beer's law is strictly valid only for monochromatic radiation. Stray light (i.e., scattered radiation), which reaches the detector without having passed through the desired beam path, molecular interactions such as hydrogen bonding, which varies with the sample concentration, and other instrumental factors such as slit width, all affect molar absorptivity and result in some deviations from Beer's law. For an accurate analysis of the concentration of an unknown sample, it is usually necessary to first create a calibration curve from standard solutions and then determine the absorbance of the sample under identical conditions. The concentration of the unknown is determined from the calibration curve. Diluted solutions (less than 2%) are recommended for this analysis.

If a calibration curve has been established previously and the instrumental conditions have not been changed, the unknown concentration can sometimes be determined by using a single calibration preparation. The concentration of the unknown is calculated by ratioing absorbances and concentrations, according to Eq. 8.

$$A_{\mathrm{std}} = c_{\mathrm{std}}$$
$$A_{\mathrm{unk}} = c_{\mathrm{unk}} \tag{8}$$

In such cases, the calibration curve of the sample should be determined periodically to make sure that the linearity of Beer's law is still valid.

For quantitative analysis of a single component, a strong absorption band that is relatively free of overlapping bands or interference is selected from the IR spectrum. The intensity of the band is measured either in units of percent transmittance or absorbance.

The intensity of the incident radiation (I_0) and the intensity of the transmitted radiation (I) can be measured by the base-line method illustrated in Fig. 10. In the FTIR spectrometer, the computer is capable of converting the transmittance into absorbance, subtracting the background or the solvent interference from the sample spectrum, generating a calibration curve, and calculating the unknown concentration.

For quantitative analysis of multiple components in a mixture where overlapping of the bands generally occurs, the number of absorption bands chosen should be equal to the number of components to be determined (n components). A series of standard mixtures (at least as many as n) containing a known amount of the substance is prepared. The resulting equations, involving the science of chemometrics, are solved by matrix algebra methods with the help of a computer. The accuracy of this type of quantitative analysis technique decreases with an increasing number of components in the mixture.

APPLICATIONS AND RECENT DEVELOPMENTS

With the continuous improvement of sampling techniques, software, and instrumental designs, more and more sophisticated FTIR spectrometers are now available. *Analytical Chemistry* biannually reviews the most recent developments in many fields of analytical techniques, including infrared spectroscopy, many times on a yearly basis.

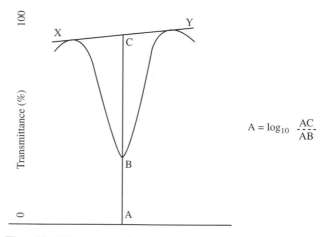

Fig. 10 Illustration of a base-line measurement method. (Adapted from Ref. 29.)

Hyphenated Techniques

Hyphenated techniques refer to the combination of one or more analytical techniques for problem solving and fundamental research. Numerous types have been reported in the scientific journals. Frequently the FTIR spectrometer is coupled with chromatographic instruments for the structural characterization of a column eluent. These systems are designed to monitor the eluent or to obtain its spectrum. Much of the development has been focused on the sampling technique and the design of the interface between the chromatographic system and the FTIR spectrometer to improve the performance of the system.

For GC–FTIR, headspace GC–FTIR, or GC–FTIR–MS, a light-pipe gas cell, direct deposition, or a matrix isolation apparatus is usually incorporated. The mobile phase is helium or nitrogen, which does not interfere. In general, the matrix-isolation technique gives a better quality of infrared spectrum and a lower detection limit. Organic material present as low as a picogram can be detected by this technique (7, 8).

For HPLC–FTIR, GPC–FTIR, or SFC–FTIR, the design of the interface is more challenging since the mobile phases used for these chromatographic systems normally have strong infrared absorbencies; thus, it is important to remove the mobile phase prior to measuring the spectrum. For the interface between the two systems flow-cells or mobile-phase elimination techniques may be used. Some recent developments point toward the elimination of mobile-phase techniques (9–11). A microbore column can help to reduce the mobile-phase volume in the system (12, 13).

FTIR Microscopy

Fourier transform infrared microscopy is the primary infrared technique for structural identification of materials at microquantities. The method is nondestructive and noninvasive. When using a proper transmittance sampling technique and a proper detector, the limit of detection can be as low as the picogram level. In the pharmaceutical industry, FTIR microscopy is used to analyze bulk drugs, excipients, and particulate contaminants (14). Recent studies have shown that by coupling FTIR microscopy with GC, HPLC, SFC, or GPC systems, the detection limit of the method is substantially improved (15, 16).

Infrared Analyzers

The combination of the fast-response FTIR spectrometer and proper sampling techniques has made the infrared analyzer the instrument of choice for the on-line monitoring of a process stream. The IR analyzer is generally compact, rugged, and easy to operate in the field or industrial production. The infrared analyzer equipped with a microprocessor or a computer is capable of identification and quantitative analysis of single or multiple components in the industrial process stream in a short time. FTIR analyzers are widely used for in-process on-line monitoring of manufacturing, waste streams, and environmental air monitoring (17–21).

SUMMARY

Infrared spectroscopy continues to be a rapidly growing analytical technique. Improvements and innovations have been made in sampling techniques and analysis software. A large variety of samples in various forms can be analyzed by IR spectroscopy. This flexibility has made infrared spectroscopy one of the most important tools in today's analytical laboratories, especially for analysis of trace contaminants.

REFERENCES

1. Duerst, R.W.; Duerst, M.D.; Stebbings, W.L. Transmission Infrared Spectroscopy. *Modern Methods of Applied Molecular Spectroscopy*; John Wiley & Sons: New York, 1998.
2. Duerst, R.W.; Stebbings, W.L.; Lillquist, Gerald, J.; Westberg, James, W.; Breneman, William, E.; Spicer, Colleen, K.; Dittmar, Rebecca, M.; Duerst, Marilyn, D. Depth Profiling and Defect Analysis. *Practical Guide to Infrared Microspectroscopy*; Marcel Dekker, Inc.: New York, 1995.
3. Willard, H.H.; Merritt, L.L., Jr.; Dean, J.A.; Settle, F.A., Jr. *Instrumental Methods of Analysis*, 7th Ed.; Wadsworth Publishing Co.: Belmont, CA, 1988.
4. Silverstein, R.M.; Bassler, G.C.; Morrill, T.C. *Spectrometric Identification of Organic Compounds*, 5th Ed.; John Wiley & Sons: New York, 1991.
5. Pouchert, C.J. Ed. *The Aldrich Library of Infrared Spectra*, 2nd Ed.; Aldrich Chemical Co.: Milwaukee, 1975.
6. Sadtler Research Laboratories. *Catalog of Infrared Spectrograms*; Philadelphia (A Continuously Updated Subscription Service).
7. Holloway, T.T.; Fairless, B.J.; Freidfine, C.E.; Kimball, H.E.; Kleopfer, R.D.; Wurrey, C.J.; Jonoby, L.A.; Palmer, H.G. Appl. Spectrosc. **1988**, *42*, 359–369.
8. Bourne, S.; Haefner, A.M.; Norton, K.L.; Griffiths, P.R. Anal. Chem. **1990**, *62*, 2448–2452.
9. Lange, A.J.; Griffiths, P.R.; Fraser, D.J. Anal. Chem. **1991**, *63*, 782–787.

10. Griffiths, P.R.; Haefner, A.M.; Norton, K.L.; Fraser, D.J.J.; Pyo, D.; Makishima, H.J. High Resol. Chrom. **1989**, *12*, 119–122.
11. Norton, K.L.; Lange, A.J.; Griffiths, P.R.J. High Resol. Chrom. **1991**, *14*, 225–229.
12. Jinno, K.; Fujimoto, C.J. Chrom. **1990**, *506*, 443–460.
13. Fujimoto, C.; Jinno, K. Trends Anal. Chem. **1989**, *8* (3), 90–96.
14. Clark, D.A.; Nichols, G. Anal. Proc. **1990**, *27*, 19–21.
15. Fraser, D.J.J.; Norton, K.L.; Griffiths, P.R. Pract. Spectrosc. **1988**, *6*, 197–210.
16. Bergin, F.J. A . Appl. Spectrosc. **1989**, *43* (3), 511–515.
17. Coates, J.P.; Rein, A.J.; Morris, K.S. Am. Lab. **1988**, *20* (2), 117–124.
18. Morris, K.S.; Rein, A.J. Am. Lab. **1988**, *20* (11), 46–52.
19. Fuller, M.P.; Garry, C.; Stanek, Z. Am. Lab. **1990**, *22* (15), 58–69.
20. Wilks, P.A. Am. Lab. **1991**, *26C–26E*.
21. McIntosh, B.C.; Vidrine, D.W.; Doyle, W.M. Am Lab. **1991**, *23* (18), 19–22.
22. Beckett, A.H.; Stenlake, J.B. *Practical Pharmaceutical Chemistry*, 3rd Ed.; Athlone Press, University of London: London, England, 1976; 2, 331–360.
23. Crooks, J.E. *The Spectrum in Chemistry*; Academic Press: New York, 1978.
24. Duerst, R.W.; Duerst, MarilynD. Transmission Infrared Spectroscopy. *Modern Techniques in Applied Molecular Spectroscopy*; Mirabella, F., Ed.; John Wiley & Sons, Inc.: New York, 1998.
25. Duerst, R.W.; et al. Depth Profiling and Defect Analysis of Films and Laminates: An Industrial Approach. *A Practical Guide to Infrared Microscopy*; Humecki, H., Ed.; Marcel Dekker, Inc.: New York, 1995.
26. Griffiths, P.R.; de Haseth, J.A. Fourier Transform Infrared Spectrometry. *Chemical Analysis*; John Wiley & Sons, Inc.: New York, 1986; 83.
27. Hannah, R.W.; Swinehart, J.S. *Experiments in Techniques of Infrared Spectroscopy*; Perkin-Elmer: Norwalk, CT, 1974.
28. Krishnan, K.; Hill, S.L. *FT-IR Microsampling Techniques*; Bio-Rad Digilab Division: Cambridge, MA, 1990.
29. Miller, R.G.J.; Stace, B.C. *Laboratory Methods in Infrared Spectroscopy*, 2nd Ed.; Heyden Press: (Wiley), New York, 1979.
30. Stewart, J.E. *Infrared Spectroscopy: Experimental Methods and Techniques*; Marcel Dekker, Inc.: New York, 1970.

SPECTROSCOPIC METHODS OF ANALYSIS—MASS SPECTROMETRY

Mike S. Lee

Milestone Development Services, Newtown, Pennsylvania

INTRODUCTION

The dramatically increased expenditures for both in-house and outsourced pharmaceutical research and development (R&D) have led to a greater dependence on technology. New technologies are constantly introduced into drug development to address throughput issues and improve development cycles. The incorporation of new technologies has resulted in fundamental change in the drug development paradigm. Recently, sample generating-based technologies such as high throughput biomolecular screening and automated parallel synthesis have shifted the bottleneck to sample analysis-based technologies.

The current focus on analytical techniques in the pharmaceutical industry emphasizes four primary figures of merit: sensitivity; selectivity; speed; and high throughput. Mass spectrometry (MS) provides each of these key attributes, and therefore, has been benchmarked an effective solution for pharmaceutical analysis in each stage of drug development (1). Perhaps more enabling than the MS-based technology itself is the diverse applications of MS in conjunction with sample preparation, chromatographic separation, and informatics. It is within this context that MS has played an increasingly vital role in the pharmaceutical industry and has become the preferred analytical method for trace-mixture analysis (Fig. 1).

A variety of MS formats are widely accepted and applied in the pharmaceutical industry. The specific MS application is often defined by the sample introduction technique. The pharmaceutical applications highlighted in this article feature two types of sample introduction techniques: dynamic and static. Dynamic sample introduction involves the use of high-performance liquid chromatography (HPLC) on-line with MS. The resulting liquid chromatography/mass spectrometry (LC/MS) format provides unique and enabling capabilities for pharmaceutical analysis. The electrospray ionization (ESI) (2) and atmospheric pressure chemical ionization (APCI) (3) modes are the most widely used. Static sample introduction techniques primarily use matrix-assisted laser desorption/ionization (MALDI) (4).

The advances in MS instrumentation (5) and role of MS within the pharmaceutical industry (1) have been recently reviewed. This article will focus on MS technologies with regard to specific applications in drug development. The intent of this article is to provide an overview of MS applications and describe the significant integration of this technology into drug development. A detailed and in-depth overview of current MS technologies and applications can be obtained from the recent proceedings of the American Society for Mass Spectrometry Conference on Mass Spectrometry and Allied Topics (www.asms.org) and the Association of Biomolecular Resource Facilities (www.abrf.org).

GENOMICS

Though the contributions of MS have been somewhat limited in the field of genomics, there has been increased participation and interest (6). Certainly, the worldwide recognition received from the Human Genome Project created a sense of urgency toward determining genetic variation.

Genomics refers to the study of genetic data to draw correlation between individual genetic inheritance and medically or biologically important parameters. For example, these parameters may involve a patient's response to a specific drug. Knowledge of the genetic basis of individual drug response may provide understanding of the observed variability in drug response arising as a result of genetically determined differences in drug absorption, disposition, metabolism, or excretion (7). Furthermore, knowledge of genetic variation may be useful during the target selection process when multiple targets are available within a specific disease state. Thus, the pharmaceutical industry has great interest in determining the genetic variation in patient populations.

Due to the existence of sequence variations, or polymorphisms, no two human genomes are identical. Single nucleotide polymorphisms (SNPs) are the most abundant genetic variation with an estimated frequency of 1 SNP per 500 basepairs. Since SNPs are so prevalent in the genome, they can act as markers that are linked with a phenotype to provide a comprehensive measure of interaction with a specific drug. The validation of

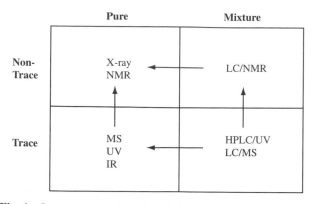

	Pure	Mixture
Non-Trace	X-ray NMR	LC/NMR
Trace	MS UV IR	HPLC/UV LC/MS

Fig. 1 Structure analysis matrix that illustrates pharmaceutical analysis preferences for four specific sample types: nontrace/pure; nontrace/mixture; trace/pure; and trace/mixture. (Courtesy of Milestone Development Services, Newtown, PA.)

a particular SNP represents an important stage for establishing SNPs as a routine clinical diagnostic marker. The validation of SNPs via MALDI-TOF MS is emerging as a valuable genotyping tool (8, 9). A schematic of a MALDI-TOF MS instrument is shown in Fig. 2.

A recent study performed by Stroh et al. (10) compared the performance of MALDI-TOF MS with restriction fragment length polymorphism (RFLP) and fluorescence polarization (FP). The study involved the analysis of known mutations of the IL-1β gene. The procedure involved amplification of patient DNA samples using standard PCR techniques followed by a primer extension step where a separate post-PCR primer is hybridized directly adjacent to the SNP site. The resulting MALDI-TOF MS data provided a direct confirmation of molecular weight for fast analysis of polymorphisms.

Knowledge of the DNA sequence flanking the SNP site allows for the optimum choice of post-PCR primer size, primer location, and dideoxy-nucleotide(s). Thus, the assay can be designed to extract complete information about the SNP regardless of its state. This emerging MS-based approach for SNP genotyping has potential to be highly automated without the requirement for fluorescent tags. Furthermore, "multiplexing" can be attained by selecting post-PCR primers of varying lengths to dedicate predetermined regions of the mass spectrum to specific SNPs.

PROTEOMICS

The study of protein structure, function, quantity, and interactions during maturation and progression of disease is referred to as proteomics. Analytical approaches that use a combination of two-dimensional (2-D) gel electrophoresis for protein separation and MS analysis for protein identification followed by database searches is a widely practiced proteomics strategy (11). The tryptic peptides extracted from gels are analyzed by MALDI-TOF MS and microcolumn or capillary LC tandem mass spectrometry (MS/MS) techniques. Typically, the MALDI-TOF MS techniques are used to quickly identify peptide fragments and confirm the presence of known proteins. Nano-scale

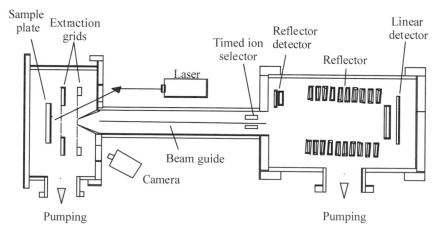

Fig. 2 Schematic of a MALDI-TOF MS instrument. MALDI-TOF samples are prepared with a matrix that contains a small organic molecule capable of absorbing ultraviolet light. A laser is used to desorb ions from the sample plate and the resulting ions are forced into the flight tube by application of the acceleration voltage from extraction grids. All ions leave the source with the same kinetic energy and travel down the flight tube toward an ion reflector. Separation is based on mass with lighter ions traveling faster than heavier ions. The ion reflector is used to correct for small kinetic energy differences between ions of the same mass resulting in improved resolution and mass accuracy. (Courtesy of Applied Biosystems, Framingham, MA.)

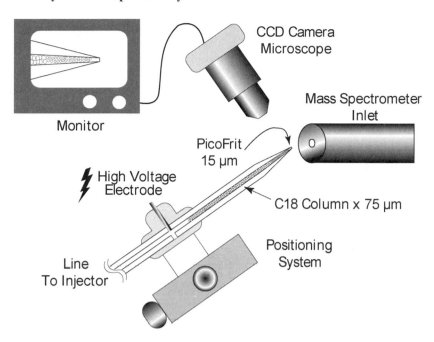

Fig. 3 Schematic of a nano-scale capillary ESI interface. This specialized LC/MS interface, operating at flow rates from 20 to 500 nL/min and using 50 to 100 μm ID columns, typically provides low femtomole sensitivity. Fully automated sample handling and preparation procedures (i.e., desalting and preconcentration) combined with specialized devices for high separation and variable nL gradient flow rates provide unique capabilities for high-throughput analysis of proteins. (Courtesy of New Objective, Cambridge, MA.)

capillary LC/MS/MS techniques (using 50–100 μm diameter columns, operating at flow rates of 20–500 nL/min) are used to further interrogate the complex protein mixture at the low femtomole level. These techniques require the use of a specialized ESI source shown in Fig. 3.

The combination of MALDI-TOF MS and capillary LC/MS/MS was recently described for the identification of disease state markers in human urine (12). In this study, urine proteins obtained from emphysema patients were separated on 2-D gels and selected spots were digested with trypsin and analyzed by MALDI-TOF. A database search using Protein Prospector identified a potential biomarker for emphysema as human alpha-1-antitrypsin (A1AT). The corresponding MALDI spectrum contained nine out of 18 peptides with masses that match the expected tryptic digest fragments for A1AT.

The same tryptic digest protein sample was analyzed by capillary LC/MS/MS using an ion trap mass spectrometer followed by a database search with SEQUEST. Figure 4 illustrates the components of an ion trap mass spectrometer. The highly automated data-dependent MS/MS analysis provided excellent sequence coverage for 11 tryptic peptides related to A1AT in a single LC/MS run. A tryptic peptide that corresponds to the A1AT sequence SVLGQLGITK observed at retention time (r_t) 30.5 min. was observed in the spectrum. The LC/MS data also

provided sequence information on unmatched MALDI peaks.

The need to detect lower concentration of protein and peptide mixtures has resulted in the increased use of hybrid quadrupole/orthogonal TOF (QTOF) MS/MS instruments (13) in conjunction with microcolumn LC. Fig. 5 shows a schematic of a QTOF instrument. This LC/MS approach provides a resolution of ca. 0.1 mass units allowing for the analysis of complex product ion spectra (14, 15). A recent publication by Chalmers and Gaskell highlights the current challenges in proteome analysis with regard to MS instrumentation (16).

NATURAL PRODUCTS DEREPLICATION

Historically, an excellent source of novel lead drug compounds is natural products. Natural product screening activities typically occur during drug discovery and involve the testing of crude extracts obtained from microbial fermentation broths, plants, or marine organisms. When activity above a certain level is detected, active components are isolated and purified for identification. This process is often time-consuming, where the physicochemical characteristics of the active components

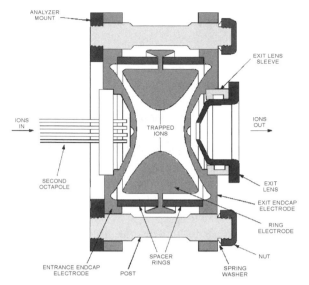

Fig. 4 Schematic of an ion trap MS instrument. This device consists of two endcap electrodes (entrance and exit) and a ring electrode. An ion trap MS separates ions based on mass-to-charge ratio (m/z). Once ions are introduced into the ion trap MS, the radiofrequency (rf) amplitude is increased so that ions are sequentially ejected (by increasing mass) and detected. This type of MS provides a routine (i.e., benchtop) and sensitive detector using either GC and LC interfaces. Furthermore, this instrument provides a unique format for multiple stages of MS analysis (MS^n). (Courtesy of Thermo-Finnigan, San Jose, CA.)

are determined, known compounds are identified (dereplication), and the novel compounds are scaled-up for more detailed investigation.

Analysis strategies that use on-line ESI-LC/MS approaches provide an integrated format for natural product dereplication by combining traditional fraction collection, sample preparation, and multi-component analysis into a single step. In this way, crude extracts are screened without extensive purification and chemical analysis. Furthermore, less material is required due to the sensitivity of the technique and chromatographic resolution is retained.

The key to natural products analysis using this approach is dependable molecular weight determination. This information is used with existing natural product databases that contain information on the bioactive compounds, the physical descriptions of the microorganisms from which they come, their spectrum of activity, the method of extraction and isolation, and physical data (i.e., molecular weight, UV absorption maxima). Molecular weight is the most critical information for initial searches because of its link to structural specificity. This information is used to make pivotal decisions on whether or not to proceed to more time-consuming isolation steps based on novelty of the compound. In recently reported studies (17, 18), LC/MS is used to increase sensitivity and accelerate analysis. These features serve to significantly reduce labor. A recent review described LC/MS-based approaches for

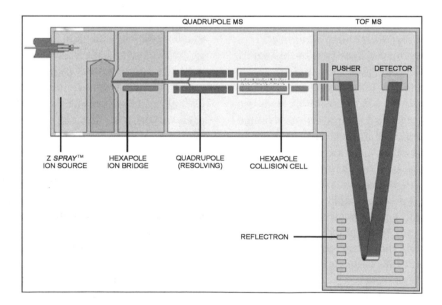

Fig. 5 Schematic of a QTOF MS instrument. Ions formed in the source region are introduced into a quadrupole mass filter (see Fig. 7) that separates ions based on mass-to-charge ratio (m/z). Selected ions are then transferred into the TOF MS for detailed analysis (i.e., high resolution capabilities). (Courtesy of Micromass, Manchester, UK.)

the characterization of natural product mixtures in conjunction with high-throughput screening (19).

The instrumental configuration of the LC/MS system developed by Ackermann et al. (17) features an HPLC, UV detector, fraction collector, ESI-tandem quadrupole (MS/MS), and MALDI-TOF MS. Filtered fermentation broths were extracted with butanol or ethyl acetate, and eluted on a gradient C18 reversed-phase HPLC separation. The eluent was split 1:10 between a tandem quadrupole MS/MS instrument (scanning 250–2000 amu/3 sec in the full scan mode) and a single wavelength UV detector (254 or 230 nm). One-min fractions were collected after the UV detector. Of these fractions, 20–50 μL is used for MALDI-TOF analysis, and the remainder is concentrated for microbiological testing. The LC/UV chromatogram was compared to the bioactivity assay histogram to highlight the peaks that contain activity. The molecular weights of the active peaks were obtained for novelty assessment of the compounds.

Similar approaches that use on-line LC/MS and LC/MS/MS techniques have been recently described for natural products dereplication (20, 21). Approximately,000 natural product extracts can be screened annually for in vivo and in vitro activity using LC/MS-based systems. A standard approach for dereplication involves a comparison of retention time, full scan mass spectra (i.e., molecular weight information), and MS/MS spectra with those from known biologically active standards. Thus, previously identified components are rapidly eliminated and do not require time-consuming structure elucidation studies. The savings of effort allow researchers to focus efforts on novel chemistries. Samples of novel compounds can then be infused into an ion trap mass spectrometer, and a multiple stage mass analysis (MS^n) fragmentation map is generated.

COMBINATORIAL CHEMISTRY

Recent reviews (22, 25) describe MS-based methods ranging from the analysis of complex molecular libraries (26) to open-access formats for drug discovery and development (27). High throughput criteria were central to each application.

An important development in the quest for high throughput combinatorial library analysis was the multiple ESI interface described by Wang et al. (28). This novel ESI interface enabled effluent flow streams from an array of four HPLC columns to be sampled independently and sequentially using a quadrupole MS instrument. The interface featured a stepping motor and rotating plate assembly. The effluent flow from the HPLC columns was connected to a parallel arrangement of electrospray needles co-axial to the mass spectrometer entrance aperture. The individual spray tips were positioned 90° relative to one another in a circular array. Each spray position was sampled multiple times per second by precise control of the stepping motor assembly.

The parallel sample analysis format using a multiplexed LC/MS interface with an orthogonal time-of-flight (TOF) MS was described by de Biasi et al. (29). This approach illustrated the high-throughput capabilities of a multiplexed ESI interface in combination with an MS format that accommodates fast chromatography methodologies. The system featured a four-way multiplexed electrospray interface attached directly with the existing source of the TOF-MS instrument. A rotating aperture driven by a variable speed stepper motor permitted the sampling of the spray from each electrospray probe tip. The data files were synchronized with the corresponding spray.

As the preparation of large libraries for lead discovery became routine, the burden placed on analysis techniques focused mainly on throughput and quality (30). However, biological assay requirements typically required pure compounds. Thus, the focus shifted toward the use of automated high throughput purification methods applied to libraries of discrete compounds (31). Reverse-phase analytical and preparative HPLC formats in conjunction with MS techniques have been critical for the high throughput purification approaches for parallel synthesis libraries. A variety of approaches that featured the use of gradient methods, short columns, and high flow rates have been described (32). Highly automated LC/MS approaches for purification at the multimilligram level were described for a quadrupole system by Zeng et al. (33). These methods featured the use of short columns that were operated at ultra high flow rates. Preparative columns were operated at flow rates in excess of 70 ml/min to match the linear velocity of the short analytical columns (4.0 ml/min). Analytical LC/MS analyses of compound libraries were achieved in 5 min for chromatographically, well-behaved compounds. Slightly longer preparative LC/MS analysis times (8–10 min/sample) were required for compounds that exhibited poor chromatographic peak shapes and/or for compound mixtures the required higher resolution separations. The fraction collection process is initiated in real-time once the reconstructed ion current is observed for a specific m/z value that corresponds to the compound of interest. This design permitted the collection of one sample per fraction. Thus, the need for very large fraction collector beds and postpurification screening and pooling was eliminated. Unattended and automated operation of this system led to the purification of overcompounds (mg quantities) per day.

BIOAFFINITY SCREENING

With the integration of highly automated parallel synthesis techniques into drug discovery programs, hundreds of thousands of compounds are now screened against a particular biological target. Once activity is determined for a mixture, the identification of the active component(s) is necessary. A recent study described the use of bioaffinity selection LC/MS methods for the identification of active mixture component(s) (34). This approach features an integrated bioaffinity-based LC/MS screening method to separate and identify compounds from mixtures.

A mixture of compounds is incubated with the target protein and the components bound to the protein are selected by using a size exclusion chromatography (SEC) "spin column." In this experiment, the unbound compounds are retained on the column. The bound components are eluted and identified with LC/MS. Increased specificity is obtained by dissociating the bound compounds and performing a second equilibration incubation with the protein. This procedure preferentially selects for the compounds with higher affinity, and results in an enhancement of the quantitative LC/MS response. Iterative stages of incubation, size-exclusion, and LC/MS allow the tighter binding components to be enriched relative to weaker binding components.

In this study, the peroxisome proliferator-activated receptor (PPARγ), which is a target for anti-diabetic drugs (construct molecular weight of 32,537 Da), is incubated with 10 ligands that range in molecular weight from 283 to 587 units. A spin column of 6000 Da cutoff is used for SEC purposes. The retained mixture of components is analyzed by fast perfusive chromatography (35, 36), using a standard full-scan LC/MS strategy. This analysis procedure allows for the identification and quantitation of the protein and the ligands, compared to their responses prior to incubation. The ligand-protein complex that dissociated under the reversed-phase chromatographic conditions is selectively detected.

This analysis scheme provided a quick measurement of binding affinity, and serves as a screening tool during drug candidate selection. Spreadsheets were constructed and used to calculate the binding affinity of the components. In the example described above, two incubation cycles followed by the SEC separation provided an enhancement of strong binders to weak binders. This LC/MS-based method provides a unique approach to obtain information

in situations when lower concentrations of tighter binding ligands are present in the same mixture with higher concentrations of weaker binding ligands. Furthermore, this method is more efficient than synthetic deconvolution procedures and does not require the use of radioligands.

Combinatorial chemistry initiatives have created a tremendous challenge for activities that deal with the screening of these mixtures for activity against a specified target (37). MS-based approaches that use affinity selection (38), encoding methodologies (39–41), pulsed ultrafiltration (42), and anti-aggregatory approaches (43) have been described.

The use of MS formats that provide accurate mass capabilities have been recently illustrated for screening combinatorial libraries (44–47). The unambiguous confirmation/identification of combinatorial library components from small quantities of material have been illustrated using a hybrid quadrupole/orthogonal TOF (QTOF) (44, 45) and Fourier transform ion cyclotron resonance (FTICR) (47) mass spectrometry. A schematic of a FTICR-MS system is shown in Fig. 6. Accurate isotope patterns or "isotopic signature" and unique mass differences between isobaric compounds can be obtained using these two MS formats.

OPEN-ACCESS SYSTEMS

Chemists now routinely use open-access MS systems in the same way that they previously used thin-layer chromatography (TLC) to monitor reaction mixtures for the desired product and to optimize reaction conditions. In practice, medicinal chemists require only molecular weight data, and are comfortable with a variety of MS ionization methods to obtain this information. However, confidence in the actual method and procedure is a requisite. Today, molecular mass measurement has quickly become a preferred means of structure confirmation over NMR and IR during the early stages of synthetic chemistry activities (i.e., drug discovery), where sample quantities are limited.

In the open-access LC/MS procedure described by Pullen et al. (48), the samples are directly introduced from solution for ease of automation and sample preparation. Chemists prepare samples in solvent to a suggested concentration range, then log the samples into the system. The sample log-in is done at any time during the continuous automated queue. Autosampler vials are used to hold the samples, and autosamplers are used to directly deliver samples in solution to the mass spectrometer. The system uses a standard method to analyze the samples in

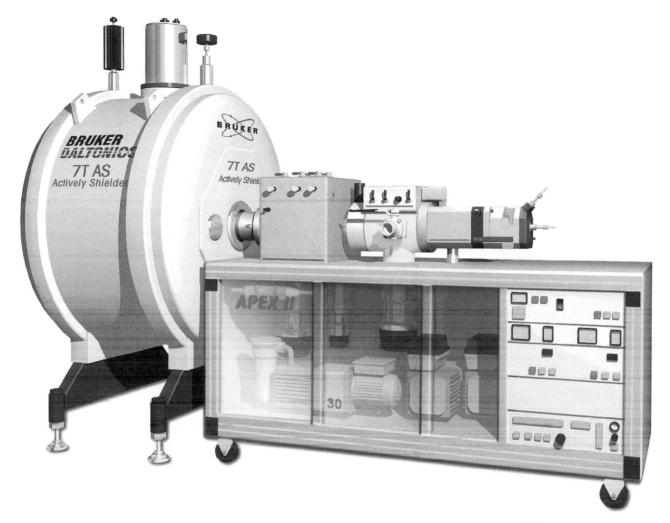

Fig. 6 Schematic of a FTICR MS instrument. This type of MS consists of an ion cyclotron resonance (ICR) analyzer cell that is situated in the homogeneous region of a large magnet. The ions introduced into the ICR analyzer are constrained (trapped) by the magnetic field to move in circular orbits with a specific frequency that corresponds to a specific mass-to-charge ratio (m/z). Mass analysis occurs when radiofrequency (rf) potential is applied (pulsed) to the ICR analyzer so that all ions are accelerated to a larger orbit radius. After the pulse is turned off, the transient image current is acquired and a Fourier transform separates the individual cyclotron frequencies. Repeating this pulsing process to accumulate several transients is used to improve the signal-to-noise ratio. (Courtesy of Bruker Daltonics, Billerica, MA.)

queue, average spectra according to a preset scheme, and print out a spectrum for the chemist. Fail-safe procedures for untrained users and instrument self-maintenance at start-up and shutdown were also developed.

Taylor et al. (49) further demonstrated the value of open-access LC/MS systems for generating a widened scope of pharmaceutical analysis applications, including: 1) characterization of synthetic intermediates and target compounds; 2) reaction monitoring; 3) reaction optimization; 4) analysis of preparative HPLC fractions; and 5) analysis of TLC plate spots. The availability of these methods led to the increased use of LC/MS for structural analysis. The short analysis time and reliable structure

confirmation resulted in the use of LC/MS as a first choice for structure characterization for synthetic chemistry applications.

Open-access LC/MS formats have spawned new dimensions in access and data management. The use of a direct exposure probe (DEP) for automated sample introduction has been developed for quick (ca. 3 min) molecular weight determination of new lead compounds and quantitative analysis (50). Figure 7 illustrates an automated direct probe system for molecular weight determination. Versatile software packages for data manipulation and processing has been a popular approach for integrating analysis and information (51–53). These software programs are efficiently implemented with stand-alone computers and servers that are networked with open-access mass spectrometer data systems. In this configuration, the data are generated, visualized, processed, and automatically reported for the chemist. The program compares a template of predicted molecular ions with the actual ions generated by ESI and APCI for the quick analysis of synthetic products, intermediates, reactants, reagents, and contaminants. A list of observed ions along with known artifact ions is generated and used to provide a measure of the quality-of-fit to the predicted product(s).

Open-access MS systems provide an effective means for maintaining the high-throughput characterization of synthetic compounds. These systems offer an efficient laboratory- to bench-scale integration of sample generation and analysis activities. Advances in analytical instrumentation and electronic communication have also

played a major role in the emergence and acceptance of MS as a front-line tool for structure characterization.

IN VIVO DRUG SCREENING

The application of APCI-LC/MS techniques for the rapid determination of protein binding and pharmacokinetics in drug discovery were recently described by Allen et al. using a single quadrupole instrument (54). A "cocktail" approach consisted of four experimental compounds and a control compound dosed orally at 1 mg/kg with plasma samples obtained at 0.5, 1, 2, 4, and 8 h post dose. To insure reproducibility, the control compound was tested with each cocktail. This approach generated timely systemic exposure (AUC and Cmax)

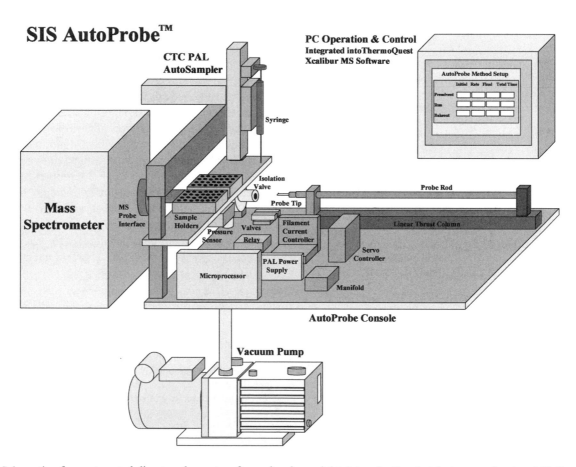

Fig. 7 Schematic of an automated direct probe system for molecular weight determination that features an ion trap MS. Samples are dissolved in a suitable solvent and injected via an automated syringe system onto the DEP wire. The probe is injected into the MS via an automated isolation valve system and the temperature is ramped to the programmed temperature. After sample analysis the probe is removed from the source and heated to a high temperature to clean the DEP wire in preparation for the next sample. This type of integrated, open-access MS-based application provides routine, unattended support for medicinal chemistry needs such as reaction monitoring and the optimization of reaction conditions. (Courtesy of Scientific Instrument Services, Ringoes, NJ.)

data on 44 test compounds in three work days, using two laboratory scientists.

The use of LC tandem quadrupole MS/MS-based screening approaches for quantitative bioanalytical measurements allow a large, chemically diverse, range of potential drug candidates to be analyzed quickly and confidently. A schematic of a tandem quadrupole MS/MS instrument is shown in Fig. 8. The development of unique LC/MS-based systems for in vivo pharmacokinetic screening reduces the analysis to a manageable number of samples, and results in a cost-effective approach to evaluate new lead compounds. Approaches to this type of methodology will likely vary, according to the behavior of the molecules of interest, standard operating procedures (SOPs), performance capabilities of the mass spectrometer, and integration of automated sample preparation, and data analysis procedures. Success will likely be dependent on the above parameters, as well as on the degree of tolerance to which the specific screen is set.

The simultaneous pharmacokinetic assessment of multiple drug candidates in one animal has been termed "n-in-one" or "cassette dosing." As discussed for the previous example, this parallel approach results in an increased productivity for bioanalysis during drug discovery. Beaudry et al. (55) recently investigated the extension of this methodology to study larger numbers of compounds in each mixture, and to integrate sample preparation with the LC/MS/MS system for increased efficiency.

The number of analytes studied in parallel was extended to 63 plus an internal standard. The increased number of analytes was made possible due to improvements to the collision region of the MS/MS system that provide increased sensitivity and reduced "memory effects." In addition, robotic systems for sample handling and on-line (solid phase extraction) SPE of plasma samples were integrated with the LC/MS/MS system. An isocratic reversed-phase HPLC method provided a cycle time of 4.5 min per sample. The on-line sample preparation and short analysis resulted in an increased sample throughput that required less time from the scientist. The method produced good performance, in terms of extraction efficiency, linearity, and limit of detection (LOD), and has the capability of analyzing 320–960 samples per day. The strategic emphasis of this approach is on providing high throughput LC/MS methods for evaluating large numbers of drug candidates during drug discovery to eliminate poor pharmacokinetic performers.

METABOLIC STABILITY SCREENING

The use of fast gradient elution LC/MS techniques on a single quadrupole instrument was described for high throughput metabolic stability screening (56). The method uses as HPLC column-switching apparatus to desalt and analyze lead candidates incubated with human liver microsomes. Substrates were selected whose in vivo clearance is controlled predominantly by phase I oxidative metabolism as opposed to phase II metabolism or renal

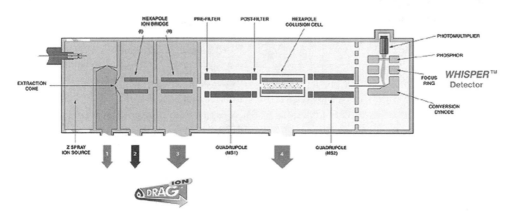

Fig. 8 Schematic of a tandem quadrupole MS/MS instrument. A tandem quadrupole MS/MS instrument consists of two quadrupole MS filters, MS1 and MS2, separated by a collision cell. Each quadrupole MS filter consists of four cylindrical or hyperbolic shaped rods. A unique combination of direct current (dc) potential and radiofrequency (rf) potential is applied to each pair of rods (one pair 180° out of phase with the other). A mass spectrum results by varying the voltages at a constant rf/dc ratio. A variety of scan modes (e.g., full scan, product ion, precursor ion, neutral loss) provide unique capabilities for quantitative and qualitative structure analysis. (Courtesy of Micromass, Manchester, UK.)

clearance. In this way, the resulting data could be resolved into four categories of metabolic stability: high ($\geq$60%); moderate ($\geq$30–59%); low ($\geq$10–29%); and very low ($<$10%).

The rapid structure identification of metabolites is a powerful complement to previously described quantitative approaches. The utility of an automated metabolite identification approach, using LC/MS/MS with an ion trap mass spectrometer has been demonstrated (57). In this study, MS^n analysis is automated to provide maximum structural information in combination with predictive strategies for biotransformation. Automated data-dependent scan functions are used to generate full scan, MS/MS, and MS^n mass spectra of metabolites within a single chromatographic analysis. This feature is unique and avoids the multiple (2–4) injections that are necessary with other MS/MS configurations (e.g., tandem quadrupole). Along with the significant savings in time, detailed structure information is generated, which enables a comprehensive analysis of substructure relationship to be constructed for each metabolite. These automated studies provide unique advantages during drug discovery, and provide an early perspective on the metabolically labile sites, or "soft spots" of a drug candidate. This knowledge is useful during lead optimization activities, and can lead to the initiation of proactive research efforts that deal with metabolism-guided structural modification and toxicity.

METABOLITE PROFILING AND IDENTIFICATION

The application of LC/MS-based techniques for the structure identification of drug metabolites has played a significant role in drug development. The early identification of drug metabolites provides valuable insights into the pathways of metabolism and biotransformation. Once metabolites are identified/confirmed, metabolism-guided structural modification during the drug discovery stage is initiated to facilitate the selection of drug candidates for subsequent development.

The identification of metabolite structures with LC/MS and LC/MS/MS techniques using quadrupole-based MS instruments are an effective approach due to their ability to analyze trace mixtures from complex samples of urine, bile, and plasma. The key to structure identification approaches is based on the fact that metabolites generally retain most of the core structure of the parent drug (58, 59). Therefore, the parent drug and its corresponding metabolites would be expected to undergo similar fragmentation and to produce mass spectra that indicate major substructures.

Kerns et al. demonstrated the application of LC/MS and LC/MS/MS standard method approaches in preclinical development for the metabolite identification of buspirone, a widely used anxiolytic drug (60). The success of this method relies on the performance of the LC/MS interface and the ability to generate abundant ions that correspond to the molecular weight of the drug and drug metabolites. The production of abundant molecular ions is an ideal situation for molecular weight confirmation because virtually all the ion current is consolidated into an adduct of the molecular ion (i.e., $[M + H]^+$, $[M + NH_3]^+$).

Full-scan mass spectra generally contain an abundant $[M + H]^+$ ion signal with little detectable fragmentation. Product-ion spectra are obtained to reveal product ions and neutral losses that are associated with diagnostic substructures of the buspirone molecule. To assist with the MS/MS structure identification, the gross substructure of buspirone is categorized into *profile groups* (61). Profile groups directly correlate specific product ions and neutral losses with the presence, absence, substitution, and molecular connectivity (62) of specific buspirone substructures and their modifications. The profile groups of buspirone are identified with abbreviations that correspond to the three specific substructures: azaspirone decane dione (A), butyl piperazine (B), and pyrimidine (P). Substituted substructures are designated with a subscript (s), and a dash (–) denotes substructure connectivity. Thus, the buspirone molecule is represented by A–B–P. The A_s–B–P designation refers to metabolite structures that contain the azaspirone decane dione, butyl piperazine, and pyrimidine substructures with substitution on the azaspirone decane dione substructure. The profile group categorization within a corresponding database allows the rapid visual recognition of primary substructures affected by metabolism.

Metabolite structure databases can be easily constructed and contain information on the structure, molecular weight, UV characteristics, RRT, and product ions of metabolites obtained from rat bile, urine, and liver S9 samples. Using this format, Kerns et al. reported the predominant buspirone metabolite profile groups as A_s–B–P, A–B–P_s, and A_s–B–P_s. These profile groups indicate azaspirone decane dione and pyrimidine as metabolically active sites of attack and the presence of multiple substitution sites on each of these substructures.

IMPURITY PROFILING AND IDENTIFICATION

Synthetic impurities are of particular concern during process research and safety evaluation activities. Often, impurities are the result of synthetic by-products or starting materials of the scale-up process. Impurities provide a comprehensive indicator of the chemical process and are diagnostic of overall quality. Process chemists use this information to guide process optimization. Knowledge of the identity and relative amount of impurities is used to diagnose process reactions so that changes in reagents and reaction conditions leads to better yields and higher quality material.

With an increasing number of novel lead candidates that enter into preclinical development, considerable resources are needed to identify impurities. LC/MS-based approaches provide integrated sample clean-up and structure analysis procedures for the rapid analysis of impurities. This advantage was demonstrated during the preclinical development of TAXOL® (18). LC/MS played an important role for the identification of impurities contained in extracts and process intermediates from *Taxus brevifolia* and *T. baccata* biomass. Because drugs derived from natural sources often have a very diverse set of structural analogs, it is important to determine which analogs are carried through the purification process and ultimately appear as impurities. This task presents a unique challenge during the early stages of drug development due to the highly complex nature of the samples.

Kerns and coworkers described a structure identification strategy that incorporates LC/MS and LC/MS/MS techniques using quadrupole-based instruments for rapid, sensitive, and high-throughput impurity analysis (18). This approach integrates traditional steps of sample preparation, separation, analysis, and data management into a single instrumental method. The resulting multidimensional data include retention time, molecular weight, UV, and substructure information. A structure database is developed for each candidate and is used to rapidly identify the same impurities in new samples. Structures are proposed based on using the drug candidate as a structural template and, with the use of a standard method approach, consistency for comparison of results throughout the preclinical development process is ensured.

Nearly all of the impurities contained the characteristic paclitaxel core substructure as indicated by the characteristic product ion at m/z 509 with variations due to modifications. Many of these taxanes contained a side-chain similar to paclitaxel, with variations occurring on the terminal amide of the side chain. The product ions that differed from the characteristic side-chain ions of paclitaxel (m/z 286) by values indicative of specific substructures were used to identify these terminal amide variations. A comparison with the paclitaxel substructural template indicated structural differences beyond the position of the amide group in the side-chain substructure.

When a new impurity was encountered during chemical process research, retention time and molecular weight information were compared to the database for rapid identification. This approach is similar to the procedure described for natural product dereplication. If the compound is not contained in the structure database, then the corresponding LC/MS/MS analysis is performed to obtain substructural detail and the proposal of a new structure.

A standard reversed-phase HPLC method was used for all the samples that are associated with a drug candidate to reduce time-consuming method development/method refinement procedures. Standard reversed-phase methods typically involve a 20–30 min cycle time and provide information for a wide range of compounds. The incorporation of a standard method strategy allows the use of autosampling procedures and standard system software for data analysis.

During the development of TAXOL®, 90 taxane impurities were rapidly identified and added to the structure database. This MS/MS information was routinely obtained for impurities down to the 100 ng level (injected), and required approximately 2–3 h for the analysis of each sample. The compounds are structurally categorized with profile group terminology. The LC/MS-based methods were significantly faster than the previously used analytical methods based on scale-up, isolation, fractionation, and individual structural analysis. Software tools capable of sample tracking, interpretation, and data storage facilitate the structure profiling of impurities, degradants, and metabolites (63). Key pharmaceutical analysis elements that deal with sample preparation, real-time analysis decisions, databasing, distribution/visualization of results (Fig. 9) and prediction of fragmentation are now highly integrated.

DEGRADANT PROFILING AND IDENTIFICATION

During the course of drug development, the bulk drug and drug formulation are studied under a variety of stress conditions such as temperature, humidity, acidity, basicity, oxidization, and light. Qin et al. described the utilization of stressing conditions that may cause degradation (64). The resulting samples may be used to validate analytical monitoring methods and to serve as predictive tools for future formulation and packaging studies.

A traditional approach to study degradant formation involves similar time-consuming scale-up and preparation steps as described for metabolite and impurity analysis. Similarly, this area of pharmaceutical analysis

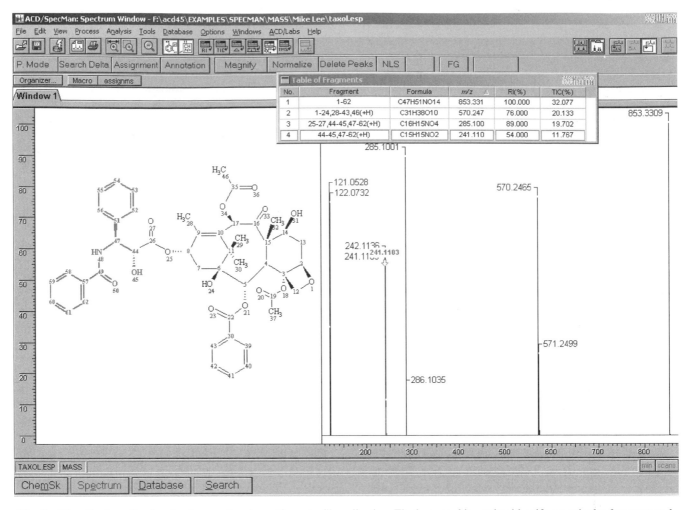

Fig. 9 Visualization of molecular fragments using a "lasso tool" application. The lasso tool is used to identify a particular fragment and, if a signal corresponding to its mass is present in the spectrum, the fragment is highlighted and the corresponding assignment is added to an assignment table. (Courtesy of Advanced Chemistry Development, Toronto, Ontario, Canada.)

has experienced the issues associated with faster drug development cycles. Rourick and coworkers recently described proactive approaches to obtain degradant information with quadrupole LC/MS methods during the preclinical development stage (65). The corresponding structural information provides insight for decisions on which leads to further develop for clinical testing. The early structural information on degradants of a drug candidate offers a unique capability for synthetic modification to minimize degradation. Structural information can also facilitate planning of preclinical drug development in process research, formulation development, and safety assessment.

The strategy for impurity and degradant identification described by Rourick et al. subjects lead candidates to various development conditions followed by LC/MS and

LC/MS/MS analysis protocols. A structure database is constructed from the corresponding results and is used to reveal unstable regions within the drug structure as well as to ascertain which candidate or homologous series of drug candidates may be the most favorable for further development. High capacity and throughput speed are necessary so that many lead candidates may be evaluated. Applicability of the method to a wide range of compound classes is desirable. Once the drug candidate enters clinical development and manufacturing, the structure database is useful for the rapid identification of impurities and degradants in samples generated during these stages of development.

The method exposes drug candidates to forced degradation conditions, (e.g., acid, base, heat, and moisture) as a *predictive profile*. The coordinated use of LC/MS and

LC/MS/MS provide structure identification for speed, sensitivity, and high throughput. Standard methods, useful for 80% of the compounds, are applied. Various types of structural data are obtained for elucidation purposes (e.g., retention time, molecular weight, MS/MS), and unknown compounds are elucidated with the candidate drug as a structural template. The LC/MS analysis provides retention time and molecular weight data, whereas LC/MS/MS provides substructural detail for structure identification. Drug candidates are incubated under drug processing, storage, and physiological conditions that were expected to occur throughout drug lifetime.

Using this approach, 10 degradants of cefadroxil, an orally effective semisynthetic cephalosporin antibiotic, were elucidated in a 2-day study. The use of standard LC/MS methods provided consistency from sample to sample throughout the development process, and allowed for the construction and use of a structural database for the rapid identification of impurities and degradants during development. The reversed-phase HPLC conditions provided a general measure of the polarity of each compound, useful for interpretation of substructural differences between related compounds. Due to the mass-resolving capability of the mass spectrometer, chromatographic resolution of co-eluting or unresolved components was not required. Abundant protonated molecule ions, $[M + H]^+$, provided reliable molecular weight information, and product-ion spectra generated valuable substructure information for each degradant. The product-ion spectrum of cefadroxil was used as a template for interpretation; specific product ions and neutral losses were compared to the spectra obtained from the unknown degradants. Product ions common to each spectrum provided evidence of substructures unchanged by the degradation conditions and differences were indicative of structural variations.

QUANTITATIVE BIOANALYSIS—SELECTED ION MONITORING

The quantitative analysis of targeted components in physiological fluids is a major requirement in clinical development. In 1991, Fouda et al. (66) pioneered the use of APCI-LC/MS on a single quadrupole instrument for the quantitative determination of the renin inhibitor, CP-80,794, in human serum. Because the pharmacological action is below 200 pg/ml, a quantitative assay in the low pg/ml range was required to monitor the drug's pharmacokinetic and pharmacodynamic properties. Also,

the structure of the CP-80,794 molecule lacked a significant chromophore for UV detection with conventional HPLC methods. Furthermore, the low volatility and thermal instability precluded analyses with GC/MS methods.

Quantitative LC/MS assays in clinical development generally involve four intensive steps: sample preparation; assay calibration; sample analysis; and data management. In the method developed by Fouda and coworkers, human serum samples were prepared with a liquid–liquid extraction procedure. Assay calibration involved the use of human serum samples fortified with CP-80,794 at 11 concentrations (6 replicates per concentration) ranging from 0.05 to 10 ng/ml. The LC/MS analysis involved the use of the SIM mode to monitor the molecular ions $[M–H]^-$ that correspond to the drug (m/z 619) and internal standard (m/z 633). In this particular LC/MS application, the negative ion mode was highly sensitive for this class of compound. Samples were loaded onto an HPLC autosampler and 80 μL aliquots are injected onto the column at 4-min intervals. The elution times of the drug and internal standard were 3.1 and 3.4 min, respectively.

At the time, this application provided a powerful benchmark for the use of quadrupole LC/MS-based methods in the pharmaceutical industry and paved the way for the tremendous growth of MS-based applications in support of clinical development. This particular assay successfully supported several clinical studies with sensitive and reliable results. This performance was benchmarked on more than 4000 clinical samples, and led to a widened scope of MS application for quantitative bioanalysis (67–71).

QUANTITATIVE BIOANALYSIS—SELECTED REACTION MONITORING

The use of selected reaction monitoring (SRM) methods for quantitative bioanalysis represents increased dimensions of mass spectrometry analysis. A SRM method that features a tandem quadrupole MS/MS instrument for the quantitative analysis of an antipsychotic agent, clozapine, in human plasma was recently described by Dear et al. (72). Preclinical development studies of clozapine in rats and dogs used HPLC with fluorescence detection (FLD). With this method, a better limit of quantitation (LOQ) of 1 ng/ml was obtained. As the compound moved into the clinical stages of development, a more sensitive method of analysis was required to obtain rapid metabolic information in support of drug safety evaluation studies. As a result, a standard LC/MS/MS method was developed for the quantitative analysis of clozapine (I) and four metabolites (II-V) in human plasma.

The LC/MS/MS strategy deployed is similar to previously described approaches for protein, natural products, metabolite, and impurity identification. An ionization technique that generates abundant molecular ion species with very little fragmentation is desirable. The product-ion spectrum is obtained to generate the substructural template of the molecule. Abundant and structurally unique transitions (molecular ion → product ion) are identified from the spectrum, and are used in the corresponding SRM experiment for quantitation. The SRM experiment provides a high degree of selectivity and better LOD than full-scan or SIM experiments for the analysis of complex mixtures (73, 74). The selectivity of MS/MS reduces the requirements for complete chromatographic resolution of each component. Therefore, LC/MS/MS experiments for quantitation typically emphasize short analytical run times to provide high sample throughput.

The inter- and intra-assay precision (% C.V.) of this method were reported to be less than 8% across the range of the limits of quantification (0.05–10 ng/ml). The accuracy (% bias) for all spiked control concentrations did not exceed ±4%. Same-day turnaround of results for over 100 samples was possible and was used to support an acute dose tolerance and pharmacokinetic study that involved the analysis of 1600 samples.

PEPTIDE MAPPING IN QUALITY CONTROL

Quality control involves a carefully designed series of analysis and protocols. The purpose of this activity during the manufacturing stage of drug development is to ensure the production of safe, high quality drug products. These measures are helpful for the producers of the product as well as the regulators (i.e., FDA). In this way, adherence to protocols and procedure are carefully monitored on a routine basis. When any uncertainty in the manufacturing process occurs, procedures are referenced and data are analyzed to determine the specific stage of manufacturing to begin examining. Thus, the responsibility of drug manufacturers and regulating agencies are to determine *when* and *how* a process went awry. The ability to do so in an efficient, straightforward manner is helpful to both parties, and ultimately, the consumer. Thus, the ability to provide this information is highly dependent on the manufacturer's ability to control the process.

The use of LC/MS in a manufacturing quality control environment for biologicals was reported by Chang et al. (75). Their approach involved three steps.

First, the expected cleavage sites (in this case, trypsin) within the amino acid sequence of the protein somidobove are indicated. This "tryptic map" serves as a template for the expected peptide fragments. Second, an analytical method using chromatography columns and conditions that provide the best resolution and reproducibility is developed. An opportunity exists to optimize the analysis based on chromatography, digestion, and LC/MS performance. Finally, the resulting LC/MS data are profiled, according to amino acid sequence, peak number, and $[M + H]^+$. Other properties such as relative retention time can also be added in this format.

IMPURITY IDENTIFICATION IN QUALITY CONTROL

Regulatory authorities strictly scrutinize the leachables (e.g., plasticizers, impurities) that may come from medical devices and drugs. It is the responsibility of the drug or medical device company to identify the leachables and to provide adequate testing of their toxicity. Monitoring methods must be developed and validated to effectively control toxic leachables during the manufacture of high quality pharmaceuticals.

As a result, materials for medical devices and drug products must be tested for leachable components. Once a known toxic compound is discovered, it must be identified for the assessment of toxicity, followed by the monitoring of levels using validated methods as required by the FDA. This identification procedure could be a time-consuming process with traditional methods that are based on fractionation and individual component analysis.

Tiller et al. demonstrated an analytical strategy with on-line LC/UV/MS and LC/MS/MS to rapidly obtain structural information for leachables from a drug-delivery device (76). Similar to proteomics-based applications, the analysis strategy makes use of "data-dependent" analysis, wherein the mass spectrometer first obtains molecular ions using full-scan techniques, and makes real-time decisions about MS/MS product-ion spectra that must be obtained. In this way, molecular weight and substructural information are both obtained for many components during a single HPLC run.

Many components were readily observed from the ESI-LC/MS chromatogram, and several polyester leachables were identified. The ESI LC/MS chromatogram revealed 15 components, compared to the three components that were observed in the 220 nm UV chromatogram. This difference illustrates the capability of ESI-LC/MS to provide a more universal detection when the analytes

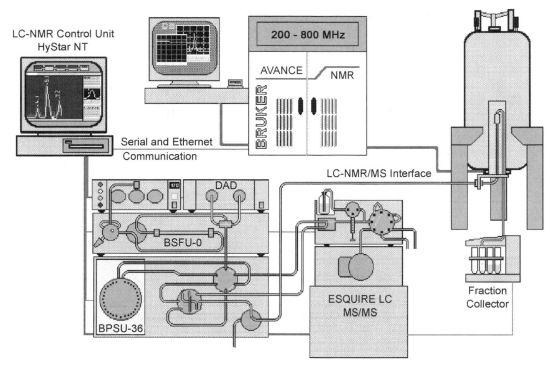

Fig. 10 Schematic of an LC/NMR/MS system. In this configuration, NMR is used to provide structural, stereochemical, or ligand binding information while MS is used to provide molecular weight information. (Courtesy of Bruker Daltonics, Billerica, MA.)

do not contain strongly UV-absorbing substructures (e.g., aromatic). The MS-based method proved to be highly efficient because molecular weight and substructural information via the full-scan and product-ion experiments, respectively, could both be obtained for the sample components.

CONCLUSIONS AND FUTURE PROSPECTS

The understanding and application of MS in the pharmaceutical industry has experienced tremendous growth due to unprecedented sample requirements (i.e., trace mixture analysis) and commercial pressure (i.e., faster development time-lines). Today, MS is an essential component of the modern pharmaceutical laboratory as well as an important complement to traditional methods of analysis.

An expanded role for highly sensitive assays for both quantitative and qualitative analysis will likely continue. Novel pharmaceutically relevant formats and systems that expand current approaches as well as create low-flow, miniaturized formats (77–79) are envisioned. Continued advances in integrated approaches that feature MS will generate significant interest with regard to pharmaceutical analysis. For example, the use of integrated systems that feature NMR/MS have been described for applications that involve LC/NMR/MS (80,81) and MS/NMR (82). A schematic of an LC/NMR/MS system is shown in Fig. 10. In these configurations, NMR is used to provide structural and stereochemical information (80, 81) or to verify binding/interaction (82) while MS is used to provide molecular weight information. New challenges that deal specifically with probing mechanism of action will likely generate the need for a broader application of MS as well as spur the development of novel technologies for sample preparation, chromatography, and information management.

REFERENCES

1. Lee, M.S.; Kerns, E.H. Mass Spectrom. Rev. **1999**, *18*, 187–279.
2. Fenn, J.B.; Mann, M.; Meng, C.K.; Wong, S.F.; Whitehouse, C.M. Science **1989**, *246*, 64–71.
3. Bruins, A.P.; Covey, T.R.; Henion, J.D. Anal. Chem. **1987**, *59*, 2642–2646.
4. Hillenkamp, F.; Karas, M.; Beavis, R.C.; Chait, B.T. Anal. Chem. **1991**, *63*, 1193A–1203A.
5. Burlingame, A.L.; Boyd, R.K.; Gaskell, S.J. Anal. Chem. **1998**, *70*, 647R–716R.

6. Kelleher, N.L. Chem. Biol. **2000**, *7*, R37–R45.
7. Wolf, C.R.; Smith, G. Pharmacogenetics. Br. Medical Bull. **1999**, *55*, 366–386.
8. Ross, P.; Hall, L.; Smirnov, I.; Haff, L. Nat. Biotechnol. **1998**, *18*, 1347–1351.
9. Haff, L.A.; Smirnov, I.P. Genome Res. **1997**, *7*, 378–388.
10. Pezzullo, L.II.; Hall, S.K.; Affourtit, J.P.; Seymour, A.B.; Stroh, J.G. Proceedings of the 48th ASMS Conference on Mass Spectrometry and Allied Topics, Long Beach California, 2000; 1552.
11. Yates, J.R. J. Mass Spectrom. **1998**, *33*, 1–19.
12. Gale, B.L.; Bleibaum, J.L.; MacKenzie, R.T.; Martin, R.L.; Straub, K.M. Proceedings 48th ASMS Conference Mass Spectrometry and Allied Topics, Long Beach, California, 2000; 62.
13. Morris, H.R.; Paxton, T.; Dell, A.; Langhorne, J.; Berg, M.; Bordoli, R.S.; Hoyes, J.; Bateman, R.H. J. Rapid Commun. Mass Spectrom. **1996**, *10*, 889–896.
14. Stevenson, T.I.; Loo, J.A. Proceedings of the 47th ASMS Conference on Mass Spectrometry and Allied Topics, Dallas, Texas, 1999; 215.
15. Buko, A.; Tang, Q.; Trevillyan, J.; Chiou, G. Proceedings of the 47th ASMS Conference on Mass Spectrometry and Allied Topics, Dallas, Texas, 1999; 248.
16. Chalmers, M.J.; Gaskell, S.J. Curr. Opin. Biotechnol. **2000**, *11*, 384–390.
17. Ackermann, B.L.; Regg, B.T.; Colombo, L.; Stella, S.; Coutant, J.E. J. Am. Soc. Mass Spectrom. **1996**, *7*, 1227–1237.
18. Kerns, E.H.; Volk, K.J.; Hill, S.E.; Lee, M.S. J. Nat. Prod. **1994**, *57*, 1391–1403.
19. Strege, M.A. J. Chromatogr. B **1999**, *725*, 67–78.
20. Gilbert, J.R.; Lewer, P. Proceedings of the 46th ASMS Conference on Mass Spectrometry and Allied Topics, Orlando, Florida, 1998; 21.
21. Janota, K.; Carter, G.T. Proceedings of the 46th ASMS Conference on Mass Spectrometry and Allied Topics, Orlando, Florida, 1998; 557.
22. Burdick, D.J.; Stults, J.T. Methods Enzymol. **1997**, *289*, 499–519.
23. Fitch, W.L. Mol. Divers. **1998-99**, *4*, 39–45.
24. Süβmuth, R.D.; Jung, G. J. Chromatogr. B Biomed. Sci. Appl. **1999**, *725*, 49–65.
25. Swali, V.; Langley, G.J.; Bradley, M. Curr. Opin. Chem. Biol. **1999**, *3*, 337–341.
26. Dunayevskiy, Y.; Vouros, P.; Carell, T.; Wintner, E.A.; Rebek, J., Jr. Anal. Chem. **1995**, *67*, 2906–2915.
27. Cepa, S.; Searle, P. Proceedings of the 46th ASMS Conference on Mass Spectrometry and Allied Topics, Orlando, Florida, 1998; 283.
28. Wang, T.; Cohen, J.; Kassel, D.B.; Zeng, L. Comb. Chem. High Throughput Screen **1999**, *2*, 327–334.
29. de Biasi, V.; Haskins, N.; Organ, A.; Bateman, R.; Giles, K.; Jarvis, S. Rapid Commun. Mass Spectrom. **1999**, *13*, 1165–1168.
30. Van Hijfte, L.; Marciniak, G.; Froloff, N. J. Chromatogr. B Biomed. Sci. Appl. **1999**, *725*, 3–15.
31. Weller, H.N. Mol. Divers. **1998-99**, *4*, 47–52.
32. Weller, H.N.; Young, M.G.; Michalczyk, S.J.; Reitnauer, G.H.; Cooley, R.S.; Rahn, P.C.; Loyd, D.J.; Fiore, D.; Fischman, S.J. Mol. Divers. **1997**, *3*, 61–70.
33. Zeng, L.; Wang, X.; Wang, T.; Kassel, D.B. Comb. Chem. High Throughput Screen **1998**, *1*, 101–111.
34. Davis, R.G.; Anderegg, R.J.; Blanchard, S.G. Tetrahedron **1999**, *55*, 1653–1667.
35. Regnier, F.E. Nature **1991**, *350*, 634–635.
36. Afeyan, N.B.; Fulton, S.P.; Regnier, F.E. J. Chromatogr. **1991**, *544*, 267–279.
37. Schriemer, D.C.; Hindsgaul, O. Comb. Chem. High Throughput Screen **1998**, *1*, 155–170.
38. Kaur, S.; McGuire, L.; Tang, D.; Dollinger, G.; Huebner, V. J. Prot. Chem. **1997**, *16*, 505–511.
39. Geysen, H.M.; Wagner, C.D.; Bodnar, W.M.; Markworth, C.J.; Parke, G.J.; Schoenen, F.J.; Wagner, D.S.; Kinder, D.S. Chem. Biol. **1996**, *3*, 679–688.
40. Hughes, I. J. Med. Chem. **1998**, *41*, 3804–3811.
41. Wagner, D.S.; Markworth, C.J.; Wagner, C.D.; Schoenen, F.J.; Rewerts, C.E.; Kay, B.K.; Geysen, H.M. Comb. Chem. High Throughput Screen **1998**, *1*, 143–153.
42. van Breeman, R.B.; Huang, C.-R.; Nikolic, D.; Woodbury, C.P.; Zhao, Y.-Z.; Venton, D.L. Anal. Chem. **1997**, *69*, 2159–2164.
43. Park, S.; Wanna, L.; Johnson, M.E.; Venton, D.L. J. Comb. Chem. **2000**, *2*, 314–317.
44. Blom, K.F.; Combs, A.P.; Rockwell, A.L.; Oldenburg, K.R.; Zhang, J.H.; Chen, T. Rapid Commun. Mass Spectrom. **1998**, *12*, 1192–1198.
45. Lane, S.J.; Pipe, A. Rapid Commun. Mass Spectrom. **1999**, *13*, 798–814.
46. Fang, A.S.; Vouros, P.; Stacey, C.C.; Kruppa, G.H.; Laukien, F.H.; Wintner, E.A.; Carell, T.; Rebek, J., Jr. Comb. Chem. High Throughput Screen **1998**, *1*, 23–33.
47. Speir, J.P.; Perkins, G.; Berg, C.; Pullen, F. Rapid Commun. Mass Spectrom. **2000**, *14*, 1937–1942.
48. Pullen, F.S.; Kerkins, G.L.; Burton, K.I.; Ware, R.S.; Teague, M.S.; Kiplinger, J.P. J. Am. Soc. Mass Spectrom. **1995**, *6*, 394–399.
49. Taylor, L.C.E.; Johnson, R.L.; Raso, R. J. Am. Soc. Mass Spectrom. **1995**, *6*, 387–393.
50. Scientific Instrument Services. *AutoProbe*^TM *Application Note*; Ringoes: New Jersey, 2000.
51. Whitney, J.L.; Kerns, E.H.; Rourick, R.A.; Hail, M.E.; Volk, K.J.; Fink, S.W.; Lee, M.S. Pharm. Tech. **1998**, May,76–82.
52. Tong, H.; Bell, D.; Keiko, T.; Siegel, M.M. J. Am. Soc. Mass Spectrom. **1999**, *10*, 1174–1187.
53. Richmond, R.; Gorlach, E.; Seifert, J.M. J. Chromatogr. A **1999**, *835*, 29–39.
54. Allen, M.C.; Shah, T.S.; Day, W.W. Pharm. Res. **1998**, *15*, 93–97.
55. Beaudry, F.; Yves Le Blanc, J.C.; Coutu, M.; Brown, N.K. Rapid Commun. Mass Spectrom. **1998**, *12*, 1216–1222.
56. Ackermann B.L.; Ruterbories K.J.; Hanssen B.R.; Lindstrom, T.D. Proceedings of the 46th ASMS Conference on Mass Spectrometry and Allied Topics, Orlando, Florida, 1998; 16.
57. Lopez, L.L.; Yu, X.; Cui, D.; Davis, M.R. Rapid Commun. Mass Spectrom. **1998**, *12*, 1756–1760.
58. Perchalski, R.J.; Yost, R.A.; Wilder, B.J. Anal. Chem. **1982**, *54*, 1466–1471.
59. Lee, M.S.; Yost, R.A.; Perchalski, R.J. Annu. Rep. Med. Chem. **1986**, *21*, 313–321.

60. Kerns, E.H.; Rourick, R.A.; Volk, K.J.; Lee, M.S. J. Chromatogr. B **1997**, *698*, 133–145.

61. Kerns, E.H.; Volk, K.J.; Hill, S.E.; Lee, M.S. J. Rapid Commun. Mass Spectrom. **1995**, *9*, 1539–1545.

62. Lee, M.S.; Klohr, S.E.; Kerns, E.H.; Volk, K.J.; Leet, J.E.; Schroeder, D.R.; Rosenberg, I.E. J. Mass Spectrom. **1996**, *31*, 1253–1260.

63. Williams, A.; Lee, M.S.; Lashin, V. Spectroscopy **2001**, *16*, 38–49.

64. Qin, X.Z.; Ip, D.P.; Chang, K.H.; Dradransky, P.M.; Brooks, M.A.; Sakuma, T. J. Pharm. Biomed. Anal. **1994**, *12*, 221–233.

65. Rourick, R.A.; Volk, K.J.; Kerns, E.K.; Lee, M.S. J. Pharm. Biomed. Anal. **1996**, *14*, 1743–1752.

66. Fouda, H.; Nocerini, M.; Schneider, R.; Gedutis, C. J. Am. Soc. Mass Spectrom. **1991**, *2*, 164–167.

67. Wang-Iverson, D.; Arnold, M.E.; Jemal, M.; Cohen, A.I. Biol. Mass Spectrom. **1992**, *21*, 189–194.

68. Ayrton, J.; Dear, G.J.; Leavens, W.J.; Mallett, D.N.; Plumb, R.S. Rapid Commun. Mass Spectrom. **1997**, *11*, 1953–1958.

69. Kaye, B.; Herron, W.J.; Macrae, P.V.; Robinson, S.; Stopher, D.A.; Venn, R.F.; Wild, W. Anal. Chem. **1996**, *68*, 1658–1660.

70. Olah, T.V.; McLoughlin, D.A.; Gilbert, J.D. Rapid Commun. Mass Spectrom. **1997**, *11*, 17–23.

71. Ayrton, J.; Plumb, R.; Leavens, W.J.; Mallett, D.; Dickins, M.; Dear, G.J. Rapid Commun. Mass Spectrom. **1998**, *12*, 217–224.

72. Dear, G.J.; Fraser, T.J.; Patel, D.K.; Long, J.; Pleasance, S. J. Chromatogr. A **1998**, *794*, 27–36.

73. Johnson, J.V.; Yost, R.A. Anal. Chem. **1985**, *57*, 758A–768A.

74. Kusmierz, J.J.; Sumrada, R.; Desiderio, D.M. Anal. Chem. **1990**, *62*, 2395–2400.

75. Chang, J.P.; Kiehl, D.E.; Kennington, A. Rapid Commun. Mass Spectrom. **1997**, *11*, 1266–1270.

76. Tiller, P.R.; El Fallah, Z.; Wilson, V.; Juysman, J.; Patel, D. Rapid Commun. Mass Spectrom. **1997a**, *11*, 1570–1574.

77. Schultz, G.A.; Corso, T.N.; Prosser, S.J.; Zhang, S. Anal. Chem. **2000**, *72*, 4058–4063.

78. Li, J.; Wang, C.; Kelly, J.F.; Harrison, D.J.; Thibault, P. Electrophoresis **2000**, *21*, 198–210.

79. Li, J.; Kelly, J.F.; Chernushevich, I.; Harrison, D.J.; Thibault, P. Anal. Chem. **2000**, *72*, 599–609.

80. Holt, R.M.; Newman, M.J.; Pullen, F.S.; Richards, D.S.; Swanson, A.G. J. Mass Spectrom. **1997**, *32*, 64–70.

81. Shockcor, J.P.; Unger, S.E.; Savina, P.; Nicholson, J.K.; Lindon, J.C. J. Chromatogr. B Biomed. Sci. Appl. **2000**, *748*, 269–279.

82. Moy, F.J.; Haraki, K.; Mobilio, D.; Walker, G.; Powers, R.; Tabei, K.; Tong, H.; Siegel, M.M. Anal. Chem. in press.

SPECTROSCOPIC METHODS OF ANALYSIS–NEAR-INFRARED SPECTROMETRY

Emil W. Ciurczak
Purdue Pharma LP, Ardsley, New York

INTRODUCTION

In recent years, there has been an increased interest in near-infrared (NIR) spectrometry. New instrumentation and algorithms have made the technique more powerful yet simple to use. The physics of NIR allow the samples to be analyzed as-is with, essentially, no preparation. NIR absorbance bands originate in the mid-infrared (MIR) region, but absorbencies are far lower (than those in the MIR), detectors are quieter, and light sources are stronger. The depth of penetration of the NIR light is such that pure materials may be analyzed, allowing whole tablets and bulk materials to be assayed quickly and easily.

Near-infrared radiation is the region of the electromagnetic spectrum between the visible and the (traditional) infrared. The nominal wavelengths for NIR are between 650 and 2500 nm (15,400 to 4000 cm^{-1}). The MIR or traditional infrared derives from the fundamental stretching, bending, and rotating motions of the molecule in question. Its wavelength range is between 2500 and 25,000 nm (4000 to 400 cm^{-1}).

Several aspects of a typical NIR spectrum derive directly from the physics of the region:

1. As the absorptivities in the NIR are 10–1000 times lower than that in the mid-range IR, the peaks are concomitantly smaller. This allows concentrated or pure samples to be scanned.
2. All the higher (1st through 6th) overtones of the O–H, N–H, C–H, and S–H bands from the IR are seen in the (much smaller) NIR region. This, in addition to combination bands (e.g., C=O stretch + N–H bend in protein), gives rise to a crowded spectrum with severely overlapping bands.
3. With lower absorptivities, the radiation penetrates deeper into a sample of either a pure material or mixture. Without dissolving, grinding, or diluting with an inert salt, the integrity of the compound is maintained. Thus, crystallinity, polymorphic form, particle size, and ratio or surface to lattice moisture is maintained.

With these differences from the mid-range IR, standard IR and UV/Vis/NIR instruments could not be counted on to produce satisfactory analyses of nonconventional pharmaceutical samples.

HARDWARE

Initially, work in the NIR was performed on instruments primarily designed for ultraviolet or visible analyses. The NIR portion of the spectrum was an afterthought in many instruments commercially available at that time: Beckman, Cary, Coleman, Perkin-Elmer, Shimadzu, Unicam, and Zeiss. The earliest instruments dedicated to NIR were based upon interference filters. The work performed by Karl Norris of the U.S. Department of Agriculture (Beltsville, MD) was initially done on the UV/Vis/NIR instruments mentioned previously. He established a number of important wavelengths associated with grains and other agricultural products. This group of "useful" wavelengths was then used to guide the wavelengths of the filters first used in the NIR instruments. Later, filters were added for tobacco and textile industries.

The first commercial instrument dedicated to NIR was developed by Dickey-John and presented in 1971 at the Illinois State Fair. The technology was licensed by Technicon and introduced soon thereafter. Technicon then developed its own scanning monochromator-based instrument. This was followed by instruments from Pacific-Scientific (now FOSS-NIR Systems) and LT Industries, to name a few companies.

In the late 1980s and early 1990s, interferometer-based instruments were introduced by companies already producing IR equipment: Nicolet, Bomem, Perkin-Elmer, and others. Often, these FT-NIR instruments were merely adapted FT-IRs that were already in existence and were not suited for pharmaceutical samples: pure raw materials, blends and granulations, tablets and capsules, and larger plastic containers.

A number of instrument suppliers as well as engineering specialty houses are able to install in-line NIR hardware in

Encyclopedia of Pharmaceutial Technology

Table 1 Typical applications of NIR in pharmaceutical production

Quantitative	Qualitative
Moisture in pure substances	Identification of pure substances
Moisture in freeze-dried materials	Identification of mixes
Mean particle size of pure substances	Qualification of pure substances
Mean particle size of mixtures/granulations	Qualification of mixes
Assay/uniformity of blends	Identification of clinical dosage forms
Content uniformity of tablets/capsules	Identity of packaging materials
Level of coating	
Prediction of dissolution times	
Tablet hardness	
Degradation products (tablets)	
Polymorphism	
Crystallinity	

production settings. For up-to-date listings and manufacturers, a newcomer (or even experienced user) should scan the Internet, attend meetings such as PittCon, IFPAC, and more specialized conferences such as the International Diffuse Reflectance Conference (Chambersburg, PA on even-numbered years) or the International NIR Conferences (Europe and Asia on various years).

SOFTWARE

Software, per se, was not available for NIR until the 1980s. Technicon (Tarrytown, NY) and Pacific Scientific (Silver Spring, MD) offered software for their scanning monochromator-based (holographic grating) instruments. The software ran their instruments, collected the spectra, and performed simple calculations. At that time, the only algorithms for NIR used multiple linear regression as the core math treatment ("step-up search" and "best-combination"). Spectral treatments such as smoothing and derivatives were available in the late 1980s, but little in the way of "higher math" treatments.

Throughout the 1980s, researchers were developing private software packages for principle components analyses (PCA) and partial least squares (PLS). These matrix-based algorithms have been commercially available for over a decade from the instrument vendors or from third-party vendors. The PCA and PLS algorithms supplied by instrument vendors are more pragmatic and tend to change more slowly than those provided by vendors whose primary function is to provide software. Recently, artificial neural networks (ANNs or NNs) have attracting attention. These are best discussed in a text devoted to the subject and have not yet been used in industrial settings.

Third-party software vendors perform an important part in supplying software for equation development. These vendors exist solely for providing arithmetic tools for the analyst. Instrument vendors are good at providing software to run their instruments and collect quality spectra. The strong point of software providers is their ability to write software solely for analysis. These programs work, in many cases, better than the software instrument companies because they are single-purposed and not multifunctional (i.e., complex and prone to longer development times and, therefore, bugs.) A listing of these vendors would be at best, ephemeral. Large conferences would be the place to start looking for current suppliers.

The first commercial qualitative analysis software was introduced in 1984 (1, 2) by Technicon. Based on Mahalanobis distance, the program used the absorbances of materials at wavelengths chosen by the software to classify them. This was first applied to incoming raw materials. Since then, virtually every manufacturer of hardware also supplies software capable of performing either qualitative or quantitative analyses. As will be touched on in applications, identification and quality assessment of incoming raw materials is commonplace in the industry.

APPLICATIONS

Owing to the late development of fast, small, and inexpensive computers, little work was performed on pharmaceutical samples until the 1980s. In 1966 (3), many pharmacologically active amine salts were investigated both in solid state and in solution. Two drugs were quantified in 1967 (4): allylisopropylacetureide and

Table 2 Some types of NIR instrumentation and suppliers

Instrument type	Representative manufacturers
Interference filter	Bran & Leubbe
	Dickey-John, Churchill
	Factory of L.I. (Hungary)
	Foss Electric
	General Analysis Corp.
	Infrared Engineering
	Moisture Systems Corp.
	Oxford Analytical, Inc.
	Percon GmbH
	Perten
	Trebor Industries
Scanning grating	Bran &Leubbe
	EG&G Princeton Applied Research
	Foss-NIRSystems
	Guided Wave, Inc.
	Hitachi Instruments, Inc.
	L.T. Industries
	Shimadzu
	Trebor Industries
	Tecator AB
	Varian
Interferometer-based	Bran & Leubbe
	Bomem, Inc.
	Buchi
	Mattson Instruments
	Midac Corp.
	Nicolet Instrument Corp.
	Perkin-Elmer Corp.
Accousto-optic tunable filter	Bran & Leubbe
	Brimrose Corp.
	EG&G Princeton Applied Research
	Infrared Fiber Systems
	L.T. Industries
	Rosemont
Diode-array	EG&G Princeton Applied Research
	KES Analysis
	Perten

phenacetin were dissolved in chloroform and simultaneously quantified at 1983 and 2019 nm, respectively.

Water was determined in several matrices (5) in 1968. Solid samples were analyzed for hydrous and anhydrous forms of strychnine sulfate, sodium tartrate, and ammonium oxalate mixed with KCI and compressed into disks containing 100 mg KCI and 25 mg drug. The water band at ~1940 nm was used for the hydrate analysis.

Since the middle 1980s, there has been an ever-expanding list of applications, both qualitative and quantitative, of NIR in pharmaceuticals. These applications are as follows:

1. Particle Size. Since the first reports of particle size measurement by NIR in 1985 (6) and 1986 (7), numerous researchers have reported using NIR for particle size assessment, both in pure samples and mixes (e.g., 8, 9).

2. Hardness. As NIR spectra are affected by physical and chemical changes within a sample, physical parameters such as hardness may be measured. In 1997, a paper by Morrisseau and Rhodes (10) was published wherein hardness from 2 to 12 kg was estimated by NIR. Several other workers have reported success in measuring hardness: Ebube et al. in 1999 (11) and Kirsch and Drennen (12) have done some quality work on the topic.

3. Polymorphism crystallinity. One of the earliest reported uses of NIR for polymorphism was for the polymorphs of caffeine in 1985 (13). In 1987, Gimet and Luong (14) used NIR to ascertain changes in crystallinity during processing.

   Differentiation between polymorphs was performed by pattern recognition in 1995 by Aldrich et al. (15). The actual control of a process was reported in 1998 by DeBraekeleer et al. (16), where they described using PCA, SIMPLISMA, and orthogonal projections to correct for temperature variation during the monitoring of polymorph conversion. This is a real-time, in-line procedure.

   Several recent papers have also highlighted NIR for polymorphism (17–20). The advantage of NIR for reading polymorphic changes is that the C–C, C–O, and other non-H bonds are not visible. The N–H and O–H bands dominate the spectrum, making crystal changes obvious for qualitative analysis.

4. Enantiomers/structural isomers. The particular optical isomer of a drug being used in a formulation is quite important. Foe example, quinine is used to treat malaria; quinidine, its optical isomer, is used for heart arrhythmia. In 1985, Ciurczak (21) observed that although pure D- and L-amino acids gave identical spectra, the racemic mixtures (DL-) produced an entirely different spectra. Some work was presented by Ciurczak (22) in 1986, which was later expanded and published (23) by Buchanan et al. in 1988, where the enantiomer ratio was determined via NIR.

   Mustillo and Ciurczak (24) presented a paper discussing the spectral effect of optically active solvents on enantiomer mixes. This information was used as a technique to screen for polar modifiers in normal-phase chromatography of racemic mixtures (25).

In 2000, the enantiomeric composition of ibuprofen in solid-state mixtures was performed by Agatonovic-Kurstrin et al. (26).

Structural or geometric isomers as well as nearly identical molecules may be discriminated by NIR. Some early work was performed by Kradjel and Ciurczak (27) and presented in 1985. Work has been performed where the type of polyvinylpyrrolidone is determined by NIR (28) The only differences between types are polymerization conditions.

5. Identification Quality Assessment. In a first of its kind paper, Rose in 1982 showed that a number of structurally similar penicillin-type drugs could be identified and determined by NIR. (29). At Sandoz, Ciurczak in 1984 reported using Mahalanobis distance-based algorithms for the identification of raw materials (30). Ciurczak also reported the use of spectral matching (SM) and principle component analysis (PCA) for raw materials (31) and suggested a method for introducing variations into samples for more robust equation development in 1986 (32). NIR has been in use for raw material ID since then in companies worldwide.

6. Blend Uniformity. An early presentation (33) of the potential for following a dry blend through its stages of mixing by Ciurczak was expanded and published in 1990 (34). A fiber probe was used on a mixture, probing at several locations to several depths. The spectra were the compared with a fully blended sample, using both a SM and a PCA program.

Another similar paper was published by Blanco et al. in 1999 (35). They also used a fiber optic probe on stopped blenders and showed for yet another blend that NIR is a useful tool. Further work was reported on blend uniformity in 1996 by Drennen et al. (36), where samples were thieved and assayed for hydrochlorothiazide by refection NIR.

Workers at Pfizer patented an automated system specifically designed for a "V-Blender." Its development is described in 1996 in a paper by Sekulic et al. (37). This design calls for a single-fiber probe to be permanently inserted in the shaft of the blender. This device was used by DeMaesschalck et al. in 1998, and a paper was published in this work. The significance of this paper was that workers outside Pfizer also used this device successfully.

A study that used both ports along the body of a blender and a two-dimensional imaging technique to measure homogeneity is described in (38). This approach uses multiple measurement points and the speed of NIR. The paper also describes a two-dimensional imaging of the surface to assess uniformity.

Papers by DeMaesserchalck et al. (39) and Berntsson et al. (40) are significant in that they disucss the mathematical treatments involved in following blend uniformity and in-line analysis of active.

7. Moisture. In NIR, as in the MIR, water has the strongest absorption of light. It stands to reason that moisture in solid products would be an important assay. For instance, Warren et al. (41) used NIR to determine the amount of water in glycerides. Transmission spectra of standard propylene glycol and glycerin were used to calibrate and measure for the water content.

Correlation of total, bound, and surface water in raw materials was the topic of a paper by Torlini and Ciurczak in 1987 (42). The NIR was calibrated by Karl Fischer titration, differential scanning calorimetry (DSC), and thermal gravimetric analysis (TGA) for the various water types. NIR could distinguish surface from bound water, whereas standard loss on drying (LOD) could not.

In a recent paper, Derksen et al. (43) showed how NIR could be used to determine the moisture content through the glass vials for freeze-dried samples with varying amounts of active.

In-line moisture of a granulation was discussed by Rantanan et al. (44) in 2000. A binder was added in a solution and the granulation evaluated for residual moisture. Derivatives were used to minimize the particle size effects. Although the measurements were performed (initially) with a full scanning instrument, the authors were able to use fixed wavelength instruments for routine usage. This is an important introduction to simple process control.

Ciurczak discusses similar simple mono-wavelength devices in a recent article (45), where he shows "spark plug" type of mini-infrared source-detector combination. This device should soon be available in the NIR range for similar applications.

8. Clinical Supplies. A rapidly growing use for NIR is the discrimination between clinical dosage forms and placebos that are made to look identical to them. Normally, unmarked tablets or capsules are arranged in a specific manner in blister packs. The identity of which is the active is kept from both the patient and the attending doctor (thus the term "double-blind").

An early application of NIR to clinical samples was published by Aldrich et al. (46) in 1994. Using a custom fiber optic assembly, samples were scanned directly through the polymeric material of the blister packs. This demonstrated the power of discrimination of NIR.

In two papers, Ritchie et al. (47, 48) described an approach for performing NIR qualitatively with an eye

S

to cGMPs (current good manufacturing practices). As clinical lots are often ad hoc formulations, it is difficult to gather enough lots to generate a discriminant equation prior to an actual clinical trial. They developed a procedure whereby equations are quickly generated for a particular study, based on that placebo and active, used for the study, then discarded. Thus, a full validation procedure is shortened to half-day per study.

9. Content Uniformity/assay. The question most often asked is when NIR will be able to be used as a release test. In the earliest NIR assays, tablets and capsules were not analyzed intact. Prior to scanning, the active was extracted and scanned in a clear liquid. The first use of NIR for tablets was reported in 1968 (49). Sherken assayed the meprobamate content in tablet mixtures and commercial preparations. Allen (50) used NIR to analyze a three-component mix: carisoprodol, phenacetin, and caffeine. The powder was extracted with chloroform and scanned in the NIR. Several other publications took advantage of the "dissolve and scan" approach (51, 52).

The first published analysis for powders was written in 1981 (53) by Becconsall et al. It described the analysis of propranolol and magnesium carbonate mixes. In 1987, Ciurczak and Torlini (54) published on the analysis of solid and liquid dosage forms using reflectance and transflectance, respectively.

In 1987, Chasseur assayed cimetidine granules (55). This was the first reported use of a synthetically produced extended range for calibration; calibration samples were produced with a range of content from 70 to 130% of label. In 1987, Osbome (54) used NIR to assay for nicotinamide in vitamin premixes.

In 1988, Jensen et al. used NIR to analyze amiodarone tablets (57). The approach was somewhat primitive: the tablets were scraped of their coating and glued to an aluminum plate. Reflectance was used and six wavelengths were needed to analyze the tablets.

Two chapters of collections were published in the early 1990s wherein solid dosage from analysis was discussed. Based on a presentation at the Fourth International Conference on NIRS (58), Stark used a newly developed diode-array spectrometer scanning between 520 and 1800 nm to analyze specimens. Samples were placed on glass slides and the light collected at a fixed angle. Intact acetaminophen, ibuprofen, and antacid tablets were collected.

In a second chapter (59), Monfre and DeThomas wrote about the calibration of a NIR instrument for the analysis of a prescription vasodilator. Individual tablets were used, but still needed to be crushed for analysis. The important part of the calibration was that no synthetic tablets were produced to extend the range. Using only production tablets ranging from 96% to 102% of label claim, the NIR results were within 0.5 mg of the HPLC values.

Borer et al. used NIR to evaluate the key sources of variation in tablet analysis in 1998 (60). The effects of active variation as well as instrumental variations were evaluated statistically. Factors such as the opening (light beam width), derivative segment size, days between measurement and calibration of the instrument, and tablet orientation were found to be significant. This study tends to affirm the value of transmission measurements where the tablet orientation and optical configurations are fixed.

NIR was used to determine the effects of changes in magnesium stearate concentration and variations in compression pressure on tablet analysis (61). Various types of Avicel (microcrystalline cellulose), varying mostly in particle size, were compressed into tablets with or without magnesium stearate as lubricant by using various compression pressures. Various mathematical treatments were used to either measure the differences or obviate their effects on the analysis.

CONCLUSIONS

The above list of applications is not intended to be a comprehensive listing of all workers or findings in the field of NIR. Rather, it is an overview and can be used as a starting point for informational purposes. By performing a citation search on the authors cited here, the people who have used their work as a basis of current research can be known and will give the analyst an extended list of authors to follow-up for additional discoveries.

REFERENCES

1. Mark, H.L.; Tunnell, D. Anal. Chem. **1985**, *57*, 1449.
2. Ciurczak, E.W. Annual Symposium on NIRA. 7th Technicon: Tarrytown NY, 1984.
3. Sinsheimer, J.E.; Keuhnelian, A.M. J. Pharm. Sci. **1966**, *55*, 1240–1244.
4. Oi, N.; Inaba, E. Yakugaku Zasshi **1967**, *87*, 213–215.
5. Sinsheimer, J.E.; Poswalk, N.M. J. Pharm. Sci. **1968**, *57*, 2006–2010.
6. Ciurczak, E.W. Proceedings of the 1st Pan American Conference, October, 1985, San Juan, PR.
7. Ciurczak, E.W.; Torlini, R.P.; Demkowitz, M.P. Spectroscopy **1986**, *1* (7), 36.
8. Ilari, J.L.; Martens, H.; Isaksson, T. Appl. Spectrosc. **1986**, *45* (5), 722.

9. O'Neil, A.J.; Jee, R.D.; Moffat, A.C. The Analyst **1999**, *124*, 33–36.
10. Morisseau, K.M.; Rhodes, C.T. Pharm. Res. **1997**, *14* (1), 108.
11. Ebube, N.K.; Thosar, S.S.; Roberts, R.A.; Kemper, M.S.; Rubinovitz, R.; Martin, D.L.; Reier, G.E.; Wheatley, T.A.; Shukla, A.J. Pharm. Develop. Tech. **1999**, *4* (1), 19–26.
12. Kirsch, J.D.; Drennen, J.K. J. Pharm. Biomed. Anal. **1999**, *19*, 351–362.
13. Ciurczak, E.W. Proceedings FACSS October 1985, Philadelphia, PA.
14. Gimet; Luong, T.J. Pharm. Biomed. Anal. **1987**, *5*, 205–211.
15. Aldrich, P.K.; Evans, C.L.; Ward, H.W.; Colgan, S.T.; Gemperline, P.J. Anal. Chem. **1996**, *68* (6), 997.
16. DeBraekeleer, K.; Cuesta Sanchez, F.; Hailey, P.A.; Sharp, D.C.A.; Pettman, A.J.; Massert, D.L. J. Pharm. Biomed. Anal. **1998**, *17*, 141.
17. Caira, M.R. *Topics in Current Chemistry*; Springer Verlag: Berlin, 1998.
18. Blanco, M.; Coello, J.; Iturriaga, H.; Maspoch, S.; Perez-Maseda, C. Anal. Chim. Acta **2000**, *407*, 247–254.
19. Patel, A.D.; Luner, P.E.; Kemper, M.S. Internat. J. Pharmaceut. **2000**, *206*, 63–74.
20. Bauer, H.; Herkert, T.; Bartels, M.; Kovar, K.-A.; Schwarz, E.; Schmidt, P.C. Pharm. Ind. **2000**, *62* (3), 231–235.
21. Ciurczak, E.W. Proceedings FACSS October 1985, Philadelphia, PA.
22. Ciurczak, E.W. Proceedings of the 26th Annual Conference Pharmaceutical Analysis August, 1986, Merrimac, WI.
23. Buchanan, B.R.; Ciurczak, E.W.; Grunke, A.; Honigs, D.E. Spectroscopy **1988**, *3* (9), 54.
24. Mustillo, D.M.Ciurczak, E.W. Proceedings of the Eastern Analytical Symposium November Somerset NJ
25. Ciurczak, E.W.; Dickinson, T.A. Spectroscopy **1991**, *6* (7), 36.
26. Agatonovic-Kustrin, S.; Beresford, R.; Razzak, M. Anal. Chim. Acta **2000**, *417*, 31–39.
27. Kradjel, C.; Ciurczak, E.W. Proceedings of the 1st Pan American Chemical Conference, October 1985, San Juan PR.
28. Kreft, K.; Kozamernik, B.; Urleb, U. Int. J. Pharmaceut. **1999**, *177*, 1–6.
29. Rose, J.J.; Prusik, T.; Mardekian, J.J. Parenter. Sci. Technol. **1982**, *36* (2), 71.
30. Ciurczak, E.W. Proceedings of the 7th Annual Symposium on NIRA Technicon, Tarrytown, NY, 1984.
31. Ciurczak, E.W. Proceedings of the AAPS National Meeting November 1990, Las Vegas, NV.
32. Ciurczak, E.W. Proceedings of the 9th Annual Symposium on NIRA Technicon, Tarrytown, NY, 1986.
33. Ciurczak, E.W. Proceedings of the AAPS National Meeting November 1990, Las Vegas, NV.
34. Ciurczak, E.W. Pharm. Tech. **1991**, *15* (9), 141.
35. Blanco, M.; Coello, J.; Eustaquio, A.; Iturriaga, H.; Maspoch, S. The Analyst **1999**, *124*, 1089–1092.

36. Wargo, D.J.; Drennen, J.K.J. Pharm. Biomed. Anal. **1996**, *14* (11), 1414.
37. Sekulic, S.S.; Ward, H.W., II; Brannegan, D.R.; Stanley, E.D.; Evans, C.L.; Sciavolino, S.T.; Hailey, P.A.; Aldrich, P.K. Anal. Chem. **1996**, *68*, 509–513.
38. El-Hagrasy, A.S.; Morris, H.R.; D'Amico, F.; Lodder, R.A.; Drennnen, J.K. J. Pharm. Biomed. Anal. in press.
39. De Maesschalck, R.; Cuesta-Sanchez, F.; Massart, D.L.; Doherety, P.; Hailey, P. Appl. Spectrosc. **1998**, *52* (5), 725–731.
40. Berntsson, O.; Danielsson, L.-G.; Johansson, M.O.; Folestad, S. Analyt. Chim. Acta **2000**, *419*, 45–54.
41. Warren, R.J.; Zaembo, J.E.; Chong, C.W.; Robinson, M.J. J. Pharm. Sci. **1970**, *59* (1), 29.
42. Torlini, R.P.; Ciurczak, E.W. *Proceedings of PittCon* March, 1987;, Atlantic City.
43. Derksen, M.W.J.; van de Oetelaar, P.J.M.; Maris, F.A. J. Pharm. Biomed. Anal. **1998**, *17*, 473–480.
44. Rantanan, J.; Rasanen, E.; Tenhunen, J.; Kansakoski, M.; Mannermaa, J-P.; Yliruusi, J. Eur. J. Pharm. Biopharm. **2000**, *50*, 271–276.
45. Ciurczak, E.W. Spectroscopy **2001**, *16* (1), 17–18.
46. Aldrich, P.K.; Mushinsky, R.F.; Andino, M.M.; Lewis, C.L. Appl. Spectrosc. **1994**, *48*, 1272–1276.
47. Ritchie, G.E.; Mark, H.L.; Ciurczak, E.W. 9th *Diffuse Reflectance Conference*, August 1998; Chambersburg, PA.
48. Ritchie, G.E.; Tso, C.; Ciurczak, E.W. Proceedings of PittCon March 2000, New Orleans, LA.
49. Sherken, S. J. Assoc. Offic. Anal. Chem. **1968**, *51*, 616–618.
50. Allen, L. J. Pharm. Sci. **1974**, *63*, 912–916.
51. Zappala, A.F.; Post, A. J. Pharm. Sci. **1977**, *66*, 292–293.
52. Corti, P.; Dreassi, E.; Corbini, G.; Lonardi, S.; Gravina, S. Analusis **1990**, *18*, 112–116.
53. Becconsall, J.K.; Percy, J.; Reid, R.F. Anal. Chem. **1981**, *53*, 2037–2040.
54. Ciurczak, E.W.; Torlini, R.P. Spectroscopy **1987**, *2* (3), 41–43.
55. Chasseur, J.C. Chim. Oggi. **1987**, *6*, 21–27.
56. Osborne, B.G. Analyst **1987**, *112*, 313–315.
57. Jensen, R.; Peuchant, E.; Castagne, I.; Roux, G. Spectrosc. Int. J. **1988**, *6*, 63–72.
58. Stark, E. *Making Light Work: Advances in Near-Infrared Spectroscopy*; Murray, I., Cowe, I., Eds.; VCH: Weinheim Germany, 1991; 27–34.
59. Monfre, S.L.; DeThomas, F.A. *Near-Infrared Spectroscopy: Bridging the Gap between Data Analysis and NIR Applications*; Hildrum, K.I., Ed.; Ellis-Hornwood: Chichester UK, 1992; 435–440.
60. Borer, M.; Zhou, X.; Hays, D.M.; Hofer, J.D.; White, K.C.J. Pharm. Biomed. Anal. **1998**, *17*, 641–650.
61. Ebube, N.K.; Thosar, S.S.; Roberts, R.A.; Kemper, M.S.; Rubinovitz, R.; Martin, D.L.; Reier, G.E.; Wheatley, T.A.; Skukla, A.J.

SPECTROSCOPIC METHODS OF ANALYSIS—ULTRAVIOLET AND VISIBLE SPECTROPHOTOMETRY

R. Raghavan
Jose C. Joseph
Abbott Laboratories, Abbott Park, Illinois

INTRODUCTION

Many compounds of pharmaceutical interest are colorless. In the early part of the 20th century, analytical methods were developed using color-forming reactions and measurement of color for quantitation. With the development of instrumentation and based on an understanding of optics, ultraviolet and visible spectrophotometric techniques advanced further. However, with rapid development of atomic absorption spectroscopy, plasma atomic spectroscopy, and GC and HPLC techniques, the interest in spectrophotometry waned in the late 1980s and in 1990s. HPLC methods and HPLC instruments advanced further. As a result, rapid scan techniques and microprocessor control of such instruments led to the development of sophisticated UV–vis spectrophotometric detectors. With renewed interest in the application of UV–vis spectrophotometric techniques, a whole new generation of spectrophotometers with microprocessor instrument control, data acquisition, data handling, and data smoothing are currently available.

BASIC CONCEPTS AND DEFINITIONS

Electromagnetic Radiation

Spectrophotometry involves the measurement of the chemical species using light energy. Light is a form of radiation called electromagnetic radiation. Electromagnetic radiation spans a very large region involving very low energy waves (<0.0012 kJ/mol) to extremely energetic cosmic radiation ($>1.2 \times 10^8$ kJ/mol). This energy can be related by the equation $E = h\nu$, where h is a constant known as Planck's constant (equal to 6.62×10^{-24} J/s), ν is the frequency, which is related to the velocity of propagation of radiation as waves; and $\nu = c/\lambda$, where λ is the wavelength of radiation, which is the distance between either of two crests or two troughs of such a wave. Electromagnetic radiation is continuous; however, it is separated into different regions with differing energies.

The instruments and techniques needed to measure radiation are different in different regions of radiation. It should be noted that this artificial separation resulted from historical development of understanding radiation phenomenon. Table 1 lists the different regions of elctromagnetic radiation.

The human eye responds to radiant energy between 150 and 310 kJ/mol (350–780 nm, wavelength). For each color observed, there is a complementary color; this complementary color corresponds to the wavelength of light that is absorbed by the material. Table 2 shows the approximate relationship between color characteristics and wavelength. The wavelength region of interest for pharmaceutical analysis is between 200 and 800 nm (UV and visible region).

Absorption of Light

When light of a particular wavelength passes through a dilute solution in an appropriate container (quartz, glass, or plastic cells), the light may interact with matter in a number of ways. A portion of the light may be absorbed and the rest passed through unaffected but redirected. The redirection phenomenon is known as scattering. The absorbed energy may be emitted with energy of lower wavelength. This process is known as emission. In UV–vis spectrophotometry, the difference between the incident and emerging beam of light is measured. This property, known as absorption, is used in quantitative and qualitative characterization of molecules of pharmaceutical interest. If the intensity of an incident beam of radiation is monitored and compared with that of an emerging beam, there is attenuation in the emergent beam. This attenuation is caused by 1) reflection at the air/cell surface interface; 2) absorption by the cell wall; 3) reflection at the cell/liquid interface; 4) absorption by solute; 5) absorption by solvent; 6) scatter by solution; and 7) refraction or dispersion by cell.

Therefore, to observe only the effect caused by the substance of interest, all other factors have to be eliminated. This is normally achieved by the use of two matched cells. By comparison of the energy of the incident

Encyclopedia of Pharmaceutical Technology

Table 1 Electromagnetic spectrum

Radiation (rays)	$\approx$Frequency (Hz)	Wavelength (m)	Energy (kJ/mol)
Cosmic rays	$>10^{20}$	$<10^{-12}$	$>1.2 \times 10^8$
Gamma rays	$10^{19.5}-10^{20}$	$10^{-12}-10^{-11}$	$1.2-12 \times 10^7$
X-Rays	$10^{16.5}-10^{19.5}$	$10^{-11}-10^{-8}$	$12,000-1.2 \times 10^7$
UV	$10^{15}-10^{16.5}$	$10^{-8}-0.38 \times 10^{-7}$	$310-12,000$
Visible	$10^{14.6}-10^{15}$	$0.38 \times 10^{-7}-0.8 \times 10^{-7}$	$150-310$
Infrared	$10^{11}-10^{14.6}$	$0.8 \times 10^{-7}-10^{-3}$	$0.12-150$
Microwave	10^7-10^{11}	$10^{-3}-10^{-1}$	$0.0012-0.12$
Radio	$<10^7$	$<10^{-1}$	<0.0012

and emergent beams from these matched cells, the extent of light absorbed by the sample of interest (or analyte) can be expressed in terms of a quantity called "absorbance."

Beer Lambert's Law (or Beer's Law)

Instruments used for UV–vis spectra measure the intensity of incident (I_o) and emerging light (I). It is related to absorbance as follows: $A = -\log(I/I_o) = -\log(T)$. T is called transmittance. The instruments can display data as either percent of transmittance or, more commonly, as absorbance A. According to Beer's law, absorbance is proportional to the concentration of the absorbing species and the length of the path through which light travels: $A = abc$, where a is a constant called the absorption coefficient or absorptivity; a is dependent on the wavelength and the unit of concentration, c, and b is the path length in centimeters. When c is expressed as mol/L (M) $A = \epsilon bc$, where ϵ is called the molar absorptivity. Beer's law is applicable under the following conditions:

Table 2 Visible spectrum characteristics

Wavelength (nm)	Color absorbed	Color observed
380–420	Violet	Green-yellow
420–440	Violet-blue	Yellow
440–470	Blue	Orange
470–500	Blue-green	Red
500–520	Green	Purple
520–550	Green-yellow	Violet
550–580	Yellow	Violet-blue
580–620	Orange	Blue
620–680	Red	Blue-green
680–780	Purple	Green

- The incident radiant beam is monochromatic (monochromatic light is light of a single wavelength or better, light of a wavelength within a very narrow range, in terms of what is experimentally feasible).
- The incident radiation travels through equidistant parallel paths through the sample.
- There is no chemical reaction occurring followed by absorption of radiant energy.
- The sample solution is homogeneous and, thus, there is no loss of radiant energy through scattering or by other reflection processes.
- Each molecule absorbs independently and is not affected by other molecules in solution. (Note: This may not be true for high solute concentration).

The common terms, symbols, and definitions of terms, per International Union of Pure and Applied Chemistry (IUPAC) in absorption measurement are given in Table 3.

Applicability of Beer's Law

The direct proportionality between absorbance and concentration for a fixed path length must be established experimentally for a given instrument under specified set of conditions. If this relationship is linear within the specified range of concentrations, the system is said to obey Beer's law. Departure from this direct proportionality arises from both instrumental and chemical reasons.

In Beer's law, c is the total analytical concentration of the absorbing species in a particular molecular state. If there is a disturbance in the concentration of this particular species as a function of solvent concentration, these deviations can be eliminated by appropriate choice of experimental conditions.

Sometimes, in organic acids and bases, the extent of hydrolysis or ionization can be affected as a function of pH. Then, the pH of the analyte should be chosen such that it is

Table 3   Spectrophotometric nomenclature (IUPAC)

Name	Symbol	Definition
Transmittance	T	P/P_0
Absorbance	A	$\log_{10} P/P_0$
Path length	b	—
Absorptivity	a	$A/bc*$
Molar absorptivity	ϵ	$A/bc\#$
Wavelength unit	nm	$10^{-9}\,\text{m}$
Absorption max	λ_{max}	Wavelength of maximum absorption

b is in cms; $c*$ units other than moles per liter; # moles per liter. Other terms used in the older literature are given in Raghavan and Joseph (1997) under Bibliography.

three units more or three units less than the pK_a of the monoprotic acid. Otherwise, the absorbance measurement can be made at a wavelength at which molar absorptivities of both species are identical. The wavelength at which the absorbencies are identical is known as isosbestic point. At this wavelength, the molar absorptivity of the two species is the same and, thus, measurements at this wavelength do not deviate from Beer's law. At millimolar concentrations at which absorbance measurements are made, the refractive index of the sample and that of the reference do not differ considerably. However, if the concentration is increased, as in derivative spectrophotometry, refractive index may be altered and, as a result, deviation from Beer's law may become significant. The second type of deviation from Beer's law occurs under derivative and dual wavelength spectrophotometric conditions. Deviation from Beer's law is negligible if:

- instrumental deviations are minimal;
- the solvent absorption is negligible in comparison with the analyte absorbance;
- the analyte concentration is within a specified range;
- there is no chemical interaction between solute molecules or between solute and solvent molecules; and
- the temperature is maintained constant, especially for flow injection analysis and reaction rate measurements.

Deviations from Beer's law caused by instrumental parameters are discussed later.

COMPONENTS OF THE SPECTROPHOTOMETER

List of Instrument Components and Functions

A spectrophotometer measures the change in light intensity when light passes through a liquid sample or other medium. Therefore, appropriate light source(s) is needed. The light source gives out radiation consisting of a whole range of wavelengths and different intensities. Therefore, these different wavelengths should be separated. The light thus separated has to be passed through the analyte sample. To monitor the emerging beam, knowledge of incident beam is gathered from a reference solution containing all the matrix elements except that of the analyte. The emerging light needs detection, and an appropriate display system is needed for proper presentation of data. These different components and their functions are presented briefly in Table 4.

Light source

Two light sources, one for each region, are commonly used. For the visible region, a tungsten filament lamp sealed inside a quartz envelope containing a small amount of iodine is used. The source is operated at 3500 K. This type of lamp has excellent stability and a useful life of more than 10,000 h. For the entire UV region, a deuterium arc discharge lamp is used. This lamp consists of a quartz envelope filled with deuterium gas at a pressure of <0.01 atm (2–3 mm) and two electrodes separated by a small distance. When electrically discharged by passing a current through the electrodes, light is emitted as a result of ionization of gas and produces a continuous emission spectrum below 375 nm. This lamp has a useful life of more than 1000 h. A typical spectrophotometer contains both types of lamps, with a mechanical source selector that automatically switches between the two lamps as necessary. (It should be noted that mercury-vapor lamps are normally used as light sources for UV detectors of high-performance liquid chromatographs. Because a majority of organic compounds of pharmaceutical interest absorbs at 254 nm, and this lamp has an intense line spectrum at 253.7 nm, this lamp finds wide use in HPLC detectors).

Monochromators and filters

In forward optic spectrophotometers, electromagnetic radiation of a specified wavelength is passed through sample solutions. Because radiation from source is polychromatic (consists of light of all wavelengths), the various wavelengths of radiation must be separated within a narrow range to form a monochromatic beam before it is passed through the cell and directed on to the detector. Two types of wavelength selectors are used. These are 1) filters, which provide a limited wavelength selection with a high bandwidth, and 2) monochromators, which provide continuous variation of wavelengths with narrow bandwidths. Monochromators serve two basic functions, namely, they isolate the narrow bandwidth of wavelengths very close to the specific

Table 4 Components of a spectrophotometer and their functions

Component	Functions of the component
Power supply	Regulates and provides constant power needed for the light sources
Light source	Provides electromagnetic radiation over a range of wavelengths; the intensity may vary as a function of wavelength
Monochromator	Selects a narrow band of wavelength of choice
Entrance and exit slits	These slits are part of a monochromator to select a narrow beam of light
Sample port	This port accommodates a cell containing sample analyte and any other reference cells
Detector	The detector consists of a photosensitive device, which converts radiation energy into electrical energy yielding an output signal; this may consist of electronic circuitry and microprocessors and other components to amplify the initial signal received from the radiant energy
Digital read-out/computer	The digitized signals from the detector are stored in a computer for data-handling and for graphical display or print-out later

(selected) wavelength and automatically adjust exit slits such that the intensity of the light at the chosen wavelength is maximum, and light of other wavelengths is minimal or preferably, negligible. In addition, the monochromator lends itself to rapid scans of the entire spectral region of interest. The monochromator is a system consisting of combinations of lenses, a dispersion device (a prism or more commonly a grating), slits, and filters.

The entrance and exit slits of a monochromator isolate narrow portions of the light beam and direct them on to the grating. The slit width may be varied automatically by instruments to increase or decrease radiant power reaching the sample and detector. The grating is automatically driven by what is called a sine-bar mechanism, in which the bar that holds the grating is attached to a stepper motor-driven micrometer screw. Thus, the instrument covers a range of approximately 200–900 nm, with wavelength variation of ±0.2 nm.

The grating is used to split polychromatic light into a series of monochromatic radiation of selected wavelengths. The diffraction grating used in UV–vis spectrophotometer is a very simple optical device that consists of parallel grooves. Most gratings in spectrophotometers are prepared holographically by coating a flat glass plate with a photosensitive material. An interference pattern is then generated by the use of laser beams. When the photosensitive layer is developed, glass plates are left with perfectly grooved patterns. To make the grating reflective, a thin film of aluminum is vacuum-deposited on its surface. A protective layer of silicon dioxide is deposited on top of this aluminum layer to keep it from tarnishing. Given the use of lasers, and holographic techniques, a precision level of <0.001 nm can be attained for these gratings.

When polychromatic radiation is incident upon the grating, it is rotated, resulting in a specific wavelength of light being allowed to pass through the slit and then onto the sample or detector depending on the nature of the spectrophotometer. Such rotation of the grating results in scanning a series of wavelengths each time with a specified wavelength. Thus, polychromatic light is split into monochromatic light. Gratings, therefore, provide stable, parallel, and highly monochromatic light, and stray radiation is greatly reduced in holographically generated grating monochromators. For UV–vis spectrophotometers, the gratings used normally have 1000–3000 lines per millimeter. Thus, a single grating, as a dispersion device, is adequate to cover the entire range between 200 and 900 nm.

Cells

Sample cells are available in a variety of shapes and sizes that can be used for many different applications. The most common is a rectangular-shaped cell, made of quartz, with dimensions of $12 \times 12 \times 45$ mm, with an inside length of 1 cm, and holds approximately 4 ml of solution. Cylindrical cells are normally 20 mm in diameter with a path length ranging from 5 to 200 mm. Because glass and plastic materials absorb in the UV region, quartz cells are required for measuring spectra below 340 nm, but cheaper glass cells or disposable plastic cells are adequate for the visible region. Cells with built-in water jackets are available for maintaining constant temperature for kinetic studies. Flow-through cells for flow injection and HPLC applications typically have cell volumes between 0.5 and $2 \mu l$, with a path length of approximately 1 cm. For limited samples, typically with a cross-sectional area of 2×2.5 mm, holding at least $60 \mu l$ of sample is available. With special ultramicrocells, samples volume as low as $5 \mu l$ can be used.

The cell windows should be maintained clean with no scratches and adhering liquids. The placement of the cuvettes is very important. Otherwise, cell walls can block the radiation beam, resulting in irreproducible erroneous results. Cells should always be stored in matched pairs, dry, and preferably inside a protective container. Catalogs provide figures and a list of the different types of cells available commercially.

Detectors

A detector is a device in which light intensity is transformed into an electrical signal. An ideal detector should have the following characteristics:

- high sensitivity irrespective of wavelength;
- very low drift in sensitivity, if any, over the entire wavelength range;
- high signal-to-noise ratio;
- no dark signal (or, if any, it should be very low);
- rapid response time;
- linear response to radiant power; and
- ease in calibration and standardization.

Even though no detector meets the entire criteria, many commercially available instruments, come very close to ideal with respect to performance characteristics.

Typically, light is allowed to fall on a metal coated with a light-sensitive substance. When light falls on this substance, electrons are released. By maintaining a potential difference of approximately 100 V, the released electrons from the cathode travel to the anode, producing a photocurrent. The resulting photocurrent thus generated is proportional to the intensity of light and is amplified, digitized, and measured. The measured current is plotted as a function of wavelength. However, in a majority of spectrophotometers, photomultiplier tubes are used to produce secondary amplification. The secondary amplification is produced such that for every primary electron generated, secondary electrons are attracted to a secondary electrode called a dynode. By using 8 to 10 dynodes, that are suitably oriented, connected in series, and having increasing positive potential, a million-fold amplification in photocurrent is attained. Very efficient silicon diodes are also used in many newer instruments.

Semiconductor silicon diodes

Semiconductor silicon diodes, called photodiodes, with special conductance properties are generally used in diode array spectrophotometers. Photodiodes are very useful because scan times of the order of a few milliseconds and thus many scans may be obtained in a very short time. In addition, the data obtained, being digital, can be further processed to generate spectra with a very high degree of resolution and accuracy.

Charge coupled device detectors

These solid state detectors are multichannel devices. They have large number of photon-detecting registers. The registers are semiconductor capacitors that have been formed on a silicon chip. These detectors, which can detect very low levels of light, are primarily used in probe-type, near-infrared, and visible spectrophotometers and in fluorometers.

Read-out devices

The electrical signal from the detector is fed into an instrument with read-out capabilities. These read-out systems may be direct-reading or null point systems. In direct-reading systems, the output of the detector is allowed to drive a sensitive meter. In the null point systems, the detector output is balanced by a reference circuit. Because of the imbalance in the current, a servomotor is activated, and this stops when the two circuits are balanced. The extent of movement of the motor directly gives a digital readout. Most popular digital read-out device provide a visual numerical display using light-emitting diodes or tubes. These are directly controlled by the signal from the detector. These digital read-out devices have very rapid response. Current spectrophotometers and photometers are microprocessor-controlled instruments with digital read-out capabilities.

INSTRUMENTATION

The components of a spectrophotometer can be arranged in one of two ways as shown in Fig. 1.

The two arrangements differ only in the relative arrangement of the sample and the monochromator. However, the complexity, the quality, and the speed at which data are acquired and presented are very different. A brief account of these is given below.

Forward Optic Spectrophotometers

Forward optic spectrophotometers are either single-beam or double-beam spectrophotometers. The single-beam instruments can be either very simple or expensive depending on the sophistication desired or needed. Simple single-beam instruments have poor stability and excessive drift. These advantages are eliminated in systems equipped with a high-resolution monochromator with adjustable slits, controlled by microprocessors for rapid data acquisition and evaluation of data.

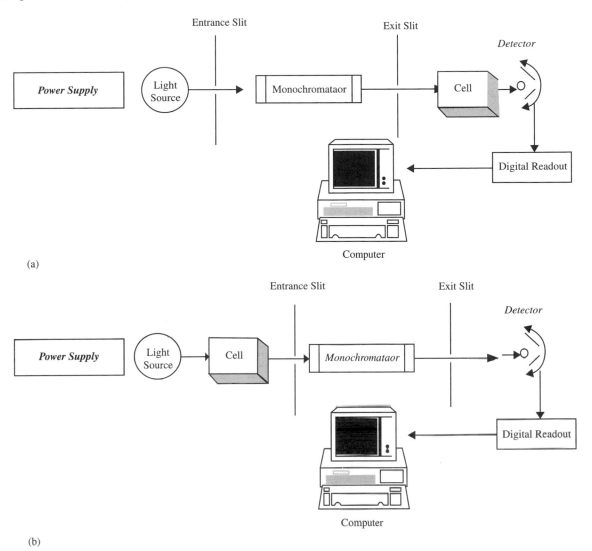

Fig. 1 (a) Components of a typical UV–vis spectrophotometer (forward optics). (b) Components of a reverse optics spectrophotometer.

There are two different types of double-beam systems. One such double-beam system, referred to a double-beam-in-time, is shown in Fig. 2a and the other, known as double-beam-in-space, is shown in Fig. 2b.

In the double-beam-in-space system the components of a single beam are exactly duplicated except for the light source. In this system, the primary light beam is split into two beams with a mirror. One of the beams passes through a reference cell containing the solvent alone, whereas the second beam passes through the sample cell. The signal from the detector of the reference cell is subtracted from that of the sample cell, and the absorbance is plotted against the wavelength.

The dual-beam, single-deflector system is referred to as a double-beam-in-time spectrophotometer. In this

system, the primary beam is split into two beams by a mechanical chopper; the chopper is a rotating wheel with alternate silvered and cut sections. The rotating chopper, in addition to splitting the beam, introduces a dark beam into each beam so that the detector records a series of alternating dark-reference dark-sample signals. Using an appropriate chopping frequency and a synchronizing signal, the three signals are measured within 10–50 ms. As a result, this configuration, more easily being amenable to microprocessor control, is used in many rapid scan spectrophotometers.

The double-beam instruments compensate for

- fluctuations in the radiation output signal;
- drift in the detector and amplifier; and

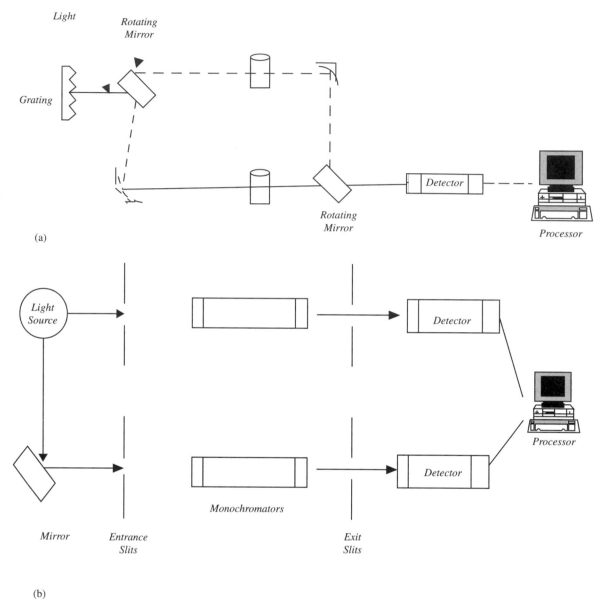

Fig. 2 (a) Block diagram of a double-beam-in-time spectrophotometer (single-detector system with a beam-splitter); a chopper motor can be used in place of the mirror. (b) Block diagram of a double-beam-in-space spectrophotometer.

- wide variations in the intensity of the light source as a function of wavelength.

Reverse Optic Spectrophotometers–Photodiode Array Detectors

The photodiode array detectors are based on reverse optics as shown in Fig. 1b. In this mode, a pair of vibrating mirrors passes the polychromatic light through either the reference cell or the sample cell. The emerging light dispersed by a dispersion grating (in the monochormator) reaches the diode array detector consisting of a linear array of miniature diodes. The number of such photodiodes may vary between 256 and 4096 per array, with 2048 being the most common. Many such diodes can be formed along the length of a silicon chip. Typically each chip is 1- to 6-cm long, and the widths of the individual diode may vary from 15 to 50 μM. The monochromatic slit width is adjusted to correspond to the width of one of the silicon diodes. Therefore, the output signal of each diode corresponds to

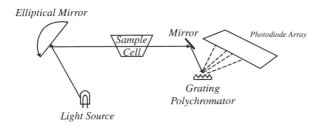

Fig. 3 Schematic of a photodiode-array detector.

the radiation of a different wavelength. By scanning the output of each diode sequentially, a spectrum can be obtained. Because the electronic processing is very rapid, the entire spectrum in a specified range can be acquired in less than 5 ms. The analog signals from the photodiodes are digitized and transferred to a computer. Many different types of multichannel detectors and other diode array detectors are commercially available. These rapid scanning detectors are used for

- analysis of multiple components in a mixture;
- following reactions pathway of short-lived intermediates in reaction kinetics;
- process control by continuous monitoring;
- measuring the dissolution rate of tablets; and
- obtaining spectra of a mobile solution (detection in HPLC).

These new instruments containing several microprocessors with appropriate hardware and software control the following:

- autosampling, which involves loading cell holders and measuring number of samples sequentially;
- automatic mixing, adding reagents, if necessary, diluting, and other sample preparations;
- setting up operating conditions such as selecting a lamp, filter, wavelength drive, and data acquisition mode;
- controlling autocalibration, automatic baseline noise storage, and baseline subtraction;
- multiple data handling characteristics such as spectrum smoothing, data graphical display, and data and peak expansion;
- addition and subtraction of spectra, creation of overlapped spectra for comparison and the like;
- control-associated hardware peripherals such as printers, plotters, etc.; and
- self-test procedures and record keeping of lamp use, maintenance records, etc. to comply with GLP regulations.

PERFORMANCE PARAMETERS OF A SPECTROPHOTOMETER

Specification and List of Parameters

The performance of a spectrophotometer is dependent on a number of parameters that affect the quality of the data, namely, wavelength accuracy, photometric (absorbance) accuracy, spectral bandwidth variations, extent of stray light, and linear response of the instrument. The performance parameters can be evaluated from the specifications provided by the manufacturer. A standard list of specifications of a typical double-beam spectrophotometer is provided in Table 5.

A brief outline of the specification terms, the values of which determine the performance parameters of the instrument, are presented below.

Wavelength Accuracy and Wavelength Calibration

The wavelength accuracy corresponds to the accuracy with which wavelengths measured in different instruments can be compared. In many spectrophotometric procedures, the analyte is quantitated by comparing the absorbance of the analyte with that of a reference standard. The standard is usually prepared at virtually the same concentration of the analyte and absorbance measured at the λ_{max} of the chromogenic species. This approach is satisfactory for most filter photometers because comparisons are made at a fixed wavelength and with the same spectral bandwidth. However, when continuous choice of wavelength is available, as in many grating spectrophotometers, the accuracy and reproducibility of wavelength as well as the intensity of analyte absorbance have to be verified. This is accomplished by wavelength calibration. For wavelength calibration, holmium oxide glass, usually supplied by the instrument manufacturer, is used. Holmium oxide glass, when scanned between 280 and 650 nm, give very short principal peaks at 241.5, 279.3, 287.6, 333.8, 360.8, 418.5, 536.4, and 637.5 nm. Wavelength accuracy can also be checked using the emission lines from a low-pressure mercury source or deuterium lamp. The spectral bright lines used for this check are 486.0 and 656.1 nm.

For broader bandpass filters, neodymium glass filters are available for additional wavelength calibration in the visible region. Special NIST reference materials referred to as SRM (standard reference materials) numbers are available for calibration and verification from the National Institute of Standards and Technology. Information about these standards can be accessed

Table 5 Standard list of specifications for a typical spectrophotometer

Specification	Typical value for a double-beam instrument
Wavelength range (nm)	190–900 nm
Wavelength accuracy (nm)	±0.3 nm at slit width of 0.2 nm
Wavelength repeatability (nm)[a]	±0.1 nm
Wavelength scanning speed	Fast, medium, slow, and super slow
Bandwidth (nm)	0.1–7.5 nm (variable and selectable)
Resolution (nm)	±0.1 nm
Stray light (%)	<0.015% at 220 and 340 nm
	<0.0003% at 220 and 340 nm (drift instrument)
Photometric accuracy (AU)[b]	±0.002 in 0–0.5 AU
	±0.004 in 0.5–1.0 AU
Photometric repeatability[c]	±0.001 in 0–0.5 AU (with NIST 930 D filter)
U (AU)	±0.002 in 0.5–1.0 AU
	±0.3%T (0–100%T)
Photometric mode	Absorbance (Abs), transmittance (%), reflectance (%), and energy (E)
Base-line correction	Selectable with storage firm ware
Drift (AU/h)	<0.0004 after warm up
Response time or time constant	≈0.1–5 s
Photometric range (AU)	−4.0–5.0
Baseline flatness[d] (AU)	Within ±0.001 Abs
Scan speed	50 nm/min to ≈2100 nm/min

[a]Wavelength repeatability is a measure of the precision of the wavelength measured.
[b]AU = Absorbance units.
[c]Photometric repeatability refers to the precision of measured absorbance especially using a standard.
[d]Baseline flatness refers to the average deviation from 0.0 AU for a blank versus blank spectrum in the wavelength range in which the spectrum is taken. *Note*: This may be dependent on scan speed.

directly from the Internet (http://www.i-nist.gov/itl/div898/index.html).

Wavelength Repeatability and Bandwidth

Spectral Bandwidth (SBW)

Wavelength repeatability is a measure of the precision of wavelength measured. The bandwidth refers to the width of an emission band (from the monochromator) at half peak height. This value, normally provided by the manufacturer is accepted. Using a mercury vapor lamp one can also check the spectral width. A number of well defined emission lines at 243.7, 364.9, 404.5, 435.8, 546.1, 576.9, and 579 nm can be used to check spectral bandwidth. However, the accuracy of the absorbance measured is dependent on the ratio of spectral bandwidth to the normal bandwidth (NBW) of the absorbing species. Most active pharmaceutical compounds have a normal bandwidth of approximately 20 nm or greater. With a SBW/NBW ratio of 0.1 or less, absorbance can be measured with an accuracy of 99.5% or greater.

Resolution

Spectral resolution is a measure of the separation between two adjacent wavelengths. The two adjacent peaks are said to be resolved when the minimum absorbance between the two peaks is 80% or lower of the maximum absorbance. Most double-beam spectrophotometers have resolution below 0.5, typically 0.1. However, many diode array and rapid scan spectrophotometric detectors have resolution between 1 and 2 nm.

Photometric Accuracy

Photometric accuracy is determined by comparing measured absorbance to a certified absorbance of accepted standards. Solutions of potassium dichromate are recommended for evaluation of photometric accuracy. [See Raghavan and Joseph (1997) under Bibliography] details about these standards. However, instrumental noise, drift, and stray light influence both photometric accuracy and precision. A discussion of these follows.

Noise

Noise in UV–vis spectrophotometry refers to uncertainties caused in the measurement of the absorbance signal. Essentially, there are two sources of noise. One is dependent on the source intensity (Schott noise) and the other independent of it. The effect of noise in spectrophotometric measurement can be significantly reduced if the concentration of the analyte is adjusted such that measured absorbance is between 0.3 and 1.2 absorbance units. A significant source of noise in double-beam instruments arises when sample and reference cells are not positioned properly. Minor imperfections in the cells cause reflections and scattering losses, which vary as a result of variations in the exposure of cell windows to the beam of light.

Drift

Photometric accuracy is also affected by drift. Drift is caused by changes in lamp intensity between measurements. This effect is nullified by subtracting the background absorbance of the analyte at a reference wavelength in a nonabsorbing region of the spectra. This process of "internal referencing" improves accuracy considerably. If the drift varies as a function of wavelength, two reference wavelengths, one before and one after the wavelength of interest, but in nonabsorbing regions, are chosen. This drift is assumed to be linear, and the drift calculated by linear fit at the wavelength of interest is subtracted.

Stray light and slitwidth

The spectral bandwidth is directly proportional to the slit width. When the slit width is narrowed, the bandwidth is less and thus the spectral purity increases. However, as the slit width is reduced, the signal-to-noise ratio also decreases proportionately, causing poorer precision. A slit width of 2 nm is adequate for most bands. A slit width of 0.5–1 nm is preferable for sharp bands. In HPLC detectors, to maximize the sensitivity, the slit width is automatically kept at 5 nm unless a rapid scan is carried out. During rapid scan, the slit width is normally changed to 1 nm. Stray light is any radiation identified by the detector outside of the narrow band of the wavelength selected by the monochromator. Scattering and diffraction inside the monochromator introduce stray light. Stray light is usually expressed as a ratio (or percent) of stray light into the sample compartment or into the detector housing. In the specification, stray light is given to be 0.015% at 220 and 340 nm. Many currently available double-beam instruments have very low stray light values. Stray light values below 0.1% gives absorbance measurement errors below 0.5%, when the absorbancies measured are approximately 0.5 AU. Stray light becomes significant for quantitative measurement if the measurement is below 220 nm or above 330 nm because the source intensity is low in these regions. Manufacturers typically give stray light data at 220 and 340 nm. Stray light contributions increase with the age of the instrument. Therefore, the extent of stray light contribution needs to be assessed when necessary.

Factors that Influence Spectra

The position and intensity of the different bands in a spectrum depends on a number of factors. The effects of some of these may be considerable.

Solvent effects

The position and intensity of the different bands in a spectrum depend on the nature and conditions of the solvent used. In addition to electronic excitation, which causes absorption, vibrational and rotational energy level changes occur when light is absorbed. As a result, when spectrum is generated in the vapor phase vibration and rotation, fine structure is observable. However, in a solvent medium, because of thermal agitation and different types of interaction of the solute with the solvent, the position of λ_{max} may differ from solvent to solvent. In general, in polar solvents, interaction degrades the spectrum into broad bands because of molecular, electronic, and hydrogen-bond interactions. In aqueous solution, pH, concentration of analyte, ionic strength, and temperature can alter the position and intensity of maxima observed.

Deviation from Beer's law: Instrumental factor

The radiation entering a sample cell is a narrow band of polychromatic radiation. Thus, the effective molar absorptivity is an average of multiple wavelengths. As a result, the positive deviations from Beer's law may occur at low concentrations, wheras negative deviations may occur at higher wavelengths. Nonlinear behavior may also occur as a result of varying path length. When radiant beam is reflected at the solution/wall interface back into the solution, the beam traverses multiple paths. Thus, the net effective path length is increased and, therefore, the absorbance increases. This becomes pronounced (~0.3%) at low concentrations.

APPLICATION OF SPECTROPHOTOMETRIC MEASUREMENTS

In pharmaceutical analysis, spectrophotometric measurements are normally used for quantitative determination of known constituents. They are also used for qualitative analysis of compounds. These are addressed briefly. [See Gilpin and Pachla (1997, 1999) for extensive review of these methods.]

Qualitative Analysis

UV–vis spectrum of an analyte in solution is usually broad with very few narrow bands and shoulder. However, based on the nature of specific functional groups present in a molecule, some general spectral behavior was observed. Based on these studies and with the aid of quantum mechanical calculations, empirical relationships between structure and functional groups have been established. The terms commonly used in defining spectra are shown in Table 6.

Organic Functional Groups and Structure Elucidation

In a molecule, the absorption of ultraviolet or visible light represents the excitation of bonding electrons. Therefore, from the position of λ_{max} and also from the intensity, the structure of functional groups present can be inferred. UV–vis spectroscopy can be used as a powerful tool to supplement identification of functional groups by other techniques. The electrons present in the ground state (lower energy state) of a molecule are excited to higher energy states by the absorption of light energy. This energy that is absorbed is measured. Some typical chromaphoric groups and their spectral characteristics are presented in Table 7.

The presence of an absorption band at a particular wavelength is a strong indication that a particular chomophore is present in the molecule. When additional functional groups are added, the characteristics change. For example, C–C double bond in butadiene absorb approximately at 214 nm. When a third double bond is conjugated, the absorption maximum is shifted to a longer wavelength by 30 nm. Also, alkyl substitution at a carbon atom leading to branching increases by another 5 nm. Empirical relationships, known as Woodward–Feiser rules, help predict the position of λ_{max} in organic molecules. These empirical rules are applied to assign structures of organic molecules or distinguish between some isomeric compounds. Organic chemists use spectral data as an additional powerful tool to assign structures of organic compounds. [For a review of structure/spectra relationships, see Thomas (1997) in Bibliography.]

Spectra of Inorganic Ions

In the case of inorganic anions, generally excitation from a nonbonding lower energy state to an excited state (n to π^* transitions) is observed. For example, NO_3^- shows absorption at 313 nm. Chromate and dichromate ions have well-defined spectral absorption, which is used in calibration. However, from such data, conformation of identity is not possible. Inorganic cationic species, which are colored, usually exhibit very characteristic spectrum. These compounds with very well-defined absorption spectra are transition and inner transition metal cation coordination complexes. For example, a solution of copper is pale blue in aqueous slightly acidic medium, whereas in ammoniacal medium it is strong blue. These are attributed to splitting of "d" orbitals in the presence of ligands that complexes with the metal ion: one set of three d orbitals is called t_{2g} and the other set is known as e_g orbitals.

In aqueous solutions containing copper, the metal ion is octahedraly coordinated, i.e., the metal ion is at the center,

Table 6 Spectral characteristics of some organic functional groups

Species/functional groups	λ (nm)	ε (L mol^{-1} cm^{-1})
Satd. hydrocarbons	<200	—
Alkenes, alkynes, aromatic compounds, aromatic heterocyclic, highly conjugated aliphatics such as carotenes	200–500	~10^4–10^5
Ethers, amines sulfides, alkyl halides	150–260	100–1000
Ketones, aldehydes, amides, esters, acids (—COOH), nitrates, N-hetrocyclics such as pyridine	250–600	10–100

Table 7 Definition of spectral terms

Spectral term	Definitions and comments
Chromophore	A functional group, when present in a molecule, shows absorption in the region between 200 and 800 nm
Auxochrome	An additional functional group in the molecule, which causes shift to longer wavelengths
Hypsochromic (blue) shift	Shift of λ_{max} to shorter wavelengths
Bathochromic (red shift)	Shift of λ_{max} to longer wavelengths
Hyperchromic	Increase in intensity of absorption
Hypochromic	Decrease in intensity of absorption

and it is surrounded by six ligands, one at each apex of an octahedron. As a result of these coordinating ligands, the d orbital electrons, which are at the axis of the approaching ligand, experience forces of repulsion and attain higher energy state compared with those orbitals that are far removed from the axis of approach. The five equi-energic d orbitals are split into two sets of equi-energy orbitals. The magnitude of the separation between the two energy states depends on the ligand field established by the ligands. In copper, of the nine d electrons, a set of six electrons occupy the lower energy state t_{2g} orbitals, and the other three occupy the excited state e_g orbitals. The e_g orbitals can accommodate four electrons. By absorbing visible light, an electron from the ground state can be promoted to the vacant excited state e_g orbital. This results in the characteristic absorption of many metals ions. EDTA, which is used in many pharmaceutical preparations, forms a hexa-coordinated complex, thus stabilizing and solubilizing metals. The example cited is for octahedral splitting. Similarly, in a tetrahedral field, the ligands can occupy the apex of a tetrahedron, and in a square planar complex, the corners of square plane. The tetrahedral and square planar complexes give rise to similar but different splitting of the d orbitals. Depending on which of these different ligand fields are formed different spectral patterns are observable for the same metal ion.

Charge Transfer Complexes

A third type of electronic transition that causes light absorption in the visible region is attributed to the formation of charge-transfer complexes. One example is the formation of the color blue by I_3^- when starch is used as an indicator in iodimetric titrations. A second example is the reaction between Fe^{3+} and thiocyanate ion SCN^-. In this case, an electron is transferred from a donor (SCN^-) to the acceptor (Fe^{3+}). The net effect is an internal redox reaction-forming Fe^{2+} and SCN radical. This type of internal redox reaction is generally reversible. However,

occasionally such charge transfer complexes may undergo irreversible redox reactions resulting in photochemical oxidation and reduction reactions. the formation of similar charge-transfer complexes in organic molecules results in the characteristic absorption in the UV region that can be used for qualitative analysis.

Qualitative Identification

The direct measurement of UV–vis spectra is rarely used for confirmation of identity of a component. However, the comparison of analyte spectrum obtained on a chromatographically separated component to that of a reference compound under identical chromatographic conditions is extensively used for identification and chromatographic purity of the eluting peak. Diode array/rapid scan spectrophotometers are very commonly used for this purpose. A perfect point-to-point comparison of spectra of two or more compounds is possible with the use of the proper computer algorithm. Under chromatoagraphic conditions, the approach is to first establish that a particular drug or chemical substantially contains a single chromatographic component. Spectral data generated are then used for identity and for establishing the chromatographic purity of the analyte of interest. A second approach is to deduce identity by comparing the ratio of absorbance at peak maximum versus absorbance at peak minimum. *USP* 24 specifies such an identification procedure for cisplatin and methyldopate. For cisplatin, an absorbance ratio of 4.5 ($\lambda_{301}/\lambda_{246}$) is specified. However, in methyldopate hydrochloride, absorbance difference between a reference standard and the bulk drug at the same concentration should not differ by more than 3.0%.

Quantitative Analysis

Absorption spectroscopy finds extensive use in every field in which the quantitation of chemical component is required. The characteristics of the spectrophotometric methods include the following:

- extensive applicability to a large number of systems;
- very high sensitivity (ppm to ppb levels can be determined);
- by the choice of wavelength, solvent, pH conditions, and added reagents, selectivity, which is normally poor, can be assured;
- excellent accuracy. Relative uncertainties of 0.5–3.0% can be easily obtained (under certain conditions, with appropriate precautions, errors can be minimized to 0.1%);
- very easy and convenient; and
- on-site data acquisition with certain type of probe spectrophotometers using hand held (palm) computers.

Application to Naturally Absorbing Species

Virtually all organic and many inorganic compounds absorb in the region between 210 and 700 nm. The conventional methods generally involve the following steps.

Selection of solvents

Any solvent exhibiting solubility of a few 10ths of a milligram to milligrams per milliliter is adequate for the purpose. Choice of the solvent is important such that it is transparent, i.e., background absorbance is extremely small. Organic solvents of spectrophotometric quality that is guaranteed to very small background absorbance are commercially available. Only these solvents are recommended for use. For aqueous solutions, the common variables such as pH, temperature, ionic strength of the medium, and the presence of interferants should be adequately controlled.

Selection of wavelength

Usually, from a spectral scan, the wavelength corresponding to the absorption maximum is selected. At λ_{max}, sensitivity is maximum and, over a narrow region close to the maximum, the absorbance is constant. Therefore, minor wavelength differences do not alter the response, and also the absorbance at λ_{max} is less sensitive to instrumental uncertainties. However, if adequate sensitivity exists, measurements can be made at λ_{min}, if interfering absorbance is negligible at λ_{min}.

Both reference and sample cells should be matched, properly cleaned, and rinsed before use. To eliminate lint and films from the outer surface of the cells, swipe cleaning with a lens paper soaked in methanol or

acetonitrile is recommended. When all these conditions are met and precautions are observed, quantitation is facilitated by comparison measurement. The reference standard concentration (C_s) is adjusted very close to the expected analyte concentration (C_u). Then standard (A_s) and sample (A_u) absorbencies are measured: $(A_u/A_s) \times C_s = C_u$.

This direct measurement can be used routinely for in-process assay of pharmaceutical formulations. The formulations during in-process conditions are not likely to contain potential degradants and thus, normally, the degradant interference is absent. Sometimes interference can be eliminated by solvent extraction of the impurities or of the analyte itself. Use of suitable nonabsorbing additives, which selectively reacts or masks the interference, can eliminate interference.

Method of standard additions

The method of standard additions may take one of several forms. If the matrix interference is constant and small, the sample is diluted to a known volume and the absorbance is measured. Then multiple volumes of a reference standard of the analyte at a known concentration are added and diluted to the same volume. The absorbance of each of the sample thus prepared is measured. From a plot of volume added versus absorbance and by extrapolation to zero volume of addition, the concentration of the analyte can be determined. Fig. 4 shows a plot of calculated absolute weight of a drug added to a fixed volume of solution as a function of measured absorbance. The x coordinate value of 4.08 corresponding to zero absorbance indicates the weight of drug in the sample.

Analysis of mixtures

The total absorbance of a solution is the sum of absorbance of the individual components in a mixture. For example, for a 1-cm cell, the total absorbances

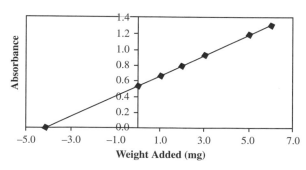

Fig. 4   Plot of weight added versus absorbance.

measured at each of two wavelengths are related to concentration as follows:

$$A_{\lambda 1} = A_1 + A_2 = \varepsilon_1 c_1 + \varepsilon_2 c_2$$
$$A_{\lambda 2} = A_1' + A_2' = \varepsilon_1' c_1 + \varepsilon_2' c_2$$

Then a known concentration of each analyte is prepared. The absorbance of these solutions are measured at each of the two wavelengths. Solving the two simultaneous equations, two equations for c_1 and c_2 are obtained. Then the known values of individual concentrations and calculated values of the four molar extinction coefficients are substituted in the derived equations to arrive at the unknown concentrations of the two components in the mixture. Multicomponent analysis is normally used in the dissolution testing of tablets. Standard hardware and software components for multicomponent dissolution testing based on compendial method are available from instrument manufacturers.

Derivative Spectroscopy

The UV–vis spectrum is a display of absorbance as a function of wavelength $A = f(\lambda)$. At the absorbance maximum, the derivative $dA/d\lambda = 0$; the second-order derivative $d^2A/d\lambda^2$ is a negative maximum. For all even-order derivatives, the spectra show well-defined peaks, and these can be used for analyte determination. The advantages of derivative spectroscopy are as follows.

- Positions of local maximum are precisely defined in the derivative plot compared with the diffuse absorption maximum. As a result, distinguishable derivative spectra are obtained for different compounds, even though normal spectra are likely to be very similar.
- Overlapping spectra, which could not be resolved by conventional techniques, are easily resolved.
- In quantitative analysis, selectivity and sensitivity are increased.
- Combined with algebraic calculations, derivative spectroscopy can be easily adopted for multicomponent analysis.

Difference Spectrophotometry

This technique uses information obtained as the difference of two absorbance measurements when two components having very close λ_{max} values are present in a sample or when there is matrix interference in the sample, the sample at the same concentration is introduced into the reference and sample cells. Then, composition of one of the cells is

modified by changing pH, or by adding a suitable reactant or by changing the temperature of the solutions. The difference in the absorbance is measured. For example, at pH 3.0, a particular species absorbs, and its absorbance is measured. By changing the pH to 7.0, the absorbance changes at the same wavelength. However, the contribution to absorbance of the interference remains the same regardless of pH. Then the difference between the absorbances measured cancels the absorbance owing to the matrix. This difference ΔA is proportional to the concentration.

In turbid or cloudy solutions, in which absorbance is affected by scattering of the sample, two absorbance measurements are made: one at λ_{max} and the other at a different wavelength where the analyte does not absorb. Then, the difference being proportional to concentration of the analyte, the analyte concentration can be calculated. Difference spectrophotometry is used in the determination of constituents in tablets, complex pharmaceutical preparations, plant extracts, syrups, biological matrices such as blood and serum, injectable oil preparations, and the like. For this technique, in addition to other general requirements such as well-matched cells that are positioned accurately, the solution should be made homogeneous, and the instrumental stray radiation at the wavelength of interest should be extremely small.

Application to Nonabsorbing Species

The limitations of naturally absorbing species for the determination of analyte concentration more often suffer from poor selectivity, sensitivity, and interference in mixtures of components. In such cases, the target analyte is reacted with a suitable reagent that results in a product, that usually absorb at longer wavelengths either in the UV or, more often, in the visible region. An appropriate reagent is selected to meet one or more of the following needs:

- to quantitate spectrophotometrically inactive compounds. These compounds usually have active functional groups such as hydroxy group, amino groups, and the like, which react to yield spectrally active products.
- to increase selectivity. When multiple components, each of which has absorbance in the wavelength maximum of the analyte are present, suitable chemical reaction selective to the analyte, is selected so the effect of the absorbing components is eliminated.
- to increase sensitivity. In many cases, the analyte may have natural absorption. However, that may not be adequate to determine at a required level (ppb or ppm

levels). In pharmaceutical manufacturing, it may be necessary to establish that the active analyte has been cleaned of the manufacturing systems below a certain level. In these cases, sensitivity enhancements are possible using an appropriate chemical reaction to yield a product with high molar absorptivity. For example, in cisplatin, although it has good absorbance sensitivity at approximately 210 nm, the sensitivity is good only for few tenths of milligrams per milliliter of cisplatin and not adequate for trace-level determination. However, by reacting cisplatin with diethyldithiocarbamate (DDTC), platinum DDTC complex with high molar extinction coefficient is obtained. Increasing the concentration using a column-switching technique and chromatographic separation, a detection limit of 0.2 ppb was attained. [See Raghavan and Mulligan (2000) and Raghavan et al. (2000).] It is not always necessary to add chemical reagents. An oxidation product may be generated on electrochemical oxidation of an analyte or by using pulsed photochemical activation, species thus generated may be more spectrally amenable for quantitation. However, if reagents are chosen for reaction, the following need to be considered for successful sensitivity and/or selectivity optimization:

- appropriate reagent concentration, solvent, and composition of the mixture; ionic strength, pH, and temperature of the reaction mixture;
- adequate reaction time for completion or for reproducible response that is proportional to the concentration of the analyte; and
- similar treatment of reagent blanks to allow for matrix changes that might affect the reaction.

Excellent reviews of application of spectrophotometric methods based on chemical reactions are available in the literature (see Bibliography).

Measurement of Color

Color comparison tubes

In pharmaceutical formulations, pale yellow color may be imparted by the excipients or as a result of formation of colored degradants, or feebly colored products may be generated intentionally as in limit tests for heavy metals. In such cases for visual testing glass color comparison tubes, Nessler tubes, of uniform cross-section and flat bottoms are used. These tubes should be matched as closely as possible in internal diameter and length. The tubes are viewed downward through the solutions against a white background. The color intensity of the unknown is compared with two successive standards, one above and one below the level of the unknown. The color is reported to be less than the most intense color standard with which it is compared. To meet compendial color requirements, special instruments are commercially available.

Probe-Type Spectrophotometers

Many dip-type UV–vis spectrophotometers, use fiber optic sampling technology coupled with highly sensitive charge coupled device (CCD) array detectors. The probe is immersed directly in the sample being measured. Then radiation from a light source is transmitted through an optic fiber to the tip. The light travels through the 0.5 cm through the sample and reflects off the back surface of curved mirror over another 0.5 cm through the sample and then back to an input filter. The sample absorbs part of the light and reflects back a small portion of the light that carries the spectral information of the sample. This reflected light travels back through suitably oriented fibers back to CCD array detectors. The spectrum is displayed through the use of the appropriate device. Direct measurement of concentrated solutions is made possible by amplifying the weak reflected light. As a result, this lends itself to on-line monitoring. Many remote filter optic sampling options for measurements not only on liquids but also on powder and solid objects are available. These spectrophotometers are miniaturized so that they can be hand-held and transportable for on-site measurements. Probe-type spectrophotometers are also useful for spectrophotometric titrations.

Spectrophotometric Titrations

The absorbance of a selected species is monitored as a function of volume of titrant added. The resulting absorbance data are plotted against volume of titrant. These titration curves have different shapes, depending on the absorbance characteristic of the analyte, added reagent, or the product formed. However, in all cases, the slope changes gradually near the equivalence point. Extrapolation of the two linear sections before and after the titration equivalance point yields an intersection point. The titrant volume corresponding to this intersection point is the equivalence point of the titration. Of the analyte, reagent added, or product in the solution, any one or two of these can be spectrally active. Therefore, a total of six possible titrant shapes are possible. Because the titration represents a series of analytical measurements, analytical accuracy is very high.

A variation of these titrations is used to determine stoichiometry and formation constant(s) of complexes. In these methods, typically the metal concentration and total volume of solutions are kept constant, but the ligand-to-metal ion ratio is continuously varied. From a plot of absorbance versus mole fraction, the stoichiometry between the metal and ligand can be obtained. Numerous variations of this method are adopted to obtain stoichiometry and formation constants or binding constants in many biochemical determinations.

VALIDATION OF SPECTROPHOTOMETRIC METHODS

The UV–vis spectrophotometric methods require validation of the method for the analysis of pharmaceutical compounds. Once the method is developed, data regarding precision, accuracy, linear response behavior, limit of quantitation, limit of detection, selectivity, and ruggedness are generated. These terms are very well-defined in many compendial monographs and in ICH, USP, and FDA guidelines. These are not addressed further. However, it should be emphasized that without appropriate validation data and reasonable understanding of how the method results will be affected by minor day-to-day variation of experimental parameters, routine generation of acceptable data may be difficult.

BIBLIOGRAPHY

1. Banwell, C.N.; McCash, E.M.; *Fundamentals of Molecular Spectroscopy*, 4th Ed.; McGraw-Hill: New York, 1994.
2. Burtis, C.A., Ashwood, R.E., Eds. *Tietz Textbook of Clinical Chemistry,* 3rd Ed.; W. B. Saunders Co.: Philadelphia, 1999.
3. Clark, B.J.; Frost, T.; Russell, M.A. *UV Spectroscopy: Techniques, Instrumentation, Data Handling*; Chapman & Hall: London UK, 1993.
4. George, W.O.; Willis, H.A. *Computer Methods in UV, Visible and IR Spectroscopy*; Royal Society of Chemistry: Cambridge, UK, 1990.
5. Gilpin, R.K.; Pachla, L.A. Pharmaceutical and Related Drugs. Anal. Chem. **1997**, *69* (12), 145R–163R.
6. Gilpin, R.K.; Pachla, L.A. Pharmaceutical and Related Drugs. Anal. Chem. **1999**, *71* (12), 217R–233R.
7. Görög, S. *Ultraviolet and Visible Spectrophotometry in Pharmaceutical Analysis*; CRC Press, Inc.: New York, 1995.
8. Görög, S.; Bihar, M.; Csizér, É.; Dravetz, F.; Gazdag, M.; Herényi, B. Estimation of Impurity Profiles of Drugs and Related Materials. Part 14: The Role of HPLC/Diode-Array UV Spectroscopy in the Identification of Minor Components (Impurities, Degradation Products, Metabolites) in Various Matrices. J. Pharm. Biomed. Anal. **1995**, *14*, 85–92.
9. Owen, T. *Fundamentals of Modern UV–Visible Spectroscopy, A Primer*, Hewlett-Packard Publication Number, 12-5965-5123E; Hewlett-Packard Company: Germany; 1996.
10. Perkampus, H.H., Ed. *UV-VIS Atlas of Organic Compounds*, 2nd Ed.; VCH Publishers: 1992.
11. Raghavan, R.; Joseph, J.C. *Ultraviolet and Visible Spectrophotometry in Pharmaceutical Analysis*; Swarbrick, J., Boylan, J., Eds.; Marcel Dekker, Inc.: New York, 1997; 15, 293–339.
12. Raghavan, R.; Mulligan, J.A. Low-Level (PPB) Determination of Cisplatin in Cleaning Validation (Rinse Water) Samples. I an Atomic Absortion Spectrophotometric Method. Drug Dev. Ind. Pharm. **2000**, *26* (4), 423–428.
13. Raghavan, R.; Burchett, M.; Loffredo, D.; Mulligan, J.A. Low-Level (PPB) Determination of Cisplatin in Cleaning Validation (Rinse Water) Samples. II. A High-Performance Liquid Chromatographic Method. Drug Dev. Ind. Pharm. **2000**, *26* (4), 429–440,
14. Silverstein, R.M.; Weber, F.X.; Silverstein, R.M. *Spectrometric Identification of Organic Compounds*; John Wiley & Sons: New York, 1997.
15. Skoog, D.A.; Holler, F.J.; Nieman, T.A. *Principles of Instrumental Analysis*, 5th Ed.; Saunders College Publishing: Chicago, 1998; 299–351.
16. Soares, O.D.D.; Costa, J.L.C. Spectrophotometers Intercomparison for Spectrocolorimetric Scale Harmonization. Rev. Scientific Instruments **1999**, *70* (12), 4471–4481.
17. Sykes, P.A.; Shiue, H-C.; Walker, J.R.; Bateman, R.C., Jr. Determination of Myoglobin Stability by Visible Spectroscopy. J. Chem. Ed. **1999**, *76* (9), 1283–1284.
18. Talsky, G., Ed. *Derivative Spectrophotometry;* VCH Publishers: New York, 1994.
19. Thomas, M. Ultraviolet and Visible Spectroscopy. *Analytical Chemistry by Openlearning*; Ando, D.J. Ed.; John Wiley & Sons: New York, 1997.
20. Thomas, M. Ultraviolet and Visible Spectroscopy. *Analytical Chemistry by Openlearning*; Ando, D.J. Ed.; John Wiley & Sons: New York, 1997.
21. *United States Pharmacopeia, 24th Ed., National Formulary,* 19th Rev. The Unites States Pharmacopeial Convention Inc.: Rockville MD, 1999, General Chapter 851.
22. Williams, R. Application of Fourier Transform Spectrometry in the Ultraviolet, Visible, and Near-IR. Appl. Spectrosc. Rev. **1989**, *25*, 63–79.

STARCHES AND STARCH DERIVATIVES

Ann W. Newman

SSCI, Inc., West Lafayette, Indiana

Ronald L. Mueller

GlaxoSmithKline, King of Prussia, Pennsylvania

Imre M. Vitez
Chris C. Kiesnowski

Bristol-Myers Squibb Pharmaceutical Research Institute, New Brunswick, New Jersey

INTRODUCTION

Starch is one of the most commonly used excipients in the pharmaceutical industry due to its disintegration and binding properties. A number of sources of starch are commercially available, with corn starch being the most common. An overview of starches and starch derivatives and their use in the pharmaceutical industry is presented.

DESCRIPTION

Molecular Structure

Starch is a polymeric material with a molecular formula of $(C_6H_{10}O_5)_n$, where n ranges from 300 to 1000. Common starches contain two types of D-glucopyranose polymers called *amylose* and *amylopectin*. Amylose is a linear polymer of α-D-glucopyranosyl units linked $(1 \rightarrow 4)$ as shown in Fig. 1a. These molecules can be comprised of 100 to over 1000 glucose units. Amylopectin is a branched polymer of α-D-glucopyranosyl units containing $(1 \rightarrow 4)$ linear linkages and $(1 \rightarrow 6)$ linkages at the branch points, as shown in Fig. 1b. This polymer is three or more times larger than amylose. Most naturally occurring starches contain approximately 30% amylose, however, specific starches and their properties are determined by the size and amount of each type of polymer molecule present in the material. Attractive forces between the polymeric molecules form the starch granules. The linear portions tend to associate into micelles, which bind the molecules together to form a somewhat ordered structure. Models of this structure have been proposed (1), and it is known that the structure is rigid and insoluble in water.

Types of Starch

Starch can be derived from a number of natural sources, including those listed in Table 1 (2). It is found in various parts of the plants and several extraction methods are used to isolate the material. The most common type of starch used in the pharmaceutical industry is corn, although studies with other types of starch have been performed (3–6).

The most common preparation of starch is wet milling, although dry milling is also performed. A series of milling, separation, concentration, and washing steps result in a suspension of starch granules (7). After processing, cornstarch is a white powder with a pale yellow tint. Bleaching is required to achieve absolute whiteness.

A number of starch modifications are used in pharmaceutical applications. Pregelatinized or compressible starch has been chemically or mechanically processed to rupture all or part of the granules in water. It is then dried to yield an excipient material suitable for direct-compression formulations. Sterilizable maize starch contains magnesium oxide (not greater than 2.2%) and has been chemically or physically treated to prevent gelatinization on exposure to moisture or steam sterilization. Soluble starch results when potato or maize starch has been chemically treated to destroy the gelatinizing ability of starch.

General Properties

Starch is a fine white powder that is odorless and tasteless. It is composed of very small spherical or elliptical granules. The botanical origin of the starch material determines the granule shape and size, and these characteristics are summarized in Table 1. It is insoluble in alcohol, most solvents, and cold water. Alkaline solutions, however, will degrade starch and its polysaccharide components. Starch

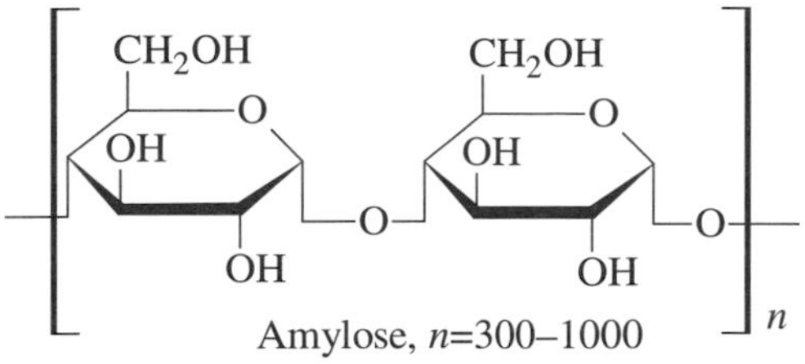

Amylose, n=300–1000

(a)

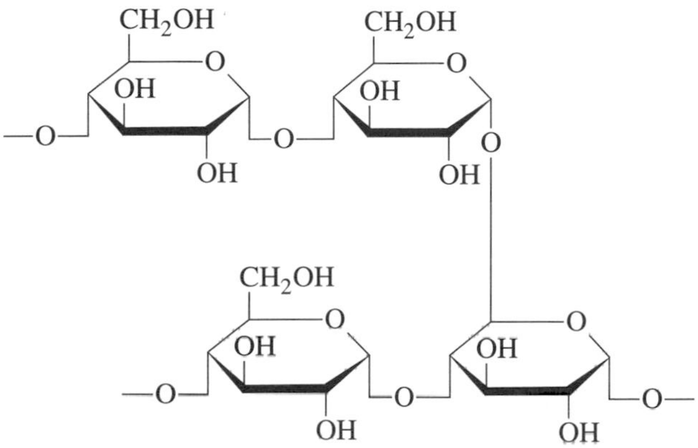

Segment of Amylopectin Molecule

(b)

Fig. 1 (a) Linear amylose starch molecule. (b) Branched amylopectin starch molecule.

is relatively resistant to enzymes other than α-amylose and amyloglucosidase.

When starch is suspended in water and heated to a critical point called the gelatinization temperature, water will penetrate the granules and swell them to produce a viscous mass. With the rising temperature, the hydrogen bonds that hold the micellar structural units and the water molecules in an aggregated state tend to dissociate. The dissociated water molecules are then able to penetrate the weakened starch structure and gradually hydrate the many hydroxyl groups along the length of the starch molecule. Gelatinization temperatures vary from starch to starch, but range from 60 to 75°C (2). Starch granules lose their characteristic shape as gelatinization proceeds.

The reaction of starch with iodine is a common identity test for starch. A dilute solution of iodine stains starches a blue to bluish red color. It is believed that the amylose portion complexes with iodine by forming a helix around it (7). This blue color has been used both as a qualitative and quantitative test for starch in various systems.

The National Formulary (8) contains numerous assays for starch including botanical characteristics, identification, microbial limits, pH, loss on drying (LOD), residue on ignition (ROI), iron, oxidizing substances, sulfur dioxide, and organic volatile impurities.

PHYSICAL PROPERTIES

Structural Information

Starch is a semicrystalline polymer. The linear amylose molecules are amorphous in nature, but the branched

Table 1 Sources and characteristics of various starches

Type of Starch	Extracted from	Granule shape	Granule size (μm)
Corn (Maize)	Seed	Round or polygonal	5–25
Tapioca	Root	Round or oval	2–25
Potato	Root	Egg-shaped	15–100
Wheat	Seed	Round or elliptical	2–10 or 20–35
Sago	Stem	Oval or egg-shaped	20–60
Arrowroot	Root	Oval	15–70
Rice	Seed	Polygonal	3–8
Barley	Seed	Round or elliptical	2–6 or 20–35
Waxy sorghum	Seed	Round or polygonal	6–30
Sweet potato	Root	Polygonal	10–25
Waxy maize	Seed	Round or polygonal	5–25

(From Ref. 2.)

Table 2 Crystallographic data for A and B type starch

Property	A type[a]	B type[b]
Lattice	Monoclinic	Hexagonal
a (nm)	2.124	1.85
b (nm)	1.172	1.85
c (nm)	1.069	1.04
α (°C)	90	90
β (°C)	90	90
γ (°C)	123.5	120
Space group	B2	—
Density	1.48	—
Volume	2.218 nm^3	—

[a](From Ref. 11.)
[b](From Ref. 12.)

amylopectin portion has been reported as partially crystalline. It is believed that the crystalline regions in the starch granule are interspersed in a continuous amorphous phase (1, 9, 10).

X-ray diffraction studies have shown that starch exists in three crystal forms designated as A, B, and C (10). These forms are dependent on the botanical source of the starch. Pattern A is observed for cereal grain starches, whereas pattern B is characteristic of tuber, fruit, and stem starches. Pattern C is intermediate between the A and B patterns and has been attributed to mixtures of A and B type crystallites. The A type pattern is commonly observed for cornstarch.

Single crystal X-ray diffraction data for the crystalline portion of A type starch have been reported and the crystallographic data are summarized in Table 2 (11). The unit cell contains 12 glucose residues located in two left-handed, parallel-stranded double helices packed in a parallel fashion. Four water molecules are located between these helices. It has been reported that the B type starch also contains chains arranged in double helices (12). The currently accepted hexagonal unit cell dimensions are in Table 2. The A and B structures differ in crystal packing of the chains and in moisture content.

Diffuse reflectance (DR) infrared (IR), Raman, and solid-state ^{13}C cross polarization/magic angle spinning (CP/MAS) nuclear magnetic resonance (NMR) spectra were acquired for unmodified and pregelatinized cornstarch (13, 14). Differences were not evident in the spectra for the various starch samples. Solution-phase, ^{1}H-NMR studies have also been performed on amylose and model compounds (15). Spectral assignments and intramolecular hydrogen bonding suggest that the same conformation is perpetuated along the amylose chain.

Thermal Properties

Thermal analysis has also been used to characterize the structure of starch. A melting endotherm due to the crystalline portions of starch has been investigated (16), but it is not clearly resolved in all samples due to the small amount of crystalline material present in the samples. This transition is also dependent on the sample preparation and moisture content of the material. Melting points of 168–210° C have been reported (16, 17).

The glass transition temperature (T_g) in starch, measured using differential scanning calorimetry (DSC), was found to be dependent on the moisture content of the preparation and covered a temperature range of 22–130°C (18). Gelatinization studies of starch using DSC showed that concentrated starch/water suspensions produced a well-defined endotherm under select conditions. The endotherm was integrated to obtain the heat of gelatinization for various starches (19).

Microscopy

A number of excellent reviews on the microscopy of starches have been published (2, 20–23). As summarized in Table 1, the granule shape and size is characteristic of the botanical origin and can be used to identify the materials. It has been reported that the floury granules, as found for potato and tapioca starches, tend to be larger and more regular in shape (round, elliptical, or oval). Horny starches, such as corn and rice, are usually

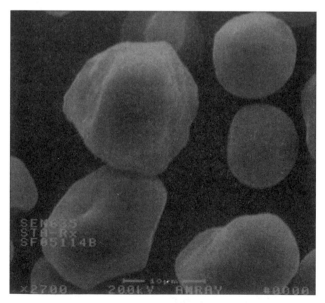

Fig. 2 Scanning electron micrograph of unmodified cornstarch granules (magnification 2700×).

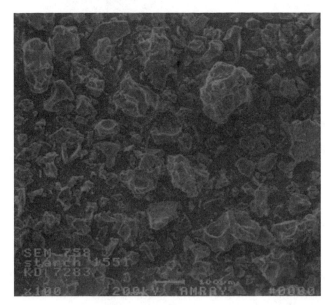

Fig. 3 Scanning electron micrograph of pregelatinized starch (magnification 100×).

described as polygonal because of the angular sides of the granules caused by the close packing of the granules in the kernel. An example is given in Fig. 2 for unmodified cornstarch. Starches are found as individual granules, but aggregated materials are also observed and are attributed to the drying conditions. Extensive heat and moisture during drying will produce a slight gelatinization of the surface of the granule and cause the granules to adhere together to form the aggregates. Pregelatinized starch exhibits an entirely different morphology, as shown in Fig. 3. The particles are irregular and the starch granules

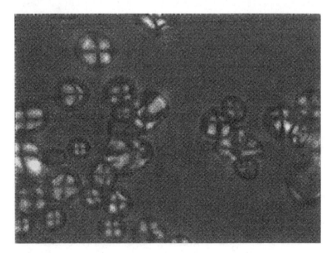

Fig. 4 Optical micrograph of unmodified cornstarch under crossed polarizers (magnification 400×).

are not evident as expected from the pregelatinization process.

When unmodified starch granules are observed using polarized light, two dark lines will form a cross or a V-shape (Fig. 4). The shape of the cross can be used to help identify the type of starch. One explanation for this feature suggests that the density and distribution of moisture throughout the granule are not uniform (2). As the granules dry, stresses are formed within the granule resulting in the bright regions observed under the polarized light. When the starch swells or is gelatinized, the cross is no longer visible with the polarizing microscope.

Micromeritic Properties

Micromeritic properties, such as particle size, surface area, density, and flow properties can affect the disintegration, handling, and tableting properties of starch materials. A number of methods for determining the particle size of various starches have been used. For bulk powder analysis, sieving is employed for large amounts of material. Another common method for particle size determination is optical microscopy because it gives a direct measurement of the individual particles (14, 24, 25). Laser light scattering analysis has also been utilized to measure the size of dry particles and suspensions (26). This analysis was found to be dependent on the model used to fit the data, and better reproducibility was obtained with samples suspended in liquid. Surface area measurements of starches have been obtained by air permeametry (27) or nitrogen adsorption (14). Relatively low surface areas ranging from approximately 0.1–0.5 m^2/g have been reported.

Bulk powder characteristics are important in understanding the handling properties of an excipient or a granulated product. A classification system to evaluate the flow properties of powders has been introduced by Carr (28, 29). A flowable powder is defined as free-flowing and tends to flow steadily and consistently, whereas a floodable powder exhibits an unstable, discontinuous, and gushing type of flow. A number of studies have investigated the bulk powder properties of starch (14, 30) and granulations made with starch (31, 32). The starch materials were found to exhibit poor to borderline flow properties.

Hygroscopicity

Starch has been classified as a moderately hygroscopic material (33). Water sorption studies have been conducted using static methods (saturated salt solutions in closed chambers) (33–35) modified inverse frontal gas chromatography (36), and automated moisture balance systems

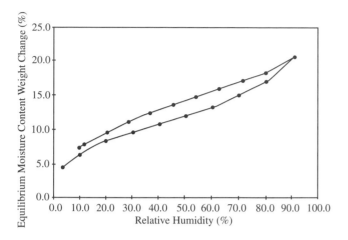

Fig. 5 Moisture isotherm for unmodified cornstarch.

(14). The isotherms are typically type II curves exhibiting hysteresis, as shown in Fig. 5. Hysteresis in starch samples has been attributed to intra- and intermolecular hydrogen bonding of water with the hydroxyl groups of the starch molecule (33, 37). The extent of hydration and swelling depends on the accessibility of the hydroxyl groups in the starch to the water, and it has been suggested that the amorphous regions are responsible for the reversible swelling of starch upon the adsorption of water (9, 37).

USES AND APPLICATIONS

Starch is widely used in the pharmaceutical industry because, among its other properties, it is readily available, inexpensive, white, and inert. Excipient compatibility studies of starch and various active drugs have been performed using thermal methods of analysis. As an example, starch has been found to be compatible with cephalexin (38) and acetylcysteine (39) using this method of excipient screening.

Starch is described as a tablet/capsule diluent, tablet disintegrant, and glidant. The function of starch can depend on how it is incorporated into the formulation. Starch will function as a disintegrant when it is added in the dry state prior to adding a lubricant. It may exhibit both binding and disintegrant properties when it is incorporated either as a paste or dry before granulation with other agents. It has been reported that starches deform mostly by plastic flow during compression, but this was found to be dependent on the particle size, size distribution, and particle shape (40).

Starch is used in many formulations for its disintegration properties. The most common explanation for the disintegration properties is the swelling of the starch granules when exposed to water, and it has been proposed that amylose is the component responsible for the disintegration properties of starch due to swelling. A second mechanism suggests that the disintegrating action of starch in tablets is due to capillary action rather than swelling. A third proposed mechanism is based on the particle–particle repulsion forces between the tablet constituents when in contact with water and the hydrophilic nature of starch (41).

A number of new applications have been reported for the use of starch in formulations. A new linear, short-chain, high surface area starch product was prepared by gelatinization followed by enzymatic degradation for use in directly compressible controlled-release systems (6). The combination of ibuprofen-starch granulates and hydroxypropyl cellulose was used to produce controlled-release formulations of ibuprofen (42). Gelatinization and freeze-drying has been used to produce cold water-swellable starch as well as a matrix forming excipient in sustained release tablets (43). Grafted starch micro-capsules are being investigated for the oral administration of vaccines to prevent degradation (44).

STARCH DERIVATIVES

Unmodified starch has proven to be an effective and inexpensive disintegrating agent, however, relatively high concentrations have been required and the flow properties have been poor. The major shortcoming of starch is that while it is effective at disintegrating tablets, it is less effective at disintegrating the granules from which the tablets are made. When other properties, such as rapid disintegration, were necessary, new materials called starch derivatives were investigated.

Starches undergo many reactions characteristic of alcohols because of the many hydroxyl groups present in the structure. Modification of the D-glucopyranosol units can occur by oxidation, esterification, etherification, or hydrolysis. The resulting starch derivatives are defined by a number of factors such as plant source, prior treatment (acid-catalyzed hydrolysis or dextrinization), amylose/amylopectin ratio or content, molecular weight distribution or degree of polymerization, type of derivative (ester, ether, oxidized), nature of the substituent group, and physical form (granular, pregelatinized) (9, 45).

The degree of substitution (DS) is a common method of characterizing starch derivatives and is a measure of the average number of hydroxyl groups on each D-glucopyranosyl unit. It is expressed as the moles of substituent per D-glucopyranosyl units, and the maximum DS is 3 since

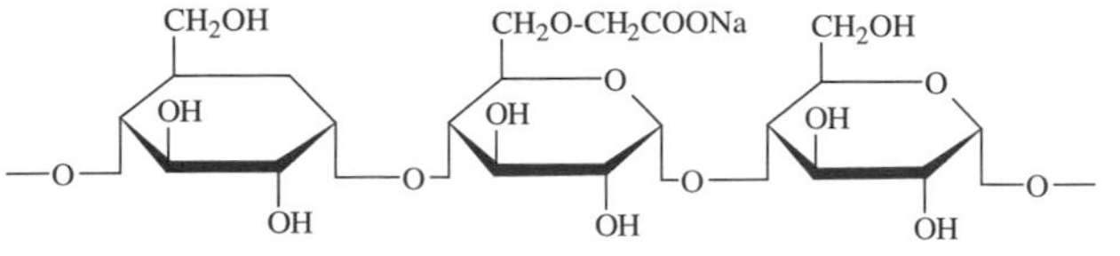

Fig. 6 Sodium starch glycolate molecule.

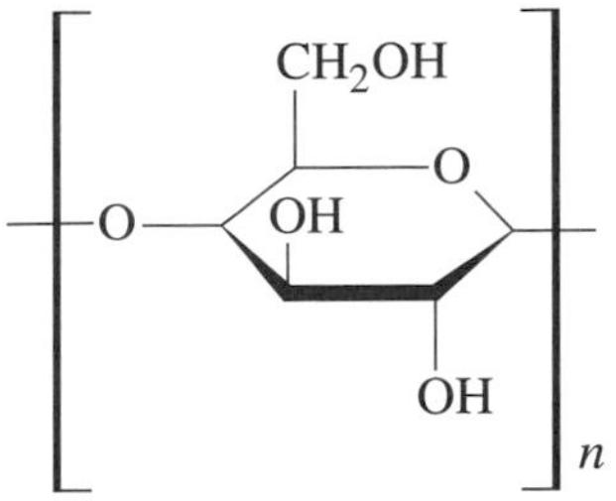

Fig. 7 Maltodextrin molecule.

three hydroxyl groups are available in the unit for substitution. Most commercially produced derivatives have a DS less than 0.2. Molar substitution is used when the substituent group reacts further with the reagent to form a polymeric substituent. It is defined as the level of substitution in terms of mole of monomeric units (in the polymeric substituent) per mole of D-glucopyranosyl unit and can be larger than 3.

Sodium Starch Glycolate

Sodium starch glycolate is the sodium salt of a poly-α-glucopyranose in which some of the hydroxyl groups are in the form of the carboxymethyl ether (Fig. 6). Starch is carboxymethylated by reacting it with sodium chloroacetate in an alkaline medium followed by neutralization with acid. Cross-linking is achieved by physical or chemical methods. The sodium starch glycolate commonly prepared from potato starch is marketed as *Explotab* and *Primojel*. It is used as a tablet and capsule disintegrant and exhibits superior disintegration properties when compared to various starches (27). Sodium starch glycolates prepared from numerous starch sources (potato, corn, wheat, rice, sago, tapioca, and enset) have exhibited variations in disintegration efficiency, which have been related to the DS, cross-linking, and purity of the materials (46, 47).

Commercial sodium starch glycolate is a white to off-white, odorless, tasteless powder. It is an amorphous material with a T_g ranging from 128 to 156°C depending on the moisture content of the sample (33). It is considered to be a hygroscopic material based on the moisture uptake observed above 50% RH. It should be stored in a closed container to prevent exposure to wide variations in humidity and temperature that may cause caking. The material is composed of oval or spherical granules in the range of 30–100 μm. Flow properties measured for this material show that it is a free flowing powder that produced formulations exhibiting excellent mechanical properties (30).

Maltodextrins

Maltodextrins are carbohydrate materials prepared by controlled acid or enzyme hydrolysis (depolymerization)

of corn starch. The D-glucose units are linked primarily by α-(1-4) bonds but have branched segments linked by α-(1-6) bonds, as shown in Fig. 7. The physical properties of these materials are determined by the degree of starch hydrolysis, which is expressed as the dextrose equivalent (D.E.) value. The D.E. is defined as the amount of reducing sugars present, which is reported as grams of D-glucose per 100 g of dry substance. A high D.E. value represents a low degree of polymerization of the maltodextrins.

The maltodextrin solids are amorphous, white, or off-white powders or granules, which are nonsweet and odorless. The materials are processed by spray drying, fluidized bed agglomeration, and roller compaction to improve their handling properties. Maltodextrins are hygroscopic above 50% RH and need to be stored below this RH in tightly closed containers. The powders will begin to gel when the materials are stored above 75% RH. The hygroscopicity of maltodextrins will increase with an increase in the D.E. value.

Maltodextrins are used as a coating agent, tablet and capsule diluent, tablet binder, and viscosity-increasing agent. They have been evaluated as a direct compression tablet excipient and were found to exhibit similar compression properties to those of other direct compression excipients (48). Studies relating the degree of polymerization and compression properties show that tablet properties such as density and tensile strength could be correlated to the degree of polymerization and the moisture content of the maltodextrins (49). Matrix pellet formulations using microcrystalline wax, maltodextrin, and various binders were used for sustained release and immediate release formulations (50).

SUMMARY

Starches and starch derivatives are important in the formulation of pharmaceutical drug substances. Various starch sources, starch modifications, and starch derivatives provide a wide range of solids, which can be used in pharmaceutical applications. The various properties exhibited by the materials can be exploited for specific uses during the formulation process.

REFERENCES

1. Lineback, D.R. Current Concepts of Starch Structure and Its Impact on Properties. J. Jpn. Soc. Starch Sci. **1986**, *33* (1), 80–88.
2. Kerr, R.W., Ed. *Chemistry and Industry of Starch;* Academic Press: New York, 1950.
3. Gadalla, M.A.F.; Abd El-Hameed, M.H.; Ismail, A.A. A Comparative Evaluation of Some Starches as Disintegrants for Double Compressed Tablets. Drug. Dev. Ind. Pharm. **1989**, *15* (3), 427–446.
4. Mitrevej, A.; Sinchaipanid, N.; Faroongsarng, D. Spray-Dried Rice Starch: Comparative Evaluation of Direct Compression Fillers. Drug Dev. Ind. Pharm. **1996**, *22*(7), 587–594.
5. Gebre-Mariam, T.; Schmidt, P.C. Characterization of Enset Starch and Its Use as a Binder and Disintegrant for Tablets. Pharmazie **1996**, *51*(5), 303–311.
6. Te Wierik, G.H.P.; Eissens, A.C.; Bergsma, J.; Arends-Scholte, A.W.; Bolhius, G.K. A New Generation Starch Product as Excipient in Pharmaceutical Tablets. III. Parameters Affecting Controlled Drug Release from Tablets Based on High Surface Area Retrograded Pregelatinized Potato Starch. Int. J. Pharm. **1997**, *157*, 181–187.
7. Whistler, R.L.; Daniel, J.R. Starch. *Kirk-Othmer Encyclopedia of Chemical Technology;* Grayson, M., Ed.; 3rd Ed.; John Wiley & Sons: New York, 1983; 21, 492–507.
8. *The National Formulary.* NF 19 United States Pharmacopeial Convention, Inc. Rockville MD, 2000; 2524–2525.
9. French, A.D.; *Starch: Chemistry and Technology;* Whistler, R.L., BeMiller, J.N., Paschall, E.F., Eds.; 2nd Ed.; Academic Press: New York, 1984; 183–247.
10. Banks, W.; Greenwood, C.T. *Starch and Its Components;* John Wiley & Sons: New York, 1975.
11. Imberty, A.; Chanzy, H.; Perez, S. The Double-Helical Nature of the Crystalline Part of A-Starch. J. Mol. Biol. **1988**, *201*, 365–378.
12. Imberty, A.; Buleon, A.; Tran, V.; Perez, S. Recent Advances in Knowledge of Starch Structure. Staerke **1991**, *43* (10), 375–384.
13. Bugay, D.E.; Findlay, W.P. *Pharmaceutical Excipients;* Marcel Dekker, Inc.: New York, 1999.
14. Newman, A.W.; Mueller, R.L.; Vitez, I.M.; Kiesnowski, C.C.; Bugay, D.E.; Findlay, W.P.; Rodriguez, C. Starch. *Analytical Profiles of Drug Substances and Excipients;* Brittain, H.G., Ed.; Academic Press: New York, 1996; 24, 523–577.
15. St-Jacquies, M.; Sundararajan, P.R.; Taylor, K.J.; Marchessault, R.H. Nuclear Magnetic Resonance and Conformational Studies on Amylose and Model Compounds in Dimethyl Sulfoxide Solution. J. Am. Chem. Soc. **1976**, *98* (15), 4386–4391.
16. Donovan, J.W. Phase Transitions of the Starch–Water System. Biopolymers **1979**, *18*, 263–265.
17. Lelievre, J. Starch Gelatinization. J. Appl. Polym. Sci. **1973**, *18*, 293–296.
18. Zeleznak, K.J.; Hoseny, R.C. The Glass Transition in Starch. Cereal Chem. **1987**, *64* (2), 121–124.
19. Stevens, D.J.; Elton, G.A.H. Thermal Properties of the Starch/Water System Part 1. Measurement of the Heat of Gelatinisation by Differential Scanning Calorimetry. Staerke **1971**, *23* (1), 8–11.
20. Sjostrom, O.A. Microscopy of Starches and Their Modifications. Ind. Eng. Chem. **1936**, *28* (1), 63–74.
21. Moss, G.E. The Microscopy of Starch. *Examination and Analysis of Starch and Starch Products;* Radley, J.A., Ed.; Applied Science Publishers, Ltd.: London, 1976; 1–32.
22. Schoch, T.J.; Maywald, E.C. Industrial Microscopy of Starches. *Starch: Chemistry and Technology;* Whistler, R.L., BeMiller, J.N., Paschall, E.F., Eds.; 2nd Ed.; Academic Press: New York, 1984; 637–647.
23. Gallant, D.J. Electron Microscopy of Starch and Starch Products. *Examination and Analysis of Starch and Starch Products;* Radley, J.A., Ed.; Applied Science Publishers, Ltd.: London, 1976; 33–59.
24. Paronen, P.; Juslin, M. Compressional Characteristics of Four Starches. J. Pharm. Pharmacol. **1983**, *35*, 627–635.
25. Juslin, M.; Kahela, P.; Paronen, P.; Turakka, L. Comparative Evaluation of Starches as Tablet Adjuvants. Acta. Pharm. Fenn. **1981**, *90*, 83–93.
26. Merkku, P.; Yliruusi, J.; Kristoffersson, E. Particle Size Determination of Some Pharmaceutical Fillers by Laser Light Diffraction Part II. Acta Pharm. Nord. **1992**, *4* (4), 265–270.
27. Smallenbroek, A.J.; Bolhuis, G.K.; Lerk, C.F. The Effect of Particle Size of Disintegrants on the Disintegration of Tablets. Pharm. Weekblad. **1981**, *116*, 1048–1051.
28. Carr, R.L. Evaluating Flow Properties of Solids. Chem. Eng. **1965**, *72*, 163–168.
29. Carr, R.L. Classifying Flow Properties of Solids. Chem. Eng. **1965**, *73*, 69–72.
30. Vennat, B.; Gross, S.; Pourrat, A.; Pourrat, H. Tablets of Hamamelis Dry Extract by Direct Compression: Comparative Study of Natural Starches and Starch Derivatives. Drug Dev. Ind. Pharm. **1993**, *19* (11), 1357–1368.
31. Kottke, M.K.; Chueh, H.-R.; Rhodes, C.T. Comparison of Disintegrant and Binder Activity of Three Corn Starch Products. Drug Dev. Ind. Pharm. **1992**, *18* (20), 2207–2223.
32. Nasipuri, R.N.; Kuforiji, F.O. Effect of Granule Size of Starch as a Direct Compression Carrier on the Physical Properties of Chlorpheniramine Tablets. Pharm. Ind. **1981**, *43* (10), 1037–1041.
33. Faroongsarng, D.; Peck, G.E. The Swelling and Water Uptake of Tablets III: Moisture Sorption Behavior of Tablet Disintegrants. Drug Dev. Ind. Pharm. **1994**, *20* (5), 779–798.
34. Sair, L.; Fetzer, W.R. Water Sorption by Starches. Ind. Eng. Chem. **1944**, *36*, 205–208.
35. Malamataris, S.; Goidas, P.; Dimiriou, A. Moisture Sorption and Tensile Strength of Some Tableted Direct Compression Excipients. Int. J. Pharm. **1991**, *68*, 51–60.
36. Paik, S.W.; Gilbert, S.G. Water Sorption Isotherms on Sucrose and Starch by Modified Inverse Frontal Gas Chromatography. J. Chromatogr. **1986**, *351*, 417–423.

37. Das, B.; Sethi, R.K.; Chopra, S.L. Sorption and Desorption of Water Vapour on Starch. Isr. J. Chem. **1972**, *10*, 963–965.

38. El-Shattawy, H.H.; Kildsig, S.O.; Peck, G.E. Cephalexin-Direct Compression Excipients: Performulation Stability Screening Using Differential Scanning Calorimetry. Drug. Dev. Ind. Pharm. **1982**, *8* (6), 897–909.

39. Kerc, J.; Srcic, S.; Urleb, U.; Kanalec, A.; Kofler, B.; Smid-Korbar, J. Compatibility Study Between Acetylcysteine and Some Commonly Used Tablet Excipients. J. Pharm. Pharmacol. **1992**, *44*, 515–518.

40. McKenna, A.; McCafferty, D.F. Effect of Particle Size on the Compaction Mechanism and Tensile Strength of Tablets. J. Pharm. Pharmacol. **1982**, *34*, 347–351.

41. Guyot-Hermann, A.M. Disintegration Mechanisms of Tablets Containing Starches. Hypothesis About the Particle–Particle Repulsive Force. Drug Dev. Ind. Pharm. **1981**, *7* (2), 155–177.

42. Palmieri, G.F.; Lovato, D.; Martelli, S. New Controlled-Release Ibuprofen Tablets. Drug Dev. Ind. Pharm. **1999**, *25* (5), 671–677.

43. Sanchez, L.; Torrado, S.; Lastres, J.L. Gelatinized/Freeze-Dried Starch as Excipient in Sustained Release Tablets. Int. J. Pharm. **1995**, *115*, 201–208.

44. Singh, M.; O'Hagan, D. The Preparation and Characterization of Polymeric Antigen Delivery Systems for Oral Administration. Adv. Drug. Delivery Rev. **1998**, *34*, 285–304.

45. Wurzburg, O.B. Starch in the Food Industry. *Handbook of Food Additives*; Furia, T.E., Ed.; The Chemical Rubber Company: Boca Raton FL, **1972**, *1*, 361–395.

46. Bolhuis, G.K.; Arends-Scholte, A.W.; Stuut, G.J.; de Vries, J.A. Disintegration Efficiency of Sodium Starch Glycolates, Prepared from Different Native Starches. Eur. J. Pharm. Biopharm. **1994**, *40* (5), 317–320.

47. Gebre-Mariam, T.; Winnemoller, M.; Schmidt, P.C. An Evaluation of the Disintegration Efficiency of a Sodium Starch Glycolate Prepared from Enset Starch in Compressed Tablets. Eur. J. Pharm. Biopharm. **1996**, *43* (2), 124–132.

48. Parrott, E.L. Comparative Evaluation of a New Direct Compression Excipient, Soludex™ 15. Drug Dev. Ind. Pharm. **1989**, *15*, 561–583.

49. Li, L.C.; Peck, G.E. The Effect of Moisture Content on the Compression Properties of Maltodextrins. J. Pharm. Pharmacol. **1990**, *42*, 272–275.

50. Zhou, F.; Vervaet, C.; Schelkens, M.; Lefebvre, R.; Remon, J.P. Bioavailability of Ibuprofen from Matrix Pellets Based on the Combination of Waxes and Starch Derivatives. Int. J. Pharm. **1998**, *168*, 79–84.

S

STATISTICAL METHODS

Charles Bon
AAI International, Wilmington, North Carolina

INTRODUCTION

Death and taxes, as the old adage goes, are the only certainties in life. Although this is an overstatement, it does emphasize the uncertain world in which the pharmaceutical scientist lives and works. Faced with "estimates" of product characteristics such as potency, content uniformity, impurity levels, and dissolution performance, the scientist must make important go/no-go decisions. These estimated values, as is true for most measured quantities, inherently vary from the true values on which correct decisions depend. Statistical methods provide tools that enable the pharmaceutical scientist to act decisively in an uncertain world. An understanding of basic statistical methods is important for all who work in the pharmaceutical field.

SOME BASIC CONCEPTS

In the developmental process for many drugs, the drug product is administered under controlled conditions to healthy, normal individuals or to the targeted patient population. This is done to characterize the rate and extent of absorption, the bioavailability, of the active drug contained in the product. The bioavailability is estimated from the measured concentrations of the drug that appear in serial blood specimens collected over a period of time after product administration. Basic statistical principles govern the behavior of the typical bioanalytical procedure used to measure these concentrations in the collected blood specimens.

The first step of a typical procedure might involve the transfer of 0.5 ml of the specimen into a screw-cap culture tube using a disposable serological pipette. Next, 100 µl of internal standard, a chemical structurally similar to the drug of interest, is added. A small volume, 1.0 ml, of a buffer solution at an appropriate pH level is added to decrease the aqueous solubility of the drug and internal standard. After thorough mixing, 7 ml of diethyl ether is added to the tube, and it is capped and shaken to extract the drug and internal standard into the organic ether phase. The tube is centrifuged to obtain a clean separation of

the aqueous and the organic phases. A 5-ml portion of the organic phase is transferred to a clean culture tube and is evaporated to dryness under nitrogen. The residual of the extract is reconstituted in 100 µl of mobile phase, an acetonitrile/methanol/buffer solution, and 10 µl is injected onto a high-pressure liquid chromatogaph (HPLC) equipped with a 3-µ, C8 column. The column effluent is monitored for ultraviolet absorbance at 280 nm, and the drug and internal standard peak area, or height, responses are determined. The drug-to-internal peak response ratio is calculated, and an estimate of the concentration of drug in each specimen is obtained through interpolation of the ratio on a calibration curve. The calibration curve is constructed from the peak response ratios of extracted calibrator specimens containing known amounts of the drug in interference-free blood.

There are several obvious sources where error can contribute to the uncertainty in the concentration estimate. If, for example, 1.0 ml of the specimen is mistakenly transferred instead of 0.5 ml, but the correct volume was used for preparing the calibrators, systematic error would have occurred. Systematic errors lead to a constant, predictable uncertainty in the estimate. To deal with a systematic error, we must recognize that it has occurred and then correct for the mistake that led to its occurrence. Statistical methods do not address systematic errors. If, however, the correct 0.5 ml-volume of specimen and 100-µl volume of internal standard were used, we still would have errors affecting the concentration estimate. These errors would be random errors. Random errors are positive and negative deviations that inherently occur in any attempt to exactly measure a quantity, in our case, specific volumes of the specimen and internal standard. We might transfer 0.498 ml of a specimen owing to an unrecognized air bubble interfering with our reading of the meniscus in the transfer pipette. Or, perhaps, 0.502 ml is transferred because of some of the specimen adhering to the outside of the pipette. Statistical methods are our tools for dealing with uncertainty resulting from random error (chance).

After the transfer of the specimen and the addition of internal standard, the drug-to-internal ratio becomes a fixed quantity. Any additional random or systematic volume errors should not affect the concentration estimate. Upon injection of the reconstituted extract onto the HPLC, however, random errors will occur that do affect the estimate. These are the result of chance deviations in the partitioning of the drug and internal standard between the mobile phase and the column. Random fluctuations in the UV detection system will also affect the concentration estimate. The influences of random errors are statistically additive. In our example, the random errors are independent of each other in that the occurrence, sign (positive or negative), and magnitude of each are unrelated to the occurrence, sign, and magnitude of the others. This is in contrast to correlated errors, which are related to each other in some predictable way.

Two important characteristics of any assay method are its accuracy and its reproducibility. Accuracy is how close an estimate is expected to be in relation to the true value for the specimen. Reproducibility relates to how repeated estimates of the same specimen vary about their average value. Both accuracy and reproducibility are usually defined for a given concentration and may differ between low and high specimen concentrations. In a good assay method, these differences should be inconsequential across the working range of the method.

The expected value of an estimate is the average of an infinite number of determinations of the estimate. These infinite determinations, taken as an aggregate, make up the population of estimates. A population does not have to be infinite in size. Some examples of finite populations are the potencies for all tablets in a given lot of a drug product or the sitting blood pressures of all patients who use a certain antihypertensive medication in the coming year. The mean (μ) of a population is a parameter of the population. The estimate of μ, obtained from a single concentration estimate for a specimen, varies from one determination to the next and is aptly referred to as a variable. If a variable conceptually takes on a continuum of values, as is the case for a concentration estimate, it is called a continuous variable. Variables that take on only certain discrete values, such as the number of tablets produced from 50 kg of active drug material, are referred to as discrete variables.

It is impossible to conduct an infinite number of extractions of a specimen to determine the accuracy of a method. As a result, we estimate the accuracy of an assay by performing a finite number of extractions (n) on the specimen. We report the accuracy as the mean ($x\cdot = \Sigma x_i/n$, $i = 1, 2, \ldots , n$) of the multiple determinations, expressed as a percent of the known concentration. The finite group of determinations is a sample from the population, and its mean is referred to as the sample mean. The sample mean is a statistic that estimates the population parameter μ. If we could obtain the means from an infinite number of same-size samples, regardless of their size, then the mean of these infinite sample means would equal μ. In statistical

terminology, we say that the sample mean is an unbiased estimator of the population mean. Unbiasedness is a desirable property for any statistic. Some statistics only become unbiased when sample sizes are large. These statistics are said to be asymptotically unbiased. Such statistics have their greatest utility when used with larger samples, such as those consisting of 20–30 determinations rather than smaller numbers such as 2–10.

Reproducibility, or precision, of a method relates to how individual estimates fluctuate around the average value. The magnitude of the fluctuation in the population is expressed by the parameter variance (σ^2). Variance is the average of the squared deviations about μ for all values x_i in the population: $\Sigma(x_i - \mu)^2/N$. An unbiased estimate of σ^2 is obtained from the deviation of each value (x_i) around the mean ($x\cdot$) for a sample taken from the population: $s^2 = \Sigma(x_i - x\cdot)^2/(n - 1) = (\Sigma x_i^2 - (\Sigma x_i)^2/n)/(n - 1)$.

The form of the equation not involving $x\cdot$ is a convenient calculating formula that avoids rounding problems that can occur when individual values are very close to the mean. It is common practice to report the standard deviation s, which is the square root of the sample variance. The standard deviation is often normalized as the percent coefficient of variation CV% by dividing it by the sample mean and expressing the result as a percent. In the analyses of pharmaceutical dosage units and in FDA regulations governing these analyses, the term relative standard deviation (RSD) is used for this calculated quantity instead of the term CV%.

Given two estimates of a statistic, one from a sample of size n and the other from a sample of size $2n$, one might expect that the estimate from the larger sample would be more reliable than that from the smaller sample. This is, in fact, supported by statistical theory. If the variance in the population is σ^2, then the variance of the sample mean for samples of size n is σ^2/n. The square root of this is the standard error of the mean. Consistent with the variance of the sample mean being $1/n$ times that of a single determination (σ^2), the standard deviation and the CV% of the sample mean are reduced by the square root of n. As a direct consequence, an assay method that relies on the mean of two independent concentration determinations has a CV $1/\sqrt{2}$ that of the same method based on a single determination. This provides an easy way to increase the precision (reduce variability) of a method. An example of this is found in radioimmunoassay in which it is common for a concentration estimate to be calculated from the mean response of two determinations of a specimen.

As noted previously, fluctuations in concentration estimates about the true value arise from multiple, independent, random errors. Each of the independent errors (σ_i^2) is statistically additive, such that the total assay error

$\sigma^2 = \Sigma\sigma_i^2$. Similarly, the CV% of the assay will be the square root of the sum of the squared CV% values for all independent sources of error in the method. It is interesting to examine the impact of this on the determination of the important pharmacokinetic measure C_{max}, the maximum concentration of a drug after administration of a drug product. For many drugs, the biological variability, the degree to which the true C_{max} value varies during replicate administrations of the product to the same individual, can have a CV of 25% or greater. If an assay method has a 10% CV and the biological variability for C_{max} is 25%, then the C_{max} estimate would have a CV of 26.9%. This is simply the square root of the sum of the two squared independent error CVs: $25^2 + 10^2$. If the precision of the assay method was improved to 5% CV, C_{max} would be estimated with a 25.5% CV. The effort required to reduce a 10% CV assay to half that level, to obtain a mere 1.4% increase in overall precision would seldom prove to be cost-effective.

A USEFUL STATISTICAL DISTRIBUTION

The normal distribution appears ubiquitously throughout science and nature. References to applications of normal theory are found throughout the pharmaceutical literature. The distribution is one of the earliest introduced, having been published in 1733 by De Moivre. Most scientists have a basic familiarity with the distribution and its characteristic bell-shaped curve (Fig. 1). Those familiar with column chromatography might recognize this shape as that of the perfect chromatographic peak. In fact, the

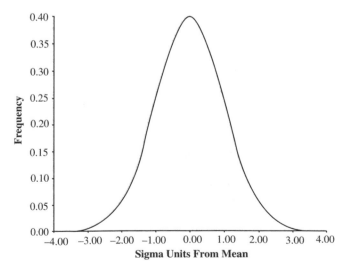

Fig. 1 The normal distribution.

principles of chromatographic peak symmetry and peak-to-peak resolution can be derived from normal theory. The normal distribution is defined by two parameters. The first, μ, defines the central location of the distribution, and the second, σ, defines the spread of the distribution about its center. The distribution has some unique properties. Its mean is the same as its median, the value at which 50% of the population are below and the remaining 50% are above. The distribution is symmetrical, its shape below its center is the mirror image of its shape above its center. Its mode, the value that occurs with the greatest frequency, also coincides with the mean and median. Approximately 68% of the distribution lies within 1σ of the mean, 95% lies within 2σ of the mean, and 99.8% lies within 3σ of the mean. The behavior of many observations in nature and many measurements in science can be approximated using the normal distribution. An important property that leads to the nearly universal application of the distribution is found in the central limit theorem. This theorem states that regardless of whether a given population is normally distributed, the distribution of the mean of randomly selected samples from the population will tend toward normality. This tendency increases as the size of the sample increases. If the population is, in reality, normally distributed, then a sample size of 1 is all that is needed. The more deviant the population distribution is from normality, the larger the sample size needs to be for its mean to be normally distributed.

It is reasonable to question whether the distribution of the estimates of a drug concentration in a blood specimen might be approximated by the normal distribution. Table 1 presents the results of repeated analyses of a specimen of interference-free plasma spiked to contain a known amount of drug. These data are taken from a comparative bioavailability study in which single doses of an unmarketed generic product and the marketed brand product of a drug were administered on separate occasions to healthy males. The values presented are the first of duplicate determinations of a quality control (QC) specimen that was included with each batch of subject specimens. This was done to verify that the in-process accuracy and precision of the assay method were consistent with the values observed during the assay validation.

A frequency histogram of the results is shown at the top of Fig. 2. The bottom of the figure shows the plot of the normal distribution with mean 207.6 ng/ml and σ 14.1 ng/ml. The shape of the histogram plot is similar to the plot of the normal distribution. The greatest deviation between the two is in the region of the center histogram. The sample distribution is higher peaked in its center, containing 42% of the values, than is the normal distribution, which has a 38% frequency at its center. The mean,

Table 1 Results of quality control specimen analyses

Batch	Conc. (ng/ml)	Batch	Conc. (ng/ml)
1	188	24	201
2	216	25	197
3	201	26	199
4	166	27	180
5	214	28	237
6	209	29	212
7	226	30	239
8	183	31	207
9	210	32	216
10	213	33	213
11	209	34	226
12	222	35	213
13	214	36	204
14	213	37	194
15	205	38	218
16	226	39	207
17	203	40	196
18	188	41	208
19	215	42	210
20	211	Mean	207.6
21	201	Median	209
22	205	Mode	213
23	206	Standard deviation	14.1

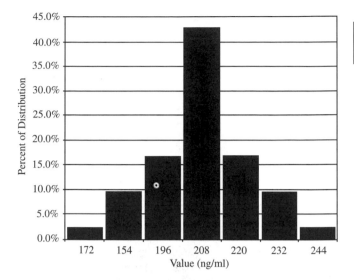

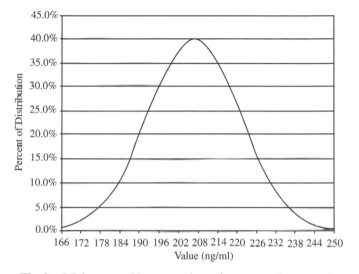

Fig. 2 QC frequency histogram plot and corresponding normal distribution.

median, and mode of the QC values are close to being equal, as would be expected if the values had come from a normal distribution.

A particularly useful form of the normal distribution is obtained by transforming each value x_i to its standard normal value. This transformation converts the distribution to one that is independent of μ and σ. The conversion is $Z_i = (x_i - \mu)/\sigma$, where Z_i is known as the standard normal deviate and is normally distributed with $\mu = 0$ and $\sigma = 1$. Tables of Z-values can be found in any elementary statistics textbook, An example is presented in Table 2. The standard normal deviate table typically provides the proportion (area under the curve) of the distribution that lies between $-\infty$ and various Z-values (the lower tail) or between various Z-values and $+\infty$ (the upper tail). The proportion of the distribution lying within a given Z range around μ is calculated by taking the difference between the tabled proportions for $+Z$ and $-Z$.

Table 3 provides the expected percentages of the standard normal distribution that lie within some selected Z ranges about μ and compares these with the percentage of the QC sample distribution that falls within these ranges. The percentages for the sample distribution are

calculated by taking the number of QC values within each range, dividing it by 42, the total number of values in the sample, and expressing this as a percent. Because μ and σ are unknown, the sample mean and standard deviation are used in the calculations. The lower limit and upper limit values, in ng/ml, for each range is calculated as: $[x - Z \cdot s]$, $[x + Z \cdot s]$.

As seen in the frequency histogram, the observed distribution of the QC values in the vicinity of the mean, between $Z = -1$ and $Z = 1$, is higher than predicted by normal theory. However, the distribution outside this region closely resembles what would be expected for a normally distributed variable. A goodness-of-fit test to determine whether a variable follows a certain statistical

Table 2 Cumulative areas under the standard normal curve ($-\infty$ to Z)[a,b]

Z	0.00	0.01	0.02	0.03	0.04	0.05	0.06	0.07	0.08	0.09
0.0	0.5000	0.5040	0.5080	0.5120	0.5160	0.5199	0.5239	0.5279	0.5319	0.5359
0.1	0.5398	0.5438	0.5478	0.5517	0.5557	0.5596	0.5636	0.5675	0.5714	0.5753
0.2	0.5793	0.5832	0.5871	0.5910	0.5948	0.5987	0.6026	0.6064	0.6103	0.6141
0.3	0.6179	0.6217	0.6255	0.6293	0.6331	0.6368	0.6406	0.6443	0.6480	0.6517
0.4	0.6554	0.6591	0.6628	0.6664	0.6700	0.6736	0.6772	0.6808	0.6844	0.6879
0.5	0.6915	0.6950	0.6985	0.7019	0.7054	0.7088	0.7123	0.7157	0.7190	0.7224
0.6	0.7257	0.7291	0.7324	0.7357	0.7389	0.7422	0.7454	0.7486	0.7517	0.7549
0.7	0.7580	0.7611	0.7642	0.7673	0.7704	0.7734	0.7764	0.7794	0.7823	0.7852
0.8	0.7881	0.7910	0.7939	0.7967	0.7995	0.8023	0.8051	0.8078	0.8106	0.8133
0.9	0.8159	0.8186	0.8212	0.8238	0.8264	0.8289	0.8315	0.8340	0.8365	0.8389
1.0	0.8413	0.8438	0.8461	0.8485	0.8508	0.8531	0.8554	0.8577	0.8599	0.8621
1.1	0.8643	0.8665	0.8686	0.8708	0.8729	0.8749	0.8770	0.8790	0.8810	0.8830
1.2	0.8849	0.8869	0.8888	0.8907	0.8925	0.8944	0.8962	0.8980	0.8997	0.9015
1.3	0.9032	0.9049	0.9066	0.9082	0.9099	0.9115	0.9131	0.9147	0.9162	0.9177
1.4	0.9192	0.9207	0.9222	0.9236	0.9251	0.9265	0.9279	0.9292	0.9306	0.9319
1.5	0.9332	0.9345	0.9357	0.9370	0.9382	0.9394	0.9406	0.9418	0.9429	0.9441
1.6	0.9452	0.9463	0.9474	0.9484	0.9495	0.9505	0.9515	0.9525	0.9535	0.9545
1.7	0.9554	0.9564	0.9573	0.9582	0.9591	0.9599	0.9608	0.9616	0.9625	0.9633
1.8	0.9641	0.9649	0.9656	0.9664	0.9671	0.9678	0.9686	0.9693	0.9699	0.9706
1.9	0.9713	0.9719	0.9726	0.9732	0.9738	0.9744	0.9750	0.9756	0.9761	0.9767
2.0	0.9772	0.9778	0.9783	0.9788	0.9793	0.9798	0.9803	0.9808	0.9812	0.9817
2.1	0.9821	0.9826	0.9830	0.9834	0.9838	0.9842	0.9846	0.9850	0.9854	0.9857
2.2	0.9861	0.9864	0.9868	0.9871	0.9875	0.9878	0.9881	0.9884	0.9887	0.9890
2.3	0.9893	0.9896	0.9898	0.9901	0.9904	0.9906	0.9909	0.9911	0.9913	0.9916
2.4	0.9918	0.9920	0.9922	0.9925	0.9927	0.9929	0.9931	0.9932	0.9934	0.9936
2.5	0.9938	0.9940	0.9941	0.9943	0.9945	0.9946	0.9948	0.9949	0.9951	0.9952
2.6	0.9953	0.9955	0.9956	0.9957	0.9959	0.9960	0.9961	0.9962	0.9963	0.9964
2.7	0.9965	0.9966	0.9967	0.9968	0.9969	0.9970	0.9971	0.9972	0.9973	0.9974
2.8	0.9974	0.9975	0.9976	0.9977	0.9977	0.9978	0.9979	0.9979	0.9980	0.9981
2.9	0.9981	0.9982	0.9982	0.9983	0.9984	0.9984	0.9985	0.9985	0.9986	0.9986
3.0	0.9987	0.9987	0.9987	0.9988	0.9988	0.9989	0.9989	0.9989	0.9990	0.9990
3.1	0.9990	0.9991	0.9991	0.9991	0.9992	0.9992	0.9992	0.9992	0.9993	0.9993
3.2	0.9993	0.9993	0.9994	0.9994	0.9994	0.9994	0.9994	0.9995	0.9995	0.9995
3.3	0.9995	0.9995	0.9995	0.9996	0.9996	0.9996	0.9996	0.9996	0.9996	0.9997
3.4	0.9997	0.9997	0.9997	0.9997	0.9997	0.9997	0.9997	0.9997	0.9997	0.9998

[a]Enter Table by Z-value to obtain cumulative area entry. As an example, area for $Z = 1.96$ (entry at row 1.9, column 0.06) is 0.9750, indicating that 97.5% of the standard normal distribution is below this Z-value, and 2.5% is above. Areas for negative Z-values are calculated by subtracting the area for the positive Z-value from 1. For example, the area for $Z = -1.96$ is calculated as $1 - 0.9750$ or 0.0250.

[b]Table values generated using the SAS System.

distribution can be constructed using a chi-square statistic (Table 4). The range of the sample values is divided into intervals, and the expected number of values (E) that should fall in each interval is calculated. It is important to keep the intervals large enough so that at least five observations are expected in each. The number of observed values (O) in the sample that falls within each interval is then determined. The chi-square statistic for this test is $\chi^2 = \Sigma[(O - E)^2/E]$. If the calculated statistic value exceeds that of the critical upper tail, chi-square value at $\alpha = 0.05$ ($p = 0.05$ testing level), we reject the hypothesis that the sample distribution is consistent with the assumed statistical distribution. If our calculated value is less than the critical value, we accept the hypothesis.

The chi-square table (Table 5) is entered according to the significance level (e.g., $p = 0.05$) and the degrees of freedom (df) for the calculated statistic. The degrees of freedom for the goodness-of-fit test are the total number of

Table 3 Distribution of results of quality control specimen analyses

±Z units about mean	Expected percent	Observed percent
3.0	99.7	100
2.5	99	98
2.0	95	93
1.5	87	88
1.0	68	74
0.7	52	64
0.5	38	55
0.2	18	24
0.1	8	12

intervals less one. If, as in our case, population parameters for the assumed statistical distribution are not known and must be estimated from the sample, then the degrees of freedom are further reduced by the number of parameters estimated. In our example using eight intervals and estimating the mean and variance of the normal distribution from the sample, there are $8 - 1 - 2 = 5$ degrees of freedom. The critical chi-square value at $\alpha = 0.05$ with 5 df is 9.24. As Table 4 shows, our calculated statistic value, 6.33, is less than the critical value. Accordingly, we accept the assumption that the QC values appear to come from the assumed normal distribution with $\mu = 207.6$ and $\sigma = 14.1$.

Normal distribution theory can be used to test whether a particular sample value is consistent with other values or with our past experience. If the mean μ and the variance σ^2 are known, then we can determine how deviant an observed value x_i, appears to be by calculating the statistic $Z = (x_i - \mu)/\sigma$ and comparing this with the table of standard normal deviates. Suppose that one of the values for our QC specimen was 170 ng/ml. Past experience has led us to believe that the results for this QC specimen are normally distributed with $\mu = 207.6$ ng/ml and $\sigma = 14.1$. Is the value of 170 ng/ml consistent with the assumption (hypothesis) that the assay is functioning properly with only random errors operative. To test this, we calculate the Z-statistic, which is equal to $(170 - 207.6)/14.1 = -37.6/14.1 = -2.77$. From the table of standard normal deviates, we see that the proportion of the normal distribution that lies within the range $-\infty$ to -2.77 (or similarly, between 2.77 and $+\infty$) is 0.0028. Therefore, the probability of encountering a value this far removed from the mean (±37.6 ng/ml) is $p = 2 \times 0.0028 = 0.0056$. Typically, when there is less than a 5% probability ($p < 0.05$) of observing a value, we would question whether our hypothesis was correct. We conclude, therefore, that either we have just observed a relatively rare event or that the assay was not working as expected. The hypothesis that the observed value deviates from its expected value owing only to random fluctuation is called the null hypothesis. If the null hypothesis is rejected, then we accept some stated alternative hypothesis. In this example, the alternative hypothesis is that the assay method was not functioning properly.

The Z-test can also be used to test if the mean $x\cdot$ from a sample of size n is consistent with the known mean μ of the population. The Z-statistic for this test is equal to $(x\cdot - \mu)/(\sigma/\sqrt{n})$, where $\sigma/\sqrt{n}$ is the standard error of the mean. The statistic is evaluated against the table of standard normal deviates just as we did in determining whether the QC value of 170 ng/ml was acceptable.

It should be noted that although it is common to use the 5% level of significance ($p < 0.05$) for testing, this level is not always appropriate. If the rejection of the 170 ng/ml QC value causes us to evaluate if the conduct and performance of the assay for a particular batch of specimens were correct, then the 5% level is probably appropriate. At this level, we would expect to have to investigate the performance of 1 in 20 of the batch runs even when everything was functioning properly. This would result in what is statistically known as a Type I error. A 5% level of extra circumspection would generally not be a problem. However, if the rejection of the 170 ng/ml value led to our dropping the value from estimates of in-process accuracy and precision, then it is not generally acceptable to erroneously exclude 5% of the values, thereby calculating estimates on the best 95% of the results. In this case, a 1% level of significance ($p < 0.01$), or even lower, would be more appropriate. At this lower level of significance, we would reject fewer values that deviated from the expected value simply owing to random error. Although this appears to be desirable, testing at a lowered level of significance also reduces our ability to reject values that differ from expected owing to true assay performance problems. This nondetection of truly aberrant values is referred to as a Type II error. Generally, the only way to decrease both Type I and Type II errors is to increase the size of the sample used in the statistical test.

THE DISTRIBUTION OF THE SAMPLE MEAN

We seldom know the population variance and, therefore, must estimate it from a sample. If the population is normally distributed or if the sample is a large one from a

Table 4 Chi-Square Goodness-of-Fit Test

Z_{low}	Z_{high}	Theoretical proportion	$x \cdot - Z_{low} * s$	$x \cdot + Z_{high} * s$	Expected (E)	Observed (O)	$(O - E)^2/E$
−4.00	−1.18	0.1190	151.2	191.0	5	5	0.000
−1.18	−0.72	0.1168	191.0	197.5	5	3	0.800
−0.72	−0.37	0.1199	197.5	202.4	5	4	0.200
−0.37	0.00	0.1443	202.4	207.6	6	7	0.167
0.00	0.37	0.1443	207.6	212.9	6	7	0.167
0.37	0.72	0.1199	212.9	217.8	5	9	3.200
0.72	1.18	0.1168	217.8	224.3	5	2	1.800
1.18	4.00	0.1190	224.3	264.1	5	5	0.000

Sum = 6.33; critical χ^2 = 9.24.

population that is not normal, then we can construct a test to determine whether the sample mean is consistent with the known, or assumed, mean. To do so, we rely on a statistic based on Student's t-distribution. The t-distribution,

Table 5 Critical values of the Chi-square and student's t Distributions[a]

DF	Chi-square values for one-sided test			t Values for one-sided test		
	0.05	0.025	0.005	0.05	0.025	0.005
1	2.71	3.84	5.02	6.31	12.71	63.69
2	4.61	5.99	7.38	2.92	4.30	9.92
3	6.25	7.81	9.35	2.35	3.18	5.84
4	7.78	9.49	11.14	2.13	2.78	4.60
5	9.24	11.07	12.83	2.02	2.57	4.03
6	10.64	12.59	14.45	1.94	2.45	3.71
7	12.02	14.07	16.02	1.89	2.36	3.50
8	13.36	15.51	17.53	1.86	2.31	3.36
9	14.68	16.92	19.02	1.83	2.26	3.25
10	15.99	18.31	20.48	1.81	2.23	3.17
11	17.28	19.68	21.92	1.80	2.20	3.11
12	18.55	21.03	23.34	1.78	2.18	3.05
14	21.06	23.68	26.12	1.76	2.14	2.98
16	23.54	26.30	28.85	1.75	2.12	2.92
18	25.99	28.87	31.53	1.73	2.10	2.88
20	28.41	31.41	34.17	1.72	2.09	2.85
25	34.38	37.65	40.65	1.71	2.06	2.79
30	40.26	43.77	46.98	1.70	2.04	2.75
35	46.06	49.80	53.20	1.69	2.03	2.72
40	51.81	55.76	59.34	1.68	2.02	2.70
50	63.17	67.50	71.42	1.68	2.01	2.68
60	74.40	79.08	83.30	1.67	2.00	2.66
∞	–	–	–	1.645	1.960	2.576

[a]Table values generated using the SAS System.

attributed to W.S. Gossett, who wrote under the pseudonym "Student," describes the behavior of the means for samples taken from a normal distribution. The t-distribution is defined entirely by the sample size n, or more typically by its degrees of freedom $n - 1$. The distribution has a shape similar to that of the standard normal distribution, bell-shaped, but for small samples is lower peaked and broader than the standard normal distribution. As the sample size increases, the distribution approaches that of the normal distribution, coinciding with it when the sample size is infinite. The t-statistic is used like the Z-statistic, for testing the consistency of a sample mean with the population mean μ. The difference between the two statistics is that for the t-statistic, σ is replaced by its sample estimate, the standard deviation s. The statistic is $t = (x \cdot - \mu)/(s/\sqrt{n})$. Table 5 provides a listing of critical t-values (think of them as t deviates) for different degrees of freedom ($n - 1$). Note that at infinite degrees of freedom, the critical t-value is simply the standard normal deviate Z.

Assume that the QC specimen was supposed to be prepared to contain 200 ng/ml of drug and that we do not know the true population variance. Is a sample mean equal to 207.6 ng/ml based on 42 determinations consistent with the true value being 200 ng/ml? This typically would be stated in the form of a null (H_0) and alternative hypothesis (H_a):

$$H_0: \quad \mu = 200\,ng/ml$$
$$H_a: \quad \mu \neq 200\,ng/ml$$

Because σ for the population is unknown, we must estimate it from the sample standard deviation s. We calculate $t = (207.6 - 200)/(14.1/\sqrt{42}) = 3.49$. Referring to Table 5 and entering it with 40 degrees of freedom, the closest-value to the $42 - 1 = 41$ degrees of freedom for our calculated statistic, we find a critical, one-sided, t-value at the 0.005 level equal to 2.70. If the calculated t-statistic value exceeds a tabled critical value ($t > t_{crit}$) or if it is less than the negation of the critical value ($t < -t_{crit}$), then the null hypothesis is rejected. In the example, the calculated value 3.49 exceeds the critical value and we reject the hypothesis that the sample comes from a population with a mean of 200 ng/ml at the 0.01 level of significance (2×0.005). We, instead, accept the alternative hypothesis that the QC specimen appears to have been prepared to contain a drug concentration different than 200 ng/ml. This is an example of a one-sample t-test.

Another application of the t-test is the two-sample t-test. This test is used to determine whether two samples come from populations with the same mean ($\mu_1 - \mu_2 = 0$) or whether the population means differ by some hypothesized amount ($\mu_1 - \mu_2 = c$). In both cases, the statistic is calculated as $t = [(x_1 - x_2) - (\mu_1 - \mu_2)]/se$, where x_1 and x_2 are the means of first sample and the second sample. The denominator of the statistic is the standard error for the difference between the two means, calculated as: $se = s_p(1/n_1 + 1/n_2)^2$, where, $s_p = [((n_1 - 1)s_1^2 + (n_2 - 1)s_2^2)/(n_1 + n_2 - 2)]^2$, s_1 and n_1 are the standard deviation and size of the first sample, and s_2 and n_2 are the standard deviation and size of the second sample. We enter the t-table with $n_1 + n_2 - 2$ degrees of freedom. If the tabled value is exceeded by our calculated value or if the calculated value is less than the negation of the tabled value, then we reject the hypothesis that the two samples are from populations with the same mean or differ by the hypothesized amount c.

Assume that we have a second set of 20 QC values from a second QC specimen, presumably prepared identically to the specimen from our previous set of values, and found a mean of 199.6 ng/ml and standard deviation 13.5 ng/ml. We can evaluate whether these results are consistent with those from 42 results on the first QC specimen. The null hypothesis for the test is that the two QC specimens have been prepared identically, $\mu_1 - \mu_2 = 0$. The alternative hypothesis would be that they are not identical, $\mu_1 - \mu_2 \neq 0$. The standard error is $se = [(41 \times 14.1^2 + 19 \times 13.5^2)/(41 + 19)]^{\frac{1}{2}}(1/42 + 1/20)^{\frac{1}{2}} = (193.566)^{\frac{1}{2}}(1/42 + 1/20)^{\frac{1}{2}} = 3.78$.

The t-statistic is $(207.6 - 199.6)/3.78 = 2.12$. Entering Table 5 with 60 degrees of freedom, we obtain a critical t-value for a one-sided test at the 0.025 level of significance equal to 2.00. As the alternative hypothesis is that the two QC specimens differ, without regard to which has the higher and which has the lower value, the test is a two-sided test. The critical table value at 0.025, one-sided, is the critical value to use for a two-sided test at 0.05. The calculated statistic exceeds this critical value, and we reject the hypothesis that the two sets of QC samples were

prepared identically. If we have the stock solutions used to prepare the two QC specimens, we would probably analyze them to see whether they have identical concentrations.

The t-distribution can also provide a tool to evaluate whether two samples on which paired determinations had been obtained appear to come from populations with the same mean (or from the same population). A paired t-test can be applied when we want to determine whether a newly trained analyst performs an assay method with the same proficiency as an experienced analyst. Suppose that each analyst processes seven different QC specimens and we obtain the following assay results, in the order (new analyst, experienced analyst): (12.6, 11.3), (3.46, 2.34), (25.4, 22.5), (10.3, 8.80), (5.89, 4.68), (16.4, 14.2), and (9.95, 8.20). The paired t-test deals with the differences for each of the paired results (new–experienced): 1.3, 1.12, 2.9, 1.5, 1.21, 2.2, and 1.75. The mean difference is 1.71, with a standard deviation of 0.641. The t-statistic is calculated by dividing this mean by the standard error (standard deviation/$\sqrt{n}$) and comparing the result with the critical t-value with $n - 1$ degrees of freedom. With the $n = 7$ pairs in the example, the calculated t-statistic is $1.71/(0.641/\sqrt{7}) = 7.06$. This exceeds the critical t-value 2.45 for the two-sided, 0.05 level of significance (the one-sided 0.025 value in Table 5) with six degrees of freedom. We conclude that a difference as large as the one observed between the two analysts would not likely be attributable to random error alone. The "new" analyst may need some additional training.

ANOTHER USEFUL DISTRIBUTION

A commonly encountered statistical distribution is the binomial distribution. This distribution deals with the behavior of binary outcomes such as the flip of a coin (heads/tails), the gender of a child (boy/girl), or the determination if a tablet has acceptable potency (pass/fail). When dealing with a sequence of independent binary outcomes, such as multiple flips of a coin or determining whether the potencies of 20 tablets are individually acceptable, the binomial distribution can be used. The probability of observing x successes in n outcomes is $C(x,n) p^x q^{n-x}$. Binomial expansion for $x = 1$ to n is $C(0,n)p^0 q^n + C(1,n)p^1 q^{n-1} + C(2,n)p^2 q^{n-2} + \ldots + C(n,n)p^n q^0$. This sum equals 1, as the probability of observing at least one of the possible outcomes is 1 (a certainty). The notation in the expansion $C(a,n)$ is the number of ways of obtaining groups of size a from n distinct items: $n!/[a!(n - a)!]$. As an example, the number of groups of size three obtainable when there are four different items is $C(3,4) = 4!/[3!(4 - 3)!] = (4 \times 3 \times 2 \times 1)/[(3 \times 2 \times 1)(1)] = 4$. Note that 0! is defined as 1. The p in the binomial expansion is the success probability for the single binary event such as observing a head with one flip of a coin. The q stands for the single-event failure probability (e.g., observing a tail) and is equal to $1 - p$.

PUTTING IT ALL TOGETHER

In the analyses of blood specimens from subjects participating in bioavailability studies, the FDA instructs laboratories to include quality control specimens (QC) at each of three known concentrations (low, mid, and high). The QC specimens are processed in duplicate with each batch of subject specimens. The acceptance criteria for the batch, based on the results of these QC specimens, is that at least four of the six values must fall within a specified range about their nominal concentrations. In addition, no more than one value at each of the three QC concentration levels can be outside its acceptance range. Combining binomial and normal distribution theory, we can estimate the number of batch runs we expect to reject because of random error.

Assume that the acceptance limit for each QC value is that it must fall within 15% of its nominal concentration. Any value meeting this criterion passes and any not meeting this criterion fails (a binary outcome). The probability of accepting a batch run based on multiple binary outcomes (QC pass/fail determinations) will be governed by the binomial distribution. The probability of a single QC value failing is equal to the probability of obtaining a concentration outside 85–115% of its nominal concentration. The concentration estimates are assumed to be normally distributed with a mean equal to 100% of the nominal concentration. The sigma value for the estimates is equal to the CV of the assay. If the assay CV is 12%, the probability of a QC value passing acceptance criteria is the probability of obtaining a Z-value between $(85 - 100)/12$ and $(115 - 100)/12$ or between -1.25 and $+1.25$. The proportion of the standard normal distribution between -1.25 and $+1.25$ is 0.7888, which is p, the probability of a single QC value passing. The value of q is $1 - 0.7888$ or 0.2112. There are three mutually exclusive ways that at least four of the six QC values can pass the acceptance criterion. All six values could pass, five of the six could pass, or four of the six could pass. These outcomes are mutually exclusive; the occurrence of any one of them excludes the possibility that either of the other two occurs. The probability of at least four of six QC values passing, then, is the sum of the probabilities of each of the three mutually exclusive ways in which this event can occur.

It should be noted that in probability calculations, when an event A can occur through any one of the mutually exclusive events B, C, D, etc., then the probability of A is the sum of the individual probabilities of B, C, D, etc. However, if A occurs only when events B, C, D, etc. all occur, then the probability of A is the product of the individual probabilities of B, C, D, etc.

Applying the binomial expansion, the probability of at least four of the six QC values passing is $C(6,6)p^6q^0 + C(5,6)p^5q^1 + C(4,6)p^4q^2 = 1(0.7888)^6 + 6(0.7888)^5(0.2112) + 15(0.7888)^4(0.2112)^2$, which equals 0.8869. For a batch to pass, however, we have the additional restriction that when only four of six values pass, no more than one of the two failures can occur at the same QC level (low, mid, or high). This restriction reduces the 15 possible ways that four of six QC values can pass to 12. This reduces the probability of the batch being accepted to $0.8869 - 3(0.7888)^4(0.2112)^2$ or 0.8351. There is an 83.5% probability of accepting a batch run, and there is nearly a 16.5% chance of rejecting it because of random error. We might consider improving the precision of the assay rather than proceeding with a method that is anticipated to erroneously reject nearly 17% of our analyses. If the CV% of the method were improved to 8%, the probability of batch acceptance increases to 0.9875, and our expected failure rate is only 1.2%. With 42 batch runs, we expect to have to repeat 1–2 batches, as contrasted with the 12% CV assay, where we expect to repeat seven batches. Here is a case in which a modest improvement in assay precision reaps big rewards.

The chi-square distribution used in the goodness-of-fit test is useful in another important statistical test. Assume that previous experience leads us to believe that the σ of an assay method is no greater than 10 ng/ml. In processing 42 batches, the observed standard deviation was 14.1 ng/ml for the QC values. Is this result consistent with the prior knowledge of the assay (H_0: $\sigma \leq 10$), or does it appear that the precision of the assay has deteriorated (H_a: $\sigma > 10$)? Application of a chi-square test can help answer this question. The appropriate statistic in this case is $\chi^2 = (n - 1)s^2/\sigma^2$, which follows a chi-square distribution with $n - 1$ degrees of freedom. In our example, we replace s in the statistic with 14.1, our sample standard deviation, and σ with our assumed upper limit of 10 for σ. The calculated statistic for this one-sided test is $\chi^2 = (42 - 1)14.1^2/10^2 = 81.51$. This calculated value exceeds the critical chi-square value 59.34 at the 0.005 level of significance and 40 (approximately 41) degrees of freedom. We conclude that the assay precision had deteriorated and would probably launch an investigation as to why.

In manufacturing a drug product, it is common to collect and analyze specimens from the mix of active and inactive ingredients, the blend. This is done to verify adequate uniformity of the blend before proceeding with the manufacturing process. The specimens are strategically collected from the blend container, for example, from the left, center, and right regions of the top, middle, and bottom of the container. Blend uniformity criteria usually require that the mean assay value for the specimens falls within an acceptable range (e.g., 95– 105%) about the label claim (100% potency) for the product. In addition, the relative standard deviation CV% for the analyses of the blend specimens must not be greater than some specified limit (e.g., 5%). Using the characteristics of the normal and the chi-square distributions, we can estimate the chances of passing blend uniformity criteria.

Suppose that prior knowledge of the manufacturing process leads us to believe that we routinely produce blends with potencies between 97 and 103% of label claim. We estimate that the variability for a "good" blend is no more than 3% CV, a composite of true blend inhomogeneity, sampling error, and analytical method variability. What is the probability of accepting a good blend? The standard error of the mean for nine specimens from the blend will be 1%, our worst-case estimate of CV for a single determination (3%) divided by the square root of the number of specimens collected (9). Assuming that the true potency of the blend is 97% (a worst-case estimate), then the probability of observing a mean from nine blend specimens that is within our acceptance range of 95–105% is the same as the probability of observing a Z-value between $(95 - 97)/1$ and $(105 - 97)/1$ or between -2 and $+8$. The proportion of the standard normal distribution contained between -2 and $+8$ is 0.977, the probability of passing the first criterion for blend acceptance. The second criterion is that the CV of the nine blend specimens must be less than 5%. With a true CV of 3%, this is the probability of observing a chi-square value less than $(n - 1)5^2/3^2 = (8)(25)/9 = 22.2$. With eight degrees of freedom, the probability of a chi-square value less than 22.2 is approximately 0.996, which is the probability of passing the second criterion. The probability of accepting the blend material is the product of the individual probabilities of passing criterion 1 and criterion 2, or 0.977×0.996, which equals 0.973. Therefore, 97% of our blend batches are expected to pass if only random error is operative.

Some have proposed widening the acceptance range (e.g., 90–110%) but requiring that all individual blend specimens fall within the widened range. Is this an easier or harder criterion to meet? The probability of a single-blend specimen being acceptable, is the probability of the standard normal deviate Z being between $(90 - 97)/3$ and $(110 - 97)/3$ or between -2.33 and $+4.33$. This probability is 0.99. For the blend to pass the first criterion,

the first specimen, the second, and the third, up through the ninth, must all, independently, be acceptable. The probability of passing this first criterion becomes 0.99^9, or 0.914. This, when combined with the probability of meeting the second criterion, results in a probability of blend acceptance being 0.914×0.996 or 0.91. Only 91% of the blends are expected to pass. The chance failure rate goes from approximately 1 in 30, based on using the mean to 1 in 11 based on using individual values, despite the widened acceptance limits.

ONE FINAL DISTRIBUTION

There is one final statistical distribution, the F-distribution, that is an important addition to the basic statistical tool chest. This distribution is used in the evaluation of two variance estimates to determine whether they are consistent with each other. The QC sample based on 42 estimates (41 degrees of freedom) had a standard deviation of 14.1 ng/ml. If we had another set of 31 QC values (30 degrees of freedom), perhaps from a second bioavailability study, with a standard deviation of 19.5 ng/ml, we might want to know whether the assay precision values for the two studies were consistent. The variance ratio statistic is s_1^2/s_2^2, where s_1 is the higher of the two standard deviations, and s_2 is the lower of the two. The calculated value of the statistic is compared with tables of critical F-values with $n_1 - 1$ numerator and $n_2 - 1$ denominator degrees of freedom. In our case, the critical $F_{30,41}$ is approximately equal to 1.74 at the 5% level of significance (see Table 6 for $F_{30,40}$, the closest value). The calculated ratio is $19.5^2/14.1^2 = 1.91$, which exceeds the critical value. The interpretation is that the assay precision for the second of the two studies differs significantly ($p < 0.05$) from that of the first (it has less precision, greater CV%).

The F-distribution has great utility in a statistical test referred to as analysis of variance (ANOVA). ANOVA is a powerful tool for testing the equivalence of means from samples obtained from normally distributed, or approximately normally distributed, populations. As an example, suppose that the following are the content uniformity values on 20 tablets from each of four different lots: lot A mean = 99.5%, standard deviation = 2.6%; lot B mean = 100.2%, standard deviation = 2.8%; lot C mean = 90.5%, standard deviation = 2.1%; and lot D mean = 100.3%, standard deviation = 2.7%.

Are any of the lots different from the other lots? To answer this question, we need to conduct a statistical test with a null hypothesis H_0: $\mu_1 = \mu_2 = \mu_3 = \mu_4 = \mu$

(all means are equal to some unknown μ), and an alternative hypothesis H_a: $\mu_1 \neq \mu$ or $\mu_2 \neq \mu$ or $\mu_3 \neq \mu$ or $\mu_4 \neq \mu$ (at least one mean is not equal to at least one of the other means). It is assumed that all lots have the same, unknown, variance, σ^2. The F-statistic involves the calculation of two variance estimates $s_1^2 = 1/(k-1)$ $\Sigma n_j (x._j - x..)^2$ and $s_2^2 = 1/(N-k) \Sigma\Sigma(x_{ij} - x._j)^2$. In the statistic, $x..$ is the grand mean across all $k = 4$ lots, n_j is the number of values from which the jth lot mean $x._j$ was determined (20 for each lot), and $N = \Sigma n_j = \Sigma\Sigma n_{ij}$ is the total number of x_{ij} values ($20 + 20 + 20 + 20 = 80$). The s_1^2 is a pooled variance estimate of how the category means vary about the grand mean, and s_2^2 is a pooled variance estimate of how the individual values within each category vary about their category mean. If the identification (grouping) of the values into categories (lots) does not affect the variance estimate, then the variance ratio s_1^2/s_2^2 will differ from 1.0 by only random error. The F-distribution describes how the ratio varies about 1.0 owing to random error when a set of values are arbitrarily grouped into categories. If the calculated statistic value exceeds the critical $F_{k-1, N-k}$ tabled value, then the null hypothesis of equal means is rejected.

In our example, $x. = \Sigma n_j x._j/N = (20 \times 99.5 + 20 \times 100.2 + 20 \times 90.5 + 20 \times 100.3)/80 = 97.625$. $s_1^2 = (1/3)[(99.5 - 97.625)^2 + (100.2 - 97.625)^2 + (90.5 - 97.625)^2 + (100.3 - 97.625)^2] = 22.689$. Because the square of the standard deviation in each lot j is $s_j^2 = \Sigma(x_{ij} - x._j)^2/(n_j - 1)$, we can calculate s_2^2 as $(1/(N-k))$ $\Sigma(n_j - 1) s_j^2 = 1/(80 - 4) [19 \times 2.6^2 + 19 \times 2.8^2 + 19 \times 2.1^2 + 19 \times 2.7^2] = 69.0$. The calculated variance ratio is $53.8/6.575 = 3.45$ and the critical 5% level $F_{3,76}$ is <2.76. The critical value 2.76 is that of $F_{3,60}$ in Table 6. This value is the closest tabled value with the desired numerator degrees of freedom (3) and denominator degrees of freedom 60, which do not exceed $N - k = 76$. As the calculated statistic value exceeds the critical F-value, we reject the null hypothesis that the means of all lots are the same. We accept the alternative hypothesis that at least one of the four means differs statistically from at least one of the other means. Looking at the four means, it appears that lot C differs from the others.

Instead of performing ANOVA, we might have considered pairing each lot mean with each of the other lot means and performing multiple two-sample t-tests to determine which ones differ significantly from the others. This approach would not be acceptable. First, it does not use all of the available information for the pooled denominator variance estimate. Second, it introduces what is known as the multiple comparison problem. The problem arises if there are multiple, separate, statistical evaluations conducted on the same set of data. When we

conduct a single test of a hypothesis at the 5% level of significance ($\alpha = 0.05$), such as H_0: $A = B$, we expect to falsely reject the hypothesis 5% of the time when A actually equals B (Type I error). We have, therefore, a 95% probability of being correct in the assessment when the null hypothesis $A = B$ is true. This is also true for the F-test of $A = B = C = D$ in ANOVA. If we were to independently perform multiple t-tests on our data with hypotheses such as $A = B$, $B = C$, $C = D$, $A = C$, etc., then for each of these 5% level tests, we have a 95% probability of obtaining a correct assessment when the null hypothesis that all means are equal is true. To correctly accept the null hypothesis of all means being equal, we must simultaneously conclude that $A = B$ and $B = C$ and $C = D$ and $A = C$, etc., from the multiple t-tests. The probability of doing so is $(0.95)(0.95)(0.95)...(0.95) = (0.95)^n$, where n is the number of pair-wise comparisons conducted by t-tests. The probability of being incorrect in this multiple pair-wise approach is $1 - (0.95)^n$, which exceeds the desired 5% level for any $n > 1$. In our case, there are $C(4, 2)$ or six possible pair-wise comparisons. The multiple pair-wise approach has a probability of an incorrect assessment, Type I error when the null hypothesis is true, equal to $1 - (0.96)^6 = 0.265$. This approach would essentially be testing at a 26.5% level of significance, rather than at the desired 5% level. For this reason, we only consider pair-wise examination of the data when the global assessment of equality of means is rejected by ANOVA. This maintains the desired 5% significance level.

For the post-ANOVA, pair-wise evaluations, there are procedures to deal with the multiple comparison problem. One such procedure is based on the F-distribution with one and $N - k$ degrees of freedom. This test also relies on the value of s_2^2 from ANOVA. The test statistic is $F = (1/s_2^2)$ $[(x._1 - x._2)^2/(1/n_1 + 1/n_2)]$, where $x._1$, $x._2$ are the means of the n_1 and n_2 values for the two lots in the pair-wise comparison. Comparing lot A and lot C: $F = (1/6.575)$ $[(99.5 - 90.5)^2/(1/20 + 1/20)] = 123.2$. This far exceeds the critical $F_{1,76}$ value at even a 1% level, which is <7.08, based on $F_{1,60}$, and we therefore reject the hypothesis that lot A and lot C means are equal. Because, the means for lot B and lot D differ from that of lot C by an even greater amount, they also are found to be statistically different from the lot C mean. By contrast, the comparison of lots A and D, with means of 99.5% and 100.3%, respectively, have an F-test value of 0.97, far less than the critical 5% value, which is <4.00.

The test of the four lots is an example of a one-way ANOVA. The one-way comes from the fact that there is only one category (lot) into which the data is classified. Often, we have more than one category (class variable) in which we need to classify data. Although our interest may

Table 6 Critical values of the F-distribution for 5% level of significance[a]

Df[b]	Numerator degrees of freedom: 1	2	3	4	5	6	7	8	9	10	11	12	15	20	25	30	40	60	100
1	161	200	216	225	230	234	237	239	241	242	243	244	246	248	249	250	251	252	253
2	18.5	19.0	19.2	19.3	19.3	19.3	19.4	19.4	19.4	19.4	19.4	19.4	19.4	19.5	19.5	19.5	19.5	19.5	19.5
3	10.1	9.55	9.28	9.12	9.01	8.94	8.89	8.85	8.81	8.79	8.76	8.74	8.70	8.66	8.63	8.62	8.59	8.57	8.55
4	7.71	6.94	6.59	6.39	6.26	6.16	6.09	6.04	6.00	5.96	5.94	5.91	5.86	5.80	5.77	5.75	5.72	5.69	5.66
5	6.61	5.79	5.41	5.19	5.05	4.95	4.88	4.82	4.77	4.74	4.70	4.68	4.62	4.56	4.52	4.50	4.46	4.43	4.41
6	5.99	5.14	4.76	4.53	4.39	4.28	4.21	4.15	4.10	4.06	4.03	4.00	3.94	3.87	3.83	3.81	3.77	3.74	3.71
7	5.59	4.74	4.35	4.12	3.97	3.87	3.79	3.73	3.68	3.64	3.60	3.57	3.51	3.44	3.40	3.38	3.34	3.30	3.27
8	5.32	4.46	4.07	3.84	3.69	3.58	3.50	3.44	3.39	3.35	3.31	3.28	3.22	3.15	3.11	3.08	3.04	3.01	2.97
9	5.12	4.26	3.86	3.63	3.48	3.37	3.29	3.23	3.18	3.14	3.10	3.07	3.01	2.94	2.89	2.86	2.83	2.79	2.76
10	4.96	4.10	3.71	3.48	3.33	3.22	3.14	3.07	3.02	2.98	2.94	2.91	2.85	2.77	2.73	2.70	2.66	2.62	2.59
11	4.84	3.98	3.59	3.36	3.20	3.09	3.01	2.95	2.90	2.85	2.82	2.79	2.72	2.65	2.60	2.57	2.53	2.49	2.46
12	4.75	3.89	3.49	3.26	3.11	3.00	2.91	2.85	2.80	2.75	2.72	2.69	2.62	2.54	2.50	2.47	2.43	2.38	2.35
13	4.67	3.81	3.41	3.18	3.03	2.92	2.83	2.77	2.71	2.67	2.63	2.60	2.53	2.46	2.41	2.38	2.34	2.30	2.26
14	4.60	3.74	3.34	3.11	2.96	2.85	2.76	2.70	2.65	2.60	2.57	2.53	2.46	2.39	2.34	2.31	2.27	2.22	2.19
15	4.54	3.68	3.29	3.06	2.90	2.79	2.71	2.64	2.59	2.54	2.51	2.48	2.40	2.33	2.28	2.25	2.20	2.16	2.12
16	4.49	3.63	3.24	3.01	2.85	2.74	2.66	2.59	2.54	2.49	2.46	2.42	2.35	2.28	2.23	2.19	2.15	2.11	2.07
17	4.45	3.59	3.20	2.96	2.81	2.70	2.61	2.55	2.49	2.45	2.41	2.38	2.31	2.23	2.18	2.15	2.10	2.06	2.02
18	4.41	3.55	3.16	2.93	2.77	2.66	2.58	2.51	2.46	2.41	2.37	2.34	2.27	2.19	2.14	2.11	2.06	2.02	1.98
20	4.35	3.49	3.10	2.87	2.71	2.60	2.51	2.45	2.39	2.35	2.31	2.28	2.20	2.12	2.07	2.04	1.99	1.95	1.91
30	4.17	3.32	2.92	2.69	2.53	2.42	2.33	2.27	2.21	2.16	2.13	2.09	2.01	1.93	1.88	1.84	1.79	1.74	1.70
40	4.08	3.23	2.84	2.61	2.45	2.34	2.25	2.18	2.12	2.08	2.04	2.00	1.92	1.84	1.78	1.74	1.69	1.64	1.59
50	4.03	3.18	2.79	2.56	2.40	2.29	2.20	2.13	2.07	2.03	1.99	1.95	1.87	1.78	1.73	1.69	1.63	1.58	1.52
60	4.00	3.15	2.76	2.53	2.37	2.25	2.17	2.10	2.04	1.99	1.95	1.92	1.84	1.75	1.69	1.65	1.59	1.53	1.48
100	3.94	3.09	2.70	2.46	2.31	2.19	2.10	2.03	1.97	1.93	1.89	1.85	1.77	1.68	1.62	1.57	1.52	1.45	1.39
∞	3.84	3.00	2.60	2.37	2.21	2.10	2.01	1.94	1.88	1.83	1.79	1.75	1.67	1.57	1.51	1.46	1.39	1.32	1.24

[a]Df are the denominator degrees of freedom.
[b]Table values generated using the SAS System.

be to determine only whether a particular class variable has meaning, it is important to include other class variables that may influence the variability of the data. ANOVA involves a null hypothesis for each classification variable that proposes that the means at each different level of the class (category) are all equal. If we reject the null hypothesis we conclude in favor of the alternative hypothesis, that at least one mean in the class differs from at least one other mean in the class. This is also a conclusion that categorizing the data by that class variable has meaning.

Assume that we have two analysts to determine the drug concentrations in plasma specimens from a bioavailability study, using our previously described analytical method. Before starting the analyses, we want to determine whether they are equally proficient with the method. We might set up the test by obtaining plasma specimens at three different concentrations of drug. We then have each analyst process in duplicate each specimen on each of two different days. The resulting drug concentration values can be categorized by three different class variables: analyst, day, and specimen. The variable analyst has two possible levels, analysts one and two. Day has two levels (days 1 and 2), and specimen has three (A, B, and C). ANOVA on the results is a three-way one, named for the three classification variables included. Our interest is in the classification by analyst, but the other two variables are necessary to properly define how the experiment was conducted. Table 7 shows the results of the experiment.

ANOVA calculations are straightforward in this example and are easily expanded to situations in which there are higher numbers of categories. The first ANOVA quantity we calculate is C, the correction factor. C is simply the square of the sum of all the individual values, divided by N, the total number of values: $(\Sigma x_{ijkl})^2/N$, where $i = 1-2$ (analysts), $j = 1-2$ (days), $k = 1-3$ (specimens), and $l = 1-2$ values for each specimen for each analyst on each day. Table 8 demonstrates the calculation of this and the other calculated ANOVA quantities. The quantity A is calculated as the sum of the squared individual values: Σx_{ijkl}^2. The ANOVA quantity for each classification variable (category) is the sum of the squared totals for each level of

the classification, divided by the number of values in each level of the classification. As seen with the variable specimen, this is the sum of the squared totals for the values for each of the specimens A, B, and C, all divided by 8, the number of values for each specimen (2 values for each of 2 days for each of 2 analysts). The principle of ANOVA is that the total sum of squares SS_{Total} is divisible into its component sums of squares for each classification variable plus random error: $SS_{Total} = SS_{Analyst} + SS_{Day} + SS_{Specimen} + SS_{Error}$. The total sums of squares are calculated as the difference between two ANOVA quantities, $A - C$. The sums of squares for each classification variable is its ANOVA quantity minus C. The sums of squares for random error is determined by difference: $SS_{Error} = SS_{Total} - SS_{Analyst} - SS_{Day} - SS_{Specimen}$. The degrees of freedom are also additive with $df_{Total} = df_{Analyst} + df_{Day} + df_{Specimen} + df_{Error}$. The total degrees of freedom are simply the total number of values less one. The degrees of freedom for each class variable are the number of levels within the class less one. The error degrees of freedom are determined by difference. Dividing each sum of squares by its degrees of freedom provides the mean square MS, which is an estimate of the population variance σ^2.

Table 7 Evaluation of the proficiency of two analysts to process plasma samples

Specimen	Day	Analyst 1	Analyst 2
A	1	52.8	57.9
A	1	52.3	57.5
A	2	53.3	58.0
A	2	52.1	57.0
B	1	42.2	45.6
B	1	42.4	44.2
B	2	41.7	43.8
B	2	40.4	44.1
C	1	56.8	64.0
C	1	57.0	64.9
C	2	59.6	62.6
C	2	57.2	61.8

Table 8 Calculation of ANOVA quantities

	Totals	No. of observations	Σ (Totals squared)/No.
All 24 values	1269.2	24	$C = 67119.53$
Days 1 and 2	637.6, 631.6	12	$T = 67121.03$
Analysts 1 and 2	607.8, 661.4	12	$K = 67239.23$
Specimens A, B, and C	440.9, 344.4, 483.9	8	$R = 68395.42$
		Square of each value	$A = 68541.24$

Table 9 Calculation of ANOVA table

ANOVA Source of variation	DF	SS	MS = SS/DF	F-ratio
Day	1	1.5000 $(T - C)$	1.5000	1.16
Analyst	1	119.7067 $(K - C)$	119.7067	92.42[a]
Specimen	2	1275.8958 $(R - C)$	637.9479	492.51[a]
Error	19	24.6108 $(A - T - K - R + 2C)$	1.2953	
Total	23	1421.7133 $(A - C)$		

[a]Indicates statistical significance ($p < 0.05$).

Table 9 shows the construction of the ANOVA table. If the variance estimate of a class variable MS_{Variable} deviates significantly from that obtained by that for random error MS_{Error}, then the null hypothesis that the means at the different levels for that variable are equal is rejected. In other words, the classification of data by that variable is explanatory of the variation observed in the data. We conduct the test by using the variance ratio test $F = MS_{\text{Variable}}/MS_{\text{Error}}$, with numerator degrees of freedom equal to those of the variable and denominator degrees of freedom equal to that of the error term. As shown in Table 9, we reject the hypothesis that the two analysts process the specimens equivalently. We also see, as we expected, that the specimen levels A, B, and C are not equal. There are no detectable differences in the values obtained over the 2 days of processing.

In the previous example, we tested the hypothesis of "equality." In reality, our interests are usually not in equality but in "comparability." We generally do not require, or even logically expect, that two lots of the same pharmaceutical product will have the exact same potency. If we had several different lots of a drug product and analyzed enough units from each (e.g., 100–200 tablets), we could detect as statistically significant even a 1% difference in the potency between the lots. Although statistically significant, such a difference would have no practical significance. We require, however, that the potencies, as with the analysts' performance on an assay, be comparable, allowing for a reasonable margin of error. Although hypothesis testing deals with tests of equality, the closely related confidence interval approach deals with comparability. The confidence interval calculation can be applied to comparisons of means from samples drawn from normal populations or from any population if the samples are large (thanks to the central limit theorem). First, we calculate the difference between two means from samples from the two population $x._1 - x._2$, which estimates the difference between the population means $\mu_1 - \mu_2$. Next, we need to calculate the standard error for this difference.

The standard error is calculated as se $= (s_p^2/n_1 + s_p^2/n_2)^{0.5}$, where n_1 and n_2 are the number of values in the first and second samples, and s_p^2 is a variance estimate (s_p^2 from t-test and s_2^2 from one-way ANOVA or MS_{Error}). We have $(1 - \alpha)$ $\times 100\%$ confidence that the true difference between the population means falls within the interval $(x._1 - x._2) \pm$ se $\times t_{\alpha/2}$, where $t_{\alpha/2}$ is the critical one-sided t-value at the $\alpha/2$ level of significance and degrees of freedom equal to those for our variance estimate s_p^2.

In ANOVA for the results from the two analysts, $MS_{\text{Error}} = 1.2953$ with 19 degrees of freedom. The means for analyst 1 was 607.8/12, or 50.65 and for analyst 2 was 661.4/12, or 55.12. The difference between the means is -4.47. The standard error se for the difference would be $(s_p^2/n_1 + s_p^2/n_2)^{0.5} = (2s_p^2/n)^{0.5} = (2MS_{\text{Error}}/12)^{0.5} = (2 \times 1.2953/12)^{0.5} = 0.465$. The critical t-value for a 95% confidence interval is the one-sided, 0.025 level value at 19 degrees of freedom, 2.095. The 95% confidence interval is $(-4.47) \pm (0.465) (2.095)$ or from -5.44 to -3.50. We have 95% confidence that the results of analyst 1 are between 6.34% ($100 \times 3.50/55.12$) to 9.88% ($100 \times 5.44/55.12$) lower than those of analyst 2 using the assay method. Because the value 0 is not included in the 95% confidence interval, we can conclude at the 5% level that there is a statistically significant difference between the two analysts, the same conclusion we had with ANOVA. However, a difference of 9.88%, the maximum confidence interval limit, might not be large enough for us to reject that the two analysts are comparable in their performance of the assay method. This is a decision that was not possible based solely on ANOVA results.

LINEAR REGRESSION

Those familiar with analytical methods probably have familiarity with "fitting a straight line" through data points. The statistical method generally used is known as linear regression or ordinary least-squares. Even the simplest scientific calculators and spreadsheet programs contain the methods for determining the slope (m) and intercept (b) of the line relating the dependent variable y (measured with random error) to the independent variable x (without random error), $y = mx + b$. The statistical form of this is $y_i = mx_i + b + e_i$, where e_i is the random error for the observation y_i at a specific value of x_i. The calculations for fitting the line are easy, with $m = [\Sigma(x_i - x\cdot)(y_i - y\cdot)]/[(x_i - x\cdot)^2]$ and $b = y\cdot - bx\cdot$, where $y\cdot$ and $x\cdot$ are the mean values for all the y_i and x_i values, respectively. It is common to have more than a single y value for each x value. A basic assumption is that the variance (error) in the determination of each y_i value is independent of its corresponding x_i value.

As previously indicated, the determination of a drug concentrations in plasma specimens requires the construction of a calibration response curve. This curve is often constructed as a straight line from the measured peak response ratios (y_i) plotted against their respective calibrator concentrations (x_i). The drug concentration in a specimen or the apparent (back-calculated) calibrator concentration is obtained from a rearrangement of the equation for the calibration line (without error) $x_i = (y_i - b)/m$. An example of a calibration curve with

back-calculated concentrations is given the first four columns of Table 10.

It is obvious that the lower end of the calibration curve does not provide an accurate representation of the calibrator concentrations, a problem that does not exist at the higher end of the curve. This problem illustrates what can happen when there is violation of the assumption of equal (homogeneous) variance for the y_i values. In bioanalytical methods, the largest component of the random error can often be attributed to volume errors, One often finds that the standard deviation of the response (y_i) is proportional to the concentration (x_i), that is, $e_i = kx_i$, where k is a constant. This violates the assumption of homogeneity of variance for y_i. To correct for this, we can use a variance-stabilizing transformation. If we divide the equation of the line by x_i, we obtain $y_i/x_i = m + b(1/x_i) + e_i/x_i$. However, $e_i/x_i = K$ is a constant, resulting in equal variance for $y_i' = y_i/x_i$. When y_i' is regressed against $1/x_i$, we obtain a line with slope equal to our desired intercept b and an intercept equal to the desired slope m. The last four columns of Table 10 demonstrate with calibrator data how this transformation provides accurate estimates for the back-calculated concentrations. The variance-stabilized line provides a slope estimate that differs only slightly from that of the original line ($0.938 \rightarrow 0.941$) and an

Table 10 Linear regression analyses of calibrator curve data

Calibrator (ng/ml) (x)	Response ratio (y)	Back[a] calculated (ng/ml)	Accuracy (%)	1/x (x')	y/x (y')	Back[b] calculated (ng/ml)	Accuracy (%)
0.250	0.321	0.134	54	4.000	1.285	0.253	101
0.250	0.311	0.123	49	4.000	1.244	0.242	97
0.500	0.545	0.373	75	2.000	1.090	0.490	98
0.500	0.59	0.419	84	2.000	1.178	0.537	107
1.00	1.042	0.902	90	1.000	1.042	1.02	102
1.00	0.994	0.851	85	1.000	0.994	0.967	97
5.00	4.981	5.10	102	0.200	0.996	5.20	104
5.00	4.466	4.55	91	0.200	0.893	4.66	93
10.0	9.911	10.4	104	0.100	0.991	10.4	104
10.0	9.247	9.65	96	0.100	0.925	9.73	97
25.0	24.132	25.5	102	0.040	0.965	25.5	102
25.0	22.448	23.7	95	0.040	0.898	23.8	95
50.0	44.061	46.7	93	0.020	0.881	46.7	93
50.0	51.171	54.3	109	0.020	1.023	54.3	109
100	101.132	108	108	0.010	1.011	107	107
100	88.314	93.9	94	0.010	0.883	93.7	94
250	227.438	242	97	0.004	0.910	242	97
250	241.472	257	103	0.004	0.966	256	103

[a]Slope = 0.938; intercept = 0.195.
[b]Slope = 0.941; intercept = 0.0834.

intercept estimate that differs more substantially ($0.195 \rightarrow 0.0834$). The approach of weighted least-squares, available in many advanced regression programs, gives the same results, using a $1/x^2$ weighting, and provides a greater choice for variance stabilization.

A FINAL WORD

The methods presented will hopefully provide a basic foundation for the application of statistics to pharmaceutical problems. Because of space limitations, the discussion has been limited to situations in which known statistical distributions could be assumed (parametric analyses). This is not always the case with real-life data. Fortunately, there are a number of nonparametric, distribution-free methods available to the pharmaceutical scientist to deal with analyses of such data. A general knowledge of statistical methods is a necessity for the pharmaceutical scientist. It is, however, also important for the scientist to realize when a problem or experimental design requires consultation with a statistician. The pharmaceutical statistician has a toolbox of methods considerably more advanced than the few basic methods presented here.

BIBLIOGRAPHY

Bolton, S. *Pharmaceutical Statistics*, 3rd Ed.; Marcel Dekker, Inc.: New York, 1997.

Brown, B.W., Jr.; Hollander, M. *Statistics: A Biomedical Introduction*; John Wiley & Sons: New York, 1977.

Chatterjee, S.; Price, B. *Regression Analysis by Example*; John Wiley & Sons: New York, 1977.

Dixon, W.J.; Massey, F.J., Jr. *Introduction to Statistical Analysis*, 3rd Ed.; McGraw-Hill Co.; New York, 1969.

Draper, N.R.; Smith, H. *Applied Regression Analysis*, 2nd Ed.; John Wiley & Sons: New York, 1981.

Kanji, G.K. *100 Statistical Tests*; Sage Publications, Inc.: Newbury Park, CA, 1993.

Li, C.C. *Introduction to Experimental Statistics*; McGraw-Hill Co.: New York, 1964.

Matthews, D.E.; Farewell, V.T. *Using and Understanding Medical Statistics*, 3rd revised Ed.: Karger AG: Basel; Switzerland, 1996, 5.

Meyer, S.L. *Data Analysis for Scientists and Engineers*; John Wiley & Sons: New York, 1975.

Snedecor, G.W.; Cochran, W.G. *Statistical Methods*, 8th Ed.; Iowa State University Press: Ames, 1989.

SAS® System. *Base SAS and SAS/STAT® Software*; Release 6.12 TS060 for Windows SAS Institute, Inc.: Cary, NC, 1989–1996.

Zar, J.H., Ed. *Biostatistical Analysis*; Prentice-Hall: Englewood Cliffs, NJ, 1974.

STERILIZATION BY MOIST HEAT

Dario Pistolesi

Fedegari Autoclavi S.p.A., Albuzzano, PV, Italy

INTRODUCTION

To sterilize something means to render it "aseptic" (from the Greek word *sepsis*, putrefaction, preceded by a privative *a*). In other words, it means to inactivate the micro-organisms that may produce this putrefactive action (in the broadest sense of the term).

Moist-heat sterilization is achieved when water vapor (or, more generically, moist heat, i.e., a suitable combination of temperature and humidity) at a definite temperature is introduced or generated (even indirectly) at the level of the micro-organisms to be inactivated and is maintained in such conditions for a definite time. As explained in detail hereafter, moist-heat sterilization proceeds as an inverse logarithmic progression. Therefore, only a treatment of infinite duration provides absolute certainty that all micro-organisms have been inactivated.

In pharmaceutical technology, to define an item as sterile, one must be able to demonstrate that on a statistical basis related to the processing conditions, no more than 1 in 10^6 units subjected to sterilization "may be" nonsterile. Therefore, the SAL (Sterility Assurance Level) of the product must be greater than (or equal to) 10^6. The obvious consequence of this situation is that although the word sterile expresses an absolute concept, the word sterilized, understood as the result of an adequate sterilization process, has a probabilistic meaning.

Current pharmacopeias, standards, and guidelines related to sterilization generally use the following type of wording:

> ... Sterilization is a special process because its efficacy cannot be verified by simple inspection and testing on the final product.... For this reason, sterilization processes have to be validated before use, the performance of the process monitored routinely and equipment regularly maintained....

Accordingly, installation qualification and operational qualification of the sterilizer and validation of the processes, combined with continuous monitoring of each individual routine process, are now considered fundamental (1). Therefore, sterility tests (i.e., microbiological tests performed on the final product) have lost much of the significance they had in the past (2), but they are still being performed. So-called parametric release (i.e., release based on the evaluation of tightly controlled physical parameters of each process, without performing sterility tests) is in fact theoretically accepted by many pharmacopoeias, but is (as stated, for example, in the *European Pharmacopoeia*) "... subject to the approval of the competent authorities ...," which are generally highly reluctant to grant such approval.

All pharmacopeias consider moist-heat sterilization as the method of choice, i.e., the method to be preferred, unless, of course, the product to be sterilized is incompatible with the characteristics of steam. The reason for this preference is the fact that moist-heat sterilization provides the best combination of flexibility, reliability, and low equipment and operating costs.

OVERVIEW

Moist-heat sterilization is achieved when a suitable combination of temperature and humidity can be introduced (or indirectly generated) at the level of the micro-organisms to be inactivated. The classic way to achieve this is by means of pressurized saturated steam at the temperature of 121°C (250°F). However, other sterilizing media (e.g., superheated water or a steam–air mixture) are also frequently used to obviate certain problems that pure steam may pose. Sometimes the load is rotated inside the chamber of the sterilizer to achieve particular results.

MOIST-HEAT STERILIZATION KINETICS (3)

Consider a system contaminated by a single microbiological species (i.e., an ampoule containing an aqueous suspension of a given micro-organism) immersed in pressurized saturated steam at constant temperature. One can demonstrate experimentally that the reaction of thermal inactivation of the micro-organism develops as a first-order chemical reaction (i.e., as a chemical decomposition reaction) in which the reaction rate is proportional at all times only to the amount of product still to be degraded. The proportionality coefficient is typical of the species and conditions of the given micro-organism. All this seems obvious for dry-heat sterilization, but not for steam sterilization, in which the water vapor molecules would appear to take part in the reaction. Actually, this bimolecular reaction is a first-order reaction, because an excess of steam is always present and its concentration can be considered constant.

The most widely used mathematical equation of the above is:

$$N = N_0 10^{-t/D} \tag{1}$$

where N_0 = initial number of micro-organisms; t = elapsed time (or sterilization time); N = number of surviving micro-organisms after exposure time t; and D = "decimal decay time," defined as the time interval required, at a specified and constant temperature, to reduce the microbial population to 1/10 of its original quantity.

At 121°C, the D-values generally oscillate between 0.2 and 1.5 min for the various microbial species that can be encountered in pharmaceutical activity. Eq. 1 allows for two important conclusions:

1. the time required to reduce the micro-organism population to any preset value is a function of the initial concentration, and
2. the effect of sterilization in the same conditions (T and t) will be very different according to the D-value of the contaminating micro-organism.

Fig. 1 shows that the same reduction ratio is achieved for different microbial species (at the same constant temperature) with an exposure time that is proportional to the D-value of each species.

Consider a batch of units (e.g., a batch of filled ampoules) with a constant initial population for each unit of 100 micro-organisms or 10^2. If $D_{121} = 1$, after 1 min at 121°C, the population will be reduced to $10^1 = 10$. After another minute, only $10^0 = 1$ micro-organism will still be surviving. After another minute, the surviving population would be $10^{-1} = 1/10$ micro-organism per unit. In biological terms, such a contamination is obviously meaningless; statistically, it means that there is a probability that $\frac{1}{10}$ of the units of the sterilized batch are still contaminated. Clearly, after another 5 min of sterilization, this probability will be reduced to $1/10^6$ or 10^{-6}. In other words, the SAL (introduced earlier) is 10^{-6}.

A more reassuring SAL, for example 10^{-9}, is very often sought. It is sufficient to extend the sterilization for just 3 additional min. The problem, therefore, is evidently not cost-related; rather, it is simply linked to the risk of subjecting the treated material to thermal degradation.

All the above considerations have been made under the assumption that the temperature is kept constant during the sterilization period. Obviously, the D-value changes when the temperature changes. When the D-values obtained experimentally for a given microbial species are plotted on a semilogarithmic chart as a function of the temperature T, a path such as the one shown in Fig. 2 is obtained.

Clearly, if D is 1.0 at 121°C, it is 0.1 at 131°C and 10 at 111°C. In other words, the value of D decreases or increases by a factor of 10 when the temperature increases

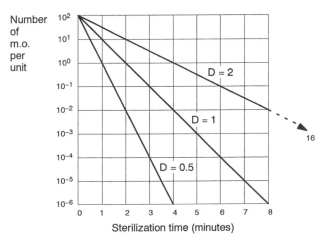

Fig. 1 Death rate curves illustrating decimal reduction concept. (From Ref. 3.)

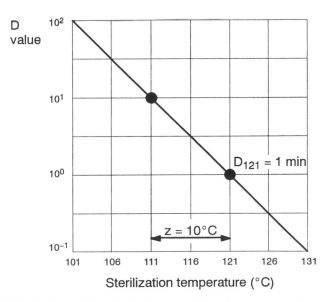

Fig. 2 Logarithm of D decreases linearly as temperature increases. (From Ref. 3.)

or decreases by 10°C. The algorithm z is defined as temperature coefficient of moist-heat sterilization, i.e., the number of degrees of sterilization temperature that causes a 10-fold variation of D or of the sterilization rate. Depending on the micro-organism being considered, the z-value varies between 5 and 15 for the 100–130°C sterilization range. The z-value is frequently assumed to be equal to 10 in the absence of precise experimental data (1).

It is evident that small temperature variations cause dramatic variations in the rate of the sterilization reaction. It is easy to calculate that a variation by only 1°C in the vicinity of 121°C causes a variation of approximately 24% in the value of D, i.e., of the sterilization rate.

F_0 or Equivalent Time

To compare the lethal effect of a sterilization performed for any given time t_x at any temperature T_x (which may vary over the time t_x), it is very useful to be able to express this lethal effect by relating it by calculation to a given reference temperature. When this reference temperature is 121°C (or, more exactly, 121.11°C, which correspond to 250°F) and z is assumed to be 10 (or 18 if the temperature is expressed in °F), the resulting algorithm is known as F_0 and is expressed by:

$$F_0 = \Delta t \sum 10^{\left(\frac{T-121}{z}\right)} \qquad (2)$$

where Δt = time interval between two successive temperature measurements; T = actual sterilization temperature in °C at the time t; and z = temperature coefficient, assumed to be equal to 10.

F_0 is known as equivalent time because its dimension is actually a time expressed in minutes. Clearly, when the values in Eq. (2) are, for example, $\Delta t = 15$ min and $T = 131$°C, F_0 is 150 min, i.e., the lethal effect is 10 times higher than that of a sterilization lasting 15 min at 121°C. If instead $\Delta t = 15$ min but $T = 111$°C, F_0 is equal to 1.5 min, i.e., the lethal effect is 10 times smaller than that of a 15-min sterilization at 121°C. An F_0 of 12 (delivered to the coldest point of the load) is generally considered sufficient for adequate sterilization in the pharmaceutical field (4).

MOIST-HEAT STERILIZATION PROCESSES

Current pharmaceutical production practice uses substantially three moist-heat sterilization processes: 1) pressurized saturated steam; 2) superheated water; and 3) steam–air mixture. Process 1 is the traditional multipurpose process, which obviously uses pure pressurized saturated steam as sterilizing medium. Processes 2 and 3 are so-called counterpressure processes; they were introduced in pharmaceutical production practice approximately 20 years ago and, respectively, use a spray superheated water and a homogeneous mixture of steam and air as sterilizing media. These processes allow the control of the pressure of the sterilizing medium independently of its temperature (which is impossible to accomplish with pure saturated steam). As explained below, these processes are used to treat solutions in containers that cannot tolerate the internal overpressure that is generated inside when sterilized with process 1.

PRESSURIZED SATURATED STEAM METHOD

This is certainly the most widely used and most versatile moist-heat sterilization method. Accordingly, it is widely used not only for sterilization of pharmaceutical products but also for laboratory and hospital sterilization and for the treatment of medical devices. Nonetheless, it has significant limitations, especially in pharmaceutical use, which are described later. The sterilizing medium is obviously pure pressurized saturated steam. The word saturated means that the steam is in thermodynamic equilibrium with its liquid form (water) at the temperature being considered.

Typical operating conditions are 121°C (i.e., 250°F) for 15 min (or even less); this temperature is matched by a saturated steam pressure of 2.05 abs bar (i.e., 205 kPa). However, higher or lower temperatures (and, therefore, pressures) are often used, with obvious appropriate adjustments of the holding time.

The term dry saturated steam is sometimes used. It should be made clear that dryness is a theoretical condition of steam and that in practice, moist saturated steam is used. This also provides assurance that the steam really is saturated and is not superheated. The use of superheated steam may in fact cause problems in process management.

However, the steam must entrain the smallest possible amount of condensate. The term steam dryness fraction defines the amount of condensate entrained by the moist steam. A dryness fraction of 0.95 means that 100 g of moist steam consist of 95 g of dry saturated steam plus 5 g of condensate, which is (or should be) at the same temperature the steam. A dryness fraction of 0.95 is considered the lower limit of adequacy for moist-heat sterilization.

The reliability of sterilization performed by means of saturated steam is based on three essential characteristics of this medium:

1. When steam condenses, it releases heat at a constant temperature and in very large amounts; 1 kg of steam condensing at 121°C (transforming into water at 121°C) releases as much as 2200 kJ (or 525 kcal).
2. The temperatures and pressures of saturated steam have a two-way correlation. Once the steam temperature is determined, so is its pressure, and vice versa. Saturated steam at 121°C inevitably has a pressure of 2.05 abs bar; saturated steam at 3.04 abs bar inevitably has a temperature of 134°C. This entails two very interesting practical possibilities: a pure saturated steam autoclave can be equally temperature- or pressure-controlled, and regardless of the parameter used for control, the second parameter can easily be used to cross-monitor the first.
3. One gram-molecular weight of water (18 g, i.e., 18 ml in the liquid state) as steam at 121°C and 2.05 abs bar occupies a volume of approximately 15 L. This means that when steam condenses at 121°C, it shrinks in volume by almost 1000 times. Consequently, additional steam spontaneously reaches the material to be sterilized. The condensate that forms can be easily removed from the autoclave chamber by means of a condensate trap or by continuous bleeding.

Apart from these three favorable characteristics, other phenomena linked to the use of pure saturated steam must be considered:

1. To perform its microbiological inactivation action, the steam must come into contact with the micro-organisms. This can occur directly or indirectly. It occurs directly when the steam makes contact, for example, with a surgical instrument located in the autoclave chamber. It occurs indirectly when the steam is generated, for example, inside a sealed ampoule that contains an aqueous solution by heat exchange with the steam in the chamber. However, it is evident that it is impossible to steam-sterilize the inside of a closed empty ampoule or its contents if they are, for example, an anhydrous oil-based solution.
2. The air initially present in the chamber and the incondensables (generally CO_2) possibly entrained by the steam have molecular weights, and therefore densities, which are 1.5–2.0 times higher than those of steam. Therefore, at the beginning of the process, the air must be removed from the chamber, and the steam must not contain incondensables. Otherwise, they tend to stratify in the lower portions of the chamber, producing unacceptable temperature gradients.

3. When closed nondeformable containers with aqueous solutions are sterilized, the pressure inside can reach values far higher than the chamber pressure. The reasons for this are explained in detail later but, in any case, the internal overpressure can reach or exceed 1.4 bar and can be intolerable for many types of container. In such cases, it is necessary or convenient to use counterpressure autoclaves (as described later).

SATURATED STEAM AUTOCLAVES

Construction

All sterilizers intended for pharmaceutical use are currently made of class AISI 316 stainless steel, including the valves and piping. Other materials may be acceptable only for service components arranged downstream of the sterilizer (e.g., the vacuum pump or the condensate trap). The service elements arranged upstream of the sterilizer (e.g., heat exchangers or water pumps) also must be made of stainless steel.

Silicone rubber or PTFE and its derivatives are generally used for gaskets (for doors, valves, etc). The chamber of these autoclaves is horizontal, with a rectangular or (rarely) cylindrical cross-section. The dimensions of these chambers can vary considerably, from approximately 100 L to 10 m^3 or more.

Doors

Doors are generally rectangular, even though the chamber is cylindrical. In this case, the doors are inscribed in the circumference. There may be one or two doors: two doors are always used when the autoclave leads into a sterile room. Two-door autoclaves are often used when this requirement does not apply, but the need is nonetheless felt to separate the loading area (where nonsterile products are placed) from the unloading area (where only already-sterilized products can be placed). The doors may be of various kinds.

Side-hinged, manually operated doors retained by radial locking bars

At present, these are the most widely used doors. The rim gasket is solid and fixed. The radial bars are moved, during closure/opening, by a central hand-wheel that is operated manually. This locking system requires lubrication, and this can entail microbiological problems, especially if the

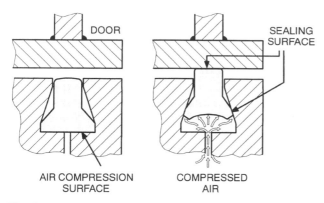

Fig. 3 Dovetail section gasket activated by compressed air. (From Ref. 5.)

door opens onto a sterile room (the closure method that uses perimetric eye-bolts is now obsolete).

Vertically or horizontally sliding, automatically operated doors

These doors have no lubrication problems, but in the horizontally sliding version (which is common for industrial-size autoclaves), they have the drawback that they occupy a considerable amount of floor space. The gasket is generally located on the chamber rabbet and is compressed toward the door by two methods: 1) the gasket is hollow and inflatable (by means of compressed air or steam); and 2) the gasket has a particular dovetail cross-section and is contained in a slot that also has a dovetail cross-section. An adequate pressure of compressed air in the rear part of the slot is sufficient to activate the seal on the door, and the release of the pressure (without requiring vacuum) is sufficient to activate the retraction of the gasket (Fig. 3).

Diagonally moving doors

These doors combine the positive features of the two precedidng types. During opening (and, in reverse, during closure), the door is automatically moved slightly upward and laterally, enough to disengage it from the mechanical systems that retain its four sides. Then the operator opens the door manually by turning it about its side hinges. The gasket is generally identical to the second one described previously.

Jacket

Saturated steam autoclaves are generally provided with a jacket, that is constituted by a second wall that more or less fully encloses the inner chamber and thus forms a secondary space around it. For the sake of brevity, the various jacket construction methods are not presented here. The purpose of a jacket is summarized as follows:

1) to preheat the autoclave initially and keep it warm during loading/unloading; 2) to preheat the load during the initial air removal phase; 3) to contribute to the drying of the load in the final vacuum phase; and 4) to reduce any condensate entrained by the steam.

Steam can be fed to the jacket-chamber assembly by: 1) Single feed in which the steam first enters the jacket, circulates inside it, flows out of it, and then enters the chamber. The reduction of condensate entrained by the steam can be achieved only with this single-feed approach. 2) Separate-feed in which, of course, two controls are provided. The jacket may be fed with plant steam, but the chamber is certainly supplied with ultraclean steam. At present, this is the solution generally used for modern autoclaves because it ensures that no microbiological or particulate contamination can reach the chamber from the jacket, which is a closed and convoluted space that is practically impossible to clean and inspect accurately.

Process

Initial air removal from the chamber

The basic reason for air removal has been addressed previously. Moreover, loads are often made of porous or packaged materials, which require reliable and rapid removal of air from the inside of the loads as well.

Today, the so-called gravity removal method is used only for special tasks. In this method, the steam enters the top part of the chamber and is distributed by a suitable sparger (theoretically on a uniform front). The air escapes through a large valve in the lower part of the chamber by way of two actions: gravity and displacement by steam. This method is rather slow and unsuitable for porous and other loads that may trap air inside recessed cavities.

A modern autoclave is generally equipped with a water-ring pump that can produce a vacuum of approximately 70 residual mbar in the chamber. Accordingly, almost 7% of the air is not removed. The following two methods are essentially used for completing air removal.

Pulsed vacuum: Once the maximum initial vacuum has been reached, the pump is stopped and steam enters the chamber until an approximate atmospheric pressure (or a higher pressure) is reached; then vacuum is produced again. Three vacuum/pressure pulses are generally sufficient to achieve suitable air removal.

Dynamic vacuum: Once the maximum initial vacuum has been reached, the vacuum pump is kept running while a 5- to 10-min. steam-injection is performed from the side of the chamber that lies opposite the vacuum drain point. Modern autoclaves can perform both methods depending on the load to be sterilized.

Heating and sterilization phases

Considerable amounts of condensate form in the chamber during the heating and sterilization phases. This condensate must be removed, and there are basically two ways to accomplish this. The first uses a condensate trap at the bottom of the chamber. This is the cheapest and simplest method, but it causes significant drops in pressure (and therefore in temperature) when the trap opens, owing to the inertia of the trap. The second method uses dynamic steam. This is the most reliable method, but it is also slightly more expensive. During the heating and sterilization phases, the vacuum pump runs continuous and extracts the condensate through a small valve. A small amount of steam of course is also extracted continuously, accordingly providing the dynamic condition of the steam.

Poststerilization phases

These phases may be very different and are clearly linked to the sterilized material and to the required results. The most common solutions are the following:

Drying–cooling final vacuum: This is produced by restarting the vacuum pump until a preset vacuum (e.g., 100 mbar) is reached. The pump is then kept running for a preset time. Porous materials (and nonporous materials also) are thus dried and cooled quickly.

Cooling by circulating cold water in the jacket: This method is used with containers that are partially filled with solutions (for example, culture media) and closed with nonhermetic closures. With such containers, drying–cooling final vacuum is not applicable because the solution would boil, and cooling by direct spray (described hereafter) may cause contamination. Steam is removed from the chamber by introducing sterile air at a pressure that is equal to, or greater than the sterilization pressure. Then cold water is circulated in the jacket. Chamber air pressurization has two purposes: to prevent boiling of the solutions and to improve heat exchanges between the load and the jacket.

Cooling by direct spraying of cold water onto the load: This method is generally used for cooling filled and sealed ampoules contained in perforated trays and generally marshaled. It is performed by spraying, or rather by nebulizing, purified water or water for injection onto the load by means of a sparger located in the ceiling of the chamber. Water nebulization produces rapid steam condensation and an equally rapid pressure drop in the chamber while the pressure inside the ampoules remains high (because the temperature of the solution decreases rather slowly). However, good-quality ampoules can withstand this treatment adequately. The water spray is generally stopped when the load temperature reaches 70–80°C. Accordingly, the load still contains enough heat energy to dry spontaneously once removed from the autoclave.

Cooling with cold water sprayed directly onto the load with air counterpressure: Very frequently, the pressure stress that occurs when using method of cooling by direct spraying of cold water, cannot be tolerated by the load. In such cases, it is possible to drain the steam from the chamber by replacing it with sterile compressed air at a pressure equal to or greater than the sterilization pressure. Cooling water is sprayed onto the load only after this replacement has been performed. However, it is obvious that this method only allows for reduction of the pressure stress of the containers in the cooling phase; the pressure stress in the sterilization phase (discussed later) is unavoidable.

Ampoule tightness tests: The purpose of these tests is to allow for rejection of ampoules that have closure defects, fractures, or cracks. These tests fall essentially into two categories: penetration of dyed solutions (usually with methylene blue) in the ampoules and poststerilization pressure stress. Details of these methods are not presented here because of space constraints.

Sterilization of the air that enters the chamber

As noted previously, in many cases it is necessary to introduce air in the sterilization chamber. This air must be sterile, otherwise it recontaminates the sterilized load or the sterile room if a two-door autoclave is connected to it. This air is generally sterilized by filtration with a system built into the autoclave. Therefore, it is necessary to:

1. Provide a filtration cartridge with suitable retention.
2. Allow in situ periodic sterilization of the assembled system by means of an automatic process of the autoclave.
3. Ensure that the filtration system and its piping maintain sterility during successive sterilization programs used for production.
4. Perform the system integrity test before and after each sterilization program of the filtration system.
5. Allow for validation of all procedures noted earlier.

Process controllers

Today, process controllers installed in autoclaves are based on programmable logic controllers (PLCs), personal computers (PCs), customized electronic solutions, or, sometimes, different combinations of the aforementioned systems. However, a very large number of autoclaves managed by old electropneumatic systems are still in operation. Modern process controllers, of course, offer previously inconceivable levels of performance. Today, temperature and/or pressure control is generally performed with a proportional-integral-derivative algorithm. Sterilization can be time-managed or F_0-managed (F_0 being accumulated by several flexible temperature probes enabled for this function). Some management systems offer exceptional flexibility in composing programs and setting parameters. Information provided in real time on cathode ray tube (CRT) or liquid crystal display (LCD) or produced/stored on paper/electronic media is highly detailed.

DIFFERENTIAL PRESSURE BETWEEN INSIDE/OUTSIDE OF A RIGID CONTAINER, PARTIALLY FILLED WITH WATER SOLUTION AND SEALED, DURING STEAM STERILIZATION

When a container in the conditions noted earlier is sterilized in a conventional autoclave that operates with pure saturated steam, during sterilization a considerable overpressure with respect to the pressure inside the autoclave

chamber is generated in the container. This is clearly attributable to the fact that the air (or gas) that was present at filling has remained in the container, whereas the air was eliminated from the autoclave chamber at the beginning of the process. Fig. 4 schematically explains the phenomenon in ideal conditions, i.e., considering air a perfect gas.

Experimentally, it turns out that the actual overpressure is higher than the theoretical one. This is attributable to various facts: the thermal expansion of water is greater than the thermal expansion of the glass of the container; the solution contains dissolved gases that come out of the solution as the temperature rises; air is not a perfect gas. Obviously, the overpressure depends on the filling temperature, the sterilization temperature, the ratio between solution volume and head volume, etc., but at 121°C, it is on average approximately 1.4 bar. Clearly, this phenomenon cannot be ignored: suffice it to note that the stopper of glass bottles with a mouth having a cross-section of approximately 4 cm² would be subjected to an expulsion force of approximately 6 kg.

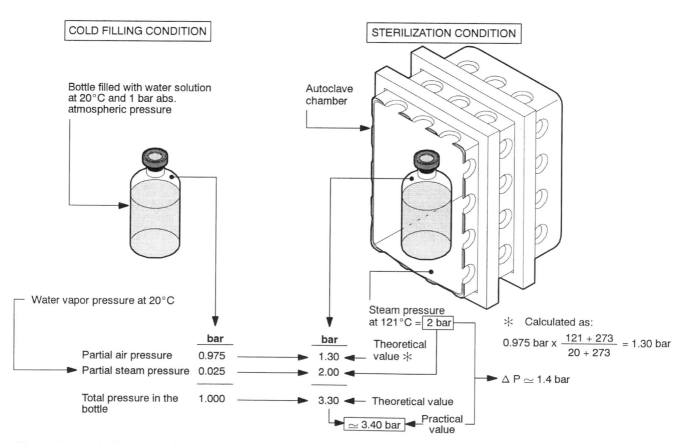

Fig. 4 Schematic description of pressures produced inside a rigid container, partially filled with water solution and sealed, during steam sterilization at 121°C. (Adapted from Ref. 5.)

These conditions therefore prohibit the use of traditional pure saturated steam autoclaves to sterilize solutions contained in a wide variety of containers such as

1. Large-volume parenterals (LVPs) in glass bottles;
2. LVPs and small volume parenterals (SVPs) in plastic containers (flexible, semirigid, rigid);
3. Prefilled glass or plastic syringes;
4. Jars and similar containers with press-on or screw caps;
5. Blisters containing various materials, for example, disposable contact lenses.

To correctly sterilize these products, it is necessary or advisable to use a counterpressure autoclave.

COUNTERPRESSURE MOIST-HEAT STERILIZATION

Moist-heat autoclaves operating with counterpressure are sterilizers capable of controlling the pressure of their sterilizing medium independently of its temperature. They are used essentially for the terminal sterilization of solutions.

Accordingly, a dual control principle is provided that acts independently on both parameters. Two methods currently in use are superheated water spray and steam–air mixture.

SUPERHEATED WATER SPRAY AUTOCLAVES

Fig. 5 is a typical diagram of these autoclaves. Alternatives are possible, but they do not alter the essential structure. The chamber is horizontal and generally cylindrical, with a single wall and rectangular door(s) inscribed in the circumference.

At the beginning of the process, after loading the product, the lower part of the chamber is filled with water of adequate chemical and bacteriological quality. The air contained in the chamber is not removed. A sanitary-type pump circulates the filling water through a heat exchanger (of the removable-plate or other sanitary

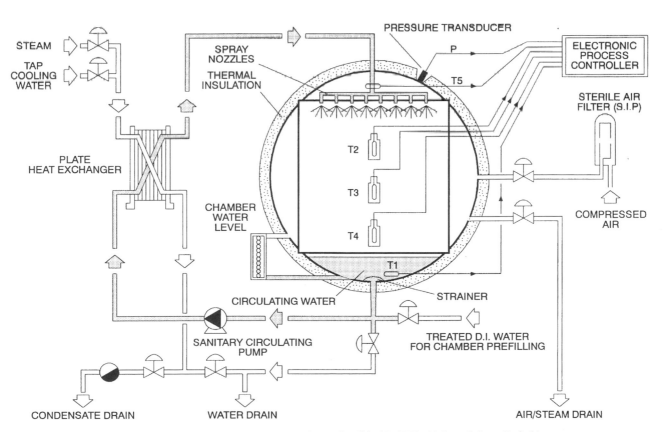

Fig. 5 Superheated water spray autoclave: simplified P.&I.D. (Adapted from Ref. 5.)

type) that is indirectly heated in countercurrent with plant steam. The water is then sprayed onto the load by a sparger located in the upper part of the chamber and equipped with a system of solid-cone spray nozzles. Uniform water redistribution in the lower layers of the load is ensured by suitable perforated racks that support the product. Sometimes additional water spray bars are located on both sides of the chamber.

Heating of the circulating water and, therefore, of the load is very gradual but quite rapid. A temperature of 121°C is typically reached in 25–30 min inside 500-ml containers; the heating rate clearly depends on the characteristics of the solution and its containers. Temperature uniformity in time and space during the sterilization phase is generally very good: much better than ± 1.0°C. The cooling phase is performed by the same circulating water, which is now sterile and continuously recirculated through the heat exchanger, in which cold water (instead of steam) now flows without contact with the sterile circulating water. The temperature inside 500-ml containers drops to approximately 80°C in 10–12 min.

This temperature is generally suitable to obtain rapid and spontaneous drying of the load once removed from the autoclave.

An appropriate partial pressure of air (sterilized by filtration) is maintained in the chamber during every phase of the process, to compensate for the overpressure inside the containers. Various methods for controlling the total chamber pressure (steam + air) can be used. With computerized process controllers, it is also possible to correlate at any time during each phase the air partial pressure to the average of the solution temperatures of two or more reference containers.

Consequently, the load suffers no thermal or pressure shocks because the differential pressure between the chamber and the containers can be reduced to zero or maintained at all times during the process in a direction that is suitable for the particular type of container during sterilization or, generally, during thermal treatments from 60 to 127°C.

Clearly, these autoclaves have some limitations in their application:

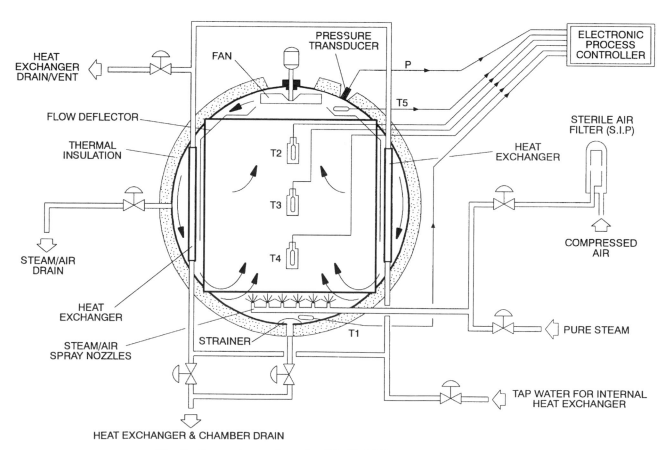

Fig. 6 Steam-air autoclave: simplified P.&I.D. (Adapted from Ref. 5.)

1. It is impossible, or illogical, to dry the load inside the autoclave by pulling vacuum in the chamber or by circulating warm air through the chamber and the load.
2. If materials that have upward-facing concave surfaces are sterilized, these surfaces will be filled with water at the end of the process. The obvious remedy is to load the material upside down.
3. When sterilizing solutions contained in PVC bags, so-called blushing can occur, i.e., the PVC can whiten because of water absorption. The time required for this blushing to disappear can be quite long, depending on the type of PVC and its plasticizer. Blushing does not occur with polypropylene (PP), polyethylene (PE), and polylaminated plastics.

These autoclaves are sterilizers that can vary considerable in size but are generally rather large (1–20 m^3 and

more). They are often provided with automated loading/unloading systems.

STEAM–AIR MIXTURE AUTOCLAVES

Figure 6 is a typical diagram of these autoclaves; possible alternatives are addressed later. The chamber is similar to that of superheated water spray autoclaves. At the beginning of the program, steam enters the chamber directly through a suitable sparger located in the lower part of the chamber. The air initially contained in the chamber is not removed. The high-efficiency fan(s) located on the ceiling of the chamber and the flow deflector system have the task of homogenizing and circulating the steam–air mixture that forms inside the chamber. This is an important

	Superheated Water Spray = SWS	**Steam–Air Mixture = SAM**
Temperature uniformity in time	Good	Good
Temperature uniformity in space	Good	Good
Total pressure control	Good	Good
Counterpressure control	Good	Good
Consumption of high quality water (WFI)	Modest, for initial filling	No
Consumption of tap water for cooling	Acceptable	Approx. 3 times higher than SWS
Consumption of compressed air	Acceptable	Acceptable
Consumption of industrial steam	Acceptable	No
Consumption of ultraclean steam	No	Acceptable
Condensate recovery	Possible and easy	Not possible
Cooling water recovery	Possible, recovered water is initially very hot	Possible, recovered water is initially very hot
Autoclave price	Acceptable	Approx. 10% higher than SWS
Total process duration	Short	Approx. 30% higher than SWS
Autoclave productivity/price	High	Approx. 30% lower than SWS
Operating principle	Quite simple and straightforward	More complex than SWS
Overall machine design	Simple	More complex than SWS
Autoclave qualification/Validation	Normal	Normal
Operating flexibility according to type of load	Suitable for any kind of container with the following remarks: – upward concavities collect water – product is unloaded wet – PVC bags may generate "blushing" effect	Suitable for any kind of container: – upward concavities collect condensate only – some kind of containers may be unloaded slightly damp – limited "blushing" effect of PVC bags
Possibility of combination with saturated steam processes	Not recommended	Feasible and moderately expensive

Fig. 7 Schematic drawing of magnetically driven fan. (Adapted from Ref. 5.)

and demanding task because the air clearly tends to stratify on the bottom. The condensate that forms is removed by continuous and spontaneous bleeding from the chamber.

The cooling phase consists of feeding compressed and sterile air to the chamber to condense and replace all the steam, while maintaining the same total sterilization pressure or possibly increasing it. Cold plant water is then fed to the internal heat exchangers, which are constituted by batteries of hollow plates arranged in the two lateral sectors of the chamber (for simplicity, only one plate is shown in Fig. 6). However, this cooling method uses two solid-gas heat exchanges, which have poor efficiency. An attempt can be made to improve efficiency by increasing the air pressure in the chamber within the limits of the product, thus increasing the density of the air and therefore its exchange efficiency. The fans of course continue to run during the cooling phase as well.

Despite this refinement, the cooling phase is significantly longer than that in superheated spray water autoclaves. A mechanically critical point of steam–air autoclaves is the tightness of the fan shaft. This problem has been completely solved in the more advanced machines by adopting magnetically driven fans (Fig. 7). The air partial pressure during the program is managed as described above for superheated water spray autoclaves, and the dimensions and loading/unloading systems are also similar.

Possible alternatives to the configuration shown in Fig. 6 are 1) horizontal fans (instead of vertical fans) located on one side of the chamber. This solution entails a more severe risk of shaft bending and vibration, which can cause wear of the delicate sealing system. More-over, it is technically more difficult to manufacture magnetically driven fans with a horizontal shaft; and 2) shell-and-tube heat exchangers (instead of plate-type exchangers).

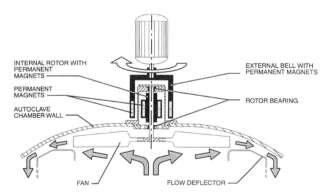

Fig. 8 Critical comparison of superheated water spray (SWS) and steam–air mixture (SAM) autoclaves. (Adapted from Ref. 5.)

With steam–air autoclaves, blushing of PVC bags is generally less intense than with superheated water spray autoclaves and essentially affects only the areas where the bags rest on the supporting racks. Among the positive features of steam–air autoclaves is the relative ease in combining the traditional pure saturated steam cycles, i.e., in manufacturing hybrid pure steam/steam–air autoclaves (in this case, the chamber is equipped with a jacket and a vacuum pump). This combination is instead not recommended for superheated water spray autoclaves, although it is offered by some manufacturers. Figure 8 is a summary comparison of superheated water spray and steam–air autoclaves.

STERILIZING A ROTATING LOAD

Currently, the pharmaceutical market more and more often requires rotating-load sterilization autoclaves. Load rotation can have essentially three goals:

1. To maintain the stability (or homogeneity) of emulsions (or suspensions) that would tend to break out because of the sterilization temperature.
2. To sterilize heat-sensitive products at high temperature, drastically reducing the sterilization time. The logic behind this principle is that, as noted, the temperature coefficient of the moist-heat sterilization reaction is very high (z is on the average equal to 10), whereas the temperature coefficient of a classic thermal degradation reaction is much lower (on the average equal to 2). Obviously, to achieve the goal, the product heating/cooling sterilization rates must be very high and uniform. Because rotation stirs the product, it indeed facilitates the penetration/removal of heat into/from the product, especially if it is dense and viscous.

    This principle is currently often used to sterilize heat-sensitive LVPs, for example, glucose solutions (especially with a high concentration of sugar) or amino acid solutions.
3. To provide the best possible testing of ampoule tightness with fast poststerilization vacuum. This testing method (presented above) achieves maximum effectiveness when the "open" defects of the ampoules are below the level of the solution. Ampoule rotation is the ideal method for achieving this condition regardless of the location of the defect on the ampoule (tip, shoulder, bottom).

Naturally, the production of this type of autoclave requires highly refined design and construction technology because 1) the load rotation system complicates

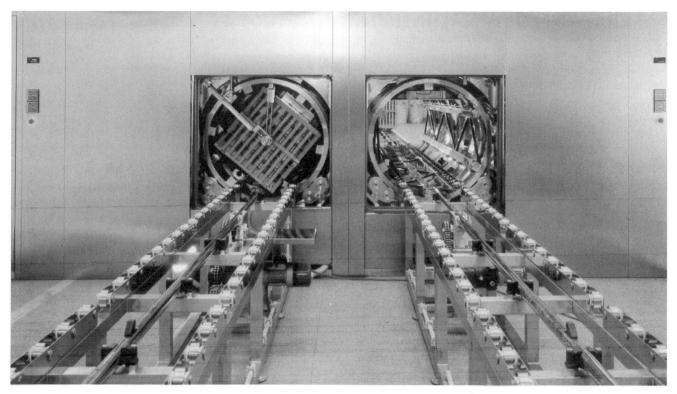

Fig. 9 Two superheated water spray autoclaves with a chamber capacity of approximately 4 m³, with a rotating load and sliding double doors. The man–machine interface of the process controller is not shown. The automated loading/unloading systems, frequently used with large sterilizers to allow faster loading and unloading operations, are shown instead. (Adapted from Ref. 5.)

construction significantly; 2) the loads to be rotated are generally bulky and heavy; 3) it is practically impossible to avoid mass displacements of the load during rotation; and 4) lubrication of the load bearing and rotating system must be avoided for hygiene-related reasons.

Finally, it is evident that the actual loading capacity of the chamber is reduced because of the presence of a cylindrical structure that must rotate inside it and support the load contained in appropriate trays with a lid (the entire system being appropriately perforated). Fig. 9 shows this cylindrical structure both when empty and when filled with the trays. These autoclaves are generally counterpressure sterilizers and the load is rotated throughout the process at an adjustable rate (1–10 rpm) and, if required, intermittently and in alternating directions.

REFERENCES

1. Carleton, F.J.; Agalloco, J.P. *Validation of Aseptic Pharmaceutical Processes*; Marcel Dekker, Inc.: New York, 1986.
2. Lavagna, S.M. *Injectables and Water for Pharmaceutical Use*; Editrice Bias: Milan, 1995.
3. Pflug, I.J. *Syllabus for an Introductory Course in the Microbiology and Engineering of Sterilization Processes*, 4th Ed.; Environmental Sterilization Service: St. Paul, MN, 1980.
4. *Validation of Steam Sterilization Cycles*. Technical Monograph No. 1 Parenteral Drug Association: Philadelphia, 1978.
5. Pistolesi, D.; Mascherpa, V. *Moist and Dry Heat Sterilization Technology*; Fedegari Autoclavi S.p.A.: Albuzzano PV, 1999; CD-ROM.

STERILIZATION BY RADIATION

Stephen G. Schulman
Phillip M. Achey
University of Florida, Gainesville, Florida

INTRODUCTION

The actions of ionizing radiations on matter and the subsequent interactions of the irradiated molecules are useful for the sterilization of pharmaceutical and surgical supplies. To take maximum advantage of the benefits derived from ionizing radiations, it is desirable to have an understanding of the fundamental processes that result in radiation damage to living and nonliving systems.

This article addresses with the effects of ionizing radiation on biological systems, beginning with the physical and chemical actions on condensed matter. After these sections, the biological responses of living systems, particularly microorganisms and viruses, to ionizing radiation are considered. A section on the current uses and government policies on the applications of ionizing radiation in areas important to the pharmaceutical industry is also included.

Description of Ionizing Radiation

Radiation energy can be either in the form of electromagnetic energy or of particle radiation. Radiation is distinguished as being either nonionizing or ionizing. Examples of nonionizing radiation include the ultraviolet, visible, infrared, and radiofrequency parts of the electromagnetic spectrum. These kinds of radiation are not addressed in this article.

A common feature of all ionizing radiation is that it is of sufficient energy to cause ionizations in the exposed material. These ionizations result in release of orbital electrons from atoms and cause disruptions of covalent bonds. Release of energy acquired by molecules in this manner will result in dramatic changes in the physical and chemical structures of the exposed materials because of the concentration and localized release of the ionizing radiation energy. By comparison, thermal heating is less efficient at causing bond rupture because of the wide distribution and diffuse release of thermal energy in matter. Whole-body exposure of a human to an amount of ionizing radiation energy equivalent to the amount of thermal energy received by drinking a cup of hot coffee will result

in the death of the individual within 30 days. Therefore, because of the potent biological action and the lack of our ability to sense exposure to ionizing radiation (unless the exposure dose rare is extremely high), it is important to practice extreme caution when working with this agent.

Another common characteristic of ionizing radiation is its ability to penetrate material. The two most commonly used forms for sterilization are energetic electron beams and electromagnetic radiation (e.g., γ-rays from cobalt-60 or cesium-137). The penetrating ability of γ-rays and X-rays is much greater than that of electrons. In either case, when developing protocols for using ionizing radiation in sterilization of material, the penetrating ability of the radiation must be considered.

PHYSICAL AND CHEMICAL ACTIONS OF IONIZING RADIATION

This section deals with the fundamental nature of the interactions of high-energy radiations with matter, from the absorption of the radiations to the eventual establishment of chemical equilibrium in the system. The process may be divided into three stages which are illustrated in Fig. 1.

1. The physical stage, consisting of the absorption of the radiant energy by the irradiated system. Its duration is of the order of 10^{-15} s.
2. The physicochemical stage, the processes that lead to the establishment of thermal equilibrium in the system. Its duration is of the order of 10^{-12} s.
3. This chemical stage, which entails diffusion and chemical reaction of the reactive species, ultimately resulting in chemical equilibrium. Its lasts upwards of 10^{-8} s, depending on the rate constants and diffusion coefficients of the reactive species.

The Physical Stage

The absorption of the energy associated with ionizing radiation by a medium results, initially, in ionization and electronic excitation. These processes occur regardless of

Encyclopedia of Pharmaceutical Technology

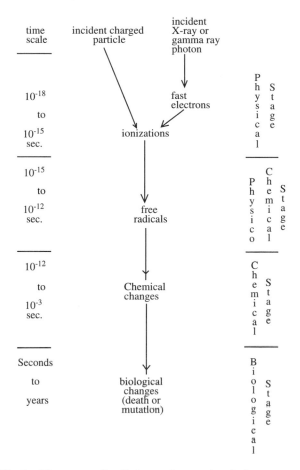

Fig. 1 The stages of radiation action on chemical systems and biological organisms.

the nature of the radiation. The mechanism of excitation and ionization by charged particles is different, however, from that effected by high-energy photons.

Charged particles

The interactions with a medium of charged particulate radiations such as protons, (β-particles, and γ-rays consist predominately of electrostatic coulomb excitation and ionization caused by ejection of atomic and molecular electrons in the medium. According to Bethe's semiclassic treatment, the energy lost to the medium, per unit length of path, by a heavy particle of charge Ze and velocity v is:

$$\frac{-dE}{dx} - \frac{4\pi Z^2 e^4 n}{mv^2} \ln \frac{2mv^2}{I} \tag{1}$$

where n is the electron density (number of electrons per unit volume) of the medium, m is the electronic mass, and I is a mean excitation potential for the medium ($I = 11.5 Zev$

for Z 30, $I = 8.8Z\ ev$ for $Z > 30$, where Z is the mean atomic number of the medium).

The term $-dE/dx$ is called the linear energy transfer (LET) of the radiation. If electrons (β-rays) are the ionizing particles, the expression for LET is slightly different:

$$\frac{-dE}{dx} - \frac{4\pi Z^2 e^4 n}{mv^2} \ln \left(\frac{mv^2}{2I} \sqrt{\frac{e}{2}} \right) \tag{2}$$

where ε is the basic of the natural logarithms.

Several important conclusions can be drawn from Eqs. 1 and 2. First, the rate of energy loss of a charged particle in a given medium is proportional to the electron in the medium. Second, because the factor v^2 outside the logarithmic term is more important than that inside, the rate of energy loss increases as the particle slows down. Third, if two particles of equal energy but different mass are compared, the heavier one will have a smaller velocity and thus a higher LET. Consequently an α-particle will produce many more excitations and ionizations per unit path length and have a shorter path length than a β-particle of the same energy.

High-energy photons

When high-energy photons such as x-rays and γ-rays pass through matter, they lose energy by way of three mechanisms: photoelectric absorption, in which the photon transfers its entire energy to an electron; Compton scattering, in which the photon transfers part of its energy to an electron; and pair production, in which the photon disappears and a high-energy electron and positron are formed. The relative importance of each of these mechanisms depends on the energy of the photon. For photons in the 100-kev to 2-MeV range, the principal mode of absorption by the medium is Compton scattering. Much higher photon energies favor pair production (at least 1.02 MeV are required to produce a pair), whereas lower energies favor photoelectric absorption. The principal effect of the absorption of high-energy photons is the production of energetic electrons that then dissipate their energies by the mechanism described by Eq. 2.

In general, the effect of transfer of energy from an energetic particle to the medium is to produce along its path a variety of electronically excited molecules, ions, and free electrons. Secondary electrons are also formed along with the ions. The electronic transitions resulting in the formation of these species occur in times [10^{-15} s] that are short compared with molecular vibration periods [10^{-14}–10^{-12} s]. The amount of energy absorbed by the irradiated system per unit mass is called the dose and is expressed in Rads, where 1 Rad ($=6.24 \times 10^{13}$ eV/gm) is the amount of radiation that will deposit 100 ergs of energy per gram of the irradiated system.

The Physiochemical Stage

This stage lasts about 10^{-14}–10^{-12} s, which is typical of the period of molecular vibrations. During this period, internal molecular rearrangements can take place.

During the physiochemical stage, the excited molecules and ions dissipate their excess energy by bond rupture, luminescence, internal conversion, and energy transfer to neighboring molecules. Also during this stage, the low-energy, secondary electrons produced during the physical stage interact with molecules in the environment resulting in the formation of free radicals.

The Chemical Stage

During this stage, the reactive intermediates (ions and radicals) produced in the previous stages diffuse away from their sites of production and undergo chemical reactions with each other and with other molecules in the environment.

In condensed systems (liquids and solids), the main reactive species produced in the physiochemical stage that react in the chemical stage are free radicals. Their primary modes of reaction are atomic abstraction, radical recombination, and addition to π-bonds.

Because most systems of interest to pharmaceutical scientists are either liquids or solids, it is useful to present some of the features of radiolysis common to liquid or solid samples.

Liquid

The irradiation of liquids results initially in the ejection of electrons with the consequent formation of ions. The ejected electrons usually lose their excess kinetic energy within the electric field of the parent ion. Most of the ion pairs formed culminate in recapture of the ejected electrons, leaving the molecules in a highly excited, electronic state that may return to the ground state by internal conversion, luminescence, or energy transfer. Alternatively, the highly excited neutral molecules may split into free radicals. Some ion pairs may be sufficiently long-lived to diffuse away from the site of production and react with the surrounding medium. The free radicals are the most important reactive species formed. Once free radicals are formed along the track of an ionizing particle, they may combine with each other or they may diffuse away from the spur and react with molecules in the bulk of

the liquid medium. Those that recombine within the spur react so rapidly that they cannot be detected by physical or chemical methods. They form stable molecular products, which are known as the molecular yield. Those radicals that diffuse away from the spur and react with the medium can be detected by physical methods such as electron spin resonance spectroscopy and by chemical methods such as compound formation with radical scavengers, e.g., iodine and diphenylpicrylhydrazyl. The compounds formed by reaction with radical scavengers are called the radical yield. The mechanisms of chemical radiation effects are frequently determined by comparison of relative molecular and radical yields. The radiation chemistry of liquids has developed along two distinct paths—that of water and aqueous solutions and that of organic liquids. The radiation chemical processes responsible for the destruction of microorganisms are probably most closely related to the former, but damage to membranes and cell walls may actually be better related to the radiation chemistry of organic liquids or even some solids.

Water and Aqueous Solution

The irradiation of pure water is believed to result in two dissociative processes. The first of these is the direct dissociation of water into hydrogen atoms and hydroxyl radicals:

$$HO \rightarrow H\cdot + OH\cdot \tag{3}$$

The second reaction is the ionization of water to yield a hydrogen ion, a hydroxyl radical, and a hydrated electron:

$$H_2O \rightarrow H^+ + OH\cdot + e^-_{aq} \tag{4}$$

The hydrated electron is a powerful reducing agent and will reduce water and the hydrogen ion according to:

$$e^-_{aq} + HO \rightarrow H\cdot + OH^- \tag{5}$$

and the hydrogen ion according to:

$$e^-_{aq} + H^+ \rightarrow H. \tag{6}$$

Because the latter two reactions result in the same products as the direct radiolysis and because the products of reduction by the hydrogen atom and the hydrated electron are identical, it is frequently impossible to determine whether the hydrated electron or the hydrogen atom is the principal reducing species in aqueous solutions. In acid solutions, it is reasonable to assume that the hydrated electron will reduce H^+ almost exclusively and that H will therefore be the predominant reducing species. However, in neutral and basic solution, the hydrated electron may be assumed to predominate. The ultimate molecular products of the radiolysis of pure water are hydrogen gas and hydrogen peroxide, formed by the reactions:

$$H\cdot + H\cdot \rightarrow H_2 \tag{7}$$

$$OH\cdot + OH\cdot \rightarrow H_2O_2 \tag{8}$$

The radiation chemistry of aqueous solutions may be considered from two points of view. The first, called the Target Theory, considers the direct effect of ionizing radiations on the solute molecules. The second approach regards transformations in the solute molecules to be attributed to interactions with the reactive intermediates formed by the radiolysis of water. Because most aqueous systems are relatively dilute, the latter approach seems statistically more reasonable. Kinetic studies of dilute aqueous systems have indeed borne out this supposition. The radiation chemistry of aqueous solutions then becomes the free radical and redox chemistry of $H\cdot$, $OH\cdot$, and e_{aq}^-.

The effectiveness of radicals in producing chemical change in aqueous systems depends on the LET of the ionizing radiation that produces these radicals. A high LET particle, such as an α-particle or a proton, will produce a large concentration of radicals along its short track. These radicals are likely to recombine, forming molecular products, before they can diffuse away from the spurs in which they are formed. Low LET particles, on the other hand, produce low radical concentration along their tracks. This minimizes the probability of recombination so that the radicals can diffuse away from the spurs and initiate chemical reactions. Protons and α-particles therefore result in high molecular yields, whereas β- and γ-rays result in high radical yields.

One of the earliest devices for the measurement of radiation dosage, the Fricke dosimeter, is based on the oxidation of the ferrous ion by OH radicals produced in the radiolysis of a dilute aqueous solution of ferrous sulfate:

$$Fe^{+2} + OH\cdot \rightarrow Fe^{+3} + OH^- \tag{9}$$

The presence of dissolved oxygen alters the nature of the redox properties of irradiated water. This is a consequence of the "radical scavenging" property of oxygen. Molecular oxygen has two unpaired electrons. One of these can form a covalent bond with a hydrogen atom, forming the hydroperoxy radical ($HO_2\cdot$). This species acts principally as an oxidizing agent; e.g.:

$$HO_2^\bullet + Fe^{+2} \rightarrow Fe^{+3} + OH_2^- \tag{10}$$

An important consequence of this is that, whereas solutions in pure irradiated water have approximately equal oxiding and reducing capabilities, the presence of oxygen in these solutions can result, in some cases, in very strong oxiding properties because of the conversion of the reducing hydrogen atom to the predominantly oxidizing hydroperoxy radical. In general, the presence of oxygen in aqueous solutions will lead to alternations of the mechanisms of radiolyses owing to the "exclusively of oxidation." Radiation damage to microorganisms tends to be far more extensive in the presence of oxygen than in its absence.

Organic Liquids

An important difference between the radiation chemistry of water and of organic liquids is that the concept of the spur (a reasonably well-defined volume in which the formation of the reactive species occurs along the track of the ionizing particle) becomes hazy. The radicals formed in water tend to recombine rather than react with the environment immediately after formation. The volume in which recombination is likely defines the spur. The radical products of irradiated organic liquids, however, are more likely to interact with their immediate environment than to undergo recombination. This is evidenced by the low molecular yields of hydrogen from irradiated organic systems.

The radiation chemistry of hydrocarbons and their derivatives has been investigated extensively. An important difference between gas phase and liquid phase radiolysis of hydrocarbons exists in that the breaking of carbon–carbon bonds is an important primary process in the gas phase, whereas in the liquid phase, the rupture of carbon–hydrogen bonds is almost exclusive. Another important difference between analogous reactions in gas and liquid phases occurs in the polymerization process. In gas phase polymerizations, the presence of radical scavengers such as iodine and benzoquinone does not appreciably alter the yields of polymeric products. In the liquid phase, however, the yields of the polymers obtained from the irradiation of materials such as vinyl chloride are seriously curtailed by the addition of radical scavengers. This indicates that polymerization in the liquid state occurs primarily by a free radical mechanism, whereas in the gaseous state, it occurs by an ionic mechanism. The irradiation of polymeric materials results in cross-linking of polymer chains and grafting of dissimilar polymeric materials. This treatment of polymers contributes considerable tensile strength and heat resistance to the irradiated polymers and is already being exploited commercially in the production of stain-resistant textiles and heat-resistant plastic containers.

Irradiation of saturated aliphatic compounds typically results in unsaturation, polymerization, and isomerization. The radiolysis of cyclohexane illustrates all three of these processes. If the radicals are very energetic, cyclohexene can be formed by the abstraction of hydrogen from a cyclohexyl radical either by a hydrogen atom or by another cyclohexyl radical. If the radicals become thermalized, recombination of radicals can occur to give bicyclohexyl. A less frequent process is rearrangement, followed by hydrogen atom capture to yield methylcyclopentane.

The irradiation of alkyl halides results in cleavage of the carbon–halogen bond. The radiolysis of methyl iodide, for example, yields ethane and molecular iodine.

Alcohols, on radiolysis in the liquid state, yield aldehydes and vicinal glycols. For example, consider the radiolysis of methanol:

$$CH_3OH \rightarrow \cdot CH_2OH + H \cdot \qquad (11)$$

$$\cdot CH_2OH \rightarrow CH_2 = O + H \cdot \qquad (12)$$

and

$$2 \cdot CH_2OH \rightarrow CH_2OHCH_2OH \qquad (13)$$

The irradiation of frozen alcohols results in deep coloration of the alcoholic glasses. Methanol turns a brilliant purple, whereas ethanol turns blue. These colored glasses are stable if kept in the dark at low temperature. Exposure to visible or ultraviolet light results in bleaching of the alcoholic glasses as well as in the elimination of the electron spin resonance signal observed in the colored glasses. The colors are believed to be caused by the absorption spectra of trapped free radicals in the glasses. The product yields from the bleached glasses are different from those of irradiated glasses that have not been exposed to light. This suggests that the trapped radicals might be photolyzed by visible and ultraviolet light.

The irradiation of aromatic compounds results in considerably lower yields of radiolysis products than does irradiation of aliphatic compounds of similar molecular weight and functional group composition. This has been attributed to effectiveness of the delocalized π-orbitals in accommodating excitation energy without permitting the molecule to dissociate. Nevertheless, some radiolysis does occur. Benzene is known to yield biphenyl, phenylcyclohexadiene, and a polymeric material of average composition $(C_6H_7)_x$, which behaves as if it were an unsaturated hydrocarbon. Dimerization and polymer formation are also characteristic of the radiation chemistry of other aromatic hydrocarbons. The resistance of polystyrene ($-(C_6H_5)$ $CH-CH_2-)_n$ to cross-linking compared with polyethylene is further evidence of the stability of aromatics to radiation effects.

Aromatic compounds frequently protect other more radiosensitive compounds from radiolysis. For example, liquid cyclohexane is protected from extensive radiolysis by the addition of a small amount of benzene. This is probably due to energy transfer from cyclohexane to benzene, followed by dissipation of the excitation energy by the aromatic π-system.

One of the most important general features of the radiation chemistry of liquids is that so much energy is deposited by the ionizing radiations, excited or reactive molecules are formed in close proximity and are likely to react with one another. This situation is not encountered in photochemistry except when lasers are used for excitation.

SOLIDS

Pharmaceutical and surgical supplies are often in the solid state when irradiated. Certainly, their containers are solid. It is therefore in order to consider some of the radiation chemistry of solids.

Because of the "fixed" positions of atoms in crystalline lattices, the effects of irradiation of solids include atomic displacements as well as electronic excitation and ionization. Although electronic alterations of materials affect their chemical behavior, atomic displacements in solids are found to have a much more pronounced effect on the physical properties of crystals. To dislodge an atom from its normal lattice position, a certain amount of energy must be transferred to the atom by an irradiating particle. Because of the large mass of the atoms, electrons and photons will be relatively ineffective in producing substantial numbers of atomic dislocations. The heavier particles, α-particles, protons, deuterons, and neutrons, will be much more effective at this process. Furthermore, unlike the primary effect of ionizing radiations in producing distal electronic disturbances through electrostatic effects, the predominant process that is required to produce atomic dislocations is direct collision.

There are two types of lattice defects that occur in all real crystals and at very high concentration in irradiated crystals. These are known as point defects and line defects. Point defects occur as the result of displacements of atoms from their normal lattice sites. The displaced atoms usually occupy sites that are not in the lattice framework; they are then known as "interstitials."

The empty lattice site left behind by the interstitial is called a vacancy. A vacancy produced by displacement of an anion or cation, along with its interstitial ion, is called a Frenkel pair, or simply a Frenkel defect. In some cases, the displaced ions are removed so far from their vacancies that they form a new layer at the crystal surface. The vacancies left behind in this case are called Schottky defects. Frenkel and Schottky defects play very important roles in the properties of solids altered by radiation damage.

Line defects (dislocations) are produced by slippage or shear of the crystal lattice. If the slippage is perpendicular to a face of the crystal so that the lattice planes on either side of the dislocation are parallel but displaced with respect to one another, the defect is called an edge dislocation. If the slippage is angular, as if produced by rotation about the shear axis so that lattice planes on either side of the defect are not perpendicular, the defect is called a screw dislocation.

There are four broad classifications of crystal types, according to the nature of the interatomic forces holding the crystal together. In metallic crystals, the atoms are thought to form a quasi-ionic lattice arrangement with the valence electrons, which bind the lattice, delocalized throughout the crystal so that they cannot be identified with any atom. Valence crystals, such as diamond, consist of a lattice in which the atoms are bonded by conventional covalent interaction throughout the lattice. This implies that a valence crystal could be considered a giant molecule. Molecular crystals (e.g., naphthalene and water) are regular arrangements of well-defined molecules that are bound together in the lattice by Van der Waals and hydrogen-bonding forces. Finally, the ultimate in electronic localization occurs in ionic crystals, in which the lattice is composed of alternating positive and negative ions held together by strong electrostatic attractions. Sodium chloride is a typical example of an ionic lattice.

Metallic Crystals

Because of the delocalization of electrons throughout the metallic crystal, no persistence of ionization or chemical decomposition can occur because a positive hole formed by an electron ejection is always refilled by an electron from the conduction band. On the other hand, sufficiently energetic radiations can cause atomic displacements. The production of interstitial atoms swells the lattice, thereby decreasing the density of the crystal.

The most obvious evidence of radiation damage in metallic crystals is decrease in electrical and thermal conductivity. This is attributable to scattering of electrons and phonons by vacancies and interstitials that destroy the order of the lattice necessary for high conductivity.

The obvious effects of radiation damage in metallic crystals can be reversed by "annealing." Heating the irradiated materials supplies the energy required to push an interstitial back into a vacancy.

Valence Crystals

The strong bonding in valence crystals results in the failure of these crystals to demonstrate, on irradiation, quasi-chemical changes such as depolymerization. Unlike metals, however, valence crystals have no conduction electrons. This permits them to retain electronic dislocations as well as atomic displacement. The trapping of dislocated electrons in the crystal by potential wells such as those created by atomic vacancies results in coloration of the normally transparent valence crystals.

Ionic Crystals

Irradiation of ionic crystals results in atomic and electronic dislocations. The trapping of displaced electrons by anion vacancies results in the absorption of visible and near ultraviolet light, which give these crystals their characteristic colors. These pseudoatomic electrons and their vacancies are called color centers.

The exposure of colored ionic crystals to visible or ultraviolet light causes the annealing of trapped electrons and results in bleaching of the colorations induced by irradiation. In some cases in which the crystal remains uncolored upon irradiation, thermoluminescence is observed in the annealing process.

The dissolution of a heavily irradiated crystal of sodium chloride in water will result in the evolution of hydrogen and chloride from the solution. The solution also turns alkaline. This is presumably owing to the reactions of trapped holes and electrons with water:

$$e^- + H_2O \rightarrow \frac{1}{2}H_2 + OH^- \tag{14}$$

$$hole^+ + Cl^- \rightarrow \frac{1}{2}Cl_2 \tag{15}$$

Trapped electrons also account for the ability of irradiated sodium chloride to initiate polymerization in acrylonitrile.

Irradiation of nitrates, chlorates, perchlorates, and bromates results in the liberation of oxygen. In $KClO_4$, irradiation results in explosion of the crystal due to the internal buildup of oxygen.

Molecular Crystals

The irradiation of substances that form crystals containing discrete molecules held together by dispersion forces results in radiolysis in the conventional sense. For example, the radiolysis of aliphatic carboxylic acids in the solid state yields hydrogen, carbon monoxide, and carbon dioxide. The relative yields of these gases depend on the strengths of the bonds involved in radiolysis and their frequency of occurrence. These considerations apply as well to liquids and gases and suggest no special solid-state effects.

Energy transfer in molecular crystals seems to be a well-established phenomenon. Irradiated crystals of anthracene containing only a trace of naphthacene show the characteristic green fluorescence of naphthacene rather than the violet of the primary constituent. If the material is dissolved in benzene, the anthracene fluorescence predominates.

The irradiation of ice results in formation of trapped hydrogen and hydroxyl radicals as well as the hydrated electron.

The irradiation of surface catalysts alters the properties of these catalysts through defect production on their surface. These defects have been observed to enhance and inhibit catalytic activity in specific cases. For example, the irradiation of silica gel enhances the rate of H_2-D_2 exchange on it.

CHEMICAL PROTECTION FROM IONIZING RADIATIONS

The effects of ionizing radiations on chemical and biological systems may be minimized by the addition of certain chemical compounds to the system to be irradiated. These compounds react either directly with the radiation or, more often, with the reactive species produced by the radiations. In so doing, they are themselves transformed into other substances, but their transformation results in the preservation of the integrity of the original chemical or biological system.

At the molecular level, there are several mechanisms that account for the protection of irradiated systems by chemical agents. These are energy and charge transfer, in which an ionized or excited molecule transfers its charge or excess energy to a protecting molecule either by collision or by resonance transfer; scavenging, in which a protecting radical scavenger reacts with radicals from the initial actions of the radiation before they can attack other molecules in the system; and complex formation, in which a protective molecule can form complexes that are either more or less susceptible to radiation damage than the original substance.

Energy and Charge Transfer

The transfer of charge or excitation energy must be fast enough to compete with dissociation processes if protection is to occur. In some cases, an activated molecule can dissociate within 10^{-14} s, the time for one molecular vibration. However, localization of energy in a particular bond usually requires $10^{-13}-10^{-9}$ s. To remove energy or charge from an activated molecule effectively, the protector should have a slightly lower ionization or excitation potential. In fluid systems, the rate of charge transfer can be limited by diffusion, in which case, the donor and acceptor must be in contact. Excitation energy, however, can be exchanged radiationlessly by molecules as much as 70 Å apart by resonance energy transfer, a dipole–dipole interaction. The process is more rapid than fluorescence and competes favorably with dissociation. Transfer processes of the resonance type are extremely efficient in crystalline materials in which the high degree of order permits excitation energy to travel in excitons that transverse the crystal in a time shorter than its vibrational relaxation time. Crystalline structure also facilitates charge transfer by providing conduction bands in which electrons can freely move about.

Energy conversions within a molecule can decrease the probability of decomposition; energy can be distributed so widely that its localization in any one bond is improbable. Aromatic compounds are protective because they can probably dissipate acquired excitation energy throughout their extensively delocalized π-systems.

Scavenging Intermediates

The addition of certain compounds that react readily with free radicals can effectively prevent these products of ionizing radiations, from causing secondary damage in the system. Molecular iodine is a very effective radical scavenger forming iodocompounds with radicals and leaving behind iodine atoms to do further scavenging, e.g.:

$$CH_3^\bullet + I_2 \rightarrow CH_3I + I^\bullet$$

$$CH_3^\bullet + I_3 \rightarrow CH_3I + I^\bullet$$

Oxygen is a diradical that enhances radiation damage by forming radicals with other radicals. An example is the scavenging of hydrogen atoms by molecular oxygen to form the hydroperoxy radical.

Complexes

Certain compounds may exert protective action by forming molecular complexes with the original molecules of the system. These complexes might be less sensitive to radiolysis or attack by radicals, or they may be better able to transfer charge and excitation energy than the original compound. For example, the radiolytic degradation of polyisobutylene is reduced by copolymerization with styrene. The radiation resistance of the porphyrin ring is enhanced by complexing it with vanadium and other metals.

The most obvious application of chemical protection from ionizing radiations is to biological systems. For a protective agent to be biologically practical, it must be nontoxic at protective concentrations, widely distributed, and remain intact for long periods before irradiation. Many substances have been applied to this problem. To date, the most effective have been compounds such as cysteine because of the scavenging property of the –SH group and the ease of oxidation of the –NH$_2$ group.

Adventitious impurities in pharmaceutical and surgical supplies may act as energy transfer acceptors, scavengers, or complexants and make radiation sterilization more difficult owing to radioprotective action.

MOLECULES OF BIOLOGICAL SIGNIFICANCE

There are two distinct theories of the actions of ionizing radiations on the compounds of living cells that result in chemical transformation that leads to mutation or cell death. The first is the target theory. This approach regards only those events that produce direct ionizations in biologically significant molecules as being important. The evidence for this is that in many cases, the amount of damage to a given organism varies logarithmically with the dose of radiation. This implies that the amount of damage possible in a cell is proportional to the number of radiosensitive molecules remaining undamaged and, therefore, capable of reacting. The other theory is based on an indirect relationship between the incident radiation and the affected, biologically significant molecules. In this approach, the solvent, water, interacts with the radiation, forming ions and radicals. These reactive species, in turn, react with the biologically significant molecules causing radiation damage. Radiation biology, under this approach, is simply a branch of the radiation chemistry of aqueous solutions. There is evidence that both the target and indirect processes occur.

In this section, the effects of ionizing radiations on molecules known to have biological significance and the relationship of the radiation chemistry of these molecules to radiation effects observed in living organism are considered.

Carbohydrates

The irradiation of aqueous solutions of carbohydrates has the same effect as it does on alcohols. The hydroxyl groups are attacked to yield carbonyl compounds. Under anoxic conditions, dimer products and, ultimately, polymers are also formed. The primary alcohol groups of carbohydrates are especially radiosensitive. Mannitol is readily oxidized to mannose and sorbitol to glucose. Although oxidation of primary alcohol groups is favored by aerobic conditions, high yields from the oxidation of secondary alcohol groups are favored by anoxic conditions.

The irradiation of polysaccharides results predominately in their degradation. This explains why fruits and vegetables become soft on irradiation. This degradation is observed to occur both in solution and in the dry state.

Amino Acids and Peptides

The irradiation of amino acids results in transformation of both the amino and the carboxylic functions. In the dry state, glycine is decarboxylated to methylamine on irradiation; in dilute aqueous solution, however, the amino group is hydrolyzed to give glyoxylic acid, acetic acid, and formaldehyde. In solutions of concentration greater than 2%, methylamine again becomes an important product. The other amino acids are similar to glycine in their radiolytic behavior. Alanine, for example, gives ethylamine and CO$_2$ in the dry state and pyruvic acid and ammonia in aqueous solution.

The aromatic amino acids, when irradiated in aqueous solution, show effects that are typical of aromatic compounds and amino acids. Phenylalanine is deaminated in aerated solutions with the formation of a ketone. The aromatic ring remains relatively stable to radiolytic decomposition.

The irradiation of peptides results in a chemistry similar to that of the amino acids but also in the breakage of the peptide bond. In aqueous solution, all irradiated peptides give ammonia whether or not free amino groups are present.

The thiol and disulfide containing amino acids degrade to keto acids with the evolution of CO$_2$ and H$_2$S, when irradiated in the dry state, In solution, however, the thiol and disulfide groups are excellent radical scavengers, and free radical attack on these groups precludes deamination.

The ultimate result of irradiation of thiol-containing amino acids is their oxidation to disulfides. Thus, irradiation of an aqueous solution of cysteine results in the formation of cystine. The irradiation of the disulfides results in higher oxidation products. For example, cystine gives cystine disulfoxide in aqueous solution. Reduction of disulfides to thiols is not observed.

Proteins and Enzymes

The irradiation of proteins results in the formation of free radicals at the sites of $-S-S-$ bonds. Aromatic amino acids in the proteins are also particularly susceptible to radiolysis; decarboxylation and deamination being common results of irradiation. Rupture of the peptide linkage is characteristic of the radiolysis of proteins. In the case of enzymes, the destruction of peptide linkages is accompanied by a decrease in biological activity. This decrease continues after irradiation is stopped. The mechanisms of radiolysis in the dry state and in solution are different, but the results are usually similar. One of the more important differences between these results is the degradation of proteins by dry-state irradiation compared with increase of molecular weight through cross-linking in solution. In general, the radiation chemistry of proteins and enzymes may be considered a special case of the radiation chemistry of peptides and amino acids.

Respiratory Proteins, Vitamins, and Coenzymes

Respiratory proteins

These substances are iron, porphyrin, protein complexes. Irradiation of these substances may produce effects in the porphyrin ring or in the protein, but oxidation or reduction of the iron is almost always involved. The iron in ferricytochrome-c is reduced to the ferrous state under neutral conditions. Under acid conditions, the ferric form is favored. Hemoglobin and oxhemoglobin are both oxidized from the ferrous to the ferric state, destroying the property of oxygen transport. Large radiation doses result in attack on the porphyrin ring and denaturation of the protein. When irradiated in the dry state in the absence of oxygen, hemoglobin is not oxidized, but it becomes insoluble because of protein denaturation. Myoglobin behaves in a manner similar to that of hemoglobin but is considerably more radiosensitive. Myoglobin is a copper-containing respiratory protein of molecular weight more than 10 times that of hemoglobin. In this case, attack at the protein part of the molecule predominates.

Vitamins and coenzymes

The irradiation of coenzyme I (diphosphopyridine nucleotide) results in reduction of the pyridine-carbox-amido ring. The product of this reduction is probably a dimer that is itself radiosensitive.

The B group vitamins, thiamine and riboflavin, are destroyed on irradiation in dilute aqueous solutions. Riboflavin is reduced in air-free solutions to a semiquinone form. Nicotinic acid is decarboxylated on irradiation in air-saturated aqueous solutions.

Para-aminobenzoic acid is destroyed on irradiation in aqueous solution by deamination and decarboxylation. Sulfanilamide and sulfathiazole are inactivated presumably because of deamination. The cobalt in vitamin B_{12} is reduced on irradiation from $+3$ to the $+2$ state.

The plant hormone auxin has been shown to be radiosensitive. The product of the irradiation of auxin (β-indoleacetic acid) is a polymer similar to that obtained in the radiolysis of indole.

Nucleic Acids

The nucleic acids DNA and RNA are responsible for the transmission of genetic information and protein synthesis. Both of these processes are dependent on the ordering of purine and pyrimidine bases that are bound to the main body of the molecule by phosphoric ester linkages. The main body of these molecules consists of ribose (5-carbon sugar) molecules linked together by phosphoric acid units to form a long strand. The purine and pyrimidine bases branch off from the chain at the ribose sites. The DNA molecule consists of two helically intertwined strands of nucleic acid held together by hydrogen bonding between purine pyrimidine pairs on opposite strands.

The irradiation of nucleic acids ruptures hydrogen bonds that hold DNA strands together results in deamination and dehydroxylation of purine and pyrimidine bases, fission of sugar base linkage, liberation of the purine bases, destruction of the pyrimidine bases, oxidation of the sugar moiety, and breakage of the nucleotide chain with liberation of inorganic phosphates. In the presence of oxygen, irradiation leads to the formation of hydroperoxides of the pyrimidine bases but not of the purine bases.

In general, the purine bases appear to be much more stable to radiolysis then pyrimidine bases. This is probably owing to the greater π-delocalization energy of the purines, which provides a pathway for nondestructive energy dissipation. Furthermore, the pyrimidine bases are known to undergo free radical reactions more readily than the purine bases. The order adenine $>$ guanine $>$ cytosine

> uracil > thymine has been established for the relative stabilities of the bases to radiolysis. In the presence of oxygen in aqueous solution, uracil and thymine form stable hydroperoxides, whereas cytosine forms an unstable hydroperoxide that decomposes to a variety of products.

Irradiation of DNA in the solid state at liquid nitrogen temperature yields radicals in which, electron spin resonance measurements indicate, the unpaired spin is delocalized over the entire chain and does not belong to any one unit of the giant molecule. The addition of small amounts of water to this system does not alter the nature of the DNA radicals produced, but a two-to-one excess of water results in the annihilation of the electron spin resonance signal for DNA with the appearance of a strong signal due to water radicals. It has been postulated that this protective effect is attributable to energy transfer that is made possible in an excess of water by structuring of the water, thus providing a pathway for the formation of a delocalized water radical, or exciton. Electron spin resonance studies of irradiated nucleoprotein solutions indicate that the protein takes most of the radiation damage, protecting the nucleic acid moiety.

The damages caused by ionizing radiations in nucleic acid and their components are obviously detrimental to the passage of genetic information that requires specific order of intact purine and pyrimidine bases in the DNA strands. Alterations in these bases and the DNA molecules in general can lead to mutations and lethal genes. The disruption of RNA molecules interferes with protein synthesis and can result in eventual cell death.

RESPONSE OF BIOLOGICAL SYSTEMS TO IONIZING RADIATION

Identification of the Critical Target

As noted previously, absorption of ionizing radiation energy depends on the atomic weights of the atoms of the material and the density of the material. In contrast to the absorption of ultraviolet and visible radiation, the absorption of ionizing radiation is virtually independent of the nature of the molecular structure. Thus, the release of ionizing radiation energy in biological systems is essentially independent of the molecular bonds contained in the different biological molecules. This complicates the task of identifying the critical actions of this type of radiation. A good understanding of the action of ionizing radiation on living cells requires that the biologically important events should be known.

Determination of the critical sites for killing and mutagenesis by ionizing radiation has required biological experiments designed to answer this question. Several criteria essential for a target to qualify as a critical site for radiation action include: 1) relatively large size, 2) one or only a few copies in the cell, and 3) that it should serve a critical function for the growth and survival of the cell. The first two criteria result from the statistical distribution of damaging events in the cell. From target theory, it has been shown that the physical distribution of energy released from ionizing radiation follows a Poisson statistical distribution. Therefore, the most likely targets to be damaged are those with the first two criteria. The two cellular components that best satisfy all three criteria are the genomic material (DNA) and the cytoplasmic membrane.

Evidence Supporting DNA as a Critical Target

DNA is considered as one of the plausible critical targets for radiation action because there is only one or a few copies of the genome in each cell, because it is large compared with other molecular components, and because it plays a critical role in the proliferation and survival of the cell.

The most compelling pieces of experimental evidence that DNA is a critical target for the biological action of ionizing radiation are the mutagenic effects of ionizing radiation and the existence of DNA repair-deficient mutants of bacteria and cultured mammalian cells, which display a high sensitivity to killing by ionizing radiation.

Cellular genetic information is determined by the base sequence of the genomic DNA. Any alterations in this base sequence, such as damage to the bases in DNA (see above), will result in changes to this base sequence and, thus, to potentially mutagenic events. Whether the base sequence change will result in a phenotypic change depends on exactly where the base change occurs. If it is in an essential region of the DNA for the gene coding for a protein product or some functional or structural RNA product (tRNA or rRNA), then the base change will give rise to a phenotypic mutant. Otherwise, the mutation will fall into the category of a "silent mutation," which refers to those genotypic changes that do not have any associated phenotypic changes. For either type of mutation, the DNA is the component that must undergo change for the mutagenic event to occur.

An important advance in the understanding of how radiation kills biological systems involved the discovery that certain cells were more sensitive to killing by radiation than others. This discovery was first observed with the killing of bacteria by ultraviolet radiation.

In the case of ultraviolet radiation, it was rather straightforward to establish that the biochemical damage involved in this differential sensitivity of cells was in DNA and, more specifically, that it was the result of the formation of intrastrand (or, much less frequently, interstrand) cyclobutane pyrimidine dimers. Several factors facilitated the identification of this type of damage. First, pyrimidines absorb ultraviolet light strongly at 260 nm, and the efficiency of killing by ultraviolet radiation is maximal at or near this wavelength. Second, there was available a sensitive and quantitative assay for this type of damage. Thus, it was possible to quantitatively measure this biochemical damage and establish its relation to biological killing by the ultraviolet radiation.

Several decades later (in the 1960s), the same differential sensitivity of bacteria to killing by ionizing radiation was observed, and the biochemical damage responsible for this differential sensitivity was determined to be single-strand breaks in the backbone of the DNA. DNA strand breaks can be measured by a sensitive assay, using agarose gel electrophoresis, thus affording the opportunity to quantitatively relate the production of strand breaks with cell killing. Additionally, the isolation of radiation-sensitive mutants that lacked the ability to efficiently repair strand breaks was achieved. Thus, there was good evidence that this type of damage was related to the killing action of ionizing radiation.

Evidence that the Cytoplasmic Membrane Is a Critical Target

The cytoplasmic membrane is critical for the survival of the cell. It is large, and there is only one present for each cell. Therefore, the cytoplasmic membrane has the key characteristics that make it a likely critical target for killing by ionizing radiation. Experimental evidence that the membrane plays a role in the lethal action of ionizing radiation involves the observation that oxygen increases the radiosensitivity of cells to killing by ionizing radiation. This radiosensitization by oxygen during radiation exposure is commonly called the oxygen effect and is active in the killing of bacteria, mammalian cells, and plant cells, but not viruses. Also, the biological inactivation of free DNA (either viral or transforming DNA) by ionizing radiation does not display the oxygen effect.

As a result of the different responses to the oxygen effect, it is common to refer to the killing action of ionizing radiation including a component that is oxygen-dependent and one that is oxygen-independent damage.

Each of these results in cell-killing. The oxygen-independent damage is considered to be damage that involves the DNA, and the oxygen-dependent damage is considered to be that to the cytoplasmic membrane. Typically, the efficiency of killing by ionizing radiation is two to four times greater when exposure occurs in the presence of oxygen compared with when exposure occurs in an anoxic environment. Thus, it is reasonable to predict that between 50 and 75% of the lethal action of ionizing radiation results from membrane damage. For the oxygen effect to occur, the oxygen must be present during radiation exposure.

Relative Sensitivity of Various Biological Systems to Killing by Ionizing Radiation

To design a protocol for sterilization of a solution or material by ionizing radiation, it is necessary to establish the exposure dose required to kill all living organisms present, which is the definition of the sterilization dose. There is a large amount of data that provides measures of the radiosensitivity of diverse biological systems to radiation. For pharmaceuticals, it is important to consider viruses as well as pathogenic bacteria and other pathogenic organisms when determining the exposure dose required for sterilization of a particular product. It is also necessary to consider the physical and chemical environmental factors that cause variations in radiation sensitivity when establishing sterilization doses for the material, for the reasons that have been addressed previously. In general, the most radioresistant biological systems are the viruses. Certain bacterial species (e.g., *Micrococcus radiodurans*) are as resistant as many viruses. The 37% survival dose for these radioresistant bacteria is approximately 20 kGy (2 Mrad).

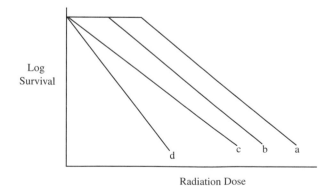

Fig. 2 Biological survival curves.

Survival Curves for Microorganisms

Ultimately, the goal of ionizing radiation treatment of pharmaceuticals is to kill all living organisms, that is, to sterilize the product. To achieve this, it is important to understand and know the survival curve response of microorganisms to killing by radiation. Fig. 2 displays the various kinds of survival curves that may be observed for microorganisms. No numbers have been assigned to the axes, because only the overall kinetic response of killing by the radiation is of interest. Curves *a* and *b* show the killing action for two hypothetical organisms with the same rate of killing but with differing repair capacities. Organisms capable of repairing lethal damage will have a characteristic threshold dose below which there is complete survival from radiation exposure. As the radiation dose increases, the repair system is not able to completely repair all radiation damage, and there is an exponential decrease in the viability of the population with increasing radiation doses. Alternatively, requirement for multiple ionization events in a critical target, or ionization events in multiple targets, can give rise to a threshold dose below which there is no observed radiation killing.

Curves *c* and *d* show the killing of organisms that lack the "shoulder" portion of curves *a* and *b*. The slope of the survival curve for organism *d* is greater than for organism *c* because organism *d* is more sensitive to radiation killing than organism *c*. Two organisms may differ in both the values of their threshold doses and in their kinetics of inactivation by radiation. It is important to keep in mind the shape and rate of inactivation of unwanted organisms when designing protocols for radiation sterilization.

USE OF IONIZING RADIATION IN THE PREPARATION OF STERILE PHARMACEUTICALS FOR HUMAN USE

At this writing, there are no approved procedures for the preparation of sterilized pharmaceuticals by exposure to ionizing radiation, although several packaging materials are approved for sterilization by doses in the 5- to 25-kGy dose region. The U.S. Food and Drug Administration (FDA) is considering rules that would permit the use of ionizing radiation in the terminal sterilization of drugs for human use. The two processes under consideration are aseptic processing and terminal sterilization for the preparation of sterile pharmaceuticals. These two methods differ in the manner by which sterilization of the product is achieved. In the case of aseptic processing, the product and the container are sterilized separately, and then final packaging of the product is carried out under aseptic

conditions. When terminal sterilization is used, the finally packaged product is sterilized. The FDA favors the terminal sterilization approach because fewer failures occur when using this technique compared with the failure rate of the aseptic processing techniques. When using terminal sterilization, the step of transfer of the product into the sterilized container under aseptic conditions is avoided, thus removing the possibility for product contamination during the transfer step. It is recognized that it will not be practical to use terminal sterilization for certain pharmaceuticals, since they might be sensitive to alteration and inactivation by the sterilizing agent, whereas they can be sterilized by filtration, when in solution.

During ongoing deliberations of which techniques should be approved by the FDA for the preparation of sterilized pharmaceuticals, the two physical methods under consideration are heat and ionizing radiation. Concerns similar to those associated with the use of ionizing radiation in food processing have been raised. After extensive discussions and hearings, the FDA has approved the commercial use of ionizing radiation for processing fruits, vegetables, poultry, beef, and spices. Before this technique is approved by the FDA as a physical agent for sterilization of pharmaceuticals, similar hearings will be required. The primary issue to be considered when developing a protocol using ionizing radiation is the establishment of the minimum and maximum allowable exposure doses. A minimum dose limit is required, to ensure that the product has been exposed to a sufficiently high dose that results in sterilization of the product. A maximum dose limit is required to avoid damage to the product resulting from unnecessarily high exposure doses. Exposure dose limits in the FDA regulations for food processing include minimum and maximum acceptable dose limits, which were established with these goals in mind.

Experiments on the action of ionizing radiation on pharmaceuticals and the killing of bacteria by ionizing radiation indicate that this treatment has the potential to be used in terminal sterilization. Reports indicate that there are no products formed in irradiated samples of penicillin G, neomycin, novobiocin, and dihydrostreptomycin, which are different from those that are formed by acidic, basic, hydrolytic, and oxidative treatments of these antibiotics. At the same exposure doses, there was a 1 million-fold reduction in the number of viable bacterial spores, which are the most radiosensitive forms of endospore forming bacteria. Thus, the use of ionizing radiation may provide an alternative to heat or chemical treatment for the sterilization of pharmaceuticals. This could provide a solution to the problem of sterilization of heat-sensitive drugs. Also, avoidance of chemical sterilization removes the possibility of contamination by residues of the chemical that was used for sterilization. It has been reported that irradiation of the antibiotic cefotaxime formed radiation products from impurities present in the cefotaxime sample. One must be aware of the role of solvents and chemicals other than the drug itself when considering radiolytic changes of a drug during sterilization.

CONCLUSIONS

The purpose of this article is to provide the pharmaceutical industry with an overview of the physical, chemical, and biological actions of ionizing radiation on molecules of interest to the industry, as well as to provide a current perspective on the prospects of the practical use of ionizing radiation as a physical agent in the sterilization of drugs for human use. Advantages of using employing ionizing radiation for pharmaceutical sterilization include:

- effectiveness on all microorganisms;
- no rise in temperature during treatment;
- consistent and reproducible protocols; and
- readily controlled and validated methods.

Although there is currently no approval by the FDA for ionizing radiation sterilization, there are active hearings being held by the agency on this matter. Considering the desire by the FDA to encourage the terminal sterilization method for sterilization of pharmaceuticals and the fact the ionizing radiation has distinct advantages over other treatment methods for use in terminal sterilization as presented above, it is expected that there will be approval of the use of this physical agent in sterilization of drugs for human use after regulatory hearings have provided sufficient information to allow identification of the appropriate conditions under which this agent can be used. Recent developments in the application of ionizing radiation for sterilization are reported on Web sites http://www.iaea.org and http://www.fda.gov.

REFERENCES

1. Alper, T. Cellular Radiobiology **1979**.
2. Barbarin, N.; Rollmann, B.; Tilquin, B. Role of Residual Solvents in the Formation of Volatile Compounds after Radiosterilization of Cefotaxime. Int. J. Pharm. **1999**, *178*, 203–212.
3. Chemical Protection from Radiation Effects. Nucleonics **1960**, *18*, 76–81.
4. Derr D., Radiation Processing What Is It? Where Is It Going? ASTM Standardization News 1993, 25–27
5. Ebert, M., Howards, A. Eds.; *Radiation Effects in Physics, Chemistry and Biology*; Year Book Medical Publishers: Chicago, 1963.
6. Pullman, B.; Pullman, A. *Quantum Biochemistry*; John Wiley & Sons: New York, 1963; 267–283.
7. Radiation Chemistry. Nucleonics **1961**, *19*, 37–68.
8. Schwarz, H.A. Radiation Chemistry. Ann. Rev. Phys. Chem. **1965**, *16*, 347–374.
9. Stock, D.A.; Achey, P.M. Repair of Single-Strand Breaks in DNA from Cultured *Leptidopteran* Cells Exposed to Gamma Radiation. *Invertebrate Cell System Applications*; Mitsuhashi, J. Ed.; CRC Press: 1989; 1, 45–61.
10. State of the Art Symposium: Radiation Chemistry. J. Chem. Ed.; **1981**, *58*, 82.
11. Swallow, A.J. *Radiation Chemistry of Organic Compounds*; Pergamon Press: London, 1960.
12. Symposium on the Development of Radiation Chemistry. J. Chem. Ed.; **1995**, *36*.
13. Tiliquin, B.; Crucq, A.S. Les Mecanismes Chimiques De La Radiosterilisation De Medicaments Solides. J. Chim. Phys. **1999**, *96*, 167–173.
14. Use of Aseptic Processing and Terminal Sterilization, the Preparation of Sterile Pharmaceuticals for Human and Veterinary Use. Federal Register, 1991; 56, No. 198, 51354–51358, October, 11, 1991.

SUPER DISINTEGRANTS: CHARACTERIZATION AND FUNCTION

Larry L. Augsburger
Huijeong A. Hahm
University of Maryland School of Pharmacy, Baltimore, Maryland

Albert W. Brzeczko
Atlantic Pharmaceutical Services, Owings Mills, Maryland

Umang Shah
Parke-Davis Division, Warner Lambert, Morris Plains, New Jersey

INTRODUCTION

Disintegrating agents are substances routinely included in tablet formulations and in some hard shell capsule formulations to promote moisture penetration and dispersion of the matrix of the dosage form in dissolution fluids. An oral solid dosage form should ideally disperse into the primary particles from which it was prepared. Although various compounds have been proposed and evaluated as disintegrants, relatively few are in common usage today. Traditionally, starch has been the disintegrant of choice in tablet formulations, and it is still widely used. However, starch is far from ideal. For instance, starch generally has to be present at levels greater than 5% to adversely affect compactibility, especially in direct compression. Moreover, intragranular starch in wet granulations is not as effective as dry starch. In more recent years, several newer disintegrants have been developed. Often called "super disintegrants," these newer substances can be used at lower levels than starch. Because they can be a smaller part of the overall formulation than starch, any possible adverse effect on fluidity or compactibility would be minimized. These newer disintegrants may be organized into three classes based on their chemical structure (Table 1).

GENERAL CHEMISTRY AND SURFACE MORPHOLOGY

Sodium Starch Glycolate

Sodium starch glycolate is a super disintegrant made from cross-linking sodium carboxymethylstarch (1). Cross-linking involves a chemical reaction with phosphorus oxytrichloride or sodium trimetaphosphate, or a physical manipulation. Carboxymethylation is performed by reacting starch with sodium chloroacetate in an alkaline medium and neutralizing with a citric or acetic acid, a process known as a Williamson ether synthesis. This synthesis yields carboxymethylation of about 25% of the glucose units. The by-products, which include sodium chloride, sodium glycolate, and sodium citrate or acetate, are partially washed out. The particle sizes of the disintegrants are increased by the substitution and cross-linking processes (3).

Sodium starch glycolates are generally spherical, a characteristic that accounts for their good flowability (4). Figure 1 shows the scanning electron photomicrographs of some of the commercially available sodium starch glycolates.

Croscarmellose Sodium

Croscarmellose sodium is derived from internally cross-linking a cellulose ether, sodium carboxymethylcellulose, which is a water soluble polymer. It is composed of repeating units of cellobiose units, with each unit consisting of two anhydroglucose units linked by 1,4-β-glucoside. Each unit also has three hydroxyl groups. The degree of substitution refers to the average number of hydroxyl groups substituted by carboxymethyl groups. Croscarmellose sodium is made from crude cellulose, which is steeped in sodium hydroxide solution (1). The cellulose is subsequently reacted with sodium monochloroacetate to form carboxymethylcellulose sodium. After completion of the substitution, the excess sodium monochloroacetate slowly hydrolyzes to glycolic acid. The glycolic acid converts a few of the sodium carboxymethyl groups to the free acid, catalyzes the cross-linkage to form croscarmellose sodium, and forms sodium chloride and sodium glycolate as the by-products.

Table 1 Classification of "super disintegrants" (partial listing)

Structural type (NF name)	Description	Trade name (manufacturer)
1. Modified starches (Sodium starch glycolate, NF)	Sodium carboxymethyl starch; the carboxymethyl groups induces hydrophilicity and cross-linking reduces solubility.	Explotab® (Edward Mendell Co.) Primojel® (Generichem Corp.) Tablo® (Blanver, Brazil)
2. Modified cellulose (Croscarmellose, NF)	Sodium carboxymethyl cellulose which has been cross-linked to render the material insoluble.	AcDiSol® (FMC Corp.) Nymcel ZSX® (Nyma, Netherlands) Primellose® (Avebe, Netherlands) Solutab® (Blanver, Brazil)
3. Cross-linked poly-vinylpyrrolidone (Crospovidone, NF)	Cross-linked polyvinylpyrrolidone; the high molecular weight and cross-linking render the material insoluble in water.	Crospovidone M® (BASF Corp.) Kollidon CL® (BASF Corp.) Polyplasdone XL (ISP Corp.)

Most of the by-products can be removed to achieve 99.5% purity by extraction with alcohol. Croscarmellose sodium may be milled to break the polymer fibers into shorter lengths and hence improve its flow properties.

Unlike sodium starch glycolate, crude croscarmellose sodium particles do not flow very well because of their twisted fibrous morphology and varying lengths. Therefore, they are cryogenically milled to improve flowability. The scanning electron photomicrographs show that the croscarmellose sodium particles are fibers with fairly sharp ends, probably because of the milling process (Fig. 2).

Crospovidone

Crospovidone is a cross-linked homopolymer of *N*-vinyl-2-pyrrolidone. The reactants, acetylene and formaldehyde, are used to form butynediol. The hydrogenation and subsequent cyclodehydrogenation of butynediol form butyrolactone. The reaction of butyrolactone with ammonia produces pyrrolidone that is then vinylated with acetylene under pressure. The linear polymerization of the vinylpyrrolidone yields polyvinylpyrrolidone, a soluble binder, while the popcorn (branched) polymerization yields crospovidone, an insoluble super disintegrant. The by-products of popcorn polymerization include vinylpyrrolidone and polyvinylpyrrolidone. Crospovidone contains less than 1.5% of the soluble material, which has been determined to be polyvinylpyrrolidone by infrared spectroscopy.

Crospovidone particles have a very different appearance from those of the other two classes of super disintegrants. Crospovidone particles seem to consist of aggregates of smaller particles that are fused together. This aggregation gives crospovidone a spongy, highly porous

appearance (Fig. 3). Scanning electron photomicrographs show that the reduction of particle size of crospovidone increases the surface area per unit weight, but decreases the intraparticulate porosity and the spongy appearance (4).

DISINTEGRANT ACTION

Although disintegrants are important components in solid dosage forms, their mechanism of action has not been clearly elucidated. The mechanisms proposed in the past include water wicking, swelling, deformation recovery, repulsion, and heat of wetting. It seems likely that no single mechanism can explain the complex behavior of the disintegrants. However, each of these proposed mechanism provides some understanding of different aspects of disintegrant action.

Water Wicking

The ability of a disintegrant to draw water into the porous network of a tablet is essential for effective disintegration. For crospovidone, water wicking has been thought to be the main mechanism of disintegration. Kornblum and Stoopak (5) observed that crospovidone swells very little, yet takes water into its network quite rapidly. Even the extensively swelling sodium starch glycolate showed improved disintegration when the molecular structure was altered to improve water uptake, as observed by Rudnic et al. (6). Unlike swelling, which is mainly a measure of volume expansion with accompanying force generation, water wicking is not necessarily accompanied by a volume increase.

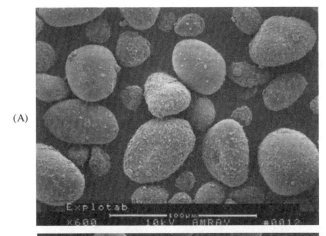

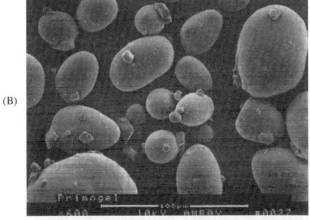

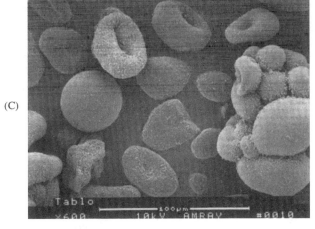

Fig. 1 Scanning electron photomicrograph of sodium starch glycolates: (A) Explotab®, (B) Primojel®, and (C) Tablo® (600× magnification).

The ability of a system to draw water can be summarized by Washburn's equation (7):

$$L^2 = \left(\frac{\gamma \cos\theta}{2\eta}\right) rt \tag{1}$$

The Washburn equation is too simplistic to apply to a dynamic tablet-disintegration process, but it does show that any change in the surface tension (γ), pore size (r), solid–liquid contact angle (θ), or liquid viscosity (η) could change the water wicking efficiency (L = length of water penetration in the capillary; t = time). For example, when Rudnic et al. (8) evaluated the disintegration efficiency of different particle sizes of crospovidone, those with the largest particle size range (50–300 µm) yielded the shortest disintegration time. Large particle size probably yielded greater pore size and altered the shape of the pore. Indeed, longer fiber length due to greater particle size could improve the efficiency of capillary uptake of water into the dosage form matrix.

Super disintegrants draw water into the matrix system at a faster rate and to a greater extent when compared to traditional starch (9). Van Kamp et al. (10), utilizing a water uptake measurement device, were able to show that tablets that demonstrate greater uptake volume and rate, such as those containing sodium starch glycolate, disintegrated more rapidly. Although the hydrophobic lubricant, magnesium stearate, seemed to negatively affect the wicking process, those containing sodium starch glycolate were less affected by the detrimental effect of mixing with the hydrophobic lubricant. Lerk et al. (11) also observed a decreased rate of wetting when disintegrants were mixed with magnesium stearate for various mixing times. The decrease in the rate of wetting was proportional to the time of mixing. Most likely, this observation reflected a greater delamination of magnesium stearate at longer mixing times.

Swelling

Although water penetration is a necessary first step for disintegration, swelling is probably the most widely accepted mechanism of action for tablet disintegrants. Indeed, most disintegrants do swell to some extent, but the variability of this property between disintegrants reduces its plausibility as a sole mechanism.

The earliest attempt to measure swelling was to measure the sedimentation volume of slurries. Nogami et al. (12) developed a reliable test to measure both swelling and water uptake. Gissinger and Stamm (13) modified this apparatus and found a positive correlation between the rate of swelling and disintegrant action for some disintegrants. List and Muazzam (14) later adapted this apparatus to measure both rate of swelling and swelling force through the application of force and displacement transducers. They found that disintegrants that generate large swelling forces are generally more effective.

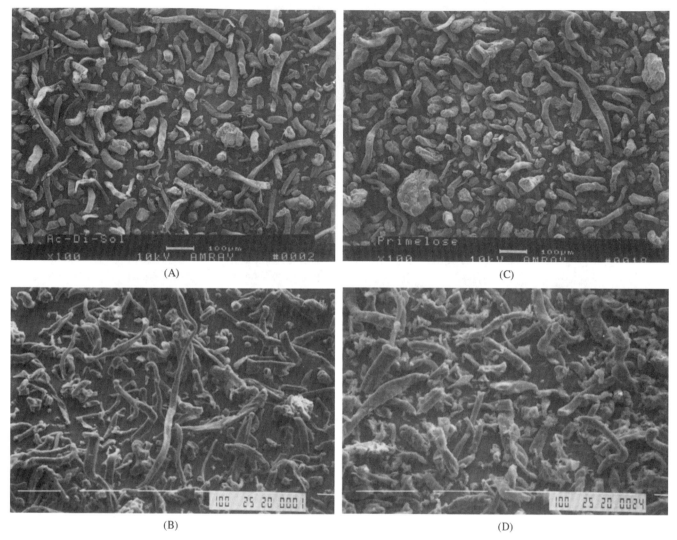

Fig. 2 Scanning electron photomicrograph of croscarmelloses: (A) AcDiSol®, (B) Nymcel ZSX®, (C) Primellose®, and (D) Solutab® (100× magnification).

For swelling to be effective as a mechanism of disintegration, there must be a superstructure against which the disintegrant swells. Swelling of the disintegrant against the matrix leads to the development of a swelling force. A large internal porosity in the dosage form in which much of the swelling can be accommodated reduces the effectiveness of the disintegrant. At the same time, a matrix that yields readily through plastic deformation may partly accommodate any disintegrant swelling if swelling does not occur at a sufficient rapidity.

The swelling of some disintegrants is dependent on the pH of the media. Shangraw et al. (3) reported that sedimentation volumes of anionic cross-linked starches and celluloses are altered in acidic media. Polyplasdone XL® and Starch 1500® were unchanged. In a separate

study, Chen et al. (15) showed that acetaminophen tablets containing Primojel® and AcDiSol® had longer disintegration and dissolution times in acidic medium compared to neutral medium. Those containing Polyplasdone XL® showed no such differences. Mitrevej and Hollenbeck (16) verified the remarkable swelling capacity of some "super disintegrants" by exposing individual particles deposited on slides to high humidities and observing their degree of swelling microscopically.

On the other hand, when Caramella et al. (17–19) evaluated different disintegrants for their ability to swell, no correlation could be observed between the maximum disintegrating force and percent of particle swelling. Because they did observe a correlation between the rate of disintegrating force development and the disintegration

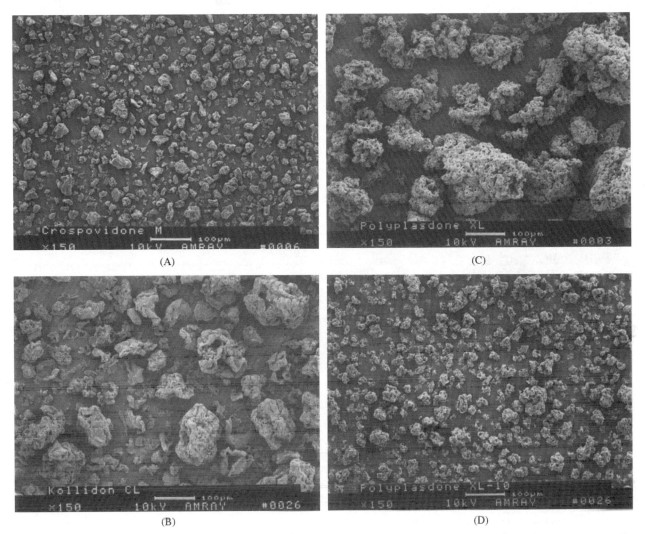

Fig. 3 Scanning electron photomicrograph of crospovidones: (A) Crospovidone M®, (B) Kollidon CL®, (C) Polyplasdone XL®, and (D) Polyplasdone XL-10 ® (150× magnification).

time, therefore, the authors suggested that the rate of development of a disintegrating force is all-important. Swelling capable of rapid force development may be preferred since a slowly developing force could hypothetically allow tablets to relieve the stress generated without bond disruption.

Deformation Recovery

The deformation recovery theory implies that the shapes of the disintegrant particles are distorted during compression, and that the particles return to their precompression shape upon wetting, thereby causing the tablet to break apart. Hess (20), with the aid of photomicrographs, showed that

deformed starch particles returned to their original shape when exposed to moisture.

Fassihi (21) concluded that at higher compression forces, disintegration may become dependent on mechanical activation of the tablet, resulting from the stored energy imparted by the compression process. He examined the disintegration times of tablets made of Emdex® powder, magnesium stearate, and 5% disintegrant. Regardless of the disintegrant used (sodium starch glycolate, microcrystalline cellulose, corscarmellose sodium, or starch), the disintegration time increased with increasing compression force, then decreased again when the compression force was above 120 MN/m^{-2}.

Research on deformation and its recovery in situ as a disintegration mechanism is incomplete. However, such a mechanism may be an important aspect of the mechanism of action of disintegrants such as crospovidone and starch that appear to exhibit little or no swelling. The efficacy of such disintegrants likely would be dependent on the relative yield strength of the disintegrant and that of the matrix in which it is compressed, since disintegration efficiency would surely depend on how much deformation is sustained by the disintegrant particles. Also, time-dependent stress relaxation could possibly be a factor in the aging of such tablets in that any deformation induced into the disintegrant, that cannot be sustained by intraparticulate bonding, gradually may recover as the matrix relaxes.

Repulsion Theory

Ringard and Guyot-Hermann (22) have proposed a particle–particle repulsion theory to explain the observation that particles that do not swell extensively, such as starch, could still disintegrate tablets. In this theory, water penetrates into the tablet through hydrophilic pores and a continuous starch network that can convey water from one particle to the next, imparting a significant hydrostatic pressure. The water then penetrates between starch grains because of its affinity for starch surfaces, thereby breaking hydrogen bonds and other forces holding the tablet together. Presently, this theory is not supported by adequate data.

Heat of Wetting

Matsumara (23) noticed that starch particles exhibit slight exothermic properties when wetted, which was thought to cause localized stress resulting from expansion of air retained in the tablet matrix. Unfortunately, this explanation, if valid, would be limited to only a few substances such as aluminum silicate and kaolinite. List and Muazzam (24) found that exothermic wetting reactions were not exhibited with all disintegrants and that even when a significant heat of wetting was generated, disintegration time did not always decrease. Caramella et al. (25) found that an increase in temperature, which should cause air expansion, did not enhance maximum force generation in several formulations. Therefore, they concluded that expansion of air in pores from heat of wetting could not be supported by the data. More recently, Luangtana-anan et al. have examined the heat of wetting of powders and tablets of magnesium carbonate and Emcompress® (26).

Magnesium carbonate tablets with significantly higher heat of wetting disintegrated more readily than the Encompress® tablets. Indeed, it would be interesting to develop a model for the mechanism of tablet disintegration using a thermodynamic approach; however, heat of wetting alone probably is inadequate to explain disintegration.

Generation of a Disintegrating Force or Pressure as a Unifying Principle

The rate of generation of a disintegrating force may be a unifying factor in the mechanisms of disintegration (19). Many proposed mechanisms may be visualized as giving rise to a force. Brzeczko (27) developed techniques to simultaneously measure the rate of liquid uptake into a tablet and the rate of generation of both axial and radial swelling forces. As indicated in Figs. 4, 5, and 6, tablet compaction contributes more to the axial pressure than to the radial pressure when super disintegrants representing the three main super disintegrant classes were studied in model tablet formulations. In all three cases, the maximum axial pressure in an anhydrous lactose matrix was well below that observed with a dicalcium phosphate dihydrate matrix when the disintegrants are compared at the same concentration. The differences in disintegrant performance in soluble and insoluble matrices could be rationalized in terms of pressure development and liquid uptake. Fig. 7 compares the maximum axial disintegrating pressure and disintegration times of the tablets containing 2% of the disintegrants in a matrix composed of dicalcium phosphate or lactose (27). As can be seen, a higher disintegration pressure favors rapid disintegration of the dicalcium phosphate-based tablets, but a slower disintegration of lactose-based tablets. Higher initial axial disintegrating pressure rates also yield shorter disintegration times for the dicalcium phosphate-based tablets, but no such correlation is seen with the lactose-based tablets, whose disintegrating pressure rates are much lower than those of the dicalcium phosphate-based tablets (see Fig. 8). Maximum water uptake and water uptake rate seem to be poor predictors of disintegration time, as seen in Figs. 9 and 10. However, lactose-based tablets show a trend toward slower disintegration with faster liquid uptake. It was suggested that faster liquid uptake leads to a faster dissolution of lactose and increased porosity to accommodate swelling and/or structural recovery.

Peppas (28) attribute the difference in disintegration rate between soluble and insoluble matrices to two proposed phenomena — an interface-controlled mechanism and a diffusion-controlled mechanism — as represented in the following equation:

$$F/F_\infty = 1 - \exp(-kt^n) \qquad (2)$$

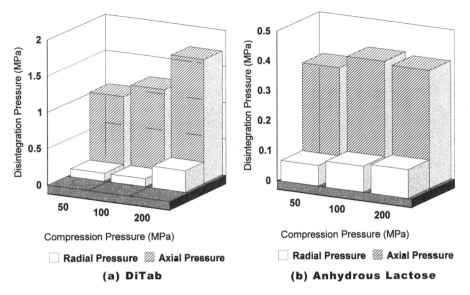

Fig. 4 The effect of compression pressure on the axial and radial disintegrating pressures of compacts made with lactose or Ditab®, and AcDiSol® (5%). (From Ref. 27.)

Here, F is the disintegration force at time t, F_∞ is the maximum force developed, k is an expansion rate constant, and n signifies which of the two mechanisms controls the disintegration. The interface controlled phenomenon involves tablet particles breaking apart from the interface of the tablet and the diffusion-controlled phenomenon involves particles diffusing away. Although it is thought that both happen simultaneously, the degree to which disintegration depends on each system can differ. For example, those tablet matrices with a relatively small n of about 0.6 are thought to be dominated by the diffusional mechanism; whereas, those with an n of greater than

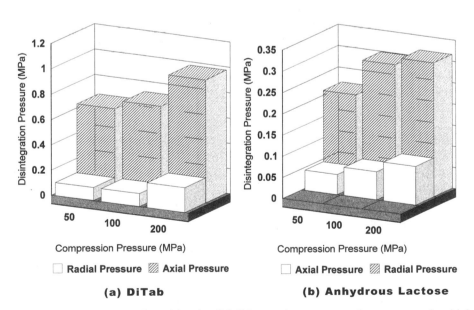

Fig. 5 The effect of compression pressure on the axial and radial disintegrating pressures of compacts made with lactose or Ditab, and Primojel® (5%). (From Ref. 27.)

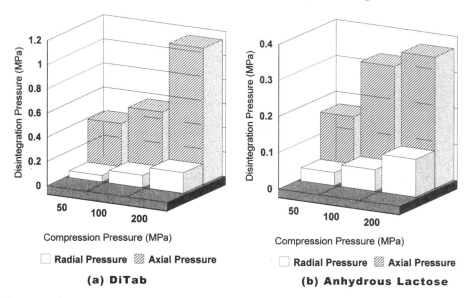

Fig. 6 The effect of compression pressure on the axial and radial disintegrating pressures of compacts made with lactose or Ditab, and Polyplasdone XL® (5%). (From Ref. 27.)

0.9 are thought to be interfacial mechanism dominant. The value of n would certainly differ based on the solubility of the matrices.

Since super disintegrants are highly hydrophilic yet insoluble in water, they would be expected to be more effective in breaking the tablet apart interfacially than controlling the diffusion per se. Indeed, Caramella et al. observed that disintegration occurred readily for tablets containing insoluble calcium phosphate; whereas, tablets containing highly soluble β-lactose disintegrated slowly. Such phenomena were explained by a lower value of n for the system containing β-lactose. In other words, the super

disintegrant's interface-controlled mechanism could not overcome the diffusion-controlled mechanism of the β-lactose (29).

FACTORS AFFECTING DISINTEGRANT ACTIVITY

Particle Size

Both the rate and force of disintegrant action may be dependent upon the particle size of the disintegrant. Smallenbroek et al. (30) found that starch grains having

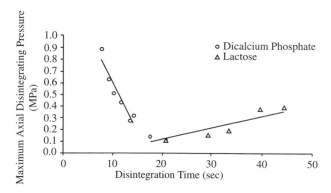

Fig. 7 Maximum axial disintegrating pressure versus disintegration time of dicalcium phosphate and lactose tablets containing 2% super disintegrants. O = Dicalcium phosphate: $r^2 = 0.92$, $p < 0.05$, significant correlation. △ = Lactose: $r^2 = 0.81$, $p < 0.05$, significant correlation. (From Ref. 27.)

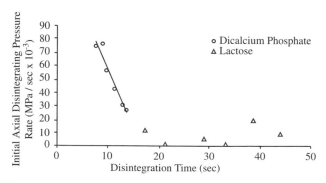

Fig. 8 Initial axial disintegrating pressure rate versus disintegration time of dicalcium phosphate and lactose tablets containing 2% super disintegrants. O = Dicalcium phosphate: $r^2 = 0.95$, $p < 0.05$, significant correlation. △ = Lactose: $r^2 = 0.10$, $p < 0.05$, no significant correlation. (From Ref. 27.)

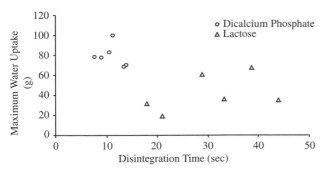

Fig. 9 Maximum water uptake versus disintegration time of dicalcium phosphate and lactose tablets containing 2% super disintegrants. $\bigcirc$ = Dicalcium phosphate: no significant correlation. $\triangle$ = Lactose: no significant correlation. (From Ref. 27.)

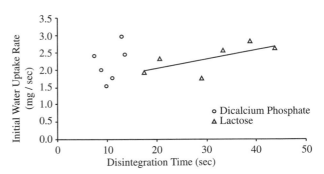

Fig. 10 Initial water uptake rate versus disintegration time of dicalcium phosphate and lactose tablets containing 2% super disintegrants. $\bigcirc$ = Dicalcium phosphate: no significant correlation. $\triangle$ = Lactose: $r^2 = 0.47$, $p < 0.05$, no significant correlation. (From Ref. 27.)

relatively large particle sizes were more efficient than the smaller particle size grades. This is probably because the continuous hydrophilic network of disintegrants is more efficiently accomplished by the bigger particles. Also, Rudnic et al. (8) found that coarser grades of crospovidone (50–100 μm, Grade B; 50–300 μm, Grade C) were more efficient than the finer particles (0–15 μm, Grade A). The differences in disintegration efficiency between Grade B and Grade C were not clear, however. When List and Muazzam (24) evaluated two different grades of crospovidone particles (100–200 μm and >315 μm), the efficiencies between the two grades were very similar (see Table 2). Results for the other disintegrants, Amberlite IRP88® and potato starch, support that coarser particle sizes allow more efficient disintegration than finer particles. For disintegrants that swell extensively, such

efficiency can be explained by the observed force development. Indeed, larger particles of sodium starch glycolate swelled more rapidly and to a greater extent than did the smaller particles (6).

Molecular Structure

Disintegrants can vary in molecular structure based on how they are manufactured or processed. Corn starch, for example, contains different ratios of two sugar fractions, amylose and amylopectin. Schwartz and Zelinske (31) concluded that the linear polymer, amylose, was responsible for the disintegrant properties associated with starch, whereas the branched polymer, amylopectin, was responsible for the gummy property.

Table 2 Effect of particle size and compression pressure on swelling pressure and disintegration time

Disintegrant	Compression pressure (bar)	Particle size (μm)	Swelling pressure (bar)	Disintegration time (s)
Amberlite IRP88®	625	<50	0.660	84
	1560	<50	1.121	30
Amberlite IRP88®	625	100–200	1.083	52
	1560	100–200	2.262	22
Potato starch	625	<50	0.165	254
	1560	<50	0.310	164
Potato starch	625	80–100	0.234	160
	1560	80–100	0.445	77
Polyplasdone XL®	625	100–200	0.898	31
	1560	100–200	1.772	14
Polyplasdone XL®	625	>315	0.760	42
	1560	>315	1.480	17

Tablet composition: 2.5% disintegrant, 1% magnesium stearate, and Emcompress®. (From Ref. 24.)

Varying the amylose to amylopectin ratio did not affect the porosities of the resulting tablets. Rudnic et al. (6) evaluated the effect of cross-linking and carboxymethyl substitution in sodium starch glycolate and concluded that the swelling of the disintegrant was largely inversely proportional to the degree of cross-linkage. Swelling also was inversely proportional to the level of substitution, but to a lesser degree. Shah et al. (32) found that carboxymethyl cellulose having high molecular weight and low levels of carboxymethylation was best for tablet disintegration.

Effect of Compression Force

Compression force affects disintegration time in different ways. First, it governs the penetration of dissolution fluids into the matrix by controlling the porosity of the compact. Low compression force can lead to relatively high tablet porosity and can allow rapid penetration of water. However, it has often been observed that tablets containing starch exhibit disintegration times that tend to pass through minimum as compression force increases (21). At low compression forces, any possible swelling or deformation recovery that may take place may be more or less accommodated by the porosity, whereas at intermediate compression forces, a maximal disintegrating effect may develop. At high compression forces, fluid penetration may be impeded by a further reduction of porosity while particle deformation of the disintegrants becomes more important. In general, List and Muazzam (14) found increased swelling pressures at higher compression forces when various amberlite resins, starches, and crospovidones were employed at the 2.5% level in dicalcium phosphate matrix tablets (see Table 2). Similar findings were reported by and Fassihi (21) and Brzeczko (27).

In two different studies Khan and Rhodes (33, 34) observed that tablets containing sodium starch glycolate disintegrate relatively slowly at low compression force, quickly at intermediate compression force, and slowly again at high compression force. However, the effects of compression force on the disintegration time of other types of disintegrants, such as cation exchange resin, calcium sodium alginate, and various forms of starches, varied widely. Perhaps the effect of compression force on the disintegration time depends on the nature of the disintegrants, such as their mechanism of disintegration and deformation characteristics.

Munoz et al. (35) found that the effect of compression pressure on disintegration time varied depending on the concentration used of the super disintegrant, Explotab®. Fig. 11 shows that shortest disintegration time could be

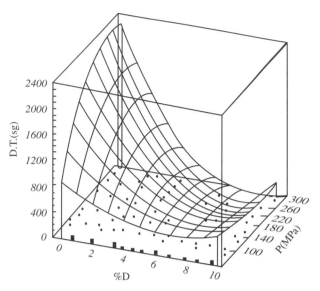

Fig. 11   Surface response of disintegration time as functions of compression pressure and percent disintegrant. (From Ref. 11.)

achieved at around 7% disintegrant concentration. At this concentration, compression force has little effect on disintegration time. The disintegration time was more affected by compression force at low disintegrant concentration, showing fastest disintegration time at intermediate compression force. This type of biphasic effect of compression force on disintegration time also was observed for AcDiSol® (36), and the surface response curve is very similar to that of Explotab®. When disintegration times were studied at 5 and 10% disintegrant, 5% AcDiSol® yielded the lowest porosity, lowest yield pressure in Heckel analysis, and shortest disintegration time. At a 10% disintegrant level, the tablets showed a slight postcompression expansion, which could explain a slightly increased disintegration time compared to the 5% disintegrant level.

The effect of compression force on disintegration efficiency seems, therefore, largely dependent on the mechanism of the disintegrant action. The effectiveness of swelling or structure recovery may well be dependent on attaining a compression force that achieves a critical porosity in the matrix. On the other hand, the capillary uptake of liquid, which is a necessary precursor to these mechanisms could be compromised if the tablet matrix is compressed to too low a porosity.

Matrix Solubility

The disintegrant mechanism seems to depend not only on the disintegrant itself but on the matrix as well. Disintegrants work most effectively in insoluble matrices

(27). Insoluble matrices, such as those containing calcium phosphate do not disintegrate adequately without disintegrants. On the other hand, tablets and capsules that primarily consist of water soluble fillers or drugs tend to dissolve rather than to disintegrate, even when disintegrating agents are present. It has been suggested that during the dissolving process, the water acts as a plasticizer (37), which can potentially reduce the development of disintegrating force. In addition, soluble materials that tend to swell can form viscous plugs, which may impede further penetration of moisture into the matrix. However, the addition of disintegrants almost predictably shortens disintegration time, despite the solubility of the matrix.

Method of Incorporation in Granulation

The method of incorporation of disintegrants in granulation has been controversial. Should the disintegrant be all extragranular, all intragranular, or divided between these two locations? Shotton and Leonard (38) reported that maize starch, sodium calcium alginate, alginic acid, and other disintegrants gave more rapid disintegration when incorporated extragranularly than when incorporated intragranularly in a sulfadiazine granulation. They also reported that the latter method gave a finer dispersion and concluded that the best compromise was to use both intra- and extragranular disintegrant.

Van Kamp et al. (39) evaluated the method of incorporation of Primojel®, AcDiSol®, and Polyplasdone XL® in prednisone tablets formed from lactose granules. Whether the incorporation of the super disintegrant was intragranular, extragranular, or evenly distributed in both sites, they found little or no difference in disintegration time, crushing strength, or dissolution of prednisone. Interestingly, their results with potato starch showed differences that did not agree with the earlier work of

Shotton and Leonard (38) in that intragranular starch was more effective than extragranular starch (see Table 3). Gordon et al. (40) reported that dissolution of naproxen, a poorly soluble drug at gastric pH levels, was faster when AcDiSol® was incorporated intragranularly, compared to when it was incorporated extragranularly or evenly distributed between the intra- and extragranular portions. Even more recently, a study reported by Khattab et al. (41) showed that the combined incorporation of intra- and extragranular disintegrating agents (sodium starch glycolate, croscarmellose sodium, or crospovidone) in a paracetamol granulation resulted in faster disintegration and dissolution than either extragranular or intragranular incorporation alone.

More studies are necessary to elucidate the effect of other factors, such as the type of binder, the type of filler, and the solubility of the matrix, which may significantly affect the effectiveness of disintegrants in different modes of incorporation. For example, Becker et al. (42) found that extragranular crospovidone was more effective in an acetaminophen tablet when the binder was maltodextrin (Licab DSH®), pregelatinized maize starch (Lycab PGS®), or low substituted hydroxypropylcellulose (L-HPC) than when polyvinylpyrrolidone or hydroxypropylmethylcellulose was the binder. In addition, the difference seen in the effectiveness of starch in different modes of incorporation between the Shotton and Leonard (38) study and the Van Kamp et al. (39) study may be related to the absence or presence of lactose, a soluble filler. Unlike the Shotton and Leonard study, Van Kamp et al. used lactose as a soluble filler, which might have reduced the relative effectiveness extragranular starch, making the intragranular incorporation more favorable.

The observations summarized in Table 4 make any attempt to generalize that one method of incorporation of disintegrant in granulation is better than another difficult.

Table 3 Effect of method of disintegrant addition in granules on the tablet properties

Disintegrant addition method	Crushing strength (kgf)			Disintegration time (s)		
	Intra	Equal	Extra	Intra	Equal	Extra
Control		6.5			664	
4% Primojel®	5.3	5.0	5.8	38	41	49
4% Ac-Di-Sol®	3.8	4.8	5.7	110	126	148
4% Nymcel zsd 16®	4.0	4.3	6.5	499	540	488
4% Polyplasdone XL®	5.8	6.0	6.1	31	40	43
20% Potato Starch	3.3	3.4	2.1	69	80	110

(From Ref. 39.)

Table 4 Comparison of different modes of incorporation of disintegrants in granules on disintegration efficiency of tablets, as reported by different investigators

Investigators	Drug (D), Binder (B), Filler	Disintegrants evaluated	Order of disintegration efficiency	Additional comments
Shotton et al.	Sulfadiazine (D) Povidone (B) No filler	Maize starch Na calcium alginate Alginic acid Microcrystalline cellulose Colloidal aluminum silicate	Extra > Intra	Extragranular incorporation yielded fastest disintegration, but intragranular incorporation yielded finer particles. Equal distribution of disintegrants is recommended.
Van Kamp et al.	Prednisone (D) Gelatin (B) Lactose (F)	Potato starch	Intra > Extra	The difference between the modes of incorporation for super disintegrants is not great.
		Primojel® Polyplasdone XL® Nymcel®	Intra > Equal > Extra Intra > Equal > Extra Extra > Intra > Equal	
Khattab et al.	Paracetamol (D) Polyvinylpyrrollidone (B) No filler	Croscarmellose Na	Equal > Extra > Intra	Overall, the equal distribution of disintegrants yielded the fastest disintegration and dissolution.
		Na starch glycolate Crospovidone	Equal > Intra or Extra Equal > Intra > Extra	

(From Refs. 38, 38, and 41.)

Table 5 Rework efficiency (%RE) of super disintegrants

Disintegrant (2%)	Relative F_s (35% porosity)[a]	Relative F_s (40% porosity)[a]	% RE[b]
Control	0.842	0.848	45
Polyplasdone XL®	0.941	0.926	64
Explotab®	0.737	0.863	86
AcDiSol®	1.045	0.951	45

[a] $\text{Re} \cdot F_s = \dfrac{\text{Maximum swelling force (1st compression)}}{\text{Maximum swelling force (2nd compression)}}$

[b] $\%RE = \dfrac{\text{AUC (1st compression)}}{\text{AUC (2nd compression)}}$

AUCs are the area under curve from the disintegration time versus compression pressure graphs.
(From Ref. 44.)

However, when all of the data are taken together, it would appear that the combined addition of disintegrants both extragranularly and intragranularly would provide the best opportunity for optimal disintegrant activity.

Effect of Reworking

The effect of recompressing a wet massed microcrystalline cellulose matrix containing super disintegrants on swelling force kinetics also has been considered (43). When the disintegrants were placed extragranularly, only Explotab® among those considered retained good efficiency after reworking. When placed intragranularly, all disintegrants had reworking efficiencies equivalent to that of the nondisintegrant control. Adding 2% disintegrant extragranularly prior to the second compression restored disintegrant behavior for Polyplasdone XL®, but only partial restoration was seen for AcDiSol®. In further work (44), reworked tablets containing 2% disintegrant extragranularly were studied. The data in Table 5 illustrate that maximal swelling forces were reduced in all cases, but there was no correlation with tablet disintegration time.

Incorporation in Hard Gelatin Capsules

The utility and performance of super disintegrants in direct-fill powder formulations for hard shell capsules filled on tamping machines are roughly analogous to those of direct compression tablet formulation. In a study where capsules were filled under controlled tamping force conditions using an instrumented Zanasi LZ 64 dosator machine, a dicalcium phosphate based formulation containing hydrocholorothiazide and different super disintegrants were tested for dissolution times (45). The croscarmelloses were found to be more effective than sodium starch glycolate in promoting hydrochlorothiazide dissolution, whereas

crospovidone was the poorest in this regard. In a follow-up multifactorial study, all main factors, including disintegrant type, compression force, level of lubricant, and filler type, were found to have significant effects on dissolution (Figs. 12 and 13) (46). In most cases at lower disintegrant concentration, increasing the tamping force improved the dissolution of hydrochlorothiazide, most likely due to reduced porosity. When the filler was changed from lactose to dicalcium phosphate, the magnitude and the order of effectiveness of the disintegrants changed.

Like the experience with tablets, the effect of disintegrants in already rapidly soluble capsule matrices is lower than that in water insoluble matrices. Perhaps doubling the concentration normally required for tablets is needed to effect efficient disintegration and significantly affect dissolution. This need for higher disintegrant concentration probably reflects the greater pore structure of capsule plugs compared to compressed tablets. At equivalent concentrations in model lactose or dicalcium phosphate-based systems, sodium starch glycolate and croscarmellose sodium were more effective than crospovidone in promoting dissolution of hydrochlorothiazide from capsules manufactured with the same tamping force (47). For either filler, disintegration times and swelling correlated well with dissolution.

NEW DISINTEGRANTS

Gellan gum and Xanthan SM® appear to have performance characteristics similar to those of super disintegrants. Gellan gum is an anionic polysaccharide of linear tetrasaccharides, and is derived from Pseudomonas elodea (48). When 4% gellan gum was incorporated in an ibuprofen tablets, its disintegration time was 4 min, which

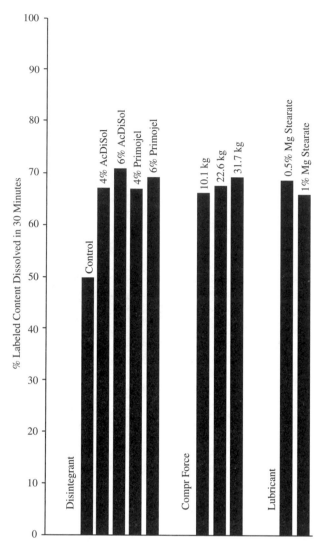

Fig. 12 The averaged effect of disintegrant, compression force, and lubricant on the release of hydrochlorothiazide from anhydrous lactose based capsules. Control = 0% disintegrant. (From Ref. 47.)

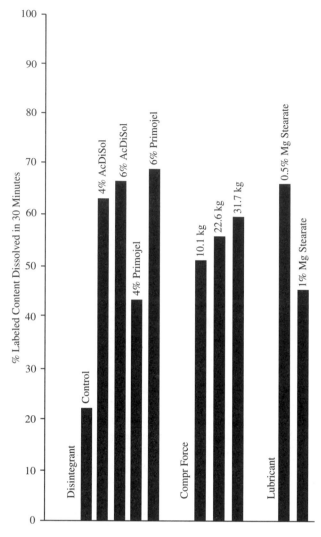

Fig. 13 The averaged effect of disintegrant, compression force, and diluent on the release of hydrochlorothiazide from dicalcium phosphate based capsules. Control = 0% disintegrant. (From Ref. 47.)

was much superior than that obtained using dried starch or Avicel PH 102® (>15 min), and comparable to those of Explotab®, AcDiSol®, and Kollidon CL® (4–7 min).

Xanthan SM® is a new USP xanthan derivative with higher hydrophilicity and lower gelling tendency (49). In aspirin tablets with 3% Xanthan SM® disintegration time was about 10 min. Increasing the concentration of disintegrant beyond 3% did not improve the disintegration time, whereas the most effective concentration of AcDiSol® was 5%, yielding a disintegration time of less than 5 min. Xanthan SM®, like AcDiSol®, has low solubility in water, but is reported to swell more extensively in water.

SUMMARY

In summary, super disintegrants are excipients used to promote rapid breakdown of oral solid dosage forms to aid dissolution in vivo. Commonly used super disintegrants include sodium starch glycolate, croscarmellose sodium, and crospovidone. Super disintegrants differ from traditional starch in that they are effective at much lower concentrations. This lower concentration provides formulation scientists greater flexibility, particularly in designing direct compression tablets. However, the effectiveness of both starch and super disintegrants depends heavily upon the composition of the tablet matrix, compression pressure, and in the case of granulation, the method of incorporation.

Because of the complexities involved, the mechanism of action of super disintegrants is not well understood. Some of the proposed mechanisms include water wicking, swelling, deformation recovery, particle repulsion, and heat of wetting. Water uptake is a necessary precursor to all other mechanisms. Not all mechanisms are well supported by research. Disintegrants appear to function by multiple mechanisms, but a predominant mechanism seems to be characteristic of each disintegrant type. Regardless of their validity, all proposed mechanisms at least have the potential to generate a disintegrating force within the matrix and this appears to be a unifying concept.

ACKNOWLEDGMENT

The authors wish to express sincere appreciation and gratitude to Ms. Lynn DiMemmo, FMC Co., Princeton, N.J., for the SEM's of the super disintegrants.

REFERENCES

1. *Handbook of Pharmaceutical Excipients*, 2nd Ed.; American Pharmaceutical Association: Washington, DC, 1994; 141–144, 462–466.
2. Bolhuis, G.K.; Van Kamp, H.V.; Lerk, C.F. Effect of Variation of Degree of Substitution, Crosslinking, and Purity of the Disintegration Efficiency of Sodium Starch Glycolate. Acta Pharm. Tech. **1984**, *30*, 24–32.
3. Shangraw, R.F.; Mitrevej, A.M.; Shah, M.N. A New Era of Tablet Disintegrants. Pharm. Tech. **1980**, *4*, 49–57.
4. Shah, U.S. *Evaluation of the Functional Equivalence of Different Sources of Super Disintegrants in Pharmaceutical Tablets*; University of Maryland: Baltimore, 1996; 16–26, 92–112.
5. Kornblum, S.S.; Stoopak, S.B. A New Tablet Disintegrating Agent: Cross-Linked Polyvinylpyrrolidone. J. Pharm. Sci. **1973**, *62*, 43–49.
6. Rudnic, E.M.; Kanig, J.; Rhodes, C.T. The Effect of Molecular Structure on the Function of Sodium Starch Glycolate in Wet Granulated Systems. Drug Dev. Ind. Pharm. **1983**, *9*, 303–320.
7. Washburn, E.W. The Dynamic of Capillary Flow. Phys. Rev. **1921**, *17*, 273–283.
8. Rudnic, E.M.; Lausier, J.M.; Chilamkarti, R.N.; Rhodes, C.T. Studies of the Utility of Cross-Linked Polyvinylpyrrolidone as a Tablet Disintegrant. Drug Dev. Ind. Pharm. **1980**, *6*, 291–309.
9. Grai, E.; Ghanem, A.H.; Mahmoud, H. Studies of the Direct Compression of Pharmaceuticals. Pharm. Ind. **1984**, *46*, 279–284.
10. Van Kamp, H.V.; Bolhuis, G.K.; De Boer, A.H.; Lerk, C.F.; Lie-A-Huen, L. The Role of Water Uptake on Tablet Disintegration. Pharm. Acta Helv. **1986**, *61*, 22–29.
11. Lerk, C.F.; Bolhuis, G.K.; Smallenbroek, A.J.; Zuurman, K. Interaction of Tablet Disintegrants and Magnesium Stearate during Mixing. II. Effect on Dissolution Rate. Pharm. Acta Helv. **1982**, *57*, 282–286.
12. Nogami, H.; Nagai, T.; Fukuoka, E.; Sonobe, T. Disintegration of the Aspirin Tablets Containing Potato Starch and Microcrystalline Cellulose in Various Concentrations. Chem. Pharm. Bull. **1969**, *17*, 1450–1455.
13. Gissinger, D.; Stamm, A. A Comparative Evaluation of the Properties of Some Tablet Disintegrants. Drug Dev. Ind. Pharm. **1980**, *6*, 511–536.
14. List, P.H.; Muazzam, U.A. Swelling —The Driving Force Behind Disintegration. Pharm. Ind. **1979**, *41*, 1075–1077.
15. Chen, C.R.; Lin, Y.H.; Cho, S.L.; Yen, S.Y.; Wu, H.L. Investigation of the Dissolution Difference Between Acidic and Neutral Media of Acetaminophen Tablets Containing Super Disintegrant and a Soluble Excipient. Chem. Pharm. Bull. **1997**, *45*, 509–512.
16. Mitrevej, A.; Hollenbeck, R.G. Photomicrographic Analysis of Water Vapor Sorption and Swelling of Selected Super Disintegrants. Pharm. Tech. **1982**, *6*, 48–50.
17. Caramella, C.; Columbo, P.; Conte, U.; Gazzaniga, A.; LaManna, A. The Role of Swelling in the Disintegration Process. Int. J. Pharm. Tech. Prod. Mfr. **1984**, *5*, 1–5.
18. Caramella, C.; Columbo, P.; Conte, U.; LaManna, A. Swelling of Disintegrant Particles and Disintegrating Force of Tablets. Labo-Pharma. Probl. Tech. **1984**, *32*, 115–119.
19. Caramella, C.; Columbo, P.; Conte, U.; LaManna, A. Tablet Disintegration Update: The Dynamic Approach. Drug Dev. Ind. Pharm. **1987**, *13*, 2111–2145.
20. Hess, H. Tablets Under the Microscope. Pharm. Tech. **1978**, *2*, 38–57, 100.
21. Fassihi, A.R. Mechanisms of Disintegration and Compactibility of Disintegrants in a Direct Compression System. Int. J. Pharm. **1986**, *32*, 93–96.
22. Guyot-Hermann, A.M.; Ringard, J. Disintegration Mechanisms of Tablets Containing Starches. Hypothesis About the Particle–Particle Repulsive Force. Drug Dev. Ind. Pharm. **1981**, *7*, 155–177.
23. Matsumara, H. Studies on the Mechanism of Tablet Compression and Disintegration. IV. Evolution of Wetting Heat and Its Reduction by Compressional Force. Yakugaku Zasshi **1959**, *79*, 63–68.
24. List, P.H.; Muazzam, U.A. Swelling —A Driving Force in Tablet Disintegration. Pharm. Ind. **1979**, *41*, 1075–1077.
25. Caramella, C.; Ferrari, F.; Conte, U.; Gazzaniga, A.; LaManna, A.; Colombo, P. Experimental Evidence of Disintegration Mechanisms. Acta Pharm. Tech. **1989**, *35*, 30–33.
26. Luangtana-anan, M.; Catellani, P.L.; Colombo, P.; Dinarvand, R.; Fell, J.T.; Santi, P. The Role of Bond Weakening by Liquids in the Disintegration of Tablets. Eur. J. Pharm. Biopharm. **1992**, *38*, 169–171.
27. Brzeczko, A.W. *Ph.D. Dissertation; A Critical Evaluation of Tablet Disintegration Processes*; University of Maryland: Baltimore, 1989; 129–172, 237–255.
28. Peppas, N.A. Energetics of Tablet Disintegration. Int. J. Pharm. **1989**, *51*, 77–83.
29. Caramella, C.; Colombo, P.; Conte, U.; Ferrari, F.; Gazzaniga, A.; LaManna, A.; Peppas, N.A. A Physical Analysis of the Phenomenon of Tablet Disintegration. Int. J. Pharm. **1988**, *44*, 177–186.

30. Smallenbroek, A.J.; Bolhuis, G.K.; Lerk, C.F. The Effect of Particle Size of Disintegrants on the Disintegration of Tablets. Pharm. Weekbld. **1981**, *116*, 172–175.

31. Schwartz, J.B.; Zelinski, J.A. The Binding and Disintegrant Properties of the Corn Starch Fractions: Amylose and Amylopectin. Drug Dev. Ind. Pharm. **1978**, *4*, 463–483.

32. Shah, N.H.; Bekersky, I.; Jarowski, C.I. *Carboxymethylcellulose: Effect of the Degree of Polymerization and Substitution on Tablet Disintegration and Dissolution. III. Urinary Salicylate from Rapid and Controlled Release Formulas*; Program and Abstracts, APhA. Acad. Pharm. Sci. Mtg., IPT Section, Nov 17, 1983; American Pharmaceutical Assoc. Washington, DC, 1983; 34–35.

33. Khan, K.A.; Rhodes, C.T. Disintegration Properties of Calcium Phosphate Dibasic Dihydrate Tablets. J. Pharm. Sci. **1975**, *64*, 166–168.

34. Khan, K.A.; Rhodes, C.T. Effect of Variation in Compaction Force on Properties of Six Direct Compression Tablet Formulations. J. Pharm. Sci. **1976**, *65*, 1835–1837.

35. Munoz, N.; Ferrero, C.; Munoz-Ruiz, A.; Velasco, M.V.; Jimemez-Castellanos, M.R. Effect of Explotab® On the Tabletability of a Poorly Soluble Drug. Drug Dev. Ind. Pharm. **1998**, *24*, 785–791.

36. Ferrero, C.; Munoz, N.; Velasco, M.V.; Munoz-Ruiz, A.; Jimemez-Castellanos, R. Disintegrating Efficiency of Croscarmellose Sodium in a Direct Compression Formulation. Int. J. Pharm. **1997**, *147*, 11–21.

37. Murthy, K.S.; Ghebre-Sellassie, I. Current Perspectives on the Dissolution Stability of Solid Oral Dosage Forms. J. Pharm. Sci. **1993**, *82*, 113–126.

38. Shotton, E.; Leonard, G.S. Effect of Intragranular and Extragranular Disintegrating Agents on Particle Size of Disintegrated Tablets. J. Pharm. Sci. **1976**, *65*, 1170–1174.

39. Van Kamp, H.V.; Bolhuis, G.K.; Lerk, C.F. Improvement by Super Disintegrants of the Properties of Tablets Containing Lactose, Prepared by Wet Granulation. Pharm. Weekbld. Sci. Ed. **1983**, *5*, 165–171.

40. Gordon, M.S.; Chatterjee, B.; Chowan, Z.T. Effect of the Mode of Croscarmellose Sodium Incorporation on Tablet Dissolution and Friability. J. Pharm. Sci. **1990**, *79*, 43–47.

41. Khattab, I.; Menon, A.; Sakr, A. Effect of Mode of Incorporation of Disintegrants on the Characteristics of Fluid-Bed Wet-Granulated Tablets. J. Pharm. Pharmacol. **1993**, *45*, 687–691.

42. Becker, D.; Rigassi, T.; Bauer-Brandl, A. Effectiveness of Binders in Wet Granulation: A Comparison Using Model Formulations of Different Tabletability. Drug Dev. Ind. Pharm. **1997**, *23*, 791–808.

43. Gould, P.L.; Tan, S.B. The Effect of Recompression on Disintegrant Efficiency in Tablets Prepared by Wet Granulation. Drug Dev. Ind. Pharm. **1985**, *11*, 441–460.

44. Gould, P.L.; Tan, S.B. The Effect of Recompression on the Swelling Kinetics of Wet Massed Tablets, Containing 'Super' Disintegrants. Drug Dev. Ind. Pharm. **1985**, *11*, 1819–1836.

45. Botzolakis, J.E.; Small, L.E.; Augsburger, L.L. Effect of Disintegrants on Drug Dissolution from Capsules Filled on a Dosator-Type Automatic Capsule-Filling Machine. Int. J. Pharm. **1982**, *12*, 341–349.

46. Botzolakis, J.E.; Augsburger, L.L. The Role of Disintegrants in Hard-Gelatin Capsules. J. Pharm. Pharmacol. **1984**, *36*, 77–84.

47. Botzolakis, J.E.; Augsburger, L.L. Disintegrating Agents in Hard-Gelatin Capsules. Part I: Mechanism of Action. Drug Dev. Ind. Pharm. **1988**, *14*, 29–41.

48. Antony, P.J.; Sanghavi, N.M. A New Disintegrant for Pharmaceutical Dosage Forms. Drug Dev. Ind. Pharm. **1997**, *23*, 413–415.

49. Rizk, S.; Barthelemy, C.; Duru, C.; Guyot-Hermann, A.M. Investigation on a New Modified USP Xanthan with Tablet-Disintegrating Properties. Drug Dev. Ind. Pharm. **1997**, *23*, 19–26.

BIBLIOGRAPHY

Buckton, G. The Role of Compensation Analysis in the Study of Wettability, Solubility, Disintegration, and Dissolution. Int. J. Pharm. **1990**, *66*, 175–182.

Caramella, C.; Colombo, P.; Conte, U.; Ferrari, F.; La Manna, A. Water Uptake and Disintegrating Force Measurements: Towards a General Understanding of Disintegration Mechanisms. Drug Dev. Ind. Pharm. **1986**, *12*, 1749–1766.

Carstensen, J.T.; Chowan, Z.T. Correlation Between Tablet Disintegration and In Vitro Dissolution. Drug Dev. Ind. Pharm. **1980**, *6*, 569–571.

Kanig, J.L.; Rudnic, E.M. The Mechanisms of Disintegrant Action. Pharm. Tech. **1984**, *8*, 50–63.

Mahmoud, H.M.; El-Shaboury, M.H. Effect of Certain Tablet Ingredients on the Penetration Rate of Powder Beds. **1985**, *94*, 125–131.

Nogami, H.; Fukuzawa, H.; Nakai, Y. Studies on Tablet Disintegration. I. The Effect of Penetrating Rate on Tablet Disintegration. **1963**, *11*, 1389–1398.

Pesonen, T.; Paronen, P.; Ketolainen Disintegrant Properties of an Agglomerated Cellulose Powder. Int. J. Pharm. **1989**, *57*, 139–147.

Shangraw, R.F.; Mitrvej, A.; Shah, M.N. A New Era of Tablet Disintegrants. Pharm. Tech. **1980**, *4*, 49–57.

SURFACTANTS IN PHARMACEUTICAL PRODUCTS AND SYSTEMS

Owen I. Corrigan
Anne Marie Healy
University of Dublin, Trinity College, Dublin, Ireland

INTRODUCTION

Surface-active agents (surfactants) are substances which, at low concentrations, adsorb onto the surfaces or interfaces of a system and alter the surface or interfacial free energy and the surface or interfacial tension. Surface-active agents have a characteristic structure, possessing both polar (hydrophilic) and nonpolar (hydrophobic) regions in the same molecule. Thus surfactants are said to be amphipathic in nature. The wide range of uses for surfactants in pharmaceutical products and systems is the subject of this article.

PHYSICOCHEMICAL BACKGROUND

Surface and Interfacial Tension; Surface and Interfacial Free Energy

Atoms and molecules at surfaces and interfaces possess energies significantly different from those of the same species in the bulk phase. The term "surface" is usually reserved for the region between a condensed phase (liquid or solid) and a gas phase or vacuum, while the term "interface" is normally applied to the region between two condensed phases.

In the case of a liquid–gas interface, molecules of the liquid in the boundary can only develop attractive cohesive forces with molecules situated below and adjacent to them. They can develop attractive adhesive forces with molecules of the gaseous phase. However at the gas–liquid interface, these adhesive forces are quite small. The net effect is that molecules at the surface of the liquid have potential energies greater than those of similar molecules in the interior of the liquid and experience an inward force toward the bulk of liquid. This force pulls the molecules of the interface together and the surface contracts.

Thus, the surface of a liquid behaves as if it were in a state of tension—the surface tension (γ)— due to the contracting force acting in all directions in the plane of the surface.

In order to extend the surface of a liquid it is necessary to bring molecules from the interior to the surface against the inward pull. The work required to increase the surface area by unit area is termed the *surface free energy*.

At the interface between two condensed phases, the dissimilar molecules in the adjacent layers facing each other have potential energies greater than those of similar molecules in the respective bulk phases. This is due to the fact that cohesive forces between like molecules tend to be stronger than adhesive forces between dissimilar molecules. Thus the interfacial tension is the force per unit length existing at the interface between two immiscible or partially miscible condensed phases and the interfacial free energy is the work required to increase the interface by unit area.

Adsorption Phenomena

Adsorption may be defined as the process of enrichment of one or more substances at a surface (1) or as the taking up of one substance at the surface of another (2). It can occur at any type of interface. However, in the context of pharmaceutical systems the interfaces where surfactant adsorption is important are the gas–liquid, liquid–liquid, gas–solid, and liquid–solid interfaces.

Adsorption at liquid–liquid and liquid–gas interfaces

Considering a system of two immiscible phases (e.g., heptane and water), a surface-active molecule that is adsorbed at the interface between the two liquids will tend to orient itself with its hydrophilic end toward the more polar liquid (water), and its hydrophobic end toward the less polar liquid (heptane). Thus the surfactant molecules replace water and/or heptane molecules of the original interface. The interaction across the interface is then between the hydrophilic group of the surfactant and the water molecules on one side of the interface, and between the hydrophobic group of surfactant and heptane on the other side of the interface. These interactions are much stronger than the original interactions between the unlike

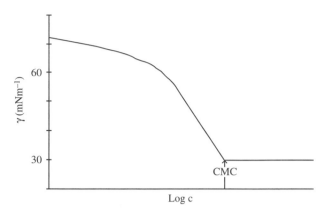

Fig. 1 Schematic plot of surface or interfacial tension (γ) versus logarithm of the surfactant concentration (c).

molecules of heptane and water; therefore the interfacial tension is significantly reduced by the adsorption of surfactant at the interface (i.e., the inward pull for each phase at the interface is reduced).

Air consists of molecules that are mainly nonpolar. Surface tension reduction by surfactants at the air–aqueous interface occurs due to adsorption of surfactants at the interface, with the hydrophilic end of the surfactant oriented toward the liquid. The presence of the surfactant molecules reduces the net inward pull toward the bulk liquid, and therefore reduces the surface tension.

The effect of a surfactant on the lowering of surface tension is shown in Fig. 1. The surface tension is lowered even at low concentrations of surfactant. As the surfactant concentration is increased, the surface layer becomes saturated with surfactant molecules, and micelles form within the bulk liquid as an alternative way of shielding the hydrophobic portions of the surfactants from the aqueous environment; the surface tension tends to a constant value. Micelles are small aggregates of surfactant in which the surfactant molecules are arranged in such a way that the hydrophobic ends are shielded from the surrounding aqueous environment. The concentration at which micelles first appear in solution is termed the critical micelle concentration (CMC).

Adsorption at solid–liquid interfaces

Adsorption of surfactant from an aqueous solution onto a solid surface may involve specific chemical interaction between the surfactant (adsorbate) and the surface (adsorbent).

Common interactions that can occur (3) include:

1. An ion-exchange process
2. An ion-pairing interaction
3. Acid–base interaction via either hydrogen bonding between substrate and adsorbate or Lewis acid–Lewis base reaction
4. Adsorption by polarization of π electrons, where the adsorbate contains electron-rich aromatic nuclei and the adsorbent has strongly positive sites
5. Adsorption by dispersion forces, i.e., London–van der Waals dispersion forces acting between adsorbate and adsorbent
6. Hydrophobic bonding.

Contact Angles and the Wetting of Solids

A drop of liquid when placed on a flat, homogeneous solid surface, comes to equilibrium, assuming a shape which minimizes the total free energy of the system. The angle between the liquid and the solid is called the contact angle (θ), the angle being measured through the liquid (Fig. 2). The contact angle may be calculated if the surface and interfacial tensions are known from Young's equation given in Eq. 1 or 2.

$$\gamma_{SA} = \gamma_{SL} + \gamma_{LA} \cos \theta \qquad (1)$$

or

$$\cos \theta = \frac{\gamma_{SA} - \gamma_{SL}}{\gamma_{LA}} \qquad (2)$$

where γ_{LA} is the surface tension of the liquid, γ_{SL} is the interfacial tension existing between the solid and liquid phases, and γ_{SA} is the surface tension (or surface free energy) of the solid. If $\theta < 90°$, wetting of the solid is said to take place. If $\theta > 90°$, wetting does not take place.

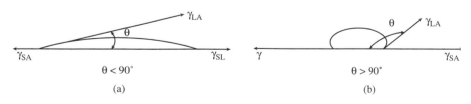

Fig. 2 Contact angles. In (a), $\theta < 90°$, and wetting of the solid occurs; in (b), $\theta > 90°$, and wetting does not take place.

The term "wetting" refers to the displacement from a surface of one fluid by another. It is most commonly applied to the displacement of air from a liquid or solid surface by water or an aqueous solution. The term "wetting agent" is applied to any substance that increases the ability of water or an aqueous solution to displace air from a liquid or solid surface.

For good wetting, $\cos \theta$ should be as close as possible to 1; that is, θ should be as close as possible to 0. From Young's equation, it can be seen that if γ_{LA} or γ_{SL} was minimized, $\cos \theta$ would be maximized, and wetting would be promoted.

Contact angles of water on powders of pharmaceutical importance are usually measured by preparing disks of the powder by compression or melting. However, compaction may change the surface, so making the measured result of little relevance. Contact angles on finely divided solids can also be determined by packing the powder into a tube and measuring the penetration of liquids into the packing.

Three types of wetting phenomena have been described (4): adhesional wetting, spreading wetting, and immersional wetting.

The way in which a particular system behaves depends on the interfacial energies between the solid substrate and any contacting liquid, and between the liquid and the second fluid (air). By manipulating these factors, the wetting process can be controlled. This may be achieved by the use of surfactants.

Modification of the wetting process by the use of surfactants

The effect of surfactants on the wetting process is a result of their adsorption at various interfaces with a resulting alteration of interfacial tensions. As has been noted from Young's equation, the wetting process is promoted if either γ_{LA} or γ_{SL} or both are reduced with γ_{SA} remaining unchanged. Surfactants almost always cause a reduction in γ_{LA}, however, the same cannot be said for γ_{SL} and the effect on the interfacial tension depends on the nature of the adsorption. Thus the addition of a surface-active agent to the system does not always promote wetting, and spreading may in fact be made more difficult (4).

If adsorption of the surfactant molecules at the solid–liquid interface occurs in such a manner that they are oriented with their polar ends toward the substrate and hydrophobic ends toward the liquid, the wettability of an aqueous solution is reduced. This orientation of surfactants molecules at the surface occurs if they are adsorbing to ionic or polar substrates (ion-exchange or ion-pairing mechanism). However, at higher concentrations of surfactant, the surfactant ions adsorb by hydrophobic

interaction with the already adsorbed layer, thus exposing their hydrophilic ends to the solution in such a way that the surface becomes more readily wetted. Thus, the contact angle may first increase and subsequently decrease following the addition of more surfactant to a solution. In contrast, where adsorption occurs onto nonpolar surfaces by, for example, van der Waals attraction, the surfactant molecules are oriented with their hydrophilic groups toward the liquid, the hydrophilicity of the substrate is increased, and it becomes more wettable.

The adsorption of surfactants onto solid surfaces is important with respect to their detergent properties, their use as wetting agents in solid pharmaceutical dosage forms, and as stabilizers for suspension formulations. The mode of action of surfactants in each of these systems is discussed further below.

Micellization

As mentioned previously, surfactant molecules have the ability to form micelles in aqueous solution. These micelles are colloidal-sized clusters of molecules. Micellization is an alternative to interfacial adsorption for removing hydrophobic groups from contact with the aqueous environment, thereby reducing the free energy of the system. In micelles, the hydrophobic groups are directed toward the center of the surfactant aggregate. In cases where there is little distortion of the surrounding solvent by the hydrophobic group, there is little tendency for micellization to occur, such as in water when the hydrophobic group of the surfactant is short or in the case of nonaqueous solvents.

One of the most important applications of micellization in the context of pharmaceuticals is their ability to solubilize drugs of poor aqueous solubility.

Micelles are dynamic species; there is a constant rapid interchange of surfactant molecules between the micelle and the bulk solution. Micelles cannot, therefore, be regarded as rigid structures with a defined shape, although an average micellar shape may be considered.

The main types of micelles recognized (3) are:

1. Small spherical
2. Elongated cylindrical, rodlike micelles with hemispherical ends (prolate ellipsoids)
3. Large, flat lamellar micelles (disklike extended oblate spheroids)
4. Vesicles, more or less spherical structures, consisting of lamellar micelles arranged in one or more concentric spheres.

In nonaqueous solvents, surfactants may form "inverted micelles" where the hydrophilic heads of the surfactant molecules are present in the center of the micelle with the hydrocarbon chains extending outward into the solvent. Dipole–dipole interactions hold the hydrophilic heads of the surfactant molecules together in the core, and in certain cases hydrogen bonding between head groups can also occur.

Micellar shape can be affected by changes in temperature, concentration and the presence of added electrolyte to the liquid phase. Changes in any of these factors may affect micellar size, shape, and aggregation number (number of surfactant monomers in the micelle).

Phase Behavior of Surfactants

Equilibrium phase structures

As the concentration of a surfactant solution is increased, structures of the types depicted in Fig. 3 may be encountered (5). At concentrations well above the CMC,

a more ordered structuring of the solution occurs. Two main types of liquid crystalline phases may be identified: the middle phase, M, exhibiting a hexagonal array of indefinitely long, mutually parallel rods; and the neat phase, G, with a lamellar structure. The liquid crystalline hexagonal phase, like the micellar phase, can exist either in a normal or reverse orientation. The order of phase structures formed upon increasing surfactant concentration generally follows a well defined sequence (Fig. 4) with a "mirror plane" through the lamellar phase in such a way that normal phase structures can be considered to be "oil-in-water" and the reverse structures to be "water-in-oil" (5).

Modified phase structures

In addition to the equilibrium phase structures mentioned above, nonequilibrium surfactant phase structures exist that are also finding applications in drug delivery. Vesicular forms of surfactants are generally formed by dispersing lamellar phases in an excess of water (or nonaqueous polar

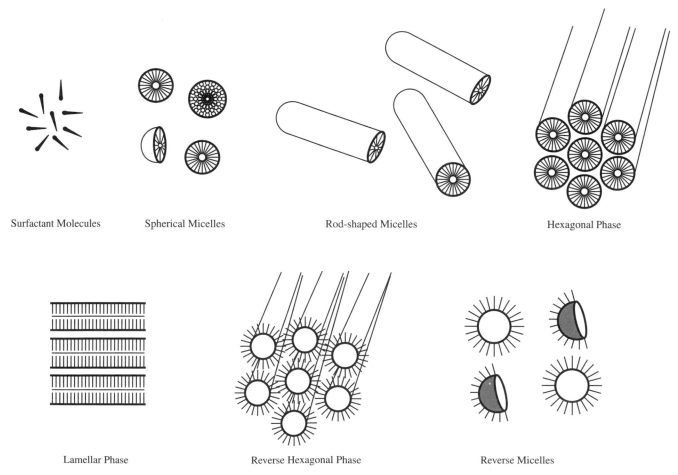

Surfactant Molecules   Spherical Micelles   Rod-shaped Micelles   Hexagonal Phase

Lamellar Phase   Reverse Hexagonal Phase   Reverse Micelles

Fig. 3 Equilibrium phase structures of surfactant molecules. (From Lawrence, M.J. Chem. Soc. Rev. **1994**, *23* (6), 417–424, reproduced by permission of the Royal Society of Chemistry.)

Increasing surfactant concentration

'oil-in-water' 'mirror plane' 'water-in-oil'

H_2O Micelle (L_1) < Hexagonal (H_1) < Lamellar (L_0) < Reversed Hexagonal (H_2) < Reversed Micelle (L_2) Solid

Cubic (I_1)   Cubic (V_1)   Cubic (V_2)   Cubic (I_2)

Fig. 4 Idealized phase sequence in surfactant-water systems. (From Lawrence, M.J. Chem. Soc. Rev. **1994**, *23* (6), 417–424, reproduced by permission of the Royal Society of Chemistry.)

solvents such as ethylene glycol or dimethylformamide) or, in the case of reversed vesicles, in an excess of oil. With most surfactants, vesicles are nonequilibrium structures that will eventually re-equilibrate back into the lamellar phases from which they originated. Vesicles are structural analogs of liposomes (discussed later); they are approximately spherical structures and have the ability to "solubilize" both lipid soluble and water soluble agents.

Several of the phase structures produced by surfactants have potential as carriers and vehicles for drugs and also as targeting systems, used to direct the drug to a specific site in the body (5).

SURFACTANT CLASSIFICATION

Surfactant molecules may be classified based on the nature of the hydrophilic group within the molecule. The four main groups of surfactants are defined as follows:

1. *Anionic surfactants*, where the hydrophilic group carries a negative charge, such as carboxyl ($RCOO^-$), sulphonate (RSO_3^-) or sulphate ($ROSO_3^-$).
   Examples of pharmaceutical importance include potassium laurate, $CH_3(CH_2)_{10}COO^- K^+$, and sodium lauryl sulphate, $CH_3(CH_2)_{11}SO_4^- Na^+$.
2. *Cationic surfactants*, where the hydrophilic group carries a positive charge (e.g., quaternary ammonium halides, $R_4N^+Cl^-$). Examples of pharmaceutical importance include cetrimide, a mixture consisting mainly of tetradecyl (ca. 68%), dodecyl (ca. 22%), and hexadecyltrimethylammonium bromides (ca. 7%), as well as benzalkonium chloride, a mixture of alkylbenzyldimethylammonium chlorides of the general formula $[C_6H_5CH_2N^+(CH_3)_2R]Cl^-$, where R represents a mixture of the alkyls from C_8H_{17} to $C_{18}H_{37}$.
3. *Ampholytic surfactants (also called zwitterionic surfactants)*, where the molecule contains, or can potentially contain, both a negative and a positive charge, (e.g., the sulfobetaines, $RN^+(CH_3)_2CH_2CH_2SO_3^-$). Examples of pharmaceutical importance include

N-Dodecyl-*N*,*N*-Dimethylbetaine, $C_{12}H_{25}N^+(CH_3)_2CH_2COO^-$.
4. *Nonionic surfactants*, where the hydrophile carries no charge but derives its water solubility from highly polar groups such as hydroxyl or polyoxyethylene (OCH_2CH_2O—) groups. Examples of pharmaceutical importance include polyoxyethylated glycol monoethers (e.g. cetomacrogol), sorbitan esters (Spans®) and polysorbates (Tweens®).

Tables 1–4 in the article *Surfactants in Pharmaceutical Products and Systems* in Volume 14 of the first edition of this encyclopedia (6), together with the references cited therein, give listings of some of the surfactants most commonly used in pharmaceuticals, along with the purpose(s) for which they are usually employed.

SURFACTANT USES IN PHARMACEUTICAL PREPARATIONS

Because of their unique functional properties, surfactants find a wide range of uses in pharmaceutical preparations. These include, depending on the type of product, improving the solubility or stability of a drug in a liquid preparation, stabilizing and modifying the texture of a semisolid preparation, or altering the flow properties of a granulate, thus aiding in the processing of the final tablet dosage form. In addition to their use as excipients to improve the physical and chemical characteristics of the formulation, surfactants may be included to improve the efficacy or bioperformance of the product. The properties of surfactants are such that they can alter the thermodynamic activity, solubility, diffusion, disintegration, and dissolution rate of a drug. Each of these parameters influence the rate and extent of drug absorption. Furthermore, surfactants can exert direct effects on biological membranes thus altering drug transport across the membrane. The overall effect of inclusion of a surfactant in a pharmaceutical formulation is complex and may be beyond those initially intended.

Surfactants may reduce the effectiveness of antimicrobials or preservatives included in a formulation (7). They also have the capacity to damage biological membranes.

LIQUID SYSTEMS

Solutions

Surfactants as solubilizing agents

Solubilization can be defined as "the preparation of a thermodynamically stable isotropic solution of a substance normally insoluble or very slightly soluble in a given solvent by the introduction of an additional amphiphilic component or components" (4). The amphiphilic components (surfactants) must be introduced at a concentration at or above their critical micelle concentrations. Simple micellar systems (and reverse micellar) as well as liquid crystalline phases and vesicles referred to above are all capable of solubilization. In liquid crystalline phases and vesicles, a ternary system is formed on incorporation of the solubilizate and thus these anisotropic systems are not strictly in accordance with the definition given above (4).

Solubilization by micelles

The location of a solubilized molecule in a micelle is determined primarily by the chemical structure of the solubilizate. Solubilization can occur at a number of different sites in a micelle:

1. On the surface, at the micelle–solvent interface,
2. Between the hydrophilic head groups,
3. In the palisades layer, i.e., between the hydrophilic groups and the first few carbon atoms of the hydrophobic groups that comprise the outer regions of the micelle core,
4. More deeply in the palisades layer, and
5. In the micelle inner core.

In aqueous systems, nonpolar additives such as hydrocarbons tend to be intimately associated with the hydrocarbon core of the micelle. Polar and semipolar materials, such as fatty acids and alcohols are usually located in the palisades layer, the depth of penetration depending on the ratio of polar to nonpolar structures in the solubilizate molecule.

In reverse micelles (formed in nonpolar solvent systems containing surfactant), polar additives may be solubilized in the core where a polar interaction of head groups occurs.

A preferred location of the solubilizate molecule within the micelle is largely dictated by chemical structure. However, solubilized systems are dynamic and the location of molecules within the micelle changes rapidly with time. Solubilization in surfactant aqueous systems above the critical micelle concentration offers one pathway for the formulation of poorly soluble drugs (7). From a quantitative point of view, the solubilization process above the CMC may be considered to involve a simple partition phenomenon between an aqueous and a micellar phase. Thus the relationship between surfactant concentration C_m and drug solubility C_{tot} is given by Eq. 3.

$$C_{tot} = C_s + PC_sC_m \tag{3}$$

where C_s is the drug solubility in the absence of surface-active agent and P is the distribution coefficient of drug between the micelle and bulk phases. A plot of C_{tot} versus C_m is linear with a slope of PC_s, which is the solubilizing capacity of the micelle (8).

The effect of altering the pH of the vehicle, in the case of a partly ionized drug will be to alter the apparent partition coefficient. Thus the effect of increasing the pH of a vehicle containing an acidic drug is to reduce the proportion of drug in the micellar phase. If the surfactant is a weak electrolyte, it may induce a concentration-dependent change in pH thus altering drug partitioning and solubility (9).

In general the solubilizing capacity for surfactants with the same hydrocarbon chain length increases in the order anionic < cationic < nonionic, the effect being attributed to a corresponding increase in the area per head group, leading to looser micelles with less dense hydrocarbon cores which can accommodate more solute.

The solubilizing capacity for a given surfactant system is a complex function of the physicochemical properties of the two components which, in turn, influence the location or sites where the drug is bound to the micelle. The molar volume of the solubilizate together with its lipophilicity are important factors, the former reducing and the latter increasing solubilization (9).

Many pharmaceutical products contain a number of solutes potentially capable of being solubilized within the micellar phase. Thus competition can occur between solutes resulting in an altered solubilizing capacity. Furthermore, the addition of a second highly solubilized component to form a mixed micellar system may greatly alter the structure, size and solubilizing capacity of the system, thereby greatly enhancing drug solubility.

Solubilization has been used for many years in the formulation of phenolic antiseptic and disinfectant solutions. In the case of Cresol and Soap Solution (Lysol) and Chloroxylenol Solution B.P., soap micelles are used to solubilize the phenolic substances. The soap (anionic surfactant) is formed by reaction of potassium hydroxide with a suitable oil such as linseed oil (in Cresol and Soap Solution) or castor oil (in Chloroxylenol Solution). The solubilizing potential of surfactant solutions for hydrophobic species has also been exploited in the design of cholelitholytic solvents for gallstone dissolution with some limited success.

Stability of drugs in solubilized systems

Solubilization of a drug by incorporation into micelles may affect its stability (7). In the micelle, the molecular environment of the drug molecules changes their proximity and orientation with respect to each other, which may affect activity. In a micelle, the drug molecules may be protected from attacking species such as hydronium or hydroxide ions and the stability of the drug may be increased. The difference in environment between the micellar and bulk aqueous phases may be such that reaction rates may be radically changed by the transfer of solute to micelles. Micellar systems may be used to deliberately alter the rates and directions of chemical reactions (7).

AB block copolymer micelles

It is well known that block copolymers in a selective solvent (a good solvent for one block but a nonsolvent for the other) form a micellar structure through the association of the insoluble segments (10). In contrast with micelles formed from low molecular weight surfactants, block copolymer micelles dissociate slowly to free polymeric chains. They have a greater capacity for solubilizing aromatic molecules and express lower CMCs. The AB block copolymers are considered useful vehicles for hydrophobic drugs.

Only a few block copolymers form micellar structures in aqueous milieu. One example is a series of polyethylene oxide/polypropylene oxide/polyethylene oxide block copolymers known as Pluronics (tradename) or poloxamers. The poloxamers have been used widely in pharmaceuticals, particularly as emulsifiers for intravenous lipids (7). At low concentrations, poloxamer monomers are thought to form monomolecular micelles by a change in configuration in solution (7). At higher concentrations, aggregation of the monomolecular micelles occurs. The aggregates so formed show the ability to solubilize drugs and increase the stability of solubilized materials. Poloxamers have low toxicity and their solubilization capabilities might prove useful in the delivery of hydrophobic drugs, although multimolecular micelle formation with core-shell structure is uncertain under physiological conditions (11).

Other block copolymers have been prepared and studied as formulation adjuvants for hydrophobic drugs, e.g., poly(ethylene oxide)/poly(aspartic acid) and poly (ethylene oxide)/poly(β-benzyl-L-asparate) block copolymers have been used with adriamycin (12, 13).

Suspensions

If a suspension is to be produced by a dispersion technique (as opposed to precipitation techniques), surfactants may be used in the formulation to aid dispersion of the solid particles in the liquid. This is particularly important if the powder is not readily wetted by the liquid vehicle. Surfactants can reduce the interfacial tension between the solid particles and the liquid vehicle. The advancing contact angle is reduced, and wetting of the solid particles promoted. Such a system is said to be deflocculated. The inclusion of a surface-active agent to improve powder wettability can often improve the bioavailability of the formulation.

The forces at the surface of a particle affect the degree of flocculation and agglomeration in a suspension. Particles dispersed in a liquid medium may become charged in one of two main ways. Ionic species present in solution may be adsorbed at the surface or, alternatively charges on the surface may arise due to ionization of groups (such as carboxyl groups for example) which may be located at the surface. The surface charge will influence the distribution of ions in the aqueous medium surrounding the solid particles. The result is the formation of what is known as an "electric double layer." If the surface charge is positive, immediately adjacent to the surface will be a region of tightly bound solvent molecules and negative counterions. Thus, the first layer is tightly bound, while the second layer (which still contains an excess of negative ions) is more diffuse (14). As two particles approach each other in aqueous medium, a weak attractive force exists just beyond the range of the double-layer-repulsive forces. This region is responsible for the particle interaction termed "flocculation."

Flocculated particles are weakly bonded, settle rapidly, do not form a cake and so are easily resuspended. For this reason it is frequently desirable to promote flocculation in a suspension.

The inclusion of surfactants in the formulation is one way of achieving what is known as "controlled flocculation." Surfactants can cause dispersed solids to flocculate by a number of different mechanisms (3). The first is where there is an electrostatic attraction of surfactant ions to oppositely charged sites on the particle surface, resulting in a lowering of the electrical energy barrier to the close approach of two particles to each other. Flocculation may also occur by a bridging mechanism. A long (usually polymeric) surfactant molecule containing functional groups at various sites may adsorb onto sites on the surface of adjacent particles, holding the particles together in a loose arrangement. Alternatively if the surfactant molecules adsorb in such a manner that the molecule extends into the liquid phase, interaction of the extended portions of surfactant molecules adsorbed to different particles result in bridging of those particles.

Another method of employing surfactants to achieve flocculation is to first treat the particles with an ionic surfactant to disperse them. A readily soluble electrolyte is then added which has the effect of compressing the electrical double layer surrounding each particle, allowing flocculation to occur. Subsequent dilution of this type of system will redisperse it (due to a decrease in electrolyte concentration).

Emulsions

Emulsification is one of the most important applications of surface-active agents in pharmaceutical systems. The phenomenon has been extensively studied and many books and chapters of books have been devoted to the subject.

Macroemulsions are either oil in water (o/w) or water in oil (w/o). The type of emulsion formed depends largely on the emulsifying agent used; the process and relative proportions of the oil and water phases are less important. In general, o/w emulsions are produced by emulsifying agents that are more soluble in the water phase than in the oil phase, and w/o emulsions are produced by emulsifying agents that are more soluble in the oil phase. It is also possible to form a multiple emulsion. For example, a small water or aqueous solution droplet may be enclosed in a larger oil droplet which is itself dispersed in an aqueous phase. Such a system is referred to as a "water-in-oil-in-water" (w/o/w) emulsion. It is also possible to from an o/w/o emulsion.

Many medicinal agents which have an unpalatable taste or texture can be made more acceptable for oral administration when formulated as emulsions. Mineral-oil-based laxatives, oil soluble vitamins and high-fat nutritive preparations are frequently administered in the form of o/w emulsions. It has been shown that in some cases the absorption of drugs may be enhanced if formulated as emulsions (15). Emulsions (o/w) have also been used for the intravenous administration of lipid nutrients. Radiopaque emulsions have been used as diagnostic agents in X-ray examinations.

Emulsification is widely used in pharmaceutical products for external application such as lotions and creams, and in aerosol products to form foams. Semisolid emulsified formulations are discussed below.

Based on the size of the dispersed particles or droplets, emulsions may be classified (16) into

1. Macroemulsions, droplets ~0.1–50 μm, opaque emulsions
2. Microemulsions, droplets 10–100 nm, transparent dispersions.

Stabilization of the dispersion of one immiscible liquid in another requires the addition of an emulsifying agent which is commonly a surfactant or a mixture of surfactants.

In the formation of an emulsion, one of the two immiscible liquids is broken up into droplets which are dispersed in the other liquid. The dispersion of one liquid in another immiscible liquid leads to a large increase in interfacial free energy because of the increase in the area of the interface. The emulsifying agent stabilises the emulsion by adsorbing at the liquid–liquid interface as an oriented interfacial film. This film reduces the interfacial tension between the liquids and also decreases the rate of coalescence of the dispersed droplets by forming mechanical, steric and/or electrical barriers around them.

A strong mechanical barrier lessens the chance of droplets coalescing on collision. For maximum mechanical stability, the interfacial film of the adsorbed surfactants should be close packed with strong lateral interactions. For this reason, a mixture of two or more surfactants is commonly used as the emulsifying agent, such as a combination of a water-soluble surfactant and an oil-soluble surfactant. In pharmaceutical (o/w) systems a mixture of a sorbitol ester (Span®) with a polyoxyethyleneated sorbitol ester (Tween®) is often used. The water soluble Tween tends to a have a greater interaction with the aqueous phase, its hydrophilic group extending further into the water than that of the nonoxyethyleneated ester. This is believed to facilitate interaction of the hydrophobic groups of the molecules, as they can approach each other more closely in the interfacial film.

The interfacial film can also stabilize the emulsion by producing repulsive electrical forces between approaching droplets. This repulsion is due to surface charge on the droplets. The surface charge effect is believed to be important only in the case of o/w emulsions. The source of surface charge is the hydrophilic head of the surfactant molecules which is oriented toward the aqueous continuous phase. In emulsions containing ionic surfactant molecules, the charge on the disperse phase droplets is due to the amphipathic ion. In the case of nonionic surfactants, the charge may arise either from adsorption of ions from the aqueous phase or from frictional contact between droplets and the aqueous phase. In the latter case, the phase with the higher dielectric constant is positively charged (3).

Microemulsions

Microemulsions consist of large or "swollen" micelles, containing an internal phase similar to that found in a solubilized solution (16). Unlike macroemulsions, they appear as clear, transparent solutions. They tend to be more thermodynamically stable than macroemulsions and can have essentially infinite lifetimes assuming no change in composition, temperature and pressure. This is in contrast to macroemulsions which, although they may remain stable for long periods of time, will ultimately undergo phase separation to attain a minimum in free energy. Microemulsions can generally be obtained by gentle mixing of the ingredients of the emulsion. In this respect, they differ from macroemulsions which require intense agitation for their formation. Microemulsions are usually prepared with more than one surfactant or using a mixture of surfactant and cosurfactant (e.g., a polar compound of intermediate chain length).

Microemulsions have been studied as drug delivery systems, in particular for topical and transdermal drug delivery (17, 18).

Microspherical particles prepared by emulsification processes

Emulsification–evaporation processes are widely used in the preparation of polymer based microspherical drug-loaded particulates. For example, hydrophobic drug-loaded PLA (polylactic acid) or PGLA (polylactide-co-glycolide) biodegradable microspheres are often prepared from emulsions containing a non aqueous dispersed phase of dichloromethane containing the drug and polymer in an aqueous continuous phase. For the preparation of hydrophilic drug loaded microspheres a double-emulsion process may be necessary. The nature of the surfactants used to stabilize the emulsion phases can greatly influence the size, size distribution, surface morphology, loading, drug release, and bioperformance of the final multiparticulate product.

Aerosols

Surfactants are found in both solution and suspension formulations of metered dose inhalers (MDIs). The most common surfactants found in pressurised aerosol preparations include sorbitan trioleate (Span 85), oleic acid, and lecithins at concentrations of 0.1–2.0% (w/w). These agents are nonvolatile liquids which dissolve in the propellant blend. Their function in the formulation is to provide lubrication for the metering valves and, in the case of suspension formulations, to maintain the disperse nature of the drug.

The three surfactants commonly used in chlorofluro-carbon (CFC)-based MDI formulations are insoluble in the CFC-replacement propellants, hydrofluoroalkane (HFA) 134a and HFA 227. Possible formulation alternatives involve the use of an adjuvant such as ethanol to aid dissolution of the surfactant or a novel surfactant. Several companies have investigated novel materials among which are fluorosurfactants, polyoxyethylenes and drugs coated with surfactant (19).

Controlled flocculation in metered-dose aerosol suspensions

Controlled flocculation is a widely used technique for stabilizing suspended systems. The aim is to alter particle surface charge or to achieve particle separation via steric hindrance with the help of appropriate stabilizing excipients. However this is particularly difficult to achieve in nonpolar systems such as suspensions in CFC (or HFA) propellants. Controlled flocculation to optimise the stabilisation of MDIs has been recommended by Ranucci et al. (20) but disputed by Hickey et al. (21).

Liposomes

Liposomes are single- or multilayered phospholipids vesicles. They are roughly spherical in shape and consist of lipid bilayers alternating with aqueous regions.

Liposomes have shown potential as drug delivery systems. The exact location of a drug molecule in a liposome depends on its physicochemical composition and the composition of the lipids. Water soluble drugs may be included in the aqueous phase, and oil-soluble drugs may be added to the membrane-forming phospholipid. An extensive account of the pharmaceutical use of liposomes is found in the article "*Liposomes as Pharmaceutical Dosage Forms*," by Y. Barenholz, and D.J.A., Crommelin, Volume 9 of the first edition of this encyclopedia (22).

SEMISOLID SYSTEMS

Surfactants are major constituents of pharmaceutical, cosmetic, and food semisolid formulations, many of which are emulsions, either oil in water (o/w) or water in oil (w/o). They are included for their stabilizing, wetting, solubilizing, detergent and penetration-enhancing properties.

Water-in-oil emulsions traditionally contain surfactants of natural origin such as cholesterol, wool fat, wool alcohols, lanolin, divalent salts of fatty acids soaps, calcium oleate and/or synthetic agents of low hydrophilic-lipophilic balance (HLB) (indicating high lipophilicity), such as Spans (fatty acid esters of sorbitan). An example of such a product is Oily Cream B.P. which consists of a 1:1 mixture of wool alcohols and water.

Oil-in-water creams, for topical use, generally contain mixed emulsifiers/surfactants; one of which is a water soluble surfactant with a high HLB, the other being an amphiphile, usually a long chain fatty alcohol (e.g., of chain length C_{14} to C_{18}) or acid (e.g., palmitic or stearic). The water soluble surfactant may be anionic (e.g., sodium lauryl sulphate), cationic (e.g., cetrimide), or nonionic (e.g., cetomacrogol, Tweens).

These mixed-surfactant systems are used not only for their ability to form complex condensed films at the liquid–liquid interface, enhancing the stability of the emulsion, but also because of their ability to impart "body" to the product, resulting in a semisolid product rather than a liquid. Mixed emulsifiers control the consistency of a cream by forming a viscoelastic network throughout the continuous phase of the emulsion. The network results from the interaction of the mixed emulsifier with water, forming a liquid crystalline phase.

Foams

Emulsification is used in aerosol products to produce foams which are generally formulated as o/w emulsions. The liquified propellant forms the disperse phase of the emulsion, and the medication is usually in the aqueous continuous phase. On discharge from the pressurised container, the propellant vaporizes to form bubbles which remain trapped within the aqueous phase giving rise to a foam. These are referred to as "stable foam" products. Nonaqueous stable foams may also be formulated, where the water is replaced by various glycols such as polyethylene glycol. "Quick breaking foams" result when the propellant is in the external phase. The product is emitted as a foam and collapses into a liquid.

Biological Effects on Percutaneous Absorption

Surfactants—traditionally common constituents and stabilizers of topical vehicles, ranging from hydrophobic agents such as oleic acid to hydrophilic sodium lauryl

sulphate—have been tested as penetration enhancers to improve transdermal drug delivery. Ionic surfactants are thought to enhance transdermal absorption by disordering the lipid layer of the stratum corneum and by denaturation of keratin. The use of penetration enhancers in general, and surfactants in particular, in transdermal therapeutic systems has been reviewed by Walters (23).

SOLID DOSAGE FORMS

Surface-active agents have been widely shown to enhance drug dissolution rates. This may be due to wetting effects, resulting in increased surface area, effects on solubility and effective diffusion coefficient or a combination of effects. Consequently surfactants have been included in tablet and capsule formulations to improve wetting and deaggregation of drug particles and thus increase the surface area of particles available for dissolution.

This wetting effect is found to be operative at concentrations below the CMC. The effect of surfactants on the dissolution of solids is complex. In addition to effects on the available surface area, surfactants in concentrations above the CMC can increase drug solubility and hence the effective concentration gradient. However they also reduce the effective rate of drug diffusion as a consequence of drug solubilization within micelles. Models to quantify the effect of surfactant concentration on drug dissolution have been developed (24). For solids whose dissolution is under significant surface control, surfactants may further influence the dissolution process. In this regard the enhancing effect of surfactants on the dissolution rate of cholesterol has been widely studied (25).

Hard Gelatin Capsules and Tablets

Wetting agents

Surfactants are used in capsule (26) and tablet formulations as wetting agents to aid dissolution.

Lubricants, anti-adherents, and glidants

The primary function of tablet lubricants is to reduce the friction arising at the interface of tablet and die walls during compression and ejection. Lubricants also possess antiadherent (prevention of sticking to the punch and, to a lesser extent, to the die wall) and glidant (improvement of flow characteristics of powders or granulates) characteristics and are useful in the processing of hard gelatin capsules.

Magnesium stearate is used extensively as a lubricant in tablet manufacture. It is an example of a "boundary lubricant," that is, the polar regions of the molecule adhere to the metal surface of the die wall (in tablet manufacture). Adsorption of magnesium stearate to the powder or granule surfaces also prevents agglomeration of the feed material and aids flow.

Lubricants may be classified as water-soluble or water-insoluble. The latter are generally more effective than water-soluble lubricants and can be used at a lower concentration (27). Common water-insoluble lubricants (which are surfactants) include magnesium stearate, calcium stearate, sodium stearate, and stearic acid; water-soluble lubricants include sodium lauryl sulphate and magnesium lauryl sulphate.

Sodium lauryl sulphate is used in the production of hard gelatin capsules where it is added to the gelatin solution during the preparation stage. The stainless steel molds are lubricated prior to dipping into the gelatin solution and sodium lauryl sulphate is added to reduce the surface tension of the mix and cause the mold pins to wet more uniformly (28).

Solid Dispersion Systems

The bioavailability of hydrophobic drugs can be increased by strategies designed to enhance the dissolution rate of the drug. This has been achieved in many cases by forming a solid dispersion of the drug in a suitable carrier, often a hydrophilic polymer such as polyethylene glycol (PEG) or polyvinylpyrrolidone (PVP). The drug is dispersed in the carrier by coprecipitation from a suitable solution containing both drug and carrier, by melting both components together, or by some other process involving a phase change. By using relatively high concentrations of carrier and a rapid precipitating process, the drug may form as an amorphous or molecularly dispersed high energy phase in the carrier. A number of workers have used surfactants as the carrier material to achieve this enhanced dissolution effect. Among the surfactants employed are polyoxyethylene stearate, Renex 650, poloxamer 188, Texafor AIP deoxycholic acid, and Tweens and Spans. Surfactants have also been added to conventional drug–polymer solid dispersions to further improve drug release properties. Sjokvist et al. (29) found that the incorporation of sodium dodecyl sulphate (1–2%) in griseofulvin (3–10%)-PEG solid dispersions eliminated any traces of crystalline drug, griseofulvin being present as a solid solution. Other three-component solid dispersions containing surfactants have also been reported such as Tween 20-Griseofulvin-PEG and Tween 20-Oxodipine-

PEG (30). Problems have been reported however as to the physical stability of surfactant containing systems, dissolution rates decreasing over a 12-month period (31).

Matrix Systems

Drug release from nondisintegrating inert matrices, fabricated from hydrophobic carriers such as polyethylene, is improved by the presence of surfactants in the dissolution medium. Drug release was shown to be a function of the pore size distribution of the matrix and the permeation pressure of the release media defined by its surface tension and contact angle. Inclusion of dioctyl sodium succinate, which reduced the contact angle below 90°, greatly enhanced drug release; increasing the concentration of polysorbate in the range of 0.001–0.1% had the same effect (32). Surfactants have also been included in matrix-type drug delivery systems to aid penetration of the dissolution medium thus increasing the rate and extent of drug release.

Suppositories

Several nonionic surface-active materials have been developed as suppositories vehicles. Many of these bases, known as water-dispersible bases, can be used for the formulation of both water-soluble and oil-soluble drugs (33). The surfactants most commonly used are the polyoxyethylene sorbitan fatty acid esters (Tweens), the polyoxyethylene stearates, and the sorbitan fatty acid esters (Spans). These surfactants may be used alone, blended, or with other suppository base materials to yield a wide range of melting points and consistencies.

Surface-active agents are widely used in combination with other suppository bases. The inclusion of these agents in the formulation may improve the wetting and water-absorption properties of the suppository. In addition, emulsifying surfactants help to keep insoluble substances suspended in a fatty base suppository (33).

The inclusion of a surfactant in the suppository formulation may enhance the rectal absorption of drugs. The effect has been attributed to the formation of mixed micelles. It has been suggested that the presence of the micelle facilitates the incorporation of the lipid component of the mixed micelle into the biological membrane. This lipid then enhances the fluidity and permeability of the membrane to the poorly absorbed drug. It appears that the colorectal mucous membrane is more sensitive to the effects of mixed micelles than the gastrointestinal membrane of the small intestine.

Surfactant Influence on Drug Absorption from the Gastrointestinal Tract

In the context of oral dosage forms containing surfactants, these agents may play a role in reducing the rate of gastric emptying and retarding the movement of drug to the absorption site by increasing the viscosity of the formulation. This is thought to be especially true of polyoxyethylene derivatives. Bile salts, which are physiological surfactants, have been shown to affect the rate of gastric emptying. The presence of bile salts in the stomach has also been shown to affect ionic movement across the gastric mucosa, thus increasing the movement of hydrogen and chloride ions out of the lumen.

Surfactants may also affect the rate and extent of drug absorption by exerting an influence on the permeability of the biomembrane. Competitive binding of the surfactant to the membrane protein is considered to be partially responsible for enhanced drug absorption in many cases. Alternatively, the enhancement may be due to allosteric rearrangement of the membrane protein which is triggered by the binding of one or more permeating species.

Nakanishi et al. (34) studied the effect of a range of surfactants on the rectal absorption of sulphaguanidine and found absorption to be increased. The increase was associated with histological changes in rectal membrane, increasing the rectal permeability. The same authors found that surfactants such as sodium deoxycholate and sodium dodecyl sulphate used together with the chelating agent EDTA could increase the rectal absorption of macromolecules such as inulin, insulin, and albumin.

The membrane effects of surfactants are explained by a combination of membrane-surfactant binding, disruption of membranes through solubilization into lipoproteins, proteins, and mixed micelles, protein–protein interactions, and selective solubilization of some membrane components by the surfactant. The structure of the surfactant may play a role in determining the range and extent of the influence of a particular surfactant on drug absorption. It appears that the greatest effect is achieved by molecules having a C12–C16 hydrocarbon chain, polyoxyethylene chain lengths between 10 and 20, and molecular areas between 1.0 and 1.6 nm^2 (4). These effects, in the case of drugs of low aqueous solubility, are in addition to the higher absorption rate, arising from an increase in drug solubility (35, 36).

Surfactants, at high concentrations, exhibit some toxicity and have the ability in many cases to disrupt a membrane. Both ionic and nonionic surfactants have been shown to assist the breakdown of the mucous layer covering the epithelium and at high concentrations are thought to interfere with the membrane itself, which may lead to disruption of membrane metabolism, particularly with regard to enzyme systems associated with the membrane. Adverse reactions to drug formulation agents including surfactants have been reviewed by Weiner and Bernstein (37).

DIRECT ACTIONS OF SURFACTANTS

Detergents

Detergents are surfactants that are used for the removal of foreign matter from a solid surface. The process involves many of the actions specific to surfactant molecules. The surfactant requires good wetting properties to ensure good contact with the solid surface. It must also have the ability to remove dirt into the bulk liquid. This is achieved by a lowering the dirt–liquid and solid–liquid interfacial tensions, thus reducing the work of adhesion between the dirt and the solid and enabling the dirt to be readily detached. Once detached, adsorption of surfactant at the dirt particle surface prevents deposition, allowing the dirt to be washed away. If the dirt is oily it may be emulsified or solubilized by the surfactant.

Antimicrobial Activity

Significant antimicrobial effects have been associated with cationic surfactants, in particular the quaternary compounds. The action mechanism of quaternary surfactants involves disruption of the cell membrane, protein denaturation, and enzyme inhibition. Quaternary compounds are able to lyse cells at relatively low concentration, resulting in leakage of cell contents into the surrounding medium. Quaternary ammonium and some phosphonium surfactants are used as topical disinfectants in commercial dermatological products, in surgical hand scrubs, and in the irrigation of skin wounds. The most commonly used quaternary compounds employed for their antimicrobial effects are cetylpyridinium chloride, benzalkonium chloride, benzethonium chloride and cetyltrimethylammonium bromide (38). Other surfactants, containing more than one quaternary (or positively ionizable group) are among the most active substances known in terms of antimicrobial activity. Included in this group are dequalinium acetate and chlorhexidine gluconate which have been used in throat lozenges and mouthwashes. The lysis of cells can also occur in the presence of anionic surfactants, although these are in general weaker in their antimicrobial activity. A wide range of anionics, in particular sodium lauryl sulphate and its homologs, finds wide application in mouthwashes (38).

Respiratory Distress Syndrome (RDS)

In 1959, surfactant deficiency was identified as the major pathogenic factor in respiratory distress syndrome in infants (39). Pulmonary surfactant is a complex mixture of phospholipids, neutral lipids, and specific proteins which spread as a monolayer at the air-liquid interfaces of the lung and lower surface tension at end-expiration thus preventing alveolar collapse. If the amount or quality of endogenous surfactant is inadequate, inspiratory pressure and the work of breathing must increase in order to re-expand the alveoli with each breath and permit adequate gas exchange. As the infant grows tired, progressive respiratory failure occurs.

Phosphatidylcholine is the major component of endogenous surfactant, constituting about 60% of total phospholipids, and dipalmitoylphosphatidylcholine (DPPC) is the primary surface-tension lowering phospholipid.

The surfactant replacement therapy treatment used may be either "natural" or "artificial." Natural surfactants are derived from bovine or porcine animal lungs or human amniotic fluid. Synthetic or artificial surfactants are composed of DPPC and spreading agents such as unsaturated phosphatidylglycerol or tyloxapol and hexadecanol (40).

NATURALLY OCCURRING SURFACTANTS

Of the naturally occurring surfactants, the bile salts and phospholipids are of particular importance.

Phospholipids

The phospholipids are widely found in biological membranes and can be used as emulsifiers especially for intravenous fat emulsions, and as a key component of liposomes. The elucidation of factors governing the solubilization of drugs in phospholipid dispersions can provide some clues as to the biological role of interactions with lipid systems in vivo (4). Phospholipids have been discussed above and in reference (22) in the context of liposomes.

Bile Salts

Bile salts are carboxylic acids (C22–C28) with a cyclopentenophenanthrene nucleus containing a branched chain of 3–9 carbon atoms ending in a carboxyl group. Structurally they form micelles which are different from the conventional spherical micelles synonymous with amphiphiles having a distinct hydrocarbon chain. The hydrophobic feature of the bile salts is associated with one surface of the steroid nucleus, and consequently intermolecular association is much more restricted. Primary and secondary micelles have been proposed, the former consisting of two to four molecules, the latter being composed of aggregates of the primary micelles. The CMC is less distinct and is highly dependent on the structure of the specific bile salt, in particular the number of hydroxy groups and their orientation.

Many studies have been completed in order to assess the effect of bile salts on the bioavailability of poorly soluble drugs. Bile salts for example, have been shown to enhance the absorption of sulphaguanidine and urogastrone. Bile salts may also play a role in enhancing the transport of a compound from the lumen of the intestine to the systemic circulation. Such absorption involves overcoming the resistance of the aqueous boundary layer and the membrane epithelium to the passage of the drug.

Bile salts readily form mixed micelles with lipid-like molecules such as lecithins or fatty acids. These mixed micelles are structurally very different from the simple micelles and generally have a much greater solubilizing capacity for hydrophobic molecules, both biological and synthetic. The solubility of DDT, a nonpolar, water insoluble molecule, for example, in bile salt micellar solution can be increased to a far greater extent by the addition of unsaturated long chain fatty acids, probably because of mixed micelle formation.

Saponins

Saponins are glycosides found in certain plants which are characterized by their property of producing a frothing aqueous solution. The term "saponin" is derived from the Latin "sapo" meaning soap. Plant materials containing saponins have been used for a long time in many parts of the world for their detergent properties, for example, in Europe, the root of *Saponaria officinalis* and in South America the bark of *Quillaja saponaria* (41).

The saponin structure is either of the steroidal (commonly tetracyclic triterpenoids) or pentacyclic triterpenoid type. Triterpenoid saponins are found, for example in Quillaia bark and in liquorice root. Quillaia B.P. is defined as the dried inner part of the bark of *Quillaja saponaria* and other species of *Quillaja* and is used as an emulsifying agent. Liquorice, the root of which also contains triterpenoid saponins, has long been used in pharmacy as a flavoring agent, demulcent, and mild expectorant.

Iscoms

Iscoms (Immune-stimulating complexes) are stable complexes of cholesterol, phospholipid, and Quil A (derived from *Quillaja saponaria*) in size ranges from 40 to 100 nm. They are promising carriers for antigens in subunit vaccines. Iscoms are considered to be multimicellar structures, shaped and stabilized by hydrophobic interactions, electrostatic repulsion, steric factors and possibly hydrogen bonds (42). Protection has been achieved after immunization with iscom-based vaccines, against viruses like the Epstein–Barr virus (43) and the measles virus (44).

SURFACE ACTIVITY OF DRUGS

A large number of drug molecules exhibit surface activity, that is, they tend to accumulate at interfaces, depress surface tension and associate to form aggregates in solution. Although the hydrophobic groups of most drugs are aromatic, they still behave like typical surfactants (which possess flexible hydrophobic chains), inasmuch as these aromatic groups have a high degree of flexibility. (Drugs that exhibit association characteristics typical of surface active agents and may reduce surface tension are reviewed in Ref. 4.)

Most of the drugs form micelles at concentrations that they do not attain in vivo. It is therefore their surface activity, rather than their self-association tendency which is more important biologically. Surface-active drugs will tend to bind hydrophobically to proteins and other macromolecules and to associate with other amphipathic substances such as bile salts, phospholipids, and receptors. As with other surface-active agents, surface-active drugs may interact directly with biological membranes. The possible biological implications of surface activity is discussed by Attwood and Florence (4) in relation to the phenothiazine tranquillisers and local anesthetics.

REFERENCES

1. Rupprecht, H.; Lee, G. Adsorption at Solid Surfaces. *Encyclopedia of Pharmaceutical Technology*, 1st Ed; Swarbrick, J., Boylan, J.C., Eds.; Marcel Dekker, Inc.: New York, 1988; 1, 73–114.
2. Myers, D. Surfaces and Interfaces: General Concepts. *Surfaces, Interfaces, and Colloids: Principles and Applications*; VCH Publishers Inc.: New York, 1991, 7–24.
3. Rosen, M.J. *Surfactants and Interfacial Phenomena*; Wiley Interscience: New York, 1989.
4. Attwood, D.; Florence, A.T. *Surfactant Systems. Their Chemistry, Pharmacy and Biology*; Chapman and Hall: London, New York, 1983.
5. Lawrence, M.J. Surfactant Systems: Their Use in Drug Delivery. Chem. Soc. Rev. **1994**, *23* (6), 417–424.
6. Corrigan, O.I.; Healy, A.M. Surfactants in Pharmaceutical Products and Systems. *Encyclopedia of Pharmaceutical Technology*, 1st Ed.; Swarbrick, J., Boylan, J.C., Eds.; Marcel Dekker, Inc.: New York, 1996; 14, 295–331.
7. Florence, A.T. Drug Solubilization in Surfactant Systems, Drugs and the Pharmaceutical Sciences. *Techniques of Solubilization of Drugs*; Yalkowsky, S., Swarbrick, J., Eds.; Marcel Dekker, Inc.: New York, 1982; 12, 15–89.
8. Ong, J.T.H.; Manoukian, E. Micellar Solubilization of Timobesone Acetate in Aqueous and Aqueous Propylene Glycol Solutions of Nonionic Surfactants. Pharm. Res. **1988**, *5* (11), 704–708.
9. Fahelelbom, K.M.S.; Timoney, R.F.; Corrigan, O.I. Micellar Solubilization of Clofazimine Analogs in Aqueous Solutions of Ionic and Nonionic Surfactants. Pharm. Res. **1993**, *10* (4), 631–634.
10. Riess, G.; Hurtrez, G.; Bahadur, P. Block Copolymers. *Encyclopedia of Polymer Science and Engineering*, 2nd Ed.; Mark, H.F., Bikales, N.M., Overberger, C.G., Menges, G., Eds.; Wiley-Interscience: New York, 1985; 2, 324–434.
11. Kataoka, K.; Kwon, G.S.; Yokoyama, M.; Okano, T.; Sakurai, Y. Block-Copolymer Micelles as Vehicles for Drug Delivery. J. Control. Release **1993**, *24* (1–3), 119–132.
12. Yokoyama, M.; Miyauchi, M.; Yamada, N.; Okano, T.; Sakurai, Y.; Kataoka, K.; Inoue, S. Polymer Micelles as Novel Drug Carrier—Adriamycin-Conjugated Poly(Ethylene Glycol) Poly(Aspartic Acid) Block Copolymer. J. Control. Release **1990**, *11* (1–3), 269–278.
13. Kwon, G.S.; Naito, M.; Yokoyama, M.; Okano, T.; Sakurai, Y.; Kataoka, K. Physical Entrapment of Adriamycin in AB Block Copolymer Micelles. Pharm. Res. **1995**, *12* (2), 192–195.
14. Martin, A.N.; Bustamante, P. *Physical Pharmacy: Physical Chemical Principles in the Pharmaceutical Sciences*, 4th Ed.; Lea and Febiger: Philadelphia, 1993, 386–388, 541–542.
15. Carrigan, P.J.; Bates, T.R. Biopharmaceutics of Drugs Administered in Lipid-Containing Dosage Forms I: GI Absorption of Griseofulvin from an Oil-in-Water Emulsion in the Rat. J. Pharm. Sci. **1973**, *62*, 1476–1479.
16. Eccleston, G. *Encyclopedia of Pharmaceutical Technology*, 1st Ed.; Swarbrick, J., Boylan, J.C., Eds.; Marcel Dekker, Inc.: New York, 1992; 5, 137–188.
17. Osborne, D.W.; Ward, A.J.I.; O'Neill, K.J. Microemulsions as Topical Drug Delivery Vehicles I. Characterization of a Model System. Drug Dev. Ind. Pharm. **1988**, *14* (9), 1203–1219.
18. Linn, E.E.; Pohland, R.C.; Byrd, T.K. Microemulsions for Intradermal Delivery of Cetyl Alcohol and Octyl Dimethyl PABA. Drug Dev. Ind. Pharm. **1990**, *16* (6), 899–920.
19. Bowman, P.A.; Greenleaf, D. Non-CFC Metered Dose Inhalers: The Patent Landscape. Int. J. Pharm. **1999**, *86* (1), 91–94.

20. Ranucci, J.A.; Dixit, S.; Bray, R., Jr.; Goldman, D. Application of Controlled Flocculation to Metered Dose Aerosols Suspensions. Pharm. Res. **1987**, *4* (2 suppl.), S-25.

21. Hickey, A.J.; Dalby, R.N.; Byron, P.R. Effects of Surfactants on Aerosol Powders in Suspension, Implications for Airborne Particle Size. Int. J. Pharm. **1988**, *42*, 267–270.

22. Barenholz, Y.; Crommelin, D.J.A. Liposomes as Pharmaceutical Dosage Forms. *Encyclopedia of Pharmaceutical Technology*, 1st Ed.; Swarbrick, J., Boylan, J.C. Eds.; Marcel Dekker, Inc. New York, 1994; 9, 1–39.

23. Walters, K.A. Penetration Enhancers and Their Use in Transdermal Therapeutic Systems. *Transdermal Drug Delivery*; Drugs and the Pharmaceutical Sciences; Hadgraft, J., Guy, R.H., Eds.; Marcel Dekker, Inc.: New York, 1989; 35, 197–246.

24. Higuchi, W.I. Diffusional Models Useful in Biopharmaceutics. Drug Release Rate Processes. J. Pharm. Sci. **1967**, *56*, 315–324.

25. Higuchi, W.I.; Su, C.C.; Park, J.Y.; Gulari, E. Mechanism of Cholesterol Gallstone Dissolution. Analysis of the Kinetics of Cholesterol Monohydrate Dissolution in Taurocholate/Lecithin Solutions by the Mazer, Benedek, and Carey Models. J. Phys. Chem. **1981**, *85* (2), 127–129.

26. Newton, J.M.; Rowley, G.; Törnblom, J-F.V. Further Studies on the Effect of Additives on the Release of Drug from Hard Gelatin Capsules. J. Pharm. Pharmac. **1971**, *23* (suppl.), 156S–160S.

27. Banker, G.S.; Peck, G.E.; Baley, G. Tablet Formulation and Design. *Pharmaceutical Dosage Forms: Tablets*; Lieberman, H.A., Lachman, L., Eds.; Marcel Dekker, Inc.: New York, 1980; 1, 61–107.

28. Jones, B.E. Gelatin Additives, Substitutes and Extenders. *Hard Capsules: Development and Technology*; Ridgway, K., Ed.; The Pharmaceutical Press: London, 1987, 54.

29. Sjokvist, E.; Nyström, C.; Aldén, M. Physicochemical Aspects of Drug Release, 13. The Effect of Sodium Dodecyl-Sulfate Additions on the Structure and Dissolution of a Drug in Solid Dispersions. Int. J. Pharm. **1991**, *69* (1), 53–62.

30. Veiga, M.D.; Escobar, C.; Bernad, M.J. Dissolution Behavior of Drugs from Binary and Ternary Systems. Int. J. Pharm. **1993**, *93* (1–3), 215–220.

31. Sjokvist-Saers, E.; Nyström, C.; Aldén, M. Physicochemical Aspects of Drug Release, 16. The Effect of Storage on Drug Dissolution from Solid Dispersions and the Influence of Cooling Rate and Incorporation of Surfactant. Int. J. Pharm. **1993**, *90* (2), 105–118.

32. Singh, P.; Desai, S.J.; Simonelli, A.P.; Higuchi, W.I. Role of Wetting on the Rate of Drug Release from Inert Matrices. J. Pharm. Sci. **1968**, *57* (2), 217–226.

33. Coben, L.J.; Lieberman, H.A. Suppositories. *The Theory and Practice of Industrial Pharmacy*, 3rd Ed.; Lachman, L., Lieberman, H.A., Kanig, J.L., Eds.; Lea & Febiger: Philadelphia, 1986; 564–588.

34. Nakanishi, K.; Masada, M.; Nadai, T. Effect of Pharmaceutical Adjuvants on the Rectal Permeability to Drugs. IV. Effect of Pharmaceutical Adjuvants on the Rectal Permeability to Macromolecular Compounds in the Rat. Chem. Pharm. Bull. **1984**, *32*, 1628–1632.

35. O'Reilly, J.R.; Corrigan, O.I.; O'Driscoll, C.M. The Effect of Simple Micellar Systems on the Solubility and Intestinal-Absorption of Clofazimine (B663) in the Anesthetized Rat. Int. J. Pharm. **1994**, *105* (2), 137–146.

36. O'Reilly, J.R.; Corrigan, O.I.; O'Driscoll, C.M. The Effect of Mixed Micellar Systems, Bile-Salt Fatty-Acids, on the Solubility and Intestinal-Absorption of Clofazimine (B663) in the Anesthetized Rat. Int. J. Pharm. **1994**, *109* (2), 147–154.

37. Weiner, M.; Bernstein, I.L. *Adverse Reactions to Drug Formulation Agents*; Marcel Dekker, Inc.: New York, 1989.

38. Rieger, M.M. Surfactants. *Pharmaceutical Dosage Forms: Disperse Systems*, 2nd Ed.; Lieberman, H.A., Rieger, M.M., Banker, G.S., Eds.; Marcel Dekker, Inc.: New York, 1996; 1, 211–286.

39. Avery, M.E.; Mead, J. Surface Properties in Relation to Atelectasis and Hyaline Membrane Disease. Am. J. Dis. Child. **1959**, *97*, 517–526.

40. Fujiwara, T.; Maeta, H.; Chida, S.; Morita, T.; Watabe, Y.; Abe, T. Artificial Surfactant Therapy in Hyaline-Membrane Disease. Lancet **1980**, *1*, 55–59.

41. Evans, W.C. Saponins, Cardioactive Drugs and Other Steroids. *Trease and Evans' Pharmacognosy*, 14th Ed.; WB Saunders Company Ltd.: London, 1996; 293–309.

42. Kersten, G.F.A. Aspects of Iscoms. Stuctural, Pharmaceutical and Adjuvant Properties; Ph.D. Thesis, University of Utrecht, 1990; 93–104.

43. Morgan, A.J.; Finerty, S.; Lövgren, K.; Scullion, F.T.; Morein, B. Prevention of Epstein-Barr (EB)Virus-Induced Lymphoma in Cottontop Tamarins by Vaccination with the EB Virus Envelope Glycoprotein GP 340 Incorporated into Immune-Stimulating Complexes. J. Gen. Virol. **1988**, *69*, 2093–2096.

44. de Vries, P.; van Binnendijk, R.; van der Marel, P.; van Wezel, A.L.; Voorma, H.O.; Sundquist, B.; UytdeHaag, F.G.C.M.; Osterhaus, A.D.M.E. Measles Virus Fusion Protein Presented in an Immune-Stimulating Complex (iscom) Induces Haemolysis-Inhibiting and Fusion-Inhibiting Antibodies, Virus Specific T Cells and Protection in Mice. J. Gen. Virol. **1988**, *69*, 549–559.

SUSPENSIONS

Robert A. Nash

Consultant, Mahwah, New Jersey

INTRODUCTION

A suspension is a particular class or type of dispersion or dispersed system in which the internal or suspended phase is dispersed uniformly by mechanical agitation throughout the external phase (called the suspending medium or vehicle). The internal phase, consisting of a homogeneous or heterogeneous distribution of solid particles having a specific size range, is maintained uniformly throughout the suspending vehicle with the aid of a single or a particular combination of suspending agent(s). In addition, unlike in a solution, the suspended particles exhibit a minimum degree of solubility in the external phase. In a colloidal suspension, the solids are less than about 1 μm in size. In a coarse suspension, they are larger than about 1 μm. The practical upper limit for individual suspendable solid particles in coarse suspensions suspensions is approximately 50–75 μm. When one or more types of solid particles that constitute the internal phase are pharmaceutically useful and/or physiologically active, the system is known as a pharmaceutical suspension.

In an emulsion, the particles of the internal phase are spherical or liquid droplets that are dispersed throughout a liquid external phase. Even though the particles may be liquid only at elevated temperatures (50–80°C) and semisolid or rigid at room temperature, as long as they appear spherical on careful microscopic examination, they are generally considered to be emulsified rather than suspended. Thus, a clue to the presence of a suspended particle is its lack of sphericity or its definitive lattice structure. Exceptions to this general rule are spherical microspheres and related spherical solid microparticles.

CLASSIFICATION

Martin and Bustamante (1) list three general classes of pharmaceutical suspensions: orally administered (sometimes referred to as mixtures), externally applied (topical lotions), and injectable (parenteral).

Oral Suspensions

The solids content of an oral suspension may vary considerably. For example, antibiotic preparations may contain 125–500 mg of active solid material in a 5-ml (teaspoonful) dose, whereas a drop concentrate may provide the same amount of insoluble drug in a 1- or 2-mL dose. Antacids and radiopaque suspensions contain relatively high amounts of suspended material for oral administration. The vehicle may be a syrup, a sorbitol solution, or a gum-thickened, water-containing artificial sweetener because in addition to ingredients, safety, taste, and mouthfeel are important formulation considerations. In the case of limited shelf life (low chemical stability of the insoluble drug), the dosage form may be prepared as a dry granulation or powder mixture that is reconstituted with water prior to use.

Topical Suspensions

Historically, the externally applied "shake lotion" is the oldest example of a pharmaceutical suspension. Calamine Lotion USP, as well as other dermatological preparations, is closely associated with the technical development of the pharmaceutical suspension (2). Because safety and toxicity considerations are most readily dealt with in terms of dermatological acceptability, many useful suspending agents were first introduced in topical formulations (3). In addition, the protective action and cosmetic properties of topical lotions usually require the use of high concentrations of the dispersed phase, often in excess of 20%. Therefore, topical lotions represent the best example of suspensions that exhibit low settling rates (4). Various pharmaceutical vehicles have been used in the preparation of topical lotions, including diluted oil-in-water or water-in-oil emulsion bases, determatological pastes, magmas, and clay suspensions.

Parenteral Suspensions

The solids content of parenteral suspensions is usually between 0.5 and 5.0%, except for insoluble forms of penicillin, in which concentrations of the antibiotic may exceed 30%. These sterile preparations are designed for intramuscular, intradermal, intra-lesional, intra-articular, or subcutaneous administration. The viscosity of a parenteral suspension should be low enough to facilitate injection. Common vehicles for parenteral suspensions include preserved 0.9% saline solution or a parenterally acceptable vegetable oil. The primary factor governing the selection of injectable ingredients is safety. Ophthalmic suspensions that are instilled into the eye must be prepared in a sterile manner. The vehicle is employed is essentially isotonic and aqueous in composition.

UTILITY OF SUSPENSIONS

A suspension is often chosen as pharmaceutical dosage form for drugs insoluble in water and aqueous fluids at the dosage required for administration and when attempts to solubilize the drug would compromise stability and safety. For oral administration, the taste of a bitter or unpleasant drug can often be masked by choosing an insoluble form of the active drug.

An aqueous suspension is a useful oral dosage form for administering insoluble or poorly soluble drugs. The large surface area of the dispersed drug particles often facilitate absorption. Unlike drug particles contained in tablets or capsules, the dissolution of drug particles in suspension and subsequent absorption commence upon dilution in gastrointestinal fluids. Finely divided particles dissolve faster and have higher relative solubilities than do similar macroparticles.

The parenteral suspension is an ideal dosage form for prolonged or "depot" release. In the administration of a drug as an aqueous or oleaginous suspension into subcutaneous or muscular tissue, the drug is deposited at the injection site. The depot acts as a reservoir, slowly releasing drug at a rate related to both the intrinsic aqueous solubility of the drug form and the type of suspending vehicle, either aqueous or oily for the purpose of maintaining prolonged systemic absorption of the drug from the injection site.

HYDROPHILIC/HYDROPHOBIC SOLIDS

Insoluble solids, regardless of particle size, that have a relatively low interfacial tension and are readily wetted by water are called *hydrophilic* solids. These solids include clays (bentonite, kaolin, talc, magnesium aluminum silicate); bismuth salts, barium sulfate, carbonates, hydroxides, or oxides of calcium, magnesium, zinc, and aluminum; and titanium dioxide. The hydrophilicity of a powder surface can be investigated with the help of moisture absorption studies in which the solid particles are exposed to varying relative humidities. Insoluble powders that absorb moisture below relative humidities of 70–80% at room temperature are said to be hydrophilic solids.

Fine insoluble solids that are not easily wetted by water and have a relatively high interfacial tension are referred to as *hydrophobic* solids. These include a large number of low-density organic materials and pharmaceutical substances, such as charcoal and sulfur. The hydrophobic nature of the latter group is accentuated by entrapped air adsorbed on the surface of these particles. Hydrophobic materials may be wetted by oils and semipolar liquids and are called lipophilic solids; conversely, hydrophilic materials behave like lipophobic solids in oils.

Hydrophilic solids can be suspended easily in water without the aid of a water-dispersible surfactant or wetting agent, and conversely hydrophobic solids can be suspended in oils and nonpolar vehicles without the use of lipid-soluble surfactants. The crystal density of hydrophilic solids usually ranges from 1.5 to 6.9 g/cm^3, whereas the crystal density of hydrophobic solids usually ranges from 0.9 to 2.2 g/cm^3.

PARTICLE SIZE CONSIDERATIONS

The mean particle diameter and the particle size distributions of suspended insoluble drugs are important considerations in formulating stable pharmaceutical suspensions. Hiestand (5) defines the lower limit of coarse suspensions as those containing particles larger than 0.1 μm. Except for a number of clays, oxides, charcoal, and pigments, the average particle size of most drugs and pharmaceutical rarely falls below 1 μm. Although most submicron inorganic excipients appear to behave like hydrophilic solids, most insoluble drugs and pharmaceutical excipients are usually soft, organic, essentially crystalline hydrophobic solids ranging in particle size from several microns to several hundred or more.

Drug particle size is an important factor influencing product appearance, settling rates, drug solubility, in vivo absorption, resuspendability, and overall stability of pharmaceutical suspensions. Insoluble drug particles are seldom uniform spheres or cubes, even after size reduction and classification. Wide distributions in particle size often lead to high-density suspensions. Systems with widely differing particle shapes (plates, needles, filaments, and prisms) frequently produce low-density slurries. The growth over time of unprotected, slightly soluble drug solids and changes in their particle size distribution in suspension are a serious problem. Crystal growth of particles is usually attributed to one or more of the following mechanisms:

- "Oswalt ripening" or the growth of large particles at the expense of smaller ones, because of a difference in solubility rates of different size particles. For example, the increase in the solubility rate of a 0.2-μm particle, is 13%. For a 2-μm particle, it is 1%, and for particles above 20 μm, it is negligible.
- Crystal growth due to temperature fluctuations on storage is of minor importance, unless suspensions are subjected to temperature variations of 20°C or more.
- A polymorphic form may change to another more stable crystalline form; changes in crystal habit may be related to the degree of solvation or hydration.
- Crystal growth may also arise when the more energetic amorphous or glassy forms of a drug exhibit significantly higher initial solubility in water than the corresponding crystalline forms.
- Size reduction by crushing and grinding can produce particles whose different surfaces exhibit high and low solubility rates. This effect can be related to differences in the free surface energy introduced during comminution (grinding).

Crystal growth and changes in particle size distribution can generally be controlled by employing one or several of the following procedures and techniques.

1. Selection of particles with a narrow range of particle sizes, such as microcrystals between 1 and 10 μm.
2. Selection of a stable crystalline drug form that usually exhibits lower solubility in water. The crystalline form that is physically most stable usually has the highest melting point.
3. High-energy milling should not be used during particle size reduction. Microcrystals are best formed by controlled precipitation techniques or shock cooling.
4. A water-dispersible surfactant wetting agent dissipates the free surface energy of particles by reducing the interfacial tension between the solid and the suspending vehicle.
5. A protective colloid, such as gelatin, gum, or a cellulosic derivative, is used to form a film barrier around the particles, inhibiting dissolution and subsequent crystal growth.
6. The viscosity of the suspending vehicle is increased to retard particle dissolution and subsequent crystal growth.
7. Temperature extremes during product storage (freeze–thaw conditioning) must not occur.

8. Supersaturation favors the formation of needlelike crystals and should be avoided.
9. Rapid or shock cooling and high agitation favor the formation of thin, small crystals and should be avoided. Slow crystallization by evaporation yields compact crystals.
10. Experimentation with different crystallizing solvents is recommended to change crystal size and shape.
11. Impurities and foreign substances during crystallization affect the reproducibility and aggregation potential of many drug particle systems.
12. Constant crystallizing conditions are essential. Batch-to-batch variation in crystal size and shape is often associated with poor control of processing and crystallization procedures.

Variations in assay results can be avoided by the preparation of homogeneous, well-mixed, or nonsettling fine particle suspensions (size 1–10 μm). Particle size reduction results in slow, more uniform settling rates. The bioavailability of drugs is improved by reducing the size of suspension particles. Furthermore, drug particles smaller than 20 μm produce less pain and tissue irritation when injected parenterally. However, fine particles may have a deleterious effect on chemical stability because of their high dissolution rate.

Particle Size Reduction

Drug solids are easy to grind. Reduction to a particle size of about 50–75 μm usually produces a free-flowing powder. Solids containing particles smaller than 50 μm tend to aggregate or agglomerate in the dry state. Furthermore, below 10–50 μm, the increased free surface energy, as evidenced by the cohesion of small particles, becomes a factor interfering with further size reduction. The powder may become damp, especially if there is a tendency to attract moisture. Material tends to "ball up," which indicates that the agglomerated masses are larger than the individual particles contained within.

As the pores between powder particles become smaller with decreasing particle size, increases in surface area facilitate liquid penetration. Aggregates behave like hydrophobic solids, entrapping air and becoming difficult to wet.

The most efficient method of producing fine particles is by dry milling prior to manufacture of the suspension. Dispersion equipment, such as colloid mills or homogenizers are normally used to wet-mill finished suspensions to break up poorly wetted fine particle aggregates or agglomerates. Among the several methods of producing small, reasonably uniform drug particles are micropulverization, fluid energy grinding, controlled precipitation, and

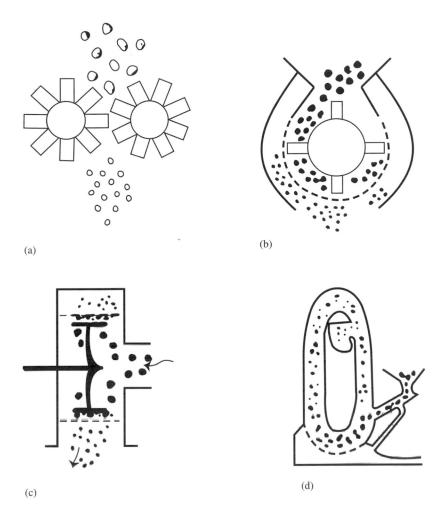

Fig. 1 The four basic types of size reduction equipment used to produce fine solid particles: (a) Crushers and shredders. (b) Hammermills. (c) Colloid mills. (d) Fluid energy mills.

spray drying. Figure 1 illustrates the four basic types of size reduction equipment used in the pharmaceutical industry to produce fine powder particles.

Micropulverization

Micropulverization is one of the most rapid, convenient, and inexpensive methods of producing fine drug powders. The milling equipment includes hammermills, micropulverizers, universal mills, end-runner mills, and ball mills. Micropulverizers are highspeed attrition or impact mills specially adapted for fine grinding. Some mills are fitted with classifiers to facilitate particle separation by centrifugation. Because ultrafine particles smaller than 10 μm are rarely produced, buildup of electrostatic charge on the surface of milled powder is encountered only occasionally. The main disadvantage of micropulverization is the large distribution of particle sizes

produced, normally in the range of 10–50 μm or higher. Nevertheless, these powders are satisfactory for the preparation of most oral and topical suspensions.

Fluid energy grinding

The process of fluid energy grinding, also referred to as jet milling or micronizing, is the most effective method for reducing particles below 10 μm. The ultrafine particles are produced by the shearing action of high-velocity streams of compressed air on particles in a confined space. The main disadvantage of fluid energy grinding is the high electrostatic charge built up on the surfaces of the milled powder, which makes powder classification and collection exceedingly difficult. However, because it is important that a majority of drug particles in parenteral suspensions are below 10 μm, fluid energy grinding is the most convenient method for their production.

Controlled crystallization

A solvent that dissolves a solid readily at room temperature may serve as a crystallizing medium when mixed with another solvent in which the compound is only sparingly soluble. A solution that is nearly saturated at a temperature about 10°C below the boiling point of the solvent combination is prepared in a temperature ranging between 60 and 150°C. Separation of microcrystals from such hot concentrated solutions is commonly induced by cooling and stirring. However, when supersaturation is obtained by agitation and shock cooling of the hot solution and through the rapid introduction of another cold miscible solvent in which the drug is only sparingly soluble, formation of minute crystalline particles (nucleates) proceeds without appreciable crystal growth, and uniform microcrystals of the drug are thus obtained. In addition, ultrasonic methods have been used during shock cooling to promote microcrystal formation.

Spray drying

Particles of microcrystalline size can also be obtained by spray-drying procedures, resulting in a porous, free-flowing, easily wetted, essentially monodispersed powder. With proper control of process variables, spherical particles are obtained that may be coated with agents to aid suspension and promote stability. However, the process is not normally considered for the preparation of ultrafine powders.

PHYSICAL ASPECTS

Stability of Suspensions

The chemical stability of a drug in suspension is controlled by the fact that the rate of degradation is related to the concentration of the drug in aqueous solution rather than to the total concentration of the drug in the product. Generally, a suspended drug decomposes only in solution as the solid phase gradually dissolves; that is, a solution concentration equal to the solubility of the drug is maintained. Drug degradation in a suspension usually follows zero-order kinetics, with the rate constant solely dependent on the saturation solubility of the drug in solution. Reducing the solubility of the suspended drug decreases the rate of degradation. The constancy of potency may be improved by selecting a pH value or range where the drug is least soluble or by replacing the drug with a less soluble derivative or salt. Decomposition in suspensions may also be described as a diffusion-controlled process or by catalysis initiated by environmental factors such as oxygen, light, and trace metals.

As a rule, the problem of suspension stability is complicated by the fact that pharmaceutical suspensions are affected at least as much by physical as by chemical factors.

Because a suspension exists in more than one state (liquid and solid), there are different ways in which the system can undergo chemical or physical change. Some of the more obvious difficulties involved in stability predictions are based on the fact that simple hydrostatic relationships (Stoke's law, etc.) used to define settling rates assume a spherical, deflocculated, free-falling particle that is not affected by particle–particle or particle–vehicle interactions. Suspensions that exhibit non-Newtonian flow are difficult to define in terms of the basic stability relationships. In addition, suspensions that are described in terms of a single representative particle do not reflect the influence of the entire particle size distribution.

Chemical stability predictions are sometimes complicated by the difficulty of determining the pH value of suspensions, which often changes because of surface coating of electrodes and differences between bulk-suspension and supernatant-vehicle readings. Accelerated elevated temperature stability testing often has a pronounced adverse effect on viscosity, particle solubility, and size distribution.

Deflocculated Suspensions

The empirical method of producing pharmaceutical suspensions is based on an attempt to prepare a stable deflocculated dispersion of a drug in a suitable suspension vehicle. In the past, a series of suspensions was often prepared using different concentrations of a favored suspending agent to identify the formulation that would produce the most homogeneous looking ("smooth") and stable suspension. The finished preparation was usually passed through a homogenizer or colloid mill to improve the final dispersion. Smooth looking viscous suspensions were produced; however, after some time, the drug particles settled slowly, forming a tightly packed sediment that was almost impossible to resuspend even with vigorous shaking. Primary particles or small aggregates, reaching the bottom of the container during sedimentation (settling), slipped past each other and produced compact layers of solids. The interparticle interaction in such compact sediments is relatively high because the interparticle distances are small, and the weak van der Waals forces of attraction, which decreases exponentially with distance, are appreciable. Such conditions frequently lead to the undersirable phenomenon of "caking or claying" and require extensive agitation for resuspension.

The physical instability of these early deflocculated suspensions led to other methods of producing physically stable pharmaceutical suspensions. For example, the density of the vehicle was made to equal or approach the crystal density of the suspended drug particles. If the drug particles are small enough and the vehicle sufficiently viscous, the particles remain suspended indefinitely in accordance with Stokes' law. Because the crystal density of most organic drug particles lies somewhere between 1.1 and 1.5 g/cm^3, the only liquid vehicles for oral use with densities (at 25°C) high enough to be considered are Sorbitol Solution USP (1.29 g/cm^3), Syrup USP (1.31 g/cm^3), and high-fructose corn syrup (1.41 g/cm^3). In practice, however, it is extremely difficult to prepare oral suspensions by the matched-density technique alone because dilution with water and other liquids reduces the vehicle density. Nevertheless, the use of high-density liquids as suspending vehicles often has a beneficial effect on physical stability.

The approximate settling velocities for nonflocculated particles of various average size were determined in the range of 0.2–200 μm at density differences between solid particles and the suspending liquid of 0.2 and 2.0 g/cm^3, respectively, with an absolute viscosity of the suspending liquid between 1 and 1000 centipoise (cP or mPa s). Terminal settling rates were calculated by a method described by Carpenter (6) for two concentrations of suspended solids, namely less than 2 and 20% vol. According to the analysis, permanent-type suspensions, which exhibit a settling viscosity of less than 0.14 cm per year at 25°C, can be obtained with a suspending liquid of a viscosity of ca 1000 cP, a density difference of 0.2 g/cm^3 or less and an average particle size of the suspended solid of 0.2 μm. This is a difficult set of criteria for most pharmaceutical suspensions to meet.

Because the distribution of particle sizes in most pharmaceutical suspension is generally above 1 μm, deflocculated or peptized systems settle very slowly in stages, with the larger particles settling more rapidly than smaller ones. Ultimately, they form a tight, dense sediment that is difficult to resuspend. When viewed under a microscope, the dispersed suspension consists of individual particles, showing no apparent association.

Deflocculated suspensions are produced by three methods.

Mutual repulsion to large ζ-potential

This is best achieved by the adsorption of an electrolyte (KCl) or polyelectrolyte dispersant (sodium hexametaphos-phate) on the surface of suspended particles to create a strong mutual repulsion between the microsize suspended particles. For example, moderate stability is achieved when the ζ-potential is between ±30 and ±60 mV, and good to excellent physical stability is achieved when the ζ-potential is between ±60 and ±100 mV. As the size and density of the suspended particles increase beyond 1 μm and 1.0 g/cm^3, respectively, the effect of ζ-potential becomes less important.

Adsorption of a smaller hydrophilic or lyophilic colloid on larger suspended particles

When a strongly hydrated hydrophilic protective colloid, such as gelatin, is adsorbed on the surface of the suspended particles, the affinity for water exceeds the mutual attraction of adjacent particles for each other. The protective colloid and hydrogen-bonded water molecules form a protective hydration layer around each suspended particle.

Steric hindrance due to adsorption of an oriented nonionic surfactant or polyelectrolyte

Adsorption of a nonionic polymer (gum or cellulosic) or surfactant (polysorbate 80) of sufficient chain length creates steric hindrance and prevents adjacent suspended particles from coming close enough to join each other. Steric stabilization has the advantage over electrostatic stabilization in that it is relatively insensitive to the presence of electrolyte in the aqueous vehicle.

Because many pharmaceutical suspensions are not capable of reaching a state of complete electrostatic repulsion and producing and maintaining deflocculated particles, the technique has been regarded as unworkable by many investigators (1, 5).

Flocculated Suspensions

Matthews and Rhodes (8), Haines and Martin (7), Hiestand (5), and Econow and co-workers (9, 10) are credited with establishing the "structured particle" concept or flocculated pharmaceutical suspension. The following definitions should prove useful in avoding confusion among three closely related terms: flocculation, agglomeration, and coagulation. The term aggregation can apply to all three.

Flocculation refers to the formation of a loose aggregation of discrete particles held together in a networklike structure by physical adsorption of macromolecules, bridging during chemical interaction (precipitation), or when the longer-range van der Waals forces of attraction exceed the shorter-range forces of repulsion. The floccule referred to as a "stable floc" usually contains varying amounts of entrapped liquid medium or vehicle within the networklike structure (Table 1).

Table 1 Suspension characteristics

Type	ζ-Potential	Relative settling rate	Sediment volume in vials at equilibrium	Drainage from vial	Resuspendability
Agglomerated or coagulated	0	Nonuniform	Low (lumpy)	Poor	Poor (may cake)
Overflocculated	0	Very high	Very high	Poor	Good
Slightly over flocculated	0	High	Moderate to high	Fair	Good
Slightly underflocculated	0	Moderate	Moderate	Good	Good
Underflocculated	0 to +10 mV	Slow	Moderate to low	Good	Fair
Deflocculated or peptized	+10 to +30 mV	Nonuniform	Low (stratified)	Good	Poor (cakes difficult to resuspend)

In agglomeration, a large number or mass of particles are closely bound together as aggregates in a dry (air) or liquid state. Coagulation or severe overflocculation refers to the massing of particles in a liquid state alone and sometimes in the form of a fluid gel structure. Aggregated particles of overflocculated systems, including adsorbed surface films, are in surface contact with each other, and each mass or coagula acts as a unit. The particles of such coagulated systems are held together by strong film-to-film bonds. Coagulated suspensions, like deflocculated suspensions, tend to "cake" on standing.

Soon after milling and suspension, unless steps are taken to prevent it, microsize particles tend to grow with time. Because the solubility rate of unprotected particles (Ostwald ripening) is higher than that of large crystals, crystal growth is favored until a more thermodynamically stable distribution of particles sizes is achieved. This phenomenon tends to promote "caking and cementing together" of particles.

The creation of a protective coat or boundary layer (with a hydrophilic colloid) about such particles offers the best protection to crystal growth. Because protective barriers may or may not flocculate, the substrate particles, the sign (positive or negative), and the charge potential on the particle surface (including a double layer) govern the choice between flocculation or dispersion (deflocculation).

The processes involved in the formation of suspensions are shown in Fig. 2. The flocculated state (C) may be reached either directly by wetting and dispersing hydrophobic particles (A) with a suitable flocculating surfactant, or indirectly by first wetting and dispersing to produce a dispersed or peptized particle (B) with a suitable surfactant and then flocculating with a suitable agent such as a hydrophilic colloid or polyelectrolyte.

In contrast to peptized or deflocculated particles, flocculated suspensions (C), which are considered pharmaceutically stable (although colloidally unstable), can always be resuspended with gentle agitation. Severe overflocculation, on the other hand, caused by the addition of too much flocculating agent or by prolonged exposure to extreme thermal conditions (freeze–thaw cycles) tend to produce agglomerated or coagulated irreversible systems (E). The term plaque (platelike) is used to describe essentially flat agglomerates, whereas the term coagula (clumplike) is reserved for thicker, three-dimensional particle masses. In the absence of a protective colloid, the process of crystal growth is indicated by the arrow connecting (A) to (D). Some authors (11) refer to the "stable floc" as the partially flocculated state. Simply stated, the greater the number of particle-to-particle contact points in the cluster, the higher the degree of flocculation.

The main advantages of the stable floc are as follows.

The aggregates tend to break up easily under the application of moderate shear stress, such as gentle agitation of a bottle or vial, or by the flow through a small orifice (hypodermic needle and/or syringe) and reform an extended network of particles after the force is removed. Flocculation, therefore, imparts a structure to the suspension with virtually no increase in viscosity (Fig.3).

In contrast to peptized or deflocculated systems, the stable floc settles rapidly, usually to a high sediment volume, and may be easily resuspended even after standing for prolonged periods of storage time. The settling rate is not rapid and maintain content uniformity with reasonable periodic agitation. The stable floc can be produced by employing aseptic techniques, using vehicle components that are safe for intramuscular injection.

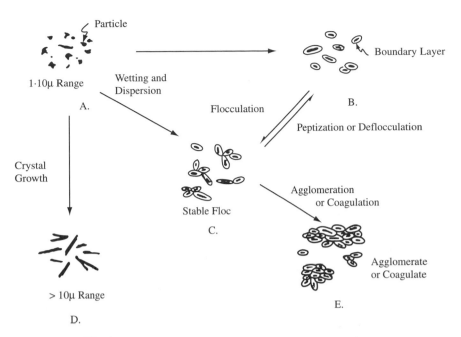

Fig. 2 Processes involved in the formation of suspensions.

Flocculated pharmaceutical suspensions are prepared using several methods. The choice depends on the properties of the drug and the class of suspension desired. The following examples illustrate how suspensions may be prepared by controlled flocculation procedures:

1. The wetting agent, polysorbate 80 (not more than 0.1–0.2% w/v of the final concentration), is dissolved in approximately half the final volume of aqueous vehicle. An anionic surfactant, such as Docusate Sodium USP, may be used as a wetting agent. This agent is, however, sensitive to pH and electrolyte concentration.

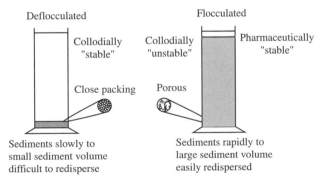

Fig. 3 Characteristics of flocculated and deflocculated suspensions. (From Ref. 5.)

2. Ultrafine particles of the drug at the desired final concentration are uniformly and carefully spread over the surface of the vehicle, and the drug is permitted to be wetted undisturbed for as long as 16 h (overnight).

3. The wetted slurry is passed through a fine wire mesh screen (100 mesh size for ca 120 μm or larger) to remove poorly wetted powder. A single pass through a colloid mill can achieve the same result.

4. The slurry concentrate of the drug is agitated gently with an impeller-type mixer.

5. Small amounts of a 10% w/v solution of aluminum chloride hexahydrate are added dropwise, to the drug slurry from a buret or dropping pipette until the flocculation endpoint is reached (zero ζ-potential). To determine the endpoint, small samples are withdrawn and transferred to a graduated cylinder, an equal amount of vehicle is added to each, and the cylinders are gently shaken and permitted to stand undisturbed. The sample with the highest ratio of sediment to total suspension volume, exhibiting a clear supernate and good drainage characteristics is considered to be at the appropriate endpoint. Usually, no more than about 0.1–0.2% aluminum chloride hexahydrate is be required to achieve the flocculation endpoint. A 10% solution of calcium choride dihydrate may also be used as the flocculating agent. In this case, 1–2% of the calcium salt may be required for stable floc formation. If the drug fails to flocculate in the

presence of polyvalent aluminum or calcium ions, the water-insoluble drug particles are considered to be positively charged, and the procedure is repeated, this time using a polyvalent anionic flocculating agent such as 10% w/v sodium hexametaphosphate or 10% trisodium citrate.

6. After the flocculation endpoint has been established and verified, the other components (preservative, colorant, flavor, buffer, etc.) are added, dissolved in the liquid vehicle, and the slurry is brought to final volume with liquid vehicle.

Another popular method of preparing an oral suspension consists of suspending the drug in a solution of a hydrophilic colloid (gelatin or gum) or a diluted magma of bentonite, attapulgite, or colloidal magnesium aluminum sililcate. The concentration of flocculating agent suspended in water, sorbitol, or syrup solution is between 0.1 and 1%. Overflocculation may be reversed by the careful addition of small amounts of a suitable surfactant or polyvalent deflocculating agent. Because clays cannot be used in injectable products, two other methods are described here.

One method, specially useful for preparing physically stable "noncaking" suspensions, consists of titrating concentrated aqueous solutions of soluble salt forms of acidic or basic drugs with a corresponding solution of a strong acid or a strong base. The water-insoluble free acid or base is precipitated at the pH of minimum solubility of the drug. The concentrations of the reacting solutions and the order of addition may be varied to produce an acceptable stable floc. If necessary, the electrolyte thus formed during precipitation may be reduced through slurry decantation or filtration to adjust tonicity and/or to maintain physical and chemical stability. This procedure can also be carried out under aseptic conditions.

A stable floc may also be produced by dispersing insoluble particles in a turbid or hazy vehicle consisting of finely dispersed or emulsified semipolar, liquid droplets, which cause the droplets to be adsorbed on the surface of the insoluble drug particles, resulting in a stable floc. Turbid aqueous vehicles have been prepared by the interaction of nonionic surfactants and preservatives. The concentration of surfactant and preservative required for haze formation may be reduced by the addition of small amounts of sorbitol to the vehicle.

Structured Vehicle

Another technique for the preparation of a stable suspension is based on the concept of the "structured vehicle," in which the viscosity of the preparation, under static conditions of very low shear, on storage approaches infinity. The vehicle is said to behave like a "false body" that is able to maintain the suspended particles in a state of more or less permanent suspension.

Structured vehicles are usually not considered for the preparation of parenteral suspensions because, owing to their high viscosity, such systems lack sufficient syringe ability for ease of use.

Bingham-Type Plastic Flow

Vehicles that exhibit the unusual property of Bingham-type plastic rheological flow are characterized by the need to overcome a finite yield stress before flow is initiated. Permanent suspension of most pharmaceutical systems requires yield-stress values of at least 2–5 Pa (20–50 dyn/cm^2). Bingham plastic flow is rarely produced by pharmaceutical gums and hydrophilic colloids. *National Formulary* (NF) carbomers exhibit a sufficiently high yield value at low solution concentration and low viscosity to produce permanent suspensions. The carbomers, however, require a pH value between 6 and 8 for maximum suspension performance. The polymer is essentially incompatible with cationic resins, certain polyvalent ions, and high concentrations of electrolytes.

Thixotropic Flow

Thixotropy is a rheological property that results in yield stress on standing. Thixotropic flow is defined as a reversible, time-dependent, isothermal gel–sol transition. Thixotropic systems exhibit easy flow at relatively high shear rates. However, when the shear stress is removed, the system is slowly reformed into a structured vehicle. The usual property of thixotropy results from the breakdown and buildup of floccules under stress. A small amount of particle settling takes place until the system develops a sufficiently high yield value. The primary advantage of thixotropic flow is that it confers pourability under shear stress and viscosity and sufficiently high yield stress when the shear stress is removed at rest.

The concentrations of Bingham-type and thixotropic suspending agents required to achieve a yield stress of 10 Pa (100 dyn/cm^2) is shown in Table 2.

Suspending agent systems such as a pseudoplastic (sodium carboxymethylcellulose) in combination with a clay (hydrated colloidal magnesium aluminum silicate) or blends and coprecipitates of sodium carboxymethyl-cellulose and microcrystalline cellulose exhibit some thixotropic flow characteristics. Other pseudoplastics such as hydroxyethylcellulose or hydroxypropyl methyl cellulose may be required to overcome possible in compatibilities with sodium carboxymethylcellulose.

Emulsion Base

An emulsion base or a waxy-type self-emulsifier to develop structure or "false body" in suspension systems is widely used in both pharmaceutical and cosmetic systems. A dilute emulsion system is not often considered for suspension purposes because of the potential complexities involved in mixing emulsion and suspension systems. The drug particles are dispersed in the primary emulsion component prior to dilution with other vehicle components. Emulsifiers that exhibit Bingham plastic or thixotropic flow characteristics should have acceptable formulating properties (taste, stability, etc.).

FORMULATION OF SUSPENSIONS

During the preparation of physically stable pharmaceutical suspensions, a number of formulation components are used to keep the solid particles in a state of suspension (suspending agents), whereas other components are part of the liquid vehicle itself and have other functions in the dosage form.

1. *Components of the suspending system*
   Wetting agents
   Dispersants or deflocculating agents
   Flocculating agents
   Thickeners

2. *Components of the suspending vehicle or external phase*
   pH control agents and buffers
   Osmotic agents
   Coloring agents, flavors, and fragrances
   Preservatives to control microbial growth

Table 2 Concentration of suspending agents in water at 25°C required to achieve a yield value of 10 Pa

Agent	Concentration (%)
Carbomer 941	0.1
Carbomer 934	0.2
Carrageenan	0.5
Carboxymethylcellulose	2.0
Xanthan gum	2.0
Algin	3.5
Magnesium aluminum silicate	5.0
Hydroxyethylcellulose	5.0
Guar gum	5.0
Tragacanth gum	5.0

(From B.F. Goodrich Specialty Chemicals, Cleveland, Ohio.)

Wetting Agents

Wetting agents are surfactants that lower the interfacial tension and contact angle between solid particles and the liquid vehicle. When the insoluble powder is added to a liquid vehicle containing a wetting agent, penetration of the liquid phase into the powder will be sufficiently rapid to permit air to escape from the particles. The resulting wetted particles either sink en masse or separate with low-shear agitation. The best range for wetting and spreading by nonionic surfactants is between a hydrophile–lipophile balance (HLB) value of 7 and 10, although surfactants with values higher than 10 are often used for this purpose. Common wetting agents and surfactants include: 1) anionic type (docusate sodium and sodium lauryl sulfate); and 2) nonionic type (polyoxyalkyl ethers, polyoxylakyl phenyl ethers, polyoxy hydrogenated castor oil, polyoxy sorbitan esters, and sorbitan esters).

Deflocculants and Dispersing Agents

Unlike surfactants, these agents do not appreciably lower surface and interfacial tension; thus, they have little tendency to create foam or wet particles. Most deflocculants, however, are not generally considered safe for internal use, and as a result the only acceptable dispersant for internal products is lecithin or a lecithin derivative (naturally occurring mixture of phosphatides and phospholipids). Because lecithins vary in water solubility and dispersibility characteristics, proper control of product specifications must be maintained to obtain reproducibility.

Flocculating Agents

Primary flocculating agents are simple neutral electrolytes in solution that are capable of reducing the ζ-potential of suspended charged particles to zero. Small concentrations (0.01–1%) of neutral electrolytes, such as sodium or potassium chloride, are often sufficient to induce flocculation of weakly charged, water-insoluble, organic nonelectrolytes. In the case of highly charged, insoluble polymers and polyelectrolyte species, similar concentrations (0.01–1%) of water-soluble divalent or trivalent ions, such as calcium salts, alums, sulfates, citrates, and phosphates, may be required for floc formation, depending on particle charge (positive or negative). These salts are often used together as pH buffers and flocculating agents.

Thickeners, Protective Colloids, and Suspending Agents

Protective or hydrophilic colloids, such as gelatin, natural gums, and cellulosic derivatives, that are adsorbed on insoluble particles, increase the strength of the hydration layer formed around suspended particles through hydrogen bonding and molecular interaction. Because these agents do not reduce surface and interfacial tension, they function best in the presence of a wetting agent. Many of these agents are protective colloids in low concentration (<0.1%) and viscosity builders in higher concentrations (>0.1%). Suspending agents commonly used in pharmaceutical suspensions include:

- *Cellulosics*: sodium carboxymethylcellulose, microcrystalline cellulose (including coprecipitates and blends of the two), hydroxyethylcellulose, hydroxypropyl cellulose, hydroxypropyl methylcellulose, methylcellulose, starch, sodium starch glycolate, and powdered cellulose
- *Clays*: attapulgite, bentonite, magnesium aluminum silicate, kaolin, silicon dioxides
- *Gums*: acacia, agar, algins, carrageenan, guar, pectin, tragacanth, xanthan
- *Polymers*: carbomers, polyvinyl alcohol, povidone, polyethylene oxide
- *Sugars*: dextrin, maltitol, sucrose
- *Others*: aluminum monostearate, emulsifying waxes, gelatin

The other agents used in pharmaceutical suspensions (pH control agents, buffers, osmotic agents, stabilizers, vehicles, colorants, flavors, fragrances, and preservatives to control microbial growth) are not discussed in this article.

STERILE SUSPENSIONS

Sterile suspensions (injectable and ophthalmic) have characteristics that are not commonly shared by other suspension systems, such as ease of resuspension, drainage, absence of foreign particulate matter and pyrogens, and syringeability in the case of injectable suspensions.

The preparation of a sterile suspension is a difficult manufacturing procedure. It requires strict attention to detail during the final recrystallization of the active drug substance, size reduction, and sterilization of the active drug substance and the suspending vehicle, aseptic wetting of the sterile drug powder with a portion of the sterile vehicle, aseptic dispersion and milling of the bulk sterile suspension, and aseptic filling of the finished suspension into sterile containers.

Various procedures for the manufacture of sterile suspensions have been reported by Akers et al. (12), Grimes (13), and Portnoff (14). At present, there is no pharmaceutically acceptable chemical agent that can be added to the finished suspension to make it both sterile and safe. Therefore, an elaborate program of sterility checks at critical phases of the operation is required.

An important property of a good parenteral suspension is syringeability; the ability of a parenteral solution or suspension to pass easily through a hypodermic needle, especially during the transfer of a product from vial to hypodermic syringe prior to injection. Increases in vehicle viscosity, vehicle density, and size and concentration of suspended particles make the transfer more difficult.

The most important of these features is probably viscosity. Fortunately, in the case of parenteral suspensions, viscosity is the easiest parameter to control. The preparation of a stable floc contributes little to the overall viscosity of the system (the so-called Einstein relationship) and does not adversely influence syringeability. Although the individual particles are held loosely together in large multiple aggregates, they are easily broken up and reformed during the passage from vial to syringe and syringe to injection site.

Drainage, or the ability of the suspension to break cleanly away from the inner walls of the primary container-closure system, is another important characteristics of a well-formulated parenteral suspension. Deflocculated to flocculated systems show this property, whereas overflocculated systems show some degree of poor drainage, also called "buttermilk appearance," a term that aptly describes this unsightly condition. Silicone coated containers, vials and plugs with dimethicone improve drainage and help reverse the tendency toward poor drainage by slightly overflocculated systems.

Resuspendability, or the ability to distribute settled particles with a minimum of shaking, is an important characteristic of parenteral suspensions. Stable, flocculated parenteral suspensions that have been undisturbed for long periods of storage time are easily resuspended.

COSMETIC SUSPENSIONS

Cosmetic suspensions are available in two types. The first comprises pigmented products that are suspended in essentially aqueous vehicles (liquid makeup, eyeliners, mascara, and blusher). These products have a high solids content, high density, impalpable powders, and pigments permanently suspended in a primary oil-in-water emulsion-type base or a complex system of hydrophilic cellulose derivatives, clays, and/or polymeric film formers, in which the gelling and suspending properties of the vehicle often are reinforced by a small amount of a Bingham-type plastic such as carbomer.

The second type comprises pigment-containing nail enamels. The coloring tints, pigments, pearls, and lakes are suspended with the aid of an organophilic, thixotropic gellant, such as stearalkonium hectorite in a nonaqueous vehicle, containing butyl acetate, ethyl acetate, and isopropyl alcohol solvents in which the primary plasticized nitrocellulose and toluene sulfonamide—formaldehyde resin film formers are dissolved. Nail enamel is an excellent example of a permanent suspension in a nonaqueous vehicle.

TEST METHODS FOR PHARMACEUTICAL SUSPENSIONS

Tingstad (15) reviewed test methods for determining the physical stability of pharmaceutical suspensions. The procedures outlined are designed to determine the state of flocculation of a formulation. Because there is more than one method of preparing stable suspensions, the following test methods and performance criteria were found useful for determining the stability of both flocculated and dispersed systems.

Appearance

The appearance in a graduated glass cylinder or transparent glass container is noted. The following questions were addressed: At equilibrium, is the color and appearance of the sediment uniform? Are there breaks or air pockets in the sediment? Is the residual drainage

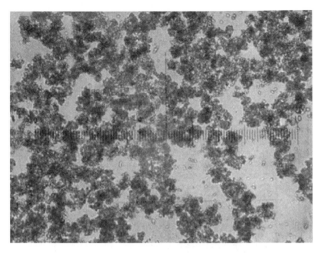

Fig. 4 Photomicrograph of a flocculated steroid suspension.

above the sediment uniform and minimal, or is there coagulated material adhering to the inside walls of the container?

Photomicroscopic Examination

The microscope can be used to estimate and detect changes in particle size distribution and crystal shape. Its usefulness can be enhanced by attaching a Polaroid-type camera to the microscope to permit rapid processing of photomicrographs (Fig. 4). These can be used, for example, to distinguish between flocculated and nonflocculated particles and to determine changes in the physical properties and stability. Sufficient fields and samples should be examined to make these determinations. Dilutions for microscopic examination should be made with supernatant external phase rather than with purified water. Individual particle size distributions can be accurately determined, using suitable electron instrumentation, for example, a Coulter Multisizer II (an electrical sensing zone instrument from Coulter Scientific Instruments, Hialeah, FL) or the Elzone 280 PC systems (Particle Data, Elmhurst, IL). General methods for particle size analysis are given in Fig. 5.

Color, Odor, and Taste

These characteristics are especially important in orally administered suspensions. Variation in color often indicates poor distribution and/or differences in particle size. Variations in taste, especially of active constituents, can often be attributed to changes in particle size, crystal

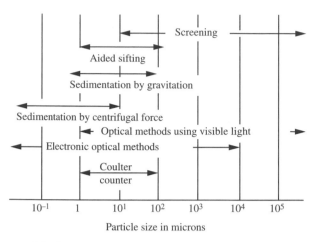

Fig. 5 General methods for particle size analysis.

habit, and subsequent particle dissolution. Changes in color, odor, and taste can also indicate chemical instability.

Sedimentation Rate, Sediment Volume, and Resuspendability

Simple, inexpensive, graduated cylinders (100–1000 mL) are useful for determining the physical stability of suspensions. They can be used to determine the settling rates of flocculated and nonflocculated suspensions and the sediment height at equilibrium. The falling height of the liquid—sediment interface of the suspension is determined as a function of time, and the sedimentation rate test is repeated periodically during storage. The sediment volume at equilibrium should be sufficiently large to support uniform resuspension with gentle agitation. The equilibrium sediment volume should be similar and reproducible batch after batch.

Volumetric graduated cylinders are used to determine the "*F*" or flocculation ratio, a value that represents the ratio of the sediment volume to the original suspension volume at a given time. It is used to measure the relative degree of flocculation and physical stability of suspensions. A sufficiently wide graduated cylinder should be used to overcome the "wall effect" which often influences the settling rate and equilibrium sediment volume of flocculated suspensions. Small graduated cylinders have a tendency to support suspensions because of the adhesive forces acting between the inner surface of the container and the suspended particles.

Viscosity

A Brookfield viscometer with a helipath attachment (Stoughton, MA) is a useful rheological instrument for measuring the settling behavior and structure of pharmaceutical suspensions and for characterizing the properties and stability of flocculated suspensions. The viscometer should be properly calibrated to measure the apparent viscosity of the suspension at equilibrium at a given temperature to establish suspension reproducibility. Apparent viscosity, like pH, is an exponential term, and therefore the log-apparent viscosity is an appropriate way of reporting the results.

Density

Specific gravity or density of the suspension is an important parameter. A decrease in density often indicates the presence of entrapped air within the structure of the suspension. Density measurements at a given temperature should be made using well-mixed, uniform suspensions; precision hydrometers facilitate such measurements.

pH Value

The pH value of aqueous suspensions should be taken at a given temperature and only after settling equilibrium has been reached, to minimize "pH drift" and electrode surface coating with suspended particles. Electrolyte should not be added to the external phase of the suspension to stabilize the pH, because neutral electrolytes disturb the physical stability of the suspension.

Freeze—Thaw Cycling

This is a useful guide to the physical stability of suspensions. If freeze—thaw cycling or elevated temperature exposures are chosen for physical stability testing, companion samples of a closely related marketed suspension should be included in the testing protocol for comparison purpose because pharmaceutical suspensions are not normally designed to withstand temperature extremes during storage (15–30°C optimum).

Drug Content Uniformity

This important testing procedure is best performed using either "unit of use" volume (e.g., 5 mL of oral liquid or a spray actuation of an oral inhalation product) or sampling from a well-mixed dispensing container from the top, middle, and bottom of the suspension.

Dissolution Testing

This technique (16) is still evolving. The favored approach at present is to submerge a small, known amount of suspension inside a secured Durapore (polyvinylidene fluoride) membrane pouch (Millipore Products, Bedford, MA) of suitable porosity in "teabag" fashion in a suitable dissolution medium using the USP Method 1 Paddle Apparatus (17). Optimization of experimental conditions (rate of agitation, volume and type of medium, temperature, etc.) must be established to achieve reproducible results.

Particle Size Measurement

Recently (18–20), with respect to the importance of particle size distribution in terms of particle characterization and product physical stability testing, there has been interest in newer light-scattering methods for particle detection called photon correlation spectroscopy (PCS). PCS methods can be applied to both micro-and nanosuspensions.

The information thus obtained from the use of such equipment includes mean particle size, particle size distribution, particle concentration, molecular weight estimation, polydispersity, particle shape, hydrodynamic interactions, and aggregation mechanisms.

In addition (21), there are several experimental options available for particle size measurement alone. They include single particle optical sensing (SPOS), laser diffraction (LD), and ultrasound attenuation (UA).

Other Procedures

Assays for potency, preservative effectiveness, compatibility with primary container-closure system, off-torque, simulated use testing, etc., should be handled in a manner similar to that used for conventional liquid solutions, with the provision that the container is well-mixed prior to sampling.

NANOSUSPENSIONS

Pharmaceutical nanosuspensions (22) are usually very finely dispersed solid drug particles in an aqueous vehicle for either oral and topical use or for parenteral and pulmonary administration. The key difference from conventional suspensions is that the particle size distribution of the solid particles in nanosuspensions is usually less than 1 μm, with an average particle size range between 200 and 600 nm.

The techniques used for preparing nanoparticles are similar to those used to prepare more conventional drug particles and include controlled precipitation, ball milling using glass or zirconium oxide pearls, and high-pressure homogenization.

Nanosuspensions can be sterilized for parenteral use by using conventional steam sterilization in an autoclave, γ-irradiation, or membrane microfiltration in certain situations.

The key to long-term physical stability of aqueous nanosuspensions is the selection of a suitable water-soluble surfactant or polymer as an external particle stabilizer to prevent particle growth. Several potential stabilizers are lecithin, phospholipids, poloxamers, and polysorbates.

The physical stability of nanosuspensions may be monitored with the use of electron microscopic analysis.

The major advantage of pharmaceutical nanosuspensions is their ability to increase the in vivo absorption of highly–water-insoluble drugs by dramatically reduced particle size.

REFERENCES

1. Martin, A.; Bustamante, P. *Physical Pharmacy*, 4th Ed.; Lea & Febiger: Philadelphia, 1993; 477–484.
2. Marcus, A.D.; DeKay, H.G. New Developments in Calamine Lotion. J. Am. Pharm. Assoc., Pract. Ed. **1950**, *11*, 227–229.
3. Boylan, J.C. The Development of Semi-Solid Dosage Forms: An Overview. Drug Dev. Commun. **1976**, *2*, 320.
4. Robinson, M.J. Third Annual National Industrial Pharmaceutical Research Conference, Land O'Lakes: WI, 1961.
5. Hiestand, E.N. Theory of Coarse Suspension Formulation. J. Pharm. Sci. **1964**, *53*, 1–18.
6. Carpenter, C.R. Calculate Settling Velocities for Unrestricted Particles on Hindered Settling. Chem. Engr. **Nov. 1983**, *4*.
7. Haines, B.A.; Martin, A.N. Interfacial Properties of Powdered Material. J. Pharm. Sci. **1961**, *50*, 228–232, 753–759.
8. Matthews, B.A.; Rhodes, C.T. Use of DLVO Theory to Interpret Pharmaceutical Suspension Stability. J. Pharm. Sci. **1970**, *59*, 521–525.
9. Ecanow, B.; Gold, B.; Ecanow, C. Newer Aspects of Suspension Theory. Am. Perfum. Cosmet. **Nov. 1969**, *84*, 27–31.
10. Ecanow, B.; Webster, J.; Blake, M.I. Conductivity Studies of Suspension Systems in Different States of Aggregation. J. Pharm. Sci. **1982**, *71*, 456–457.
11. Michaels, A.S.; Bolger, J.C. The Plastic Flow Behavior of Flocculated Kaolin Suspension. Ind. Eng. Chem. Fundam. **1962**, *1*, 153–162.

12. Akers, M.J.; Fites, A.L.; Rabinson, R.L. Formulation Design and Development of Parenteral Suspensions. J. Parenter. Sci. Technol. **1987**, *41*, 88–96.

13. Grimes, T.L. Scaleup and Manufacture of Sterile Suspensions, APhA 133rd Annual Meeting, San Francisco, March 19, 1986.

14. Portnoff, J.B. The Development of Sterile Suspensions—Case Study, APhA 133rd Annual Meeting, San Francisco, March 19, 1986.

15. Tingstad, J.E. Physical Stability Testing of Pharmaceuticals. J. Pharm. Sci. **1964**, *53*, 955–962.

16. Stout, P.J.; Howard, S.A.; Mauger, J.W. Dissolution of Pharmaceutical Suspensions. *Encyclopedia of Pharmaceutical Technology*; Swarbrick, J., Boylan, J.C., Eds.; Marcel Dekker, Inc.: New York, 1991; 4, 169–192.

17. United States Pharmacopeia 24, The Pharmacopeial Convention, Rockville, MD 2000, 4.

18. Castanho, M. *Light Scattering and Photon Correlation Spectroscopy*, NATO ASI Series, High Technology, 1997; 40, 31–36.

19. Constantinides, P.P.; Yiv, S.H. Int. J. Pharm. **1995**, *115*, 225.

20. Ruth, H. Saint Int. J. Pharm. **1994**, *116*, 253.

21. Nicoli, D. Am. Lab. **Jan. 2000**.

22. Miiller, R.H.; Jacobs, C.; Kayser, O. Nanosuspensions. *Pharmaceutical Emulsions and Suspensions*; Nielloud, F., Marti-Mestres, G., Eds.; Marcel Dekker, Inc.: New York, 2000.

23. Banker, G.S.; Rhodes, C.T. *Modern Pharmaceutics*, 2nd Ed.; Rev. Exp., Marcel Dekker, Inc. New York, 1989, 339–353.

24. *Handbook of Pharmaceutical Excipients,* 3rd Ed., APhA and Pharmaceutical Press: London, 2000.

25. Martin, A.; Bustamante, P. *Physical Pharmacy*, 4th Ed.; Lea & Febiger: Philadelphia, 1993; 477–484.

26. Nash, R.A. Pharmaceutical Suspensions. *Pharmaceutical Dosage Forms, Dispersed Systems*; Lieberman, H.L., Rieger, M.M., Banker, G.S., Eds.; Marcel Dekker, Inc.: New York, 1988; 1, 151–198.

27. Zografi, G.; Swarbrick, J.; Schott, H. Disperse Systems. *Remington's Pharmaceutical Sciences*; Gennaro, A.R., Ed.; Mack Publishing Co.: Easton PA, 1990; 257–309.

TABLET COMPRESSION: MACHINE THEORY, DESIGN, AND PROCESS TROUBLESHOOTING

Michael J. Bogda

Barr Laboratories, Inc., Pomona, New York

INTRODUCTION

The most common method of drug delivery is the oral solid dosage form, of which tablets and capsules are predominant. The tablet is more widely accepted and used compared to capsules for a number of reasons, such as cost, tamper resistance, ease of handling and packaging, ease of identification, and manufacturing efficiency. Over the past several years, the issue of tamper resistance has resulted in the conversion of most over-the-counter drugs from capsules to predominantly all tablets.

Pharmaceutical products have been manufactured into compressed tablets for many years. During the 1950s, much research was devoted to the physics of compression (1, 2). Since that time, the pharmaceutical industry has attained a much greater understanding of the compression process, which resulted in the development of more robust pharmaceutical formulations (3–5). This has been achieved by the use of instrumented tablet presses and sophisticated data collection systems combined with the development of mathematical models.

During this time, a significant portion of the development work has been conducted on older equipment, which has been retrofitted to measure compression and ejection-force signals. Recent advances in the design of tablet compression equipment has resulted in higher-efficiency machines designed to optimize compression efficiency, minimize tablet weight variation, and provide greater flexibility, allowing the production of a greater range of products. However, the modern sophisticated machines still employ the same general concepts of operation: die fill, tablet compression, tablet ejection, and tablet scrape-off. Therefore, studies conducted on older equipment designed to evaluate the compression characteristics of materials, can offer significant insight into material behavior. However, modern machines provide greater accuracy and efficiency as follows:

- Improved material feed systems.
- Improved cam design and material of construction.
- Multistage compression.
- Isolated design for quick cleaning and changeover.

- Improved force-measurement techniques.
- Introduction of electronics to provide force control.
- Integration of on-line weight, thickness, and hardness test units providing weight feedback control to the force control unit, and
- High-speed single-tablet sorting to reject out-of-specification tablets.

Therefore, optimal product development can typically be performed on these machines that offer improved compression designs and material feed systems.

This article provides the basic information necessary to understand the general process of tablet formation. General machine design characteristics and tablet press nomenclature are presented. Tablet press control systems and process automation are discussed, followed by process and product troubleshooting on tablet compression equipment.

THE PROCESS OF TABLET FORMATION

The quality of a compressed tablet is determined by material fill characteristics and compression behavior. During compression, the rate at which tablets can be produced can be limited due to nonuniform material fill characteristics. Pending successful and reproducible material fill (die fill), the powder mass must form a coherent compact that stays intact upon ejection out of the die. Therefore, tablet press performance can be limited due to poor fill characteristics and/or poor compression behavior.

Die fill characteristics depend upon material flow properties that are primarily affected by particle size and shape. Additionally, high interparticle friction can have a detrimental effect on die fill characteristics due to powder bridging and nonuniform flow characteristics. A nonuniform particle size distribution may also lead to material segregation resulting in uniformity problems. Tablet presses employ volumetric filling of the material into the die cavity. Most high-speed tablet presses are equipped with force feeders, which use rotating paddles to promote

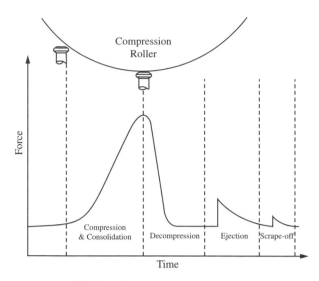

Fig. 1 The compression process.

uniform die fill characteristics. For certain materials, attention must be paid to ensure that the action of the power feeder does not cause overmixing or segregation of the material.

Upon proper die fill, one must consider whether the material will form a tablet. The tableting characteristics of powders depend on the viscoelastic properties of the material. The process of compaction has been defined as "the compression and consolidation of a two-phase system due to an applied load." (6). The quality of the compact depends on the compression and consolidation of the powder mass, decompression of the compact, ejection from the die, and subsequent scrape-off from the lower punch. A schematic representation of the compression process is shown in Fig. 1. Because these viscoelastic properties are time dependent, both the magnitude and the rate of application (and release) of the compression force affect tablet quality.

Compression and Consolidation

During compression, the bulk volume of the material is reduced, resulting in the displacement of the gaseous phase (air) (6). Further increasing the force leads to particle deformation and rearrangement. At this point, the three principal modes of deformation are as follows:

1. *Elastic deformation*: A spontaneously reversible deformation of the compact in which, upon removal of the load, the powder mass reverts back to its original form. Most materials undergo elastic deformation to some extent. Compression of rubber would be by elastic deformation.

2. *Plastic deformation*: After exceeding the elastic limit of the material (yield point), the deformation may become plastic, that is, the particles undergo viscous flow. This is the predominant mechanism when the shear strength between the particles is less than the tensile or breaking strength. Plastic deformation is a time-dependent process.

3. *Brittle fracture*: Upon exceeding the elastic limit of the material (yield point), the particles undergo brittle fracture if the shear strength between the particles is greater than the tensile or breaking strength. Under these conditions, the larger particles are sheared and broken into smaller particles.

The compression process includes these three mechanisms. The individual characteristics of the material under investigation determine the extent to which each is active. Since some of these deformation characteristics are time-dependent, machine characteristics can have a major effect on tableting performance. These characteristics determine the rate of force application, dwell time (i.e., the time of maximum compression force, which depends on the punch head flat diameter and the tangential velocity), and the rate of decompression (see Fig. 1).

Typically for materials that undergo plastic deformation, as machine speed is increased there is less time for stress relaxation. Under these conditions, the tablets may cap and laminate. However, capping and lamination can be eliminated or minimized by slowing down the compression process (reducing the machine speed), lowering the rate of force application (larger compression roller diameter), or increasing the time of compression (multistage compression).

The final tablet properties are also affected by the consolidation (i.e., bonding) mechanisms of the powder which is influenced by its chemical nature, the surface area of the contact points, contamination (including film coatings such as magnesium stearate), and interparticle distance. The predominant consolidation mechanisms are listed below (7–10):

- *Mechanical theory*: As the particles undergo deformation, the particle boundaries intertwine to form mechanical bonds.
- *Intermolecular forces theory*: van der Waals forces bond the molecules together at the newly sheared surfaces of the particle boundaries. Microcrystalline cellulose is believed to undergo significant hydrogen bonding during tablet compression (11).
- *Liquid-surface film theory*: Thin liquid films form which bond the particles together at the particle surface. The energy of compression produces melting or solution at the particle interface followed by subsequent

solidification or crystallization thus resulting in the formation of bonded surfaces. Due to the applied pressure, the particles may melt or dissolve. As the pressure is released, solidification and crystallization occur.

The intermolecular forces theory and the liquid-surface film theory are believed to be the major bonding mechanisms in tablet compression. Many pharmaceutical formulations require a certain level of residual moisture to produce high quality tablets. The role of moisture in the tableting process is supported by the liquid-surface film theory.

During tablet formation, as load is applied to the powder mass, plastic deformation and brittle fracture create clean surfaces that are brought in intimate contact by the applied load. These surfaces bond together by a number of mechanisms such as those listed earlier. Plastic deformation is believed to create the greatest number of clean surfaces. Because it is time-dependent, higher rates of force application should lead to the formation of less new clean surfaces, resulting in weaker tablets. Additionally, because tablet formation is dependent upon the formation of clean new surfaces, high concentrations or overmixing of materials that form weak bonds result in weak tablets. Magnesium stearate, for example, forms weak bonds and easily wets surfaces. Therefore, over-lubrication or overmixing of magnesium stearate may lead to weak tablets.

Fragmentation (the creation of new clean surfaces) continues at the same time at which bonding and densification occur. A high quality tablet can be formed only when the process of bonding and densification exceeds fragmentation. The rates at which these functions occur are dependent upon the rate at which the forces are applied.

During compression, the powder compact typically undergoes a temperature increase (12, 13), which depends on frictional effects that are dependent, in turn, on the specific material characteristics, the lubrication efficiency, the magnitude and rate of application of the compression forces, and the machine speed. Typical temperature increases are between 4 and 30°C (14). As the tablet temperature rises, stress relaxation and plasticity increase, while the elasticity decreases and strong tablets are formed (15). Therefore, compression of material, at elevated temperature with increased ductility should result in stronger tablets.

It is believed that under certain conditions precompression is beneficial because it helps to remove entrapped air (16) and extends dwell time, thereby increasing the degree of stress relaxation and plastic deformation (17) as well as

the number of bonds, thus increasing tablet strength. Additionally, by extending the time of compression, precompression may provide a gradual loading and unloading of force. However, recent studies (18) suggest that a high level of precompression (higher than that of the main compression) may improve the tableting character-istics more than conventional tableting where main compression exceeds precompression. It is theorized that this effect is due to the high initial compression force that raises the tablet temperature, thereby increasing ductility and allowing greater plastic deformation. Application of the lower second compression force increases the formation of particle–particle bonds while minimizing particle-bond rupture, resulting in stronger tablets.

Decompression

After the compression and consolidation of the powder in the die, the formed compact must be capable of withstanding the stresses encountered during decompres-sion and tablet ejection (19). The rate at which the force is removed (dependent on the compression roller diameter and the machine speed) can have a significant effect on tablet quality. The same deformation characteristics that come into play during compression play a role during decompression.

After application of the maximum compression force, the tablet undergoes elastic recovery. While the tablet is constrained in the die, elastic recovery occurs only in the axial direction. If the rate and degree of elastic recovery are high, the tablet may cap or laminate in the die due to rapid expansion in the radial direction only. If the tablet undergoes brittle fracture during decompression, the compact may form failure plains due to the fracturing of the surfaces. Tablets that do not cap or laminate are able to relieve the developed stresses by plastic deformation. Since plastic deformation is time-dependent, stress relaxation is also time-dependent. Therefore, tablet fracture is affected by rates of decompression (machine speed) since the compact may not have sufficient time to relieve the internal stresses created during decompression. Formulations which contain significant concentrations of microcrystalline cellulose typically form good compacts due to its plastic deformation properties. However, if the machine speed and the rate of tablet compression are significantly increased, these formulations exhibit capping and lamination tendencies.

The rate of decompression can also have an effect on the ability of the compacts to consolidate (form bonds). Based on the liquid-surface film theory, the rate of crystallization or solidification should have an effect on the strength of the bonded surfaces. The rate of crystallization is affected by the pressure (and the rate at which the pressure is removed). High decompression rates should result in high rates of crystallization. Typically, slower crystallization rates result in stronger crystals. Therefore, if bonding occurs by these mechanisms, lower machine speeds (lower rates of decompression and crystallization) should result in stronger tablets.

Ejection

After decompression, the tablet remains in the die until it is ejected. During this time, a residual die wall force is exerted by the tablet on the die wall. Tablet ejection is defined by three stages (6):

1. The initial ejection peak force required to break the tablet adhesion to the die wall. This force is the highest force encountered during ejection and occurs over a very short period of time.
2. The force required to push the tablet up the die wall, which is typically lower than the ejection peak force. However, inadequate lubrication or damaged dies may result in slip-stick behavior where the tablet continues to adhere and break adhesions to the die wall surface. These conditions typically result in tablet failure.
3. Declining forces as the tablet emerges from the die.

Inadequate lubrication typically results in high ejection forces and possibly tablet failure. Ejection forces below 200 N are optimal, although forces up to 400 N are common. Ejection forces ranging between 400 and 800 N are considered high. Forces exceeding 800 N result in excessive heat build-up and could lead to machine damage and product failure. Inadequate lubrication can also result in striations along the tablet side wall, and picking and sticking.

Tablets that undergo significant elastic recovery upon decompression may exhibit capping upon ejection out of the die. Under these circumstances, the tablet builds up significant stress while in the die, which can only be relieved in the axial direction. As the tablet emerges from the die, its top portion can expand in both the radial and axial directions while the portion remaining in the die is confined. Shear stresses develop along the edge of the die and result in tablet failure.

Scrape-Off

Tablet scrape-off occurs immediately after ejection. Figure 2 illustrates a tablet stripper on a rotary tablet press. Typical forces during tablet scrape-off are 2 N or less. Scrape-off forces of 6 N or higher result in tablets

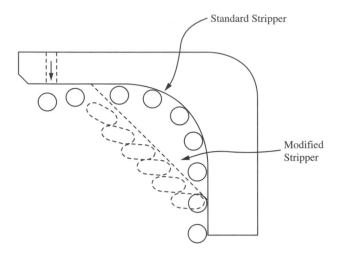

Fig. 2 Tablet stripper.

sticking to the lower punches and subsequently picking or, under extreme circumstances, shearing the bottom of the tablet. Frequently, shearing of the lower portions of the tablet due to scrape-off problems is mistaken for capping. However, this can be easily distinguished by examining the lower punches and rotating the press manually.

At high machine speeds, scrape-off problems may be encountered due to tablets backing up at the point of discharge. Under many circumstances, specially modified tablet strippers have proven to be beneficial for shaped tablets by discharging the tablets off the die table as quickly as possible (see Fig. 2).

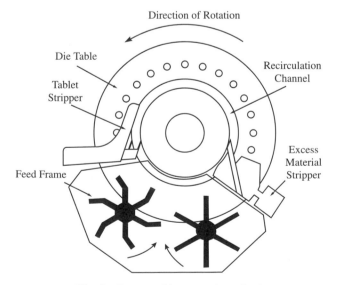

Fig. 3 Rotary tablet press (top view).

ROTARY TABLET PRESS DESIGN

Pharmaceutical tablets are generally produced on rotary tablet presses (Fig. 3), where upper and lower punches reside in the upper and lower turret, respectively. The dies are inserted in the die table and secured by die lock screws. The upper and lower turret and the die table are precisely aligned. The movement of the punches is controlled by cam tracks and compression rollers. As the entire assembly rotates, the upper and lower punches move along the cam tracks to accomplish die fill, tablet compression, ejection, and scrape-off.

Tablet Compression

Tablet compression can be separated into the two distinct yet equally important phases of die fill-weight adjustment and tablet formation as shown in Fig. 4. As die fill begins, the lower punch face is initially flush with the die table surface as the lower punch enters the overfill cam at the entry of the feeder. The lower punch travels under the feeder and is pulled down by the overfill cam. At this point the lower punch has passed through approximately 50% of the feeder and the die cavity contains more material than required.

After overfilling the die cavity, the lower punch is adjusted to a constant height as it passes into the weight-regulation unit. The constant height, known as the fill depth, is measured as the distance between the lower punch face and the die table surface. Since die fill is volumetric, the constant height of the lower punch in the weight-regulation unit provides a constant volume of material. Therefore, the fill depth is affected by the density of the granulation. Variation of granulation density between batches results in different fill depths, whereas variable granulation density within a batch results in fluctuating fill depth requirements.

As the lower punch passes from the fill cam to the weight-regulation cam, the excess material is pushed back into the feeder and scraped off at the top of the die table by the excess material stripper and directed into a recirculation channel. On many modern presses, the lower punch is lowered by approximately 2–4 mm relative to the top of the die table after the excess material stripper. This lowers the material away from the top of the die table, minimizing uncontrolled loss as the upper punch enters into the die cavity after scrape-off. Under these circumstances the upper punch does not contact the top of the material until it enters into the die, minimizing material loss and weight variation. Additionally, lowering the slug of material away

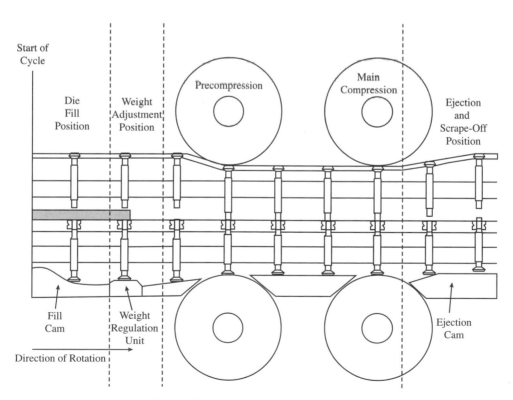

Fig. 4 Rotary press (sequences of compression).

from the die table surface reduces material loss due to the centrifugal force of the rotating die table.

Overfilling of the die cavity is necessary to achieve uniform tablet weights and to optimize machine running conditions. However, at times excessive overfilling can lead to other problems such as excessive wear for abrasive raw materials, particle size reduction for friable granulations, material segregation, and overmixing of lubricant. Therefore, the effect of different machine running conditions must be evaluated for each different product separately.

The material that is directed into the recirculation channel is subsequently introduced back into the feeder at the tablet stripper or at the inside edge of the feeder. It is worth noting that the paddle in the feeder at the point of material entry rotates in the opposite direction as the turret to aid in die fill and induce flow back into the feeder.

Frequently the maximum machine speed may depend on die fill characteristics due to excess tablet weight variation at high machine speeds. However, because the compression characteristics of most pharmaceutical products exhibit viscoelastic properties, the press speed may also have a major effect on the compressibility of the material. For this reason, the ability to compress a tablet adequately is often the overriding factor to consider in tablet compression.

The process of tablet formation begins as the upper punch is lowered directly into the die cavity after the excess material stripper. As mentioned previously, it is advantageous if the slug of material is lower than the die table surface as the upper punch enters to minimize uncontrolled material loss and weight variation. After the upper punch enters into the die, the upper and lower punches begin to move toward each other as the punches ride along cam tracks toward the precompression rollers. At the precompression stage, the initial (and typically the lower) compression force is applied. Traditionally, tablet presses were equipped to apply a 20 kN maximum precompression force using relatively small compression rollers (approximately 100-mm (4-in.) diameter rollers). However, to improve flexibility, many modern rotary tablet presses are equipped with identical precompression and main compression force capabilities, allowing the application of 80–100 kN forces using 250–300-mm-diameter compression rollers.

After application of the precompression force, the punches move toward the main compression rollers where the final (main) force is applied. As the punches impact the rollers, the compression force increases until the punch head flat is tangent to the compression roller and maximum force is applied (see Fig. 1). The applied compression force is a measured value and depends on the distance between the punches and the quantity of material in the die. After main compression, the upper punch is pulled out of the die cavity while the lower punch impacts the ejection cam to begin the ejection process. As the die table continues to rotate, the lower punch raises the tablet out of the die cavity to eject the tablet to the point of scrape-off.

Press Design and Layout

Modern rotary tablet presses are typically designed in separate machine sections (press zones). Typical sections to provide separation and isolation of the compression area from the other components are as follows:

- Upper cam section
- Compression section
- Lower cam section
- Lower mechanical section
- Electrical section

With the proper separation of these areas, only the compression zone is exposed to material, thus reducing cleaning and change-over time of the tablet press. In addition to the machine sections, an understanding of other machine subsystems is necessary, such as the lubrication system and the diagnostic systems (safety systems) to achieve optimal machine performance.

Modern rotary tablet presses are either single-sided or double-sided. A single-sided machine has one feeding station, one set of precompression and main compression rollers, and one discharge station. These machines produce one tablet per punch station per die table revolution. A double-sided machine has two feeding stations, two sets of precompression and main compression rollers, and two discharge stations, and produces two tablets per punch station per die table revolution. The double-sided machine operates identically to the single-sided machine with the exception that the excess material from the first feeding station passes into the second feeding station. A double-sided machine has a higher output than a single-sided machine. Its pitch circle diameter is also greater, which could result in weight uniformity and compressibility issues.

Bilayer tablet presses employ the same general design concepts as single-sided machines. Typically, a double-sided machine can be converted to a bilayer machine by replacing various cams. The material for each layer is introduced separately into each feeder and is removed from the die table to prevent contamination.

Upper cam section

The upper cam section is typically shrouded and sealed to prevent exposure of material. It consists of the upper cam track, all upper compression rollers, and all adjustments to the position of the upper compression rollers. The primary components of the upper cam section are as follows:

1. *Upper punch removal/dwell cams*: The upper punches are loaded and removed from the machine at this location. These cams typically reside directly above the material feeder. In many press designs, the upper punch dwell cam is designed to measure the tightness of the upper punches in the turret. A spring loaded cam designed to raise the upper punch slightly (1–4 mm) is connected to a proximity sensor. If the punches are too tight then the spring-loaded cam falls instead of raising the upper punches, thus tripping the proximity sensor and shutting down the machine. In alternative press designs, the upper punch tightness is measured in the upper-punch pull-up cam, typically by a strain gauge measurement of the lifting force.

2. *Upper punch lowering cam*: The upper punches are lowered into the die cavity by the upper-punch lowering cam. This cam is typically CAD optimized to minimize the acceleration and velocity of the upper punch as it enters into the die cavity. In this way, the upper punch travels in a smooth and controlled manner as it enters the die cavity, thus improving weight uniformity.

3. *Upper precompression and main compression rollers insertion depth adjustments*: Insertion depth for both precompression and main compression is adjusted in the upper cam section. The insertion depth determines the location of tablet formation in the die cavity relative to the top of the die table as shown in Fig. 5. It is measured as the distance at which the upper punch enters into the die at the tangent between the upper punch head and the compression roller. Insertion depth can be varied between 2 and 6 mm on most machines and is typically maintained between 3 and 4 mm. For precompression and main compression, the insertion depth should be maintained at approximately the same position. On most modern rotary tablet presses, the adjustments for precompression and main compression insertion depth are independent. However, on many older designs, the precompression roller is attached to the main compression roller assembly and its position is measured relative to the main compression roller position. In this way, the ratio of precompression to main compression remains constant as machine adjustments are made.

4. *Upper punch pull-up cam*: After compression, the upper punch enters into the upper-punch pull-up cam, which removes the upper punch from the die cavity. This cam

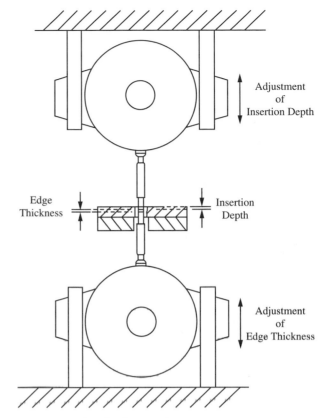

Fig. 5 Rotary tablet press layout.

provides an excellent location to measure the upper punch pull-up force that determines the tightness of the upper punches. Compared to the upper punch dwell cam, this location has the advantage of determining the punch tightness not only in the turret but also in the die cavity. Detection of tight punches at this location prevents almost all possibility of machine damage.

5. *Cam material of construction*: Both the upper and lower cam sections use cams to guide the punches while the turret rotates. These cams are typically made of various materials such as steel, bronze, or alloy. Most of the cam tracks in the turret are designed to smoothly guide the punches. Many modern rotary tablet presses use polymer composite cams for nonimpact points. These cams have excellent qualities in that they provide superior abrasion resistance and have self-lubricating properties minimizing cam and tool wear, heat generation, and noise, and ultimately resulting in increased machine speeds. However, cams that undergo impact (e.g., ejection cam) and stress (e.g., weight-regulation cam) require metal construction with good impact resistance. For this purpose, an aluminum–bronze alloy provides superior abrasion resistance and excellent impact strength.

Compression section

The compression section contains all components that are exposed to the material, such as the material hopper, the feeder, the excess material stripper, the upper and lower turrets, the die table, and the tablet stripper. Additionally, the dust-collection shrouds are located in the compression section. Proper shrouding of this area ensures that none of the upper and lower punch heads, compression rollers, and cam tracks are exposed to material. Proper maintenance and setup of the compression section is critical for optimal press performance. The primary components of the compression section are explained in the following section:

Material hopper: The material hopper is an integral part of the feeding system as shown in Fig. 6. Typically, it is capable of holding approximately 5–10 kg of material. Low level sensors are mounted in the hopper to signal an alarm, shut off the machine or activate a feeding mechanism to deliver more material when the product falls below this level. The material hopper should be symmetrical with steep discharge angles to promote mass flow and prevent funnel flow (rat holing) in the granulation. The discharge outlet of the hopper should be as large as possible reaching into the feeder to prevent material bridging.

On many machines the base of the hopper is equipped with a valve to shut off material flow to the feeder if necessary. Depending on the nature of the granulation, the hopper valve can contribute to material bridging. For materials with very poor flow characteristics, a slide valve may be preferable to a butterfly valve.

Older generation machines typically employ large hoppers, but more recent designs offer options to install only a straight chute in place of a large overhead hopper. This design minimizes poor flow behavior and segregation due to funnel flow.

Gravity feed frame: Older machines typically employ gravity feed frames which rely on gravitational and turret rotational forces to achieve die fill. These feed frames provide good performance for materials with good flow properties but are typically limited to slow machine speeds. On the other hand, gravity feeders do not agitate the product and impart no energy. Therefore, they offer advantages for products where material segregation and overmixing are of concern. For example, products that are sensitive to overblending of magnesium stearate (i.e., exhibit capping when overblended) may exhibit improved compressibility by using a gravity feeder as opposed to a force feeder.

Force feeder: Force feeders are typically multi-chamber and multipaddle feeders as shown in Fig. 6. These feeders are critical to allow optimal press performance at high machine speeds with minimal weight variation. For products with good flow properties, the feeder should move the material from the overhead hopper to the dies with minimal mixing. Most force feeders contain two or three chambers and paddles. The three chamber/paddle system typically performs better than the two chamber/paddle designs. The top paddle and feed chamber are connected directly to the hopper and move the material from the overhead hopper to the filling chambers located directly above the die cavities. The top chamber eliminates the effect of the head pressure on material flow, thus providing uniform die fill regardless of the quantity of material in the hopper. Alternate systems offer level sensors that are designed to provide a constant quantity of material to the feeding chambers, thus also eliminating the effect of head pressure on material flow.

The force feeder chambers contain material baffles that function to prevent the material from randomly packing in the chambers, which results in nonuniform fill. Optimal systems provide minimal energy input and minimal particle mixing while providing uniform fill. The speed of the paddles can be sychronized with the die table speed minimizing tablet weight variation. The appropriate paddle speed can be determined by using a force-control system that displays the standard deviation of the compression force. The optimal feeder speed is determined by adjusting the feeder speed to achieve the lowest standard deviation in the compression force, which corresponds to the least weight variation.

A rectangular paddle design is typically used to minimize powder mixing in the feeder. However, for materials with poor flow characteristics (bridging in the hopper) due

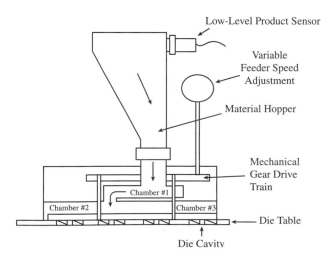

Low-Level Product Sensor

Variable
Feeder Speed
Adjustment

Material Hopper

Mechanical
Gear Drive
Train

Chamber #1

Chamber #2   Chamber #3

Die Table

Die Cavity

Fig. 6   Material feeding system.

to interparticle friction, a round (or wedge) paddle design can improve flow by forcing interparticle slippage. Under these circumstances, round paddles provide a mixing effect with possible impact on uniformity, compressibility, and dissolution.

The feeder height above the die table surface is very important to minimize product loss and prevent scaling of low melting materials. The feeder height is usually maintained between 0.05 and 0.10 mm (0.002–0.004 in.). Very fine particles may require a feeder height of 0.025 mm (0.001 in.).

Excess-material stripper: The excess-material stripper is located immediately after the feeding system and scrapes off the excess material on the die table after weight adjustment. It is often overlooked during setup although it is one of the most critical components of the tablet press. A brass stripper is employed, which sits flush on the die table under spring tension. The material is scraped off just before the lowering cam. The brass stripper directs the excess material into the recirculation channel. A tail-over-die covers the die cavity after scrape-off to the point of upper punch entry. This design minimizes uncontrolled material loss due to flinging of material out of the die cavity at high rotational speeds.

Precompression and main compression rollers: After die fill and scrape-off, the punches rotate to the precompression station where an initial force is applied to the compact. The tablet is frequently partially formed during the precompression stage. Subsequently, the upper and lower punches move together under the main compression rollers where the final tablet is formed. The main compression roller is usually larger than the precompression roller. However, latest advances suggest that similar sizes for precompression and main compression rollers with the ability to apply similar loads may result in optimal tablet formation. The compression rollers are made of premium tool steels and are surface hardened.

Because the compression characteristics of powders are time-dependent (the exact extent of this dependency depends on the primary modes of deformation), the final tablet properties depend not only on maximum compression forces but also on the rate at which these forces (rate of deformation) are applied and removed. On a rotary tablet press, the rate of deformation is determined by the tangential velocity of the punch and the compression roller diameters. The tangential velocity of the punch is a product of the press speed and the die table circumference (i.e., die table rpm × 3.14 × pitch circle diameter). As the tangential velocity increases, the rates of compression and decompression increase while the overall compression time decreases. The roller diameter affects both the rate of compression and decompression. As the diameter increases, the rates of compression and decompression decrease.

Optimal compression efficiency is achieved on machines that offer multistage compression with high precompression and main compression force flexibility (typically 100 kN maximum). The roller diameters should be as large as possible to provide the lowest possible rates of compression and decompression. If compression problems exist, the longest time for compression should be allowed by running at low press speeds and running on machines with a small pitch-circle diameter.

As mentioned previously, for certain types of products, precompression at a force level higher than that of main compression may increase tablet hardness. The author has found that for materials that primarily undergo brittle fracture, application of a precompression force higher than the main compression force can result in a higher tablet hardness. However, this is typically not the case for materials with elastic properties (e.g., products prone to capping and lamination) because these products require gradual application of force to minimize elastic recovery and allow stress relaxation.

Most heavy tonnage machines (80–100 kN capability for precompression and main compression) have no mechanical linkage between the upper and lower compression rollers. Therefore, for these machines, movement of the upper punch insertion depth does not result in an equal movement of the lower compression roller position. The compression rollers are typically mounted to a block assembly that is adjusted by an eccentric or a vertical slide adjustment (see Fig. 5). An eccentric adjustment typically results in a slight off-center alignment as the roller moves through all of its possible positions, whereas a vertical slide adjustment always maintains the roller along the center line. On older rotary tablet presses the rollers are attached to a rocker arm with one side fixed to the machine roof or base. On the upper compression roller, the other side of the rocker arm is mechanically linked to the lower roller rocker arm. In this way, adjustment to insertion depth results in simultaneous adjustment of both the upper and lower roller positions. As with the eccentric roller adjustment, rocker arm position adjustment results in a slight off-center alignment as the roller moves through all of its possible positions.

Although most rotary tablet presses operate by maintaining fixed roller positions during compression, some designs incorporate a compression compensator system in which the counterforce for compression is air pressure. This system compresses to a constant force and allows roller movement when the preset force is achieved. Under these conditions, potential exists to increase the time that the force is maintained near its peak value (approximately 90% of maximum). Compression to a constant force should theoretically provide a more uniform tablet hardness and more uniform dissolution profiles while allowing a greater variation in tablet thickness.

Tablet stripper: The tablet stripper scrapes off the tablets from the lower punch and directs them down the discharge chute. On high-speed machines, special attention must be paid to the tablet takeoff to prevent tablet backup; modifications are necessary for shaped tablets, as shown in Fig. 2. On high-speed machines it is critical to move the tablets off the die table as quickly as possible. Under some circumstances, repositioning of the Plexiglas cover on the tablet stripper to provide minimal clearance between the tablet and the cover may prevent shingling of tablets. The height of the lower punch at the point of scrape-off should always be checked to verify that it is not below the die table surface. Typically the lower punch should protrude approximately 1–2 mm from the die table surface at the point of scrape-off. For deep concave tablets, a protrusion height above 2 mm may be necessary.

Tablet presses equipped with single-tablet rejection capabilities reject tablets at the point of scrape-off. Based on the compression force of the punch station, single tablets are sorted by using a compressed-air blow off or a mechanical fast gate. On single-sided machines (36 stations) both systems work well for both large and small tablets. However, double-sided, high-speed machines may present difficulties for large tablets at high press speeds.

Material recirculation: Material is recirculated from the center of the turret into the feed frame. Some press designs include recessed recirculation channels to minimize particle attrition and prevent excess material loss to the vacuum system. It is critical not to recirculate too much material because this can result in low product yields and can have a detrimental effect on the powder's physical properties, which could result in poor compressibility, uniformity, and final properties (e.g. reduced dissolution rate).

The point of re-entry of the granulation into the feeder corresponds to the location where the lower punch enters into the fill cam when it is flush with the die table surface. Therefore, the material from the recirculation channel is typically the material in contact with the lower punch face and is the first material to be filled for each die cavity. The effect of the material in the recirculation channel should always be evaluated when compression problems occur, which can be associated with the lower punch. An example would be a case where a granulation exhibits picking only on the lower punch and not routinely on all tablet presses. Additionally, this granulation is slightly underlubricated, very friable, and undergoes minimal brittle fracture.

Previous experiments showed that, as particle size decreases, ejection force and picking tendencies increase. It was determined that, for this product, excessive material recirculation resulted in a reduction in particle size and an increase in picking tendencies. However, the picking problem was seen only on the lower punches because the reduced particle size material came into direct contact only with the lower punches. The problem was minimized by reducing the amount of material in the recirculation channel and redirecting the material from the recirculation channel to incorporate it into the bulk of the material in the feeder, thus preventing it from contacting the lower punch directly.

Dust extraction: Adequate dust extraction is necessary to maintain high-speed operation for extended periods of time. The entire compression area should be shrouded to minimize dust infiltration into other press areas. Effective dust extraction minimizes dust and oil contamination on the surface of the tablets, which could produce black specs. Insufficient dust extraction results in excessive material build-up on the lower and upper punches leading to tight punches. However, the proper balance of dust extraction without high levels of material loss must be determined. If the dust extraction level is too high material could be extracted from the die cavities and the recirculation channel. Furthermore, the dust extraction systems preferentially removes the fine particles. Therefore, if the granulation is a direct-compression blend where the active constituent is of fine particle size, minimum dust extraction levels combined with minimal recirculation may be necessary to prevent a loss of active constituents (resulting in possible low assay).

Lower cam section

The lower cam section is completely sealed from the compression section. It houses the lower compression rollers, the entire lower cam track that guides the lower punches as the turret rotates, and all adjustments for the lower precompression and main compression roller positions. Additionally, any motors necessary for automatic machine adjustment are contained in this section.

Fill cam: The fill cam is designed to lower the punch to overfill the die cavity. Lower-punch fill cams are typically available in a variety of sizes that are changed depending on the final fill depth as determined by the weight regulation cam. Press manufacturers recommend a fill cam in which the weight regulation cam operates in the approximate center of the fill cam. Typical fill cams have a range of approximately 10 mm with an increment range of 4 mm (e.g., 0–10, 4–14, 8–18, and 12–22 mm). Special-order or very shallow fill cams are also available (e.g., 0–6 mm). Alternatively, some manufacturers offer a greater selection of cams with a narrower range and lower increment (e.g., 5.5 mm range with an increment of 2 mm). These cams should offer greater precision in fill in certain cases. However, with the narrower range, minor changes in the granulation density could result in the necessity to change fill cams throughout the course of the run.

Flexibility in fill cam options offers advantages for specific problem areas. For example, if a material is very abrasive, a shallow fill cam should be chosen to minimize the amount of material that is removed from the feeder and subsequently returned to the feeder and the recirculation channel. A deep fill cam can cause overpacking of the feeder, which could result in jamming, temperature increases, and overmixing of granulation or lubricant.

Weight regulation cam: The lower punch travels from the fill cam to the weight regulation cam, which determines the final volume of material that remains in the die cavity after scrape-off. Proper design and operation of this unit is essential to ensure uniform tablet weights. In general, the unit should operate in a manner to ensure smooth punch travel minimizing punch chatter as the lower punch is raised to a precise and constant height.

The weight-regulation unit consists of several critical components that determine its efficiency of operation as shown in Fig. 7. The lower punch rides on the dosing rail that maintains the lower punch at a constant height at the final fill depth. In order to minimize vertical movement (and subsequently punch chatter) the head of the lower punch is held tight against the lower dosing rail by the holding-down cam which is spring loaded. To ensure that the holding-down cam is tight against the head of the lower punch, a 1–5 mm (0.04–0.20 in.) gap should be maintained between this cam and the lower dosing cam

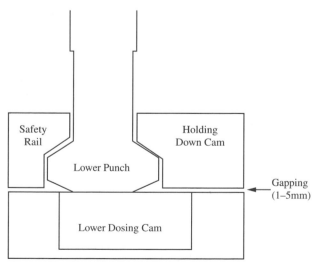

Fig. 7 Weight regulation unit.

when the lower punch rests on the dosing cam. During press setup, the fit can be easily checked by placing a lower punch in the weight regulation unit and verifying the absence of vertical movement of the punch. This function is critical to minimize tablet weight variation at high speeds. On many press designs, the weight regulation unit contains a safety cam on its inside.

The lower dosing rail and holding-down cam should always be made of a tough, abrasion-resistant material; aluminum–bronze alloy is highly recommended. The condition of the dosing rail and the holding-down cam should be checked every 6 months to ensure optimal performance. If significant wear is observed, the cams should be replaced or, in the case of the holding-down cam, reworked to provide a tight fit.

As the lower punch leaves the dosing unit, it is pulled down slightly (approximately 2 mm) by the lowering cam. Periodically the condition of the lowering cam should be checked to ensure proper lowering of the punch in order to minimize weight variation.

Many modern presses are equipped to measure the tightness of the lower punches. This function is critical to minimize machine damage as well as cam wear. As mentioned above, excessive cam wear increases tablet weight variation. Lower-punch tight sensors are typically mounted in either of the two locations. The transition cam from the fill cam to the weight regulation unit is an ideal location to measure lower punch tight forces because it is designed to raise the level of the lower punch to the final dosing height. In addition, the lowering cam can measure the counterforce to pulling down the lower punch.

Lower punch brakes: Most rotary tablet presses are equipped with lower-punch brakes that are Teflon tipped and spring loaded to apply constant pressure to the lower punches. Alternatively, some manufacturers apply pressure to a friction belt that provides resistance on the lower punches. The lower-punch brakes act as a "retention" system for holding the lower punches in place during press setup. More importantly, these systems help to minimize lower-punch chatter at high press speeds thus minimizing tablet weight variation. Some press manufacturers use the lower punch seals to retain the lower punches.

Precompression and main compression rails: The precompression rail provides the transition support for the lower punch from the weight regulation unit to the precompresison roller, while the main compression rail provides the transition support from the precompression roller to the main compression roller. The optimal press designs provide positive support with these cams by ensuring that the lower punch head flat is always in contact with the rail surface. In this way, there is no abrupt vertical movement of the lower punch as it passes to the compression rollers. Vertical movement of the lower punch before precompression and between the compression stations can cause the introduction of air into the bottom of the compact, resulting in capping at the lower-punch face. Many presses rely on the lower punch brakes or seals to prevent this type of movement. Under these conditions, vertical movement of the lower punches will gradually occur as these components wear causing periodic compression problems.

Adjustment of lower precompression and main compression roller thickness: The position of the lower compression rollers is adjusted from the lower cam section. As shown in Fig. 8, the position of the lower rollers relative to the upper rollers (i.e., insertion depth) determines the tablet edge thickness. Typically, the machine-control panel shows edge thickness on the indicator. However, adjustment of the edge thickness actually results in adjustment of the lower roller position only. For machines that have no mechanical link between the upper and lower compression rollers, the tablet edge thickness indication on the control panel is only valid at the specific insertion depth that was set during edge thickness calibration. However, for some of the electronic, fully automated machines, the machine automatically moves the lower compression roller during the insertion depth adjustment to maintain the same tablet edge thickness.

Ejection rail: After compression the lower punch impacts the ejection rail (or on some machines an ejection roller). Upon impact the tablet is broken free from the die

side wall and begins to move up the die as the machine rotates. The ejection rail should be made of a tough, abrasion resistant material such as aluminum bronze alloy.

Scrape-off rail: After riding up the ejection rail, the lower punch rides on the scrape-off rail to provide a constant height for tablet scrape-off. The height of the lower punch scrape-off can be adjusted to optimize the single tablet rejection height or the tablet scrape-off height.

Force overload system: Most tablet presses are equipped with force overload systems designed to prevent machine and punch damage. As stated previously, the compression force is not a set value, rather a measured value obtained from the fixed punch distance and the quantity of material in the die. On most tablet presses, a maximum allowable compression force can be set. This force setting is actually the counterforce to the measured compression force. If the compression force exceeds this counterforce, the compression assembly will back-off thus reducing the force. Most tablet presses use a hydraulic, air, or spring-loaded system on the lower compression assemblies (both precompression and main compression). In these systems the hydraulic or spring systems are calibrated to the measured force in the die and move instantaneously during an overload condition. Some of the more recent rotary tablet presses use strain gauges to measure the actual compression force for force overload (as opposed to force control). In these systems, the machine mechanically moves the compression assembly when the measured force is exceeded. Therefore, since these systems do not react as quickly as hydraulic, air, or spring systems they typically include a safety margin to initiate an overload condition prior to reaching the actual set value (e.g., 95% of maximum entered value).

Lower mechanical section

The lower mechanical section houses the main drive motor, the gearbox, the hydraulic pump, the lubrication pump, and the signal wire distribution. Proper venting and cooling of the lower mechanical section is essential to prevent machine damage and minimize heat generation. This section should be equipped with a cooling system for products that are sensitive to heat generation (e.g., contain low melting point components that are prone to picking and sticking).

Electrical section

The electrical section contains all electrical controls and components (e.g., programmable controllers, relays, contacts, and fuses), the signal wire distribution, and the

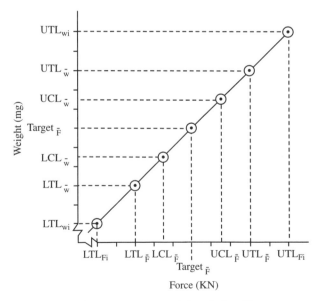

Fig. 8 Force versus weight relationship.

integrated or remote force control systems. On many machines the electrical section is connected to the front of the press, thus minimizing space requirements. However, modern fully automated machines use computers that may be sensitive to machine vibration, dust, and heat. Therefore, these electronics should be located remotely from the machine.

Lubrication system

Most high speed rotary tablet presses employ automatic lubrication systems during operation. Effective punch lubrication is essential for the movement of the punches in the turret, in the cam tracks, and under the compression rollers. Punch-lubrication systems allow high speed operation over extended periods of time while minimizing cam and tool wear and reducing heat generation.

The lubrication pump is typically maintained in the lower mechanical section and allows variation of both the lubrication interval and time duration. The quantity of oil delivered is normally determined by the oil distribution nozzles connected to the distribution manifolds. The upper punches are usually lubricated on the punch head flat via a felt pad located in the upper punch dwell cam or the upper punch lowering cam. On many modern designs the upper punch barrel is also lubricated. The punch barrel is lubricated via radially drilled holes in the turret that transports oil to the punches by rotational forces, or by overlubricating the punch neck and allowing gravity to transfer the oil down the barrel. Because the upper punch shaft has the greatest area of contact with the upper turret, lubrication of the punch shaft is critical to allow high-speed operation. Poor lubrication of this area can result in heat generation and metal expansion, ultimately causing machine seizure and severe damage.

The lower punches are lubricated at the punch neck. Oil distribution lines are frequently provided to lubricate both sides of the punch neck. Subsequently, gravitational forces distribute the oil over the head of the punch. The lower punch barrel is typically lubricated by radially drilled holes in the turret.

All presses equipped with punch-lubrication systems require oil and dust seals to prevent oil contamination in the product and dust contamination in the turret punch sockets. These seals are normally double lipped, designed to strip oil on one side and powder on the other. As mentioned previously, some press designs use the lower punch seals to retain the lower punches.

Inadequate punch lubrication can lead to excessive heat generation, which could affect tablet properties. An example is a granulation that primarily undergoes elastic and plastic deformation. This product was normally run on a tablet press without an automatic lubrication system. Production requirements resulted in batch campaigning. At the beginning of the production campaign, the punches were lubricated and placed into the machine. Over the course of the first batch, the product was easily maintained within tablet hardness and thickness specifications. However, as the campaign transitioned into batches two and three, tablet hardness tended to increase while the thickness remained constant. Machine adjustments were made to maintain the hardness and thickness within specification, but in the end the hardness could not be maintained below the maximum limit without exceeding the thickness specification. At this point the machine was inspected and the lower punches were observed to be warm. They were removed, cleaned, lubricated, and placed back in the machine. Upon resuming production, the tablets returned to their original characteristics. In this case, the lack of a punch lubrication system combined with batch campaigning (extended running conditions) resulted in a temperature increase in the machine. For this elastic material, the increased temperature resulted in greater plasticity and more stress relaxation, improving the compressibility of the product. Although under many circumstances this effect would be beneficial, in the present case the improved compressibility resulted in out-of-specification product. The problem was resolved by removing the punches after each batch for cleaning and lubrication.

Instrumentation

Modern rotary production tablet presses are typically equipped to measure precompression and main compression forces. Additionally, measurement and monitoring of tablet ejection force can prove to be beneficial for specific problem products and for production troubleshooting. However, for most pharmaceutical products proper product development and optimization work eliminate the need to instrument a production machine for ejection force. Rotary tablet presses can also be equipped to measure both upper punch and lower punch pull-down forces. These measurements are primarily made to detect tight-running punches and are necessary on production machines only if the machine monitoring system uses direct force measurement for these functions. Tablet scrape-off force can also be measured, but this is only recommended on development machines. Scrape-off forces are typically below 6 N. Therefore, instrumentation of a tablet stripper requires highly sensitive instrumentation that is easily damaged.

Precompression and main compression forces are normally measured for the upper punches (20, 21). These forces are typically measured using strain gauges arranged in a full wheatstone bridge (22). Strain gauges are basically resistors applied to the metal surface in a specific orientation. Under load, the member deflects and the strain changes the resistance of the gauge. The change in resistance is proportional to the applied force. However, due to design differences, some machines measure the lower compression forces as opposed to upper compression forces. The compression force should be measured as close to the compression event as possible. For the most accurate and reproducible readings, the strain gauge should be in line with the compression event as opposed to off center at a remote location. This is easily accomplished on most rotary tablet presses by using a shear pin to support the compression rollers. However, the pin must not be rotated when the position of the compression rollers is changed. Therefore, this system is ideally suited for machines that change roller position by a vertical slide mechanism as opposed to an eccentric mechanism. Shear pins are typically custom manufactured, where quality depends not only on the pin design but also on the strain gauge receptivity and arrangement.

Many modern rotary tablet presses use off-the-shelf load cells for force measurement. These load cells are highly accurate, durable, and easily replaced and calibrated. However, the final accuracy and repeatability of force measurement in the machine not only depend on the quality of the load cell, but also on the design of the compression assembly and the placement of the load cell within the assembly.

Machines that utilize rocker arms with a mechanical linkage between the upper and lower compression assemblies are normally instrumented by applying a strain gauge to the upper rocker arm or to the mechanical linkage connecting the assemblies. The point of strain gauge application is "necked-down" to increase the sensitivity of the member. These instrumented members should be calibrated in the machine to account for the effect of other machine members on the measured force.

The force measurement system (strain gauges or load cells) should be calibrated on a yearly basis or after the compression assembly has been disassembled for any reason. The calibration should be made in the machine to assure accuracy. It is typically performed using a modified punch assembly and a calibrated load cell that are rotated under the compression roller to produce a load. The output of the machine force measurement system is compared to the output of the calibrated load cell. Many machine manufacturers use this single-point calibration to modify the strain gauge factor so that the two outputs are the same

at this load level. Subsequently, different load levels are tested and the error between the machine force measurement system and the calibrated load cell is determined. Alternatively, loads can be applied to the system ranging from the minimum to maximum compression forces. The outputs from the calibrated load cell and the machine force measurement system are recorded and a linear regression is performed on the data to calculate a new strain gauge factor across the entire force measurement range. Subsequently, different load levels are tested and the error between the readings is calculated.

PRESS CONTROL AND AUTOMATION

Conventional rotary tablet presses are controlled by periodically taking tablet samples from the discharge chute and checking their tablet weight, thickness, and hardness. If the tablet weight is outside of the established control limit, the operator increases or decreases the weight by adjusting the fill depth (increasing fill depth increases tablet weight and decreasing fill depth reduces tablet weight). If either the tablet hardness or thickness requires adjustment, the operator typically adjusts the tablet edge thickness on either main compression or precompression. Since there is normally an inverse relationship between the tablet hardness and thickness, the operator usually reduces edge thickness to increase tablet hardness (or decrease thickness) or increases edge thickness to decrease tablet hardness (or increase thickness).

Force and weight control systems use the same basic concepts as conventional machines. Force control systems monitor the tablet compression force and adjust the fill depth to maintain a constant force. Force control systems alone compensate for flow and density variations in the granulation, providing a constant fill quantity. Weight control systems, on the other hand, work in conjunction with the force control system as a secondary control loop and replace the manual function of the machine operator, periodically removing tablet samples to test tablet weight, thickness, and hardness. If the weight control system indicates that the tablet weight must be adjusted, the force control setpoint or the tablet edge thickness is altered resulting in a change in the fill depth from the force control system.

Force Control

During tablet compression, the distance between the rollers remains constant unless a machine adjustment is made to change tablet hardness or thickness. Additionally, all

Table 1 Tablet weight-control points and tolerance limits

Item	Description	Specification (mg)
UTL_{W_i}	Upper tolerance limit of individual tablet weight	105.0
$UTL_{\overline{W}}$	Upper tolerance limit of average tablet weight	103.0
$UCL_{\overline{W}}$	Upper control limit of average tablet weight	101.5
$Target_{\overline{W}}$	Target of average tablet weight	100.0
$LCL_{\overline{W}}$	Lower control limit of average tablet weight	98.5
$LTL_{\overline{W}}$	Lower tolerance limit of average tablet weight	97.0
LTL_{W_i}	Lower tolerance limit of individual tablet weight	95.0

tooling dimensions (tooling length and die cavity size) are constant within established standards. Under these conditions, for a specific material of uniform density, if the same volume of material is delivered to each die, the maximum measured compression force for each punch station is the same. If, on the other hand, different volumes of material are delivered to each die, the maximum measured compression force for each punch station is different. On this basis, adjustment of fill depth (fill volume) to maintain a constant compression force should result in a constant tablet weight. This concept is the general basis of all rotary tablet press force control systems.

The force control systems assume a linear relationship between tablet weight and compression force for a particular granulation, tooling set, and machine tablet edge thickness (i.e., distance between compression rollers). By establishing the relationship between compression force and tablet weight at a specific machine tablet edge thickness (as shown in Fig. 8), a force control system is able to maintain a constant tablet weight by maintaining a constant compression force. Additionally, a force control system is capable of monitoring every compression force and rejecting tablets when the forces exceed specific established limits (for both average forces and individual

forces), thereby essentially monitoring every tablet weight.

The first step in using a force control system is to establish the force versus weight relationship to allow calculation of the appropriate force control set points which correspond to the desired weight control points. Table 1 gives example of weight control points and tolerance limits for a theoretical product.

The tablet press is initially run at target conditions to make the product within specifications. For example, the tablets are made at target conditions of 100 mg at an average compression force of 10 kN. After establishing this point, the fill depth is adjusted to either increase or decrease the tablet weight and the corresponding compression force is measured. In the present example, the tablet weight was increased to 103 mg and the average measured compression force was approximately 13 kN. This procedure should be repeated for several different tablet weights. The data are used for regression analysis to calculate the required force set points that correspond to the weight control points as shown in Fig. 8 and Table 2.

As an alternative to performing regression analysis, fill depth can be adjusted to achieve each average weight

Table 2 Force setpoints

Item	Description	Specification (kN)
UTL_{F_i}	Upper tolerance limit for individual compression force	15.0
$UTL_{\overline{F}}$	Upper tolerance limit for average compression force	13.0
$UCL_{\overline{F}}$	Upper control limit for average compression force	11.5
$Target_{\overline{F}}$	Target for average compression force	10.0
$LCL_{\overline{F}}$	Lower control limit for average compression force	8.5
$LTL_{\overline{F}}$	Lower tolerance limit for average compression force	7.0
LTL_{F_i}	Lower tolerance limit for individual compression force	5.0

requirement and the resultant compression force can be recorded and set.

During normal production with the force control system in operation as specified above, the tablet press will operate to maintain the constant compression force of 10 kN by adjusting the fill depth (see Fig. 9). Most force control systems do not require the user to input the upper and lower force control limits for average compression force that are typically set by the manufacturer within tighter tolerances than those demanded by the weight requirements. The control system typically calculates the average compression force every revolution and compares it to the force set point. If the average measured compression force varies from the set point of 10 kN (outside of the tolerance set by the manufacturer) then the force control system adjusts the fill depth to return the force to 10 kN. If the compression force is outside the average tolerance limits (below 7 kN or above 13 kN), the machine will shut down and reject the tablets. This condition should correspond to average tablet weights outside of the 97.0–103.0 mg limits. Typically, the force control system is capable of adjusting the fill depth to maintain the compression force well within the tolerance limits. However, if the material has poor flow characteristics and exhibits bridging followed by surging, the system may be unable to compensate quickly enough to prevent these out of control conditions.

During the entire operation, if any of the individual measured compression forces goes outside of the individual tolerance limits of 5 kN or 15 kN (corresponding to individual tablet weights below 95 mg or above 105 mg), these individual tablets are rejected at the point of tablet scrape-off. Some machine designs are not effective at sorting individual tablets reliably and reject multiple tablets if this condition occurs. For most machine designs, the user can specify a maximum number of individual tablets that can be sorted per punch location or

per batch before the machine shuts down. Exceeding these maximum limits may indicate a problem punch or excessive weight variation for the batch, possibly related to a setup problem.

As described, a force control system maintaining a constant compression force will adequately compensate for variations in granulation density, thus providing more uniform tablet weights. However, operation of this system still requires an operator to periodically check tablet weight, thickness, and hardness. If during a weight check the operator determines that the average tablet weight has gone beyond the control limit, while the average compression force is still being maintained at its set point, the operator must take one of the following actions:

- The system is placed in manual mode (shut-off force control system) and the tablet weight adjusted back to target by increasing or decreasing the fill depth as necessary. Once the weight is within requirements, the force control set point is changed (and all other limits by the same amount) to the current value that is displayed and the machine is returned to the automatic mode.
- While in the automatic mode, the force control set point is increased or decreased to increase or decrease the tablet weight, respectively. For example, by increasing the force set point, the control system increases fill depth to achieve the higher compression force requirement thus increasing tablet weight. The machine is allowed to stabilize and tablet weight is checked. Adjustments are made until tablet weight is within specifications.
- While in the automatic mode, the machine tablet edge thickness is increased or decreased to increase or decrease the tablet weight, respectively. For example, by increasing the machine tablet edge thickness, the measured compression force is decreased. The force control system will then increase fill depth to return the compression force to its previous value thus increasing tablet weight.

Minor changes in the force to weight relationship over the course of a compression run are common. These may be due to changes in the compressibility of the granulation or to changes in the machine over the course of the run (such as temperature changes).

Tablet presses that use a compression compensator system, which in turn compress to constant compression forces and allow roller movement, operate by the same control theories as those presented for force control. However, these systems measure roller displacement as opposed to compression force and relate it to tablet weight.

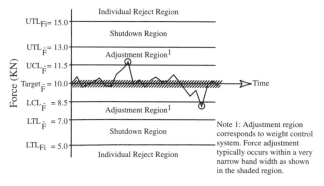

Fig. 9 Force control system.

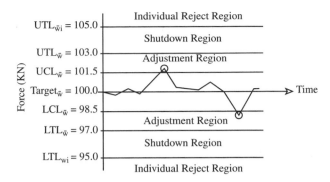

Fig. 10 Weight control system.

Weight Control

Weight control, as a secondary control loop to force control, allows automation of the tableting operation. The weight control system (Fig. 10) maintains the same limits as those presented for force control (Fig. 9). The machine assumes the place of the operator and periodically samples the tablet press to determine the tablet weight. The sampling requirements should be set to the same interval and number of tablets as those required for manual operation. Most weight feedback systems measure individual tablet weights and calculate the average weight for feed back purposes.

In the example given above, it is assumed that the weight feedback system will measure 10 individual tablet weights every 15 min. The force control system is in operation and is maintaining the average compression force at 10 kN. If during each 15 min. check, the average weight of 10 tablets is within the average control limits (see Fig. 10), no machine adjustments from the weight control system will be made. Alternatively, if the average tablet weight goes beyond the average control limits (above 101.5 mg or below 98.5 mg) the weight control system will initiate a change in one of the following ways depending on the machine:

Increase or decrease the force control setpoint to increase or decrease the tablet weight, respectively. The new force control set point is calculated by means of the machine manufacturer's control algorithm. Typically after adjustment to the new force control set point, the weight control system should resample and verify that the average tablet weight is now within the average control limits.

Increase or decrease the machine tablet edge thickness to increase or decrease the tablet weight, respectively. The new machine tablet edge thickness setting is calculated by the manufacturer's algorithm. After the new setting has been made and the fill depth adjusted to maintain constant compression force, the weight control system should resample and verify that the average tablet weight is now within the average control limits.

The weight control systems that change the force control setpoint result in a change of the compression force throughout the run with a relatively constant tablet thickness. On the other hand, by changing the machine tablet edge thickness, the compression force remains relatively constant throughout the run while the tablet thickness varies. Since these adjustments are usually relatively small, both methods of machine adjustment typically produce similar results.

If during any check the average tablet weight exceeds the average tolerance limits (below 97 mg and above 103 mg) or an individual tablet exceeds the individual tolerance limits (below 95 mg and above 105 mg), the machine will shut off and reject the tablets. It is important to note that individual tablet weights exceeding the tolerance limits indicate that the tablet rejection system is not functioning properly.

Control and Monitoring of Weight/Thickness/Hardness

Tablet presses equipped to measure tablet weight, thickness, and hardness use the same concepts for force and weight control as presented here. These systems offer the additional flexibility of testing and controlling both tablet thickness and hardness. However, most machine manufacturers and tablet manufacturers have found that additional control of either tablet thickness or hardness is both difficult and costly. It is cost effective to only monitor tablet thickness or hardness and shut-off the machine if tolerance limits are exceeded. In this way, fully automated operation is possible without operator testing.

TROUBLESHOOTING

A proper understanding of a material's compression characteristics combined with a knowledge of tablet compression equipment allows efficient troubleshooting of production problems. Although there is no substitute for a robust granulation, a product can be optimized by examining all of the different machine factors that can affect performance. By applying a variety of the concepts discussed here, a large variety of processing problems can be eliminated.

Tablet Weight Variation

Excessive tablet weight variation can be caused by a variety of factors. For many granulations, the inherent poor flow characteristics of the material may be the rate limiting step, and simply slowing down the machine may reduce weight variation. Additionally, optimization of the feeder paddle speeds to minimize the standard deviation in the compression force should help to minimize weight variation. If weight variation is excessive, the following machine components should be examined:

- The tightness of the *hold-down cam* should be examined to verify that it is not excessively worn and is holding the lower punch tight against the dosing cam. If the previous product resulted in tight lower punches, premature wear may have occurred on this cam, causing increased weight variation.
- The condition of the *lower punch pull-down cam* should be examined to verify that it is not overly worn and that it drops the lower punch to pull the material in the die cavity below the die table surface.
- Both the condition and position of the *excess material stripper* should be examined to assure that it sits snug and level on the die table surface for complete scrape-off.
- Different types of *feeder paddles* can be used to promote flow (e.g., round feeder paddles are used for materials that exhibit bridging). The feeder speed should be optimized to minimize force and weight variation.
- The best *fill cam size* is that where the fill depth is centered in its range.
- A minimum amount of *material recirculation* is necessary to provide steady flow and fill. Too much recirculation can result in material back-up and reduction in the granulation particle size. The recirculation channel must be free of obstructions (i.e., broken tablets).
- If large tablets are being produced requiring deep fill depths, then *insertion depth* should be increased. Otherwise, as the punches pass from a deep fill to a shallow insertion depth, the uncompressed granulation will be pushed out of the die cavity resulting in material loss.

Product Yield

Product yield can be affected by a number of factors. Unfortunately, yield problems are not noticed until after the loss occurs. However, by paying attention to the following areas during setup, these problems can be minimized:

- Excessive material loss can be avoided by ensuring that the *excess material stripper* is flush against the die

table. Otherwise the material will be sucked into the dust extraction system.
- The *feed frame height* should be maintained between 0.05 and 0.10 mm (0.003–0.004 in.). For very fine particle size granulation, the clearance should be reduced to 0.025–0.05 mm (0.001–0.002 in.).
- The *fill cam size* should be reduced to minimize overfilling and material recirculation.
- Material in the *material recirculation* channel should be maintained at a minimal level. As more material is recirculated, the likelihood for loss is greater. The piece guiding the material from the recirculation channel to the feeder must be properly positioned.
- If the *insertion depth* is too shallow relative to the fill depth, material will be pushed out of the die and lost to the dust extraction system.
- Excessive *feeder speeds* cause excess material recirculation and increase material loss.
- It may be necessary to reduce *press speed*. As the press speed is increased, the turret rotational forces will sling more material to the outside of the turret from both the recirculation channel and the die cavity.

Low Hardness

Tablet hardness is affected by many factors. For troubleshooting purposes, it should be determined if the low hardness is due to capping or noncompressibility. For formulations that exhibit low hardness without capping, the following guidelines are helpful:

- For *multi-stage compression*, a machine should be equipped for both precompression and main compression with large diameter rollers.
- The *ratio of precompression to main compression* should be adjusted. For tablets that exhibit no capping problems, both precompression and main compression forces should be maximized.
- *Press speed* is reduced in order to increase total compression time.
- Formulations sensitive to lubricant levels may exhibit low hardness due to overmixing in the feeder. If the formulation contains a significant quantity of magnesium stearate or there is a shift in particle size thus extending the lubricant differently, overmixing can reduce tablet hardness. In this case, the *feeder speed should* be reduced to a minimum.

Capping and Lamination

Tablet capping and lamination typically create the most difficult problems, due to a variety of causes. Identification of the cause often leads to the solution. The basic concepts to alleviate these problems center on minimizing elastic behavior while promoting plastic deformation. Depending on the exact nature of the problem, this can be achieved from a formulation perspective by modifying the formula to incorporate a plastically deforming matrix, by adding components to enhance bonding, or by increasing the moisture level. Alternatively, from a machine perspective the following guidelines should be followed:

- The *rate of force application* should be reduced by applying the compression force as gradually as possible. This can be accomplished by lowering the press speed or using a machine with a small pitch circle diameter.
- The *ratio of precompression to main compression* should be modified with gradual application of the precompression force followed by main compression. A precompression force that is too high can be harmful.
- The effect of reducing the *compression force* should be evaluated. In many circumstances, overcompression of a granulation will result in failure.
- A machine with large *compression-roller diameters* should be used to minimize the rate of force application.
- *Die cavity wear* must be investigated and the condition of the die cavities examined. If the dies are very worn, slip-stick behavior may occur during tablet ejection resulting in tablet failure.
- *Curled/damaged punches* promote tablet capping. Under these conditions the tools should be reworked or replaced.

Picking and Sticking

Tablet picking and sticking problems are typically related to formulation issues. However, in small scale manufacturing these problems do not occur frequently. Regardless, once a product is approved, it is difficult to make significant formulation changes. To minimize these problems the following areas should be considered:

- *Heat of compression*: Excessive heat generation during compression will increase the picking tendency of a low melting material. Use of cooling systems for the compression section or lower mechanical section may be helpful.
- *Press speed*: Lowering press speed and compression force reduces heat generation. Lower press speeds extend the contact time between the material and the punch face.
- *Precompression force*: Elimination of precompression may prevent picking. For example, some materials pick if the compression force is too low. Therefore, application of precompression at low forces may result in tablet picking.

- *Tool condition*: The condition of press tooling should always be evaluated when picking occurs. Polishing the punches and application of various coatings to the tools may help to eliminate picking for certain materials.
- *Start-up conditions*: Start-up should always be close to optimum conditions to prevent fouling the punch faces. If maintaining the force above a minimum is necessary to prevent picking, starting up near aim conditions of compression force prevents initial picking.
- *Tablet stripper*: The point of impact of the lower punches should be repositioned relative to the tablet stripper. Under many circumstances the stress of impact on the stripper can cause failure and sticking in logos.

Tablet Jams and Chipping

Tablet jams and chipping at the stripper reduce tablet quality and may contaminate the feeder resulting in weight variation. High speed machines typically have greater problems than slower machines. These problems are solved by focusing on the tablet stripper and lower punch ejection height.

- *Scrape-off height*: For many tablet types (e.g. deep concave tablets) the height of the lower punch at the point of scrape-off must be increased to ensure that the tablet is removed completely from the die when it impacts the tablet stripper.
- *Modified tablet stripper*: For shaped tablets, a modified tablet stripper that removes the tablets from the die table quickly prevents tablet back-up and breakage.
- *Height of plastic cover*: If the tablets exhibit layering or shingling, the height of the stripper cover should be lowered to just accommodate one tablet between the cover and the die table.
- *Tablet stripper*: The impact point of the stripper can cause chipping. Both the height and position of the tablet stripper must be checked. Damaged punches must be replaced or repaired.
- *Air assist*: If tablet jams cannot be eliminated by modifying the tablet stripper, an air assist blow-off at the tablet stripper may solve the problem.
- *Static eliminator*: In the production of lightweight tablets in a low humidity environment, static electricity may cause tablet back-up. In this case, installation of a static eliminator will improve tablet discharge.

SUMMARY

Optimal manufacturing of tablets requires good equipment and materials. The equipment is only a tool to achieve the final goal of high quality tablets. However, if the materials have marginal flow and compressibility problems, machine flexibility allows the production of the highest quality product possible.

REFERENCES

1. Higuchi, T.; Arnold, R.D.; Tucker, S.J.; Busse, L.W. J. Am. Pharm. Assoc. **1952**, *41*, 93–96, Sci. Ed.
2. Train, D. J. Pharm. Pharmacol. **1956**, *8*, 745–761.
3. Nystrom, C. Drug Dev. Ind. Pharm. **1993**, *19*, 2143–2196.
4. Wray, P.E. Drug Dev. Ind. Pharm. **1992**, *18*, 627–658.
5. Hoblitzell, J.R.; Rhodes, C.T. Drug Dev. Ind. Pharm. **1990**, *16*, 469–507.
6. Marshall, K. Compression and Consolidation of Powdered Solids. *The Theory and Practice of Industrial Pharmacy*, 3rd Ed.; Lea & Febiger: Philadelphia, 1986.
7. Parrot, E.L. Compression. *Pharm. Dosage Forms: Tablets*, 2nd Ed.; Marcel Dekker, Inc.: New York, 1990; 2.
8. Goetzel, C.G. *Treatise of Powder Metallurgy*; Interscience Publishers, Inc.: New York, 1949; 1, 259–312.
9. Heistand, E.N. Int.: J. Pharm. **1991**, *67*, 217–229.
10. Hiestand, E.N.; Smith, D.P. Int. J. Pharm. **1991**, *67*, 231–246.
11. Reier, G.E.; Shangraw, R.E. J. Pharm. Sci. **1966**, *55*, 510–514.
12. Hanus, E.J.; King, L.D. J. Pharm. Sci. **1968**, *57*, 677–684.
13. Rankell, A.S.; Higuchi, T. J. Pharm. Sci. **1968**, *57* (4), 574–577.
14. *Fette Technical Bulletin 8004*; Fette America Inc.: Rockaway, NJ.
15. Esezobo, S.; Pilpel, N. J. Pharm. Pharmacol. **1986**, *38*, 409–413.
16. Gunsel, W.C.; Kanig, J.L. Tablets. *The Theory and Practice of Industrial Pharmacy*, 2nd Ed.; Lea & Febiger: Philadephia, 1976.
17. Hiestand, E.N.; Peot, C.B.; Ochs, J.E. J. Pharm. Sci. **1977**, *66*, 510–519.
18. Bateman, S.D.; Rubinstein, M.H.; Thacker, H.S. Pharm. Tech. Int. **June 1990**, *30–36*.
19. Rippie, E.G.; Morehead, W.T. J. Pharm. Sci. **1994**, *83*, 708–715.
20. Watt, P.R. *Tablet Machine Instrumentation in Pharmaceutics: Principles and Practice*; Ellis Horwood: Chichester, UK, 1988.
21. Oates, R.J.; Mitchell, A.G. J. Pharm. Pharmacol. **1994**, *46* (4), 270–275.
22. Schmidt, P.C.; Vogel, P.J. Drug Dev. Ind. Pharm. **1994**, *20*, 921–934.

TABLET EVALUATION USING NEAR-INFRARED SPECTROSCOPY

Christopher T. Rhodes
Karen Morisseau
University of Rhode Island, Kingston, Rhode Island

INTRODUCTION

Near-infrared spectroscopy (NIRS) continues to grow in importance as a useful analytical technique. It offers unique potential as a rapid, nondestructive method of quantitative and qualitative evaluation. NIRS has been used extensively in the food and agricultural industries for many years to determine moisture, protein, and starch content in grains (1). The pharmaceutical industry has been cautiously slow to accept NIRS as a commonly used technique, probably because of the absence of primary absorption bands. In recent years, an increasing amount of academic research is being carried out on the theory behind NIR. The use of NIRS for pharmaceutical applications has grown owing, in part, to technological advances in instrumentation and software.

Several reviews (2–7) have been published recently, attesting to its increasing popularity. Textbooks (8) relating to pharmaceutical uses of NIRS are becoming more common. Literature references pertaining to pharmaceutical uses date back to the early 1980s (9, 10). However, earlier NIR articles exist and were not taken seriously by the pharmaceutical industry at the time. In 1966, Sinsheimer and Keuhnelian (11) reported quantitative NIRS work with pharmaceutically active compounds pressed into pellets.

NIRS involves the multidisciplinary approaches of the analytical chemist, statistician, and computer programmer. The word chemometrics refers to the application of mathematical or statistical methods to measurements made on chemical systems of varying complexity. Chemometrics is defined (12) as the chemical discipline that uses mathematical, statistical, and other methods that apply formal logic to design or select optimal measurement procedures and experiments, and to provide maximum relevant chemical information by analyzing chemical data.

Chemometrics has found widespread use in the interpretation of analytical data and is relied on for the development of NIRS methods.

In pharmaceutical applications, NIRS is more often used as a secondary analytical technique than as a primary tool. As a secondary method, a reference method is required to determine the reference component values that are to be used in the NIR calibration. The mathematical expression relating the component property (or properties) to absorbance is called a calibration model (also referred to as an algorithm). Using sophisticated spectral software, the analyst can correlate sample spectra to laboratory data, develop a calibration model, and apply that model to similar, new samples to predict constituent properties.

THEORY

The NIR region of the electromagnetic spectrum is from 800 to 2500 nm. The segment from 1100 to 2500, known as the Herschel region (13), is the range most often used in the analysis of pharmaceutical products. In the NIR region, the radiation can penetrate compacted materials such as tablets, providing a vast amount of spectral information about the sample.

The NIR region of the spectrum contains overtones and combination bands that are primarily attributed to hydrogen vibrations (OH, CH, NH). These overtones and combination bands are much weaker than the fundamental vibrations, thus, the molar absorptivities are much smaller than those of the corresponding infrared bands. Smaller molar absorptivities allow the use of undiluted samples and penetration of solid samples with good results.

There are several notable differences among the near-infrared region and other infrared regions of the electromagnetic spectrum. Conventional infrared instruments usually operate in the near-, mid-, or far-infrared regions, depending on the energy source and the detectors used. The wavelength range used for the NIR is just beyond the visible end of the spectrum and is referred to in terms of nanometers. Other regions of the spectrum are referred to in terms of wave numbers. Thus, the near-infrared region is $14{,}300$–$4000\,\mathrm{cm}^{-1}$, the midinfrared range is 4000–$200\,\mathrm{cm}^{-1}$, and the far infrared is from 200–$10\,\mathrm{cm}^{-1}$.

INSTRUMENTATION

NIRS instruments are typically designed as either transmittance or reflectance, with some allowing the user to switch from one to the other. The difference between the two instrument configurations lies in the positioning of the sample and the detector(s). In transmittance mode, the sample is placed between the monochromator and the detector so that the entire pathlength of the sample is integrated into the measurement. Transmittance measurements require higher frequency energy (800–1400 nm) because of the greater depth of penetration into the sample (14). In reflectance mode, the monochromatic light is illuminated directly onto the sample, and the reflected light is collected by detectors positioned at 45° angles to the sample.

Advances in instrumentation have resulted in a wide array of choices for analysts. These include instruments for specific applications with custom sample holders as well as general multiuse types. In the past 10 years, various patents have been issued for sample holders (15), sample supports (16), and a fiber optic system for dissolution (17).

An extensive product review of recent NIR technology was published by Noble (18). Enormous progress has been achieved in chemometrics and computing power, making many new applications possible. There are dozens of manufacturers of NIR spectrophotometers in the United States. There are many vendors of sampling components and software packages for data analysis. Research data of the most recent instrumentation and software are available directly on the World Wide Web, as most manufacturers maintain a Web site. There are numerous Internet (19) sites that provide links to professional spectroscopy societies, publishers of spectroscopy journals, and patents (20) related to pharmaceutical uses of NIR.

The US FDA's Division of Drug Analysis sponsored a cooperative study among manufacturers of NIRS instruments and pharmaceutical manufacturers to analyze a series of tablets, hard and soft gelatin capsules, and powders. One goal of the study was to demonstrate that a near-infrared scan was not unique among manufacturers. Another reason for the study was to establish FDA guidelines for the Instrument Qualification and Performance Verification of NIR instruments used in pharmaceutical analysis. Nine manufacturers participated in the study and represented makers of numerous types of monochromators (acousto-optical tunable filter or AOTF, dispersive and Fourier transform-NIR or FT-NIR). Ciurzcak (21) reported a detailed account of the study to compare instrument performance in similar products, thus providing some comparative information to potential buyers of NIR equipment. Ciurczak concluded that the quality of the spectra depends on the monochromator, and there is a range of noise variability in both FT-NIR and dispersive-type instruments. Examination of the spectra appearing in the report indicated differences in photometric noise and in spectral resolution (in certain regions) among instruments. One of the manufacturers, Analytical Spectral Devices, Inc., Boulder, CO, was identified in the study as the source of the donated spectra for the report and also provided their data over the Internet.

DATA ANALYSIS AND CALIBRATION

Obtaining Sample Spectra

The process of scanning a sample is quite simple and very rapid. The sample holder and surface must first be gently cleaned of debris and a reference (usually an internal ceramic Coor's standard) scan taken. The sample may then be placed in the sample holder, which may hold one or more of a specific type of sample. The sample is positioned, the lid closed, and the scan taken. Scan times are usually approximately 40 s. If multiple scans of the same sample are needed, the sample may be removed and rescanned. Instrument software facilitates the process and allows the spectra to be named and stored in data files.

Calibration

Calibration models are developed to determine the relationship between calibration set spectra and the constituent value of interest for those samples. Calibration involves taking spectra from many samples varying over the measurement range and also measuring the desired parameters. A rugged chemometric model for a complex sample may require hundreds to thousands of samples taken from all possible situations, in and out of specification, that it may encounter. Samples selected for calibration must contain all of the variables affecting the chemical and physical properties of the samples to be analyzed. To characterize each source of variation, it is recommended that 15 to 20 samples be run for each variable. Application of a math treatment, such as second derivative, prepares the raw spectral data for use in a regression and subsequent development of a calibration equation. This type of treatment results in a data file that will yield more information more easily than a raw data file.

Because NIR bands are mixtures of overtones and combinations, the intensity of the absorbance at particular wavelengths do not necessarily respond linearly to a change in concentration. In the case of a mixture, band mixing may further disrupt any linear relationship between the intensity and the concentration. These are the reasons why the simple application of Beer's law $A = ebc$, where A = absorbance, e = absorptivity, b = path length, and c = concentration to NIR bands may not generate equations suitable for quantitation. Multiple regression techniques help avoid this problem. Linear calibration methods such as multiple linear regression (MLR), principal component analysis (PCA), and partial least-squares regression (PLS) are routinely used in NIR analyses. The choice of regression technique is subjective, depending on many factors. For further description of these techniques, see the introduction to multivariate calibration methods by Thomas (22). Other chemometric techniques useful in NIRS methods include BEAST bootstrap error-adjusted single-sample technique (BEAST), a nonparametric clustering algorithm used by Lodder and co-workers (23) to detect capsule tampering by NIRS. Qualitative NIR methods use pattern-recognition techniques to "train" the computer to identify an unknown material. Residual variance methods and discriminant analyses (Mahalanobis distance) were described by Mark and Tunnell (24), and were compared by Gemperline and Boyer (25). Gerhausser and Kovar (6) reported strategies for optimization of spectral libraries and compared two pattern-recognition methods to identify 117 drug substances.

Validation

Regardless of the mathematics used to interpret NIR spectra, the method must still undergo a validation process. The principal elements of ensuring linearity, accuracy, selectivity, and reproducibility of a quantitative method are required.

The validation process determines the amount of error owing to variation among the values in the population. It is used to check for the existence of a relationship between the calibration set and the validation set. Manufacturers of NIRS instrumentation include software packages that allow the operator to predict analytical results on data files that have been stored, thus allowing for validation of the calibration equation and testing for errors in the developed calibration. This enables calibration equation performance testing in terms of precision. The validity of these models depends on the ability of the calibration set to accurately represent the samples in the prediction set.

One source of prediction error is the inherent accuracy and precision of the reference analytical method used. If the reference method produces erroneous values that are consistently high or low, this bias will be reflected in

the prediction results. Other sources of prediction error relate to the reproducibility, stability, and repeatability of the NIR instrument. Reproducibility (precision) is validated by making repeated measurements of the same sample and removing it between runs. Small changes in conditions may occur owing to multiple insertions of a sample onto the instrument. Stability refers to similar changes that may occur over a longer period (hours or days). Repeatability refers to the instrument's ability to generate consistent measurements under the same conditions (without removing the sample from the instrument) over a relatively short period (seconds or minutes). All of these factors must be addressed to ensure the validity of the NIR calibration model.

Regulatory Issues

The American Society for Testing and Materials (ASTM) recently published an official document (27) providing a guide to spectroscopists for the multivariate calibration of infrared spectrometers. The scope of the publication, entitled *Standard Practices for Infrared Multivariate Quantitative Analysis* includes a description of multivariate calibration methods for the determination of physical or chemical characteristics of materials. This document is the first official standard for the application of chemometric multivariate analysis to near-infrared and infrared instruments.

Regulatory bodies around the world have given approval for NIR methods for a variety of purposes. In June 1995, the Medicines Control Agency (MCA) granted approval to Glaxo Wellcome in the United Kingdom for a NIR method for the identification and assay of Zovirax® (acyclovir) tablets. This is believed to be the first official approval for NIR granted by the MCA as an assay method for tablets.

In Norway, Wieders Farmasoytiske A/S received approval for the use of NIR as an alternative method for identification, assay, and determination of moisture content of paracetamol (acetaminophen) tablets. The Norwegian Medicines Control Authority approved the method in December 1996.

Other regulatory approvals are described in later sections of this chapter.

CURRENT METHODS OF TABLET EVALUATION

Official standards for the evaluation of tablets are given by the *U.S. Pharmacopeia* (USP) and other compendia and include uniformity of dosage units (weight variation, content uniformity) and disintegration testing. Unofficial tests include those for mechanical strength (hardness, crushing strength) and resistance to abrasion (friability). A major disadvantage of current compendial methods of tablet evaluation is that they are time-consuming and destructive in nature. Once a test is performed on a sample, the integrity of that sample is usually lost (with the exception of weight testing) and no additional testing may be done on it. For example, a traditional quantitative analysis such as high-performance liquid chromatography (HPLC) typically calls for the tablet to be ground, followed by dissolution and dilution in a suitable medium. A significant amount of time and labor is required to run each sample in duplicate or triplicate. Other traditional methods of tablet evaluation also involve time-consuming sample preparation, such as KBr dilution for mid-infrared analysis.

The mechanical strength of a tablet plays an important role in the development and control procedures. Crushing strength is the most widely used test of mechanical strength. It is defined as the compression force that, when applied diametrically to a tablet, just fractures it (28). Tablet hardness depends on the weight of material and the space between the upper and lower punches at the moment of compression. Inconsistent hardness values are likely to result from variation in these parameters. The fundamentals of powder compression are given in a report by Leuenberger and Rohera (29).

The Erweka hardness tester measures horizontal crushing strength by applying a load at 90° to the longest axis. This type of hardness tester is subject to two sources of inherent error: 1) the possibility of an incorrect zero, and 2) a scale that does not accurately indicate the true load applied. Other commercially used instruments include the Strong-Cobb, Monsanto, and Pfizer hardness testers. Variations in crushing strength values obtained from different types of hardness testers may be attributed to inaccuracies in instrument scale values, incorrect zero adjustment, and varying methods of applying the load. This necessitates calibration when comparing results from different types of testers. The physical dimensions and shape of the tablet may also contribute to the property of crushing strength.

The conventional methods of hardness testing for tablets also involve a subjective operator error. The scale on the Erweka hardness tester is divided into segments of 0.25-kg units. Very often, the sample under evaluation may produce a reading that falls between two divisions, and it is up to the operator to decide on the result.

Tablet-coating processes are commonly used in the pharmaceutical industry. Aqueous film coatings composed of cellulose derivatives and other polymers are useful for the control of dissolution of drug from the tablet. Gravimetric analysis and HPLC are often used to determine the endpoint of the coating process.

ADVANTAGES OF NIRS TABLET EVALUATION

NIRS is a nondestructive method, thus, 100% inspection of batches is theoretically possible, allowing better control of product uniformity. NIR is also noninvasive, enabling subsequent evaluation of the same tablets by another method. Samples may be retained for further analysis by NIR or other methods, allowing a direct correlation between tests. Economic benefits are obvious for manufacturers, who may increase profits per batch because of the need for fewer retained samples. NIRS is particularly useful in the early stages of product development when the supply of the new drug is limited.

NIR analysis is rapid, requiring less than one minute to analyze a single sample. Also, NIR analyses do not require the use and ultimate disposal of organic solvents, thereby reducing environmental waste. Advances in instrumentation, fiber optics, and software offer many options. Portable NIRS units are not uncommon.

Accelerated degradation samples may be analyzed and returned to the associated storage condition at each of the appropriate time intervals, thus drastically reducing the number of samples taken from the batch.

Measurement of powders can take place directly through the unopened glass jar or vial because glass does not absorb in the NIR region. Direct measurement through the container further reduces sampling errors, which may be introduced when a sample is withdrawn.

Multiple components of a sample may be analyzed simultaneously. A single spectrum can be obtained and compared with several different calibration sets at the same time, allowing the measurement of several constituents at one time. This saves considerable time and labor.

LIMITATIONS OF NIRS TABLET EVALUATION

The initial calibration process for a substance or a product can be quite detailed. A calibration equation is needed for each constituent in the sample. NIR calibrations must be formulation-specific. The accuracy of the NIR method cannot be better than the reference method from which it was built. Ruggedness of the models improves when all expected types of variation are included in the model. Careful selection of representative samples is imperative to the successful performance of the calibration. The choice of mathematical models depends highly on the character of the sample.

Another issue is that of transferability of the calibration model among instruments. This has been a significant obstacle to more widespread use of NIR methods. Transferability is especially important to multisite facilities, because it is needed to avoid time-consuming recalibration procedures. Calibration errors may occur among instruments because of slight differences in instrument response, especially if full-spectrum multivariate models are used. Shenk and Westerhaus (30) addressed the problem and proposed a standardization algorithm, which was modified by others (31, 32).

Physical attributes of the tablets can affect the calibration process. For example, scored tablets and those of differing geometries may produce more variable NIR spectra than flat, unscored tablets. Work in our laboratory (33) demonstrated a difference in NIR hardness testing of scored Avicel®-based chlorpheniramine tablets. Mixed calibration models composed of flat and concave tablets gave variable hardness prediction results, supporting the assertion that calibration models should contain samples of homogeneous composition.

Borer and coworkers (34) published a useful evaluation of sources of variability encountered in the NIR analysis of drug products. Analysts involved in NIRS method development should consider this report. Parameters included in the study included.

1. instrument settings (number of scans averaged per spectrum, iris opened or closed, frequency of reference spectrum collection);
2. data treatment (segment value used for second-derivative calculation); and
3. library design (total number of samples, number of days required to complete the library).

BULK DRUG PROPERTIES

Raw Material Identification

NIRS is useful for the analysis of both raw materials and finished dosage forms. Qualitative determination of pharmaceutical raw materials using NIRS was reported as early as 1982 (35). The largest variations in commercially produced excipients and actives appear to be in moisture content and particle size (36, 37). These parameters may be monitored by NIRS with relative ease. Incoming substances may be tested for immediate identity confirmation on the receiving dock by inserting a fiber optic probe directly into the barrel. Spectral data for each lot of material purchased may be saved and added to the growing spectral reference library.

The use of NIRS as an identification method involves the establishment of a comprehensive library containing the spectra of many compounds. The sample is scanned and identified by finding the most similar item in the library. Comparison of the sample spectrum to the library reference spectrum is achieved by calculating (via computer) the cosine of the angle between the vectors of both spectra. This value is called the spectral match value (SMV) and may range from -1 to $+1$, with $+1$ being a perfect match. Plugge and Van Der Vlies (38) utilized the SMV for a NIR method of identification of ampicillin trihydrate. In their work, an SMV of 0.9980 was established as a minimum value for positive identity of ampicillin. The conformity index or CI is also calculated to establish the degree of conformity of a batch to specifications. Conformity testing detects deviations from normal processing by comparing the average batch spectra with the library of a representative collection of approved batches of the same material.

Particle Size

The measurement of particle size is a key issue in the formulation of many pharmaceutical products. Particle size distribution is known to directly influence physical properties of powders, such as dissolution rate, powder flow, bulk density, and compressibility. Conventional methods of particle size measurement include sieve analysis and laser diffractometry (39).

Ciurczak and associates (40) reported a NIR method of determination of particle size of pure, granular substances. The method is based on theories of reflected light, in which reflectance increases as the particle size decreases. The reference method was a low-angle laser light-scattering (LALS) particle sizer (Malvern). The researchers found linear results for particles above 85 mm, but less accurate results for smaller particles.

O'Neil et al. (41) described a NIRS method for measuring the median particle size of numerous compounds and excipients. Malvern data and NIR reflectance spectra of sieved fractions and bulk samples were used to construct multiple linear regression (MLR) and quadratic least-squares fit calibration models. The same group (42) reported success in measuring the cumulative percentage frequency particle size distribution of microcrystalline cellulose (Avicel) using NIRS. This study compared the use of three-wavelength MLR and principal component regression (PCR), each model using Malvern and NIR reflectance data. The PCR model produced smaller SEPs, suggesting a more robust model than the MLR.

Frake and co-workers (43) extensively evaluated numerous chemometric techniques for the NIRS prediction of mass median particle size determination of lactose monohydrate. Models evaluated in zero order (untreated) and second derivative were MLR, PLS (partial least squares), and ANN (artificial neural network). The researchers concluded that there is more than one way to treat data and achieve a good calibration model. The group also confirms previous observations that derivitization of data does not remove "particle size effects" (previously thought to contribute to baseline shift).

Other researchers (44) have also reported NIR particle size studies.

Polymorphism and Racemization

Many drugs have the ability to form several distinct crystalline forms or polymorphs. Although the polymorphs are chemically identical, they are different arrangements of molecules and may exhibit different properties. Each polymorph may possess different energy levels and ultimately affect the dissolution rate of the compound. The infrared spectra of polymorphs may be expected to vary owing to different arrangement of functional groups (hydrogen bonding and polarization may be affected). Traditional methods for the identification of polymorphism are differential scanning calorimetry (DSC) and X-ray crystallography. However, these technique are destructive, and thus multiple runs of the same sample are not possible. Ciurzcak (45) reported a NIR method of identification of the polymorphs of caffeine. Aldridge and co-workers (46) reported a NIR method of detection of polymorphism in which pattern-recognition methods were used to discriminate between the desired polymorphic form of a drug substance and another undesired polymorph. A significant outcome of this work was the successful transfer of the calibration between six other NIR instruments without the use of multivariate calibration transfer algorithms.

Gimet and Luong (47) used NIRS to determine whether the processing of a granulation resulted in racemization. Others (48) have also reported the differential identification of optically active forms.

Moisture Content

The classic methods of water determination are Karl Fischer (KF) titration, gas chromatography (GC), and loss on drying (LOD). Using near-infrared methods, the presence of water is indicated by a major NIR absorption band at approximately 1920–1950 nm. The absorption maximum and peak shape depend on the degree of hydrogen bonding occurring within the environment where the water is located. The stronger the hydrogen bond, the longer the wavelength of the NIR absorption maxima. A second band attributed to water may appear at approximately 1450 nm and is attributed to bound water.

The NIRS determination of moisture content has been documented by numerous researchers (49–51). Plugge and Van Der Vlies (52) described a NIR method for ampicillin, which measures eight quality control criteria:

- identity,
- water content,
- crystallinity,
- ampicillin content.
- fraction of anhydrous ampicillin,
- residual reagent,
- residual organic solvents, and
- residual starting material.

DeThomas and VonBargen (53) patented a NIR fiber optic system for the measurement of moisture or "a constituent" in a powder. Berntsson, and associates (54) described a NIRS method to determine at-line moisture content in bulk hard gelatin capsules. Capsules were equilibrated at various humidities, and reference moisture content was determined by loss on drying.

Zhou and co-workers (55) at Eli Lilly and Company developed a NIRS method to determine moisture content in a freeze-dried drug product using gas chromatography (GC) as the reference method. A standard error of prediction (SEP) as low as 0.07% w/w was obtained using the NIR method in the range of 0.1–5.7% water. At very low water levels, the workers found the GC method to be more precise than the NIR method.

Corti and co-workers (56) developed a NIRS method to determine the water content of crushed ranitidine chlorhydrate tablets. KF titration was used as the reference method. Higher NIRS errors were found with the samples having a water content of less than 1%.

Dziki and coworkers (57) used NIRS to monitor the mobility of water within the sarafloxacin crystal lattice. The study involved the veterinary product sarafloxacin in an aqueous granulation process. A failed lot of the product was indistinguishable from an acceptable lot using X-ray powder diffraction, midinfrared spectroscopy, differential scanning calorimetry (DSC), and TGA. NIRS detected intermediate stages of water absorption in the granulation and enabled the process to be controlled.

An interesting report on NIR measurement of water in skin was published recently by Martin (58) at Helene

Curtis, Inc. NIRS measurements indicated four types of water contained in the skin. The workers presented tentative assignments for the absorption bands:

- lipid bilayers (1875 nm)
- secondary and primary water on protein groups (1909 and 1923 nm), and
- bulk water beneath the stratum corneum (1890 nm).

Studies were performed in vivo on two volunteers as well as in vitro using porcine skin. Although not directly related to tablet evaluation, the work is notable for its contribution to the transdermal delivery of drugs, potential NIR prediction of drug penetration through the skin, and conclusions regarding moisturizer use on the skin.

PRODUCT EVALUATION

Identification and Potency

Reports describing NIR methods of identification of solid and liquid dosage forms have increased in the literature during the 1990s (59–62). Earlier work has been reviewed elsewhere (see Introduction). Virtually all new NIR methods include product identification in the assay. Gottfries and co-workers (63) reported a NIR method for the measurement of metaprolol in controlled-release tablets. In their work, a comparison was made between the diffuse reflectance and transmission modes. The workers found better prediction of tablet strength using transmission mode and reasoned that reflectance spectra are more sensitive to the inhomogeneity of the material.

Ebube and coworkers (64) reported a NIR method that can distinguish between three Avicel® products owing to the varying particle sizes. The method was also designed to predict tablet hardness and lubricant concentration. Regardless of the small sample sizes used, good results were obtained.

North, Young and Leng et al. (65) recently presented an interesting comparison of NIR diffuse reflectance and transmittance for the analysis of tablets. Tablets used were of different drug content and size as well as coated and uncoated. Both methods produced excellent resolution of two tablet strengths. Uncoated and coated tablets produced different spectra by reflectance, but only a minimal difference was seen by transmission. Of two drug peaks seen in the reflectance spectra, only one band was observed in transmission because no transmission through the tablet occurred in the region of the second peak. Both methods produced difference in spectra as a result of difference in tablet size and surface curvature.

Merckle and Kovar (66) reported an assay of effervescent tablets (intact and powdered) by NIRS in transmittance and reflectance modes. Results of quantitative determination of acetylsalicylic acid (ASA) and ASA in combination with ascorbic acid and/or paracetamol were comparable in both transmittance and reflectance modes. Corti and associates (67) described a NIR transmittance analysis of coated tablets, using both whole and milled tablets.

Brashear and coworkers (68) developed a diffuse reflectance NIRS method to quantify lomefloxacin and polyethyleneglycol (PEG) within a polymeric implant. The properties of pore-forming excipients such as PEG are known to affect the rate of drug release from a matrix.

Sondermann and Kovar (69) described a study using NIRS for the identification of "ecstasy" street samples. Ecstasy tablets may contain either N-Methyl-3,4-Methylendioxyamphetamine (MDMA) or N-Ethyl-3,4-Methylendioxyamphetamine (MDE) as well as other amphetamine derivatives. In addition, various excipients were present, and nonstandardized production procedures contributed to inhomogeneous tablets. The authors researchers included a broad range of excipients in their calibration work and succeeded in constructing three PLS models for identification.

Identity testing of blister packaged tablets/supplies for clinical trials

A noninvasive NIR method was reported by Dempster and et al. (70) for the identification of tablets within blister packages. The method identified and discriminated various potencies of an experimental drug, placebo tablets, and clinical comparator tablets.

Aldridge and coworkers (71) described a NIRS method for nondestructive identification of blister-packaged tablets. The NIR method drastically reduced the assay time required by the previous TLC method. The TLC method required a full day to analyze 40 tablets, compared with the NIR method, which analyzed 10 tablets in 7 min.

Detection of adulteration

Lodder, Selby and Hieftje et al. (72) reported a NIR method of detection of capsule tampering. Several nonprescription products were selected for the study and tested with and without the addition of various adulterants. The NIR method provided a rapid, noninvasive way to screen products for known foreign substances. One limitation of the NIR method is the inability to predict which substances might be present in a product. Although the NIR spectra of many adulterants may be present in the spectral library, there is the possibility that a new, unknown substance could be added to a product and not detected as an error in the NIR product spectrum.

Product development

In the drug-discovery field, chemists can use NIR to monitor the progress of reactions. Hearn and coworkers (73) reported a NIR method to monitor the preparation of compounds for screening as antituberculosis drugs. The reaction of isonicotinic acid hydrazide (INH) with carbonyl compounds in the preparation of Schiff bases was followed. Forbes and coworkers (74) described a NIR conformance test method to assay and identify two chemical intermediates used in the manufacture of Loracarbef, a carbacephalosporin.

Bauer, Dziki and Quick et al. (75) used NIRS to investigate the problem of dissolution failure in an erythromycin tablet formulation. The technique enabled the group to identify the presence of a dehydrated dihydrate produced during formulation. The dihydrate was found to gradually bind with magnesium hydroxide in the tablet formulation, thus delaying the process of dissolution. The use of NIR facilitated the development of a humidifying process that reversed the binding and increased the dissolution rate.

Quality Control Parameters

Tablet hardness

It has been shown (76, 77) that the NIR signal varies with a change in compression force. In other words, changes in tablet hardness result in an alteration in the NIR spectra of the sample. Presumably, increasing the compression force during the tableting process causes the tablet to be smoother as well as harder, thus causing less light scattering, leading to a greater absorbance and higher baseline. NIR hardness testing of tablets can be performed at the same time as other parameters such as identity, moisture content, and coating thickness.

Further work by Kirsch and Drennen (78) on NIR hardness testing has explored the use of various mathematical models for calibration. Other researchers have also reported NIR methods for the measurement of tablet hardness (64, 79).

Tablet coating

NIRS has been used to determine tablet-coating and core thickness. Kirsch and Drennen (80) evaluated the use of NIR at-line to monitor film coating in a Wurster column. The method was successful at predicting coating thickness of two coating formulations at various intervals during the process and was less time-consuming than wet chemical methods. Earlier work by Kirsch and Drennen (81) described a NIR method to determine film-coating parameters of theophylline tablets. Increasing coating thickness, corresponded to increased NIR absorbance in certain regions of the spectrum. Calibration models were developed for tablet hardness, coating thickness and the prediction of time to 50% dissolution.

Buchanan and coworkers (82) at Merck reported a NIR method for evaluating a new coating-thickness manufacturing process. A precision film-coating process was tested whereby an immediate-release drug-active coating surrounded an extended-release active-drug core. The NIR method enabled the evaluation to proceed more quickly and less expensively than did the reference HPLC method. The implementation of the NIR method allowed rapid evaluation of tablets and assisted in identifying "dead zones" in the Wurster column, thus allowing immediate correction and revision of the process.

Determination of degradation products

Drennen and Lodder (83) reported a nondestructive NIRS method to monitor the decomposition of aspirin. In contrast to the multi step HPLC assay for salicylic acid and the USP identity tests for aspirin, the NIR method involved a 90-s scan of individual intact aspirin tablets. The workers correlated changes in spectra to the mass of water absorbed, the mass of salicylic acid formed, and the time the tablets spent in a hydrator.

Shimoyama and coworkers (84) reported a NIR analysis of photodegradation of poly(methyl methacrylate) using an in situ fiber optic device. This type of technology from a related discipline is notable as a potential application for pharmaceutical systems.

Characterization of powder blends and blend homogeneity

Powder blending is a fundamental step in the process of manufacturing pharmaceutical products. Only a homogeneous mixture can be properly subdivided to provide uniform doses of the active ingredients. The current procedures for monitoring blend uniformity require that the blending process be stopped at defined intervals to obtain samples of the blend. The samples are collected from different locations in the blending vessel using a sample thief. The samples are then sent to a laboratory and analyzed using traditional methods such as HPLC or UV until the active components are within specification for that formulation. This approach requires a significant amount of time and labor and may be subject to errors induced by sampling methods.

NIRS has been shown by several researchers to be useful for evaluating the powder-mixing process. Wargo and Drennen (85) demonstrated the use of a NIR method to determine homogeneity of powder blends.

In 1995, the European Patent Office granted a patent to Dr. Paul K. Aldridge, Pfizer Central Research, Groton, CT, for an apparatus (86) for mixing and detecting on-line homogeneity. The apparatus involves the use of a diffuse-reflectance fiber optic probe interfaced on-line with a V-blender. Sekulic and co-workers (87) at Pfizer described the use of this apparatus for on-line monitoring of powder blend homogeneity. An 8-quart twin-shell V-blender was interfaced with a fiber optic probe at the axis of rotation. Spectra were collected at prescribed intervals, and data analysis was performed using a series of commercial software. Variability in the NIR spectra as a function of time was measured, and it was shown that this variability reached a minimum level sooner than what traditional blending times suggest. DeMaesschalck et al. (88) used the NIR on-line method described in article by the Sekulic and associates to design an approach for deciding when the blend is homogeneous. They calculated the average standard deviation between spectra taken at each time and used the dissimilarity between each new measurement and the ideal mixture spectrum to monitor changes in the mixture during the blending process.

Scientists at Merck were issued a U.S. patent in 1996 for a method (89) of measuring the homogeneity of tablets using NIR. It can be used to monitor the pharmaceutical material during the tableting process (powder mix, granular mix, and compressed tablets).

CONCLUSIONS

NIRS has proven to be a fast, reliable, and cost-saving method for numerous applications in the pharmaceutical industry. It is no longer the esoteric method it was once believed to be. The pharmaceutical industry has learned a great deal about NIRS from the agricultural and food industries. Concepts and techniques have been borrowed and fitted to the needs of pharmaceutical scientists. Users in all disciplines face common issue, such as calibration transfer, moisture contamination, particle size, and the rigors of calibrating multiple constituents.

NIRS possesses a great and, as yet, incompletely exploited potential in the area of identity testing of drug substances. It has already begun to replace traditional compendial methods of quality control. It has gained recognition from the FDA. and other regulatory agencies, a signal to skeptics that NIRS is a solid alternative to traditional methods of analysis. Aggressive workers in the field are moving to develop and receive approval for NIR

methods that bypass the traditional reference methods. A greater understanding of the mathematics involved with NIR analyses has contributed to the wider use of NIR methods. Small companies that wish to use NIR analyses may find it wise to contract out their work to groups with more expertise because initial startup can be expensive and initial calibration work may be time-consuming.

We confidently predict that NIRS will rapidly become an established and standard method for many types of pharmaceutical analyses.

REFERENCES

1. Osborne, B.G.; Fearn, T. *Near Infrared Spectroscopy in Food Analysis*; Longman Scientific & Technical: United Kingdom, 1986; 2.

2. Morisseau, K.M.; Rhodes, C.T. Proven and Potential Uses of Near-Infrared Spectroscopy for the Evaluation of Tablets; Tableting and Granulation Year Book. *Pharm. Tech. Suppl.* 6–11.

3. Morisseau, K.M.; Rhodes, C.T. Pharmaceutical Uses of Near-Infrared Spectroscopy. Drug Dev. Ind. Pharm. **1995**, *21*, 1071–1090.

4. Corti, P.; Dreassi, E. Near Infrared Reflectance Analysis: Features and Applications in Pharmaceutical and Biomedical Analysis. Farmaco. **1993**, *48* (1), 3–20.

5. MacDonald, B.F.; Prebble, K.A. Some Applications of Near-Infrared Reflectance Analysis in the Pharmaceutical Industry. J. Pharm. Biomed. Anal. **1993**, *11*, 1077–1085.

6. Axon, T.G.; Brown, R.; Hammond, S.V.; Maris, S.J. Focusing Near Infrared Spectroscopy on the Business Objectives of Modern Pharmaceutical Production. J. Near Infrared Spectrosc. **1998**, *6*, A13–A19.

7. Workman, J.J., Jr.; Review of Process and Non-Invasive Near-Infrared and Infrared Spectroscopy. Appl. Spectrosc. Reviews, May 1 **1999**, *34*, 1–2, 1–89.

8. Ciurczak, E.W.; Drennen, J.K. *Near Infrared Spectroscopy in Pharmaceutical and Medical Applications, Practical Spectrosc. Series*; Gadamasetti, K.G., Ed.; Marcel Dekker, Inc.: New York, in press.

9. Rose, J.J.; Prisick, T.; Mindakia, J. J. Parent. Sci. Tech. **1982**, *26*, 71–78.

10. Ciurczak, E.W.; Torlini, R.P. Analysis of Solid and Liquid Dosage Forms Using Near-Infrared Reflectance Spectroscopy. Spectrosc. **1987**, *2* (3), 41–43.

11. Sinsheimer, J.E.; Keuhnelian. Am J. Pharm. Sci. **1996**, *55*, 1240.

12. Massart, D.L.; Vandeginste, B.G.M.; Deming, S.N.; Michotte, Y.; Kaufman, L. Data Handling in Science and Technology. *Chemometrics: A Textbook*; Vandeginste, B.G.M., Rutan, S.C., Eds.; Elsevier Publishing: New York, 1988; 2, 5.

13. Willard, H.H.; et al. Infrared Spectroscopy. *Instrumental Methods of Analysis*, 7th Ed.; Wadsworth Publishing Company: Belmont, 1988; 287.

14. Workman, J.J., Jr.; Burns, D.A. Commercial NIR Instrumentation. *Handbook of Near-Infrared Analysis*; Burns, D.A., Ciurczak, E.W., Eds.; Marcel Dekker, Inc.: New York, 1992; 37–51.

15. Lodder, R.A. Sample Holders or Reflectors for Intact Capsules and Tablets and for Liquid Microcells for Use in Near-Infrared Reflectance Spectrophotometers, US Patent 165,751, November 21, 1989.

16. Drennen, J.K. Near-Infrared Reflectance Spectrometer System and Related Sample Cell and Sample Support, US Patent 898,454, May 25, 1993.

17. Soloman, S. Non-Destructive Identification of Tablet and Tablet Dissolution by Means of Infrared Spectroscopy, US Patent 338,909, October 21, 1997.

18. Noble, D. Illuminating Near-IR. Anal. Chem. **1995**, *67* (23), 735A–740A.

19. — http://kerouac.pharm.uky.edu/asrg/cnirs/ir_spec.htm (accessed May 2000).

20. — http://leden.tref.nl/~mderksen/patents.html (accessed May *2000).*

21. Ciurczak, E.W. Pharmaceutical Mixing Studies Using Near-Infrared Spectroscopy, Tableting and Granulation Yearbook; Pharm. Tech. Supp. **1997**, *18–28.*

22. Thomas, E.V. A Primer on Multivariate Calibration. Anal. Chem. **1994**, *66* (15), 795A–804A.

23. Lodder, R.A.; Selby, M.; Hieftje, G.M. Detection of Capsule Tampering by Near-Infrared Reflectance Analysis. Anal. Chem. **1987**, *59*, 1921–1930.

24. Mark, H.L.; Tunnell, D. Qualitative Near-Infrared Reflectance Analysis Using Mahalanobis Distances. Anal. Chem. **1985**, *57*, 1449–1456.

25. Gemperline, P.J.; Boyer, N.R. Classification of Near-Infrared Spectra Using Wavelength Distances: Comparison to the Mahalanobis Distance and Residual Variance Methods. Anal. Chem. **1995**, *67*, 160–16.

26. Gerhausser, C.I.; Kovar, K.A. Strategies for Constructing Near-Infrared Spectral Libraries for the Identification of Drug Substances. Appl. Spectrosc. **1998**, *51*, 1504–1510.

27. American Society for Testing and Materials (A.S.T.M). *Standard Practices for Infrared Multivariate Quantitative Analysis*; Practice E1655-00, A.S.T.M: West Conshocken, Pennsylvania, 1995; 1–25.

28. Marshall, K.; Rudnic, E.M. Tablet Dosage Forms. *Modern Pharmaceutics*, 2 edn; Banker, G.S.; Rhodes, C.T., Eds.; Marcel Dekker, Inc.: New York, 1990; 355–425.

29. Leuenberger, H.; Rohera, B.D. Fundamentals of Powder Compression. Pharm. Res. **1986**, *3* (1), 12–22.

30. Shenk, J.S.; Westerhaus, M.O. Crop Sci. **1991**, *31*, 1694–1696.

31. Bouveresse, E.; Massart, D.L. Modified Algorithm for Standardization of Near-Infrared Spectrophotometric Instruments. Anal. Chem. **1995**, *67*, 1381–1389.

32. Wang, Y.; Kowalski, B.R. Appl. Spectrosc. **1992**, *46*, 764–771.

33. Morisseau, K.M. *The Effect of Compression Force on the Near-Infrared Spectra of Tablet Dosage Forms*; University of Rhode Island, 1996; 130–242, Doctoral dissertation.

34. Borer, M.W.; Zhou, X.; Hays, D.M.; Hofer, J.D.; White, K.C. Evaluation of Key Sources of Variability in the Measurement of Pharmaceutical Drug Products by Near Infrared Reflectance Spectroscopy. J. Pharm. Biomed. Anal. **1998**, *17*, 641–650.

35. Rose, J.R. Quantitative and Quanlitative Analysis with NIRA. Proceeding of the 2nd Annual Symposium on NIRA, Technicon, Tarrytown, New York, July, 1982.

36. Ciurczak, E.W. NIR Analysis of Pharmaceuticals. *Handbook of Near-Infrared Analysis*; Burns, D.A., Ciurczak, E.W., Eds.; Marcel Dekker, Inc.: New York, 1992; 549–563.

37. Burger, T.; Fricke, J. NIR Radiative Transfer Investigations to Characterise Pharmaceutical Powders and Their Mixtures. J. Near Infrared Spectrosc. **1998**, *6*, 33–40.

38. Plugge, W.; Van Der Vlies, C. Near-Infrared Spectroscopy as an Alternative to Assess Compliance of Ampicillin Trihydrate with Compendial Specifications. J. Pharm. Biomed. Anal. **1993**, *11* (6), 435–442.

39. Aulton, M.E. Pharmaceutics: The Science of Dosage Form Design. Churchill Livingstone: Edinburgh, 1988.

40. Ciurczak, E.W.; Torlini, R.P.; Demkowicz, M.P. Determination of Particle Size of Pharmaceutical Raw Materials Using Near-Infrared Reflectance Analysis. Spectroscopy **1986**, *1*, 36–39.

41. O'Neil, A.J.; Jee, R.D.; Moffat, A.C. The Application of Multiple Linear Regression to the Measurement of the Median Particle Size of Drugs and Pharmaceutical Excipients by Near-Infrared Spectroscopy. Analyst **1998**, *123*, 2297–2302.

42. O'Neil, A.J.; Jee, R.D.; Moffat, A.C. Measurement of the Cumulative Particle Size Distribution of Microcrystalline Cellulose Using Near Infrared Reflectance Spectroscopy. Analyst **1999**, *124*, 33–36.

43. Frake, P.; Gill, I.; Luscombe, C.N.; Rudd, D.R.; Waterhouse, J.; Jayasooriya, U.A. Near-Infrared Mass Median Particle Size Determination of Lactose Monohydrate, Evaluating Several Chemometric Approaches. Analyst **1998**, *123*, 2043–2046.

44. Dredàn, J.; Zelkò, R.; Antal, I.; Bihari, E.; Ràcz, I. Effect of Particle Size and Coating Level on the Diffuse Reflectance of Wax Matrices. J. Pharm. Pharmacol. **1998**, *50*, 139–142.

45. Ciurczak, E.W. In Proceedings of FACSS, Philadelphia, 1985.

46. Aldridge, P.K.; Evans, C.L.; Ward, H.W., II; Colgan, S.T. Near-IR Detection of Polymorphism and Process-Related Substances. Anal. Chem. **1996**, *68*, 997–1002.

47. Gimet, R.; Luong, A.T. J. Pharm. Biomed. Anal. **1987**, *5*, 205.

48. Buchanan, B.R.; Ciurczak, E.W.; Grunke, A.; Honigs, D.E. Spectroscopy **1988**, *3*, 54.

49. Kamat, M.; Lodder, R.A.; DeLuca, P.P. Near-Infrared Spectroscopic Determination of Residual Moisture in Lyophilized Sucrose Through Intact Glass Vials. Pharm. Res. **1989**, *6*, 961–965.

50. Sinsheimer, J.E.; Poswalk, N.M. Pharmaceutical Applications of the Near-Infrared Determination of Water. J. Pharm. Sci. **1968**, *57*, 2007–2010.

T

51. Zhou, X.; Hines, P.; Borer, M.W. Moisture Determination in Hygroscopic Drug Substance by Near Infrared Spectroscopy. J. Pharm. Biomed. Anal. **1998**, *17* (2), 219–225.

52. Plugge, W.; Van Der Vlies, C. The Use of Near Infrared Spectroscopy in the Quality Control Laboratory of the Pharmaceutical Industry. C. J. Pharm. Biomed. Anal. **1992**, *10*, 797–803.

53. DeThomas, F.A.; VonBargen, K.P. System for Measuring the Moisture Content of Powder and Fiber Optic Probe Therefore, US Patent 931,783, January 11, 1994.

54. Berntsson, O.; Zackrisson, G.; Ostling, G. Determination of Moisture in Hard Gelatin Capsules Using Near-Infrared Spectroscopy: Applications to At-Line Process Control of Pharmaceuticals. J. Pharm. Biomed. Anal. **1997**, *15*, 895–900.

55. Zhou, X.; Hines, P.A.; White, K.C.; Borer, M.W. Gas Chromatography as a Reference Method for Moisture Determination by Near Infrared Spectroscopy. Anal. Chem. **1998**, *70*, 390–394.

56. Corti, P.; Dreassi, E.; Corbini, G.; Lonardi, S.; Viviani, E.; Mosconi, L.; Bernuzzi, M. Application of Near Infrared Reflectance to the Analytical Control of Pharmaceuticals: Assay of Ranitidine Chlorhydrate and Water Content in Tablets. Pharm. Acta Helv. **1990**, *65*, 28–32.

57. Dziki, W.; Bauer, J.F.; Szpylman, J.J.; Quick, J.E.; Nichols, B.C. The Use of Near-Infrared Spectroscopy to Monitor the Mobility of Water Within the Sarafloxacin Crystal Lattice. J. Pharm. Biomed. Anal. **2000**, *22*, 829–848.

58. Martin, K. In Vivo Measurements of Water in Skin by Near Infrared Reflectance. Appl. Spectrosc. **1998**, *52*, 1001–1007.

59. Bradfield, K.B.; Forbes, R.A. Development and Validation of an Analytical Method for Identification of Granulated Nicarbazin by Near Infrared Reflectance Spectroscopy. J. Near Infrared Spectrosc. **1997**, *5*, 41–65.

60. Jedvert, I.; Josefson, M.; Langkilde, F. Quantification of an Active Substance in a Tablet by NIR and Raman Spectroscopy. J. Near Infrared Spectrosc. **1998**, *6*, 279–289.

61. Han, S.M.; Faulkner, P.G. Determination of SB-216469-S During Tablet Production Using Near-Infrared Reflectance Spectroscopy. J. Pharm. Biomed. Anal. **1996**, *14*, 1681–1689.

62. Eustaquio, A.; Graham, P.; Jee, R.D.; Moffatt, A.C.; Trafford, A.D. Quantification of Paracetamol in Intact Tablets Using Near-Infrared Transmittance Spectroscopy. Analyst **1998**, *123* (11), 2303–2306.

63. Gottfries, J.; Depui, H.; Fransson, M.; Jongeneelen, M.; Josefson, M.; Langkilde, F.W.; Witte, D.T. Vibrational Spectrometry for the Assessment of Active Substance in Metoprolol Tablets: A Comparison Between Transmission and Diffuse Reflectance Near-Infrared Spectrometry. J. Pharm. Biomed. Anal. **1996**, *14*, 1495–1503.

64. Ebube, N.K.; Thosar, S.S.; Roberts, R.A.; Kemper, M.S.; Rubinovitz, R.; Martin, D.L.; Reier, G.E.; Wheatley, T.A.; Shukla, A.J. Application of Near-Infrared Spectroscopy for Nondestructive Analysis of Avicel Powders and Tablets. Pharm. Dev. Tech. **1999**, *4*, 19–26.

65. North, N.; Young, K.; Leng, M. A Comparison Between NIR Diffuse Reflectance and Transmittance for the Analysis of Pharmaceutical Tablets, 8th FOSS/NIRSystems European Pharmaceutical User Group Meeting, SmithKline Beecham, Harlow, UK, October 1–8, 1997.

66. Merckle, P.; Kovar, K.A. Assay of Effervescent Tablets by Near-Infrared Spectroscopy in Transmittance and Reflectance Mode. J. Pharm. Biomed. Anal. **1998**, *17* (3), 365–374.

67. Corti, P.; Ceramelli, G.; Dreassi, E.; Mattii, S. Near Infrared Transmittance Analysis for the Assay of Solid Pharmaceutical Dosage Forms. Analyst **1999**, *124*, 755–758.

68. Brashear, R.L.; Flanagan, D.; Luner, P.E.; Seyer, J.J.; Kemper, M.S. Diffuse Reflectance Near-Infrared Spectroscopy as a Nondestructive Analytical Technique for Polymer Implants. J. Pharm. Sci. **1999**, *88* (12), 1348–1353.

69. Sondermann, N.; Kovar, K.A. Screening Experiments of Ecstasy Street Samples Using Near Infrared Spectroscopy. For. Sci. Int. **1999**, *106*, 147–156.

70. Dempster, M.A.; Jones, J.A.; Last, I.R.; MacDonald, B.F. Near-Infrared Methods for the Identification of Tablets in Clinical Trial Supplies. J. Pharm. Biomed. Anal. **1993**, *11*, 1087–1092.

71. Aldridge, P.K.; Mushinsky, R.F.; Andino, M.M.; Evans, C.L. Identification of Tablet Formulations Inside Blister Packages by Near-Infrared Spectroscopy. Appl. Spectrosc. **1994**, *48*, 1272–76.

72. Lodder, R.A.; Selby, M.; Hieftje, G.M. Detection of Capsule Tampering by Near-Infrared Reflectance Analysis. Anal. Chem. **1987**, *59*, 1921–1930.

73. Hearn, M.J.; Celi, P.; Chanyaputhipong, P.Y.; Chi, W.; Kang, J.O.; Katz, A.; Shah, R.; Thai, M.; Ung, P. Using Near Infrared Spectroscopy to Monitor the Preparation of Compounds for Screening as Antituberculosis Drugs. J. Near Infrared Spectr. **1995**, *3*, 19–23.

74. Forbes, R.A.; Persinger, M.L.; Smith, D.R. Development and Validation of Analytical Methodology for Near-Infrared Conformance Testing of Pharmaceutical Intermediates. J. Pharm. Biomed. Anal. **1996**, *15*, 315–327.

75. Bauer, J.F.; Dziki, W.; Quick, J.E. Role of an Isomorphic Desolvate in Dissolution Failures of an Erythromycin Tablet Formulation. J. Pharm. Sci. **1999**, *88* (11), 1222–1227.

76. Kirsch, J.D.; Drennen, J.K. Determination of Film-Coated Tablet Parameters by Near-Infrared Spectroscopy. J. Pharm. Biomed. Anal. **1995**, *13*, 1273–1281.

77. Morisseau, K.M.; Rhodes, C.T. Near-Infrared Spectroscopy as a Nondestructive Alternative to Conventional Tablet Hardness Testing. Pharm. Res. **1997**, *14* (1), 108–111.

78. Kirsch, J.D.; Drennen, J.K. Nondestructive Tablet Hardness Testing by Near-Infrared Spectroscopy: A New and Robust Spectral Best-Fit Algorithm. J. Pharm. Biomed. Anal. **1999**, *19*, 351–362.

79. Guo, J.H.; Skinner, G.W.; Harcum, W.W.; Malone, J.P.; Weyer, L.G. Application of Near-Infrared Spectroscopy in the Pharmaceutical Solid Dosage Form. Drug Dev. Indust. Pharm. **1999**, *25* (12), 1267–1270.

80. Kirsch, J.D.; Drennen, J.K. Near-Infrared Spectroscopic Monitoring of the Film Coating Process. Pharm. Res. **1996**, *13*, 234–237.

81. Kirsch, J.D.; Drennen, J.K. Determination of Film-Coated Tablet Parameters by NIR Spectroscopy. J. Pharm. Biomed. Anal. **1995**, *13*, 1273–1281.

82. Buchanan, B.R.; Baxter, M.A.; Chen, T.S.; Qin, X.Z.; Robinson, P.A. Use of Near-Infrared Spectroscopy to Evaluate an Active in a Film Coated Tablet. Pharm. Res. **1996**, *13*, 616–621, 1996.

83. Drennen, J.K.; Lodder, R.A. Nondestructive Near-Infrared Analysis of Intact Tablets for Determination of Degradation Products. J. Pharm. Sci. **1990**, *79*, 622–627.

84. Shimoyama, M.; Matsukawa, K.; Inoue, H.; Ninomiyaa, T.; Ozaki, Y. Non-Destructive Analysis of Photo-Degradation of Poly(Methyl Methacrylate) by Near Infrared Light-Fibre Spectroscopy and Chemometrics. J. Near Infrared Spectrosc. **1999**, *7*, 27–32.

85. Wargo, D.J.; Drennen, J.K. Near-Infrared Spectroscopic Characterization of Pharmaceutical Powder Blends. J. Pharm. Biomed. Anal. **1996**, *14* (8), 1415–1423.

86. Aldridge, P.K. Pfizer, Inc. Apparatus for Mixing and Detecting On-Line Homogeneity. European Patent Publication **1993**, A*1*, 631–810.

87. Sekulic, S.S.; Ward, H.W.; Brannegan, D.R.; Stanley, E.D.; Evans, C.L.; Sciavolino, S.T.; Hailey, P.A.; Aldridge, P.K. On-Line Monitoring of Powder Blend Homogeneity by Near-Infrared Spectroscopy. Anal. Chem. **1996**, *68* (3), 509–513.

88. DeMaesschalck, R.; Sanchez, F.C.; Massart, D.L.; Doherty, P.; Hailey, P.A. On-Line Monitoring of Powder Blending with Near-Infrared Spectroscopy. Appl. Spectrosc. **1998**, *52* (5), 725–731.

89. Richmond, E.W.; Buchanan, B.R.; Baxter, M.A.; Duff, A.; Tully, O.M.; Thornton, S.A. Method and System for Determining the Homogeneity of Tablets, US Patent 296,833; April 2, 1996.

90. Williams, P., Norris, K., Eds. *Near-Infrared Technology in the Agricultural and Food Industries*, American Association of Cereal Chemists: St. Paul, MN, 1987.

91. Burns, D.A., Ciurczak, E.W., Eds. *Handbook of Near-Infrared Analysis*, Marcel Dekker, Inc.: New York, 1992.

TABLET FORMULATION

Larry L. Augsburger
University of Maryland, Baltimore, Maryland

Mark J. Zellhofer
University Pharmaceuticals of Maryland, Inc., Baltimore, Maryland

INTRODUCTION OBJECTIVES OF TABLET FORMULATION

The best new therapeutic entity in the world is of little value without an appropriate delivery system. Tableted drug delivery systems can range from relatively simple immediate-release formulations to complex extended- or modified-release dosage forms. The most important role of a drug delivery system is to get the drug "delivered" to the site of action in sufficient amount and at the appropriate rate; however, it must also meet a number of other essential criteria. These include physical and chemical stability, ability to be economically mass produced in a manner that assures the proper amount of drug in each and every dosage unit and in each batch produced, and, as far as possible, patient acceptability (for example, reasonable size and shape, taste, color, etc. to encourage patients to take the drug and thus comply with the prescribed dosing regimen).

The discovery of new therapeutic entities always initiates excitement, but the contributions of the formulation specialist are either not well understood or are often taken for granted and thus remain "unsung." However, the drug and its delivery system cannot be separated. The general design criteria for tablets are given as follows

1. Optimal drug dissolution and, hence, availability from the dosage form for absorption consistent with intended use (i.e., immediate or extended release).
2. Accuracy and uniformity of drug content.
3. Stability, including the stability of the drug substance, the overall tablet formulation, disintegration, and the rate and extent of drug dissolution from the tablet for an extended period.
4. Patient acceptability. As much as possible, the finished product should have an attractive appearance, including color, size, taste, etc., as applicable, in order to maximize patent acceptability and encourage compliance with the prescribed dosing regimen.

5. Manufacturability. The formulation design should allow for the efficient, cost-effective, practical production of the required batches.

That tablets can be formulated to uniquely meet these criteria accounts for their emergence as the most prevalent oral solid dosage form. Although several different types of tablets may be distinguished, they are mostly made by compression, intended to be swallowed whole and designed for immediate release. This paper presents a systematic approach to the design and formulation of immediate-release compressed tablets.

MODERN TABLET FORMULATION DESIGN AND MANUFACTURE

Tablet dosage forms have to satisfy a unique design compromise. The desired properties of rapid or controlled disintegration and dissolution of the primary constituent particles must be balanced with the manufacturability and esthetics of a solid compact resistant to mechanical attrition.

Excipients are critical to the design of the delivery system and play a major role in determining its quality and performance (1). They may be selected to enhance stability (antioxidants, UV absorbers), optimize or modify drug release (disintegrants, hydrophilic polymers, wetting agents, biodegradable polymers), provide essential manufacturing technology functions (binders, glidants, lubricants), enhance patient acceptance (flavors), or aid in product identification (colorants). Thus a tablet formulation is not a random combination of ingredients, but rather a carefully thought out, rational formulation designed to satisfy the above criteria.

A long list of possible excipients is available to the formulation scientist, but certain external factors such as cost, functional reliability, availability, and international acceptance govern their selection. For example, although the official compendia provide standards for identity and purity of excipients, monographs may not provide tests to assure their functionality. For instance, the NF monograph for Compressible Sugar provides no test for compressibility. The monograph for Lactose USP does not address the many particle size and tableting grades meeting monograph standards. The NF monograph for Pregelatinized Starch refers to grades that are "compressible and flowable in character," but provides no specifications or tests for these properties. Nor do the monograph tests for disintegrants and lubricants necessarily relate to their functionality. The need to provide functionality tests or tests for properties clearly related to functionality may be as important as controlling identity and purity (2). This point has been made even more apparent in recent years with the emergence of multiple sources of such modern excipients as direct-compression filler-binders and the various classes of "super" disintegrants.

A major problem currently being faced by multinational firms and others who market in the international arena, is the lack of universal acceptability of excipients in different countries. The selection of excipients for international markets is often a compromise between functional efficacy, local restrictions, and cost and availability in the countries where the product is to be made. In recent years, the globalization of the pharmaceutical industry has brought about an intense interest in developing harmonized pharmacopeial excipient standards, Good Manufacturing Practices (GMP) for excipient manufacture, and safety evaluation guidelines for new excipients to eliminate or avoid trade barriers between different countries (3). The International Pharmaceuticals Excipients Council (IPEC), which consists of producers, users, and pharmaceutical scientists, was launched in 1991 to assist regulatory authorities in the United States, Japan, and Europe with harmonization. The separate organizations later formed in the United States (IPEC-Americas), Europe (IPEC-Europe), and Japan (JPEC) are now known as TriPEC and include, as of 1993, more than 100 excipient and pharmaceutical firms (3).

PREFORMULATION

The objective of preformulation studies is to develop a portfolio of information about the drug substance to serve as a set of parameters against which detailed formulation design can be carried out. Preformulation investigations are designed to identify those physicochemical properties of drug substances and excipients that may influence the formulation design, method of manufacture, and pharmacokinetic-biopharmaceutical properties of the resulting product.

Following is a generalized preformulation protocol appropriate for tablet dosage forms. For certain tests, it is assumed that the drug substance is multisourced (a previously new chemical entity whose patent has expired and which is available to the generic market) for which a USP monograph exists.

Identity and Purity

The study of any drug substance must start with the determination of identity and purity. Such tests are necessary to identify degradents and contaminants and may include organoleptic tests for color, odor, and taste. Purity tests can be found in the USP for almost all marketed compounds. Alternative methods can be employed only if they are validated against the USP procedure. Tests other than potency, which can help to identify or determine the purity of compounds, are melting point, specific rotation, pH, heavy metals, residue on ignition, etc. Impurities can occasionally affect stability, and metal contamination can catalyze chemical reactions. Impurities can also alter the color of drug substances. Techniques can be utilized to give a quantitative estimate of impurities such as the impurity index (II) and the homogeneity index (HI). An ordinary impurity test can be found in the USP that estimates impurities by thin-layer chromatography (TLC).

Crystal Properties and Polymorphism

Many drug substances appear in more than one polymorphic form. The form is determined by certain conditions during the crystallization step. Occasionally drug substances are precipitated in such a way that molecules do not organize themselves in any set pattern, resulting in an amorphous powder. It is also possible for solids to entrap solvents stoichiometrically to form solvates.

Even though they are chemically identical, the different polymorphic forms of a compound are associated with different free energies, and, therefore, have different physical properties that can impact significantly on product performance (4). These include differences in solubility and dissolution rate (affecting bioavailability), solid-state stability (affecting potency), deformation characteristics (affecting compactibility), and particle size and shape (affecting powder density and flow properties). The form with the lowest energy is more stable than the others. Although the other polymorphs are thus energetically unfavored, if kept dry, they may persist indefinitely and are called "metastable." A metastable form may be preferred, particularly for its ability to dissolve more rapidly.

Polymorphic transformation can take place during pharmaceutical processing, such as particle size reduction, wet granulation, drying, and even during the compaction process (5). Tests employed to determine crystal properties include differential thermal analysis (DTA), differential scanning calorimetry (DSC), and X-ray diffraction (4). See also the article Thermal Analysis of Drugs and Drug Products by D. Giron in this encyclopedia.

Particle Size, Shape, and Surface Area

Probably no characteristics of a drug substance are more important than particle characteristics in determining its performance in a formulation. This is particularly true in those cases where the drug is a poorly soluble nonelectrolyte or a free acid form with poor solubility at low pH values. Such drugs are likely to exhibit dissolution-rate-limited absorption, and if dissolution does not take place rapidly enough, a therapeutic concentration in the body fluids may never be achieved, the peak plasma concentration may be significantly delayed, or much of the drug may bypass that region of the gastrointestinal (GI) tract where absorption is best. Particle size reduction (e.g., micronization) is often utilized to enhance dissolution rate. Small particles present a larger surface area per unit weight to the dissolution media and hence dissolve more rapidly than large particles. Particle size and surface area are two of the most important properties determining the solubility rate of a drug and thus potentially its bioavailability. There are numerous examples of bioavailability problems and bioinequivalence due to the inappropriate particle size of the drug substance.

Particle size and shape also play an extremely important role in the homogeneity of powder blends and the unblending of powders in a mixer. Segregation in handling or during the compaction process has a significant effect on the content uniformity of the finished products. Particle size can also affect the stability of a drug substance in that it governs the surface area available for oxidation and hydrolysis. Surface area is critical for interaction with excipients in tablet dosage forms and can greatly affect stability. Methods to determine particle size and shape include light microscopy, scanning electron microscopy, sieve analysis, and various electronic sensing-zone particle counters. Methods available for surface area measurement include air permeability and various gas adsorption techniques.

Bulk Powder Properties

Bulk powder properties are extremely important in pharmaceutical processing (6). Knowledge of the true and bulk densities of the drug substance as well as of the excipients is extremely useful in

- Providing perspective as to the size of the final tablet and the size and type of processing equipment needed,
- Anticipating problems in the physical mixing of powders and the homogeneity of intermediate and final products because significant differences in true densities can result in segregation,
- Anticipating problems in flow properties, since that property is affected by density, and
- Identifying differences in different lots and raw materials from different suppliers because different polymorphic forms can be expected to exhibit different true densities.

A comparison of true particle density, apparent particle density, and bulk density can provide information on total porosity, interparticle porosity, and intraparticle porosity. Methods include true particle density measurements via helium pycnometry, mercury intrusion porosimetry, and poured and tapped bulk density.

The influence of sorbed moisture on chemical stability and the flow and compaction of powders and granulations is well established. The moisture content and hygroscopicity of excipients is particularly important as total product processing as well as finished product stability can be affected. Hygroscopicity, moisture-sorption isotherms, and equilibrium moisture content can be determined by thermogravimetric analysis and Karl Fisher titration methods.

The compactibility of relatively large-dose drug substances and formulations is another important property. Compactibility is of less concern for smaller-dose drugs for which direct compression fillers may be able to compensate for a lack of ability to form mechanically strong compacts. An instrumented tablet press (7) or compaction simulator (8) may be used to assess the relationship between the mechanical strength of the compact and the force (or pressure) employed to form the tablet. This relationship is the easiest of all compaction measurements to establish and provides important information on the ability of the material to form practical compacts. Measures of compact mechanical strength include hardness (or crushing force), tensile strength, and friability. Other more complex studies, more easily and perhaps best done using a compaction simulator, include measurement of the work or energy of compaction, pressure–density (Athy–Heckel) analysis, strain-rate sensitivity, and elastic recovery (9).

The Athy–Heckel analysis can provide information on deformation mechanism and give an estimate of the mean yield pressure of the material (10). A comparison of yield pressures determined at different punch speeds can give information on the strain-rate sensitivity of the material (11). If the major components of the formulation (including the drug) are strain-rate sensitive, the tablets produced on a high-speed production press may exhibit lamination or capping. Excessive elastic recovery may also indicate such tablet failure. The Hiestand indices (bonding and brittle fracture) may be used to assess the compactibility of materials under laboratory conditions (12).

For the evaluation of flow properties the following test methods may be used:

- Angle of repose
- Minimum orifice diameter,
- Carr index,
- Flow rate, and
- Direct observation of weight variation during tableting runs.

The ultimate goal of flow analysis is to identify the powder or powder blend that provides the least weight variation in the finished tablet. The more fluid the powder is, the more efficiently and reproducibly it should fill the die cavities of a tablet press. This more efficient and reproducible die fill should be reflected in increased tablet weights and reduced intertablet weight variation (13).

Solubility and Permeability

In many cases, the rate of dissolution in gastrointestinal fluids is the rate-limiting step in absorption. The bioequivalence requirements established by the FDA define low solubility as "... <5 mg/mL in water, and slow dissolution rate to be <50% in 30 minutes" (14). However, the solubility of a drug should be considered together with its dose; that is, even a very poorly soluble drug having a sufficiently small therapeutic dose may completely dissolve under physiological conditions. Thus, Amidon et al. (15) have defined a "high solubility" drug as one which at the highest human dose is soluble in 250 ml (or less) water throughout the physiological pH range (1–8) at 37°C. A "low solubility" drug is thus one which requires more than 250 ml of water to dissolve the largest human dose at any pH within the physiological range. The likelihood of having bioavailability problems requires both a consideration of the dose and a solubility volume of the drug and its permeability. Amidon et al. (15) created a Biopharmaceutics Drug Classification System (BCS) based on estimates of these two parameters:

1. Class I: High solubility and high permeability
2. Class II: Low solubility and high permeability
3. Class III: High solubility and low permeability
4. Class IV: Low solubility and low permeability

A jejunal permeability of at least $2–4 \times 10^{-4}$ cm/s, measured in humans by an intubation technique, is considered "high permeability." For many substances, this permeability corresponds to a fraction absorbed of 90% or better. The classification system provides a logical basis for estimating the risk of bioavailability problems. For example, Class I drugs (e.g., propranolol HCl, metoprolol tartrate) are expected to exhibit few bioavailability problems. On the other hand, Class II drugs (e.g., piroxicam) are more likely to exhibit dissolution-rate-limited absorption problems. Class III drugs (e.g., atenolol) are more likely to be prone to absorption (permeability) rate-limited absorption. Class IV drugs (low solubility–low permeability) present formidable obstacles to bioavailability. An in vitro–in vivo correlation (IVIVC) is expected only in the case of Class II drugs. An *IVIVC* could be expected for Class I drugs if the dissolution rate is slower than the gastric emptying the rate. With a sufficiently rapidly dissolving Class I drug, little or no *IVIVC* is expected because gastric emptying (not dissolution) would be the rate limiting step. Little or no *IVIVC* is expected for Class III or Class IV drugs.

The FDA has adopted the BCS in developing a guidance that provides relaxed policies on scale-up and postapproval changes of immediate-release oral solid dosage forms (SUPAC-IR). For certain changes, requirements depend on the drug class, with the most liberal policies for Class I drugs, less liberal policies for Classes II and III drugs, and the least liberal policies for Class IV drugs. First issued as a draft on Nov. 29, 1994 for comment (16, 17), a revised version was published in the *Federal Register* on Nov. 30, 1995.

The intrinsic dissolution rate (IDR) of drugs is frequently measured in preformulation tests by the rotating disk method or Wood's apparatus (18). An automated IDR system, based on a modification of a standard dissolution apparatus, allows for attachment to the stirrer of a die in which the pure drug has been compressed with the tablet face flush with the bottom surface of the die (19). The IDR may be used to detect different polymorphs as well as to judge the risk of a drug exhibiting dissolution-rate-limited absorption. Kaplan (20) suggested that an IDR of higher than 1 mg $\text{cm}^{-2}\text{min}^{-1}$ indicated that dissolution-related absorption problems were unlikely, whereas an IDR lower than 0.1 mg $\text{cm}^{-2}\text{min}^{-1}$ indicated dissolution-rate-limited absorption.

Drug-Excipient Compatibility Studies

A knowledge of the interaction of drugs and excipients is essential in the initial formulation of a product. It may also be necessary later on during processing scale-up, when problems arise, to determine if incompatibilities exist which affect manufacturing or stability. Drug-excipient interactions are often directly related to the moisture present in one or another of the components or to the humidity to which the formulation is exposed during processing or storage. These studies are always carried out at accelerated temperature and humidity conditions, even though it must be recognized that some interactions are physical (melting and volatilization) and not chemical and that accelerated aging may not be predictive. Tests for excipient-drug interactions are usually conducted on blends of the pure drug and excipient in ratios similar to those in the final dosage form. For example, excipient-to-drug ratios are higher for filler-binders than for lubricants and disintegrating agents. These studies are often performed with the help of a factorial or fractional-factorial experimental design (21). Powders are physically mixed and may be granulated or compacted to accelerate any possible interaction. Samples can be exposed in open pans or sealed in bottles or vials to mimic product packaging. Evaluation of samples includes

1. Visual inspection for changes in color or texture.
2. Both HPLC and TLC are commonly employed with unstressed samples being used as controls. In general, only qualitative results are important initially.
3. Differential thermal analysis is applied and the appearance or disappearance of one or more peaks is noted. Isothermal microcalorimetry can also be employed as well as a thermal activity monitor (TAM) technique.

Compatibility studies are essential in characterizing both raw materials and finished formulations. It has been argued that binary drug-excipient screening studies are inefficient, unrealistic, and ignore processing variables. A better approach may be to carefully select potential excipients based on known chemistry and published compatibility data, and perform miniformulation stability studies (22).

Formulation Design

Based on the preformulation information, decisions can be made regarding formulation design and process strategy. Initial guidance may be provided by the proposed dose. Relatively low-dose drugs can often be tableted by direct compression, a term that is applied to the process by which tablets are compressed directly from blends of the active

ingredient and suitable excipients. No wet or dry granulation is required, although the drug may occasionally be sprayed out of solution onto one of the excipients to ensure uniform dispersion of drug in very low dosage. Larger doses of poorly compactible drugs may be granulated prior to tableting. The process steps required and the choice of excipients are often governed by other properties of the drug.

Analysis of Critical Variables and Formulation Development

Based on the analysis of the preformulation data, likely excipients are selected and small batches may be produced. The number and size of the batches depend on the availability of the drug substance. The batches are intended to assess the feasibility of the formulation, including the types and levels of excipients, as well as the process and its operational variables, such as order of addition, mixing times, compression force, granulation time, etc. The goal is to develop a formulation and process that meets the criteria set forth earlier under Objectives.

MANUFACTURE

Traditionally, tablets have been made by granulation, a process that imparts two primary requisites to formulations: compactibility and fluidity. Both wet granulation and dry granulation (slugging or roll compaction) are used (Table 1). Regardless of whether tablets are made by direct compression or granulation, the first steps, milling and mixing, are the same; the subsequent steps differ.

The wet massing of powders is typically carried out in high-shear mixers prior to wet screening. The wet granules are often dried in fluidized-bed equipment, enhancing the efficiency of the process. Alternatively, wet granulation may be carried out in fluid-bed drier-granulators in which the liquid phase is sprayed onto fluidized powders while the hot air flow dries the granules. This process reduces the number of handling steps and the time and space needed for granulation; it can be automated. The advantages and disadvantages of wet granulation are given in Table 2. See also Granulations by H.G. Kristensen and T. Schaeffer, Vol. 7 (1st Ed.), pp. 121–160, of this encyclopedia.

Regardless of the granulation method, the comparative simplicity of the direct compression process offers obvious advantages, such as

1. Economy
2. Elimination of heat and moisture

Table 1 Typical unit operations involved in wet granulation, dry granulation, and direct compression

Wet granulation	Dry granulation	Direct compression
Milling and mixing of drugs and excipients	Milling and mixing of drugs and excipients	Milling and mixing of drugs and excipients
Preparation of binder solution	Compression into slugs or roll compaction	Compression of tablets
Wet massing by addition of binder solution or granulating solvent	Milling and screening of slugs and compacted powder	
Screening of wet mass	Mixing with lubricant and disintegrant	
Drying of the wet granules	Compression of tablets	
Screening of the dry granules		
Blending with lubricants and disintegrant to produce "running powder"		
Compression of tablets		

3. Optimization of tablet disintegration
4. Stability

The most obvious advantage of direct compression is its greater economy, owing to reduced processing time, less equipment and space required, less process validation, and lower energy utilization. Generally, only blending and compression are required, although prior micronization of the drug may be needed. Unlike wet granulation, processing does not require heat or moisture, which can be detrimental to drug stability. Moreover, direct compression avoids the high pressures associated with slugging or roll compaction. In addition, disintegration is optimized because directly compressed tablets produce primary particles upon disintegration, rather than granules, which must deaggregate to liberate primary particles. Finally, direct compression tablets often exhibit fewer long-term problems of chemical stability or changes in dissolution.

Although there are many significant advantages of direct compression over granulation, there also are important limitations:

1. Uniform blending and prevention of unblending of low-dose drugs
2. Fillers often are costlier than fillers used in granulation
3. Physical properties and functional specifications are more critical; properties of raw materials must be defined and carefully controlled
4. Limitations in producing colored tablets
5. Dust problems
6. Limitations in the dilution capacity of fillet-binders
7. More sensitive to lubricant softening and overmixing than granulations

Limitations in the dilution capacity of excipients can make the direct compression of large-dose, poorly compactible drugs impractical. Lubrication is often

Table 2 Advantages and disadvantages of wet granulation

Advantages	Disadvantages
Enhances fluidity and compactibility. suitable for high-dose drugs with poor flow and/or compactibility	Each unit process brings its own set of complications
Reduces air entrapment	The large number of unit processes increases the chances of problems
Reduces dustiness	Difficult to control and validate
Provides for the addition of a liquid phase (wet granulation) suited to dispersion of low-dose drugs in solution to ensure content uniformity	Potential adverse effects of temperature, time, and rate of drying on drug stability and distribution during drying
Enhances wettability of powders through hydrophilization (wet granulation)	Overall more costly than direct compression in terms of space, time, and equipment requirements
Permits handling of powders without loss of blend quality	

a compromise between the amount and type needed for adequate lubrication and their adverse effect on compactibility. Content uniformity is of greater concern in direct compression tableting, particularly with low-dose drugs. Since the drug is not "locked" into granules, direct compression blends are subject to unmixing in subsequent processing steps. In addition, drugs are often micronized prior to blending to enhance their dissolution rate, and the resulting high surface-to-mass ratios may lead to difficulty in flowing and mixing due to surface interactions. Another important limitation is that unlike granulation, which tends to compensate for variability in excipients, direct compression is heavily dependent upon reproducible properties of the excipients (and the drug). Raw material standards must be carefully defined and address functionality. Lot-to-lot variations in both the drug and the excipients must be avoided. The cost of raw materials and their testing is higher in direct compression.

Thus, direct-compression tableting requires careful attention to the choice of excipients, appropriate flow properties, and blend homogeneity, and to the interplay of formulation and process variables that can affect both compactibility and drug dissolution. See also Direct Compression Tableting by R.F. Shangraw, Vol.4, (1st Ed.) pp. 85–106, of this encyclopedia.

Excipients

The design of the formulation and selection of excipients is especially critical in tablet dosage forms. Products can vary from a relatively simple aspirin tablet containing aspirin and starch to more complex systems that might contain fillers, binders, disintegrating agents, glidants, lubricants, and coating agents. Modified release introduces even more complexity. The appropriate selection of excipients and their concentration are clearly critical to both the ability to manufacture tablets as well as to their performance as a drug delivery system. Since others have illuminated the various excipient classes in great detail, references are provided in Table 3.

Manufacturability

Excipients function to provide compactibility, lubrication, flow properties, disintegration efficiency, wetting, etc. Poor choice of excipients may give rise to poor characteristics (hardness, appearance), which can be important in packaging, storage, and patient acceptance. Problems with excipients may arise from variations in source or lot, particularly in formulations made by direct compression. Examples of excipient problems include variation in performance between Hoc cellulose and microcrystalline cellulose relative to particle size, flow, and compactibility,

or different polymorphic forms of sorbitol (α, β and γ) resulting in tablet hardening. Differences in lactose particle size and modification (spray-dried or anhydrous) can provide differences in surface areas over which a lubricant is distributed. Anhydrous lactose hydrates at high humidities with increase in size.

Biopharmaceutics

The formulation of a tablet can affect its bioavailability. Particular care should be given to low-dose poorly soluble drugs, especially those that are micronized. Drugs with low water solubility should never be formulated solely with insoluble fillers, including calcium salts (calcium sulfate, calcium phosphate) which are only soluble at very low pH. Differences in solution rate between hydrated and nonhydrated forms of calcium salts as well as between dibasic and tribasic forms may also be important. In some cases, excipients complex with drug substances such as calcium salts with tetracycline. Varying the ratio of soluble to insoluble fillers in tablets can significantly alter the dissolution pattern of poorly soluble drugs (weak acids and nonelectrolytes), but has little effect on weak bases, which are soluble in gastric fluids.

The type and amount of disintegrating agent can also be important. Differences in source (corn, potato, rice) as well as variations in amylopectin–amylose ratios result in variable disintegration times. The fact that starch included within granules is not as effective as starch added between granules has led to tablets with good disintegration but poor dissolution. Incorporation of super-disintegrants (crospovidone, croscarmellose, sodium starch glycolate) has improved dissolution from both direct-compression and wet-granulation formulations. Both croscarmellose and sodium starch glycolate can complex with small amounts of cationic drugs in water, but not in physiologic fluids (23).

The type and amount of binder used in granulations affects dissolution rates. Many binders are hydrophilic polymers whose solubility and solubility rate depend upon molecular weight. Quality control tests such as viscosity may be necessary as part of raw material testing of polymeric substances. However, an advantage of the granulation process is that it results in a wetting of drug surfaces, which enhances drug dissolution once the granules have disintegrated. Wetting agents such as sodium lauryl sulfate can significantly improve the dissolution of drugs of poor water solubility formulated into direct compression tablets.

Perhaps the greatest source of concern in excipients is with lubricants, particularly magnesium stearate, which is not only hydrophobic but also has a laminar crystal structure. When blended with other ingredients, it tends to

Table 3 Excipients literature

Excipient class	References (1st Ed.)
General	Rudnic, E.; Kottke, M. Tablet Dosage Forms. In *Modern Pharmaceutics*, 3rd Ed.; Banker, G., Rhodes, C., (Eds.); Marcel Dekker, Inc.: New York, 1996; 333.
Diluents and fillers	Czeisler, J.; Perlman, K. *Encyclopedia of Pharmaceutical Technology*; Swarbrick, J., Boylan, J., (Eds.); Marcel Dekker, Inc.: New York, 1991; Vol. 4, 37.
Binders	Kristensen, H. *Encyclopedia of Pharmaceutical Technology*; Swarbrick, J., Boylan, J., (Eds.); Marcel Dekker, Inc.: New York,1988; Vol. 1, 415.
Disintegrants	Shangraw, R.; Mitrevej, A.; Shah, M. Pharm. Tech. 1980; *4* (10), 49. Augsburger, L.L.; Brzeczko, A.W.; Shah, U.; Hahm, H. Encyclo of Pharm *Technology*; Swarbrick, J., Boylan, J., (Eds.); Marcel Dekker, Inc.: New York, 2001;. Vol. 20, Suppl. 3.
Lubricants and glidants	Zanowiak, P. *Encyclopedia of Pharmaceutical Technology*; Swarbrick, J., Boylan, J., (Eds.); Marcel Dekker, Inc.: New York, 1994; Vol. 9, 87.
Film coating agents	Radebaugh, G. *Encyclopedia of Pharmaceutical Technology*; Swarbrick, J., Boylan, J., (Eds.); Marcel Dekker, Inc.: New York, 1993; Vol. 6, 1.
Controlled-release agents	Chien, Y. *Encyclopedia of Pharmaceutical Technology*; Swarbrick, J., Boylan, J., (Eds.); Marcel Dekker, Inc.: New York, 1990; Vol. 3, 281.
Coloring agents	Woznicki, E.; Schoneker, D. *Encyclopedia of Pharmaceutical Technology*; Swarbrick, J., Boylan, J., (Eds.); Marcel Dekker, Inc.: New York, 1990; Vol. 3, 65.
Flavor modifiers	Adjei, A., et al. *Encyclopedia of Pharmaceutical Technology*; Swarbrick, J., Boylan, J., (Eds.); Marcel Dekker, Inc.: New York, 1993, Vol. 6, 101.

make them hydrophobic by delaminating to coat their surfaces. The problems with magnesium stearate are thus highly process dependent. For example, blending time differences of as little as 2 min can significantly alter the dissolution pattern of finished tablets. Because direct-compression formulations have a higher specific surface area, the same amount of magnesium stearate blended for the same length of time makes direct-compression tablet matrices more hydrophobic than matrices made from granulations. The degree of shear imparted by different mixers during processing significantly affects the distribution of magnesium stearate (24). The characteristics of magnesium stearate vary from supplier to supplier and sometime within the same supplier (25). It is essential to draft raw material specifications and strictly adhere to Standard Operating Procedures (SOPs) during the manufacture of products containing this lubricant. Establishing purchasing specifications beyond those listed in the *National Formulary*, such as bulk and tap density, powder fluidity, particle size, surface area, degree of hydration, and morphology is desirable.

THE EFFECTS OF MANUFACTURING PROCESSES ON FORMULATIONS

Numerous unit processes are involved in making tablets, including particle size reduction and sizing, blending, granulating, drying, compaction, and (frequently) coating. Various factors associated with these processes can seriously affect content uniformity, bioavailability, or stability. Some of these are given in the following list:

1. Particle Size Reduction
   —Nonuniform particle size can lead to segregation problems
   —Development of electrostatic forces inhibits complete blending
   —Changing the crystalline state can affect solubility
2. Blending
   —Nonhomogeneous distribution of drug substance is the result of poor blending or unblending
   —Overblending of lubricant lowers dissolution rates and affects compactibility
3. Granulation
   —Nonhomogeneous distribution of binder and drug substance gives drug-rich or drug-poor fines
   —Decomposition of drug substance due to residual moisture
   —Uneven granule size (too many or to few fines) leads to compaction or uniformity problems
4. Tableting
   —Uneven compaction pressures affect dissolution
   —Loss of mix quality in hopper and feed frame gives poor content uniformity
   —Additional shearing of lubricant in feed frame lowers dissolution rates

5. Coating
  —Nonuniform or incomplete coverage of tablets and beads results in different dissolution patterns

When validating new equipment or procedures, the sampling techniques must reflect the quality of the material being tested, the blend of powders, moisture in granulation, or coating integrity.

Another potential source of problems in manufacturing is reprocessing or reworking. Reworking may be required when finished products fail to meet hardness, content uniformity, disintegration, dissolution, or appearance specifications. Reworking procedures must be in writing and are often part of New Drug Applications (NDAs) and Abbreviated New Drug Applications (ANDAs). Although practiced less today than in past years, given the high cost of some drug substances, reworking continues to be justified, but may involve the following problems: overdistribution of lubricant leading to poor compactibility and dissolution; distribution of particles of coating in the reprocessed tablet may lower the dissolution rate; and loss in compactibility due to work hardening of direct-compression fillers, particularly at higher initial compaction pressures. Reworking is less likely to cause dissolution problems with water-soluble drugs.

SYSTEMATIC FORMULATION DEVELOPMENT

Previously, pharmaceutical experimenters were rarely afforded the luxury of using expanded experimental designs. Time and manpower constraints, imposed by an ever-quickening pace to market, have prevented the thorough examination and full understanding of most commercial formulations. Although the pace of formulating pharmaceutical systems has not lessened recently, a rapid turnaround means formulators must quickly gather information and base final decisions on that information. The window for error is narrower, and the formulator can no longer afford to use empirically gathered data to obtain the critical dosage form information needed for a marketable formulation. Systematic development approaches are also desirable to provide data in anticipation of the use of SUPAC (scale up and postapproval changes) regulatory policies by providing for the establishment of a research database that can help justify such changes to regulatory agencies.

Enormous progress has been made in the direction of systematic formulation development through the use of such statistical tools as multivariate analysis and response surface methodology, and artificial intelligence.

Experimental Design

In the long term, an efficient experimental design saves time and avoids costly mistakes, and some pharmaceutical firms have departments devoted to the preparation of experimental designs and their analysis. If a statistician is not available, a myriad of commercial experimental-design software packages are on the market (SAS, JMP, STATGRAPHICS, DESIGN EXPERT) with which a formulator can design experiments on a personal computer. These same packages can also aid in data analysis and presentation.

The early phase of such a statistical experimental design approach may include screening designs such as two-level full or fractional factorial designs or Plackett-Burman designs. The number of experimental runs is reduced by intentionally confounding some experimental effects. Ultimately, the screening design narrows the number of potential variables for further study.

The latter phase of such as a central experimental design approach might include response surface methodologies to optimize a formulation such as a central composite or Box-Behnken design. Such methods allow experimenters to assess the effects of several variables at one time without having to study every possible unique combination of variables. This way, a systematic identification of critical variables and an optimization of the formulation and process can be obtained. Response surfaces are generated, which give formulators a graphic demonstration of the effect of variables on various responses, such as drug dissolution. The designs and models available to experimenters are numerous and the proper choice depends on the number of variables and the possible responses. General references for experimental design can be consulted as well as design software manuals, if a statistician is not available for advice.

Artificial Intelligence Approaches

Among the artificial intelligence approaches that have been used to provide support for the formulation process are expert systems and artificial neural networks. An expert system (ES) is an intelligent computer program that attempts to capture the expertise of specialists who have knowledge and experience in a well-defined domain. They are designed to simulate an expert's problem solving process. Developed more than 20 years ago for other applications, expert systems are a relatively new idea in pharmaceutical technology. In rule-based systems, the knowledge is highly structured and often represented as a set of rules that express the relationship between several pieces of information in the form of conditional statements. These statements specify actions to be taken or advice to be followed. Such systems can shorten development time, simplify formulations, provide the rationale for decisions taken in arriving at a formulation, serve as excellent teaching tools for novices, and accumulate and preserve the knowledge and experience of experts. ESs suffer from the limitation that they are not creative. They can only deal with situations that have been anticipated. They must be designed to handle every contingency. Examples include expert systems developed for formulating tablets (26), for process troubleshooting (27), and for the selection of a mixer (28).

Used in other disciplines for about 40 years, artificial neural networks (ANNs), like ESs, have only recently been applied to pharmaceutical development. ANNs are computer-based programs that attempt to simulate certain functions of the biological brain, such as learning, generalizing, or abstracting from experience. They have the ability to discern relationships or patterns in response to exposure to facts ("learning."). ANN models may be viewed simply as multiple nonlinear regression models. Through ANNs, the data and information generated during experimental work may be transformed relatively easily into knowledge that would enable the formulator to at least construct a few domain specific rules, even though confined, for future cases. However, ANN effectiveness is limited by the training data selected. One limitation is that, in most cases, ANNs lack explanation capability and there is difficulty in obtaining justification for results. Examples of applications to product development include predicting model granulation and tablet characteristics from knowledge of material and process variables (29), and predicting drug release from immediate release formulations (30). The development of a hybrid system, i.e. an Expert Network, that integrates ANNs and ESs has the potential of taking advantage of the strengths of both ANNs and ESs and avoiding the weaknesses of either (31, 32).

Formulation Development

Whether working in a large established laboratory or a small research organization, formulators are well advised to take an overall look at the development process to assess the most rational approach to their particular needs and resources. Among many approaches to rational tablet formulation, the strategy used by researchers at the

University of Maryland in collaboration with FDA scientists (33) examines the drug product development process in light of the SUPAC guidance.

This generalized plan focuses on the assessment the possible influence of formulation and processing variables on bioavailability and manufacture. The research protocol is best visualized by the flow chart in Fig. 1. The model begins with the preformulation stage wherein information is obtained on the physico-chemical and biopharmaceutic properties of the drug. One outcome of the preformulation study should be the identification of the biopharmaceutic class (BCS) in which the drug falls since this will provide important guidance in making formulation decisions. For multi-sourced drugs, the different sources are considered. The preformulation study results in a portfolio of information, which provides guidance in formulation design and in the development of appropriate hypotheses to be tested and the critical variables studies that follow.

In the critical variables analysis phase, a statistical experimental design is created (e.g., factorial, Box–Behnken) intended to assess critical formulation and process variables in relatively small-scale manufacture. In these studies, the ranges of composition variables are chosen to at least encompass those noted in the recommendations of the AAPS–FDA Workshop on Scale-up of

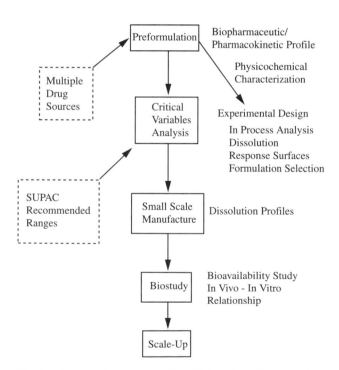

Fig. 1 A research model used in a University of Maryland and FDA collaborative research program. (From Ref. 33.)

Immediate Release Oral Solid Dosage Forms or SUPAC. This phase is usually preceded by a development phase during which variables and levels to be studied are determined and the exact method of manufacture is established. Experimental formulations are assessed at least in terms of dissolution performance, content uniformity, and weight variation. On the basis of these studies, the specific formulations to be manufactured for biostudy are selected.

In the small-scale clinical manufacturing phase, formulations are manufactured under GMP conditions for possible clinical testing. These will be manufactured on a larger scale than those in the previous phases. An experimental design is chosen; however, if some of the variables can be eliminated based on the earlier experiments, the number of formulations produced may be reduced.

The intent of the biostudy phase is to establish an in vitro–in vivo relationship. If an appropriate correlation can be established, dissolution may serve as a surrogate for biostudies in the interpretation of what is significant and what is not among the variables studied.

In the scale-up phase, larger runs of formulations are manufactured. The formulations are selected to determine if the larger scale will enhance the significance of certain variables.

The statistical analysis of the data provides the opportunity to predict changes in dissolution performance resulting from incremental changes in one or more formulation or process variable at a time (e.g., the level of an excipient or the time of mixing).

The development model presented here may differ from some formulation research programs in that biostudies may not be performed on small-scale batches. The major advantage of early biostudies is the potential for early IVIVC and subsequent surrogate use of dissolution testing in further work. Scale-up and pilot-plant roles in formulation changes, while not covered thoroughly here, are reviewed by Racz (34).

REFERENCES

1. Chowhan, Z.T. Excipients and Their Functionality in Drug Product Development. Pharm. Tech. **1993**, *17* (9), 72.
2. Czeisler, J.L.; Penman, K.P. Diluents, *Encyclopedia of Pharmaceutical Technology*, 1st Ed.; Swarbrick, J., Boylan, J.C., Eds.; Marcel Dekker, Inc.: New York, 1991; 4, 40–43.
3. Blecher, L.; Ohmae, T.; deJong, H.J. Tri-PEC: Reports from IPEC-Americas, JPEC, and IPEC-Europe. Pharm. Tech. **1994**, *18* (8), 53.
4. Raleblian, J.; McCrone, W.J. Pharmaceutical Applications of Polymorphism. Pharm. Sci. **1969**, *58*, 911.
5. Matsumoto, T.; Nobuyoshi, K.; Iliguchi, S.; Otsuka, M.J. Effect of Temperature and Pressure During Compression on Polymorphic Transformation and Crushing Strength of Chlorpropamide Tablets. Pharm. Pharmacol. **1991**, *43*, 74.
6. Brittain, H.G. Raw Materials. Drug Devel. Ind. Pharm. **1989**, *15*, 2083.
7. Schwatz, J.B. The Instrumented Tablet Press: Uses in Research and Production. Pharm. Tech. **1981**, *5* (9), 102.
8. Hunter, B.M.; Fisher, D.G.; Pratt, R.W.; Rowe, R.C. A High Speed Compression Simulator. J. Pharm. Pharmacol. **1976**, *28*, 65.
9. Maganti, L.; Celik, M. Compaction Studies on Pellets I. Uncoated Pellets. Int. J. Pharm. **1993**, *95*, 29.
10. Muller, F.X.; Augsburger, L.L. The Role of the Displacement-Time Waveform in the Determination of Heckel Behavior Under Dynamic Conditions in a Compaction Simulator and a Fully Instrumented Rotary Tablet Machine. J. Pharm. Pharmacol. **1994**, *46*, 468.
11. Roberts, R.J.; Rowe, R.C. The Effect of Punch-Velocity on the Compaction of a Variety of Materials. J. Pharm. Pharmacol. **1985**, *37*, 377.
12. Hiestand, E.; Smith, D.P. Indices of Tableting Performance. Powder Tech. **1984**, *38*, 145.
13. Augsburger, L.L.; Shangraw, R.F. Effect of Glidants in Tableting. J. Pharm. Sci. **1966**, *55*, 418.
14. Fed. Reg. *21CFR, Ch. 1*; (4/1/87 Ed.) Part 32; 320.
15. Amidon, G.L.; Lennernas, H.; Shah, V.P.; Crison, J.R. A Theoretical Basis for a Biopharmaceutic Drug Classification: The Correlation of In Vitro Drug Product Dissolution and In Vivo Bioavailability. Pharm. Res. **1995**, *12*, 413.
16. INTGUIDE.1R9. *FDA Center for Drug Evaluation and Research*: Rockville, MD, 1994.
17. Lucisano, L.J.; Franz, R.M. FDA Proposed Guidance for Chemistry, Manufacturing, and Controls Changes for Immediate-Release Solid Dosage Forms: A Review and Industrial Perspective. Pharm. Tech. **1995**, *19* (5).
18. Wood, J.H.; Syarto, J.E.; Letterman, H.J. Improved Holder for Intrinsic Dissolution Rate Studies. Pharm. Sci. **1965**, *54*, 1068.
19. Koparkar, A.D.; Augsburger, L.L.; Shangraw, R.F. Intrinsic Dissolution Rates of Tablet Filler-Binders and their Influence on the Dissolution of Drugs from Tablet Formulations. Pharm. Res. **1990**, *7*, 80.
20. Kaplan, S.A. Biopharmaceutical Considerations in Drug Formulation Design and Evaluation. Drug Metab. Rev. **1972**, *1*, 15.
21. Jacobs, A.L. Determining Optimum Drug/Excipient Compatibility Through Preformulation Testing. Pharm. Manuf. **1985**, *2* (6), 43.
22. Monkhouse, D.C.; Maderich, A. Whither Compatibility Testing. Drug Devel. Ind. Pharm. **1989**, *15*, 2115.
23. Hollenbeck, R.G.; Mitrevej, K.; Fan, A. Estimation of the Extent of Drug-Excipient Interactions Involving Croscarmellose Sodium. Pharm. Sci. **1983**, *72*, 325.
24. Bolhuis, G.K.; deJong, S.W.; Lerk, C.F. The Effect of Magnesium Stearate Admixing in Different Types of Laboratory and Industrial Mixers on Tablet Crushing Strength. Drug Devel. Ind. Pharm. **1987**, *13*, 1547.
25. Danserean, R.; Peck, G.E. The Effect of the Variability in the Physical and Chemical Properties of Magnesium

Stearate on the Properties of Compressed Tablets. Drug Devel. Ind. Pharm. **1987**, *13*, 975.

26. Rowe, R.C. An Expert System for the Formulation of Tablets. DTI Manuf. Intel. Newsletr. **1993**, *14*, 13–15.

27. Murray, F.J. The Application of Expert Systems to Pharmaceutical Processing. Pharm. Tech. **1989**, *13* (3), 100–110.

28. Lai, F.K.Y. A Prototype Expert System for Selecting Pharmaceutical Powder Mixers. Pharm Tech. **1988**, *12* (8), 22–31.

29. Kesavan, J.G.; Peck, G. Pharmaceutical Granulation and Tablet Formulation Using Neural Networks. Pharm. Dev. Tech. **1996**, *1* (4), 391–404.

30. Ebube, N.K.; McCall, T.; Chen, Y.; Meyer, M.C. Relating Formulation Variables to In Vitro Dissolution Using an Artificial Neural Network. Pharm. Dev. Tech. **1997**, *2* (3), 225–232.

31. Turban, E. *Expert Systems and Applied Artificial Intelligence*; Macmillan Publishing Co.: New York, 1992.

32. Caudill, M. Expert Networks. *Neural Network PC Tools*; Academic Press: New York, 1990; 189–214.

33. Augsburger, L.L.; Shangraw, R.; Lesko, L.; Williams, R. An Approach Toward Establishing a Scientific Foundation for Interpreting Regulations and Workshop Reports on Scale-Up and Post Approval Changes. Pharm. Res. **1994**, *11* (10), S-161.

34. Racz, I. *Drug Formulation*; John Wiley & Sons: New York, 1989; 25–27.

BIBLIOGRAPHY

American Pharmaceutical Association and the Royal Pharmaceutical Society of Great Britain. *Handbook of Pharmaceutical Excipients*, 3rd Ed.; American Pharmaceutical Association and Pharmaceutical Press: Washington, 2000.

Armstrong, A.M.; James, K.C. *Understanding Experimental Design and Interpretation in Pharmaceutics*; Ellis Horwood Ltd: Chichester, UK, 1990.

Franz, R.M.; Browne, J.; Lewis, A. Experimental Design, Modeling, and Optimization Strategies for Product and Process Development, *Pharmaceutical Dosage Forms: Disperse Systems*, 2nd Ed.; Lieberman, H.L., Rieger, M., Banker, G., Eds.; Marcel Dekker, Inc.: New York, 1996; 1, 427–514.

Peck, G.E.; McCurdy, V.E.; Banker, G.S. Tablet Formulation and Design, *Pharmaceutical Dosage Forms: Tablets*, 2nd Ed.; Lieberman, H.L., Lachman, L., Schwartz, J., Eds.; Marcel Dekker, Inc.: New York, 1989; 1, 75–130.

Polderman, J. *Formulation and Preparation of Dosage Forms*; Elsevier/North-Holland: New York, 1977; 3–28.

TABLET MANUFACTURE

Norman Anthony Armstrong
Cardiff University, Cardiff, United Kingdom

INTRODUCTION

The compressed tablet is by far the most widely used dosage form, having advantages for both producer and user. However, the manufacture of tablets can be a complex process, since only a few raw materials inherently possess those properties which are necessary for the production of tablets of satisfactory quality. Hence some preliminary treatment and/or incorporation of excipients in the formulation is usually needed. Tablet manufacture is a paradox. Considerable ingenuity and formulation expertise are required to transform a mass of particles into a low porosity mass. Yet, after the tablet has been ingested, the requirement then is usually for the tablet to release its active ingredient as rapidly as possible, and further ingenuity is needed to bring this about.

Tablets are solid preparations each of which contains a single dose of one or more active ingredients. They are obtained by compressing uniform volumes of particles, and are almost always intended for oral administration.

The earliest reference to a dosage form resembling the tablet is to be found in tenth century Arabic medical literature. Drug particles were compressed between the ends of engraved ebony rods, force being applied by means of a hammer. Details of the tabletting process, as it is now known, were first published in 1843 when William Brockedon was granted British Patent 9977 for "manufacturing pills and medicinal lozenges by causing materials when in a state of granulation, dust or powder, to be made into form and solidified by pressure in dies." In this case, too, force was applied by a hammer. Potassium bicarbonate was the first pharmaceutical substance to be so treated.

The use of compressed pills, as they were then known, increased rapidly. It is likely that the term "tablet" for this dosage form was first used in the United States in the 1870s. Power-driven presses replaced Brockedon's hammer, and by 1874 there existed both rotary and excentric presses, which in their mode of operation were fundamentally similar to those in use at the present time. The tablet lent itself to mass manufacture by mechanical means, in contrast to the slower labour-intensive production of older solid dosage forms such as the pill. It is impractical for individual pharmacists to produce small quantities of tablets on a commercial scale, and this led to the concentration of pharmaceutical manufacture in relatively few industrial sites.

A monograph for Glyceryl Trinitrate Tablets was included in the British Pharmacopoeia of 1885, but no other tablet monograph appeared there until 1945. This was not due to lack of popularity of the dosage form itself, but rather the absence of suitable methods of quality control that were applicable to tablets.

The tablet did not meet with universal approval. In 1895 an editorial in the Pharmaceutical Journal in the United Kingdom described the tablet as "one of the evils suffered by legitimate pharmacy," and predicted that tablets "have had their day" (1). Notwithstanding such a prediction, the usage of tablets has continued to increase. The 2000 edition of the British Pharmacopoeia contains 320 monographs for tablets, far in excess of any other dosage form.

The tablet is the most popular dosage form because it provides advantages for all concerned in the production and consumption of medicinal products. Though the initial capital outlay for the manufacturer of tablets is considerable, they can be produced at a much higher rate than any other dosage form, tablet presses capable of producing about one million tablets per hour being available. Furthermore, the fact that the tablet is a dry dosage form promotes stability, and in general, tablets have shelf lives measured in years. They are also convenient to transport in bulk, since they contain relatively small proportions of excipients unlike, for example, oral liquids.

From the viewpoint of the pharmacist, tablets are easy to dispense, while the patient receives a concentrated and readily transportable and consumed dosage form. Furthermore, if properly prepared, tablets provide a uniformity of dosage greater than that of most other medicines, and appropriate coating can mask unpleasant tastes and improve patient acceptance.

The tablet also provides a versatile drug delivery system. Though most tablets are intended to be swallowed intact, the same basic manufacturing process, associated with appropriate formulation, provides medicines for sublingual, buccal, rectal, and vaginal administration, together with lozenges, soluble, dispersible, and effervescent tablets. In addition, techniques that can delay or otherwise modify the release of the active ingredient from the tablet are available.

Naturally tablets only possess these advantages if they are properly formulated and manufactured. A well-prepared tablet should possess the following qualities:

1. It should, within permitted limits, contain the stated dose of drug.
2. It should be sufficiently strong to withstand the stresses of manufacture, transport, and handling so as to reach the patient intact.
3. It should deliver its dose of drug at the site and at the speed required.
4. Its size, taste, and appearance should not detract from its acceptability by the patient.

TABLET COMPRESSION

All tablets are made by a process of compression. Solid, in the form of relatively small particles, is contained in a die and a compressing force of several tonnes is applied to it by means of punches. The shape of the die governs the cross-sectional shape of the tablet, and the distance between the punch tips at the point of maximum compression governs its thickness. The conformation of the tablet faces, usually flat or convex, is a reflection of those of the punches.

The tip of the lower punch moves up and down within the die, but never actually leaves it. The upper punch descends to penetrate the die and apply the compressive force. It is then withdrawn to permit ejection of the tablet, brought about by an upward movement of the lower punch.

There are two types of tablet press. The excentric press has one die and one pair of punches. The rotary press has a larger number of dies which are fitted, with their corresponding punches, into a rotating turret.

Irrespective of the type of press that is used, the process of tablet compression can be divided into three stages, as shown in Fig. 1.

Stage 1, Filling

The lower punch falls within the die, leaving a cavity into which particulate matter flows under the influence of gravity from a hopper. Though tablets are usually described in terms of weight, the die is filled by a volumetric process. The volume is determined by the depth to which the lower punch descends in the die. Unless this volume is filled reproducibly on each occasion, then

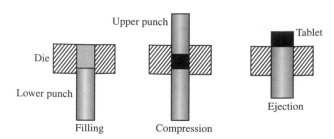

Fig. 1 Cycle of operations of an excentric tablet press.

the mass of the tablet will vary, and with it the drug content of each tablet. Therefore, uniform filling is essential. However, it must be borne in mind that the die cavity has a cross-section of only a few millimetres, and only a fraction of a second is available for filling each die. It therefore follows that the particles must flow easily and reproducibly.

Stage 2, Compression

The upper punch descends, and its tip enters the die, confining the particles. The distance separating the punch faces decreases, either by movement of the upper punch alone (as in excentric presses) or by movement of both punches (as happens in rotary presses). The porosity of the contents of the die is progressively reduced, and the particles are forced into ever-closer proximity to each other. This process is facilitated by the particles fragmenting and/or deforming. Once the particles are close enough together, interparticulate forces then cause the individual particles to aggregate, forming a tablet. The magnitude of the force is governed by the minimum distance separating the punch faces. Therefore, a second essential property of the particles is that they cohere under the influence of a compressive force. It is also essential that this coherence be maintained when the compressing force is removed.

Stage 3, Ejection

The upper punch is withdrawn from the die, and so the force being applied to the tablet is removed. The effect of this might be to cause the deformed particles to return to their former shape, which would result in a decrease in interparticulate contact and hence tablet strength. It is essential that this does not occur. As the upper punch leaves the die, the lower punch moves upwards, pushing the tablet before it. During the compression stage, the particles are forced into intimate contact with the interior die wall. It follows that attempts to remove the tablet will be opposed by frictional forces and so successful ejection demands lack of adhesion between the tablet and the die wall.

Therefore in summary, for a particulate solid to be successfully transformed into tablets, three key properties need to be present:

1. Good particle flow.
2. The ability of the particles to cohere under the influence of a compressing force. This coherence must be retained after the compressing force has been removed.
3. The ability of the tablet to be ejected from the die after the compressing force has been removed.

Few powders possess all these essentials and some possess none of them. Thus, before successful tabletting can take place, some preliminary treatment with the addition of one or more excipients is almost invariably needed.

METHODS OF TABLET PRODUCTION

The pretreatment that is usually necessary takes the form of granulation. The process of granulation is essentially one of size enlargement, and it serves several purposes in the tablet manufacturing process:

1. It improves flow by increasing particle size, since large particles flow more readily than small ones.
2. It improves compression characteristics, adding to the cohesive strength of the tablet.
3. Once a homogeneous mixture has been achieved, segregation is prevented, since particles that are stuck together cannot separate.
4. It reduces dust.

Both wet and dry granulation techniques are available.

Tablet Manufacture by Wet Granulation

This is the traditional method of pretreatment of solids prior to tabletting. Despite its complexity and inherent disadvantages, even now about half the tablets produced worldwide are manufactured by this process. Its essence is that particles of active ingredient, with a diluent if necessary, are stuck together using an adhesive, the latter usually being water-based. The result is a granular product which flows more readily and has an improved ability to cohere during compression.

A flow diagram of the wet granulation process together with appropriate excipients is shown in Fig. 2.

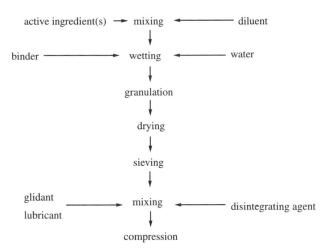

Fig. 2 The wet granulation process of tablet manufacture.

The diluent

The first stage in the wet granulation process is often a dry mixing stage in which the active component is mixed with a diluent. Many drugs need to be administered in doses of only a few milligrams or even less, yet a tablet that weighs less than about 50 mg is difficult for the patient to handle conveniently. It is therefore necessary to increase the bulk of such a tablet with a diluent. Some commonly used diluents are listed in Table 1.

The ideal diluent would be both chemically and physiologically inert, and would not interfere with the bioavailability of the active ingredient. It should also be inexpensive and be easily tabletted since, if the proportion of active ingredient is small, the overall tabletting properties of the mixture are largely governed by those of the diluent.

Lactose is by far the most frequently used diluent for solid dosage forms. An inexpensive disaccharide obtained as a by-product of the cheese industry; it is available in a number of forms, though α-Lactose monohydrate is the variety that is normally used as the diluent in tablets made by wet granulation. It is freely albeit slowly soluble in water and as such it is a suitable diluent for active ingredients of low water solubility. Lactose is a nonreducing sugar, and is reasonably inert. It can take part in the Maillard reaction when mixed with substances containing primary amine groups, giving highly colored products, and thus its use is contraindicated in such formulations (2).

Probably the second most commonly used diluent in the wet granulation process is dibasic calcium phosphate. This substance is virtually insoluble in water and hence is always used in conjunction with a disintegrating agent. Its properties have been reviewed by Carstensen and Ertell (3).

Table 1 Tablet diluents

Diluent	Comments
Calcium carbonate	Insoluble in water (Cal-Carb[R], Millicarb[R], Pharma-Carb[R], Sturcal[R])
Calcium phosphate, dibasic	Insoluble in water, good flow properties, available in dihydrate and anhydrous forms (Cyfos[R], Calstar[R], Calipharm[R], Emcompress[R])
Calcium phosphate, tribasic	Insoluble in water (Tricafos[R], Tri-Cal[R], Tri-Tab[R])
Calcium sulfate	Insoluble in water (Cal-Tab[R], Compactrol[R])
Cellulose, microcrystalline	Good compression properties, may not need lubricant, can act as disintegrant (Avicel[R], Emcocel[R], Vivacel[R])
Cellulose, microcrystalline silicified	Combination of microcrystalline cellulose and silica (Prosolv[R])
Cellulose, powdered	(Elcema[R], Solka-Floc[R])
Dextrates	(Emdex[R])
Dextrose	Hygroscopic, reducing sugar (Tabfine[R])
Fructose	(Fructofin[R])
Lactitol	(Finlac[R])
Lactose monohydrate	The most commonly used diluent. Inexpensive, takes part in Maillard reaction (Fast-Flo[R], Lactochem[R], Microtose[R], Pharmatose[R], Tablettose[R], Zeparox[R])
Magnesium carbonate	
Maltitol	(Maltisorb[R], Maltit[R])
Maltodextrin	(Glycidex[R], Lycatab[R], Maltrin[R])
Maltose	(Advantose[R])
Mannitol	Freely soluble in water, negative heat of solution and therefore cool taste, popular for chewable tablets, noncariogenic (Pearlitol[R])
Sodium chloride	Freely soluble in water, used in solution tablets
Sorbitol	
Starch	Also acts as disintegrating agent, may give soft tablets
Starch, pregelatinized	Also acts as disintegrating agent. (Lycatab[R], Pharma-Gel[R], Pre-Jel[R], Sepistab[R], Starch 1500[R], Starx 1500[R])
Sucrose	Freely soluble in water, sweet taste, hygroscopic, used in lozenges in conjunction with lactose
Sugar, compressible	(Dipac[R], Nutab[R])
Sugar, confectioner's	
Sugar spheres	(Nu-Core[R], Nu-Pareil[R])
Talc	
Xylitol	Negative heat of solution, cool taste (Xylifin[R], Xylitab[R])

Proprietary names are given in parentheses.

Mixing

The purpose of the mixing stage is to ensure that the powder blend and hence the resulting tablets are homogeneous in content. A random mixture is defined as one where the probability of sampling a given type of particle is proportional to the number of such particles in the total mixture. Thus, the aim is to produce a mixture such that when a sample is removed, the relative proportions of the components of that sample are the same as in the mixture as a whole.

Unlike molecules in a fluid, which in time will mix spontaneously by a diffusion mechanism, powder particles do not mix spontaneously but remain in their relative positions. Therefore before mixing can occur, energy must be put into the system. This causes the powder bed to dilate or expand, the particles separate from one another and this leads to relative motion among them.

It might be intuitively expected that the randomness of a mixture will progressively increase with time, but this is not always the case. Under certain conditions, an optimum mixing time occurs, beyond which the mixture shows a tendency to separate back into its components. This process is known as segregation. Segregation is particularly likely to occur in mixtures where the components differ markedly in size, with differences in shape and density as secondary factors. It is especially likely to occur if regular patterns of movement are set up in the mixing device, and for this reason, mixers are designed so that an irregular mixing motion occurs (4).

Although in general a size difference between components can lead to segregation, a situation where there is a large difference in sizes between components may be beneficial. In such circumstances, small particles of one component can become trapped in irregularities in the surface of the larger component. These are not random mixtures, as the particles of the two components cannot behave independently. This concept is called "ordered mixing" and it has found applicability in the manufacture of solid dosage forms containing small quantities of highly potent active ingredients (5) (see the article on Blenders and Blending in this encyclopedia).

Granulation

The underlying process of size enlargement in wet granulation is achieved by either one or both of two different mechanisms. Firstly, adjacent solid particles may be stuck together using an adhesive. Such substances are known as binders or granulating agents. Secondly, dissolution of the solid in the granulating liquid can occur, followed by evaporation of the liquid phase of the latter. This will result in the deposition of dissolved material on particle surfaces, forming so-called crystal bridges. The occurrence of this mechanism will depend on the solubility of the solids in the liquid phase. Thus, sucrose will form crystal bridges with an aqueous granulating fluid, whereas calcium phosphate will not.

The process and underlying mechanisms of granulation have been fully described by Sherrington and Oliver (6). Details of commonly used binders are given in Table 2. They are often natural or synthetic polymers and are usually added as aqueous solutions or dispersions. Alternatively, they can be mixed with the other solids in the formulation in the dry state, water then being added.

If the active ingredient is unstable in the presence of water, then a granulation process using nonaqueous liquids can be used. The usual granulating system in such cases is povidone dissolved in isopropanol. The extra costs and environmental problems posed by the use of a volatile and flammable liquid are disincentives to the use of nonaqueous granulation.

The traditional piece of granulating apparatus is the shear granulator. Its function is to homogeneously incorporate an adhesive and viscous liquid such as starch paste into a mass of dry powder to form agglomerates. It follows that a considerable shearing force needs to be exerted. The mixed solids are loaded into the bowl of the mixer, and the liquid added with agitation. The damp solid is then forced through a relatively coarse screen (about 1–2 mm), often by means of oscillating bars, to give discrete granules. The progression of the granulation process can be monitored by measuring the electrical power consumption by the granulator, and hence optimum granulation times can be established. Ertell et al. have shown that the size of the granulator and the mixing time can be major influences on the physical properties and dissolution rate of the resulting tablets (7).

As described above, the wet granulation process is a long and hence expensive procedure, which has been improved by the introduction of high-speed mixer granulators. These have agitator and chopping blades, which enable mixing, wet massing, and granulation to take place in the same piece of apparatus. In such devices, the granulation process takes place extremely rapidly, and hence the establishment of optimum granulation times is even more important.

A further technique is fluid-bed granulation. Air is passed into the powder bed from below. This causes the particle, of powder to form a suspension in the air and gives effective mixing. The granulating fluid is then sprayed over the particles, which adhere on collision and they are then dried in the heated air stream.

The wet granulation process, apparatus, and pharmaceutical applications have been comprehensively reviewed by Kristensen and Schaefer (8) (see the article on Tablet Granulation in this encyclopedia).

Drying

After the process of granulation, the product exists as a wet mass from which the liquid must be removed, since the presence of water leads to the impairment of flow properties, and perhaps to chemical instability. Water is usually removed by evaporation for which energy is needed. This is normally provided as heat, though microwave energy is being increasingly used for drying in tablet manufacture.

The essential constituents of an effective piece of drying equipment are a heat supply to increase the temperature and thereby reduce relative humidity, a device for removal of evaporated water and a means of minimizing the distance that water molecules must diffuse before they can be evaporated.

The fluidized bed drier is the most commonly used device for drying tablet granules. The solid is fluidized from below by a jet of hot air, and so each granule becomes separated from its neighbors. The air provides an effective means of heat transfer, as well as of removing water vapor. The speed of the drying process is governed by the distance that water molecules must diffuse before they arrive at the evaporative surface. Since the wet granules are present as individual units, the maximum distance over which diffusion occurs is equal to the radius of a granule. Hence, fluidized bed drying is a rapid process.

Table 2 Binders used in the wet granulation process

Binder	Concentration in the granulating fluid (% w/v)	Comments
Acacia mucilage	Up to 20	Yields very hard granules
Alginic acid	1–5	
Carbomer	5–10	(Carbopol^R)
Carboxymethylcellulose calcium	5–15	(Nymcel^R)
Carboxymethylcellulose sodium	5–15	(Nymcel^R)
Cellulose, microcrystalline		(Avicel^R, Emcocel^R, Vivacel^R)
Powdered cellulose		(Elcema^R, Solka Floc^R)
Ethyl cellulose	1–3	(Aquacoat^R)
Gelatin	5–20	Forms gel in cold water, therefore warm solution used, strong adhesive
Glucose, liquid	Up to 50	Strong adhesive, hygroscopic
Guar gum	1–10	
Hydroxyethyl cellulose	2–6	(Cellosize^R)
Hydroxypropyl cellulose	2–6	(Klucel^R, Methocel^R)
Hydroxypropyl cellulose—low-substituted	5–25	
Hydroxypropylmethyl cellulose	2–5	(Methocel^R, Pharmacoat^R)
Magnesium aluminum silicate	2–10	(Pharmasorb^R, Veegum^R)
Maltodextrin	2–10	(Glucidex^R, Lycatab^R, Maltrin^R)
Methylcellulose	1–5	(Celacol^R, Methocel^R)
Polydextrose		(Litesse^R)
Polyethylene oxide	5	(Polyox^R)
Povidone	0.5–5	Also known as PVP or polyvinylpyrrolidone. Soluble in water and some organic solvents, can be used for nonaqueous granulation, very commonly used, synthetic material (Kollidon^R, Plasdone^R)
Sodium alginate	1–3	(Manucol^R)
Starch paste	5–25	Very commonly used
Starch, pregelatinized	5–10	(Lycatab^R, Pharma-Gel^R, Pre-Jel^R, Sepistab^R, Starch 1500^R, Starx 1500^R)
Sucrose (syrup)	Up to 70	Hygroscopic, tablets may harden on storage
Water		Suitable for solids that are freely soluble in water

Proprietary names are given in parentheses.

The temperature of the bed can be precisely controlled, and a free-flowing product results. The resemblance to fluid-bed granulation will be apparent, and apparatus based on the fluidized bed principle is available in which mixing, granulation, and drying take place in the same chamber.

Although the apparent turbulence of the air stream may give rise to interparticulate collisions and hence attrition, this is not usually a severe problem. However, the rapid movement of particles in a hot, dry atmosphere can lead to the development of static electrical discharges. Suitable precautions must therefore be taken, especially if flammable liquids have been used in the granulation process.

A more traditional means of drying is the tray drier. Hot air flows over a series of shelves on which the wet material is spread. Compared to the fluidized bed drier, the solid–air interface is smaller, and water molecules may have to diffuse through the whole thickness of the solid layer before the evaporative surface is reached. Thinner layers give quicker evaporation, but this would reduce the overall capacity of the drier. Thus, the drying process is slower in a tray drier than in a fluidized bed drier.

As water diffuses through the bed of solid, it will carry with it any components of the formulation that are soluble in it. This will lead to a nonuniform distribution of these components in the solid. This is not usually a problem with

Table 3 Tablet glidants

Glidant	Concentration in tablet (%)	Comments
Calcium silicate	0.5–2	
Cellulose, powdered	1–2	(Elcema[R], Solka Floc[R])
Magnesium carbonate	1–3	
Magnesium oxide	1–3	
Magnesium silicate	0.5–2	
Silicon dioxide, colloidal	0.05–0.5	Excellent glidant (Aerosil[R], Cab-o-Sil[R])
Starch	2–10	
Talc	1–10	Insoluble in water but not hydrophobic

Proprietary names are given in parentheses.

fluidized bed drying, but with tray drying, significant differences in composition can occur between the upper and lower surfaces of the solid bed. This can give rise to nonuniform drug content and, if the migrating species is colored, variation in the appearance of the product (9, 10).

Microwaves are being increasingly employed in the pharmaceutical industry for drying purposes. The incident microwave radiation (frequencies of 2450 and 960 MHz are used) causes electrons in substances such as water to resonate, which in turn generates heat and causes the water to evaporate. The water vapor is removed under vacuum, and hence the product dries rapidly at a relatively low temperature. As the bed of solid is stationary, particle attrition does not occur, and dust formation is minimized (see the article on Drying and Driers in this encyclopedia).

Second mixing stage

When the drying process is complete, it is likely that the product will have cohered into relatively large masses, especially if tray drying has been used. The dried material is therefore passed through a sieve (usually 250–700 μm) to break up aggregates and to give a relatively uniformly sized granule. A second mixing stage now follows in which several important ingredients of the formulation are added.

The glidant

The formation of granules from the original powder particles may have improved flow sufficiently for uniform die filling to be achieved. However, if flow is still not good enough, a glidant (also known as an anticaking agent) can be added to improve flow still further.

The most frequently used glidant is colloidal silicon dioxide, which has a mean size of about 20 nm. It is thought to act by lodging in the surface irregularities of the granule, forming a more rounded structure and hence reducing interparticulate friction. Colloidal silica has the added advantage of acting as a moisture scavenger.

Residual water in the formulation is bound to the silica, thereby providing a drier environment for the other ingredients.

Methods of assessing glidant action have been reviewed by Augsburger and Shangraw (11). Lerk et al. showed that a concentration of 0.2% colloidal silica in a tablet formulation had no effect on tablet crushing strength. However, higher concentrations reduced crushing strength especially when associated with prolonged mixing times (12).

Some commonly used glidants are shown in Table 3.

The lubricant

When the tablet formulation is compressed, the sides of the tablet are brought into intimate contact with the die wall. The tablet must then be ejected from the die, involving the movement of the side of the tablet relative to the die wall. Therefore, friction between the tablet and the die wall must be overcome. With materials such as lactose, friction resistance can be considerable, and it may be impossible to remove the tablet from the die without damage to the tablet or to the tablet press. Therefore, a lubricant is almost invariably included in a tablet formulation. A lubricant is a substance that deforms easily when sheared between two surfaces, and hence when interposed between the tablet and the die wall, provides a readily deformable film (13).

Details of some tablet lubricants are shown in Table 4.

Inadequate lubrication can often be recognized by vertical scratches on the sides of the tablet. It may also lead to a build-up of solid on the punch faces, which in turn gives a matt, dimpled appearance to the face of the tablet, a phenomenon known as picking.

In practice, magnesium stearate is by far the most frequently used tablet lubricant, and is extremely effective. Its activity, as with other metallic salts of fatty acids, is believed to derive from adhesion of the polar metallic portion of the molecule to the powder particle surface.

Table 4 Tablet lubricants

Lubricant	Concentration in tablet (wt%)	Comments
Calcium stearate	0.5–2	Water insoluble
Fumaric acid	5	Water soluble
Glyceryl behenate	0.5–4	Water insoluble
Glyceryl palmitostearate	0.5–5.0	Water insoluble (Precirol[R])
Hydrogenated vegetable oil	1–6	Water insoluble, may be used in conjunction with talc (Lubritab[R], Sterotex[R])
Magnesium lauryl sulfate	1–2	Soluble in warm water
Magnesium stearate	0.25–5	Water insoluble, excellent lubricant, reduces tablet strength, prolongs disintegration and dissolution times
Polyethylene glycol 4000 or 6000	2–5	Soluble in water, moderately effective, also known as macrogols (Carbowax[R])
Sodium lauryl sulfate	1–2	Water soluble, moderate lubricant, but good wetting properties, often employed in conjunction with stearates (Empicol[R], Stearowet C[R])
Sodium stearyl fumarate	0.5–2.0	Sparingly soluble in cold water, soluble in hot water (Pruv[R])
Starch	2–10	Moderate lubricant
Stearic acid	1–3	Water insoluble
Talc	1–10	Insoluble in water but not hydrophobic. A moderate lubricant
Zinc stearate	0.5–2	Water insoluble

Proprietary names are given in parentheses.

As a consequence, the hydrocarbon portion of the molecule becomes oriented away from the surface (14). Thus, a nonpolar layer is presented to adjacent powder particles and structures such as the press tooling. It is from the formation of this nonpolar layer that the advantages and disadvantages of the use of magnesium stearate in a tablet arise.

To act as an effective lubricant in a tablet, the lubricant must be dispersed over the surface of the powder particles or granules. The more complete this layer, the more effective the lubricant action will be. However, this has two deleterious consequences. The first is that each powder particle presents a hydrophobic and hence water repellent exterior. It is well known that the presence of a lubricant based on fatty acids slows disintegration and dissolution, and has been shown to cause bioavailability problems.

The second consequence is that direct contact between powder particles is, at least in part, replaced by contact between adjacent hydrocarbon layers. Since these by definition have low shear strength, it is not surprising that interparticulate bonding is reduced and hence the tablet structure is weakened. Reduction in tablet strength is particularly marked with substances such as microcrystalline cellulose that undergo deformation on compression, since although the particles may change shape, the hydrocarbon layer remains intact. Substances which fragment on compression suffer a smaller reduction in strength, since new surface, uncontaminated by lubricant, is created as the particles break up. This new surface can then take part in interparticulate bonding (15).

All these factors, both positive and negative, are consequences of the attrition of particles of lubricant and their spreading around the exterior surface of the other components of the tablet. Therefore, any processing factor that can affect lubricant attrition or the completeness of the film might be expected to influence tablet disintegration, dissolution, bioavailability, and physical strength. The mixing process is extremely important here, and mixing time, mixer type, and batch size (16) have all been shown to influence tablet properties. Thus, there is a need to establish a minimum lubricant concentration and an optimum mixing time within which adequate lubrication is achieved without the development of undesirable tablet characteristics. To ensure batch-to-batch uniformity, the parameters of the mixing process such as type of mixer, batch size, and mixing time must be kept as constant as possible. A mixing time of 2–5 min usually suffices to give adequate lubrication (17).

The water repellent properties of hydrocarbon based lubricants can be countered to a certain extent by the inclusion of a wetting agent such as sodium lauryl sulfate into the formulation. Such materials themselves can have a limited lubricant action. Mixtures of stearates and lauryl sulfates are commercially available.

Sodium stearyl fumarate has been used as an alternative for magnesium stearate. It has about the same lubricating effect, and causes similar tablet strength reduction and prolongation of disintegration time (18).

Lubricants based on fatty acids, because of their low water solubility, are unsuitable for tablets which must be dissolved in water before use. Polyethylene glycol 6000 (macrogol 6000) is soluble in water, but its lubricant activity is limited. Magnesium lauryl sulfate has been suggested as a water-soluble substitute for magnesium stearate. In addition to its lubricant action, this substance, like sodium lauryl sulfate, is an effective wetting agent (19).

It must be stressed that the functions of a glidant and lubricant in a tablet formulation are totally different. A few materials, e.g. talc, can act as both glidant and lubricant, but usually two different excipients are needed. Thus, although colloidal silicon dioxide is an excellent glidant, it has no lubricant activity. Conversely, magnesium stearate, despite its popularity as a lubricant, can hinder rather than promote flow.

The disintegrating agent

Strongly coherent particles are essential for the production of robust tablets, which will have high physical strength and low porosity. However, before it can be absorbed in the gastrointestinal tract, the active ingredient must dissolve, and a physically strong tablet is an impediment to dissolution. Therefore, tablet formulations often include a disintegrating agent, which when it comes into contact with water, disrupts the tablet structure and leads to fragmentation. A larger surface area is thus exposed to the dissolving fluid and dissolution is facilitated. Tablets which contain a large proportion of solids that are freely soluble in water have less need of a disintegrating agent, since such tablets tend to erode from their exterior surfaces rather than disintegrate.

Details of some tablet disintegrating agents are given in Table 5.

For many years, starch was the disintegrating agent of choice. Recently, however, so-called "super disintegrants" have been introduced, which markedly reduce tablet disintegration time. Such substances include croscarmellose, crospovidone, polacrilin potassium, and sodium starch glycolate (20).

The disintegrating agent may be mixed with other powders prior to wetting with the granulating fluid (intragranular) or at the second mixing stage (extragranular), or both. Shotton and Leonard found that while extragranular disintegrating agents caused the tablet to disintegrate quicker, intragranular disintegrants not only broke down the tablet but also the constituent granules, giving a finer product (21).

The mechanism of action of disintegrating agents has been the subject of some debate (22). Some substances such as starch swell when they come into contact with water, and disruption of the tablet structure has been attributed to this. However, other effective disintegrants do not swell in this way, and are believed to act by providing a network of hydrophilic pathways inside the tablet through which water can diffuse. Irrespective of the precise mechanism of disintegration, it is clear that water uptake into the tablet must be the first step in the disintegration process (23).

Addition of wetting agents such as sodium lauryl sulfate or sodium docusate can assist this water penetration by lowering the surface tension, and they are often used in conjunction with hydrophobic lubricants such as magnesium stearate (see the article on Tablet Disintegrants and Disintegration in this encyclopedia).

Tablet Manufacture by Dry Granulation

Although widely used, the wet granulation method of tablet manufacture suffers from several disadvantages. Water is the usual granulating fluid, and this exposes tablet ingredients to the danger of hydrolysis. Furthermore, the granulating fluid has to be removed, usually by heating. In addition to the energy costs that are incurred, the elevated temperature will accelerate any hydrolytic reaction that might be taking place.

Dry granulation is an alternative method that can be used, and this process is shown in Fig. 3. The components of the formulation are compressed in the dry state. If sufficient bonding strength cannot be achieved by compression alone, a binder is added, also in the dry state.

The initial compression stage can take place by one of two methods. The first uses a conventional tablet press, a process often referred to as "slugging." Because the components of the formulation will not have the necessary attributes for producing good tablets, the tablets produced at this stage (the slugs) will not be of acceptable quality, especially as regards to appearance and weight uniformity. The slugs are then broken down to form a granular product, which after sieving can then be compressed again to give satisfactory tablets. Malkowska and Khan showed that the ease of compressibility of the formulation at the second compression was inversely proportional to

Table 5 Tablet disintegrating agents

Disintegrating agent	Concentration in tablet (wt%)	Comments
Alginic acid	2–10	
Carbon dioxide		Created in situ in effervescent tablets
Carboxymethylcellulose calcium	1–15	(Nymcel[R])
Carboxymethylcellulose sodium	1–5	(Nymcel[R])
Cellulose, microcrystalline	Up to 10	Directly compressible, some lubricant properties (Avicel[R], Emcocel[R], Vivacel[R])
Cellulose, powdered	5–15	Solka Floc[R]
Croscarmellose sodium	0.5–5	(Ac–di–Sol[R], Solutab[R])
Crospovidone	2–5	(Kollidon CL[R], Polyplasdone XL[R])
Docusate sodium	0.5–1	Acts primarily as a wetting agent
Guar gum	2–8	
Hydroxypropyl cellulose—low-substituted	5–25	
Magnesium aluminum silicate	2–10	(Veegum[R])
Methylcellulose	2–10	
Polacrilin potassium	2–10	Cation exchange resin (Amberlite IRP88[R])
Poloxamer	5–10	
Povidone	0.5–5	(Kollidon[R], Plasdone[R])
Sodium alginate	2.5–10	(Manucol[R])
Sodium glycine carbonate		Source of carbon dioxide for effervescent tablets
Sodium lauryl sulfate	0.5–2	Primarily a wetting agent but aids disintegration (Empicol[R])
Sodium starch glycolate	2–8	(Explotab[R], Primojel[R])
Starch	2–10	Potato and maize starches are most frequently used
Starch, pregelatinized	5–10	(Lycatab[R], Pharma-Gel[R], Pre-Jel[R], Sepistab[R], Starch 1500[R], Starx 1500[R])

Proprietary names are given in parentheses.

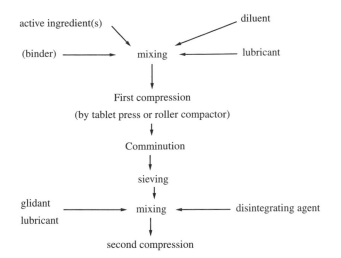

Fig. 3 The dry granulation process of tablet manufacture.

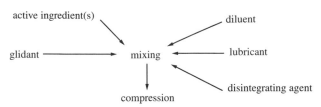

Fig. 4 The direct compression process of tablet manufacture.

the pressure used at the slugging stage, implying that slugging at high pressure should be avoided (24).

A second method of compression is to use a roller compactor. The powder mixture is passed between two contra-rotating cylindrical rollers to form a cake, which as before is broken down to a product of granular size and then recompressed. Both methods require the addition of a lubricant prior to the first compression stage, though more lubricant will probably be needed before the second compression.

Tablet Manufacture by Direct Compression

Both wet and dry granulation methods of tablet manufacture are complex multistage processes, but are necessary to convert the components of the formulation into a state that can be readily compressed into acceptable tablets. If, however, a major component of the formulation already possesses the necessary degree of fluidity and compressibility, granulation would be unnecessary. This is the basis of the direct compression method of tablet manufacture (25).

The key component here is the diluent. This must not only possess those properties which are necessary for satisfactory tablet formulation, but also retain those properties when mixed with the other constituents of the formulation such as the active ingredient.

The process of direct compression is shown in Fig. 4. The ingredients are mixed together and then compressed. Almost invariably a lubricant must be added, and a glidant and a disintegrating agent included when necessary. The process does not involve the use of a liquid, and hence a drying stage with its attendant energy costs is avoided.

Details of some direct compression diluents are given in Table 6. The majority of these are available from only one supplier, though the two most frequently used—spray-dried lactose and microcrystalline cellulose—are available from several sources.

In view of the apparent simplicity of this method of tablet manufacture and the number of suitable diluents that are commercially available, it is perhaps surprising that techniques of tablet manufacture involving granulation are still so widely used. Direct compression can, of course, only be used when a diluent is required by the formulation, i.e., the active ingredient must be relatively potent. Direct compression can offer significant savings in energy, equipment, and material handling costs. Against this must be set higher ingredient costs, since direct compression diluents are more expensive than other diluents.

There are, however, other factors which must be considered. In wet granulation, the properties of the individual drug and diluent particles are, at least to a certain extent, hidden by the binder, whereas in direct compression, the original particles are still present. Therefore, in the latter technique, a premium is placed on batch-to-batch consistency of particulate properties such as size and shape for both drug and diluent. In a direct compression formulation, the components can behave as individual particles, and therefore there is a danger that these can segregate after mixing and prior to compression. In a granulation process, the particles are bound together and so segregation is less likely to happen. Furthermore, the reduction in dust formation brought about by granulation cannot occur in direct compression.

The true direct compression process as described earlier almost invariably applies to formulations containing potent active ingredients and where the direct compression properties derive from the diluent. A few substances do possess adequate flow and cohesive properties without the need for pretreatment. These are usually crystalline inorganic salts such as sodium chloride and potassium chloride. Direct compression forms of less potent active ingredients are available e.g., paracetamol and ascorbic acid. These can be directly compressed into tablets, perhaps after the addition of a lubricant. However, such

Table 6 Direct compression tablet diluents

Diluent	Proprietary name	Comments
Calcium phosphate, dibasic	Emcompress^R, Di-Tab^R	Good flow properties, high density, insoluble in water
Calcium phosphate, tribasic	Tri-Tab^R	Insoluble in water
Calcium sulfate	Compactrol^R	Insoluble in water
Cellulose, microcrystalline	Avicel^R, Emcocel^R, Vivacel^R	Highly compressible, low bulk density, acts as disintegrant
Cellulose, powdered	Elcema^R	
Dextrates	Emdex^R	
Lactitol	Finlac^R DC	
Lactose		
Anhydrous alpha	Pharmatose DCL30^R	Good flow properties
Anhydrous beta	Pharmatose DCL21^R	
Spray-dried	Fast-Flo^R, Zeparox^R, Pharmatose DCL11^R	
Lactose-cellulose coprocessed mixture	Cellactose^R	
Maltodextrin	Lycatab^R, Maltrin^R	Fairly soluble in water, slight lubricant effect
Mannitol	Pearlitol^R	Freely soluble in water, negative heat of solution
Sorbitol	Neosorb^R	
Starch, pregelatinized starch	Starch 1500^R, Starx 1500^R	Disintegrant
Sucrose–maltodextrin coprecipitate	Des-Tab^R, Dipac^R, Nu-Tab^R	Good flow properties, moisture sensitive
Xylitol	Xylitab^R	Freely soluble in water, negative heat of solution

substances are more accurately described as "pre-granulated," in that the granulation process—either wet granulation or precompression—has been carried out by the excipient manufacturer (see the article on Direct Compression Tabletting in this encyclopedia).

THE BEHAVIOR OF PARTICLES UNDER A COMPRESSIVE LOAD

All tablet manufacture can be regarded as the application of pressure to a population of particles enclosed in a confined space. An understanding of particle behavior under such conditions is therefore the key to understanding the formation and properties of tablets.

Application of a Force to Particles in a Die

Attractive forces exist between any two solid bodies. These forces may be nonspecific, e.g., van der Waal's forces, or may be more specific in nature, e.g., brought about by molecules exhibiting intermolecular hydrogen bonds. However, irrespective of their nature, it is these forces acting among a large population of particles that enable a coherent tablet to be formed (26). Their magnitude depends directly on the particle mass and inversely on the square of the distance separating the particles. It follows, therefore, that with small particles of small mass, a tablet will only be formed when adjacent particles are forced into intimate contact with each other. This contact is brought about by the application of force.

A representation of what may happen to an individual particle when a force is applied to it can be obtained by considering what happens to a spring when subjected to a load that is applied and then removed. This is shown in Fig. 5. Although the analogy of a powder under compression to a spring undergoing elongation is not exact, it does provide useful comparisons. The load is termed the stress and the change in length the strain.

Initially there is a rectilinear relationship between stress and strain, and if the stress is removed, the spring returns to its original length. This is elastic behavior and is completely reversible. The spring is said to obey Hooke's law and the reciprocal of the slope of this portion of the curve is Young's Modulus for the spring.

If the stress is further increased, eventually a point is reached when the straight-line relationship is lost. This is

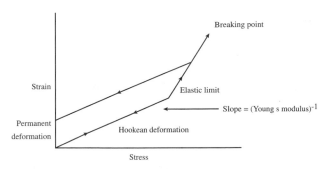

Fig. 5 Stress–strain relationships.

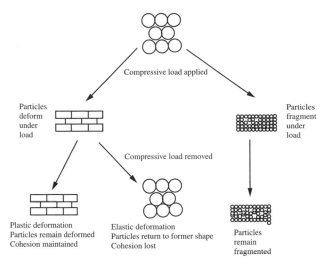

Fig. 6 Elasticity and plasticity in a particulate mass.

termed the elastic limit. If stresses in excess of the elastic limit are applied and then removed, the spring will not return to its original length. Thus, a fraction of the change in length is permanent or irreversible, and this is termed plastic behavior. Further increase in load will result in more and more plastic deformation until eventually the load is so great that the breaking point of the spring is reached and it snaps. Now, consider now a number of particles constrained in the die of a tablet press and to which a progressively increasing force is applied. A series of events can then occur, perhaps sequentially but there is a greater likelihood that some overlap will occur.

The particles will undergo rearrangement to form a less porous structure. This will take place at very low forces, the particles sliding past each other. This stage will usually be associated with some fragmentation, as the rough surfaces move relatively to one another and asperities are abraded away.

The particles have now reached the stage where relative movement becomes impossible, although the porosity of the powder bed may still be considerable. A further increase in applied force can then induce elastic deformation, plastic deformation, or fragmentation. Which of these alternatives predominates will depend on the properties of the material involved, but the net result will be a further decrease in porosity, and an increase in interparticulate contact.

If only elastic deformation has occurred, then when the compressing force is removed, the particles will return to their former shape. The additional interparticulate contact caused by compression will be lost and a coherent tablet will not be formed Fig. 6.

If, however, the elastic limit has been passed, then as the force is removed, not all the increased interparticulate contact will be lost, cohesion will be retained and a tablet will be formed. Thus, from the point of view of forming a robust tablet, substances with low elastic limits, which undergo plastic deformation at low compressive forces, are preferable to more elastic bodies.

If consolidation of the powder mass is brought about by fragmentation, then a large number of points of interparticulate contact are created, from which the strength of the tablet derives. In this case, removal of the compressing force should have no effect on tablet strength, since there is no way the fragments can recombine into the original particles. However, purely fragmentary consolidation is unlikely to have occurred, and so the effect of removal of the force on deformed particles must still be considered.

Force Transmission through a Powder Bed

Consider as before a group of particles in the die of an excentric tablet press. Force is applied by means of the descending upper punch and because the lower punch is passive, the force will be transmitted to it through the powder bed. The distribution of force within the powder bed was investigated by Train, who embedded force transducers (q.v.) in a relatively large mass of powder (27). He found that the diminution of force did not proceed uniformly on descent through the bed, but formed a much more complex pattern. This was caused by the forces being transmitted to and reflected from the die wall. Significant features are zones of high force at the periphery near the moving punch, and much lower in the powder mass on its vertical axis. On the other hand, low force zones occur on the same axis but much nearer to the moving punch Fig. 7. Train's findings were later confirmed by Charlton and Newton using gamma-ray attenuation (28).

The consequences of such a force distribution on tablet strength can be profound. Particle deformation, whether elastic or plastic, will be proportional to the force applied,

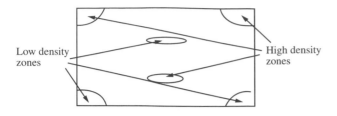

Fig. 7 Density distribution in a compact prepared on an excentric tablet press.

and as has been discussed, this deformation is an essential preliminary to the formation of the interparticulate bonds on which tablet integrity depends. Thus, the porosity of the tablet, and hence its strength, will vary within the tablet. The weakest points in the tablet structure will be those that receive the lowest force i.e., on the face of the tablet adjacent to the stationary punch and on the central axis near to the moving punch. Thus, because of its nonuniform density, some parts of a tablet are stronger than others.

It should be noted that this discussion assumes that only one punch is actively applying the force to the powder mass while the other is stationary and passive. This is true in the case of an excentric press, but with a rotary tablet press, both punches move and hence both exert forces on the powder bed. The force distribution so obtained is thus different from that shown in Fig. 7, and results in two low density zones near the faces of the tablet and a high density zone in approximately the centre of the powder mass.

The effect of the removal of the compressing force must now be considered. Elastic recovery will occur to a greater or lesser extent, which will result in a reduction in the strength of interparticulate bonds and an overall weakening of the tablet. It therefore follows that if a tablet is to be disrupted by elastic recovery, this is most likely to occur at its weakest point. This is just below the top surface, and is the phenomenon often encountered in tablet manufacture known as lamination or capping. With this explanation in mind, some effects associated with capping, and some causes and pragmatic solutions to the problem can now be explained.

Capping was for many years considered to be due to the entrapment of air in the tablet, and even the production of tablets in vacuo which still capped did little to dispel this theory. Neither did this suggestion explain why air should cause the fracture just below the face of the tablet. However, by considering the nonuniform density distribution in the tablet, it can be seen that the weakness is not caused by the presence of air per se, but rather the relative absence of solid in those parts of the tablet that have high porosity (29). As compression proceeds, it follows that the pores in the tablet structure are filled with air at

a progressively elevated pressure, and this will obviously assist disruption of the tablet when the compressing force is removed. Thus, any factor which obstructs the expulsion of air from the powder mass during compression will exacerbate capping, though it is not the fundamental cause. Such factors include the clearance between punch and die, the speed at which the force is applied, and the presence of small particles, which makes passage of air through the tablet more tortuous (30).

Any applied stress that exceeds the breaking strength of the tablet will also cause the tablet to break at its weakest point. A number of stresses occur when the tablet is removed from the die after compression. The die may become worn at the point in the die where the tablet is compressed, i.e., the die is fractionally wider at this point than elsewhere. Thus, when the tablet is ejected, it is forced through an aperture, the diameter of which is slightly less than that of the tablet itself. This will obviously stress the tablet, and the interparticulate bonds may be overcome at their weakest point. Also as the tablet is extruded from the die, elastic expansion will occur not just in an axial but in a radial direction. The latter occurs progressively, i.e., one segment of tablet is free to expand while the one below is still constrained by the die. Bond disruption will be an inevitable consequence.

CHARACTERIZATION OF THE COMPACTION PROCESS

A range of parameters has been devised which attempts to describe the process of powder compaction, both to elucidate principles and also to enable predictions to be made regarding compaction properties. The majority of these depend on the availability of methods of accurately measuring applied force and punch position.

Measurement of Applied Force and Punch Movement

The aim of any tabletting process is to produce tablets that are of satisfactory quality. Virtually all tablet properties e.g., porosity, physical strength, disintegration time, dissolution time are dependent in some way on the force that is applied by the punches to the particles in the die.

Considerable research on tablet properties was performed for many years, but until a method of accurately measuring compression force was available, meaningful studies could not be carried out.

The key to progress in this field was the introduction of the so-called instrumented tablet press by Higuchi and others in the mid 1950s (31), in which force transducers were fitted to the press to measure the applied load. This revolutionized research into the tabletting process and in addition has lead to the development of presses with automatic tablet weight control, since the mass of particles in the die governs the force detected by the transducer (32) (see the article on Automation of Tablet Presses in this encyclopedia).

A force transducer is also known as a strain gauge. In its simplest form, the strain gauge is a network of wires through which an electric current is passed. The wires are bonded very securely to a component of the press, e.g., the upper punch. If a force is applied to the punch, it deforms. The magnitude of the deformation (the strain) is governed by a combination of the magnitude of the force (the stress) and the value of Young's modulus for the material from which the punch is made. The wire of the strain gauge is also deformed, and hence its electrical resistance changes. If the gauge is incorporated into a Wheatstone bridge circuit, then a small change in voltage results. The size of the signal from the strain gauge is proportional to the amount of deformation, which in turn is a function of the applied force. Hence, after amplification and appropriate calibration, the voltage changes can be expressed in terms of the applied force. Signals from the transducers can be fed into an oscilloscope or chart recorder, or stored electronically and subsequently manipulated by computer.

A further advance was the fitting of displacement transducers to tablet presses. These too give out an electrical signal, the magnitude of which is governed by the position of a sensing device in relation to a fixed reference point, and in this way punch movement can be measured. As before, these signals can be amplified, recorded, and stored. If the outputs of the force and displacement transducers are combined, the applied force at a given point in time, and punch position at the same instant can be established.

Instrumentation of rotary presses is more difficult than that for an excentric press if transducers are to be fitted directly to the punches. Since the turret of the press rotates, a fixed connection between transducers and the recording device is impracticable. Alternatives to fixed connections are slip rings and radiotelemetry. A further option is to fit transducers to points of the press remote from the punches and which do not rotate. Techniques for fitting transducers to both excentric and rotary tablet presses, their calibration, and applications of the information derived from instrumented presses have been reviewed by Watt (33).

Fig. 8 shows the output from force and displacement transducers fitted to both punches of an excentric tablet press. The upper punch describes an approximately sinusoidal path as it descends to penetrate the die (point

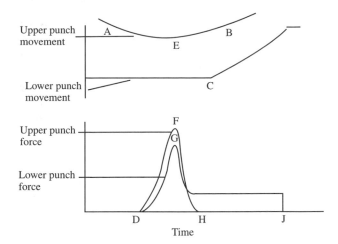

Fig. 8 Force and displacement data from an instrumented excentric tablet press.

A) and then rises after the compression event has taken place, leaving the die at point B. The lower punch remains motionless during the compression event and then rises to eject the tablet from the die (point C).

As the upper punch enters the die and comes into contact with the particles, the height of the bed of particles is reduced and hence porosity decreases. Initially porosity reduction is brought about by particle rearrangement. This requires a very low force which is probably not detectable by the force transducers, the output of which remains zero. The upper punch then encounters a resistance to its motion (point D) as further consolidation by rearrangement becomes impossible. Hence, the output of the upper punch force transducer rises, slowly at first and then more rapidly. Particles are deformed and/or fragmented during this stage to form a coherent tablet. Force is transmitted to the lower punch, and a similar rise is detected by transducers there. As maximum upper punch penetration is achieved (point E), force maxima are detected on both punches (points F and G), that on the lower punch being less than that on the upper.

Once the maxima have occurred, the upper punch begins to rise, and the force detected on both punches falls. That on the upper punch returns to zero as contact is lost between the ascending punch and the top surface of the tablet (point H). That on the lower punch does not fall to zero until ejection is complete (point J). The greater the ejection force, the greater the need for a lubricant in the formulation.

The reason why the lower punch maximum force is less than that of the upper punch is because a fraction of the force applied by the upper punch is transmitted to the die wall, where it results in die wall friction. This is reduced by the presence of a lubricant. Hence, the ratio between lower punch maximum force and upper punch maximum force, often called the R value, is used as the basis of comparison between lubricants (34). R has a maximum value of unity and lubricants based on stearates usually exhibit R values greater than 0.95.

The time that elapses from point D to point F is known as the consolidation time. This is the time interval when a force is detectable at the upper punch. The contact time is the period when the upper punch is in contact with the original particles or the tablet (point D to point H). The residence time is the period when a force is detected at the lower punch (point D to point J), which ends on tablet ejection.

Transducer output from a rotary tablet press differs in two aspects. Firstly, the lower punch plays an active role in the compression event and moves upwards as the upper punch moves downwards. The second difference is small but important. Because of the sinusoidal movement of the upper punch in an excentric press, the punch speed is only zero at the instant when it reverses direction (point E). Punches on a rotary press have a flat area on the punch head. As the punches pass under or over the pressure rolls, the flat area dictates that there is no punch movement. The period during which this occurs is called the dwell time, and though it only lasts a fraction of a second, it can have a major effect on the consolidation process (35, 36).

Tablet Strength Profiles

The physical strength of a tablet is dependent on the extent and strength of interparticulate bonds and these in turn are related to the compressive force which is applied. Therefore, the relationship between the applied force and some parameter related to tablet strength is a good indication of the ease with which a given substance will form satisfactory tablets, and may also give an insight into the compaction mechanism of the solid and its mechanical properties.

The strength is usually assessed as the force required to fracture a tablet in a defined direction e.g., its diameter. This has traditionally been referred to as the "hardness" of the tablet, which is incorrect terminology in this context. In material science, hardness is a surface property related to resistance to indentation. Terms such as physical strength or mechanical strength are more appropriate.

The compression force is measured using an instrumented tablet press as described earlier. The physical strength of the tablet is measured with crushing apparatus such as that described in most current pharmacopoeias. The results are conventionally presented graphically with compression force as the abscissa and strength as the ordinate.

This technique is satisfactory when comparing tablets of the same size and shape, such as in-process control. However, if virtually identical tablets are not being tested, problems may arise. The force is sometimes expressed as the compression pressure, obtained by dividing the force by the cross-sectional area of the punch. This is valid if the punch has a flat surface, the area of which can be easily calculated; but in practice this is often not the case, and conversion between compression force and compression pressure involves assumptions regarding the area of the punch face, which may not be valid.

The physical strength of a tablet is also dependent on its dimensions. In the construction of a force-strength profile, all tablets will have the same cross-sectional area as the same tooling will have been used. However, as the compressive force is changed, so will the tablet height. Hence, comparisons made on the basis of breaking strength will not be truly valid.

This problem has been circumvented in part by the calculation of the tensile strength of the tablet. The most commonly used formula is shown in Eq. 1, introduced by Rudnick et al. (37) and Fell and Newton (38).

$$\mathrm{Ts} = 2P/\pi dt \qquad (1)$$

where Ts is the tensile strength of the tablet (MPa), P the crushing strength (N), d the tablet diameter (m), and t the tablet thickness (m).

This equation applies to cylindrical tablets which have a diameter and whose height is constant over the whole tablet surface. Newton et al. have attempted to extend the concept of tensile strength to tablets that are not cylindrical (39).

Confusion can often arise in the units that are used to express compression force or pressure and the strength of the tablet. Table 7 gives examples of units that have been used recently for the axes of tablet strength profiles. Comparison between different tablet formulations would be greatly facilitated if authors used and journal editors insisted on the use of the SI system of units. The SI unit of length is the meter, that of force the Newton and that of pressure the Pascal. The unit for physical strength is the Newton and that of tensile strength calculated from Eq. 1 is the Pascal.

Relationships between Tablet Porosity and Compression Force or Pressure

Fig. 8 shows the movement of both the upper and lower punches of the tablet press in relation to fixed reference points and from these data, the distance separating the two

Table 7 Some units used for the construction of tablet strength profiles

Abscissa parameter	Unit	Ordinate parameter	Unit
Force	kg	Crushing strength (hardness)	kg
	lb		Strong-Cobb units
	kN		N
	N		kp
Pressure	Kg cm^{-2}	Tensile strength	Kg cm^{-2}
	Pa		Pa
	MPa		MPa
	lbin^{-2}		

punch faces can be calculated. If both punch faces are in contact with the tablet, it follows that the distance of their separation is equal to the height of the tablet (h). Consequently, if the cross-sectional area of the die (a), the tablet weight (w) and the true density of the solid from which the tablet is made (ρ) are all known, the porosity of the tablet (η) can be calculated from Eq. 2.

$$\varepsilon = 1 - (w/ah\rho) \qquad (2)$$

For cylindrical tablets, Eq. 2 becomes Eq. 3

$$\varepsilon = 1 - (4w/\pi d^2 h\rho) \qquad (3)$$

As the applied force (or pressure) being applied at the same moment in time can also be determined from Fig. 8, it follows that a relationship between force and porosity can be constructed.

A typical relationship is shown in Fig. 9. As force is increased from zero, the porosity of the tablet falls rapidly, but then further increase in force has a progressively smaller effect. The porosity value at which the curve becomes virtually horizontal is dependent on the solid being compressed. Substances that deform plastically typically give tablets of lower porosity than those which fragment.

Many equations have been derived in attempts to provide a mathematical expression of Fig. 9. These have been reviewed by Kawakita and Ludde (40). It must be stressed that such equations are simply mathematical descriptions of the data, and they have no underlying physical significance.

The most widely used of these equations is the Heckel relationship (41):

$$\ln 1/(1 - D) = kP + A$$

where D is the relative density of the tablet and hence $(1 - D)$ is the porosity, P is the applied pressure, and k and A are constants.

This equation predicts that a graph of $\ln 1/(1 - D)$ against P should yield a straight line of slope k and intercept A. Heckel surmised that the greater the slope, the greater degree of plasticity in the solid being compressed. Hersey and Rees (42) defined the reciprocal of k to be the mean yield pressure of the solid.

Fig. 10 shows a typical Heckel diagram. Deviations from linearity often occur at low and high pressures. These are to be expected. At low pressures, reduction in porosity is largely by particle rearrangement, and thus the true consolidation mechanism, i.e., fragmentation or deformation, will be a minor component of the total consolidation process. At high pressures, porosity can become very low and hence its reciprocal becomes a very large number.

However, the real problem with Heckel plots is identifying a truly rectilinear section. When pressure–porosity diagrams were first devised, instrumented tablet presses were not widely available. The height of the tablet was measured after ejection from the die and thus the net

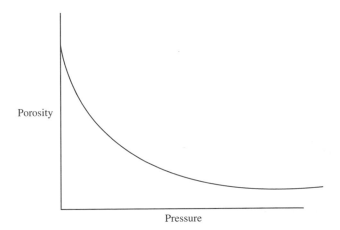

Fig. 9 A force-porosity diagram.

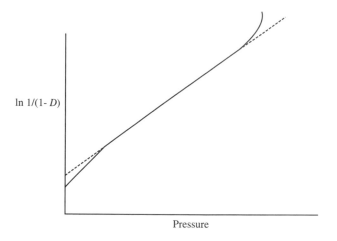

Fig. 10 Pressure and porosity data plotted according to the Heckel equation.

change in height was a combination of height reduction by consolidation and a height increase by elastic expansion. Furthermore, the typical plot comprised only a small number of points, and an apparently rectilinear zone could be identified. With improvements in instrumentation and in particular linkage to a computer, Heckel plots of several hundred points became feasible with tablet height measurements being made before ejection from the die. In the author's experience, the more points there are on a pressure–porosity diagram, the more difficult it is to identify a truly rectilinear section.

Paronen and Ilkka have surveyed the use of the Heckel and other compression equations and have drawn attention to difficulties in their interpretation (43).

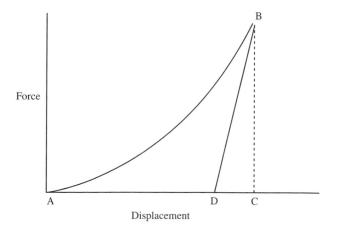

Fig. 11 A force-displacement curve.

Force-Displacement Curves

Fig. 8 shows how force and punch displacement change with time. It is therefore possible to determine both the force and displacement values at any given point in time, and from this, a force–displacement curve can be constructed. Usually the force is plotted as the ordinate and displacement as the abscissa Fig. 11.

The area enclosed by the curve has the units of force (Newtons) multiplied by distance (metres), which is dimensionally equivalent to work or energy (in Joules). Therefore, the force–displacement curve has been used to calculate the work consumed in the compression of a solid (44).

Further refinement of this technique has enabled estimates of elasticity and plasticity of the solid to be made. If the particles were totally nonelastic, then as soon as the upper punch reached its maximum penetration and began to rise again, contact would be lost with the tablet. Therefore, the force recorded by transducers fitted to the upper punch would instantly fall to zero. This clearly does not happen, as demonstrated by the upper punch force values after maximum punch penetration in Fig. 8. This can only mean that as the upper punch ascends, the tablet expands elastically, keeping in contact with the punch face. Thus, the area ABC in Fig. 11 represents the work expended on compressing the solid, and area DBC is the work delivered back to the upper punch by the expanding tablet. The difference between these two areas (i.e., ABD) has been termed the "Net work" of compression.

Use of this technique has shown that the presence of a granulating agent causes a marked increase in the plasticity of the powder mass, with a consequent increase in cohesion and tablet strength. The film of granulating agent between the particles can be regarded as a highly viscous liquid with a large yield value. Application of a force in excess of the yield value causes granules to deform, and this becomes permanent when the force is reduced to below the yield value (45). A somewhat similar mechanism is believed to account for the properties of some direct-compression tablet diluents, e.g., spray-dried lactose, which consists of small crystalline masses embedded in an amorphous and more easily deformed matrix.

The force–displacement curve has been extensively used to characterize the compression event. However, it depends on the availability of sensitive and properly calibrated transducers. Even small inaccuracies in measuring displacement at high force values can have a profound effect on the resultant value of the area under the curve. Ragnarsson has provided a very thorough review of the uses and potential pitfalls of the force–displacement curve (46).

Time-Dependent Effects

It has long been known that for some formulations, changing the speed of operation of the tablet press or changing the type of press can have a profound effect on tablet quality. Such circumstances may arise, for example, when changing from a slow excentric press in formulation development to a high speed rotary in production.

As described earlier, diagrams of transducer output against time enable parameters such as contact time and dwell time to be defined Fig. 8. Also the slope of the displacement–time diagram equals the speed of the punch and the slope of the force–time diagram is the rate of change of the force. If the operating speed of the press is altered, there is a proportional change in all of these.

Such considerations are important because the consolidation of many substances is time-dependent. Fragmentation can be regarded as a virtually instantaneous process. However, substances that undergo deformation behave in a viscoelastic manner, and the time over which the compression force is applied can be crucial. As the time over which they are compressed is reduced, such materials show less consolidation and this in turn can affect the physical strength of the tablet. For example, Armstrong and Palfrey (47) studied the effects of punch speed change on the tablet strength of four direct compression diluents. Though tablet strength was reduced in all cases, solids such as modified starch suffered the greatest reduction. Roberts and Rowe investigated the relative sensitivity of the yield pressures of a range of solids to changes in compression speed, and again found that those solids which deformed on compression showed the greatest change (48).

The rate of consolidation in an excentric press is governed by the speed at which the upper punch moves into the die. This in turn is governed by the lengths of the excentric arms of the press and its speed of operation. In a rotary press, punch speed is governed by the diameter of the die table, the diameter of the pressure roll, the geometry of the punch head, and the speed of operation. Formulae for the calculation of punch speeds at any point of the compression cycle for both types of press have been derived (49, 50).

It is important to distinguish the punch speed from the output of the press. Though rotary presses have a much higher output than excentric presses, this largely derives from their multiplicity of punch stations. It does not necessarily follow that their punch speeds during compaction are significantly greater (51).

If the work of compression in Joules is divided by the time in seconds over which compression occurs, then the power of compression (in Watts) is obtained.

An alternative method of calculating power of compression is to multiply the force by the punch speed when that force was applied. This too can be obtained from the data in Fig. 8. This permits the compression events on different presses to be compared (49).

REFERENCES

1. Editorial: The Passing of the Tablet Fad, Pharm. J. **1895**, February *12*.
2. Castello, R.A.; Mattocks, A.M. Discoloration of Tablets Containing Amines and Lactose, J. Pharm. Sci. **1962**, *51* (1), 106–108.
3. Carstensen, J.T.; Ertell, C. Physical and Chemical Properties of Calcium Phosphate for Solid State Pharmaceutical Formulations, Drug Dev. Ind. Pharm. **1990**, *16* (7), 1121–1133.
4. Campbell, H.; Bauer, W.C. Cause and Cure of Demixing in Solid–Solid Mixers, Chem. Eng. **Sept. 1966**, *179–185*.
5. Staniforth, J.N.; Rees, J.E.; Kayes, J.B. Relation between Mixing Time and Segregation of Ordered Mixes, J. Pharm. Pharmacol. **1981**, *33*, 175–176.
6. Sherrington, P.J.; Oliver, R. *Granulation*; Heyden and Sons: London, 1981.
7. Ertel, K.D.; Zoglio, M.A.; Ritschel, W.A.; Carstensen, J.T. Physical Aspects of Wet Granulation. IV. Effect of Kneading Time on Dissolution Rate and Tablet Properties, Drug Dev. Ind. Pharm. **1990**, *16* (6), 963–981.
8. Kristensen, H.G.; Schaefer, T. Granulation; Drug Dev. Ind. Pharm. **1987**, *13* (4/5), 803–872.
9. Rubinstein, M.H.; Ridgway., K. Solute Migration during Granule Drying, J. Pharm. Pharmacol. **1974**, *26*, 24P–29P.
10. Armstrong, N.A.; March, G.A. Quantitative Assessment of Surface Mottling of Colored Tablets, J. Pharm. Sci. **1974**, *63* (1), 126–129.
11. Augsburger, L.L.; Shangraw, R.F. Effect of Glidants in Tabletting, J. Pharm. Sci. **1966**, *55* (4), 418–423.
12. Lerk, C.F.; Bolhuis, G.K.; Smedama, S.S. Interactions of Lubricants and Colloidal Silica During Mixing with Excipients, Pharm. Acta Helv. **1977**, *52* (3), 33–39.
13. Bowden, F.P.; Tabor, D. *The Friction and Lubrication of Solids*, 2nd Ed.; Clarendon Press: Oxford, 1964.
14. Miller, T.A.; York, P. Pharmaceutical Tablet Lubrication, Int. J. Pharm. **1988**, *41*, 1–19.
15. De Boer, A.H.; Bolhuis, G.K.; Lerk, C.F. Bonding Characteristics by Scanning Electron Microscopy of Powders Mixed with Magnesium Stearate, Powder Tech. **1978**, *20*, 75–82.
16. Bolhuis, G.K.; Holzer, A.W. Lubricant Sensitivity. *Pharmaceutical Powder Compaction Technology*; Alderborn, G., Nystrom, C., Eds.; Marcel Dekker, Inc.: New York, 1996; 517–560.
17. Ragnarsson, G.; Holzer, A.W.; Sjogren, J. Influence of Mixing Time and Colloidal Silica on the Lubricating Properties of Magnesium Stearate, Int. J. Pharm. **1979**, *3*, 127–131.

18. Holzer, A.W.; Sjogren, J. Evaluation of Sodium Stearyl Fumarate as a Tablet Lubricant, Int. J. Pharm. **1979**, *2*, 145–153.

19. Salpekar, A.M.; Augsburger, L.L. Magnesium Lauryl Sulfate in Tabletting: Effect on Ejection Force and Compressibility, J. Pharm. Sci. **1974**, *63* (2), 289–293.

20. Shangraw, R.F.; Mitrevej, A.; Shah, M. A New Era of Tablet Disintegrants, Pharmaceutical Technology **1980, Oct.**, *49–57*.

21. Shotton, E.; Leonard, G.S. Effect of Intragranular and Extragranular Disintegrants on the Particle Size of Disintegrated Tablets, J. Pharm. Sci. **1976**, *65* (8), 1170–1174.

22. Lowenthal, W. Disintegration of Tablets, J. Pharm. Sci. **1972**, *61* (11), 1695–1711.

23. van Kamp, H.V.; Bolhuis, G.K.; de Boer, A.H.; Lerk, C.F.; Lie-A-Huen, L. The Role of Water Uptake on Tablet Disintegration, Pharm. Acta Helv. **1986**, *61* (1), 22–29.

24. Malkowska, S.; Khan, K.A. Effect of Recompression on the Properties of Tablets Prepared by Dry Granulation, Drug Dev. Ind. Pharm. **1983**, *9* (3), 331–347.

25. Bolhuis, G.K.; Chowhan, Z.T. Materials for Direct Compression. *Pharmaceutical Powder Compaction Technology*; Alderborn, G., Nystrom, C, Eds.; Marcel Dekker, Inc. New York, 1996; 419–500.

26. Nystrom, C.; Karehill, P.G. Intermolecular Bonding Forces. *Pharmaceutical Powder Compaction Technology*; Alderborn, G., Nystrom, C, Eds.; Marcel Dekker, Inc.: New York, 1996; 17–53.

27. Train, D.; Lewis, C.J. Agglomeration of Solids by Compaction, Trans. Inst. Chem. Engrs. **1962**, *40*, 235–263.

28. Charlton, B.; Newton, J.M. Application of Gamma-Ray Attenuation to the Determination of Density Distributions Within Compacted Powders, Powder Technol. **1985**, *41*, 123–134.

29. Ritter, A.; Sucker, H.B. Studies of Variables that Affect Tablet Capping, Pharm. Technol. **1980**, July, *24–34*.

30. Mann, S.C.; Roberts, R.J.; Rowe, R.C.; Hunter, B.M.; Rees, J.E. The Effect of High Speed Compression At Sub-Atmospheric Pressures on the Capping Tendency of Pharmaceutical Tablets, J. Pharm. Pharmacol. **1983**, *35*, 44P.

31. Higuchi, T.; Nelson, E.; Busse, L.W. The Physics of Tablet Compression. 3. The Design and Construction of an Instrumented Tabletting Machine, J. Am. Pharm. Assn. Sci. Ed. **1954**, *43*, 344–348.

32. Murray, F.J. Tablet Press Automation: A Modular Approach to Fully Integrated Production, Drug Dev. Ind. Pharm. **1996**, *22* (1), 35–43.

33. Watt, P.R. *Tablet Machine Instrumentation in Pharmaceutics—Principles and Practice*; Ellis Horwood: Chichester, 1988.

34. Nelson, E.; Naqvi, S.M.; Busse, L.W.; Higuchi, T. The Physics of Tablet Compression. 4. Relationship of Ejection and Upper and Lower Punch Forces during the Compressional Process, J. Am. Pharm. Assn. Sci. Ed. **1954**, *43*, 596–602.

35. Akande, O.F.; Ford, J.F.; Rowe, P.H.; Rubinstein, M.H. The Effects of Lag-Time and Dwell-Time on the Compaction Properties of 1:1 Paracetamol/Microcrystalline Cellulose Mixtures Prepared by Precompression and Main Compression, J. Pharm. Pharmacol. **1998**, *50*, 19–28.

36. Munoz-Ruiz, A.; Jiminez-Castellanos, M.R.; Cunningham, J.C.; Katdare, A.V. Theoretical Estimation of Dwell and Consolidation Times in Rotary Tablet Machines, Drug Dev. Ind. Pharm. **1992**, *18* (19), 2011–2028.

37. Rudnick, A.; Hunter, A.R.; Holden, F.C. An Analysis of the Diametral Compression Test, Mater. Res. Stand. **1963**, *3*, 283–289.

38. Fell, J.T.; Newton, J.M. Determination of Tablet Strength by the Diametral Compression Test, J. Pharm. Sci. **1970**, *59* (5), 688–691.

39. Pitt, K.G.; Newton, J.M.; Richardson, R.; Stanley, P. Material Tensile Strength of Convex-Faced Aspirin Tablets, J. Pharm. Pharmacol. **1989**, *41*, 289–292.

40. Kawakita, K.; Ludde, K.H. Some Consideration on Powder Compression Equations, Powder Technol. **1970**, *4*, 61–68.

41. Heckel, R.W. Density-Pressure Relationships in Powder Compaction, Trans. Metall. Soc. AIME **1961**, *221*, 671–675.

42. Hersey, J.A.; Rees, J.E. Deformation of Particles during Briqueting, Nature **1971**, *230*, 96.

43. Paronen, P.; Illka, J. Porosity-Pressure Functions. *Pharmaceutical Powder Compaction Technology*; Alderborn, G., Nystrom, C. Eds.; Marcel Dekker, Inc.: New York, 1996; 55–75.

44. de Blaey, C.J.; Polderman, J. Compression of Pharmaceuticals. I the Quantitative Interpretation of Force-Displacement Curves, Pharm. Weekblad **1970**, *105*, 241–250.

45. de Blaey, C.J.; van Oudtshoorn, M.C.B.; Polderman, J. Compression of Pharmaceuticals. III. Study on Sulphadimidine, Pharm. Weekblad **1971**, *106*, 589–599.

46. Ragnarsson, G. Force-Displacement and Network Measurements. *Pharmaceutical Powder Compaction Technology*; Alderborn, G., Nystrom, C. Eds.; Marcel Dekker, Inc. New York, 1996; 77–97.

47. Armstrong, N.A.; Palfrey, L.P. The Effect of Machine Speed on the Consolidation of Four Directly Compressible Tablet Diluents, J. Pharm. Pharmacol. **1989**, *41*, 149–151.

48. Roberts, R.J.; Rowe, R.C. The Effect of Punch Velocity on the Compaction of a Variety of Materials, J. Pharm. Pharmacol. **1985**, *37*, 526–528.

49. Armstrong, N.A.; Abourida, N.M.A.H.; Gough, A.M. A Proposed Consolidation Parameter for Powders, J. Pharm. Pharmacol. **1983**, *35*, 320–321.

50. Rippie, E.G.; Danielson, D.W. Visco-Elastic Stress–Strain Behavior of Pharmaceutical Tablets: Analysis during Unloading and Postcompression Periods, J. Pharm. Sci. **1981**, *70* (5), 476–482.

51. Armstrong, N.A. Time-Dependent Factors Involved in Powder Compression and Tablet Manufacture, Int. J. Pharm. **1989**, *49*, 1–13.

TARGETED DRUG DELIVERY: MONOCLONAL ANTIBODIES AS DRUG TARGETING AGENTS

Ban-An Khaw

Northeastern University, Boston, Massachusetts

INTRODUCTION

The concept of targeted drug delivery may be considered to have originated with the proposed "magic bullet" of Paul Ehrlich for specific eradication of the spirochete of syphilis at the beginning of the 20th century (1). Yet this vision of targeted drug delivery did not begin until Pressman and Keighley in 1948 (2) demonstrated that radiolabeled antibodies could be specifically targeted to rat kidneys. Thus, antibodies became specific pharmaceuticals for targeting radioisotopes to various pathological disorders for diagnosis and therapy including various tumor. The next major thrust in the advancement of targeted drug delivery, using antibodies was provided by the revolutionary publication of Kohler and Milstein on monoclonal antibody technology (3). Monoclonal antibodies have since dominated the "targeting" in the targeted drug delivery systems.

The term targeted drug delivery conjures up a vision of a) a targeting moiety, and b) the drug to be targeted. The targeting moiety can be receptors, ligands, oligonucleotides, hormones, or antibodies. The drug to be targeted could be radioisotopes, pharmaceuticals, immunochemicals, chemicals, toxins, or biologicals. Thus, the concept of targeted drug delivery becomes almost all encompassing. Yet in practice, targeted drug delivery is somewhat restricted. Literature search of the term "targeted drug delivery" invariably resulted in the reference of articles relating to antibody mediated liposomes delivery system. Yet it should also include antibody, bispecific antibody, or avidin–biotin antibody delivery system. In oncology, antibodies may provide the primary targeting device for targeted drug delivery. Similarly antibodies form the primary targeting reagents in the cardiovascular applications. This chapter will restrict targeted drug delivery to targeting with antibodies and stress their appications in the cardiovascular arena, with cursory introductory review of the most pertinent targeting aspects in oncology.

ANTIBODIES IN CANCER IMAGING

Pressman and Keighley were the first to demonstrate that radioiodinated antibodies to normal rat kidneys targeted specifically to the kidneys in vivo (2). The potential for targeted delivery of radioiostopes for tumor therapy and diagnosis was immediately recognized by many investigators. However, progress for the next decade or so was disappointing due to lack of specific targets associated with tumors, pure antibodies for in vivo trials, and appropriate radiolabels for tagging the available antibodies. Never the less, Mach et al. (4), and Goldenberg et al. (5) succeeded in using polyclonal antibodies to carcinoembryonic antigen (CEA) to image carcinomas. Subsequently these same investigators used monoclonal antibodies to show that carcinomas can be imaged with radiolabeled anti-CEA antibodies (6, 7).

Since those early days of tumor imaging with immunoglobulin fractions, or affinity purified antibody fractions radiolabeled with I-131, monoclonal antibodies, and new and improved radiolabeling methods have enabled investigators to image breast (8), colon (9), lung (10), ovarian (11), and prostate cancers (12). Melanomas (13), T-cell lymphomas (14), pancreatic cancer (15), and indeed every form of cancer have been targeted with polyclonal or monoclonal antibodies in either experimental or clinical trails. Improvements in labeling with radioisotopes, such as Tc-99m, In-111, and I-123 to antibodies, have also led to better and more efficient gamma imaging. Further improvements in radioimmuniscintigraphy include use of bispecific monoclonal antibodies (16) and multistep avidin–biotin conjugated antibodies to reduce nontarget organ activities and enhanced target to background ratios (17).

In the therapeutic arena, antibodies have also been used for immunotherapy and radioimmunotherapy. Immunotherapy itself is essentially targeted drug therapy where specific antibody may activate complement, attract inflammatory cells, and/or induce production of cytokines, or as in the case of Herceptin inhibit cell growth by binding to ErbB2 that are overexpressed in metastatic breast cancer (18). Similarly, Rituxan is an antibody that binds to overexpressed CD20 in non-Hodgkins lymphoma (19) inducing apoptosis in these cancer cells (20). On the other hand, radioimmunotherapy may under certain oncologic conditions provide greater benefit. Use of murine–human chimeric monoclonal antibodies for targeting of ovarian cancer with β emitters for therapy has also been encouraging (21).

Immunotoxins consisting of tumor associated antigen specific antibody linked to the toxic chains of ricin, abrin, or other toxins have also been tested. Although phenomenal results in cancer therapy were anticipated, the progress has been disappointing. The only unequivocal success has been the in vitro treatment of bone marrow cells to rid them of malignant cells for subsequent injection into patients with hematological malignant cancer after whole body irradiation (22). Targeting of cancer cells with immuno-conjugates of target specific antibody covalently linked with drugs, such as doxorubicin, have also been undertaken (23). Other methods for targeted drug delivery include use of immunoliposomes for delivery to specific tumors (24).

Despite these novel methods for targeted drug delivery directed with monoclonal antibodies, monoclonal antibodies have not totally met the expectations of the "magic bullet" of Paul Elrlich in oncology. Therefore, apart from diagnostic imaging with radiolabeled monoclonal antibodies and direct immunotherapy, other innovative targeted drug delivery systems have had only limited clinical success.

TARGETED DRUG DELIVERY IN THE CARDIOVASCULAR SYSTEM

As indicated above, antibodies can provide target specificity as well as function as carriers of those drugs for targeted delivery. Whether the drug to be delivered is a radioisotope for imaging or therapy, or an antimetabolyte, the prototypical model exemplified will be the radiolabeled antibodies for targeted drug delivery.

The application of antibodies in cardiovascular targeting in vivo originated with the experimental demonstration of the feasibility of using radiolabeled antimyosin antibody for diagnosis of acute myocardial infarction in 1976 (25). Since then, the use of antibodies in the cardiovascular system has encompassed imaging of myocarditis (26), heart transplant rejection (27), dilated cardiomyopathy (28), alcohol induced cardiomyopathy (29), adriamycin cardiotoxicity (30), various other cardiomyopathies (31), vascular clots (32), atherosclerotic lesions (33), and even

certain cancers such as soft tissue sarcomas (34). Yet the best characterized and studied antibody for cardiovascular diagnostic targeting is monoclonal antimyosin Fab for its exquisite specificity in the detection of myocardial cell death associated with various forms of cardiomyopathies.

Targeted Delivery of Radiolabeled Antimyosin Antibody in Acute Myoardial Infarction

To enable targeted delivery of any drug, there must be target specific structures not present on normal nontarget organs or cells that can be recognized by the targeting reagents, or neostructures must be exposed during the development of the pathological conditions. Since the cell membrane of normal cardiac cells are composed of the same lipid bilayer as that found in necrotic cells, one cannot envision a target specific cell membrane structure that is present only on the membranes of necrotic cells. However, it is reasonable to assume that structures such as the cardiac myofilaments are not exposed to the extracellular environment in viable cardiocyte, but following myocardial necrosis they would become exposed to the extracellular milieu (35). Therefore, such structures should provide new targets for delineation of the necrotic from nonnecrotic myocardium. Anticardiac myosin antibody was chosen as the model targeting moiety for the delivery of the model drug for diagnostic imaging of acute myocardial infarction (25). The above hypothesis was validated using hypoxic neonatal murine myocytes in primary cultures treated with antimyosin antibody attached covalently to 1 μm diameter polystyrene beads, where the beads prepresented potential drugs for targeting (35). Normal myocytes with intact sarcolemma prevented accumulation of antimyosin beads (Fig. 1a) whereas hypoxic myocytes with sarcolemmal lesions were targeted by antimyosin beads at the lesions sites (Fig. 1b). Upon higher magnification (×100,000), targeting of the beads can be discerned as the myofilaments are seen wrapped around the antimyosin-beads (Fig. 1c). Such specific targeting of the necrotic myocardium can also be demonstrated in vivo in experimental and clinical situations by gamma imaging technology.

To establish without equivocation that antimyosin Fab can target the necrotic myocardium with highest specificity, a mixture antimyosin antibody labeled with I-125 and normal IgG labeled with I-131 was administered by intracoronary delivery into dogs with experimental acute myocardial infarction (36). Targeting of both radiolabeled immunoglobulin species was assessed by gamma scintillation counting (36). I-125 labeled antimyosin antibody localized in the necrotic myocardium with a target to nontarget ratio of ≃ 32:1 at the infarct center, whereas

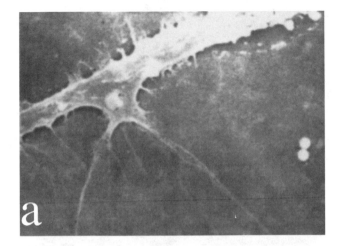

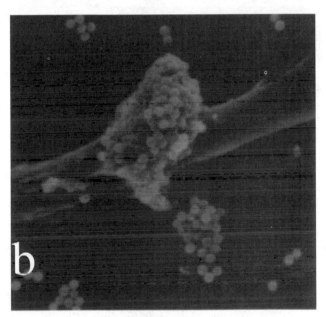

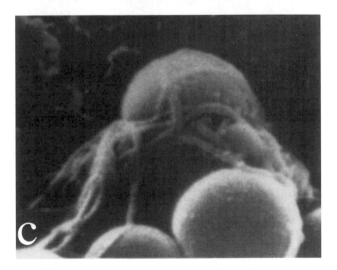

nonspecific localization was only about 6.5:1 in the same tissue samples (36). Similarly, in vivo demonstration of the specificity of antimyosin antibody for the necrotic myocardium was performed with antimyosin Fab (Fig. 2A) and nonspecific Fab radiolabeled with In-111 (Fig. 2B). Dogs with experimental acute myocardial infarction injected with In-111 labeled antimyosin Fab showed in vivo localization of the radiolabel conjugated to antimyosin Fab in the infarct. The nonspecific Fab control also radiolabeled with In-111 did not localize in the infarcted region of the myocardium in control infarcted dogs (37).

To further demonstrate the exquisite specificity of antimyosin for targeting acute myocardial infarction, two monoclonal antimyosin antibodies, one with high and the other with low affinity, were employed to visualize canine acute myocardial infarction. The low affinity antimyosin Fab (3H31E6) despite being specific for myosin, with an apparent affinity of $\simeq 6.5 \times 10^6$ L/mole, showed no in vivo targeting of the radiolabeled antibody even at 5 h after antibody administration (Fig. 2D). On-the-other-hand, with the higher apparent affinity antimyosin Fab (R11D10) (1×10^9 L/mole), the infarct may be visualized as early as 1 hour but unequivocally some time later after intravenous administration (Fig. 2C) (37). The ratios of target (T) to blood pool (B) activities of the in vivo gamma images were determined by computer planimetry to be 1.7 ± 0.38 (mean ± SD) for R11D10 Fab, which was significantly greater than that of 3H31E6 Fab (0.85 ± 0.12). The latter was the same as the T/B ratios obtained with nonspecific Fab (0.75–0.771) (37). Another monoclonal antimyosin Fab (2G42D7) with an apparent affinity similar to R11D10 also provided T/B ratio of 1.5 + 0.27 ($p = 0.13$). These studies confirmed that not only is antimyosin specific for targeting acute myocardial necrosis, the requirement of sufficiently high affinity for successful in vivo visualization makes this targeting phenomenon exquisitely target specific.

Similarly, gamma images of patients with persistently occluded left anterior descending coronary artery (LAD) and another with reperfused LAD injected with In-111 labeled monoclonal antimyosin R11D10 Fab (38) showed

Fig. 1 Scanning electron micrographs of murine neonatal primary myocytes in culture treated with antimyosin linked 1μ diameter fluorescent polystyrene beads. a) A normal myocyte showing the intact cell membrane and a lack of antimyosin-bead binding. b) A necrotic myocyte with a region of sarcolemmal disruption showing antimyosin-bead binding in that region. c) 100,000 times magnification of the region of cell membrane disruption showing antimyosin-beads wrapped around by the myofilaments that contain myosin.

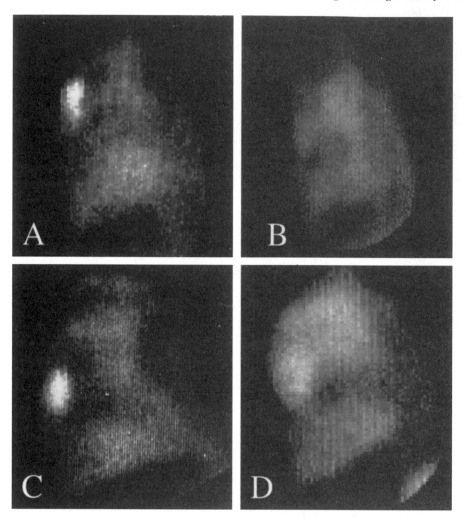

Fig. 2 Gamma images of four dogs with acute experimental myocardial infarction, injected with high affinity ^{111}In-labeled antimyosin Fab (Ka = 0.5–1 × 10⁹ L/M) (A and C), ^{111}In-labeled nonspecific monoclonal Fab (B) and the low affinity ^{111}In labeled 3H3 antimyosin Fab (Ka = 5 × 10⁶ L/M) (D). At 5 h post intravenous administration of these antibodies, only the images with high affinity antimyosin showed unequivocal infarct uptake, whereas the images with nonantimyosin specific monoclonal Fab and the low affinity antimyosin Fab showed only blood pool activity. (From Ref. 37.)

unequivocal targeting of the radiopharmaceutical in the region of the hearts corresponding to the areas subtended by the occluded coronary vessels (Fig. 3). In patients with no infarction, no targeting of radioactivity in the myocardial region was obtained.

Despite the ability of antimyosin Fab to specifically delineate acute myocardial infarction, its utility is hampered by the slow blood clearance of the Fab fragments (38). This causes delayed development of high enough target to background ratios for in vivo visualization by gamma scintigraphy, especially in clinical use to >12 h after intravenous administration. Usually, images were acquired 18–24 h after IV administration, however, small MI may require 48 h of blood clearance to enable

unequivocal diagnosis. If on the other hand, qualitative diagnostic end-point is the desired outcome, irrespective of visual confirmation of the infarct size, then infarcts may be detected rather early after intravenous antibody administration over and above the blood pool activity (39). These rate-limiting steps may be overcome by using smaller antibody fragments, such as sFv (40), CDR (41), and mimetics (42). However, by increasing the clearance rate, there is a concomitant decrease in the absolute available antibody for target localization. Therefore, we developed a new approach to improve target to background ratios in experimental myocardial infarct visualization by decreasing the background activity without affecting the target activity at any time point.

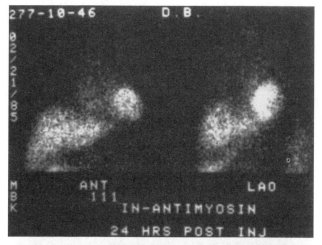

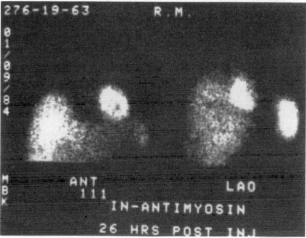

Fig. 3 Anterior and 45° LAO images of two patient with acute MI at 24 and 26 h after intravenous administration of In-111 labeled antimyosin Fab. Images of a patient with persistently occluded LAD (no reperfusion) (top) and those of a patient with successful reperfusion (bottom). (From Ref. 38.)

ENHANCING IN VIVO TARGETED DRUG DELIVERY WITH NEGATIVE CHARGE-MODIFIED MONOCLONAL ANTIBODIES

Since antibodies are basic glycoproteins, under physiological conditions they are positively charged (43). Cells and extracellular matrices, on the other hand are negatively charged due to the presence of cell membrane bound acidic residues such as sialic acids (44,45) and heparan sulfate proteoglycans (46), respectively. Therefore, the potential for nonspecific ionic interaction between the positively charged molecules and the negatively charged cell surfaces or extracellular matrices exists. Such nonspecific interaction has been utilized to deliver methotrexate–polylysine conjugates to malignant cells (47), protracted release of basic fibroblast growth factor for the salvage of the infarcted myocardium (46), as well as for the delivery of genetic constructs by lipofection or cationic liposomes (48). Alternatively, we proposed that if the basic (positively charged) antibodies were to be modified to carry a highly anionic polymer so that the isoelectric point of the modified antibody becomes low (e.g., PI < 5), then this modified antibody should have reduced nonspecific ionic interaction with nontarget cells and extracellular matrices (49). However, the affinity of the antibody at $\simeq 1 \times 10^9$ L/mole can easily overcome the repulsive ionic forces when the charge-modified antibody approaches its homologous antigen. This would permit the same targeting of the charge-modified antibody as with the noncharge modified antibody due to the same antigenic specificity and affinity, but should result in lower nontarget background activity and thereby allow earlier development of high enough target to background ratios for visualization of the target (49). Furthermore, since negatively charged diethylene triamine pentaacetic acid chelate modified polymers are used, very high specific radioactivity radiolabeled antibody preparations can be prepared.

Antimyosin Fab was covalently modified with multi-DTPA conjugated polylysine that has been made totally anionic by succinylation (50). The immunoreactivity of the negatively-charge-modified AM-Fab carrying a polymer of approximate 3.3 or 17 kD was identical to that of the unmodified AM-Fab (50). When these negative charge-modified AM-Fab preparations were labeled with In-111, a specific radioactivity of 50–100 mCi/mg AM-Fab was obtained. The specific radioactivity of the conventional AM-Fab was only 2–10 mCi/mg AM-Fab. Thus, less negative charge-modified AM-Fab was needed to deliver the same radioactivity relative to the conventional dose. When the negative charge-modified AM-Fab was administered into dogs with reperfused experimental MI, myocardial infarcts were visualized within 30 min of intravenous administration of the antibody preparation (Fig. 4), whereas the conventional In-111 labeled AM-Fab required 1–2 h of antibody circulation and clearance before infarcts were visualized.

This earlier target visualization could be, as stated previously, due to quicker development of high target to background ratios for visualization by gamma imaging, which requires a ratio of about 10:1. It could also be due to a new concept developed in our laboratory where visualization could be achieved not based on target to background ratios, but on the absolute difference in the radioactivity between target and background (51). Assuming that the same amount (500 µg) of charged

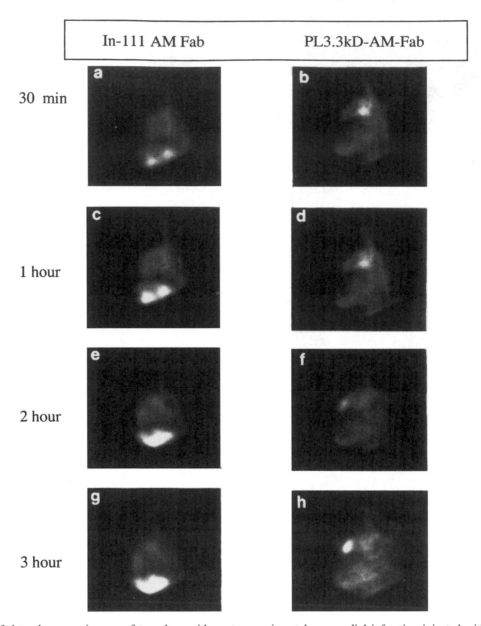

Fig. 4 Serial left lateral gamma images of two dogs with acute experimental myocardial infarction injected with negative charge-modified In-111 labeled antimyosin Fab (right panels) and conventionally In-111 labeled antimyosin Fab (left panels); a and b = 30 min images, c and d = 1h, e and f = 2h, and g and h = 3h post intravenous administration. (From Ref. 50.)

modified and unmodified antimyosin Fab radiolabeled with In-111, were injected into dogs with experimental MI, and at 5 h post injection there were 0.1718 ± 0.0201%ID/g (52) of negative-charge modified antimyosin Fab in the infarct, since the specific radioactivity of negative-charge modified antimyosin Fab was 100 mCi/mg, the absolute radioactivity in 1 g of infarct would be 85.9 μCi. On the other hand, 500 μg of unmodified antimyosin Fab with a specific radioactivity of

5 mCi/mg with 0.2041 ± 0.0204%ID/g would only have 5 μCi/g of the infarcted myocardium. Since normal myocardial activities were 0.0056 ± 0.0004%ID/g with charge-modified antimyosin Fab and 0.0263 ± 0.0037%ID/g with unmodified antimyosin Fab, the absolute background radioactivities were 2.8 and 0.658 μCi, respectively. Therefore, the difference between target and background for charge-modified antimyosin Fab would be 83.1 μCi and the ratio between

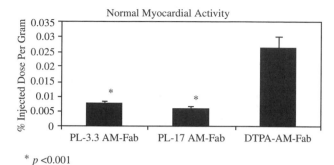

Fig. 5 Normal myocardial activity of polymer modified antimyosin Fab and conventionally In-111 labeled antimyosin Fab. (From Ref. 50.)

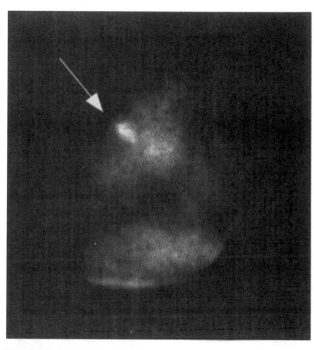

Fig. 6 Left lateral gamma image of a rabbit with a 216 mg experimental myocardial infarct visualized with In-111 labeled negative charge-modified antimyosin Fab. Arrow points to the small infarct visualized in vivo. (From Ref. 52.)

target to background would be 30.7:1. The difference in the absolute activity between target and background on the other hand for unmodified antimyosin Fab would be only 4.34 μCi and the ratio 7.6:1. Therefore, with a differential of 83 μCi/g between target to background, one should be able to clearly visualize the target quite early, whereas a differential of 4.34 μCi may not permit easy early visualization.

To determine whether earlier visualization was due to increased infarct activity or decreased nontarget organ activities, biodistribution data were also compared. Figure 5 shows that even in the normal myocardium (nontarget tissue), the radioactivity was significantly lower for 3.3 and 17 kD negative charge-modified polymer-AM-Fab than that of the conventionally labeled AM-Fab ($p < 0.001$) (50). The applicability of negative charge modification was further demonstrated in a rabbit model where an infarct as small as 216 mg was visualized by in vivo imaging within 3 h after intravenous administration (Fig. 6) (52). The percent injected dose localization in this animal was as high as 1.73% ID/g providing ≃ 86.3 μCi/g of the target. The mean maximal target to nontarget (minimal) ratio from the seven rabbits was 53.9 ± 18.4 (52).

Therefore, negative charge modification of AM-Fab not only imparted lower nontarget organ activity without affecting the target activity, it also provided antibody preparations with very high specific radioactivity enabling the use of less proteinaceous compounds for in vivo administration. Furthermore, it also showed that when high target activity is achieved, visualization was possible earlier based on the difference between target and background activities, rather than target to background ratios. Whether this process of negative charge modification will ever find clinical application may not be determined by scientific feasibility but more by

commercial considerations. Nevertheless, a murine–human chimeric antibody F(ab')$_2$ specific for proliferating smooth muscle cells associated with atherosclerotic lesions has been negatively charge modified, labeled with In-111 and shown to localize in the carotid artery atherosclerotic lesions in all nine patients studied to date (53).

Antimyosin is highly specific and sensitive for diagnosis of myocardial necrosis associated with acute myocardial infarction. Despite its requirement of approximately 24 h lag time for unequivocal diagnostic imaging, it is highly useful for diagnosis of equivocal myocardial infarction, myocardial necrosis associated with unstable angina, right ventricular infarction (54), and perioperative myocardial infarction in by-pass surgery (55).

ANTIMYOSIN IMAGING IN DIAGNOSIS OF VARIOUS CARDIOMYOPATHIES

Myocarditis

Myocarditis is a cardiomyopathy of highly variable clinical manifestations that can in more severe cases, lead to dilated cardiomyopathy and heart failure (56).

It is believed to have a viral origin but the chronic component of the etiology is believed to be autoimmnue in nature. To unify the diagnosis of the disease, the Dallas Criteria were formulated (57). The criteria mandated the presence of mononuclear cell infiltration and myonecrosis demonstrated in endomyocardial biopsies for unequivocal diagnosis of myocarditis. However, the criteria focused only at a limited phase of myocarditogenesis. Irrespective of the inflammatory obligatory component of the criteria, the presence of myonecrosis led us to propose that antimyosin immunoscintigraphy should be able to target the myonecrotic component of the disease and provide a very sensitive diagnostic indicator for noninvasive diagnosis of myocarditis. In the initial study of 28 patients with histories and clinical findings suggestive of myocarditis, In-111 antimyosin immunoscintigraphy was positive in 17 patients (61%) (Fig. 7, left panel) and negative in 11 (39%) (Fig. 7, right panel) (26). All antimyosin negative patients were also negative by endomyocardial biopsy criteria, whereas all biopsy positive patients were also positive by biopsy criteria (26). A potential complication in the use of In-111 antimyosin Fab for diagnosis of acute myocarditis is the misinterpretation of residual blood pool activity for myocardial uptake. Since myonecrosis associate with myocarditis is generally diffused and not as intense as seen in acute myocardial infarction, uptake of In-111 labeled antimyosin could also be diffused and of low contrast. Therefore, it is recommended that single photon emission tomographic imaging be performed in case of equivocation. The tomographic reconstruction images in the transverse, sagittal, and coronal views should show myocardial activities rather than blood pool activities.

Dilated Cardiomyopathy

It has been clinically suspected that active myocarditis is capable of resulting in heart failure and acute dilated cardiomyopathy. Although the exact number of cases of active myocarditis or ongoing inflammation that ultimately resulted in ideopathic cardiomyopathy is not known. Dec et al. (28) studied 74 patients (50 men and 24 women) with dilated cardiomyopathy with global ejection fraction less than 0.45 with In-111 antimyosin Fab. Thirty-nine patients (53%) were positive by imaging criteria. Of these 39, 11 patients had histologically verified myocarditis, whereas 28 showed no evidence of myocarditis on biopsy. Out of the remaining 35 patients with normal antimyosin images, 33 were also negative by endomyocardial biopsy criteria. However, two were false negative since they had biopsy verified myocarditis. Thus, the sensitivity of antimyosin imaging was 85% and the predictive value of a normal scan was 94%. However, the specificity was only 54%, using the Dallas Criteria as the gold standard. This low specificity is most probably due to the need to use a Gold Standard that is highly insensitive and because myocarditis is a disease of either right or left or both ventricles, and endomyocardial biopsies are primarily obtained from the right ventricles. Irrespective of this low specificity of antimyosin imaging for diagnosis of myocarditis, patients with abnormal antimyosin scan and biopsy results showed significant improvement in the mean ejection fraction form 0.27 ± 0.02 to 0.43 ± 0.04 within 6 months follow-up examination. Whereas, patients with normal scans and nondiagnostic biopsy results had only slight improvement in the ejection fraction from 0.19 ± 0.02 to 0.24 ± 0.03. Furthermore,

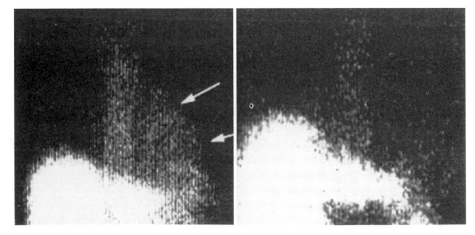

Fig. 7 In-111 Antimyosin gamma images of two patients suspected of having myocarditis: a) positive image (left panel), and b) a negative image (right panel). The arrows point the myocardial activity.

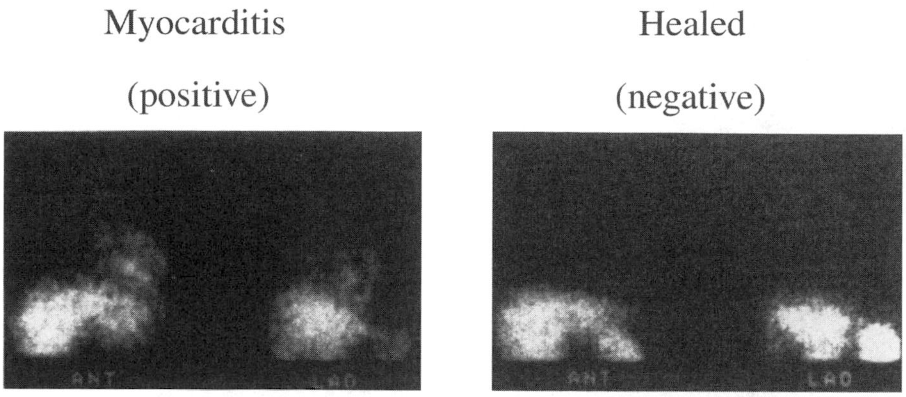

Myocarditis

(positive)

Healed

(negative)

Fig. 8 Planar anterior and LAO In-111 antimyosin gamma images of a patient with biopsy positivity for myocarditis obtained initially when the left ventricular ejection fraction was only 34% (left panels) and after 6 months of steroid therapy (right panels) when the LVEF had normalized to 55% are shown.

those patients with positive antimyosin scans and negative biopsy results showed significant improvement in ejection fraction at follow-up indicating that since spontaneous improvement in cardiac function is a recognized feature of active myocarditis, the subset of patients with antimyosin scan positivity and spontaneous improvement in the cardiac function had myocarditis, which biopsy failed to detect. Negative antimyosin imaging can also be used to follow efficacy of therapy. Fig. 8 shows that although the initial antimyosin images were positive, after 6 months of steroid therapy, the images were negative for myonecrosis component of the Dallas Criteria.

Heart Transplant Rejection

Since commencement of immunosuppressive treatments for acute heart transplant rejection is predicated on the presence of myonecrosis on endomyocardial biopsies, antimyosin imaging should also be applicable for directing therapy. Frist et al. (58) showed that antimyosin could be used to detect myonecrosis associated with acute rejection. However, they also noted that immediately after transplantation, there appeared to be a basal uptake of In-111 labeled antimyosin Fab probably due to myocardial injury associated with transplantation related procedures. Subsequently Ballester et al. showed systematically that this initial antimyosin positivity could return to baseline as quickly as 3 months after transplantation (59). Furthermore, they showed that if antimyosin uptake assessed as Heart to Lung activity ratios remained elevated for greater than 1 year after transplantation, prognosis for the patient was poor and that patient was

a prime candidate for re-transplantation. Various degrees of intensity of In-111 antimyosin uptake were shown in Fig. 9, ranging form normal antimyosin scan (A), to mild uptake (B), to moderate uptake (C), to significant uptake (D) (60).

Antimyosin imaging appears to be highly sensitive for the detection of acute heart transplant rejection. Relative to the gold standard of endomyocardial biopsy, antimyosin has a sensitivity of 95% (61), however, specificity was only 33%. This discrepancy may be due to a lack of specificity of antimyosin or to a low sensitivity of biopsy in the detection of rejection. However, sampling error of endomyocardial biopsy is a distinct possibility that may account for the discrepancy since transplant rejection is histologically a patchy process. Therefore, if antimyosin were taken as the gold standard, then the sensitivity and specificity of endo-myocardial biopsy would be 31 and 95%, respectively (61). This is consistent with the low diagnostic yield of endomyocardial biopsy reported for the diagnosis of active myocarditis (62, 63)

Other Cardiomyopathies

Due to the mechanism of targeting of antimyosin Fab, it appears that antimyosin could also be used to delineate various cardiomyopathies as long as there is an association of the disease process with irreversible myocardial injury where the integrity of the cell membrane has been compromised. Therefore, antimyosin Fab has been used successfully to demonstrate myocardial injury due to Adriamycin cardiotoxicity (64), in Rheumatic carditis (65), in Lyme carditis (66), Churg–Strauss disease (67) and Cardiac contusion (68).

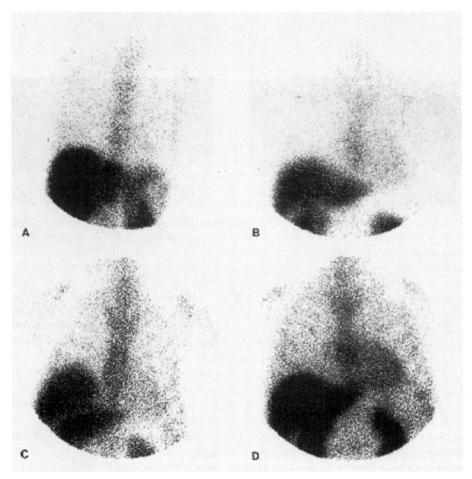

Fig. 9 Anterior gamma images of patients with various degrees of rejection detected by In-111 antimyosin imaging. A = normal scan, B = mild uptake, C = moderate uptake and D = significant uptake. (From Ref. 60.)

TARGETING VASCULAR DISORDERS WITH RADIOLABELED ANTIBODIES

Imaging Blood Clots

Attempts to image blood clots preceded the era of monoclonal antibodies. Spar et al. used polyclonal antifibrinogen antibodies to detect thrombi in vivo in the mid 1960s (69). Since the antibody reacted with fibrinogen as well as fibrin, the specificity for the detection of preformed clots was poor. Hui et al. in 1983 (70) developed monoclonal antibodies (59D8 and 64C5) specific for the β chain of the fibrin molecule. They were made to a 7 amino acid N-terminal sequence of the β chain of fibrin. Since the N-terminus of the β chain of fibrin constitutes neoantigen generated when fibrinogen is cleaved by thrombin, these monoclonal antibodies did not cross react with fibrinogen. Kudryk et al. (71) also generated a similar monoclonal antifibrin T2G1S that

also reacted with the same N-terminal of the β chain of fibrin. Although there are other monoclonal antibodies with varying specificities for fibrin, only 59D8 and T2G1S have seen clinical studies. Fig. 10 (left panel) shows a 24-h-image of the lower extremities of a normal subject, whereas Fig. 10 (right panel) shows a set of spot images in a patient with venographically documented DVT.

It appears that imaging DVT was quite easily feasible in experimental and clinical trials. Whether imaging of pulmonary emboli in a clinical situation with monoclonal antifibrin antibody would be successful is not known. Experimentally, Kanke et al. (72) showed that 64C5 monoclonal antifibrin was able to image PE. However, small PE of <50 mg were not visualized in vivo by gamma imaging despite a correlation between clot size and total antifibrin uptake. Further improvements are needed to make this method of detection of DVT or PE a clinical reality.

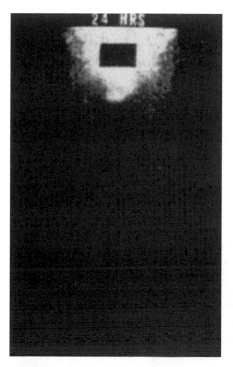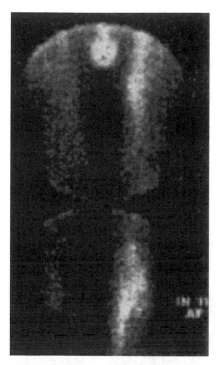

Fig. 10 Anterior gamma images of normal control (left) and patient with DVT (right) with Tc-99m labeled antifibrin Fab. Radiolabeled antifibrin uptake can be seen in the left thigh and calf regions. (From Ref. 32.)

Targeting Atherosclerotic Lesions with Radiolabeled Antibodies

Atherosclerosis is another intravascular pathological disorder that appears to be amenable to targeting with monoclonal antibodies. It was initially thought that atherosclerotic lesions possessed no unique compounds that could serve as specific targets. These lesions are composed of macrophages that had become foam cells by the ingestion of oxidized LDL, and smooth muscles cells of the synthetic phenotype. No differentiated antigens were thought to exist in the lesions. Therefore, conventional modes of diagnosis, such as arteriography or ultrasonography, were believed to suffice for providing information on the anatomical narrowing of the affected vessels. Although these methods are effective, they cannot provide pathophysiologic information that may shed light on the stability as well as the pathogenesis of the lesions.

To elucidate the potential metabolic component of the pathogenesis of atherosclerotic lesions, several approaches have been taken experimentally. Radiolabeled oxidized LDL (73) as well as antibodies to the activated macrophages (74) have been tried with some

results. A monoclonal antibody that is specific for a complex antigen produced only by the proliferating smooth muscle cells of atherosclerotic lesions was developed by Scotgen Biopharmaceuticals, Inc. (75). This IgM isotype antibody designated Z2D3 (76) was shown to be able to target experimental atherosclerotic lesions in a rabbit model (77). The IgM subclass of Z2D3 was class switched to IgG as well as genetically engineered to produce a murine–human chimeric IgG Z2D3 antibody. Fig. 11 (top panel) shows a set of gamma images of a rabbit with experimental atherosclerotic lesions targeted with In-111 labeled chimeric Z2D3 F(ab')$_2$. The lesions could be visualized in the region of the descending aorta that was the site of experimentally induced lesions. In this model, the lesions were induced by de-endothelialization of the descending aorta from the region of the diaphragm to the bifurcation of the femoral arteries (75). The rabbits were kept on 6% peanut oil, 2% cholesterol enriched chow for at least 3 months. This protocol produced lesions that are more akin to human fibrous lesions, unlike the fatty streak lesions observed in Watanabi hyperlipidemic rabbits. As controls, rabbits with similar lesions were injected with In-111 labeled charge-modified normal human IgG F(ab')$_2$ (Fig. 11, lower panels). No specific targeting was seen in vivo in

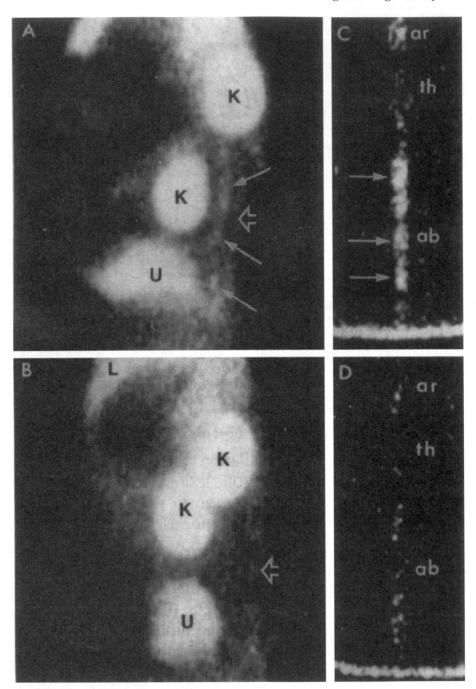

Fig. 11 Left lateral oblique images of rabbits with experimental atherosclerotic lesions induced in the descending aorta imaged with In-111 labeled murine-human chimeric Z2D3 F(ab')$_2$ (Top panels) and In-111 labeled human IgG F(ab')$_2$ (Bottom panels). The in vivo gamma images are shown in the left panels (k = kidney, U = urinary bladder activity, solid thin arrows = atherosclerotic lesions, and open larger arrow = spinal activity), and the ex vivo images of the excised aortas from the aortic arch to the femoral bifurcation are shown in the right panels.

the region of the experimental lesions. Immunohistologically, this antibody stains the region of smooth muscle cell proliferation and not the quiscent smooth muscles of the contractile phenotype of the media (Fig. 12). Ultimately, the negative charge-modified chimeric Z2D3 F(ab')$_2$ was used to determine whether

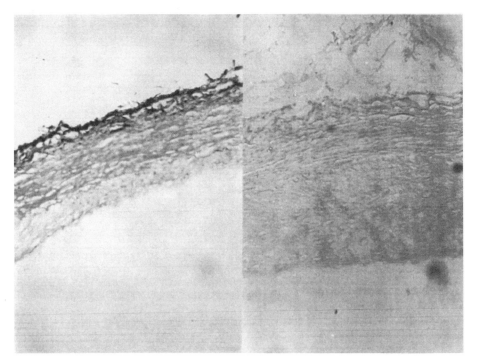

Fig. 12   Immunoperoxidase staining of frozen sections of atherosclerotic rabbit descending aorta (left panel) and normal rabbit aorta (right panel).

it could delineate atherosclerotic lesions in carotid lesions in patients (78). Using planar and SPECT imaging, it was observed that the lesions were better detected with SPECT imaging (Fig. 13) (79). Whether this antibody Z2D3 will have wide clinical application must await additional trials.

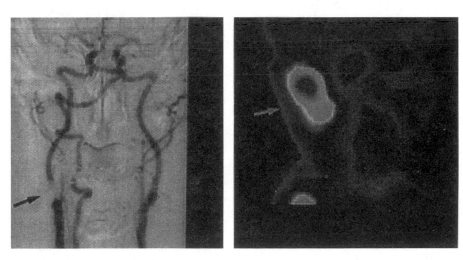

Fig. 13   Coronal tomographic image of a patient with carotid atherosclerotic lesions obtained 4 h after IV administration of In-111 labeled negative-charge modified murine–human chimeric Z2D3 F(ab')$_2$ (right panel). The arrow denotes the carotid lesion. The acrotid angiogram demonstrating a severe right internal carotid artery lesion (arrow) is shown in the left panel).

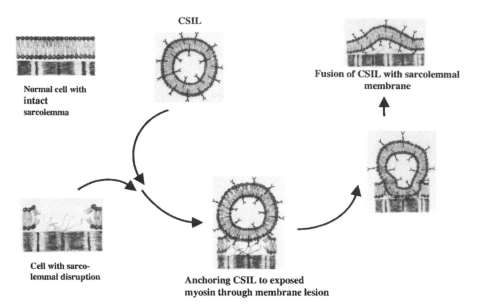

Fig. 14 Diagrammatic representation of the hypothesized mechanism of cell membrane sealing and salvage by antimyosin liposomes. (Adapted From Ref. 84.)

TARGETING CELL MEMBRANE LESION WITH CYTOSKELETAL-ANTIGEN SPECIFIC IMMUNOLIPOSOMES

Two primary kinds of cell deaths are now known to exist in the animal kingdom. Oncotic (formerly known as necrotic) and apoptotic cell deaths differ in that the former is due to external nonphysiological injury to the cell (80) and the latter "apoptosis is due to internally mandated process of suicide cell attrition or programmed cell death known" (81). Under pathological conditions of an ischemic insult to organs, such as the heart and the brain, the primary mode of cell death in the center of infarction is oncotic (82). Apoptosis plays a role in the periphery and in reperfused regions (83). Acute myocardial infarction is believed to be the result of oncosis, where development of cell membrane lesions constitute the irreversible phase. The presence of these lesions, which is initially represented by submicroscopic holes in the sarcolemma in the acute phase of myocardial injury, permits washout of intracellular macromolecules into the circulation. At the same time, certain intracellular proteins including the components of the cytoskeleton, such as myosin and vimentin, become exposed through these holes to the surroundings milieur. Appropriately labeled antibodies against intracellular cytoskeletal antigens have been used to demarcate these cell membrane lesions (25).

Therefore, we hypothesized that if these cell membrane lesions could be sealed at the time or prior to reperfusion, then viability of myocardial cells should be preserved (84). To achieve cell membrane lesion sealing, we proposed that liposomes would be the ideal agent. However, the liposomes must be provided with target recognition sites that are specific for the lesions in the cell membrane. To achieve this, a monoclonal antibody that specifically recognizes myosin of the myofilaments that constitutes the cytoskeleton of the muscle cells was used. Thus, antimyosin immunoliposomes should be able to target the cytoskeletal myosin exposed through the small lesions of the cell membrane during the process of ischemic injury before the lesions become too large for repair (Fig. 14).

Preservation of Cell Viability by Cytoskeleton-specific Immunoliposomes

Proof of concept studies were performed in vitro in cell cultures of H9C2 rat embryonic cardiocytes. Two million H9C2 cardiocytes were incubated in aliquots of 10% fetal calf serum in DMEM at 37°C, 5% CO2. After overnight incubation, the cells were washed in phosphate-buffered saline and recultured in fresh medium (with or without different liposome preparations) (84). Nitrogen was bubbled through the medium vigorously for 4 min dislodging all cells (>95%) from the bottom of the flasks. The flasks were then closed tightly to maintain hypoxia

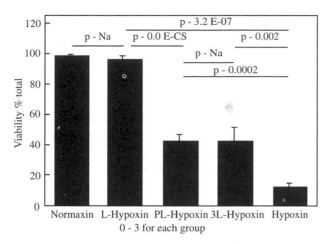

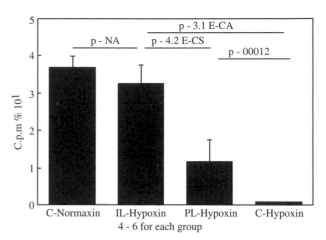

Fig. 15 Comparison of cell viability of H9C2 cardiocytes in culture by Trypan Blue dye uptake criteria. Viability of hypoxic (24 h) cells treated the IL were compared to PL or IgG-liposome. Positive control was the normoxic cultures and the negative control was hypoxic cells with no treatment. (From Ref. 84.)

Fig. 16 Comparison of cell viability of H9C2 cardiocytes by ^{3}H-Thymidine uptake criteria. Viability of hypoxic cells (24 h) treated with IL was compared to Normoxic cells (p = NS), PL treated hypoxic cells ($p < 0.01$) and untreated hypoxic cells ($p < 0.01$). (From Ref. 84.)

through overnight incubation at 37°C. H9C2 cardiocytes in hypoxic culture conditions were incubated with anti-myosin-immunoliposomes (IL), plain liposomes (PL) and control nonspecific IgG liposomes (IgL). Hypoxic and normoxic cardiocytes without liposome treatment were included as additional controls. Liposomes were prepared from a mixture of egg phosphatidylcholine and cholesterol at a molar ratio of 7:3. For incorporation of antimyosin antibody 2G42D7 into liposomes, the antibody was modified with N-glutaryl phosphatidyl ethanolamine (NGPE) (85,86) and added to the detergent-solubilized lipids. Liposome preparations containing fluorescent rhodamin-labeled lipids were also used for fluorescent microscopy and confocal microscopy (84).

At the end of the hypoxic period, viability of the cells were assessed by the Trypan Blue dye exclusion criteria. Fig. 15 demonstrated that the viability of hypoxic cells treated with IL were not significantly different form the viability of the normoxically cultured H9C2 cardiocytes. The viability of hypoxic cardiocytes treated with plain liposomes or IgG-liposomes was significantly lower than either those of immunoliposome treated hypoxic cells or normoxica cells. Since there was no difference in viability in cardiocytes treated with PL or IgG-liposomes, subsequent studies utilized only PL treatment as control. The phenomenon of preservation of cell viability with IL treatment was reaffirmed by ^{3}H-thymidine uptake studies (84). DNA replication as reflected by ^{3}H-thymidine uptake, was similar in the normoxic cells and the hypoxic cells treated with IL. However, cells treated with PL had only about 10% of ^{3}H-thymidine

uptake of either the normoxic or IL treated hypoxic cells. Hypoxic cells with no treatment at all showed almost no

Fig. 17 Epifluorescent micrographs of 24 h hypoxic H9C2 cardiocytes treated with rhodamine labeled IL (right) or rhodamine labeled PL (left). Cells treated with IL were all viable; however, they all showed attached rhidamine fluorescent indicating attachment of IL to the cells. (From Ref. 84.)

[3]H-thymidine uptake, indicative of a lack of viable cells (Fig. 16).

The sites of targeting of IL on hypoxic cardiocytes was visualized by fluorescent microscopy, using rhodamine labeled antimyosin immunoliposomes. Fig. 17 shows that only cells treated with antimyosin–rhodamine labeled IL were still confluent in the culture and that almost all cells were labeled with fluoresent liposomes. Those cells treated with rhodamine labeled PL showed extremely sparse number of cells still attached to the culture plates at 24 h of incubation, with essentially no or minimal fluorescence. Confocal microscopic examination of the cultures treated with rhodamine labeled IL showed that the cells still retained their morphology and shape with scattered fluorescent liposomes attached to the cell membranes (Fig. 18, left panel). Those cells treated with rhodamine labeled PL were shrunken and only a few random cells showed some nonspecific attachment of fluorescent PL (Fig. 18, right panel). In this study, untreated hypoxic cells were all dead and since there was no fluorescent compounds added in them, no micrographs were obtained.

It is also very important, how efficacious this protective effect can last. Therefore, we undertook a study to determine whether antimyosin IL can protect severely injured cardiocytes cultured under hypoxic conditions for 1–5 days (87). The experiment was designed as already described, however, cells were kept under hypoxic conditions during different times. Cell viability was assessed by ^{3}H-Thymidine (^{3}H-T) uptake. Untreated hypoxic cardiocytes (HC), normoxic cardiocytes (NC), and cardiocytes treated with PL were used as controls. Survival of NC increased from 100% (the mean ^{3}H-T uptake in control NC was assigned 100%) to ca. 250%

after 24 h indicative of cell replication, whereas virtually no cardiocytes survived after 24 h of hypoxia. PL added to HC provided some protection. Cell viability after 24 h was ca. 78%, which dropped to ca. 4% after 2 days of hypoxia, and to less than 1% after 3 or more days. However, when hypoxic cells were treated with IL, not only did IL conferred protection, IL also permitted cell replication. This is evidenced by the similarity in the increase of [3]HT uptake after 24 h in NC (250%) and in IL-treated HC (ca. 225%, p = NS). These data show that the protective effect imparted by IL on hypoxic cells leads to a long-term preservation of cardiocyte viability that might be especially apropos for preservation of cell viability during organ transportation for transplantation.

Preliminary In Vivo Experiments on Decreasing Infarct Size with CSIL

In our preliminary study utilizing a model of myocardial infarction in rabbits, when antimyosin IL, IgG-L, PL, or saline placebo were delivered concomitant with circumflex coronary artery occlusion for 45 min followed by reperfusion, the infarct size determined at 6 h of reperfusion, of IL treated rabbit hearts were approximately 5–10% of the control PL, IgG-L, or saline placebo treated rabbit hearts (88). Fig. 19 shows nitroblue tetrazolium stained heart sections of IL treated rabbit (top left panel) relative to PL (top right panel), IgG-L (bottom left panel), or saline placebo (bottom right panel) treated rabbit hearts. In nitroblue tetrazolium staining, normal myocardium stained as purple to dark brown, where as the infarcted myocardium is seen as light colored regions. Whether intravenously delivered IL would have any efficacy

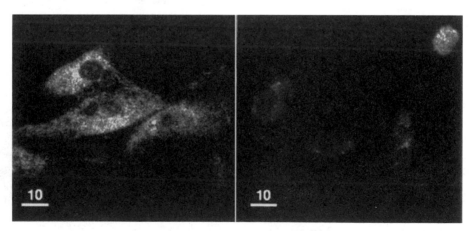

Fig. 18 Confocal micrographs of 24 h hypoxic H9C2 cardiocytes treated with rhodamine labeled IL (right) or rhodamine labeled PL (left). The micrographs are shown in pseudocolors. Cells treated with IL showed retention of membrane integrity and cell morphology (left panel). Liposomes represented as yellow colored regions are also discernable on the cells. Cells treated with PL showed presence of only dead cells with only a few cells having nonspecifically attached PL (right panel). (From Ref. 84.)

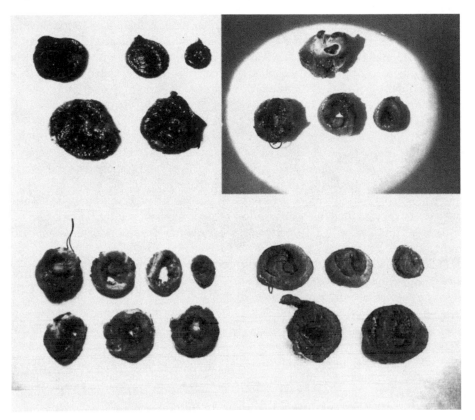

Fig. 19 Nitroblue tetrazolium stained heart sections of rabbits with acute myocardial infarction treated with PL (left panel), saline placebo (middle panel) and IL (right panel). The sites of left circumflex coronary artery occlusion can be seen in the middle and right panels to be at the 4th slices by the presence of the silk sutures. Normal myocardium is stained purple or brown, whereas the infarcted regions remain as light colored regions.

relative to direct intraatrial delivery of the liposomes is not know at this time. None the less, in acute myocardial infarction, angioplasty is an alternative method to thrombolytic reperfusion therapy, therefore, in combination with angioplasty, it may be possible to deliver the IL directly into the infarct zone at the time of angioplasty.

Fusion of Cytoskeleton-specific Immunoliposomes with Hypoxic Cells

To demonstrate that preservation of cell viability is due to fusion of IL with the cell membranes, IL were prepared with intraliposomal silver grains. The rationale was that the only way silver grains can enter the treated hypoxic cardiocytes is by fusion of the IL with the cell membrane that resulted in preservation of cardiocyte viability. If endocytosis of the IL is the process of internalization without fusion, then plain liposomes should also show internalization of the silver grains. To prepare such liposomes (84), silver nitrate was added in a buffer solution during liposome preparation by sonication.

Liposomes, purified from the nonentrapped silver nitrate by dialysis were dialyzed in 0.12 M NaCl solution and exposed to light for 1 h that led to the formation of fine electron-dense precipitate of silver oxide inside liposomes.

Figure 20 shows that only cells treated with silver grains impregnated antimyosin IL retained the cell morphology and showed internalization of the silver grains (Fig. 20, top panel). Cardiocytes treated with silver grains impregnated PL showed no viable cells. However, after extensive search one viable cell as identified. The silver grains were observed out side the cell (Fig. 20, bottom panel) (89). The size of each clump of silver grains seen in Fig. 20 top panel is consistent with the size of the liposomes that were prepared and was approximately 200–300 μm in diameter. From this study, it was not possible to determine whether silver grains would also migrate to the nucleus. Silver grains, once internalized may not be as mobile as soluble pharmaceuticals or genetic constructs. Furthermore, since no internalization of silver grains was observed with PL, the mechanism of internalization seen with IL does not appear to be due to endocytosis or pinocytosis. Therefore,

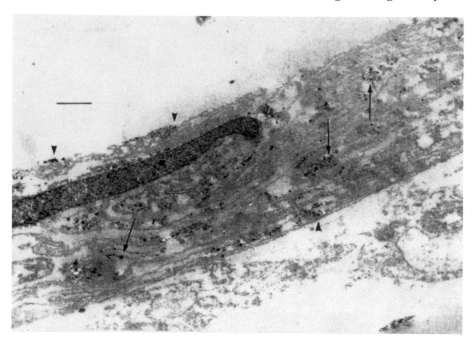

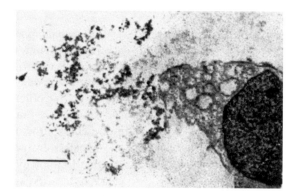

Fig. 20 Transmission electronmicrographs of hypoxic H9C2 cardiocytes treated with silver grains impregnated IL or PL. Silver grains in seen intracellularly in IL treated cells; arrows, arrow heads represents 1 μm. (From Ref. 84.)

internalization of the silver grains delivered by IL is consistent with the proposal that cytoskeleton-specific IL is able to fuse with the membrane of hypoxic cells releasing their contents into the cytoplasm.

Intracytoplasmic DNA Delivery

Since antimyosin immunoliposomes can be used to seal cell membrane lesions (84) and intraliposomally entrapped silver grains can be delivered directly into the cytoplasm (88), we also hypothesize that if we substitute genetic constructs for the silver grains, then such constructs should also be deliverable directly into the cytosol (90). Delivery of genetic constructs directly into the cytosol, bypassing the endocytic route, might result in higher efficiency of gene expression. To demonstrate this hypothesis, we initially used antimyosin sFc vector (90), then pGL2 luciferase vector (91) and finally bacterial beta galactosidase vector (92). The rationale for using three different vectors is to show that irrespective of the origin of the vectors, one murine, one insect, and one bacteria origin, they all can transfect the cardiocytes and result in very efficient gene expression. All these in vitro studies showed that vectors delivered directly into the cytoplasm were

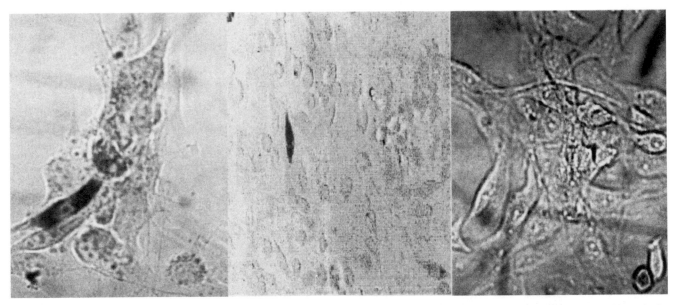

Fig. 21 Evidence of successful gene transfection with bacterial β-galactosidase vectors with IL in hypoxic cells, or with cationic liposomes or IgG-liposomes. The β-galactosidase activity was developed with X-Gal at pH 7.0. Cells treated with IL-β-galactosidase vector showed many cells with blue color. The culture was also confluent. Cells treated with cationic liposome-β-galactosidase vector showed only two cells with gene expression. The cells were also not confluent indicating cell attrition. IgG-liposome treated cells also showed no β-galactosidase expression.

expressed with very high efficiency. Comparative studies with standard cationic liposomes showed that although transfection efficiency of cationic liposomes was very efficient, due to the over-loading of the cell membrane with approximately 40,000 liposomes per cell (93), the viability of transfected cells declined dramatically. Furthermore, since internalization of the vectors is via endosomes, the factor of vector loss due to lysosomal activity was considerable as evidence by a lower number of cells expressing the gene products.

When IL was used for transfection of bacterial β-gal vector into hypoxic cells, the majority of the cells showed bacterial β-galactosidase activity when stained with X-gal color reagent. Although individual cells transfected with IL displayed less β-galactosidase activity than those few cells expressing the enzyme activity after cationic liposome transfection, the total number of cells demonstrating gene expression were at least 40 times more (94). This result is consistent with our calculation that only 3–4 copies of vectors were delivered per cell by IL transfection, whereas when cationic liposomes were used, more than 3000 copies of the vectors were delivered per cell (94). Fig. 21 shows the comparison of the photomicrographs of cells with successful expression of the β-galactosidase vector transfected with IL (A) or cationic liposomes (B) and IgG liposomes (C). Those cells treated with PL similar to IgG-L also showed no transfection.

Although the present novel method of gene transfection requires institution of an insult to the cell membrane, our studies with cell viability already showed that almost no cells were lost due to cell death in these treated cultures. Therefore, for efficient in vitro cell transfection and gene expression, this immunoliposome method would be highly desirable. Whether this method would be valuable in vivo, additional studies are necessary.

CONCLUSIONS

Monoclonal antibodies are the targeting moieties of the "targeted drug delivery systems." Whether the drugs to be targeted are radioisotopes for diagnosis or therapy, or chemotherapeutic agents such as doxoruibicin that are directly attached to the antibodies as immunoconjugates or entrapped in liposomes and targeted as immunoliposomes, the antibodies provide the most easily available and versatile targeting reagent. Although this article has concentrated on the demonstration of antibodies in targeted drug delivery in the cardiovascular system, their potential is by no means restricted to this system. The imaging and therapeutic applications described for the cardiovascular system should be ameanable to adaptation to other organ systems. A cursory discussion of monoclonal antibodies in oncological uses was provided. Although the potential trageted drug delivery applications in neurological and other systems were not discussed in this article, their utilities are by no means negligible. However, it would be the subject of another article. Therefore, only the cardiovascular application of monoclonal antibodies in targeted drug delivery has been attempted in this review.

REFERENCES

1. Ehrlich, P.; Herter, C.A. Ueber Einige Verwendungen der Naphtochinonsulfosaure. Z. Physiol. Chem. **1904**, *61*; 379–392.
2. Pressman, D.; Keighley, G. Zone of Activity of Antibodies as Determined by the Use of Radioactive Tracers: Zone of Activity of Nephrotoxic Antikidney Serum. J. Immunol. **1948**, *59*; 141–146.
3. Kohler, G.; Milstein, C. Continuous Cultures of Fused Cells Secreting Antibodies of Predefined Specificity. Nature: (London) **1975**, *256*; 495–497.
4. Mach, J.-P.; Carrel, S.; Forni, M.; Ritschard, J.; Donath, A.; Alberto, P. Tumor Localization of Radiolabeled Antibodies Against Carcinoembryonic Antigen in Patients with Carcinoma. New Eng. J. Med. **1980**, *303*; 5–10.
5. Goldenberg, D.M.; DeLand, F.H.; Kim, E.E.; Primus, F.J.; van Nagell, J.R., Jr.; Estes, N.; DeSimone, P.; Rayburn, P. Use of Radiolabeled Antibodies to Carcinoembryonic Antigen for the Detection and Localization of Diverse Cancers by External Photoscanning. New Engl. J. Med. **1978**, *298*; 1384–1388.
6. Mach, J.P.; Buchegger, F.; Forni, M. Use of Radiolabeled Monoclonal Anti-CEA Antibodies for the Detection of Human Carcinomas by External Photoscanning and Tomoscintigraphy. Immunol. Today **1981**, 2; 239–247.
7. Bischof-Delaloye, A.; Delaloye, B.; Buchegger, F. Clinical Value of Immunoscintigraphy in Colorectal Carcinoma Patients: A Prospective Study. J. Nucl. Med. **1989**, *30*; 1646–1656.
8. Rainsbury, R.M.; Westwood, J.H.; Coombes, R.C. Localization of Metastatic Breast Carcinoma by Monoclonal Antibody Chelate Labeled with In-111. Lancet **1983**, *1*; 934–938.
9. Chatal, J.F.; Saccavini, J.C.; Fumoleau, P. Immunoscintigraphy of Colon Carcinoma. J. Nucl. Med. **1984**, *25*; 307–314.
10. Kramer, E.L.; Noz, M.E.; Liebes, L.; Murthy, S.; Tiu, S.; Goldenberg, D.M. Radioimmunodetection of Non-Small Cell Lung Cancer Using Technetium-99m-Anticarcino-embryonic Antigen IMMU-4 Fab' Fragment. Preliminary Results. Cancer **1994**, *73* (3 Suppl); 890–895.
11. Epenetos, A.A.; Sheperd, J.; Britton, K.E. I-123 Radioiodinated Antibody Imaging of Occult Ovarian Cancer. Cancer **1985**, *55*; 984–987.
12. Babaian, R.J.; Lamki, L.M. Radioimmunoscintigraphy of Prostate Carcinoma. Semin. Nucl. Med. **1989**, *19*; 309–321.
13. Larson, S.M.; Carrasquillo, J.A.; Krohn, K.A. Diagnostic Imaging of Malignant Melanoma with Radiolabeled Antitumor Antibodies. JAMA **1983**, *249*; 811–812.
14. Carasquillo, J.A.; Mulshine, J.L.; Bunn, B.A. Tumor Imaging of In-111 T101 Monoclonal Antibody is Superior to Iodine-131 T101 in Cutaneous T-Cell Lymphoma. J. Nucl. Med. **1987**, *28*; 281–287.
15. Mariani, G.; Molea, N.; Bacciardi, D.; Boggi, U.; Fornaciari, G.; Campani, D.; Salvadori, P.A.; Giulianotti, P.C.; Mosca, F.; Gold, D.V. Initial Tumor Targeting, Biodistribution, and Pharmacokinetic Evaluation of the Monoclonal Antibody PAM4 in Patients with Pancreatic Cancer. Cancer. Res. **1995**, *55* (23 Suppl); 5911s–5915s.
16. Peltier, P.; Curtet, C.; Chatal, J.-F. Radioimmunodetection of Medullary Thyroid Cancer Using a Bispecific Anti-CEA/Anti-insium-DTPA Antibody and an Indium-111 Labeled DTPA-Dimer. J. Nucl. Med. **1993**, *34*; 1267–1273.
17. Pimm, M.V.; Fells, H.F.; Perkins, A.C.; Baldwin, R.W. Iodine-131 and Indium-111 Labelled Avidin and Streptavidin for Pre-Targetted Immunoscintigraphy with Biotinylated Anti-Tumour Monoclonal Antibody. Nucl. Med. Commun. **1988**, *9* (11); 931–941.
18. Brenner, T.L.; Adams, V.R. First Mab Approved for Treatment of Metastatic Breast Cancer. J. Am. Pharm. Assoc. **1999**, *39*; 236–238.
19. McLaughlin, P. Clinical Status and Optimal Use of Rituximab for B-Cell Lymphomas. Oncology **1998**, *12*; 1763–1777.
20. Nielsen, U.B.; Marks, J.S. Internalizing Antibodies and Targeted Cancer Therapy: Direct Selection from Phage Display Libraries. Pharm. Sci. Technol. Today **2000**, *3* (8); 282–291.
21. Mahe, M.A.; Fumoleau, P.; Fabbro, M. A Phase II Study of Intraperitoneal Radioimmunotherapy with Iodine-131-labeled Monoclonal Antibody OC-125 in Patients with Residual Ovarian Carcinoma. Clin. Cancer. Res. **1999**, *5* (S10); 3249s–3253s.
22. Winkler, U.; Barth, S.; Schnell, R.; Diehl, V.; Engert, A. The Emerging Role of Immunotoxins in Leukemia and Lymphoma. Ann. Oncol. **1997**, *8* (Suppl 1); 139–146.
23. Trail, P.A. Cure of Xenografted Human Carcinoma by BR96-doxorubicin Immunoconjugates. Science **1993**, *261*; 212–215.
24. Bernstein, N. Antibody-directed Targeting of Liposomes to Human Cell Lines: Role of Binding and Internalization on Growth Inhibition. Cancer Res. **1987**, *47*; 5954–5959.
25. Khaw, B.A.; Beller, G.A.; Haber, E.; Smith, T.W. Localization of Cardiac Myosin-Specific Antibody in Myocardial Infarction. J. Clin. Invest. **1976**, *58*; 439–446.
26. Yasuda, T.; Palacios, I.F.; Dec, G.W.; Fallon, J.T.; Gold, H.K.; Leinbach, R.C.; Strauss, H.W.; Khaw, B.A.; Haber, E. Indium-111 Monoclonal Antimyosin Antibody Imaging in the Diagnosis of Acute Myocarditis. Circulation **1987**, *76*; 306–311.
27. Ballester, M.; Carrio, I.; Abada, M.L. Patterns of Evolution of Myocyte Damage After Human Heart Transplant Detected by 111 In Monoclonal Antimyosin. Am. J. Cardiol. **1988**, *62*; 623–627.
28. Dec, G.W.; Palacios, I.; Yasuda, T.; Fallon, J.T.; Khaw, B.A.; Strauss, H.W.; Haber, E. Antimyosin Antibody Cardiac Imaging: Its Role in the Diagnosis of Myocarditis. J. Am. Col. Cardiol. **1990**, *16* (1); 97–104.

29. Ballester, M.; Martí, V.; Carrió, I. Spectrum of Alcohol-Induced Myocardial Damage Detected by Indium-111-Labeled Monoclonal Antimyosin Antibodies. J. Am. Coll. Cardiol. **1997**, *29* (1); 160–167.

30. Estorch, M.; Carrio, I.; Berna, L. 111 In-Antimyosin Scintigraphy After Doxorubicin Therapy in Patients with Advanced Breast Cancer. J. Nucl. Med. **1990**, *31*; 1965–1969.

31. Narula, J.; Khaw, B.A.; Southern, J. Monoclonal Antibodies in Cardiovascular Diseases. Khaw, B.A., Narula, J., Strauss, H.W., Eds.; Lea & Febiger: Philadelphia, 1994; 118–126.

32. Knight, L.C. Antifibrin Antibody for Detection of Deep Vein Thrombosis. *Monoclonal Antibodies in Cardiovascular Diseases*; Khaw, B.A., Narula, J., Strauss, H.W., Eds.; Lea & Febiger: Philadelphia, 1994; 171–186.

33. Narula, J.; Ditlow, C.; Chen, F.; Khaw, B.A. Monoclonal Antibodies for Detection of Atherosclerotic Lesions. *Monoclonal Antibodies in Cardiovascular Diseases*; Khaw, B.A., Narula, J., Strauss, H.W., Eds.; Lea & Febiger: Philadelphia, 1994; 206–215.

34. Kairemo, K.J.; Wiklund, T.A.; Liewendahl, K. Imaging of Soft-tissue Sarcomas with In-111-Labeled Monoclonal Antimyosin Fab Fragments. J. Nucl. Med. **1990**, *31*; 23–31.

35. Khaw, B.A.; Scott, J.; Fallon, J.T.; Haber, E.; Homcy, C. Myocardial Injury: Quantitation by Cell Sorting Initiated with Anti-Myosin Fluorescent Spheres. Science **1982**, *217*; 1050–1053.

36. Khaw, B.A.; Gold, H.K.; Leinbach, R.C.; Fallon, J.T.; Strauss, H.W.; Pohost, G.M.; Haber, E. Early Imaging of Experimental Myocardial Infarction by Intracoronary Administration of 131 I-Labeled Anticardiac Myosin (Fab')₂ Fragments. Circulation **1978**, *58*; 1137–1142.

37. Khaw, B.A.; Petrov, A.; Narula, J. Complementary Roles of Antibody Affinity and Specificity in In Vivo Diagnostic Cardiovascular Targeting: How Specific is Antimyosin for Irreversible Myocardial Damage. J. Nucl.Cardiol. **1999**, *6*; 316–323.

38. Khaw, B.A.; Yasuda, T.; Gold, H.K.; Leinbach, R.C.; Johns, J.A.; Kanke, M.; Barlai-Kovach, M.; Strauss, H.W.; Haber, E. Acute Myocardial Infarct Imaging with Indium-111-Labeled Monoclonal Antimyosin Fab. J. Nucl. Med. **1987**, *28*; 1671–1678.

39. Khaw, B.A. The Current Role of Infarct Avid Imaging in Cardiovascular Nuclear Medicine-I. Seminars in Nuclear Medicine. **1999**, *XXIX* (3); 259–270.

40. Nedelman, M.A.; Shealy, D.J.; Boulin, R.; Bruntm, E.; Seasholtz, J.I.; Allen, I.E.; McCartney, J.E.; Warren, F.D.; Oppermann, H.; Pang, R.H.L.; Berger, H.J.; Weisman, H.F. Rapid Infarct Imaging with a Technetium-99m-Labeled Antimyosin Recombinant Single-Chain Fv: Evaluation in a Canine Model of Acute Myocardial Infarction. J. Nucl. Med. **1993**, *34*; 234–241.

41. Calcutt, M.J.; Komissarov, A.A.; Marchbank, M.T.; Deutscher, S.L. Analysis of a Nucleic-Acid-Binding Antibody Fragment: Construction and Characterization of Heavy-Chain Complementarity-Determining Region Switch Variants. Gene **1996**, *168* (1); 9–14.

42. Saragovi, H.U.; Fritzpatrick, D.; Raktabutr, A.; Nakanishi, H.; Kahn, M.; Greene, M.I. Design and Synthesis of a Mimetic from an Antibody Complementarity Determining Region. Science **1991**, *253*; 792–795.

43. Painter, R.H.; Freedman, M.H. Isolation and Characterization of Electrophoretically Homogenous Rabbit Anti-hapten Antibody Populations. II. Survey of the Isoelectric Properties of Antihapten Antibodies Directed Against Charged and Uncharged Proteins. J. Biol. Chem. **1971**, *246*; 1742–1751.

44. Silva Filho, F.C.; Santos, A.B.S.; de Carvalho, T.M.U.; de Souza, W. Surface Charge of Resident, Elicited, and Activated Mouse Peritoneal Macrophages. J. Leukocyte Bio. **1987**, *41*; 143–149.

45. Gallagher, J.E.; George, G. Brody AR. Sialic Acid Mediates the Initial Binding of Positively Charged Inorganic Particles to Alveolar Macrophage Membranes. Am. Rev. Respir. Dis. **1987**, *135*; 1345–1352.

46. Yanagisawa-Miwa, A.; Uchida, Y.; Nakamura, F.; Tomaru, T.; Kido, H.; Kamijo, T.; Sugimoto, T.; Kaji, K.; Utsuyama, M.; Kurashima, C.; Ito, H. Salvage of Infarcted Myocardium by Angiogenic Action of Basic Fibroblast Growth Factor. Science **1992**, *257*; 1401–1403.

47. Shen, W.-C.; Ryser, H.J.-P. Conjugation of Poly-L-Lysine to Albumin and Horseradish Peroxidase: A Novel Method of Enhancing the Cellular Uptake of Proteins. Proc. Natl. Acad. Sci. **1978**, *75*; 1872–1876.

48. Gao, X.; Huang, L. Cationic Liposomes and Polymers for Gene Transfer. J. Liposome. Res. **1993**, *3*; 17–30.

49. Torchilin, V.P.; Klibanov, A.L.; Nossiff, N.D.; Slinkin, M.A.; Strauss, H.W.; Haber, E.; Smirnov, V.N.; Khaw, B.A. Monoclonal Antibody Modification with Chelate-linked High-Molecular-Weight Polymers: Major Increases in Polyvalent Cation Binding without Loss of Antigen Binding. Hybridoma **1987**, *6*; 229–240.

50. Khaw, B.A.; Klibanov, A.; O'Donnell, S.M.; Saito, T.; Nossiff, N.; Slinkin, M.A.; Newell, J.B.; Strauss, H.W.; Torchilin, V.P. Gamma Imaging with Negatively-Charge-Modified Monoclonal Antibody: Modification with Synthetic Polymers. J. Nucl. Med. **1991**, *32*; 1742–1751.

51. Narula, J.; Petrov, A.; Ditlow, C.; Pak, K.Y.; Chen, F.W.; Khaw, B.A. Maximizing Radiotracer Delivery for Scintigraphic Localization of Experimental Atherosclerotic Lesions with High-Dose Negative-Charge-Modified Z2D3 Antibody. J. Nucl. Cardiol. **1997**, *4*; 226–233.

52. Narula, J.; Torchilin, V.P.; Petrov, A.; Khaw, S.; Trubetskoy, V.S.; O'Donnell, S.M.; Nossiff, N.D.; Khaw, B.A. In-Vivo Targeting of Acute Myocardial Infarction with Negative Charge, Polymer-Modified Antimyosin Antibody: Use of Different Cross-linkers. J. Nucl. Cardiol. **1995**, *2*; 26–34.

53. Carrio, I.; Pieri, P.; Prat, L.; Tison, V.; Pedrini, L.; Moscatelli, G.; Sardi, G.; Estorch, M.; Berna, L.l.; Riambau, V.; GuJiu, M.; Pak, Ch; Ditlow, Ch; Chen, F.; Khaw, B.A. In-111 Chimeric Negative-Charged-Z2D3 PL-F(ab')₂ in the Detection of Atherosclerotic Plaques. J. Nucl. Med. **1995**, *36* (5); 133.

54. Johnson, L.L.; Seldin, D.W.; Tresgallo, M.E.; Bhatia, K.; Rodney, R.A.; Gibbons, J.F.; Esser, P.D. Right Ventricular Infarction and Function from Dual Isotope Indium-111-Antimyosin/Thallium-201 SPECT and Gated Blood Pool Scintigraphy. J. Nucl. Med. **1991**, *32* (Abstract); 1018.

55. van Vlies, B.; van Royen, E.D.; Visser, C.A.; Meyne, N.G.; van Buul, M.M.; Peter, R.T.; Dunning, A.J. Frequency of Myocardial Indium-111 Antimyosin Uptake After

Uncomplicated Coronary Artery Bypass Surgery. Am. J. Cardiol. **1990**, *66*; 1191–1195.

56. Narula, L.; Khaw, B.A.; Yasuda, T. Antimyosin Imaging for Acute Myocarditis. *Monoclonal Antibodies in Cardiovascular Diseases*; Khaw, B.A., Narula, J., Strauss, H.W. Eds.; Lee & Febiger: Philadelphia, 1994; 67.

57. Aretz, H.T.; Billingham, M.E.; Edwards, W.D.; Factor, S.M.; Fallon, J.T.; Fenoglio, J.J.; Olsen, E.G.J.; Schoen, E.J. Myocarditis: A Histopathologic Definition and Classification. J. Cardiovasc. Pathol. **1986**, *1*; 3–14.

58. Frist, W.; Yasuda, T.; Segall, G.; Khaw, B.A.; Strauss, H.W.; Gold, H.K.; Stinson, E.; Oyer, P.; Baldwin, J.; Billingham, M.; McDougall, R.; Haber, E. Noninvasive Detection of Human Cardiac Transplant Rejection with in Antimyosin (Fab) Imaging. Circulation **1987**, *76*; V81–85.

59. Ballester, M.; Obrador, D.; Carrio, I.; Caralps-Riera, J.M. Indium-111 Monoclonal Antimyosin Antibody Studies in the Diagnosis of Rejection and Management of Patients After Heart Transplantation. *Monoclonal Antibodies in Cardiovascular Disease*; Khaw, B.A., Narula, J., Strauss, H.W., Eds.; Lee & Febiger: Philadelphia, 1994; 79–98.

60. Ballester, M.; Obrador, D.; Carrio, I.; Caralps-Riera, J.M. Indium-111 Monoclonal Antimyosin Antibody Studies in the Diagnosis of Rejection and Management of Patients After Heart Transplantation. *Monoclonal Antibodies in Cardiovascular Diseases*; Khaw, B.A., Narula, J., Strauss, H.W., Eds.; Lee & Febiger: Philadelphia, 1994; 81.

61. Ballester, M.; Obrador, D.; Carrio, I.; Moya, C.; Auge, J.M.; Bordes, R.; Marti, V.; Bosch, I.; Berna, L.; Estorch, M.; Pons, G.; Camara, M.L.; Padro, J.M.; Aris, A.; Caralps, J.M. Early Postoperative Reduction of Monoclonal Antimyosin Antibody Uptake is Associated with Absent Rejection Related Complications After Heart Transplantation. Circulation **1992**, *85*; 61–68.

62. Chow, L.H.; Radio, S.J.; Sears, T.D.; McManus, B.M. Insensitivity of Right Ventricular Biopsy in the Diagnosis of Myocarditis. J. Am. Coll. Cardiol. **1989**, *14*; 915–920.

63. Becker, A.E.; Heijmans, C.D. Essed CE. Chronic Nonischemic Heart Disease and Endomyocardial Biopsies. Worth the Extra. Eur. Heart. J. **1991**, *12*; 218–223.

64. Carrio, I. Diagnosis of Doxorubicin Cardiotoxicity with Indium-111 Antimyosin Fab. *Monoclonal Antibodies in Cardiovascular Diseases*; Khaw, B.A., Narula, J., Strauss, H.W., Eds.; Lee & Febiger: Philadelphia, 1994; 99–108.

65. Narula, J.; Malhotra, A.; Yasuda, T.; Talwar, K.K.; Reddy, K.S.; Chopra, P.; Southern, J.F.; Vasan, R.S.; Tandon, R.; Bhatia, M.L.; Khaw, B.A.; Strauss, H.W. Usefulness of Antimyosin Antibody Imaging for the Detection of Active Rheumatic Myocarditis. Am. J. Cardiol. **1999**, *84* (8); 946–950.

66. Casans, I.; Villar, A.; Almenar, V.; Blanes, A. Lyme Myocarditis Diagnosis by Indium-111 Antimyosin Antibody Scintigraphy. Eur. J. Nucl. Med. **1989**, *15*; 330–331.

67. Krause, T.H.; Schumichen Cbeck, A.; Lang, B.; Hohnloser, S.; Moser, E. Scintigraphy Using ^{111}In-Labeled Antimyosin in Churg–Strauss Vasculitis with Myocardial Involvement. Nuklearmedizin **1990**, *29*; 177–179.

68. Hendel, R.C.; Cohen, S.; Aurigemma, G.; Whitfield, S.; Dalberg, S.; Pape, L.; Leppo, J. Focal Myocardial Injury Following Blunt Chest Trauma: A Comparison of Indium-111 Antimyosin Scintigraphy with Other Noninvasive Methods. Am. Heart J. **1992**, *123*; 1208–1215.

69. Spar, I.L.; Goodland, R.L.; Schwartz, S.I. Detection of Preformed Venous Thrombi in Dogs by Means of I-131-Labeled Antibodies to Dog Fibrinogen. Circ. Res. **1965**, *17*; 322–329.

70. Hui, K.Y.; Haber, E.; Matsueda, G.F. Monoclonal Antibodies to a Synthetic Fibrin-Like Peptide Bind to Human Fibrin but not Fibrinogen. Science **1983**, *222*; 1129–1132.

71. Kudryk, B.; Rohoza, A.; Ahadi, M.; Chin, J.; Wiebe, M. Specificity of a Monoclonal Antibody for the NH_2-terminal Region of Fibrin. Mol. Immunol. **1984**, *21*; 89–94.

72. Kanke, M.; Matsueda, G.R.; Strauss, H.W.; Yasuda, T.; Liau, C.S.; Khaw, B.A. Localization and Visualization of Pulmonary Emboli with Radiolabeled Fibrin Specific Monoclonal Antibody. J. Nucl. Med. **1991**, *32*; 1254–1260.

73. Roberts, A.B.; Lees, A.M.; Lees, R.S.; Strauss, H.W.; Fallon, J.T.; Taveras, J.; Kopiwoda, S. Selective Accumulation of Low Density Lipoproteins in Damaged Arterial Wall. J. Lip. Res. **1983**, *24*; 1160–1167.

74. Virgolini, I.; Muller, C.; Fitscha, P.; Chiba, P.; Sinzinger, H. Radiolabeling Autologous Monocytes with in Oxine for Reinjection in Patients with Atherosclerosis. Prog. Clin. Biol. Res. **1989**, *355*; 271–280.

75. Harrison, D.C.; Calenoff, E.; Chen, F.; Parmley, W.; Khaw, B.A.; Ross, R. In Plaque-Associated Immune Reactivity as a Tool for the Diagnosis and Treatment of Atherosclerosis. Trans. Am. Clin. Climatol. Assoc. **1992**, *103*; 210–217.

76. Khaw, B.A.; Calenoff, E.; Chen, F.; O'Donnell, S.M.; Nossiff, N.D.; Strauss, H.W. Localization of Experimental Atherosclerotic Lesion with Monoclonal Antibody Z2D3. J. Nucl. Med. **1991**, *32* (5); 1005.

77. Narula, J.; Petrov, A.; Bianchi, C.; Ditlow, C.C.; Dilley, J.; Pieslak, I.; Chen, F.W.; Torchilin, V.P.; Khaw, B.A. Noninvasive Localization of Experimental Atherosclerotic Lesions with Mouse/Human Chimeric Z2D3 Antibody Specific for the Proliferating Smooth Muscle Cells of Human Atheroma: Imaging with Conventional Antibody and Image Enhancement with Negative Charge-Modified Antibody. Circulation **1995**, *92*; 474–484.

78. Carrio, I.; Pieri, P.L.; Narula, J.; Prat, L.; Pedrini, L.; Riva, P.; Sarti, G.; Pak, Ch; Ditlow, Ch; Chen, F.; Khaw, B.A. In-111 Chimeric Negative-Charged Z2D3 PL-F(ab')$_2$ Imaging of Proliferating Smooth Muscle Cell in Atherosclerotic Lesions. J. Nucl. Med. **1996**, *37* (5); 49.

79. Khaw, B.A.; Carrio, I.; Pieri, P.L.; Narula, J. Radionuclide Imaging of the Synthetic Smooth Muscle Cell Phenotype in Experimental Atherosclerotic Lesions. Trends Cardiovas. Med. **1996**, *6*; 226–232.

80. Majno, G.; Joris, I. Apoptosis, Oncosis, and Necrosis: An Overview of Cell Death. Am. J. Pathol. **1995**, *146* (1); 3–15.

81. Kerr, J.F.R.; Wyllie, A.H.; Currie, A.R. Apoptosis: A Basic Biological Phenomenon with Wide Ranging Implications In Tissue Kinetics. Br. J. Cancer. **1972**, *26*; 239.

82. Jennings, R.B.; Schaper, J.; Hill, M.L.; Steenberg, C., Jr.; Reimer, K.A. Effect of Reperfusion Late in the Phase of Reversible Ischemic Injury: Changes in Cell Volume, Electrolytes, Metabolites, and Ultrastructure. Circ. Res. **1985**, *56*; 262–278.

83. Bailik, S.; Geenen, D.L.; Sasson, I.E.; Cheng, R.; Horner, J.W.; Evans, S.M.; Lord, E.M.; Koch, C.J.; Kitis, R.N. Myocyte Apoptosis During Acute Myocardial Infarction in

the Mouse Localizes to Hypoxic Regions but Occurs Independently of p53. J. Clin. Invest **1997**, *100*; 1363–1372.

84. Khaw, B.A.; Torchilin, V.P.; Vural, I.; Narula, J. Plug and Seal: Prevention of Hypoxic Cardiocyte Death by Sealing Membrane Lesions with Antimyosin-Liposomes. Nature Med. **1995**, *1*; 1195–1198.

85. Weissig, V.; Lasch, J.; Klibanov, A.L.; Torchilin, V.P. A New Hydrophobic Anchor for the Attachment of Proteins to Liposomal Membranes. FEBS Lett **1986**, *202*; 86–90.

86. Torchilin, D.L.; Klibanov, A.L.; Huang, L.; O'Donnell, S.; Nossiff, N.D.; Khaw, B.A. Targeted Accumulation of Polyethylene Glycol-Coated Immunoliposomes in Infarcted Rabbit Myocardium. FASEB J. **1992**, *6*; 2716–2719.

87. Khaw, B.A.; Vural, I.; Narula, J.; Haider, N.; Torchilin, V.P. Cardiocyte Viability by Immunoliposome-Cell Membrane Sealing at 1, 2, 3, 4 and 5 Days of Hypoxia Proceedings of 23rd International Symposium on Controlled Release of Bioactive Materials. Kyoto, Japan 1996, 617, 618

88. Khaw, A.B.; Vural, I.; DaSilva, J.; Torchilin, V.P. In Vivo Myocardial Preservation with Cytoskeleton Specific Immunoliposomes in Acute Myocardial Infarction Proceedings of the 27th International Symposium on Controlled Release of Bioactive Materials, in press.

89. Khaw, B.A.; Vural, I.; DaSilva, J.; Torchilin, T.P. Use of Cytoskeleton-Specific Immunoliposomes for Preservation of Cell Viability and Gene Delivery. STP Pharma Sci. **2000**, *10* (4); 279–283.

90. Khaw, B.A.; Vural, I.; Torchilin, V.P.; Haider, N.; Narula, J. Expression of Antimyosin sFv Gene in Cardiocytes: Use of Cytoskeleton-Specific Immunoliposomes for Transfection Proceedings of 23rd International Symposium on Controlled Release of Bioactive Materials Kyoto Japan 1996, 135, 136.

91. Khaw, B.A.; Vural, I.; Torchilin, V.P.; Narula, J. Intracytoplasmic Delivery of Plasmid pGL2 Vector by Cytoskeleton Specific Immunoliposome Transfection Proceedings of the 25th International Symposium on Controlled Release of Bioactive Materials 1998; 25, 178, 179.

92. Khaw, B.A.; Vural, I.; Narula, J.; Torchilin, V.P. Comparative Efficiencies of Transfection by Cationic Liposomes and Cytoskeleton Specific Immunoliposomes Proceedings of the 26th International Symposium on Controlled Release of Bioactive Materials 1999; 26, 218, 219.

93. Felgner, P.L.; Ringold, G.M. Cationic Liposome-Mediated Transfection. Nature **1989**, *337*; 387–388.

TECHNOLOGY TRANSFER CONSIDERATIONS FOR PHARMACEUTICALS[a]

Ira R. Berry

Duramed Pharmaceuticals, Inc., Somerset, New Jersey

INTRODUCTION

Technology transfer for pharmaceutical products is a program that has been followed for some time (1–11). Issues to be considered when organizing the transfer of technology from the research arena to the production and quality assurance environments are reviewed in this article. The discussion focuses on the coordination and implementation of a transfer program for a product, with emphasis given to those factors special to the pharmaceutical industry. The success of any program is highly dependent on the effectiveness of the communication preceding its implementation; therefore, the preparation and distribution of a complete document summarizing raw material and equipment requirements, manufacturing and packaging processes, process validation parameters, quality control procedures, and safe handling procedures—as well as a detailed plan of action outlining expected results and time frames—must be distributed before the scale-up experience. Input from the marketing and manufacturing centers must be integrated into the plan to ensure that the right product is developed at the right price within the desired time frame. An outline encompassing these critical aspects of a transfer program is presented.

Whether a tablet, a transdermal patch, a topical ointment, or an injectable, the transformation of a pharmaceutical prototype into a successful product requires the cooperation of many individuals. To complete the task efficiently, the transfer of a product from the research and development area to production must be organized. Planning for process commercialization is one area where tangible rewards can be realized. The successful transfer of a project to a production site from the research arena does not happen on its own. Organizing the transfer of a technology or new product from research to production may be one of the most perplexing problems that development scientists, engineers, and marketers may encounter during their careers. This article provides some

[a](Revised from Ref. 1.)

insight into the issues that should be considered during the transfer program and offers a sequence of events toward completing the task.

A major decision focuses on that point where the idea or process is advanced from a research-oriented program to one targeted toward commercialization. Generally, the cost of product development rises dramatically during the pilot scale-up and initial production batch efforts. In other words, the critical path for success is dependent on the completion of the technology transfer to the production site at an affordable cost.

The three primary considerations to be addressed during an effective technology transfer are the plan, the persons involved, and the process. A plan must be devised to organize the personnel and the process steps. Once prepared, the plan must be communicated to the involved parties in research, at the corporate level, and at the production site. The success of any program is highly dependent on the effectiveness of the communication preceding its implementation. Therefore, identifying the parties involved in the development process is one of the most important tasks to be confronted and must be completed early in the transfer process.

PERSONNEL

The proper personnel must be informed of their involvement, desired contributions, and responsibilities. This helps identify potential problem areas that may hinder the accomplishment of the challenge at hand. It is desirable to appoint a project leader or liaison from the research and development group as the focus of the communication pattern. This individual has the responsibility to coordinate the assembly of the necessary information to support the product's advancement for process development. The trap to avoid here is to assign someone to this role and not give him or her the authority commensurate with the responsibilities with which he or she has been charged. The practice of pairing a seasoned project manager as a mentor with a less-experienced future

Encyclopedia of Pharmaceutical Technology

project coordinator is recommended. In this manner, team players can be nurtured. The communication and networking skills of the successful manager can be shared across the organization. On the other hand, it is expected that individuals who do not possess the necessary talents to be effective are identified before they encounter the stressful world of project management alone and, more importantly, before they have a chance to contribute to the failure of a potentially successful product.

Through mentoring, the one-to-one contact offers the unique opportunity for the sharing of ideas, skills, and observations. If properly organized with two-way evaluations, both participants should benefit. Not all individuals, however, are suited for the role of mentor. Care should be exercised in the selection and pairing of mentors for the less experienced. Perhaps a human resource manager could assist in identifying those people with the interpersonal skills required for this teaching position.

Information from the product development area would be gathered from the formulator, analytical and microbiology testing groups, and the packaging development unit. Issues to be considered from these groups will be discussed below. A safety evaluation from the toxicology group and industrial hygienist should be completed before a scale-up effort. In today's regulatory climate, a concise and understandable summary must be provided regarding the risks associated with and procedures for proper handling of all chemical substances, whether drug actives or excipients. Failure to provide sufficient information to those not skilled in the art to make the decision to initiate a handling, weighing, or processing operation may lead to an unfortunate employee injury. Although an employee has a "right to know," employers have an obligation to provide the necessary warnings and training to minimize placing an employee at risk. The legal ramifications of improper training or notification are outside the scope of this article.

An opinion should be solicited from the patent department or a patent attorney. With the implementation of the General Agreement on Tarrifs and Trade (GATT) accord, patents take on a new meaning. The impact of this legislation is far reaching, not only in the United States, where major revisions in the patent laws have been required and implemented, but also in many foreign countries where patents may be essentially worthless or not enforceable. In general, patents have an effective life of 20 years from the date of initial filing. Additional periods of exclusivity may be allowed, on application and when certain criteria are met, that extend the effective term of a patent. In summary, care must be exercised to ensure that proper legal protection of the novel concept has been secured in those areas where desired.

The drug regulatory affairs unit must also be involved with the product transfer to specify "how much" of "what" information is needed either to submit for a drug approval or to introduce a product to the marketplace. The goal here is to collect the proper amount and kind of data necessary to support the prerequisite filings, either internal or external to the company.

The corporate office commonly involves personnel from the production planning unit, engineering group, and new product coordination section, as well as from marketing, because each of these divisions has a vested interest in the success of the venture. It is important to identify the needs of those people at the corporate level to minimize delays caused by the "we did not know that we had to do this now" club. Activities such as product label preparation, copy for advertisements and promotional pieces, and package graphics may need to be initiated during the transfer program as not to lose valuable lead times. The acceptance or approval process in some companies is very labor-intensive and therefore time-consuming. This is one area where a detailed time and event plan has been shown to yield a significant impact on timely completion of a project.

Keeping the corporate participants informed becomes a pivotal task for the project manager in obtaining the final acceptance of the product by the corporation. Therefore, any time taken with those people involved at the corporate level to explain the steps involved in the transfer program is time well spent. Like any educational process, consistency and repetition enforce learning. It is incumbent on management to foster cooperation among individuals at the functional research and corporate centers, because the loss of time is the worst enemy an organization can face.

There are a number of individuals at the manufacturing site who must work as a team to ensure the timely and efficient completion of this transfer effort. The plant manager, technical director, production planning group, manufacturing area supervisor, and quality control and quality assurance units—as well as the plant engineering, packaging and transportation supervisors—must be informed as to their responsibilities. Personnel training must also be considered if the technology is new to the site. Last but not least are the contributions that the line mechanics and chemical operators can make to the program. They perform the necessary production functions daily. Their insight and practical experience are an invaluable resource that should not be overlooked.

The success of the transfer is dependent on the ability of the project leader to motivate employees to work toward a mutually beneficial goal, namely, introducing a new product that will improve consumer health and create jobs and increased profit for the company.

MOTIVATING PARTICIPANTS

Implementation of a positive return on involvement is one mechanism by which changes in responsibilities and tasks can be implemented. Changes here include the manufacture of new products or using new procedures to produce existing products. By involving personnel in the planning of changes, in discussing the resources necessary to complete the tasks, and in creating an environment in which innovation can strive, the project manager should strive to realize the completion of the program quickly and efficiently with reliable quality at an affordable cost. At the same time, those who have worked to bring the program to completion should share a feeling of teamwork and a sense of accomplishment. Return on involvement encompasses the philosophy that employees are a key element in the successful introduction of any technology or product approval. Project managers must keep this in mind because they frequently depend on the cooperation of individuals outside their direct control to accomplish their goals.

PRETRANSFER CONSIDERATIONS

Several assumptions must be satisfied before the advancement of any product to plant scale-up trials. First, the marketing division should have examined the proposed product prototypes and agreed that the product meets their needs. Second, the intended commercial package configurations should have been selected. Although it is not uncommon to package portions of the first scale-up batch in a variety of formats, it is incumbent on the project leader to eliminate unnecessary packages to minimize the dilution of effort. Third, any constraints, such as cost or time, must be identified so that they may be given due consideration.

There is an important question to be asked, i.e., does the product meet the needs of the consumer? The development staff believes they have captured marketing's vision with their product offering; however, the marketing and sales units must concur. The decision is generally in the sales unit, because those people are responsible for making the product available to the consumer and, more important, they are responsible to see that the product meets the consumer demands, real or perceived. It is expected that any pertinent focus groups or market research studies would be completed before the scale-up effort. These studies help confirm the product concept and its viability in the marketplace.

The cost of a development program increases dramatically as the number of package configurations to be advanced to commercialization increases. Selecting the proper package sizes, closures, colors, and neck finishes is compromised by the package composition and availability, and, finally, the intended use and cost of the unit. For example, a smaller unit lasting 1 month, such as a calendar pack, makes marketing sense for oral contraceptives for several reasons. Dispensing and unit sales are generally cyclic and more predictable, allowing for better profit projections. The calendar pack and monthly cost to the consumer not only position the product toward enhanced consumer acceptance but also toward better patient compliance, especially with expensive medications. In contrast, inhalation aerosol units, because of their pattern of chronic use, frequently contain sufficient doses to last several months. Suffice it to note, it behooves the marketing unit to work with financial analysts to determine the optimal product configuration and cost profile that maximizes consumer acceptance and convenience, unit turns, profits, and resources.

Constraints always exist but occasionally are not communicated accurately or promptly. Competition in the marketplace frequently causes introduction deadlines and endproduct cost constraints that must be considered during the initial phases of a development program. On the other hand, lead times for materials and personnel resources must be appreciated when commitments are made to timelines. Without planning in advance, the task may not be possible at all. Factors that influence decisions may originate externally as well as internally. Care must be exercised to address those issues that affect the timely completion of a project.

Physicochemical properties of raw materials and the finished dosage form should be characterized before any scale-up effort. Having methodology available and validated to compare batches is essential. For example, drug-release profiles and viscosities have the potential of being altered in scale-up by manufacturing procedures and equipment. Care must be exercised to maintain the desired profiles and other product specifications. The effect of batch size and process scale-up should be monitored closely.

Formulation and/or development of advanced drug-delivery systems such as microencapsulated molecules, transdermal patches, or liposomes are frequently accomplished in the laboratory. However, large-scale production of these dosage forms may be problematic because the same conditions of manufacture may not be attainable or desirable in the plant setting. Consultation with process development personnel during the finalization of the prototype development phase is one way of minimizing scale-up difficulties.

An area occasionally overlooked by the development staff is the necessity of securing confidentiality agreements from vendors supplying technologies or services to a firm. All contractors should be required to execute a confidentiality agreement that specifically encompasses the technology and product being developed. These documents should be prepared, reviewed, and executed by the appropriate legal and executive officers of both organizations. Especially when the science or product is not well-defined and patent protection has not been secured, such as with the development of novel, specialized drug delivery systems or new chemical

		Completion Dates	
Activity		Target	Actual
1.	Formulation selected	_____	_____
2.	Site for plant trial established	_____	_____
3.	Planning meeting scheduled	_____	_____
	a. Review of development report	_____	_____
	b. Manufacturing formulation/procedures	_____	_____
	b. Handling and safety issues	_____	_____
	c. Raw material specifications and suppliers	_____	_____
	d. Packaging procedures	_____	_____
	e. Packaging component specifications and suppliers	_____	_____
	f. Testing procedures and validation	_____	_____
	g. Process validation protocols	_____	_____
4.	Date of plant trial established	_____	_____
	a. Manufacturing	_____	_____
	c. Packaging	_____	_____
	d. Quality assurance testing	_____	_____
	c. On-site review of experience	_____	_____
	d. Shipment of samples to R&D for testing	_____	_____
5.	Date of shipment delivery	_____	_____
	a. Confirmation of results	_____	_____
	b. Stability initiation	_____	_____
	c. Product evaluation	_____	_____
	Safety	_____	_____
	Efficacy	_____	_____
	Drug release	_____	_____
6.	Postproduction review meeting	_____	_____
7.	Assembly of final pilot plant documents	_____	_____
	a. Manufacturing	_____	_____
	b. Packaging	_____	_____
	c. Handling and safety procedures	_____	_____
	d. Quality control specifications and analytical methods	_____	_____
	e. Stability data	_____	_____
	f. Material safety data sheet	_____	_____
	g. Shelf-life projection	_____	_____
	h. Process validation summary	_____	_____
	i. Bibliography	_____	_____
8.	Review of validation report	_____	_____
	a. Research and Development	_____	_____
	b. Manufacturing	_____	_____
	c. Engineering	_____	_____
	d. Quality Assurance/Quality Control	_____	_____
	e. Regulatory Affairs	_____	_____
	f. Corporate	_____	_____
	g. Marketing	_____	_____
9.	Issuance of final product specifications	_____	_____
10.	First commercial batch	_____	_____

Fig. 1 Project technology transfer checklist. (Modified from Ref. 1.)

entities, this task must be completed expeditiously, and no work should be initiated until the agreements have been properly executed.

TRANSFER PROGRAM

Any development and technology transfer program should be reduced to a written document such as that shown in Fig. 1. An outline or checklist must be compiled to ensure that appropriate consideration has been given to relevant issues. This helps ensure also that all parties are approaching the task from the same perspective and priority. A manufacturing site must be designated and the appropriate personnel notified as to their involvement. The necessary information must be collected and disseminated to the involved parties. At a minimum, copies of the proposed formula, manufacturing and testing procedures, and safe handling considerations should be distributed to allow sufficient time for review and comment. A planning review session should be convened with representatives from the research, corporate, marketing, manufacturing, quality assurance, regulatory affairs, and engineering departments in attendance. Selection of the time and location of this meeting should be made to encourage maximum participation.

The meeting should be chaired by the project leader. It is his or her responsibility to determine the relevant issues to be discussed, to follow up that an agenda for the meeting is distributed, and to establish that minutes of the meeting are taken. Concerns that arise during this meeting should be noted and addressed because the purpose of the meeting is to draw from the experience of the participants to identify potential problem areas in the program. The tone of this session should be one of consensus and not one of autocratic rule. Motivation, communication, and cooperation must be stressed in the voice and actions of the project leader. This is the first step toward accomplishing the primary program objective, namely, the timely and informed transfer of a new product from the research arena to the production site. The following subjects should be discussed at the planning meeting:

- Formula—handling and safety considerations
- Raw materials
- Manufacturing equipment
- Manufacturing precautions
- Manufacturing procedures
- Packaging
- Process validation
- Specifications for raw materials, packaging components, and in-process and finished product

- Validated analytical methods
- Regulatory considerations
- Rework procedures
- Transportation

Each aspect should be reviewed to ensure that critical issues have been addressed. If an aspect is not relevant, it should be stated that it is not applicable to the program. An issue perceived as unimportant in one department may be a monumental task in another department. With new drugs and drug-delivery systems, this effort is critical to the success of a program.

FORMULA

Understanding the formula, its derivation, and its constraints is one of the first prerequisites to any development program. The feasibility of the formula may be established by reviewing the ingredients of the composition and explaining their function in the formula. It would be appropriate to review the claims and physical characteristics of the product while evaluating a sample so that the participants of a planning meeting appreciate the appearance and attributes of the product.

The safety evaluation completed by the toxicology group and/or industrial hygienist should be reviewed with the participants because they, as managers, will most likely assume the responsibility to protect the safety of employees who will work on this project. The employees' right to know must be protected further by keeping them informed of the potential risks to which they may be exposed.

Prerequisite safety information can be transmitted by draft material safety data sheets, especially for new drug actives and new drug products. Preparation of the draft document may lead to the question: Are the process handling procedures for this product necessary and appropriate? Those personnel involved in the manufacturing of drug products are cognizant of the concepts of inherent risk due to an agent's toxicity, and potential risk, due to exposure. Whether the new drug and/or product should be handled in an open environment, contained area, or in isolation must be determined by those people who are responsible for safety. In all cases, the procedures must be reviewed and approved by the individual responsible for the involved manufacturing and testing sites.

Comments about the prestability and finished product stability profiles should be presented as an overview of the new product's chemical stability. This will support the anticipated shelf life of the formula and its ability to withstand the "process shocks" normally encountered during production scale-ups. The toxicity of the finished product should be discussed. This information ensures that a decision regarding the handling of the formula has been made based on generated data and experience. A draft or tentative material safety data sheet may be one route to disseminate this information.

Constraints on specific ingredients or sources of ingredients, cost of goods, or manufacturing equipment should be reviewed. Constraints must be considered when formula optimization is undertaken; however, optimizing formulas may be best addressed in the production environment because batch size and manufacturing equipment sometimes have been shown to render viable laboratory and small-scale formulas virtually inoperative in the plant. The experience gained during the manufacture of laboratory and scale-up batches is invaluable and should be shared with the participants, especially the production and quality assurance staffs, in written reports and follow-up meetings.

Many firms use a laboratory development report to record these activities. These data can be incorporated into a full project-development history. For new drug products, development histories are needed to fulfill regulatory directives. The detail necessary in any summary report depends greatly on the magnitude of the problems encountered during development and the corporate structure in which one lives. For some multinational companies, the product-development report serves as the basis of spreading interest in a new product across global borders.

RAW MATERIALS

Sources of raw materials, especially those critical to a new product's functionality, should be identified. Availability and costs should be ascertained to aid in the planning process. Care should be taken to ensure that new drug actives and, when possible, excipients are secured from vendors with a current acceptable FDA compliance profile and a drug master file.

Testing monographs including methods to ascertain a lot's chemical and, if necessary, microbiological integrity should be provided to the selected manufacturing site in advance so that the methods may be applied to the incoming supplies. Handling of materials including storage, disposal, and employee precautions should be documented, especially for new or potentially hazardous materials. Again, material safety data sheets (MSDS) for all materials used should be available and disseminated to the plant personnel before any exposure.

MANUFACTURING

Equipment

When new drugs and drug-delivery systems are developed in the laboratory, the correlation of the necessary production equipment may be very difficult indeed. For example, the shear needed to create the desired particle size of an emulsion with the help of laboratory equipment may pose serious problems in the selection of plant equipment necessary to reproduce the attributes of the product. Recording the speed of a laboratory mixer is not sufficient by itself for this task; definition of the operating principle and equipment design is necessary to accomplish the task.

Any equipment used in drug manufacturing, including packaging, should have undergone an equipment evaluation, including installation, operational, and performance qualification, following a written protocol. This is an important step in a process-validation program. Through this effort, the operating parameters and capabilities of a given piece of equipment are documented. Furthermore, should a major component of the equipment fail, installation of a replacement part of known specifications reduces and in many cases eliminates the need for revalidation of every product processed with that equipment. The equipment itself, however, must be shown to meet its previous operating capabilities before being placed back into service.

The availability, size, and surfaces or composition of the required equipment should be specifically identified so that the scale-up effort may be representative of a production run. A preliminary compatibility screen of contact surfaces should be completed before the selection of scale-up equipment. The location of the equipment in reference to other requirements, such as services or the packaging area, may be a factor in the selection of equipment. A cleaning-validation study should be conducted to ensure that no residues of active ingredient or cleaning agent remain after cleaning and that the equipment is suitable for production use again. Alternative equipment may be considered and used; however, experience will dictate its suitability.

Precautions

Any concerns regarding the handling of equipment or product by employees should be addressed in the planning stage. This is especially important with regard to environmental (particulate contamination or sterility) or atmospheric (oxygen, moisture, or light sensitivity) problems.

Procedures

Procedures should be clear and concise. Specific descriptions should be used when possible. For example, "pass the emulsion through a suitable colloid mill (Eppenbach mill) at a setting of 0.005 inch (0.12 mm)" is preferred to a description referencing a more general description of a piece of equipment. Process-validation testing is necessary using specific equipment, as described by design and operating principle.

Procedures should be realistic, and any instructions must be scale-oriented. Specific parameters may be necessary for manufacturing areas. For example, cooling or heating times are typically equipment-dependent. Cooling 1 kg in the laboratory in 15 min may take 4 hours for a 40,000-kg batch in the plant. Similarly, filtration of small batches in the laboratory may not provide the necessary information to predict filter life or flow rates needed for large-scale manufacturing.

Based on the experience gained during the pilot scale-up effort, a process flow chart should be constructed. It helps identify steps and issues in need of process-validation review. In addition, the timing of activities toward the scheduling of manpower needs, such as for in-process testing, is generally more apparent when viewed in the context of the total process.

Process-optimization parameters as identified during the pilot scale-up effort should be monitored during the production scale-up batch. In this manner, appropriate recommendations based on experience may be integrated into the production of future batches. Many optimization experiments may be efficiently incorporated into the process-validation program.

Packaging

The description, specifications, and test methods for any packaging configuration should be available to the plant before the production scale-up. Unit functionality and fit should be included as a practical use test in any specification. The plant equipment to be used in packaging should be evaluated for feasibility, speed, and contact surface compatibility. Preliminary evaluations of surface compatibility, discussed previously, should suffice as an early indication of packaging equipment suitability.

The availability of or lead time to secure the necessary packaging components that are representative of the commercially marketed package frequently places stress on the project timeline. Package costs and possible alternative packaging can be evaluated with bulk produced from this batch. Therefore, a course of action to minimize project failure resulting from an unsatisfactory package

may be appropriate. The resultant dilution of resources and increased project expense must be weighed in accepting this course of action.

The number of various package sizes to be filled from a batch may be critical. For example, for generic drugs, entire batches must be filled for the batch to be accepted by the FDA. Although the batch may be filled into numerous package formats, care must be exercised to fill a sufficient number of each format to ensure proper equipment set-up and that the filling speeds used are representative of a full-scale production effort.

Procedures for packaging the batch including fill tolerances and precautions such as aseptic handling or nitrogen gassing should be reviewed to state the requirements for acceptance in advance. As a part of this production scale-up effort, it may be desirable to evaluate the product's bulk stability in the storage tank or storage drums to establish limits on the length of time a batch may be held before final packaging. This is especially important if the bulk product is to be manufactured at one site and transported to another site for packaging. Storage container compatibility deserves appropriate attention also.

Finally, the personnel involved in packaging should be instructed on any safety and handling issues that might affect them or compromise the product's integrity. Whether it is for the development of new package formats, such as for intranasal drug administration or transdermal patches, or for more traditional delivery systems, such as cycle packs, solutions, or aerosols, the need to educate employees involved in the processing is essential to the transfer program's success. Identifying and controlling process variables are necessary while experience is gained, and the process is optimized and validated.

PROCESS VALIDATION

Each class of product has specific issues to be addressed for process validation. In general, variable process steps such as mixing times and temperatures should be validated. Many articles have been written regarding the validation of processes affecting pharmaceutical products (12–14). Protocols to evaluate those parameters that may affect a product's integrity should be agreed on by the R&D, regulatory, production, QA, and engineering staffs. During the preparation and packaging of the pilot production batch, generation of data toward improving the efficiency of these processes, as well as minimizing batch-to-batch variations, is very important because this information will serve as documentation to support the new product's commercial feasibility. Also, the establishment of cleaning procedures and documentation of cleaning validation can be accomplished at this time.

There is no magic number of batches required to prove that a process is validated. Generally, the number of batches accepted is three. The technical complexities of and product sensitivities to variable parameters dictate how extensive a validation program is needed. Suffice it to note that the process must be controllable and reproducible and yield a product that meets the desired specifications.

QUALITY CONTROL AND QUALITY ASSURANCE

One of the purposes of the pilot production batch is to introduce the new product in its entirety to the functional areas of the site (manufacturing, packaging, and testing), that is, the release of raw materials and packaging components as well as in-process, bulk, and finished product testing should be completed at the site as if the pilot scale-up were a commercial batch.

In-process testing, bulk release before packaging, and finished product specifications are proposed. Specification limits are proposed based on the experience gained with smaller laboratory and scale-up batches. Any comments or concerns regarding the test methods and specifications should be addressed at this time. Reagents and equipment to complete the required testing must be available at the plant. A contact at the R&D analytical laboratory should be established to explain aberrant values or to answer questions.

Communication of requirements of time and manpower to the quality control department is a critical issue that must not be overlooked. Prompt attention to analysis needs does help keep the pilot production batch process moving forward. If microbiological release of bulk product is needed before packaging, the project timeline should reflect the time period (3–5 days) generally needed for this activity.

Sampling must be scheduled for release and stability testing using a statistically valid sampling program. This is especially important for stability studies. In this manner, the chosen samples are documented to be representative of the entire batch.

Batch documentation is an important factor. Preparation of master batch records in accordance with plant standard operating procedures (SOPs) should be followed by an approval of the document by the sponsoring division, usually the formulator or process development staff of the R&D unit. On completion of a batch, review of the batch records by the quality assurance group ensures compliance to GMP and that all necessary deviations from and modifications to the manufacturing records are properly explained and documented.

THE MANUFACTURING TRIAL SCHEDULING DATE

At the conclusion of the planning meeting, any actions that must be undertaken before the scale-up should be documented and a responsible party identified. At the discussion of the trial date, time constraints must be considered, along with the availability of raw materials, packaging components, plant scheduling time, and personnel. Coordination of personnel and supplies is the responsibility of the project leader. The ability to lead and negotiate another individual's priorities helps bring the trials to completion on schedule.

Finally, arrangements for transporting raw materials and packaged finished products must be made to ensure that the scale-up effort is completed on schedule and that stability studies are initiated expeditiously. Participants should leave the meeting under the impression that one person is in charge of the project, that the program has been well thought out and documented, and that commitments will be honored. Early issuance of meeting minutes will reinforce the importance of individual responsibilities and serve as notice to the participants and their superiors that their cooperation has been solicited, is needed, and is expected.

COMPLETION

In review, the activities to be completed at the manufacturing site are:

- Release of raw materials and packaging components
- Manufacture and packaging of the trial batch
- Generation of data from in-process, bulk, and finished product samples
- Process validation, including equipment qualification and reviews of batch records, processing, cleaning validation, and on-site experiences
- Shipment of finished product to the research facility for testing

An exit interview with involved plant personnel offers an opportunity for their comments to be heard. Their efforts should be acknowledged and their input seriously considered and incorporated into the manufacturing document. Any differences that cannot be resolved at this time should be noted and studied further. The art of listening and diplomacy must be used inasmuch as this forum must be one of cooperation and not one of confrontation.

At this meeting, a discussion about possible rework procedures may be appropriate. The ability to recover materials, especially expensive drug actives, is desirable. Early identification of steps where rework may be possible allows for procedures to be tested, verified, and put in place, should they be needed. For pharmaceuticals, rework procedures may be used only if they are appropriately documented, validated, and approved by the responsible corporate and government bodies. Rework procedures are not an automatic means for handling out-of-specification product lots but rather for identifying where an effort may be implemented successfully. Logistics and economics, as always, dictate whether a rework should be considered.

POSTPRODUCTION ACTIVITIES AND EVALUATION

Once the plant experience has been concluded, confirmatory analyses on duplicate samples for in-process, bulk release, and finished product previously tested at the plant site should be completed at R&D. In this manner, the proposed methods are challenged to yield similar results from different analysts in different locations. Discrepancies in values generated at this point must be investigated and resolved. Samples should be placed into the stability testing system according to the organization's procedures.

Finally, a report must be prepared and issued expeditiously summarizing the experience, reviewing each area's involvement, and proposing, if necessary, changes in the process or control methods. Timely and factual communication of project progress to the other corporate areas not directly involved in the scale-up, such as the marketing, finance, and purchasing units, draws their attention and commitment of resources. By fostering informed decision-making through directed written communication, the time required to plan or complete these activities to bring the product to market is minimized, and resource usage is optimized.

A formal postproduction trial review meeting should be held with representatives from the R&D, corporate, marketing, quality assurance, regulatory affairs, and production centers. Plans to commercialize the product or to submit documentation for government approval if this is the next step in the development scheme are outlined, contingent on the successful completion of a defined stability program. Agreement as to the suitability of all the factors involved in the preparation of the product should be the result of this meeting, with a substantiating document in the form of meeting minutes or a signed "statement of concurrence" generated and distributed.

A monograph of all pertinent sections to support the product's introduction should be assembled, reviewed, and disseminated to the appropriate parties. This document should include:

- Manufacturing formula
- Draft label copy
- Raw material tests and specifications
- Manufacturing procedure
- In-process tests and specifications
- Finished product test methods and specifications
- Packaging component specifications and drawings
- Packaging component test methods
- Stability data on bulk product
- Stability data on packaged product
- Shelf-life projection of expiration dating
- Material safety data sheet for the product
- Bibliography

A projection of shelf life should be included to document the recommendation for the expiration date. Although accelerated stability data are frequently used to support expiration dating for up to 24 months, extension of dating beyond 24 months is based on real-time test results.

A bibliography of all project reports and memos should be assembled, including the development and validation reports. Ideally, the project leader should maintain a file in chronological order of all communications and reports. Compiling the file into a bibliography is a tedious task but one that, should the need to answer a question arise, will be well worth the effort. Product development histories and testing "quirks" regularly appear in these documents and in no other place. Skilled project leaders maintain an ongoing listing as a means of tracking a project. A bibliography for a new pharmaceutical product may be voluminous, and a reference to its location may be useful. The transfer of the project is considered complete when the first commercial batch is produced under the supervision of the manufacturing site without problems.

SUMMARY

This article has reviewed issues to be considered when organizing the transfer of pharmaceutical technology from the research arena to the production environment. Critical areas affecting the manufacture, packaging, safety, and quality of pharmaceutical products are discussed in relationship to their impact by the technology transfer process. The necessity of a plan with input from the various organizational centers is emphasized. The success of the program is highly dependent on the communication and cooperation shared throughout the process.

REFERENCES

1. Popp, K.F. *Encyclopedia of Pharmaceutical Technology*; Swarbrick, J., Boylan, J.C., Eds.; Marcel Dekker, Inc.: New York, 1996; 14, 419–432.

2. Amico, L.A.; Pilot Plant Operation. *Encyclopedia of Pharmaceutical Technology*, 1st Ed.; Swarbrick, J., Boylan, J.C. Eds.; Marcel Dekker, Inc. New York, 1995; 12, 187–207.

3. Franz, R.M.; Copeland, R.D.; Lewis, L.D.; Stagner, W.C. Pilot Plant Design. *Encyclopedia of Pharmaceutical Technology*; Swarbrick, J., Boylan, J.C., Eds.; Marcel Dekker, Inc.: New York, 1995; 12, 171–186.

4. Groen, J.J. Project Management. *Encyclopedia of Pharmaceutical Technology*, 1st Ed.; Swarbrick, J., Boylan, J.C., Eds.; Marcel Dekker, Inc.: New York, 1995; 13, 121–150.

5. Owen, V.M. Technology Transfer in the Diagnostic Industry. Med. Dev. Technol. (Lond) **1994**, *5*, 23–26.

6. Popp, K.F. Drug Dev. Ind. Pharm. **1987**, *13* (13), 2339–2362.

7. Popp, K.F. Organizing the Transfer of Pharmaceuticals from Research to Production. *Specialized Drug Delivery Systems—Manufacturing and Production Technology*; Tyle, P., Ed.; Marcel Dekker, Inc.: New York, 1990; 37–50.

8. Rao, A.V.; Rajan, J.V. Transfer of Drug Technology from Laboratory to Industry. Eastern Pharmacist (India) **1985**, *28*, 63–65.

9. Testa, E.G.; Lepiti, S. Product Technology Transfer. Pharmaz. Ind. (Germany) **1981**, *43* (12), 1231–1234.

10. Upupa, N. Research, Product Development, and Pilot Plant Scale Up. Pharmacy Times (India) **1990**, *22*, 63–65.

11. Evanoff, B.J.; Hofmann, K.L., Jr. *Validation of Active Pharmaceutical Ingredients*, 2nd Ed.; Berry, I.R., Harpaz, D., Eds.; Interpharm Press: Englewood, CO, 2001.

12. Berry, I.R. Process Validation: Practical Applications to Pharmaceutical Products. Drug Dev. Ind. Pharm. **1988**, *14* (2 & 3), 377–389.

13. Berry, I.R.; Nash, R.A. *Pharmaceutical Process Validation*, 2nd Ed.; Marcel Dekker, Inc.: New York, 1993.

14. Berry, I.R.; Harpaz, D. Eds.; *Validation of Active Pharmaceutical Ingredients*, 2nd Ed.; Interpharm Press: Englewood, CO, 2001.

THERMAL ANALYSIS OF DRUGS AND DRUG PRODUCTS

Danièlle Giron

Novartis Pharma AG, Basel, Switzerland

INTRODUCTION

Thermal analysis techniques, in which a physical property is monitored as a function of temperature or time while the analyte is heated or cooled under controlled conditions, are fundamental techniques for the characterization of drugs and drug products, not only while processing or aging conditions may be simulated but while the methods gives access to thermodynamic data. Due to the different informations delivered, thermal analysis methods are concurrent or complementary to other analytical techniques, such as spectroscopy, chromatography, melting, loss on drying, assay, for identification, purity, and quantitation. They are basic methods in the field of polymer analysis and in physical and chemical characterization of pure substances as well as for mixtures. They find good applications for preformulation, processing, and control of the drug product. The introduction of automation considerably increases the advantages of these methods. New horizons are open with the availability of combined techniques and microthermal analysis.

PRINCIPLES AND EXPERIMENTAL FACTORS

Considering the number of physical parameters of a substance that may be measured, the number of techniques derived is very large. Details on most techniques are well described by Wendlandt (1). For pharmaceutical applications, the methods generally used are differential scanning calorimetry (DSC), thermogravimetry (TG) (or thermogravimetric analysis: TGA), and, to a lesser extent thermomechanical analysis (TMA). All techniques are automated and have data acquisition. Hyphenated techniques and modulated DSC are growing techniques, "state of the art" for the 21st century. Excellent books or review articles dealing with the principle, instrumentation, and applications of thermal analysis methods for pharmaceuticals are given in (1–15). As emphasized by Cheng et al. (14), tendency in the next two decades will be more precise and meaningful measurements in these techniques and new developments in obtaining the temperature dependence of a material's structure and dynamics.

Differential Scanning Calorimetry (DSC)

When a material is heated or cooled, there is a change in its structure or composition. These transformations are connected with a heat exchange. Differential scanning calorimetry (DSC) is used for measuring the heat flow into and out of the sample, as well as for determining the temperature of the thermal phenomenon during a controlled change of temperature. The first method developed by Le Chatelier in 1887 was differential thermal analysis (DTA), where only the temperature induced in the sample was measured.

The principle of DSC is as follows: two ovens are linearly heated; one oven contains the sample in a pan, the other contains an empty pan as a reference pan. If no change occurs in the sample during heating, the sample pan and the reference pan are at the same temperature. If a change such as melting occurs in the sample, energy is used by the sample and the temperature remains constant in the sample pan while the temperature of the reference pan continues to increase. Therefore a difference of temperature occurs between the sample pan and reference pan.

Manufacturers use two methods of measurements. In the first method called "heat flux DSC," the instrument measures this temperature difference (DTA). Through calibration, this temperature difference is transformed into a heat flow, dq/dt. Therefore, there is a thermal factor that may vary with temperature. In the second method, called "power compensation DSC," two individual heaters are used in order to monitor the individual heating rates of the two individual ovens. A system controls the temperature difference between sample and reference. If any temperature difference is detected, the individual heatings are corrected in such a way that the temperature is kept the same in both pans. That is, when an endothermic or exothermic process occurs, the instrument delivers the compensation energy in order to maintain equal temperature in both pans.

In the first case temperature is primarily measured, and in the second case, energy is primarily measured.

Encyclopedia of Pharmaceutical Technology

The differentiation of measuring principles is with modern instrumentation not very significant under normal applications. Due to calibration and integrated data handling, the instruments produce similar qualities of reported results.

Each instrument can deliver the same information, that is, heat flow as a function of temperature (or time). The peak shape, the resolution, and the sensitivity depend on the principle of measurement and the specification of the instrument.

For first-order transitions such as melting, crystallization, sublimation, boiling, etc., the integration of the curve gives the energy involved in the transition. For second-order transitions, the signal gives the change in the specific heat, for example, glass transitions.

Fig. 1 shows typical transitions. Melting and crystallization are first-order transitions. The extrapolated onset temperature (T_e) is the melting or boiling point. The peak temperature (T_m) is dependent on instrument and measurement parameters. The glass point is determined as inflexion point. Manufacturers represent the heat flow in different ways: the endotherms in the positive side for power compensation DSC and in the negative side for heat flux DSC. Melting, boiling, and sublimation are endothermic, which means they need energy. Crystallization is exothermic, which means that it supplies energy. Desolvatations without melting are generally endothermic. Solid–solid phase transition and decomposition may be endothermic or exothermic.

Modern instruments provide heating, cooling and isotherms between subambient temperatures (with a cooling device) and higher temperatures in the range of 1200–1500°C. In order to avoid reactions with the atmosphere the measurements are carried out under nitrogen. The major components of the systems include the DSC sensors, the furnace, the programer, and the data handling. The temperature plotted on the abscissa is the programed temperature, not the temperature of the sample.

The difference between the programed and the actual temperature of the sample is called "thermal lag." It depends on the thermal resistance of the instrument and the heating rate. In modern instruments dedicated to accurate analytical measurements for pharmaceuticals, the sensors are in direct contact with the bottom of the pans and the sample size is in the milligram range or less. Therefore this correction is not very high, but it has to be taken into consideration. Generally pure indium (>99.9999%) is used for the correction of the thermal lag.

Great efforts have been made in recent years in order to validate the different instruments not only in comparing principle and results but also in determining the critical parameters such as heating and cooling rates, particle size, weight, resolution, atmosphere, and type of pans (crimped pan, sealed pan, open pan, etc.).

The instruments include automation and data acquisition. The calibration of the instrument should be done at a yearly basis. This includes the measurement of temperature and enthalpy. Most certified standards are highly purified metals. Indium is the preferred reference standard, but it covers only one temperature. It is recommended for pharmaceuticals to include several organic substances for which the melting point or the melting enthalpy has been accurately determined. Sarge et al. (16,17) proposed several organic substances and metals. The heat determination of quartz was also recommended. Sabbah (18) published recently a broad review of data of organic substances. For pharmaceuticals, it is suitable to have certified materials covering a broad range corresponding to the thermal events of interest (19).

Tables 1 and 2 are examples of calibration of the temperature and of the calorimetric response of PE-DSC-7 instruments by using different materials (20). Very important for pharmaceutical industry is the confidence of the laboratory that delivers the reference. Since the heating rate may have an influence on the data, it is recommended to compare the melting point and the melting enthalpy of organic standards, additionally to indium, at different heating rates covering the measurement range. For very accurate determinations, it is recommended to use standards with a melting point in the range of the considered temperature in a series of measurements.

Pressure DSC

In Pressure DSC (PDSC), the sample can be submitted to different pressures, which allows to characterize substances at the pressures of processes or to distinguish overlapping peaks observed, for example, by desolvatation (21).

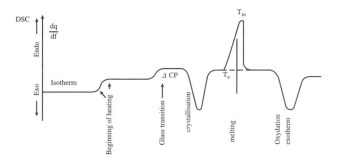

Fig. 1 Theoretical DSC scans.

Table 1 Example of calibration of Perkin-Elmer DSC-7 instruments with melting standards at 10 K min^{-1} under nitrogen

Certified substances	Onset T (°C) certificate	Instrument 1 Onset T (°C)	ΔT (°C)	Instrument 2 with intracooler Onset T (°C)	ΔT (°C)
Iodobenzene	−31.3			−32.2	0.9
H$_2$O	0.0			0.1	0.1
4-Nitrotoluene	51.5	50.4	1.1	51.2	0.3
Biphenyl	69.3	68.2	1.1	68.6	0.7
Naphthalene	80.2	79.4	0.8	80.1	0.1
Benzil	94.7	94.21	0.6	94.5	0.2
Acetanilide	114.0	113.9	0.1	113.6	0.4
Benzoic acid	122.1	122.0	0.1	121.8	0.4
Diphenylacetic acid	146.5	146.9	0.4	146.9	0.4
Indium	156.6	156.8	0.2	156.5	0.1
Anisic acid	183.1	183.6	0.5	183.2	0.1
2-Chloro-anthraquinone	210.0	210.1	0.1	210.1	0.1
Tin	231.9	232.7	0.8	232.7	0.8
Anthraquinone	284.5	285.2	0.7	284.8	0.7
Lead	327.5	328.6	1.1	—	—
Zinc	418.9	420.3	1.4	—	—

Modulated DSC

This new technique introduced in 1993 (22) has been thoroughly examined and discussed (23). Main advantages are the separation of overlapping events in the DSC scans. In conventional DSC, a constant linear heating or cooling rate is applied. In modulated DSC (MDSC), the normally linear heating ramp is overlaid with a sinusoidal function (MDSC) defined by a frequency and an amplitude to produce a sinusoidal-shaped temperature versus time function. Using Fourier mathematics, the DSC signal is split into two components: one reflecting non-reversible events (kinetic) and the other reversible events.

$$T = T_0 + bt + B \sin(\omega t)$$

$$dq/dt = C(b + B\omega \cos(\omega t)) + f'(t, T) + K \sin(\omega t)$$

where T is temperature, C the specific heat, t the time, ω the frequency, $f'(t,T)$ is the average underlying kinetic function once the effect of the sine-wave modulation has been substracted. K is the amplitude of the kinetic response to the sine-wave modulation and $(b + B\omega \cos(\omega t))$ is the measured quantity dT/dt or "reversing" curve.

The total DSC curve, the reversing curve giving reversible transitions and the nonreversing curve giving irreversible transitions (e.g. the glass transitions), is

Table 2 Examples of calorimetric measurements of standards with two different DSC-7 instruments and measurement cell at different times (A, B, C) at 10 K min^{-1} under nitrogen

Standard substance	ΔH (J/g) (Theory)	A ΔH (J/g)	A % deviation	B ΔH (J/g)	B % deviation	C ΔH (J/g)	C % deviation
Naphthalene (80.2°C)	148.6	147.1	1.0	148.6	0.0	—	—
Benzil (94.7°C)	112.0	110.1	1.7	112.8	0.7	—	—
Benzoic acid (80.2°C)	147.2	—	—	—	—	146.6	0.4
Biphenyl (69.3°C)	120.4	120.0	0.6	—	—	120.5	0.1
Diphenyl-acetic acid (146.5°C)	146.9	—	—	146.8	0.1	—	—
Indium (156.6°C)	28.7	28.63	0.2	28.8	0.35	28.7	0.1
Tin (231.9°C)	60.2	60.0	0.3	—	—	60.8	1.0

obtained. MDSC is a valuable extension of conventional DSC. Its applicability (24) is recognized for precise determination of the temperature of glass transitions and for the study of the energy of relaxation, and it depends on a number of important parameters to be studied. It has been recently applied for the determination of glass transitions of hydroxypropylmethylcellulose films (25) and for the study of amorphous lactose (26), as well as for the study of some glassy drugs (27).

Microwave thermal analysis (MWTA)

In this new technique (28), microwaves are used both to heat a material and to detect thermal transitions.

Micro-DSC

The instruments of conventional DSC allows to measure very small amounts of material. The author was able to characterize the melting peak of indium with 0.032 mg by using a DSC-7 of Perkin-Elmer. New instrument generation will permit to increase sensitivity and amount of material to be studied decrease to nanorange (29).

Microcalorimetry

Microcalorimetry is a growing technique (30,31) complementary to DSC for the characterization of pharmaceuticals. Larger sample volume and high sensitivity means that phenomena of very low energy (unmesurable by DSC) may be studied. The output of the instrument is measured by the rate of heat change (dq/dt) as a function of time with a high sensitivity better than 0.1 μW. Microcalorimery can be applied to isolated systems in specific atmospheres; or for batch mode where reactants are mixed in the calorimeter. Solution calorimetry can be used in adiabatic or isoperibol modes in microcalorimeters at constant temperature. (See the corresponding article about calorimetry of this edition.)

Thermogravimetric Analysis

In thermogravimetry (TG or TGA) the change in sample mass is determined as a function of temperature and/or time. The instrument is a thermobalance that permits the continuous weighing of a sample as a function of time. The sample holder and a reference holder are bounded to each side of a microbalance. The sample holder is in a furnace, without direct contact with the sample, the temperature of which is controlled by a temperature programer. The balance part is maintained at a constant temperature. The instrument is able to record the mass loss or gain of the

sample as a function of temperature and time [$m = f(T)$]. Most instruments also record the DTG curve, which is the rate of the mass change $dm/dt = f(T)$.

The DTG curves, allow a better distinction of overlapping steps, as demonstrated in Fig. 2, for $CuSO_4 \cdot 5H_2O$. The area under the DTG curve is proportional to the mass change, and the height of the DTG peak at any temperature gives the rate of mass change. The real advantage of DTG is to permit accurate location of the end of a desolvatation process if decomposition follows desolvatation by use of the minima in the DTG curve.

The instrument used in thermogravimetry is a thermobalance (balance controller, sample chamber, furnace, furnace controller) with data processing. In order to check the stability of the system a baseline at the highest sensitivity has to be done for all heating rates in the temperature range of analysis: The highest deviation will be observed at the highest heating rate. The thermobalance may have a vertical or horizontal construction. The sensitivity of new thermobalances attains 0.1 μg. Some manufacturers offer combined DSC/TG instruments.

The mass accuracy is generally not a problem of modern TG. Calibration of the mass with certified mass can be used as for all other balances. Electrostatics, temperature fluctuation, sensitivity of the sensor, and thermal lags have to be known, what is best done with regular calibration. For automatic TG, the pans have to be tightly closed and pierced just before the measurement; therefore, the TG curves of desolvatation may be different as for open pans. The use of a protective gas and its flow, as well as the sample mass and the heating rate play a role in the comparison of the temperature of thermal events. The influence of heating rate is examplified in Fig. 3 with $CuSO_4 \cdot 5H_2O$. The limit of detection can be calculated by determining the maximum

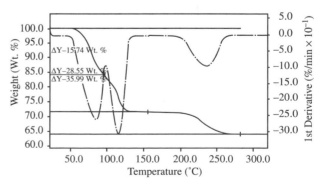

Fig. 2 TG of copper(II) sulfate pentahydrate with the heating rate 20 K min^{-1}. Use of DTG for the different steps.

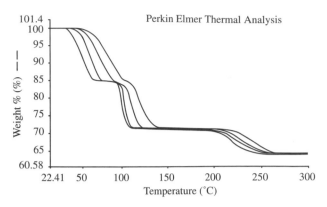

Fig. 3 TG of copper(II) sulfate pentahydrate. Influence of the heating rate. TG curves from the top: 20 K min⁻¹, 10 K min⁻¹, 5 K min⁻¹, 2.5 K min⁻¹.

of deviation of the base line in the temperature range of interest.

Table 3 shows an example of calibration performed with hydrates, which cover the starting of dehydration temperature from 50 to 120°C and the end of dehydration from approx. 150°C until to 270°C with different heating rates.

Since there is no contact between pan and furnace, the thermal lag is higher than in DSC. The standards recommended by ICTA and distributed by NBS are ferromagnetic standards exhibiting loss of ferromagnetism at their curie point temperature within a magnetic field: Nickel (354°C), Permanorm 3 (266°C), Numetal (386°C), Permanorm 5 (459°C), Trafoperm (754°C). The method does not permit the temperature measurement with high precision. These standards have been studied by several authors (32). The ICTA temperatures are within 5–10°C. McGhie et al. (33) proposed a calibration technique in which a small inert platinum weight is suspended by a fusible link composed of a calibration standard that releases the platinum weight at the temperature of melting. The Mettler instrument TGA 850 is constructed so that the melting curve of standards can be measured and used as calibration, as demonstrated in Table 4.

TG can be used with different atmospheres and under vacuum. TG has a huge number of pharmaceutical applications. Automated TG is extremely efficient to replace the loss on drying assay in drug substances, being able to separate loss of solvent from decomposition by using very small amounts of substance. Solvent entrapped or bounded as solvate is easily determined (9, 34, 35). A comprehensive article on TG has been recently written by Dunn and Sharp (36). Ozawa proposes the use of modulated TG for kinetic analysis (37).

Water sorption–desorption isotherms can be carried out by using thermobalances. Now specific instruments allow to measure water sorption–desorption isotherms at different constant temperatures (e.g., dynamic vapor sorption instrument (DVS), Surface Measurement Systems Ltd., Monarch Beach, US).

Thermomechanical Analysis

In thermomechanical analysis (TMA) the deformation of the sample under stress is monitored against time or temperature while the temperature increases or decreases proportionally to time. Changes are detected by mechanical, optical, or electrical transducers. The stress may be a compression, penetration, tension, flexure, or torsion. Generally the instruments are also able to measure the sample dimensions, a technique called thermodilatometry. The stress (F/A) expressed in N/m^2 or Pa may be a normal tensile stress σ, a tangential shearing stress τ, or a pressure change Δp; the force applied is F and A is the area.

The deformation is measured by the strain, which is the deformation per unit dimension.

Elongation $\varepsilon = \Delta L/L_0$
Volume strain $\theta = \Delta V/V_0$
Shear strain $\gamma = \Delta x/y$

For an elastic material, the Young's modulus is defined by

$$E = (F/A)/(\Delta L/L_0) \quad or \quad E = \sigma/\varepsilon$$

Creep is the gradual irreversible elongation of the sample.

Table 3 Example of calibration of loss of mass with three hydrate standards

| | **Theoretical amount water** | **Result** | | |
Substance		**5 K min⁻¹**	**10 K min⁻¹**	**20 K min⁻¹**
Sodium-tartrate dihydrate	15.7%	15.73%	15.60%	15.73%
Calcium-oxalate monohydrate	12.3%	12.55%	12.51%	12.48%
Copper-sulfate pentahydrate	36.1%	36.08%	36.03%	36.04%

Table 4 Example of calibration of the temperature of TGA 850 with melting standards

Substance	Theory	Result		
		5 K min^{-1}	10 K min^{-1}	20 K min^{-1}
Nitrotoluene	51.5°C	51.49°C	51.64°C	53.78°C
Indium	156.6°C	157.62°C	157.38°C	157.74°C
Tin	231.9°C	233.44°C	233.42°C	233.68°C

These parameters depend on the temperature. The coefficient of thermal expansion is

$$\alpha = \left[\frac{dL}{dT}\right]\left[\frac{1}{L_0}\right]$$

The instruments have a furnace, and mostly a linear variable differential transformer (LVDT) to produce an electrical signal from a linear movement. An additional unit controls the force applied. Special attachments allow the same instrument to work in different modes such as elongation, compression, penetration, or tension.

The slope of the TMA trace may also be obtained by DTMA.

$$\frac{dL}{dt} = L_0 \quad \alpha \frac{dT}{dt}$$

where dT/dt is the heating rate.

Thermomechanical methods are very useful for the determination of phase transformations such as polymorphic solid–solid transitions or glass transitions. Fig. 4 shows some theoretical curves for glass transition and polymorphic transition in extension or in penetration mode. Recently TMA has been proposed for the measurement of the internal stress of tablets of ethylcellulose of different molecular weight (38) and for measurement of swelling of polysaccharide hydrogels (39) and of polymeric films (40).

Calibration of the instrument for its response to length may be carried out with a standard length piece of metal or ceramic. The temperature can be calibrated in the same way as for DSC. Metal standards such as indium, tin, or lead are mostly used. Recent publications (41) deal with calibration and errors of TMA.

Dynamic Mechanical Analysis

In this technique, the mechanical response of a sample is measured as it is deformed under oscillating load against temperature or time. Dynamic mechanical analysis (DMA) is a further development of TMA, but the instruments are different.

DMA is mostly applied to the study of polymers. Relevant parameters are the storage modulus and the loss modulus. Generally the loss tan δ, which is the ratio of these modulus, is plotted against temperature. A recent overview of the pharmaceutical applications of DMA has been published by Craig and Johnson (42).

Torsional braid analysis (TBA) is a particular case where the sample supported by a fiberglass braid is subjected to a torsional strain.

Hyphenated Techniques (Combined Techniques)

A comprehensive characterization of the physical properties of materials often requires a multidisciplinary approach since no single technique is capable of characterizing pharmaceuticals completely.

Thermomicroscopy or hot stage microscopy is a well-established method (43, 43–45) for the microscopic observation with polarization of the sample while heating

Table 5 Study of two polymorphs with unique melting curve

Property	Crystalline form A	Crystalline form B
Melting point °C	304	311
Melting enthalpy in kcal/mol	12	11
Water uptake after 1 day 92% RH	0%	3.2% (Hydrate)
Transformation in alcohols	A	B→A

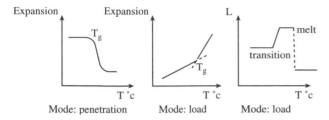

Fig. 4 Theoretical TMA curves for glass transition T_g and polymorphic transition.

or cooling, allowing to see desolvatation, melting, crystallization, eutectic formation, and even transformations in suspensions in solvents. The combination of hot stage microscopy to new technology such as high-resolution color camera, image manipulation software makes the technique very attractive for inducing metastable states, for observation of crystal habit, and for better interpretation of other methods. Thermophotometry is the measurement of the light intensity and thermoluminescence of the light emitted by the sample. FT-IR microscopy (15, 45, 46), Raman microscopy (47–49) are excellent additional tools to thermomicroscopy. Calibration of microscope, of heating unit, and of spectroscopic methods should be done. TEM (transmission microscopy) and SEM (scanning electron microscopy) with EDX have been combined to DSC for the study of solid-state reactions.

Newly born, the scanning thermal microscopy derived from atomic force microscopy brings a revolution in the instrumentation for measuring thermophysical and thermomechanical properties of the matter, and the TA instrument was awarded at Pittsburg 1998. The instrument has been applied for the characterization of Ibuprofen compacts as model substance (50).

Temperature-resolved X-ray diffraction with a heating cell is widely used (12, 51–54). Crystalline changes are clearly assigned; the X-ray diffraction patterns obtained in situ allow to predict quantitative methods if, for kinetic reasons, forms that are present at high temperatures occur at ambient conditions. Low-temperature X-ray diffraction cell has been developed for the study of frozen aqueous solutions (55). The introduction of XRD-DTA cell (56) and recently of the DSC-XRD instrument of Rigaku presented at the Denver X-ray Conference in 1999 (57) demonstrates the advantage of this direct combined technique. The observation of polymorphic transformation by using variable temperature synchrotron X-ray diffraction method is a promising technique with the new computerized ability for obtaining structural data (58).

Thermogravimetry can be coupled with DSC. Most companies offer the TG-IR (59) or the TG-MS coupling

(60). Synergic chemical analysis by coupling TG-FT-IR, TG-MS or TG-GC-MS has been recently discussed (61). Fig. 5 demonstrates the ability of TG-MS for the study of dehydration and decomposition of calcium oxalate dihydrate. The steps correspond to the dehydration into anhydrous calcium oxalate, followed by the transformation into calcium carbonate then by the formation of cacium oxide (10, 11). The sample studied in Fig. 5 contains additionally to crystal water some free water. The TG-MS shows that some amount of the CO evolved during the decomposition also transforms into CO_2.

These new emerging combined techniques enables the observation of extremely small samples with a high degree of information. They find a good place for proper screening (55) (according to the polymorphic studies required by ICH) (62) in order to choose the proper form and to justify its choice. They also permit to analyze more easily the complex matrixes of drug products.

APPLICATIONS OF THERMAL ANALYSIS TECHNIQUES FOR DRUG SUBSTANCES

The transitions observed by thermal analysis techniques are based upon the Gibbs phase rule and phase diagrams, p, T, concentration.

All transitions or reactions involving energy changes may be measured by DSC. Transitions involving mass changes are detected by TG. For a single product, specific heat, glass transition, melting, boiling, sublimation, decomposition, and phase transitions induced by polymorphism during heating are important for the choice of the salt form and for safety studies where the DSC exothermic peaks are relevant. The use of DSC for the measurement of the melting point of raw materials has been proposed (20). Hydrates or solvates, or volatile compounds in the formulations can be investigated by DSC combined with TG and TG-MS. DSC curves of mixtures of solid compounds depend upon the phase diagrams in solid state. If there is no interaction in the solid state and if there is a miscibility in the melt, an eutectic behavior is observed. This enables the purity determination of raw materials, the analysis of enantiomers, and the study of "physical interactions" in preformulation. If the compounds are not miscible in the liquid state, the DSC curve of the mixture is the addition of the DSC curves of each compounds. Interaction is observed in the solid state in case of formation of solid solution or complex formation between components or in the case of chemical reaction.

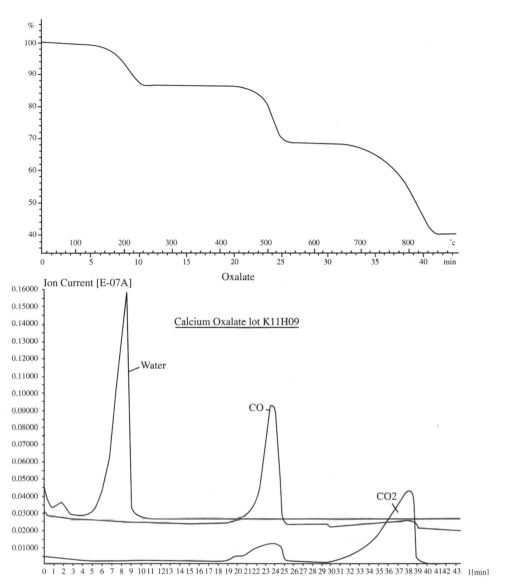

Fig. 5   TG and TG-MS of calcium oxalate monohydrate. The TG steps correspond to the dehydration followed by the formation of calcium carbonate, then calcium oxide is obtained. The evolved gas is detected by MS.

Polymorphism/Pseudopolymorphism and Amorphous State

Polymorphism is the tendency of any substance to crystallize into different crystalline states. The solid forms of the same compound are called polymorphs or crystalline modifications. On melting, they produce the same liquid. Polymorphs show the same properties in the liquid or gaseous state but they behave as different substances in the solid state. The best known example of polymorphism is carbon, which can exist in the form of graphite or as a diamond.

The amorphous state characterizes crystallization in a nonordered, random system, related to the liquid state. The name "glassy state" is given to amorphous products that liquify by undergoing a glass transition.

The expression pseudopolymorphism applies to hydrates and solvates.

Different solid phases that may occur during crystallization or galenical processes are polymorphs, amorphous phases, or solvates as the result of compound formation with the solvent (63–66).

A recent detailed review about thermal analysis of polymorphs and pseudopolymorphs (67) listed more than 300 drug substances presenting this behavior in the literature. Polymorphism of excipients and their thermal analysis has been reviewed in (68).

DSC gives not only temperature of events, but also melting energies. The Burger's rule and the energy diagrams (69–74) help considerably to approach the thermodynamic equilibrium of a polymorphic system.

For each polymorph (single compound), there is a solid–liquid equilibrium curve and a solid–gas equilibrium curve. The solid–gas curves meet at a point. If the liquid–gas equilibrium curve meets the two solid–gas curves *after* this point of intersection, there will be a solid 1, solid 2 equilibrium curve and a reversible transition point 1↔2 at a specific pressure. This is known as *enantiotropy*. At the transition point, the free energy of the two forms is the same.

The term *monotropy* applies in the case of an irreversible transition from one form to another. Monotropy is bound to the existence of metastable thermodynamic forms. The liquid–gas curve crosses the solid–gas curves for the two forms *before* their point of intersection.

Knowing the relationship between the thermodynamic quantities H (enthalpy), G (free energy), S (entropy), and T (temperature), it is often simple to represent equilibrium states by plotting the free energy G as a function of the temperature for each form. If the two curves intersect before the melting point, there is reversibility, i.e.

enantiotropy, and if the reverse is true, there is *monotropy*.

The relationship between melting enthalpies of two solid phases A and B and the heat of transition is:

$$\Delta H_t = \Delta H_A^f - \Delta H_B^f$$

Figs. 6A and 6B illustrate the plots of the functions G and H versus temperature (energy/temperature diagrams) for each polymorph and for the liquid. The thermodynamic reversibility of the solid transition between two crystalline forms is characteristic of enantiotropic systems. Each form has its thermodynamic stability range. The lower melting form is stable in the temperature range below the transition point; the higher melting form is stable in the temperature range above the transition point. In case of monotropy only one form is stable whatever the temperature range. The Burger' rule is as follows in the case of *enantiotropy*, the lower melting form has the higher melting enthalpy and the transition into the high melting form by heating is endothermic; in the case of *monotropy*, the thermodynamic stable form is the higher melting form with the higher melting enthalpy. The transformation of the unstable form into the stable form is exothermic.

Because of kinetic factors, metastable forms are encountered in temperature ranges outside the thermodynamic range. Crystallization processes generally imply the cooling of concentrated solutions or precipitation by addition of cosolvent. Depending on the relative positions of

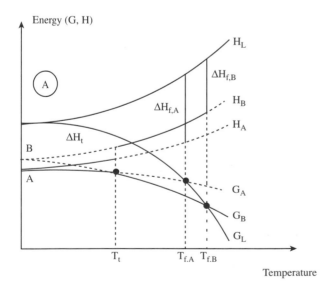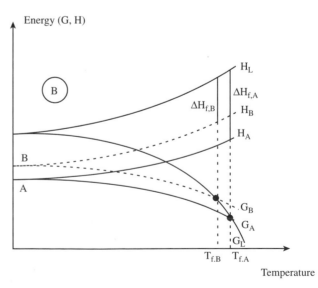

Fig. 6 Energy diagrams showing plots of enthalpy H and Gibbs free energy G, against temperature T, for the solid and liquid phases of a single compound, showing (A) enantiotropy and (B) monotropy.

the solubility curves of the metastable polymorphic forms and the metastable curve of supersaturation, the first nucleous can be a metastable form. Transformation to the stable crystalline form may or may not occur, depending on kinetic factor. Furthermore solvates exist at lower temperatures and their presence should be considered and finally due to the humidity of the air or from water activity of the solvents, hydrates may be formed. Polymorphism of solvates and hydrates is not uncommon. This phenomenon of concomittant polymorphs has been recently reviewed (75).

Fig. 7 illustrates the behavior of polymorphs A and B in case of enantiotropy (Fig. 7a) and monotropy (Fig. 7b) during heating. For all analysis where a temperature change is involved, kinetic factors have to be considered for proper interpretation of the results. The DSC scans will differ if the sample being analyzed is stable or metastable at ambient temperature. A is the stable form at ambient temperature in both cases.

In the case of *enantiotropy* (Fig. 7a), only the form A should be encountered below the transition point and the behavior upon heating is illustrated by the DSC scan 1, the endothermic transition A ⇔ B should be observed followed by the melting peak of the form B. For kinetic reasons, e.g., in case of too quick heating rate, the transition A ⇔ B does not occur and form A melts. Then two possibilities may be found: no other signal occurs (DSC scan 2) or an exothermic crystallization of B from the melt occurs and later on, the melting peak of B is observed (DSC scan 3). If the metastable form B occurs below the transition, upon heating it can be transformed into A with an exothermic transition (DSC scan 4);

thereafter, the form A transforms into the form B according to scan 1 or scan 2). Finally (scan 5), the metastable form B can melt without any transformation.

In the case of monotropy (Fig. 7b) only the form A should exist and the DSC scan should show the melting peak of the stable form A (scan 1). If the metastable form B is heated, then scan 2 or 3 may be observed: the form B transforms exothermically into the stable form A (scan 2) or the form B melts and the stable form A grows from the melt and its melting peak is observed.

In the case of racemate, the situation is more complex since one racemate polymorph can be a true racemate and the other one a conglomerate (73, 74) and one has to consider additional solid phase transitions such as peritectoids and eutectoids, which are not polymorphic transitions (76).

Very often some substances have two melting points separated by an exotherm. Such a DSC scan can correspond to a monotropy or to an enantiotropy. The sample may be a pure form or a mixture. Using different heating rates and tempering in DSC, one may be able to measure melting points and melting enthalpies and to use the Burger' rule.

The TG curve is extremely valuable for preventing misinterpretations. McCauley (77) describes the DSC curve of phthalylsulfathiazole, which presents such a DSC curve with two endothermic peaks separated by an exothermic peak. The TG curve demonstrates a strong decomposition during the first melting. The resulting degradation product then recrystallizes and melts at higher temperatures. We observed such an effect for aspartam

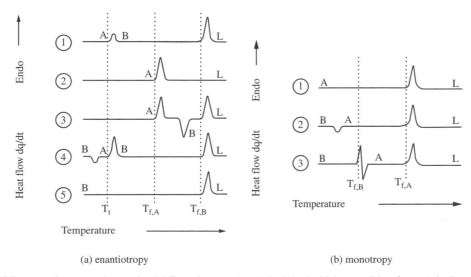

(a) enantiotropy   (b) monotropy

Fig. 7 Possible DSC curves for two polymorphs: (a) Enantiotropy A (⇔) B, B is the highest melting form, A is the stable form below the transition point. (b) Monotropy B → A, A is the highest melting form. (For explanations of the scans, see text.)

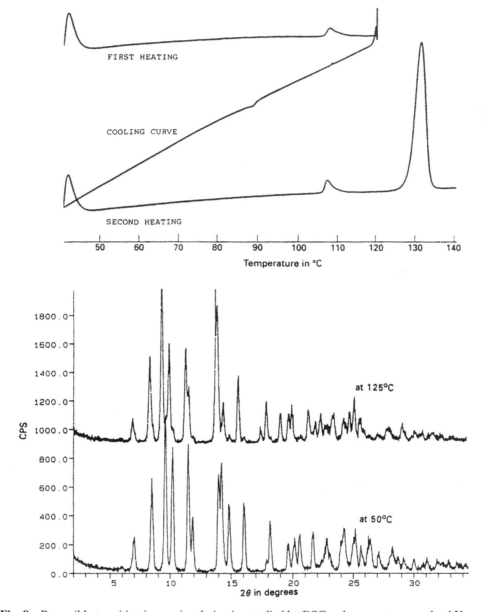

Fig. 8   Reversible transition in a purine derivative studied by DSC and temperature-resolved X-ray powder diffraction (From Ref. 67.)

(13) and for a malonate salt, which decomposed in the corresponding base (12). If an isomerization takes place, then only the analytical data of the product obtained allow us to have an accurate interpretation.

These curves illustrate the complex transitions that may occur when heating or cooling polymorphs. Therefore, combined techniques are very useful for complete interpretation of observations given by DSC as emphasized in (54). Fig. 8 illustrates a reversible enantiotropic transition followed by DSC and by temperature-resolved X-ray diffraction of a purine derivative. For this substance

six crystalline forms were found. The Burger's rule as well as the study of the supersaturated solutions and the use of combined techniques allowed us to find out that the form of Fig. 8 was the stable form below the transition point. All other forms were monotrops to this form (78).

Table 5 deals with the example of a benzisoquinoline hydrochloride for which both forms presented a melting that was followed by decomposition. No change was observed by slow heating rate. Since the melting enthalpies differed only by 10%, the proper interpretation needed the verification of the hypothesis:

enantiotropic transition. The analysis of the insoluble solid in the equilibration of both forms in alcohols (solvent mediated transition) showed that form A is always obtained, what confirmed the observation of the Burger's rule.

Amorphous State

If a physical property of a crystalline substance is plotted against temperature, a sharp discontinuity occurs at the melting point. For amorphous substances, there is no melting point, and a change of slope occurs at the so-called glass transition temperature T_g. The glass transition is characterized by a change of heat capacity. Below this temperature, the amorphous phase has certain properties of a crystalline solid (e.g., plastic deformation) and is termed "glassy." Above this temperature, the substance retains some of the properties of a liquid, e.g., molecular mobility, and is termed "rubbery." Above this temperature, the increase in molecular mobility facilitates spontaneous crystallization into the crystalline form with an exothermic enthalpy change after the glass transition. The use of amorphous forms is attractive, particularly for sparingly soluble compounds because of the enhanced solubility and dissolution rate over the crystalline state leading to increased bioavailability. However, the amorphous state is thermodynamically unstable. The glass transition temperature T_g is lowered by water or other additives, facilitating conversion to the rubbery state and hence facilitating crystallization (79). Since it may be interesting to maintain the amorphous state, the temperature of the glass transition and its behavior should be characterized. DSC and modulated DSC are commonly used. Hancock and Zografi studied intensively the amorphous state of drug substances and used the relaxation energy at the glass transition as well as the dependency of the heating rate for the study of the "fragility" of the amorphous state (80–82). Depending on the temperature, the isothermal crystallization in one or the other polymorphic form may be favored as demonstrated for amorphous indomethacine (83).

The study of the amorphous state (for drug substances and also for excipients) is based upon the changes observed in the glass transition. Fig. 9 shows the influence of the heating rate for the determination of the glass transition by DSC for the polymeric excipient Carbopol 974. It is classical to perform a first run for the elimination of water and relaxation energy and to determine the glass transition temperature T_g of the pure compound, if no degradation occurs during the first run. However, this procedure is not valid if it is desirable to study the role of the matrix.

When the amorphous material does not transform into the crystalline material, the measurement of the melting

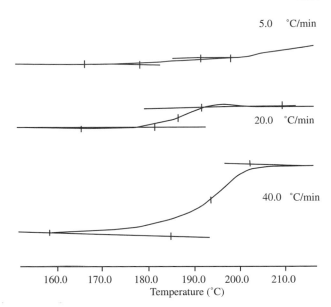

Fig. 9 Quality control of excipients by using the glass transition. Example of Carbopol 974 P. Second DSC run in order to eliminate water and relaxation: Influence of the heating rate.

peak allows to determine the degree of crystallinity of mixtures by comparing its value with the melting enthalpy of a pure crystalline material. If the amorphous sample crystallizes upon heating, then the crystallization peak may be used for the determination of the amorphous content. Such an example is given in Fig. 10. In this case it was possible to attain a limit of detection of 1%.

Pseudo-polymorphism

In the case of solvates, binary phase diagrams of temperature versus concentration of the solvent (or water) at a given pressure are useful for the understanding of the phase transitions. The characterization of solvates and hydrates need the use of both DSC and TG. Desolvatation can be complex: melting of the solvate followed by exothermic recrystallization into the anhydrous form or solid-state transformation with evaporation and possibly further endothermic or exothermic events corresponding to a cascade of phase transitions. In such complex situations, combined techniques TG-IR or TG-MS and temperature-resolved X-ray diffraction are extremely helpful since the identity of the volatile component or of possible volatile decomposition product can be identified on line (54, 67). In case of hydrates, water sorption–desorption isotherms as well as the X-ray diffraction in humid chambers are needed (54, 84).

The DSC, TG curves of solvates and hydrates are related to the phase diagrams between substance and solvent (or

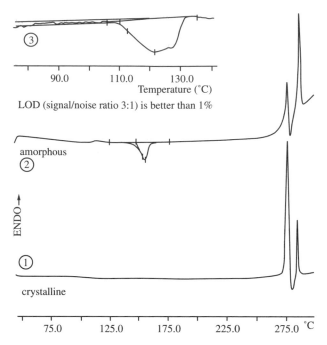

Fig. 10   Determination of amorphous content by DSC at 20 K min^{-1}. 1) Crystalline sample, 2) amorphous sample, 3) exotherm of a sample containing 4% amorphous as calculated by DSC. Calculation of the limit of detection by peak/noise ratio.

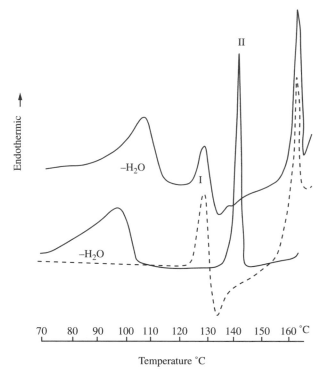

Fig. 11   Polymorphism of a trihydrate. (From Ref. 10.)

water). Eutectic are observed (85). Fusion or decomposition of the solvate may occur during heating. Therefore, one may observe the melting of the solvate followed by recrystallization into the anhydrous form or the endothermic desolvatation in the solid state. In certain cases both phenomena may overlapp. Details about experimental factors and examples can be found in (67). If the anhydrous form is metastable, further phase transitions follow the desolvatation. If several solvates or hydrates exist, the transitions observed depend on the pressure, as demonstrated by Soustelle (86) in the case of copper sulfate pentahydrate. Depending on the pressure, the direct dehydration into the anhydrous or the dehydration via the monohydrate, or the three dehydration steps trihydrate, monohydrate and anhydrous forms may be obtained. Hydrates have been the subject of several reviews (87, 88). Polymorphism of hydrates (89) is also frequent. Figure 11 shows the case for a drug substance with polymorphic behavior of the trihydrate. The anhydrous form shows a dual melting (enantiotropy). This form was very hygroscopic and transformed into the trihydrate H_I at room temperature. The DSC scan of this trihydrate shows a dehydration peak in solid state, followed by the same scan as on the original anhydrous form. After storage for several months in a tropical climate (30°C/75% RH), a second trihydrate H_{II} is obtained. The same trihydrate H_{II} is also obtained by crystallization in water or after equilibration of the original anhydrous form with saturated aqueous solution. The DSC scan of this trihydrate differs from the first one because the dehydration gives rise to a new anhydrous form. This interpretation was confirmed by X-ray Guinier de Wolff diagrams, purity analysis, Karl Fischer, and TG (10, 67).

Often the solvates (hydrates) are not detected since, according the corresponding phase diagram, at ambient temperature, they can be partly or completely dissociated. Suspensions of hydrates in water should shift the equilibrium toward the formation of the stable hydrated form. The ability of DSC measurements at subambient temperatures allow to determine phase transitions. Giron et al. (90) proposed to use the melting peak of freezable water for the analysis of suspensions of drug substances in water in combination with TG for the determination of the number of molecules of water bounded as hydrates.

Study of Transition: Kinetics

Since transitions may occur during milling, processing, and aging, thermal methods are widely used for the kinetic study of all transformations. The purpose of any kinetic study is to obtain information concerning the reaction mechanism through comparison of a series of measured fractions converted versus time. Most mechanisms in solid state are a nucleation period, a growth zone, and an unreacted core. For phase transitions of polymorphs and pseudopoymorphs, only heterogene kinetic applies (at least two modifications or two phases and a gaz). In heterogene kinetic a great number of factors should be considered as temperature gradient in the sample, particle size, activation, nucleus, or diffusion.

A summary of current kinetic methods used with thermal analysis techniques can be found in (67).

Microcalorimetric Techniques

Solution calorimetry allows us to investigate processes that involve enthalpy changes. Adiabatic microcalorimeters and isoperibol calorimeters used in batch modes or flow modes allow for the precise determination of the heat of solution. Mixing the reactants is accomplished by breaking a bulk allowing reactants to mix or by special chambers where the reactants are mixed together.

If a compound exists in two or more different crystalline or amorphous configurations with different lattice energies, the heating solution in any given solvent will differ. The difference in the heats of solution will be equal to the difference in lattice energy of the solids, provided that the solid compounds are identical chemically. For example, we measured the energy of solution in water of the two modifications of a drug substance. The difference of $9.7 \, kJ \, mol^{-1}$ was found very close to the difference of the melting energies of $9.1 \, kJ \, mol^{-1}$ measured by DSC (54). However, the DSC information is superior since the temperatures of melting of both forms are measurable. Since the lower melting form had a lower melting energy, it was the stable form and both forms were enantiotropically related. For review see Ref. 67.

Byström (91) developed a technique in order to determine the crystallinity of drug substances by isothermal microcalorimetry. Considering that micronization introduces amorphous regions not measurable by X-ray diffraction, the method should be an analytical tool

for analyzing batch-to-batch quality. The principle of the measurement lies in the transformation of the amorphous state in the crystalline one at high humidity levels. The amorphous substance adsorbs water and the glass transition is lowered, permitting the acceleration of the crystallization. The energy evolved is measured in function of time by isothermal microcalorimetry. Results were found comparable with X-ray diffraction but a quite lower limit of detection is possible (better than 1%) (54, 92, 93).

DSC Purity Analysis

The basis of any calorimetric purity method is the relationship between the melting depression of a substance and the level of impurities according to van't Hoff's law. The purity is readily calculated from the DSC curve of a single melting event of a few milligrams of the substance, without the need for reference standard of the drug substance and its impurities.

The DSC impurity analysis is described in USP. With modern equipment including robotic systems and data aquisition, the DSC purity analysis is a state-of-the-art technique for pharmaceutical development.

The determination of purity by means of DSC is based on the assumption that impurities depress the melting point of a pure material according to the eutectic phase diagram behavior.

Figure 12 shows the phase diagram for the two component mixture with the so-called eutectic point. At the eutectic point E (e.g., 40% A, 60% B), the crystals A and B melt together at the temperature T_E, below the melting temperature of the pure compounds. If a mixture of A and B (containing, e.g., 90% A) is heated, the melting of eutectic mixture (which is 40% in A) is observed initially, until all of B is melted. During the melting of the eutectic (40% A, 60% B) a part of A is melted with B, with the corresponding amount $2/3 \times 10\%$ of A, i.e., 6.66% of A.

Then as the temperature increases, pure A melts between T_E and T_m. T_m is the temperature at the end of the melting. For the corresponding DSC curve, an endotherm

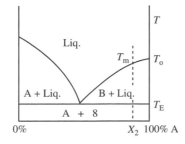
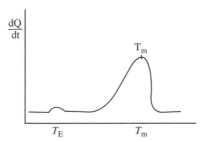

Fig. 12 Binary phase diagram with eutectic, and DSC curve of the composition x_2.

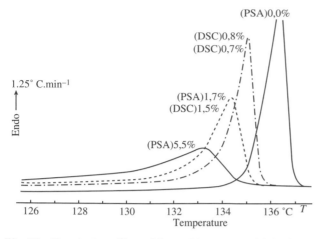

Fig. 13 Broadening effect of the melting curve of β-hydroxypropyltheophylline due to impurities. PSA = phase solubility analysis. All batches have the same TLC purity results. (From Ref. 6.)

at the eutectic temperature is observed, then the melting of crystals A occurs. The effect of impurity on the DSC curve is a melting depression and a broadening of the melting curve (Fig. 13).

The amount of impurities is calculated from the melting-point depression $\Delta T = T_0 - T_m$.

The van't Hoff's law for *diluted solutions* is

$$x = \frac{(-\Delta T \ \Delta H_f)}{R T_0^2}$$

where x is the mole fraction of impurities, ΔT the melting point depression, ΔH_f the melting point of pure material, T_m the melting of the analyte, T_0 the melting point of the pure compound, and R the gas constant.

The DSC procedure does not directly measure ΔT, but can be used to calculate it from the melting curve. At the eutectic point, all of B is in the liquid phase. During the melting of A after the eutectic point the concentration of B varies in the liquid phase. This causes the broadening of the DSC curve. With no solid solution formation, the concentration of impurity in the liquid phase at any temperature during the melting is inversely proportional to the fraction melted at that temperature, and the melting-point depression is directly proportional to the mole fraction of impurity. A plot of the observed analyte temperature T_i versus the reciprocal of the fraction melted $1/F_i$ at temperature T_i should yield a straight line with the

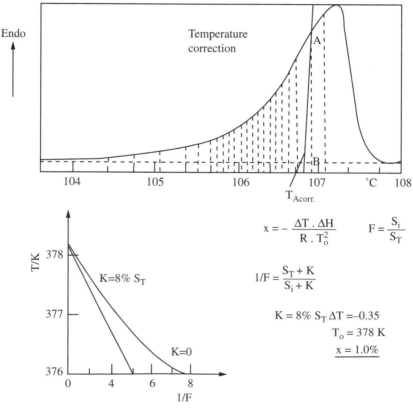

$$x = -\frac{\Delta T \cdot \Delta H}{R \cdot T_o^2} \qquad F = \frac{S_i}{S_T}$$

$$1/F = \frac{S_T + K}{S_i + K}$$

$$K = 8\% \ S_T \quad \Delta T = -0.35$$
$$T_o = 378 \ K$$
$$\underline{x = 1.0\%}$$

Fig. 14 Purity calculations by DSC.

slope equal to the melting-point depression $(T_0 - T_m)$. The theoretical melting point of the pure compound T_0 is obtained by extrapolation to $1/F_i = 0$:

$$T_i = T_0 - \frac{RT_0^2(1/F_i)}{\Delta H_f} x$$

This relation may be expressed as

$$T_i = T_0 - \Delta T(1/F_i)$$

Substituting the experimentally obtained values for ΔT, ΔH_f, and T_0 in the first equation yields the mole fraction of the total eutectic impurities, which, when multiplied by 100, gives the mole percentage of total eutectic impurities.

The temperature of each point T_i is the sample temperature, not the programmed temperature. Due to the thermal lag, a correction depending on the instrument has to be done for each point.

The melting curve is divided into small portions and each area S_i is calculated. The melted fraction F_i,

$$F_i = \frac{S_i}{S_{total}}$$

is calculated for each point and the curve T_i is plotted as a function of $1/F_i$, where T_i is the temperature at fraction F_i (Fig. 14). The slope ΔT and the ordinate T_0 can be calculated.

Partly because of the lack of the eutectic-point detection, the curve is not a straight line, and a correction factor K must be added to each fraction of the curve. Formation of solid solution or artefacts during melting may also be responsible.

$$F_i = \frac{S_i + K}{S_{total} + K}$$

Software from manufacturers mostly use iterative linearization, which gives the best value of K. Characteristics of this determination are as follows:

- Impurities are measured, which have an eutectic behavior (i.e., solubles in the liquid phase and insolubles in the solid phase).
- The sum of impurities should be $\leq 2\%$.
- The result is expressed in mol % without knowledge of impurities.
- Pure material is not needed.
- Small amounts (1–2 mg or less) of material are used.
- If decomposition occurs during melting, it can give erroneous results.
- The purity results are obtained after less than 1 h.

The influence of products parameters and instrument parameters have been discussed in detail by Giron et al.

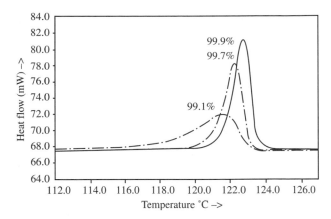

Fig. 15 Stability screening. Example of DSC purity results obtained for a drug substance sensitive to moisture. From the top to the bottom: Initial sample (purity 99.9%), sample stored under humid conditions at 50°C (purity 99.7%), sample stored under humid conditions at 80°C (purity 99.1%).

(94), who proposed a validation scheme for DSC purity method. The authors showed the advantage of the method as support to chromatographic techniques, for the monitoring of purification for the study of stability behavior of raw materials under stress conditions, for establishing purity profiles. Fig. 15 shows the DSC scans corresponding to a stability screening of a drug substance sensitive to moisture.

Enantiomers

Enantiomers are stereoisomers, which are mirror images of each another. An equimolecular mixture of two enantiomers is called a racemate. Crystalline racemates occur in three different types. The first is termed a conglomerate, that is, a mechanical mixture of crystals of pure enantiomers that is formed from two solid phases. The most common type is the racemic compound, which consists only of one crystalline phase in which the two enantiomers are present in equal quantities. The third type is the pseudoracemate in which a solid solution of the two enantiomers is present.

Conglomerates that are equimolecular mixtures of two crystalline enantiomers are easily separated by cristallization. There are two phases in the solid state and only one phase in the liquid state (miscibility). The equation of Schröder–Van Laar in its simplified form correlates the composition of mixtures to the end of fusion T^f:

$$\ln x = \frac{\Delta H_A^f}{R}\left[\frac{1}{T_A^f} - \frac{1}{T^f}\right]$$

where x is the mole fraction of the more abundant enantiomer ($0.5 \leq x \leq 1$) of a mixture that melts at T^f (in

K). ΔH_A^f and T_A^f are respectively the enthalpy of fusion and the melting point of the pure enantiomers, and R is the gas constant.

Racemic compounds, or true racemates, exhibit two eutectic points each between the pure enantiomer and the racemic compound. The shape of the DSC diagrams can vary, depending on the relative positions of temperatures of eutectics and racemic compound and on the composition of the eutectics (Figs. 16b and 16c). In the case of Fig. 16c it is difficult to distinguish by DSC a racemic compound from a conglomerate. Other methods as IR or X-ray are suitable for proper interpretation. For example, propanol hydrochloride has been described as conglomerate (95) or as racemate compound (96).

The equation of Schröder–Van Laar, which permits the calculation of the liquidus curve, may be applied to the point of the liquidus between the pure enantiomers and the corresponding eutectics ($T_A^f E_R$ and $T_A^f E_S$. For the part $E_R R E_S$, the equation of Prigogine and Defay applies:

$$\ln 4x(1-x) = \frac{2\Delta H_R^{tf}}{R}\left[\frac{1}{T_R^f} - \frac{1}{T^f}\right]$$

where x represents the mole fraction of the enantiomer in the mixture that melts at T^f and ΔH_R^f and T_R^f are respectively the enthalpy of fusion and the melting point of the racemic compound. Polymorphism can occur for the racemic compound and the enantiomers. Phase diagrams with monotropic transformation or enantiotropic transformation have been discussed (75, 76). Quite interesting is the transformation of the racemic compound into a conglomerate since this phenomenon can be used for purification via crystallization, as described for nimodipine (97). DSC is applied for the establishment of phase diagrams, for the determination of thermodynamic data (98), for the purity determination, or for the monitoring of industrial resolutions. For the establishment of phase diagrams it is suitable to add spectroscopic or crystallographic methods (99).

Two methods can be used for the purity determination: the direct method or the indirect method (75). The direct method is applied for mixtures when the phase diagram is established using Schröder–Van Laar or Prigogine–Defay equation. For enantiomers of high purity (>95%) the general DSC purity method for eutectic impurities is applicable. The same limitations remain (polymorphism, degradation, during melting). The method gives the sum of impurities without differentiation of the type of impurity. For purity > 95% the same results have been obtained using the indirect and the direct methods (100, 101).

Conglomerates are easy to purify by crystallization or by the entrainment technique described by Jacques et al. (75), which involves introducing seed crystals of the desired enantiomer into a cooling saturated solution of the racemic mixture. According to these authors, conglomerate formation is observed three times, more frequently with salts. Therefore it is advantageous to compare the behavior of salts forms. On the other hand, for a synthesis in several steps, it is useful to study the behavior of each step in order to choose the step exhibiting a conglomerate behavior resulting in an efficient enantiomeric resolution. In the case of racemic compound, the entrainment technique can be used in those cases where the eutectics are situated very close to the racemate. This underscores the value of systematic searches for derivatives that form conglomerates or at least racemic compounds whose eutectics are close to that of the racemate.

Another further way of purification is the formation of diastereomeric salts. However, partial solid solution are often observed and it is difficult to achieve high purity. Resolution via diastereomeric salt formation based on a part of the DSC curve has been discussed (102).

The change from racemates to enantiomers has implication in the galenical formulations. Propanolol-base enantiomer has a better skin permeation than racemate, what was explained by a lowering of the melting point (103). The stereospecific preformulation of ibuprofen has also been discussed. The theoretical phase diagram has been calculated from the DSC curves of the (+) enantiomer and of the racemate by using the equations of Schröder–Van Laar and Prigogine–Defay equations. Experimental data confirm the calculated data (104, 105).

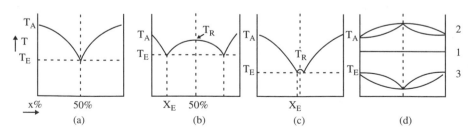

Fig. 16 Phase diagrams for enantiomers: (a) conglomerate, (b) and (c) racemic compound, (d) solid solution.

The low melting point of the enantiomer may have implications of the pharmaceutical process. Relationships between physical properties and crystal structures of chiral drugs have been discussed (106).

APPLICATION OF THERMAL TECHNIQUES FOR THE DRUG PRODUCT: PREFORMULATION, PROCESSING, AND AGING

The preformulation includes the choice of the salt form and of the polymorph of the drug substance. Melting points, solubilities, dissolution, hygroscopicity, stability, feasibility, processability, and polymorphic behavior have to be considered. The second step is to study the behavior of the drug substance with excipients (107).

Excipients

The use of thermal analysis techniques for pharmaceuticals implies the knowledge of the thermal behavior of the excipients. A great number of publications deal with polymorphic behavior of excipients and especially with the amorphous forms as prerequisite knowledge for freeze drying and milling processes.

Lactose exists in two isomeric forms α and β. It is possible to obtain the α-monhydrate, anhydrous crystalline α and β forms, as well as an amorphous form. The pharmaceutical properties of these various types are different. The hardness of tablets obtained using amorphous lactose produced by lyophilization is 10 times that obtained using crystalline forms. During milling, it has been observed that the monohydrate loses part of its water of crystallization and of its crystallinity. Heat treatment of different lactoses has permitted the discovery of an anhydrous, unstable α form and a crystal containing α and β in the ratio 1:1. Under the influence of high degrees of humidity, amorphous lactose crystallizes and anhydrous forms tend to reconvert to the monohydrate (68, 108, 109).

The thermal analysis studies of different forms of sorbitol, mannitol, glucose, magnesium stearate are reviewed in (68). Mono-, di-, and trihydrate of magnesium stearate as well as the amorphous form may be found. According to Wada et al. (110), thermal analysis is the most appropriate method for characterization of magnesium stearate.

Thermal analysis are widely used for polymers and copolymers analysis (4). Glass transitions, melting, and decomposition processes are analyzed. Since the glass transition temperature T_g is marked by changes in the thermal capacity, expansion coefficient, and rigidity, TMA technique as well as DSC may be used. T_g increases with molecular mass up to certain values. Plasticizers and water depress this temperature. Thermal stability and influence of antioxidants and fillers may be analyzed by TG or DSC, under oxygen.

The compatibility of polymers in blends is tested by comparing DSC curves of the components. Immiscible crystalline blends such as polyethylene–polypropylene show the DSC peaks of polyethylene and polypropylene. Immiscible amorphous blends exhibit two glass transitions; in miscible blends a new glass point is observed. Partially miscible blends have two glass points situated between the glass points of each polymer. Different equations such as Gordon–Taylor express the relation between the new glass transition T_g and the glass transition points T_{g1} and T_{g2} of components. W_1 and W_2 are the weight fractions and K is the ratio $\Delta C_{p2}/\Delta C_{p1}$.

$$T_g = W_1 T_{g1} + K W_2 T_{g2} / W_1 + K W_2$$

The polymers mostly used in pharmaceutical packaging are polyethylene, polypropylene, PVC, polyamide, polystyrol, nylon, cellulose acetate, polyethylene terephthtalate, and blends thereof. Copolymers and rubbers are also used. The DSC melting curve of polyethylene used for packaging purposes is characteristic. Low- and high-density polyethylene are differenciated by their melting points (111). Melting point and density of polyethylene are linearly correlated (112). Crystallinity may be determined as described above for amorphous state.

Polyethylene glycols (PEG) have been intensively characterized by thermal analytic methods. The melting points of PEG increase with the molecular weight and decreases with the content of water as a result of eutectic formation (10). Corrigan (113) studied the different DSC peaks of PEG: Once folded chain crystals and extended chain crystals are present in PEG 6000, which results in two DSC peaks. In PEG of higher molecular mass, only folded chain crystals are present. Lower molecular mass PEG contain only extended chain crystals. Craig reviewed the thermal studies of PEG, including properties in aqueous solutions (114, 115). Phase diagram of PEG 4000 was recently discussed (116). Higher molecular mass PEG are generally used in solid dispersion systems and their melting behavior is relevant for the temperature of galenical preparation (5, 117).

Glass transitions of polyvinylpyrrolidones of different molecular weight may be used as identity (10, 118). Water depresses the glass transitions and effects the physical properties of polyvinylpyrrolidone, as demonstrated by Tan and Challa (119).

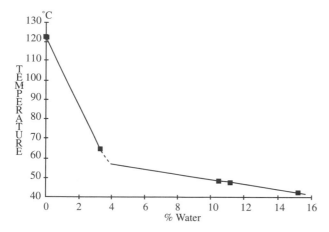

Fig. 17 Influence of the water content on the glass transition temperature of HPMC 4000 measured by DSC in sealed pans.

A large number of cellulose derivatives have been studied for food as well as for pharmaceutical applications (120–123). The measurement of the glass transition is often difficult due to the broad endotherm of dehydration of water. Figure 17 shows the effect of water on the depression of the glass transition of hydroxypropyl methylcellulose HPMC4000.

Film coating processes need the knowledge of the glass transitions for a proper film. Ethylcellulose, cellulose phthalate, polyvinylalcohols, polymethyl methacrylates have been studied and the critical parameters for film formation discussed (124–126).

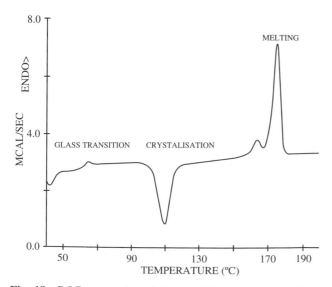

Fig. 18 DSC curve of L-polylactic acid after quenching from the melt. (From Ref. 10.)

Polysaccharides and water interaction are especially studied for their use in spray-dried products in food and in biotechnology (127–129).

Biodegradable polymers can be crystalline or amorphous. Poly-L-lactic and D,L-polyactic acids have been studied by Pitt and Gu (130). Figure 18 deals with the second run of poly-L-lactic acid after quenching. The glass transition is followed by crystallization, the melting of the crystalline form. Aging and crystallinity of biodegradable polymers have been studied by Akktar et al. (131). TG is useful for the determination of the entrapped solvent (often methylene chloride) and of moisture (5, 10). Microspheres containing biodegradable polymers are intensely analyzed by thermal analysis techniques allowing both the glass transition point of the polymer and the physico-characterization of the drug substance to be analyzed; thermal techniques generally with electron microscopy are used for the optimization of the drug loading and of the process (132). The physical aging of the polymer can be assessed in DSC by the amplitude associated with the glass transition of the matrix. This relaxation energy increases with aging. Rosilio studied the progesterone poly(D,L-lactide-co-glycolide) microspheres. Aging acts on the solid state of the drug substance loaded. Different polymorphs are obtained, depending on the copolymer composition (133).

Phase Diagrams

The thermodynamic phase diagrams are the basis for understanding DSC curves of formulation: eutectics, solid solutions, eutectics with partial solid solutions, and compound formation with congruent or incongruent melting. Figure 19 exemplifies the building of the phase diagram of propyphenazone and butesamide, using the DSC curves. In order to save the number of DSC scans, theoretical curves can be added (134). Such phase diagram was performed between a drug substance and stearic acid: no formation of the salt was observed (13). Recently thermal analysis has been used for the complex phase diagram of propanol/oleic acid for which the salt and a mesomorphic phase have been found (135).

DSC was proposed for compatibility studies comparing DSC curves of components and mixtures. Unfortunately some misinterpetation may occur. DSC curves can only reflect physical behavior. The formation of eutectic is not an incompatibility. Furthermore, water generally is not present in the mixtures at the temperatures of the melting peaks. Giron et al. (9) performed the DSC curves of a drug substance and several excipients, the initial DSC curves of the mixtures and the DSC curves of the mixtures after 1 month at 50°C/<30% RH and 50°C/75% RH. Chromatography was used for the chemical analysis

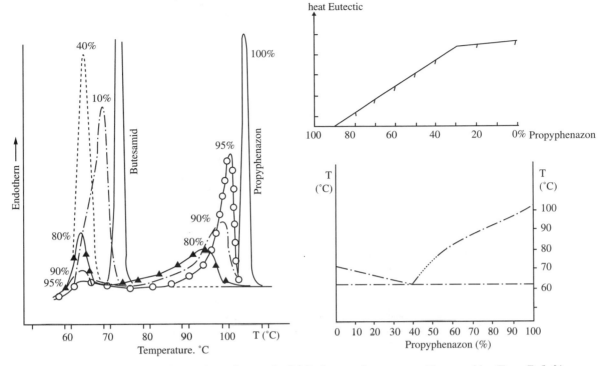

Fig. 19 Example of building a phase diagram by DSC of propyphenazone and butesamide. (From Ref. 6.)

of the drug. Figure 20 shows the comparison of the DSC curves of the mixtures. The effect of the humidity on the degradation is very striking: The drug substance is completely decomposed with calcium sulfate, avicel, and stearic acid. For talc and dicalcium phosphate, there is no degradation. The observation of the initial DSC curves for the five excipients would have wrongly given the conclusion to the same compatibility.

For such compatibility studies, isothermal microcalorimetry has been suggested (e.g., Ref. 136).

The DSC study of mixtures of drug and excipients is very useful, for the information gained (e.g., if the eutectic melts at ambient temperature). In other cases, one may target interaction with excipients as it is the case of solid dispersions, solid solutions, or complex formation. The choice of the carrier defines the characteristics of dissolution of the dispersed drug. Poorly water-soluble active ingredients are combined with water-soluble carriers in order to increase the dissolution of the active ingredient. A good water-soluble drug combined with a slightly soluble carrier leads to a retardation of drug release from the matrix. For reviews on solid dispersions, see Refs. 5 and 137. For the development of solid dispersions, the method of preparation, the type of systems, the dissolution characteristics, and the aging problems should be considered. DSC is appropriate for the study of solid dispersions by comparing DSC curves of pure compounds, of physical mixtures or

melted mixtures to the DSC curve of the solid dispersion. TG, X-Ray diffraction, and hyphenated techniques are good complements. The transitions observed are those transitions expected from the phase diagrams, or the amorphous state with glass transition or very often new metastable forms of drug substance as well as metastable forms of excipients.

The phase diagram given in Fig. 21 for darodipine–polyethylene glycol 6000 results from DSC experiments carried out by two techniques (10). The DSC of physical mixtures obtained by grinding were scanned just after the end of melting. After cooling a second scan at 5 K min^{-1} was performed. In the second technique the mixtures were dissolved in methanol and the solvent evaporated. With both techniques, the same results were obtained.

The knowledge of the phase diagram allows the choice of the temperature of the process. It can be suitable to choose higher loading than the eutectic composition. Once the solid dispersion manufactured and milled, DSC is very advantageous for checking the batch reproductibility or the stability behavior by the measurement of the melting enthalpy of the eutectic. For a solid dispersion with 40% darodipine, a standard deviation of 1.4% for the melting point of the eutectic located at 58°C and 2.4% for the heat of eutectic of 27 cal g^{-1} was found.

PEG used for solid dispersion vary from molecular weight 1000 to molecular weight 20,000. PEG of lower

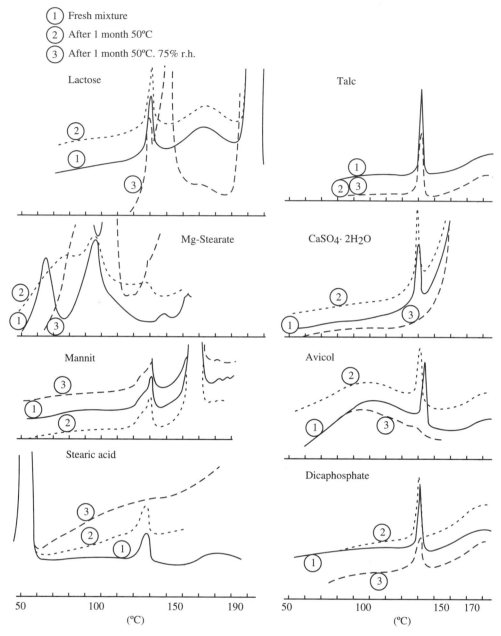

Fig. 20 DSC curves of 10% drug substance with excipients: 1: Original curves; 2: curves after 1 month at 50°C/<30% RH; and 3: 50°C/75% RH. The initial DSC curves suggest an incompatibility only with mannitol and magnesium stearate. The DSC curves (curves 3) after storage at 50°C/75% RH allow the differentiation of the excipients: degradation with stearic acid, calcium sulfate dihydrate, and avicel.

molecular weight are liquid and therefore not suitable. The quality mostly used are PEG 4000 and PEG 6000. The composition of the eutectic of most drug substances lies in small concentration of drug substance. Some monotectics (0% drug substance) have been described. The highest amount of drug is obtained with gluthetimide with an eutectic composition of 32% (5).

Solid solutions: The drug and the carrier are miscible in the solid state. Polyvinylpyrrolidones (PVP) with different molecular weights dissolve drug substances such as diazepam (138) through hydrophobic interactions. The disparition of the DSC peak of the drug substance demonstrates the formation of the solid solution.

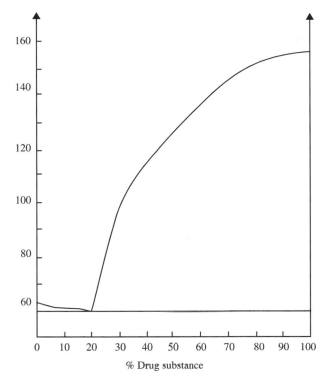

Fig. 21 Phase diagram of a solid dispersion of darodipine–PEG 6000.

Drug substance and carrier can be both in the glassy state. Total miscibility, partial miscibility, or total immiscibility has been observed. This type of system is very sensitive to temperature and moisture and crystallizations are often observed after long storage.

New derivatives of starch, mainly cyclodextrins (139) which forms inclusion compounds, are best carriers for the monitoring of the dissolution characteristics of the drug. These cyclic oligosaccharides contain six (α-CyD), seven (β-CyD), and eight (γ-CyD) α-(1,4)-linked glucose units. A great number of chemically modified cyclodextrins have been manufactured in the last decade. Complexes are formed through inclusion in the cavity or through interactions with chemical groups. In order to obtain complexation, the compounds have to bind a complex first in solution. From the usual methods of preparation, kneading, coprecipitation, freeze drying, or spray drying, often the spray-drying technique gives the best results.

Giordano et al. (140) suggested a method of calculation of the ratio guest/host. They performed DSC analysis of dispersions of different compositions with an excess of the guest molecule. The remaining energy in the melting peak of the guest molecule allows the calculation of the amount of free drug. They plot this amount for differents composition versus the total guest fraction and

compared the plot obtained with the theoretical plots for ratios 1:1, 1:2, 1:3.

In most cases the DSC peak of the drug substance disappears and no new peak is observed. With hydrocortisone butyrate (141), a new peak corresponding to the complex has been observed. For this drug, the complexation increases in the order α-CyD, β-CyD, γ-CyD, and dimethyl-β-CyD. Thermogravimetry analysis has also been used (142). The temperatures of vaporization, sublimation, or degradation of the drugs are displaced to higher temperatures, due to the complexation.

Analysis of the Drug Product

If the components are not miscible in the solid and the liquid states, their DSC peaks remain unchanged. This allows to identify components of the drug product, to follow aging problems with polymorphism and in favourable cases to quantify the drug substance and the excipients (11, 20, 143, 144).

Fatty Acids and Glycerides Derivatives

Most fats and similar compounds show polymorphism behavior, including fatty acids, fatty alcohols,

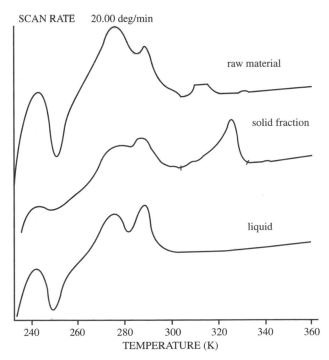

Fig. 22 DSC curves for the monitoring of fractionation of a liquid excipient. Scan rate 20 K min^{-1}.

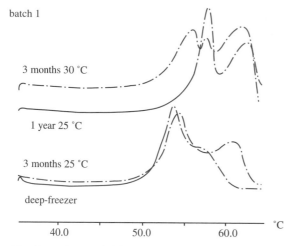

After 1 year the same DSC curve is obtained at 25 °C, 30 °C as after 2 years as demonstrated with another batch.

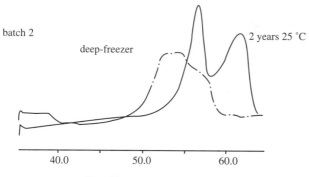

Fig. 23 Aging of precirol.

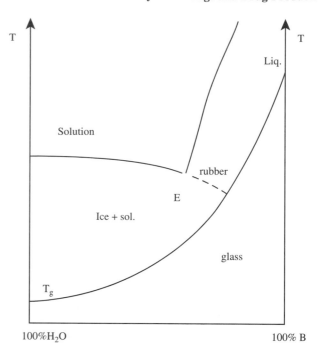

Fig. 24 Phase diagram of water and amorphous substance during freeze drying.

cetostearyl alcohols, glycerides, oils, hydrogenated or transesterified oils, and suppositories (145). This polymorphic behavior is characterized by change of melting by aging, giving rise to hardning effects of suppositories and precipitations of liquid excipients that are complex mixtures of glycerides. Examples of aging problems are given in (10). Fig. 22 is an example of the control of the fractionation of a liquid excipient, using DSC. Aging of the precirol excipient is demonstrated in Fig. 23. Sub ambient DSC was also used for the preformulations of microemulsions (11–13). The solid fat index, calculated as a percentage of the solid as function of the temperature, is very valuable for the evaluation of suppositories (146). Analysis of the drug is also possible. Chemical reaction was observed for aminophylline (147). Since most fatty acid derivatives are unsaturated, they are very sensitive to oxidation. The oxidability and the influence of antioxidants can be measured by DSC and TG, comparing the starting of the degradation (148).

Interaction with Water

The phase diagrams of drug substance and excipients with water as well as the study of the temperature of glass transition (see Fig. 24) are the basis of the choice of the conditions of freeze-dried or spray-dried formulations (149–152). The lyophilizates are well characterized by DSC and TG. The polymorphic behavior of all components can be studied by thermal techniques. For proteins, it is suitable to have excipients in the formulation that remains amorphous. Trehalose was found to be a very efficient lyoprotectant (153).

Freezable water is determined by the measurement of the melting peak of ice. This technique is currently applied for creams, and gels (154, 155). Examples of the melting peak of freezable water are given in Fig. 25. Swelling properties of modified release matrices and their interaction during dissolution have been studied (156, 157).

Monoglycerides–water systems have been characterized (158). Three classes of phases (lamellar, cubic, and hexagonal) have been determined. Water/oil systems and their aging on the phase transitions have been studied using DSC (159, 160). Thermogravimetry can be successfully used additionally (161).

Liposomes are multilayered vesicles consisting of concentric bilayers of phospholipids interdispersed with

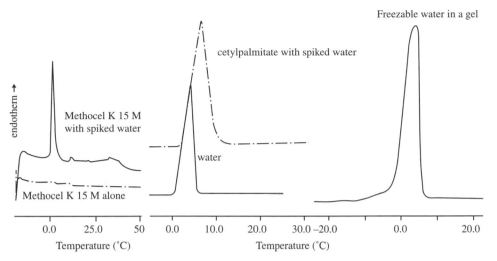

Fig. 25 Determination of freezable water, using the melting peak of ice. (a) Methocel K 15 M, (b) cetyl palmitate, and (c) pharmaceutical gel.

aqueous phases. In aqueous media, the phospholipids undergo gel, liquid crystalline transitions easy to detect by DSC. The study of the change of these transitions, temperature, peak width, and energy allows to characterize the hydrated phospholipid bilayers and to study the liposome formation with drugs (162–164). Drug targeting studies with phospholipids membranes have been proposed using DSC technique (165).

CONCLUSION

Thermal analysis methods are widely used in all fields of pharmaceutics. They are unique for the characterization of single compounds. The information correlated with the thermodynamic phase diagrams is extremely helpful for rational preformulation and development of new delivery systems. Very rapid and requiring only very small samples of material, these methods are applicable in development and also in production for quality control. The combination with spectroscopic and crystallographic data will allow better insight in complex phase changes behavior.

REFERENCES

1. Wendlandt, W.W. Thermal Analysis. *Chemical Analysis*; 3rd Ed., Elving, P.J., Winefordner, J.D., Kolthoff, I.M., Eds.; John Wiley: New York, 1986; 19.
2. Haines, P.J. *Thermal Methods of Analysis, Principles, Applications and Problems;* Blackie, Academic Professional: London, 1995.
3. Wunderlich, B. *Thermal Analysis*; Academic Press: New York, 1990.
4. Turi, E.A. *Thermal Characterization on Polymeric Materials*; 2nd Ed.; Academic Press: New York, 1997.
5. Ford, J.L.; Timmins, P. Pharmaceutical Thermal Analysis Techniques and Applications. *Series in Pharmaceutical Technology, Ellis Horwood Books in Biological Sciences*; Rubinstein, M.H. Ed.; John Wiley & Sons: New York, 1989.
6. Giron-Forest, D. Thermoanalytische Verfahren. *Pharmazeutischer Qualitätskontrolle*; Feltkamp, H., Fuchs, P., Sucker, H., Eds.; Stuttgart, Leipzig Germany, 1983; 298–310, Georg Thieme Verlag.
7. Barnes, P.A. Applications of New Methods and Instrumentation in Thermal Analysis. Thermochim. Acta **1987**, *114*, 1–8.
8. Brennan, W.P. Some Applications of Thermal Analysis as a Supplement to or Replacement for ASTM Testing Standards. Thermochim. Acta **1977**, *18*, 10–13, and 101–111.
9. Giron, D. Applications of Thermal Analysis in the Pharmaceutical Industry. J. Pharm. Biochem. Anal. **1986**, *40*, 755–770.
10. Giron, D. Thermal Analysis in Pharmaceutical Routine Analysis. Acta Pharm. Jugosl. **1990**, *40*, 95–157.
11. Giron, D. Thermal Analysis of Drugs and Drug Products. *Encyclopedia of Pharmaceutical Technology*; Swarbrick, J., Boylan, J.C., Eds.; Marcel Dekker, Inc.: New York, 1995; 15, 1–79.
12. Giron, D. Thermal Analysis, Microcalorimetry and Combined Techniques for the Study of Pharmaceuticals. J. Therm. Anal. Calorim. **1999**, *56*, 1285–1304.
13. Giron, D. Contribution of Thermal Methods and Related Techniques for Rational Development of Pharmaceuticals. P.S.S.T. **1998**, *1*, 191–262.
14. Cheng, S.Z.D.; Li, C.Y.; Calhoun, B.H.; Zhu, L.; Zhou, W.W. Thermal Analysis: The Next Two Decades. Thermochim. Acta **2000**, *355*, 59–68.

15. Thompson, K.C. Pharmaceutical Applications of Calorimetric Measurements in the New Millenium. Thermochim. Acta **2000**, *366*, 83–87.

16. Sarge, S.M.; Gmelin, E. Temperature, Heat and Heat Flow Rate Calibration of Differential Scanning Calorimeters. Thermochim. Acta **2000**, *347*, 9–13.

17. Sarge, S.M.; Hohne, G.W.H.; Cammenga, H.K.; Eysel, W.; Gmelin, E. Temperature, Heat and Heat Flow Rate Calibration of Scanning Calorimeters in the Cooling Mode. Thermochim. Acta **2000**, *361*, 1–20.

18. Sabbah, R.; Xu-wu, A.; Chickos, J.S.; Leita, M.L.; Roux, M.V.; Torres, L.A. Reference Materials for Calorimetry and Differential Thermal Analysis. Thermochim. Acta **1999**, *331*, 93–204.

19. Giron, D.; Goldbronn, C.; Piechon, P. Thermal Analysis Methods for Pharmacopea Materials. J. Pharm. Biochem. Anal. **1989**, *7*, 1421–1430.

20. Giron, D. Characterization of Pharmaceuticals by Thermal Analysis. Am. Pharm. Rev. **2000**, *3*(2), 53–61, 3 (3), 43–53.

21. Han, J.; Gupte, S.; Suryanarayanan, R. Applications of Pressure Differential Scanning Calorimetry in the Study of Pharmaceutical Hydrates. II. Ampicillin Trihydrate. Int. J. Pharm. **1998**, *170*, 63–72.

22. Gill, P.S.; Sauerbrunn, S.R.; Reading, M. Modulated Differential Scanning Calorimetry. J. Thermal. Anal. **1993**, *40*, 931–939.

23. Hohne, G.W.H. Modulated DSC. Thermochimica Acta **1999**, *330*, 45–51.

24. Coleman, N.J.; Craig, D.Q.M. Modulated DSC: A Novel Approach to Pharmaceutical Thermal Analysis. Int. J. Pharm. **1996**, *135*, 13–29.

25. McPhillips, H.; Craig, D.Q.M.; Royall, P.G.; Hill, V.L. Characterization of the Glass Transition of HPC Using Modulated DSC. Int. J. Pharm. **1999**, *180*, 83–90.

26. Craig, D.Q.M.; Barsnes, M.; Royall, P.G.; Kett, V.L. An Evaluation of the Use of Modulated Temperature DSC as a Means of Assessing the Relaxation Behavior of Amorphous Lactose. Pharm. Res. **2000**, *17*(6), 696–700.

27. Bottom, R. The Role of MTDSC in the Characterisation of a Drug Molecule Exhibiting Polymorphic and Glass Forming Tendencies. Int. J. Pharm. **1999**, *192*(1), 47–53.

28. Parkes, G.M.B.; Barnes, P.A.; Bond, G.; Charsley, E.L. Qualitative and Quantitative Aspects of Microwave Thermal Analysis. Thermochim. Acta **2000**, *356*, 85–96.

29. Olson, E.A.; Efremov, M.Y.; Kwan, A.T.; Lai, S.; Petrova, V. Scanning Calorimeter for Nanoliter-Scale Liquid Samples. Appl. Phys. Lett. **2000**, *77*(17), 2671–2673.

30. Buckton, G. Application of Isothermal Microcalorimetry in the Pharmaceutical Sciences. Thermochim. Acta **1995**, *248*, 117–129.

31. Wadsö, I. Isothermal Calorimetry. Thermochim. Acta **1999**, *294*, 1–11.

32. Charsley, E.L.; Warne, S.St.; Warrington, S.B. Thermogravimetric Apparatus Temperature Calibration Using Melting Point Standards. Thermochim. Acta **1987**, *114*, 53–61.

33. McGhie, A.R.; Chiu, J.; Fair, P.G.; Blaine, R.L. Studies on ICTA Reference Materials Using Simultaneous TG-DTA. Thermochim. Acta **1983**, *67*, 241–250.

34. Komatsu, H.; Yoshii, K.; Okada, S.; Chem. Pharm. Bull. **1994**, *42*, 1631–1635.

35. Giron, D. Goldbronn, C., Pfeffer, S. Automation in Thermogravimetry: Application in Pharmaceutical Industry Poster Presented at the 4th Symposium on Pharmacy and Thermal Analysis. Karlsruhe, 1999.

36. Dunn, J.G.; Sharp, J.H. *Treatise on Analytical Chemistry*, Kolthoff, I.M. Ed.; 2nd Ed.; Part 1 John Wiley & Sons: New York, 1993; 13, 127–267.

37. Shlieout, G.; Zessin, G. Investigation of the Internal Stress of Ethylcellulose Tablets by TMA. Pharmazie **1997**, *52*, 713–717.

38. Ozawa, T. Kinetic Analysis by Repeated Temperature Scanning. Part 1. Theory and Methods. Thermocim. Acta **2000**, *356*, 173–180.

39. Nakamura, K.; Kinoshita, E.; Hatakeyama, T.; Hatakeyama, H. TMA Measurement of Swelling Behavior of Polysaccharide Hydrogels. Thermochim. Acta **2000**, *352*, 171–176.

40. Knop, K.; Matthée, K. Quellungsmessungen Von dünnen Polymerfilmen Mittels TMA. User Com (Mettler Toledo Application) **1998**, *2*, 9–10.

41. Syler, R.; ASTM Spec. Techn. Publ. **1991**, *1136*, 22–31, Matsumari N., ASTM Spec. Techn. Publ., 1991, 1136, 32–48.

42. Craig, D.M.Q.; Johnson, F.A. DMA for Pharmaceuticals. Thermochim. Acta **1995**, *248*, 97–115.

43. Kühnert-Brandstätter, M. *Thermomicroscopy in the Analysis of Pharmaceuticals Intern. Ser. Monog. Anal. Chem.*, Belcher, R., Freiser, M. Eds.; Pergamon Press: Oxford, 1971; 45.

43a. Kühnert-Brandstätter, M. *Thermomicroscopy of Organic Compounds in Comprehensive Analytical Chemistry*; Svehla, G., Ed.; Elsevier Publisher: Amsterdam, 1982; XVI, 329–428.

44. Cooke, P.M. Chemical Microscopy. Anal. Chem. **1996**, *68*, 333R–378R.

45. Vitez, I.M.; Newman, A.W.; Davidovich, M.; Kiesnowski, C. The Evolution of Hot Stage Microscopy to Aid Solid-state Characterizations of Pharmaceutical Solids. Thermochim. Acta **1998**, *324*, 187–196.

46. Kellner, R.; Kühnert-Brandstätter, M.H.; Malissa, H. FTIR-Microscopic Investigations of Microphases and Microphase-Transitions in Organic Substances. Mikrochim. Acta **1998**, *2*, 133–137.

47. Moss, R. La Spectroscopie Raman à Transformée De Fourier Dans Un Laboratoire d'analyse Industrielle. Analusis Magazine **1994**, *22*, M17–M22.

48. Szelagiewicz, M.; Marcolli, C.; Cianferani, S.; Hard, A.P.; Vit, A.; Burkhard, A.; von Raumer, M.Ch.; Hofmeier, Ch.A.; Zilian, A.E.; Francotte, E.; Schenker, R. In Situ Characterization of Polymorphic Forms. The Potential of Raman Techniques. J. Therm. Anal. **1999**, *57*, 23–43.

49. Griesser, U.J.; Auer, M.E.; Burger, A. Micro-Thermal Analysis, FTIR-and Raman-Microscopy of (*R*,*S*)-Proxyphylline Crystal Forms. Microchem. J. **2000**, *65*(3), 283–292.

50. Craig, D.Q.M.; Royall, P.G.; Reading, M.; Price, D.M.; Lever, T.J.; Furry, J. Micro-Thermal Analysis for the Characterization of Pharmaceutical Materials. *Proc. Conf. North Am. Thermal Anal. Soc.*; 26th Omnipress: Madison Wisconsin, 1998; 610–615.

51. Epple, E.; Cammenga, H.K. Temperature Resolved X-ray Diffractometry as a Thermoanalytical Method: A

Powerful Tool for Determining Solid State Reaction Kinetics. J. Therm. Anal. **1992**, *38*, 619–626.

52. Conflant, P.; Guyot-Hermann, A.M. Contribution of X-ray Powder Diffraction Versus Temperature to the Solid State Study of Pharmaceutical Raw Materials. Eur. J. Pharm. Biopharm. **1994**, *40*, 388–392.

53. Giron, D.; Draghi, M.; Goldbronn, C.; Pfeffer, S.; Piechon, P. Study of the Polymorphic Behaviour of Some Local Anesthetic Drugs. J. Therm. Anal. **1997**, *49*, 913–927.

54. Giron, D. Investigation of Polymorphism and Pseudo-Polymorphism in Pharmaceuticals by Combined Thermo-analytical Techniques. J. Therm. Anal. Calorim. **2000**, ICTAC, in press.

55. Cavatur, R.K.; Suryanarayanan, R. Characterization of Phase Transformations during Freeze-drying by In Situ X-Ray Powder Diffractometry. Pharm. Dev. Technol. **1998**, *3*, 579–586.

56. Ashizawa, K.; Netsu Sokutei **1998**, *25*, 97–104.

57. Arii, T.; Kishi, A.; Kobayashi, Y. Coupled DSC and X-Ray Diffraction Instrument. Thermochim. Acta **1999**, *325*, 151–156, Rigaku Application Note Presented at the 48th Annual Denver X-ray Conference, 1999.

58. Caira, M.R. Crystalline Polymorphism of Organic Compunds. Top. Curr. Chem. **1998**, *198*, 163–208.

59. Materazzi, F. Application of Coupled TG-IR. To the Polymorphism of Pharmaceuticals. Appl. Spectrosc. Rev. **1997**, *32*, 385.

60. Ozawa, T. Application of TG-MS. Mass Spectrom. Soc. **1998**, *11*, 52.

61. Breen, C.; Last, P.M.; Taylor, S.; Komadel, P. Synergic Chemical Analysis—The Coupling of TG with FTIR, MS and GC-MS. Thermochimica Acta **2000**, *363*, 93–104.

62. Decision Tree: Investigating the Need to Set Acceptance Criteria for Polymorphism in Drug Substances and Drug Products International Conference on Harmonization (ICH) Guideline Specification Q6A, 1999.

63. Haleblian, J.; McCrone, W.J. Pharmaceutical Applications of Polymorphism. Pharm. Sci. **1969**, *58*, 911–929.

64. Haleblian, J.K. Characterization of Habits and Crystalline Modifications of Solids and Their Pharmaceutical Applications. Pharm. Sci. **1975**, *64*, 1269–1288.

65. Giron, D. Le Polymorphisme. Labo-Pharma-Probl. Techn. **1981**, *307*, 151–160.

66. Masse, J.; Bauer, M.; Billot, P.; Broquaire, M.; Chauvet, A.; Doveze, J.; Garinot, O.; Giron, D. Etude Du Polymorphisme Et Du Pseudopolymorphisme à L'aide Des Méthodes Thermo-Analytiques, Rappport d'une Commission SFSTP. S.T.P. Pharma Prat. **1997**, *7*, 235–246.

67. Giron, D. Thermal Analysis and Calorimetric Methods in the Characterization of Polymorphs and Solvates. Thermochim. Acta **1995**, *248*, 1–59.

68. Giron, D. Le Polymorphisme Des Excipients. STP Pharma (Hors serie) **1990**, *6*, 87–98.

69. Burger, A.; Ramberger, R. On the Polymorphism of Pharmaceuticals and Other Molecular Crystals. I. Theory of Thermodynamic Rules. Mikrochim. Acta **1979**, *2*, 259–271.

70. Burger, A.; Ramberger, R. On the Polymorphism of Pharmaceuticals and Other Molecular Crystals. II. Applicability of Thermodynamic Rules. Mikrochim. Acta **1979**, *2*, 273–316.

71. Burger, A. Thermodynamic and Other Aspects of the Polymorphism of Drugs. Pharm. Int. **1982**, *3*, 158–163.

72. Burger, A.; Henck, J.O. The Presentation of Polymorphic Systems by Energy/Temperature Diagrams. Biopharm. Pharm. Technol. **1995**, *1*, 10–11.

73. Toscani, S. An Up-To-Date Approach to Drug Polymorphism. Thermochim. Acta **1998**, *321*, 73–79.

74. Jacques, J.; Collet, A.; Wilen, S.H. *Enantiomers, Racemates and Resolutions*; John Wiley, 1981.

75. Bernstein, J.; Davey, R.J.; Henck, J.O. Concomittant Polymorphs. Angew. Chem. Int. Ed. **1999**, *38*, 3340–3461.

76. Coquerel, G. Review on the Heterogeneous Equilibria Between Condensed Phases in Binary Systems of Enantiomers. Enantiomer **2000**, *5*, 481–498.

77. McCauley, J.A. Detection and Characterization of Polymorphism in the Pharmaceutical Industry. AIChE Symp. Ser. **1991**, *87*, 58–63.

78. Giron, D.; Piechon, P.; Goldbronn, C.; Pfeffer, S. Thermal Analysis, Microcalorimetry and Combined Techniques for the Study of the Polymorphic Behavior of a Purine Derivative. J. Therm. Anal. Calorim. **1999**, *57*, 61–72.

79. Hancock, B.C.; Zografi, G. The Relationship Between the Glass Transition Temperature and the Water Content of Amorphous Solids. Pharm. Res. **1994**, *11*, 471–417.

80. Hancock, B.C.; Zografi, G. Characteristics and Significance of the Amorphous State in Pharmaceutical Systems. J. Pharm. Sci. **1997**, *86*, 1–12.

81. Shalaev, E.Y.; Zografi, G. How Does Residual Water Affect the Solid State Degradation of Drugs in the Amorphous State. J. Pharm. Sci **1996**, *85*, 1137–1141.

82. Hancok, B.; Dalton, C.R.; Pikal, M.J.; Shamblin, S.L. A Pragmatic Test of a Simple Calorimetric Method for Determining the Fragility of Some Amorphous Pharmaceutical Materials. Pharm. Res. **1998**, *15*, 762–767.

83. Andronis, V.; Zografi, G. Crystal Nucleation and Growth of Indomethacin Polymorphs from the Amorphous State. J. Non-Cryst. Solids **2000**, *271*, 236–248.

84. Kontny, M.J.; Zografi, G. Sorption of Water by Solids. Drugs Pharm. Sci. **1995**, *70*, 387–418.

85. Di Martino, P.; Piva, F.; Conflant, P.; Guyot-Hermann, A.M. Thermal Analysis and Powder X-Ray Diffraction Study of Terpin. Evidence of a Eutectic (Hydrate/Anhydrous Form). J. Thermal Anal. Calorim. **1999**, *57*, 95–111.

86. Soustelle, M. Physico-Chemical Transformation of Powders. *Powder Technology and Pharmaceutical Processes*; Chulia, D., Deleuil, M., Pourcelot, Y. Eds.; Elseveier Science: Amsterdam, 1994; 27–58.

87. Morris, K.R. Structural Aspects of Hydrates and Solvates. Drugs Pharm. Sci. **1999**, *95*, 125–181, Polymorphism in Pharmaceutical Solids; Brittain, H.G., Ed.; Marcel Dekker, Inc.: New York.

88. Kankhari, R.K.; Grant, D.J.W. Pharmaceutical Hydrates. Thermochim. Acta **1995**, *248*, 61–79.

89. McCauley, J.A.; Varsolona, R.J.; Levorse, D.A. The Effect of Polymorphism and Metastability on the Characterization and Isolation of Two Pharmaceutical Compounds. J. Phys. D, Appl. Phys. **1993**, *26*, B85–B89.

90. Giron, D.; Goldbronn, C. Use of Sub-Ambient DSC to Complement Conventional DSC And TG. J. of Thermal Anal. **1997**, *49*, 907–912, 1998; 51, 727.

91. Byström, K. Thermometric Company. Application Note 22004 **1990**, .

92. Humera, A.; Buckton, G.; Rawlins, D.A. The Use of Isothermal Microcalorimetry in the Study of Small Degrees of Amorphous Contend of Hydrophobic Powder. Int. J. Pharm. **1996**, *130*, 195–201.

93. Giron, D.; Remy, P.; Thomas, S.; Vilette, E. Quantitation of Amorphicity by Microcalorimetry. J. Thermal Anal. **1997**, *48*, 465–472.

94. Giron, D.; Goldbronn, C. Place of DSC Purity Analysis in Pharmaceutical Development. J. Thermal. Anal. **1995**, *44*, 217–251.

95. Neah, S.H.; Shinwari, M.K.; Hellmuth, E.W. Melting Point Phase Diagrams of Free Base and Hydrochloride Salts of Bevantolol, Pindolol and Propanolol. Int. J. Pharm. **1993**, *99*, 303–310.

96. Elsabee, M.; Frankerd, R.J. Solid State Properties of Drugs. DSC Of Chiral Drugs Mixtures Existing as Racemic Solid Solutions, Mixtures or Racemic Compounds. Int. J. Pharm. **1992**, *86*, 221–230.

97. Grunenberg, A.; Kell, B.; Henck, J.O. Polymorphism in Binary Mixtures, as Exemplified by Nimodipine. Int. J. Pharm. **1995**, *118*, 11–21.

98. Li, Z.; Zell, M.T.; Munson, E.J.; Grant, D.J.W. Characterization of Racemic Species of Chiral Drugs Using Thermal Analysis, Thermodynamic Calculation and Structural Studies. J. Pharm. Sci. **1999**, *88*, 337–346.

99. Rustichelli, C.; Gamberini, M.C.; Ferioli, V.; Gamberini, G. Properties of the Racemic Species of Verapamil Hydrochloride and Gallopamil Hydrochloride. Int. J. Pharm. **1999**, *178*, 111–120.

100. Pitré, D.; Nebuloni, M.; Ferri, V. Calorimetric Determination of the Enantiomeric Purity of (1R,2R)-2 Amino-1 (4-nitrophenol) 1,3 Propanediol. Arch. Phar. (Weinheim) **1991**, *324*, 325–328.

101. Pitré, D.; Nebuloni, M. Further Characterization of the Solid Form of Iopanoic Acid and Its Enantiomers. Arch. Phar. (Weinheim) **1992**, *325*, 385–388.

102. Madarasz, J.; Kozma, D.; Pokol, G.; Acs, M.; Fogassay, E. Merit of Estimation from DSC Measurements for the Efficiency of Optical Resolutions. J. Thermal Anal. **1994**, *42*, 877–894.

103. Tonitou, E.; Chow, D.D.; Lawter, J.R. Chiral Beta-blockers for Transdermal Delivery. Int. J. Pharm. **1994**, *104*, 19–28.

104. Romero, A.J.; Rodhes, C.T. Approaches to Stereospecific Preformulation of Ibuprofen. Drug Dev. Ind. Pharm. **1992**, *17*, 777–792.

105. Dwivedi, S.K.; Sattari, S.; Jamaki, F.; Mitchell, A.G. Ibuprofen Racemate and Enantiomers. Phase Diagrams, Solubility and Thermodynamic Studies. Int. J. Pharm. **1992**, *87*, 95–104.

106. Li, Z.; Grant, D.J.W. Relationship between Physical Properties and Crystal Structure of Chiral Drugs. J. Pharm. Sci. **1997**, *86*, 1073–1078.

107. Doelker, E. Physicochemical Behavior of Active Substances. Consequences for the Feasibility and Stability of Pharmaceutical Forms. S.T.P. Pharma Prat. **1999**, *9*, 399–409.

108. Buckton, G.; Darcy, P. Water Mobility in Amorphous Lactose Below and Close to the Glass Transition Temperature. Int. J. Pharm. **1996**, *136*, 141–146.

109. Figura, L.O. The Physical Modification of Lactose and Its Thermoanalytical Identification. Thermochim. Acta **1993**, *222*, 187–194.

110. Wada, Y.; Matsubyara, H. Magnesium Stearate. Thermochim. Acta **1992**, *196*, 63–84.

111. Containers <661> Physico-Chemical Tests Plastics. *USP 24*; 2000, 1933–1935.

112. Schneider, H.A.; Di Marzio, E.A. The Glass Transition of Polymer Blends. Polymer **1992**, *33*, 3453–3460.

113. Corrigan, O.I. Retardation of Polymeric Carrier Dissolution by Dispersed Drugs. Drug. Dev. Ind. Pharm. **1986**, *12*, 1777–1791.

114. Craig, D.Q.M.; Newton, J.M. Characterization of Polyethylene Glycols using Differential Scanning Calorimetry. Int. J. Pharm. **1991**, *74*, 33–41.

115. Craig, D.Q.M. A Review of Thermal Methods Used for the Analysis of the Crystal Form, Solution Thermodynamics and Glass Transition Behavior of Polyethylene Glycols. Thermochim. Acta **1995**, *248*, 189–203.

116. Sunol, J.J.; Farjas, J.; Berlanga, R.; Saurina, J. Thermal Analysis of a Polyethylene Glycol (PEG 4000): T-CR-T Diagram Construction. J. Thermal Anal. Calorim. **2000**, *61*, 711–718.

117. Ford, J.L. The Use of Thermal Analysis in the Study of Solid Dispersions. Drug Dev. Ind. Pharm. **1987**, *13*, 1741–1777.

118. Barabas, E.S.; Adeyeye, C.M. Povidone. *Analytical Profiles of Drug Substances and Excipients*; Brittain, H.G., Ed.; Academic Press: New York, 1993; 22, 555–685.

119. Tan, Y.; Challa, G.; Polymer **1976**, *17*, 739–750.

120. Sakellariou, P.; Rowe, R.C.; White, E.F.T. The Thermomechanical Properties and Glass Transition Temperatures of Some Cellulose Derivatives. Int. J. Pharm. **1985**, *27*, 267–277.

121. Ford, J.L. Thermal Analysis of Hydroxypropylmethycellulose and Methylcellulose: Powders, Gels and Matrix Tablets. Int. J. Pharm. **1999**, *179*, 209–220.

122. Kaloustian, J.; Pauli, A.M.; Pastor, J. Thermal Analysis of Cellulose and Some Etherified and Esterified Derivatives. J. Thermal. Anal. **1997**, *48*, 791–804.

123. Sanghavi, N.M.; Sheikl, F.; Fruitwala, M.; Drug Dev. Ind. Pharm. **1994**, *20*, 1923–1931.

124. Sakellariou, P.; Rowe, R.C.; White, E.T.F. The Solubility Parameters of Some Cellulose Derivatives and Polyethylene Glycols Used in Tablet Film Coating. Int. J. Pharm. **1986**, *31*, 175–177.

125. Wu, C.; McGinity, J.W. Non Traditional Plasticization of Polymeric Films. Int. J. Pharm. **1999**, *177*, 15–27.

126. Amighi, K.; Moes, A.J. Determination of Thermal Properties and Film Formation Characteristics of Different Acrylic Aqueous Dispersions Used for Film Coating. Pharm., Biopharm. Pharm. Technol. **1995**, *1*, 52–53.

127. Appelqvist, I.A.M.; Cooke, D. Thermal Properties of Polysaccharides at Low Moisture: An Endothermic Melting Process and Water–Carbohydrate Interactions. Carbohydr. Polym. **1993**, *20*.

128. Cesaro, A. Thermodynamics of Phase Equilibria in Biotechnological Polysaccharides. Indian J.Technol. **1992**, *30*, 565–577.

129. Corrigan, O.I. Thermal Analysis of Spray Dried Products. Thermochim. Acta **1995**, *248*, 245–258.

130. Pitt, G.G.; Gu, Z.W. Modification of the Rates of Chain Cleavage of Poly(e-caprolactone) and Related Polyesters in the Solid State. J. Controlled Release **1987**, *283*(4), 283–291.

131. Aktar, S.; Ponton, C.W.; Notariami, L.J.; Gould, P.L.; Pharm. Res. **1989**, *5*, 556–560.

132. Dubernet, C. Thermal Analysis of Microspheres. Thermochimica Acta **1995**, *248*, 259–269.

133. Rosilio, V. Study of Progesterone Loaded Poly (D,L - Lactide-co-Glycolide). Pharm Res. **1998**, *13*, 794–800.

134. Giordano, F.; Bettinetti, G.P. An Experimental and Theoretical Approach to the Analysis of Binary Systems. J. Pharm. Biomed. Anal. **1988**, *6*, 951–955.

135. Crowley, K.J.; Forbes, R.T.; York, P.; Nyqvist, H.; Camber, O. Oleate Salt Formation and Mesomorphic Behavior in the Propanolo/Oleic Acid Binary System. J. Pharm. Sci. **1999**, *88*, 586–591.

136. Koenigbauer, M.J. Pharmaceutical Applications of Microcalorimetry. Pharm. Res. **1994**, *11*, 777–783.

137. Serajuddin, A.T.M. Solid Dispersion of Poorly Water-Soluble Drugs: Early Promises, Subsequent Problems and Recent Breakthroughs. J. Pharm. Sci. **1999**, *88*, 1058–1066.

138. Keipert, S.; Voigt, R. Interactions between Macromolecules Excipients and Drugs. Improvement of Dissolution of Benzodiazepines Derivatives by PVP. Pharmazie **1986**, *41*, 400–404.

139. Duchêne, D. *New Trends in Cyclodextrins and Their Derivatives*; Santé Paris, 1991.

140. Giodarno, F.; Bruni, G.; Bettinetti, G.P. Solid State Microcalorimetry on Drug Cyclodextrin Binary Systems. J. Thermal. Anal. **1992**, *38*, 2683–2690.

141. Chun, I.K.; Yun, D.S.; Int. J. Pharm. **1993**, *96*, 916103.

142. Funk, O.; Schwab, L.; Frómming, K.H.; J. Inclusion Phenom. Mol. Recognit. Chem. **1993**, *16*, 299–314.

143. Giron, D.; Goldbronn, C. Use of DSC and TG For Identification and Quantification of the Dosage Form. J. Thermal. Anal. **1997**, *48*, 473–483.

144. Bucci, R.; Magri, A.D.; Magri, A.L. DSC in the Chemical Analysis of Drugs. Determination of Diclofenac in Pharmaceutical Formulations. J. Therm; Anal. Calorim. **2000**, *61*(2), 369–376.

145. Garti, N. *Crystallization and Polymorphism of Fats and Fatty Acids*; Marcel Dekker, Inc.: New York, 1988.

146. Giron, D.; Riva, A.; Steiger, M. DSC as Support for the Development of Suppositories. Thermochim. Acta **1985**, *85*, 509–512.

147. Prya-Jones, R.H. Aminophylline Suppository Decomposition: An Investigation Using DSC. Int. J. Pharm. **1992**, *86*, 231–237.

148. Riga, A.; Patterson, G.H. *Oxidative Behavior of Materials by Thermal Analytical Techniques*; ASTM Special Technical Publication 1326, 1997, ASTM.

149. Franks, F. Freeze-Drying: From Empiricism to Predictability. The Significance of Glass Transition. Dev. Biol. Stand. **1992**, *74*, 9–19.

150. Franks, F. The Glassy State in Foods. *Int. J. Food Sci. Technol.* Blanshard, J.M.V., Lillford, P.J., Eds.; 1995; 30, 89–100.

151. Liapiz, A.I.; Pikal, M.J.; Bruttini, R. Research and Development Needs and Opportunities in Freeze-Drying. Drying Technol. **1996**, *14*, 1265–1300.

152. Ross, H.; Franks, F. Stabilization of Pharmaceutical Drug Substances by Freeze-Drying: A Case Study. Drug Stab. **1996**, *1*, 73–85.

153. Mehl, P.M. Solubility and Phase Transitions in the System Trehalose/Water. J. Thermal Anal. **1997**, *49*, 817–821.

154. Junginger, H.E. Polyhydroxy Methacrylate-co-methacrylic Acid: Effect of Water, PEG 400 and PEG6000 on the Glass Transition Temperature. Polymer **1989**, *30*, 1946–1953.

155. Kodama, M.; Kato, H.; Aoki, H. Water Molecules in Subgel Phase of Dimyristoylphosphatidylethanolamine/Water. Thermochim. Acta **2000**, *352*, 213–221.

156. Katzhendler, I.; Mader, K.; Friedman, M. Structure and Hydration Properties of Hydroxypropyl Methylcellulose Matrices Containing Naproxen and Naproxen Sodium. Int. J. Pharm. **2000**, *200*, 161–179.

157. Aoiki, S.; Ando, H.; Ishii, M.; Watanabe, S.; Ozawa, H. Water Behavior During Release from a Matrix Observed Using Differential Scanning Calorimetry. J. Controlled Release **1995**, *33*, 365–374.

158. Morley, W.G.; Tiddey, G.J. Phase Behaviour of Momoglyceride-Water Systems. J. Chem. Soc. Faraday Trans. **1993**, *89*, 2823–2831.

159. Eccleston, G.M.; Beattie, L. Microstructural Changes During Storage of Systems Containing Cetostearyl Alkohol/Polyoxyethylene Alkyl Ether Surfactants. Drug Dev. Ind. Pharm. **1988**, *14*, 2499–2518.

160. Eccleston, G.M. Phase Transitions in Ternary Systems and Oil-Un-Water Emulsions Containing Cetrimide and Fatty Alkohols. Int. J. Pharm. **1985**, *27*, 311–32.

161. Regola, A.; Canesi, M.; Dolfini, A.; Gazzaniga, A. Use of Thermogravimetry in the Physicochemical Characterization of Hydrophilic Creams. Boll. Chim. Farm. **1996**, *135*, 67–71.

162. Blume, A. Biological Calorimetry: Membranes. Thermochimica Acta **1991**, *193*, 292–347.

163. Taylor, K.M.G.; Morris, R.M. Liposomes. Thermochimica Acta **1995**, *248*, 289–302.

164. Van Winden, E.C.A.; Zhang, W.; Crommelin, D.J.A. Effect of Freezing Rate on the Stability of Liposomes During Freeze-drying and Rehydration. Pharm. Res. **1997**, *14*, 1151–1156.

165. Puglisi, G.; Fresta, M.; Ventura, C.; Mazzone, G.; Vandelli, M.A. Methotrexate Interaction with a Lipid Membrane Model of DPPC. J. Thermal Anal. **1995**, *44*, 1287–1299.

TITRIMETRY

Vesa Virtanen

Orion Pharma, Kuopio, Finland

DEFINITION OF TERMS

Titrimetry or titrimetric analysis is any method of quantitative chemical analysis in which the amount of a substance is determined by measuring the volume that it occupies or the volume of a second substance that is needed to react completely with the substance being determined. Titration is a process of chemical analysis in which the quantity of some constituents of a sample is determined by adding to the measured sample an exactly known quantity of another substance with which the desired constituent reacts in a definite, known proportion. The reagent of exactly known composition used in a titration is called a standard solution.

The goal of titration is the equivalence point, where the addition of standard solution in an amount that is chemically equivalent to the substance with which it reacts. In fact, its position can be estimated only by observing physical changes associated with it in the solution. These changes manifest themselves at the endpoint of the titration.

An indicator is a supplementary chemical compound that exhibits a change in color as a result of concentration changes occurring near the equivalence point.

PRECIPITATION TITRATIONS

In these titrations, the determination of the substance is effected by precipitating it in the form of an "insoluble" compound of known composition. The equivalence point is reached when sufficient reagent to complete precipitation has been added. In practice, the insoluble reaction product formed will be very slightly soluble and to an extent that depends on the amount of solvent present as well as on the nature and amounts of other ions and compounds present.

In the simplest general case of a slightly soluble salt (AB) formed by the reaction of the oppositely charged univalent anion (A^-) and cation (B^+) of two soluble salts:

$$A^- + B^+ = AB \quad \text{and} \quad Kppn = [A^-][B^+]/[AB]$$

where Kppn is the precipitation constant. Assuming that interferences are small enough to be neglected, the concentration of the insoluble salt AB may be regarded as being constant:

$$Kppn[AB] = [A^-][B^+] = \text{constant} = S_{AB}$$

where the constant S is the solubility product. If the solution is pure, equivalent concentrations of A^- and B^+ will be present, and therefore:

$$[A^-] = [B^+] \text{ or } [A^-]^2 = [B^+]^2 = S_{AB}.$$

In this case, if the product $[A^-][B^+]$ exceeds $(S_{AB})^{0.5}$, the solution is saturated with respect to AB, and this substance separates as a precipitate (1).

Titration Curves

Titration curves are based on the negative logarithm (to the base 10) of the molar concentration of the species; p-values or p-functions are useful for deducing the properties required of an indicator as well as the titration error that its use is likely to cause.

The general shape of a titration curve for the precipitation titration of a solution containing one anion, Cl^-, is shown in Fig. 1. Curves plotted from calculated pX values are always symmetrical. A curve plotted by using experimentally obtained values for $[Cl^-]$ is not symmetrical. The lack of symmetry is due to those ions that are being adsorbed in excess by the precipitate in different amounts. This fact is not taken into account in theoretical calculations. Accurate precipitation titrimetry requires a long, steep AB section because the length of AB depends on the initial concentrations of the reactants and the value of the solubility product of the compound precipitated. An increase in analyte and reagent concentration enhances the change in pX in the equivalence point region.

Precipitation titrations can be extended to mixtures that form precipitates of different solubilities. The titration curve in Fig. 2 for a chloride/iodide mixture is a composite of the individual curves for the two anionic species. Because silver iodide has a much lower solubility than does silver chloride, the initial additions of the reagent

Encyclopedia of Pharmaceutical Technology

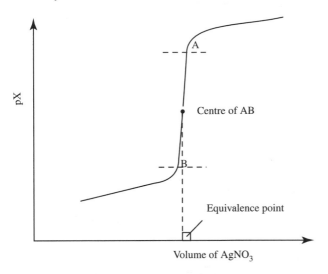

Fig. 1 A theoretical precipitation titration curve.

result exclusively in formation of iodide. Thus, two equivalence points are evident.

Endpoint Detection

The stoichiometric equivalence point should be immediately detectable. This usually requires a large change in some physical or chemical property of the solution. This point in the reaction is often located by means of a

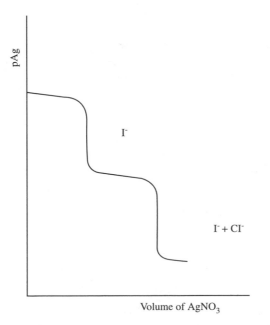

Fig. 2 Titration curve of solution with iodide and chloride.

secondary system, which provides an observable endpoint. This secondary system must be reproducible, clearly identifiable, and ideally coincident with the stoichiometric equivalence point. Because coincidence is not always achieved, the difference between the endpoint and the equivalence point should be easily measurable. Often, so-called blank solution is used for this correction. A chemical indicator produces a visually detectable change in the solution, usually color or turbidity, or may form another precipitate that has a distinctive color. The indicator functions by reacting competitively with one of the reactants or products of the titration and, therefore, its concentration must be kept low, favoring an intense color at the endpoint. For some determinations, an electro-chemical sensor provides an accurate way of locating the equivalence point.

The formation of a second, highly colored precipitate is the basis of the Mohr method of endpoint detection. Chloride and bromide ions are titrated with standard silver nitrate using chromate ion as indicator, the endpoint being indicated by the appearance of brick-red silver chromate (2).

$$Ag^+ + Cl^- \rightarrow AgCl \quad (s)$$
$$Ag^+ + CrO_4^{2-} \rightarrow Ag_2CrO_4 \quad (s)$$

Because silver chromate is more soluble, the K_{sp} value (soluble product constant) of silver chromate is not exceeded until the precipitation of Cl^- is complete. The endpoint can be corrected by using the Mohr method to standardize the silver nitrate solution against pure sodium chloride.

The Volhard method of endpoint detection involves using Fe^{3+} ions as the indicator (3). This procedure requires a suitably acidic solution to prevent precipitation of iron(III) as the hydrated oxide. It has the disadvantage that it is useful only for the reaction:

$$SCN^- + Ag^+ \leftrightarrow AgSCN \quad (s)$$

After the first excess of thiocyanate ions is added, the indicator reaction is:

$$Fe^{3+} + SCN^- \leftrightarrow Fe(SCN)^{2+} (red)$$

This means that to determine halide ion (except F^-) back titration is required. In this case, a measured aliquot of standard silver nitrate solution is added to the sample, and the excess silver ion is determined by back-titration with a standard thiocyanate solution.

An adsorption indicator is typically an organic dye, such as fluorescein and its derivatives. Most adsorption indicators are weak acids. Their use is thus confined to basic, neutral, or slightly acidic solutions in which

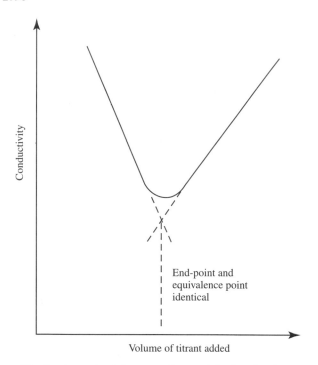

Fig. 3 A conductivity curve for precipitation titration.

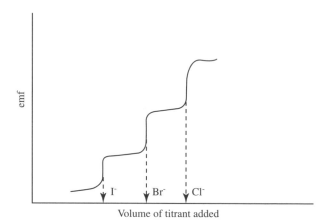

Fig. 4 Titration curves for a mixture of halides.

the indicator exists predominantly as the anion. Some cationic adsorption indicators are suitable for titrations in strongly acidic solutions. In this case, adsorption of the dye and coloration of the precipitate occur if the precipitate particles possess a negative charge.

Because the total amount of ions in solution decreases as the analyte is precipitated, the conductance of the solution must decrease. For an accurate result, the plot of conductivity against volume of titrant added has the characteristics shown in Fig. 3. This technique is suitable for both dilute and concentrated solutions as well as for colored solutions.

The electromotoric force (emf) of a cell depends on the ionic concentration of the solutions. To locate the equivalence point, the variation in emf is monitored as the concentration of the analyte changes. When the measured emf is plotted against the total volume of titrant added, the curve produced is similar to that of a titration curve Fig. 4. This technique has all the advantages of the conductometric method and gives an experimental curve from which the endpoint can be detected accurately.

Applications

Most applications of precipitation titrations are based on the use of a standard silver nitrate solution and are therefore sometimes called argentometric methods (Table 1).

NEUTRALIZATION TITRATIONS

Acid–Base Equilibria

Aqueous solutions always contain hydronium ions as well as hydroxide ions as a consequence of the dissociation of water:

$$2\ HO \leftrightarrow HO^+ + OH^-$$

Certain solutes cause changes in the concentrations of the two species, often with profound effect on the chemical characteristics of the solution.

Application of the mass law to the dissociation of water leads to $Kw = [H_3O^+][OH^-]$, where Kw is called the ion-product constant for water. At 25°C the ion-product constant has the numerical value of 1.0×10^{-14} mole^2/L^2. In pure water, the concentrations of hydronium and hydroxide ions are identical, and pure water is neutral.

A useful relationship is obtained from the negative logarithm of both sides of the ion-product constant expression. Thus:

$$-\log Kw = -\log[H_3O^+][OH^-]$$
$$= -\log[H_3O^+] - \log[OH^-]$$

Table 1 Typical applications of precipitation titrations

Analyte	Titrant	Endpoint Detection
Cl^-, Br^-, I^-	Ag^+	Potentiometric
Cl^-, Br^-, I^-	Ag^+	Precipitate
Ag^+	SCN	Fe(III), potentiometric
Cl^-, Br^-	$Hg(NO_3)_2$	Precipitate
SO_4^{2-}, MoO_4^{2-}	$Pb(NO_3)_2$	Precipitate

from which it follows that:

$$pKw = -\log Kw = pH + pOH$$

where pKw represents the negative logarithm of the ion-product constant of water. At 25°C, pKw is 14; that is, pH + pOH = 14.00.

Buffer Solutions

A buffer solution resists changes in pH as a result of dilution or small additions of acids or bases. The most effective buffer solutions contain high and approximately equal concentrations of a conjugate acid–base pair. The resistance of buffer mixtures to pH is changed by adding acids or bases. The ability of a buffer to prevent a significant change in pH is directly related to the total concentration of the buffering species and their concentration ratios. The buffer capacity of a solution is defined as the number of equivalents of strong acid or base needed to cause 1.00 L of the buffer to undergo a 1.00-unit change in pH (4).

Acid–Base Indicators

Endpoint detection in a neutralization titration is ordinarily based on the abrupt change in pH that occurs near the equivalence point. A noninstrumental method of pH measurement much used in simple titrations uses indicators. These are generally organic dyes, or weak acids or bases, that on dissociation or association undergo internal structural changes at or near the equivalence point of the neutralization, resulting in a color change.

A list of some compounds possessing acid-base indicator properties is shown in Table 2. Ethanol is the common solvent for indicator solutions.

Titration curves of simple systems

When both reagent and analyte are strong, the net neutralization reaction can be expressed as follows:

$$H_3O^+ + OH^- = 2\,HO$$

The hydronium ions in an aqueous solution of a strong acid derive from two sources: the reaction of the solute with water and the dissociation of water itself.

Titration of a strong acid with a strong alkali starts with pure acid in the start that is gradually diluted, changing increasingly to a neutral salt until only neutral salt remains at the equivalence point. Immediately beyond the equivalence point, the amount of strong alkali increases. The change in pH near the equivalence point will be sharp and large. This may or may not be at pH 7, depending on

Table 2   Some acid-base indicators

Indicator	pH range	Color change
Cresol red	0.2–1.8	red–yellow
Thymol blue	1.2–2.8	red–yellow
	8.0–9.6	yellow–blue
Bromophenol blue	3.0–4.6	yellow–blue
Methyl yellow	2.9–4.0	red–yellow
Methyl orange	3.1–4.4	red–orange
Congo red	3.0–5.0	blue–red
Bromocresol green	3.8–5.4	yellow–blue
Methyl red	4.2–6.3	red–blue
Bromocresol purple	5.2–6.8	yellow–purple
Bromothymol blue	6.0–7.6	yellow–blue
Phenol red	6.8–8.4	yellow–red
Cresol purple	7.6–9.2	yellow–purple
Thymol blue	8.0–9.6	yellow–blue
Phenolphthalein	8.3–10.0	colorless–red
Thymolphthalein	9.3–10.5	colorless–blue
Alizarin yellow GG	10–12	colorless–yellow

the degree of ionization of the acid and base, that is, their strengths as acid or base.

Titration of a weak acid such as acetic acid against strong base gives a titration curve as that shown in Fig. 5. At first, partly ionized acid is present owing to a pH too high for a strong acid. As neutralization continues, more acid ionizes and mainly ionized acid and salt are present. Therefore, the pH changes gradually; this is called the buffer effect. If a strong acid is titrated with a weak base such as ammonia, the converse occurs.

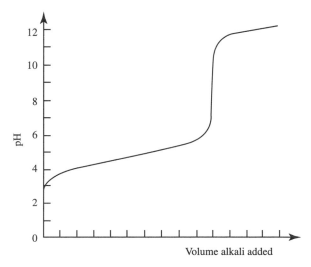

Fig. 5   A weak acid-strong base titration curve.

When a weak acid is titrated with a weak base, the titration curve shows a continuously and gradually changing pH with the addition of base. No region with a sharp shift in pH is obtained for small additions of titrant. If a sharp shift occurs, it is still less than 2 pH units and not detectable by indicators. On both sides of the equivalence point, buffers are present, and at the equivalence point, the pH depends on the relative strengths of acid and base.

Titration curves of complex systems

Complex systems include solutions containing two acids or bases, which contain or consume two or more protons, and amphiprotic substances that act as both acids and bases. A characteristic of all such systems is that two or more equilibria must be considered in describing their behavior. As a consequence, the techniques for pH data derivation are often more complex than for simple systems.

A titration curve for the titration of weak and strong acids with strong base is shown in Fig. 6. The stronger acid is neutralized first, along with some of the weaker acid. As a result, a curve more sloping is obtained. The sharp pH change of the strong acid is still obtained, although the weaker acid interferes. After all the strong acid has gone (point A), the weaker acid is titrated (point B).

Compounds with two or more acidic or basic functional groups will yield multiple endpoints in a titration, provided the acidic or basic groups differ sufficiently in strength. Computational techniques permit the derivation of reasonably accurate theoretical titration curves for polyprotic acids or bases, provided the ratio K_1/K_2 is above 103. K_1 and K_2 are dissociation constants. The titration curve of a dibasic weak acid with NaOH resembles that shown in Fig. 6.

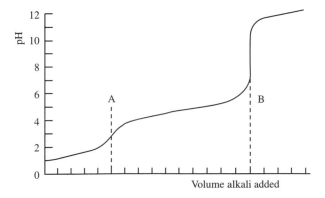

Fig. 6 Titration of a mixture of a strong and a weak acid with alkali.

The derivation of a titration curve for a polyfunctional base is similar to the previous one for acid.

Amphiprotic substance, when dissolved in a suitable solvent, behaves both as a weak acid and as a weak base. If either its acidic or its basic character predominates sufficiently, titration of the species with a strong base or a strong acid may be feasible.

Applications in Aqueous Media

Several important elements that occur in organic and biological systems are conveniently determined by methods that involve an acid-base titration as the final step. Generally, these elements are nonmetallic such as carbon, nitrogen, chlorine, bromine, sulfur, phosphorus, and fluorine. However, in addition, similar methods exist for several less commonly encountered species. In each case, the element is converted to an inorganic acid or base that can be titrated.

Numerous inorganic species can be determined by titration with strong acids or bases. For example, ammonium salts are determined by conversion to ammonia with strong base and distillation in the Kjeldahl apparatus. Also, inorganic nitrates and nitrites can be determined using Kjeldahl method (5) by reducing these species to ammonium ion.

Carboxylic and sulfonic acid groups import acidity to organic compounds. Most carboxylic acids and sulfuric acids are readily dissolved in water, and their titration with a base is straightforward. If solubility in water is not sufficient, the acid can be dissolved in ethanol and titrated with aqueous base. Aliphatic amines and many saturated cyclic amines can be titrated directly with a solution of a strong acid. Esters are determined by saponification with a measured quantity of standard base. The excess base is titrated with standard acid.

Many aldehydes and ketones can be assayed with the aid of a solution of hydroxylamine hydrochloride. The liberated hydrochloric acid is titrated with base. The total salt content of a solution is determined by converting the salt to an equivalent amount of an acid or a base by passage through a column packed with an ion-exchange resin and then titrated with either base or acid, respectively.

Applications in Nonaqueous Media

Many useful titrations can be performed in glacial acetic acid, which is used widely for the titration of aromatic amines, amides, ureas, and other weak nitrogen bases. Direct titration of most amino acids with a standard acid can be performed in glacial acetic acid.

Basic solvents such as ethylenediamine, dimethylform-amide, pyridine, and dimethylsulfoxide can be used for acids that are too weak to be titrated in water. Amine salts, inorganic salts, carboxylic acids, phenols, and imides are soluble in ethylenediamine, where they exhibit enhanced acidic characteristics.

Many sulfa drugs such as sulfanilamide, sulfathiozole, and sulfathalidine can be titrated in ethyleneamine with tetrabutylammonium hydroxide. The ability of dimethylformamide to dissolve salts, polymers, and many organic compounds accounts for its wide use as a titration solvent. Inert solvents such as acetone can be used for titration of acids, acetonitrile for both acids and bases, and ethyl acetate for amines. A suitable nonaqueous medium such as methyl isobutyl ketone makes it possible to discriminate among various mineral acids that are not leveled by the solvent as they are in water.

OXIDATION–REDUCTION TITRATIONS

Equilibrium

Oxidation of a substance (element or a compound) involves the loss of electrons. Conversely, reduction of a substance involves the gain of electrons. Thus, in oxidation–reduction system, electron transfer occurs.

In titration of iron(II) with cerium(IV):

$$Ce^{4+} + Fe^{2+} \leftrightarrow Ce^{3+} + Fe^{3+}$$

equilibrium is attained after each addition of titrant. After the first addition of cerium(IV), all four species will be present in the solution in amounts dictated by the equilibrium constant of the reaction. At chemical equilibrium of an oxidation–reduction system, the electrode potentials E for the two half-reactions are identica. Thus, at any point in the titration:

$$E_{Ce^+} = E_{Fe^+} = E_{system}$$

If the solution contains a reversible oxidation–reduction indicator as well, its potential must be the same as that for the system:

$$E_{In} = E_{Ce^{4+}} = E_{Fe^{3+}} = E_{system}$$

Titration Curves

The potential of a system can be measured experimentally by determining the emf of a suitable cell. Thus, for the titration of iron(II) with cerium(IV), the cell is:

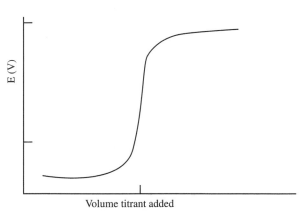

Fig. 7   Titration curve for iron(II) with cerium(IV).

$$SCE \| Ce^{4+}, Ce^{3+}, Fe^{3+}, Fe^{2+} | Pt$$

The potential of the platinum electrode versus a saturated calomel electrode (SCE) is determined by the affinity of Fe^{3+} for electrons:

$$Fe^{3+} + e \rightarrow Fe^{2+}$$

and that of Ce4+:

$$Ce^{4+} + e \rightarrow Ce^{3+}$$

In deriving Esystem data for a titration curve, either ECe4+ or EFe3+ can be used. Short of the equivalence point, the concentration of cerium(IV) is vanishingly small. The concentrations of iron(II), iron(III), and cerium(III) can be calculated from the amount of titrant added.

Applying the Nernst equation for the iron(III)/iron(II) couple gives a value for the potential of the system directly. Using the couple cerium(IV)/cerium(III) would give the same answer, but it would first be necessary to calculate a value for the concentration of cerium(IV), which in turn would require evaluation of the equilibrium constant for the reaction.

As shown in Fig. 7 there is a rapid change in the value of E as the titration is proceeded through the endpoint. In fact, the titration curve has the same general form as that of an acid–base titration. An exact value for the endpoint can be calculated using the Nernst equations for the half-reactions.

The shape of the curve for an oxidation–reduction titration depends on the nature of the system under consideration. The titration curve in Fig. 7 is symmetric about the equivalence point because the molar ratio of oxidant to reductant is equal to unity. An asymmetrical curve results if the ratio differs from this value. Solutions containing two oxidizing or reducing agents yield titration curves containing two inflection points if the standard

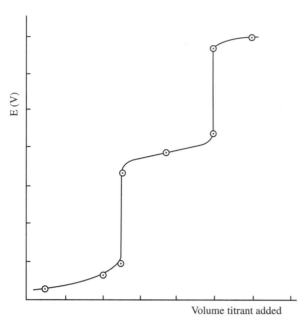

Fig. 8 Titration of iron(II) and titanium(III) with cerium(IV).

potentials for the two species are different by more than approximately 0.2 V. Fig. 8 shows the titration curve for a mixture of iron(II) and titanium(III) with cerium(IV). The first additions of cerium are used by more readily oxidized titanium(III) ion, thus, the first step in the titration curve corresponds to titanium and the second to iron.

Oxidation–Reduction Indicators

Specific indicators owe their behavior to a reaction with one of the participants in the titration. The best-known specific indicator is starch, which forms a dark blue complex with triiodide ion. Also, potassium thiocyanate is

used as a specific indicator, for example, in titration of iron(III) with solutions of titanium(III) sulfate.

Oxidation–reduction indicators

A redox indicator is essentially a compound that has oxidized and reduced forms with different, and preferably intense, colors (Table 3). The half-reaction responsible for color change in a typical oxidation–reduction indicator can be written as:

$$Indicator_{(oxidized)} + ne = Indicator_{(reduced)}$$

Applications

Standard oxidants

The powerful oxidant potassium permanganate, $KMnO_4$, is a widely used oxidizing agent. It is most commonly used with solutions that are 0.1 N or greater in mineral acid. Under those conditions, the product is manganese(II):

$$MnO_4^- + 8 H^+ + 5 e \leftrightarrow Mn^{2+} + 4 HO$$

However, the tendency of permanganate to oxidize chloride ion is a disadvantage because hydrochloric acid is such a useful solvent and, furthermore, $KMnO_4$ solutions have limited stability.

For example, determinations of Sn, H_2O_2, Fe, V, Mo, W, U, Ti, Mg, Ca, Zn, Co, Pb, Ag, K, Na, and HNO_2 potassium permanganate are used as oxidizing agents.

A sulfuric acid solution of cerium(IV) is nearly as potent an oxidizing reagent as is permanganate and can be substituted for the latter in most of the applications described with potassium permanganate. Cerium(IV) does not oxidize chloride ion at a detectable rate as does permanganate, and the reagent is indefinitely stable. On the other hand, the color of cerium(IV) is not sufficiently intense to serve as an indicator. In

Table 3 Some redox indicators

Indicator	Color change oxidized-reduced	Transition potential, V
Indigomonosulphonate	Blue—colorless	+ 0.26
Phenosufranine	Red—colorless	+ 0.28
Indigotetrasulphonate	Blue—colorless	+ 0.36
Methylene blue	Blue/green—colorless	+ 0.53
Diphenylamine	Violet—colorless	+ 0.76
p-Ethoxychrysoidine	Yellow—red	+ 0.76
Diphenylamine sulfonic acid	Red/purple—colorless	+ 0.85
Eriocaucin A	Red—yellow/green	+ 0.98
1,10-phenanthroline iron(II)	Pale blue—red	+ 1.11
2,3-diphenylamine dicarboxylic acid	Blue/violet—colorless	+ 1.12

addition, the reagent cannot be used in neutral or basic solutions.

Use of potassium dichromate is limited because of its lesser oxidizing strength and slowness of some of its reactions. This technique is used for determination of iron(II), nitrate, chlorate, permanganate, and organic peroxides, among others.

Iodine, a relatively weak oxidant, is used for the selective determination of strong reducing agents. Iodine can be used for determination of As, Sb, Sn, H_2S_2, SO_2, $S_2O_3^{2-}$, and N_2H_4, among others. Its great advantage is its ready availability as a sensitive and reversible indicator. Its disadvantages include the low stability of iodine solutions and the incompleteness of reactions between iodine and many reducing agents.

Potassium bromate is a convenient source of bromine in organic analysis. Few organic compounds react sufficiently rapidly for a direct titration, and, thus, a measured excess of the bromate is added to the sample, and after the reaction is complete, the excess bromine is back-titrated with an arsene(III) solution. Some organic compound analyzed using bromine substitution are, for example, phenol, *p*-chlorophenol, salicylic acid, acetylsalicylic acid, *m*-cresol, aniline, sulfanilic acid, and *b*-naphtol. Bromine addition is used most often in the estimation of olefinic unsaturation in fats, oils, and petroleum products.

Reductants

Because of the readiness of reducing agents to react with atmospheric oxygen, the titrations must be carried out in and the reagents must be stored under an inert atmosphere. Alternatively, a stable standard oxidizing agent can be used for titration of an aliquot of the reductant to determine the current concentration of the reducing agent.

A variety of oxidizing agents such as Cr(VI), Ce(IV), Mo(VI), NO_3^-, NH_2OH, and organic peroxides can be determined by reaction with a measured excess of standard iron(II) solution. Standard potassium dichromate is frequently used for the back-titration.

Iodide ion is a moderately effective reducing agent. In its applications, a standard solution of sodium thiosulfate is used to titrate the iodine liberated by reaction of the analyte with an unmeasured excess of potassium iodide. Some substances determined by using iodometric method are IO_4^-, IO_3^-, BrO_3^-, ClO_3^-, Br_2, Cl_2, O_2, O_3, Cu^{2+}, NO_2^-, and organic peroxide.

The water content in solids and many organic acids, alcohols, esters, ethers, anhydrides, and halides can be determined using Karl–Fischer reagent (6), composed of iodine, sulfurdioxide, pyridine, and methanol.

COMPLEX-FORMATION TITRATIONS

Metal ions can act as electron-pair acceptors, reacting with electron donors to form coordination compounds or complex ions. The donor species, or ligand, must have at least one pair of unshared electrons to form the bond. Remarkable growth in the analytical applications of complex-formation reactions is attributable to a particular class of coordination compounds called chelates. These compounds are made by the reaction of a metal ion and a ligand that contains two or more donor groups. The properties of chelates can differ markedly from the parent cation.

Titration Curves

The data necessary to plot theoretical *p*-functions versus reagent volumes require the use of formation (or stability) constants (Fig. 9). Equilibrium between a metal ion M,

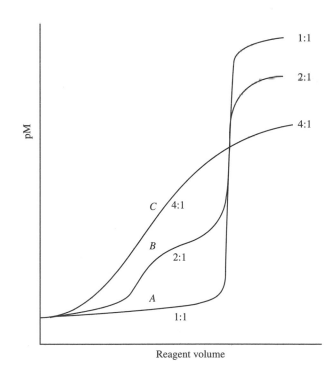

Fig. 9 Curves for complex formation titrations. Titration of the tetradentate ligand D (curve A), bidentate ligand (curve B), and unidentate ligand (curve C).

possessing a coordination number of 4, and the quadridentate ligand D can be represented by:

$$M + D \leftrightarrow MD$$

In similar manner, the equilibrium between M and bidentate B can be represented by:

$$M + 2B \leftrightarrow MB$$

Overall formation of MB2 occurs in two steps and involves the intermediate formation of MB:

$$M + B \leftrightarrow MB$$
$$MB + B \leftrightarrow MB$$

The formation constants for these individual processes are:

$$K_1 = [MB]/[M][B]$$

and

$$K_2 = [MB]/[MB][B]$$

The equilibrium constant for the overall reaction is given by the product of the individual steps:

$$K_{overall} = [MB]/[M][B]^2 = K_1 K_2$$

The complex between M and a simple, unidentate ligand A results in the overall equilibrium:

$$M + 4A \leftrightarrow MA$$

This process occurs also in a stepwise manner, and the equilibrium constant for the overall reaction is therefore numerically equal to the product of the constants for the four constituent processes.

Endpoint Detection

In some complex-formation titrations, the endpoint is noted by the formation or disappearance of a solid phase. For example, in the titration of cyanide with silver ion, the solution remains clear, but the first excess of silver causes formation of a white solid that marks the endpoint. The electron-donor groups of most common ligands tend to combine not only with metallic ions but also with protons; thus, the equivalence point in a complex-formation titration is often accompanied by a marked change in pH, which can be detected with an acid–base indicator.

Formation or disappearance of a soluble colored complex can also indicate an endpoint. Many reagents that form colored complexes with certain metals have been developed only for use as indicators in these titrations. If the cation being titrated produces a color with the indicator, the endpoint will be characterized by the disappearance of this color. When the cation does not give a colored complex, a second cation that does is introduced, and the first excess of titrant then decolorizes this complex.

Some Applications

Inorganic complexing reagents such as $Hg(NO_3)_2$, $AgNO_3$, $NiSO_4$ and KCN can be used for complex-formation titrations. Mercury(II) ion forms neutral complexes with most of the anions that precipitate with silver nitrate such as Br^-, Cl^-, SCN^-, CN^- and thiourea.

$AgNO_3$ reacts with CN^- forming $Ag(CN)_2-$. Iodine used as indicator and endpoint is detected by formation of solid AgI. $NiSO_4$ can also be used for determination of CN^- with AgI as indicator. The endpoint is also detected here by formation of AgI. KCN reacts with Cu^{2+}, Hg^{2+}, and Ni^{2+} forming $Cu(CN)_4$, $Hg(CN)_2$ and $Ni(CN)_4$. Various indicators for endpoint detection can be used (7).

Numerous tertiary amines that also contain carboxylic acid groups form remarkably stable chelates with many metal ions. Ethylenediamine tetra-acetic acid (EDTA) can be used for determination of 40 elements by direct titration using metal-ion indicators for endpoint detection (8). Direct titration procedures are limited to metal ions that react rapidly with EDTA. Back titration procedures are useful for the analysis of cations that form very stable EDTA complexes and for which a satisfactory indicator is not available. EDTA is also used for determining water hardness; the total concentration of calcium and magnesium expressed in terms of the calcium carbonate equivalent.

POTENTIOMETRIC TITRATIONS

In potentiometric titrations, the activity of one species is continuously monitored as it changes during the course of the titration, for example, in the titration:

$$AgNO_3 + NaCl \leftrightarrow AgCl + NaNO$$

where silver nitrate is added to aqueous sodium chloride. The change in activity of the Cl^- can be monitored. The potential between the reference electrode and the indicator electrode is usually measured at the start of and after the addition of small amounts of titrant. A reproducible equilibrium is of little concern. Requirements for reference electrodes are greatly relaxed. In potentiometric titrations, accuracy is higher than that in direct potentiometric measurements because measured potentials are used to

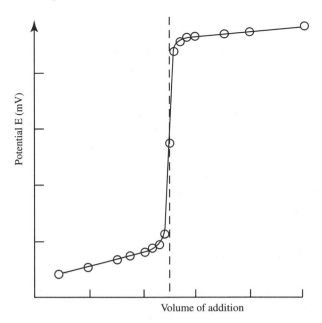

Fig. 10 Potentiometric titration curves.

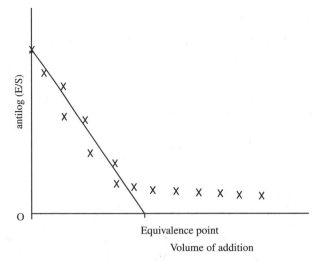

Fig. 11 Gran's plot for a potentiometric titration.

detect rapid changes in activity that occur at the equivalence point of the titration. The change in emf versu titration volume is more interesting than the absolute value of the emf. In potentiometric titrations, the influence of liquid-junction potentials and activity coefficients is minimized. The acid and alkali errors of the glass electrode occur at extremes of pH and have little effect near the interesting equivalence point.

Titration Curves and Endpoint Detection

In potentiometric titrations, the titration curve can be followed point by point, plotting as the ordinate successive values of the cell emf versus the corresponding volume of titrant added as the abscissa (Fig. 10). The titrant should be added in the smallest accurately measurable increments that provide an adequate density of points, particularly in the vicinity of the equivalence point. The greatest change in emf occurs around the equivalence point. The most straightforward method takes the midpoint in the steeply rising portion of the curve as the endpoint.

A second approach is to calculate the change in potential-per-unit change in volume in reagent ($\Delta E/\Delta V$). By inspection, the endpoint can be located from the inflection point of the titration curve. This is the point that corresponds to the maximum rate of change of cell emf per unit volume of titrant added (usually 0.05 or 0.1 mL). The first-derivative method is based on the sigmoid shaped curve.

The second-derivative method is an extension of the first-derivative method. The second-derivative of the data changes sign at the point of inflection in the titration curve. This change is often used as the analytical signal in automatic titrators.

Grans method (9,10) involves the use of the Nernst equation:

$$E = E^*; +S \log C_i$$

where

S is electrode slope, E^* is $E' \pm (0.0591/n) \log i$, and

and E' is the constant incorporating the potential of the reference electrode and the standard potential of the half-cell containing the solution under investigation and the ion selective electrode. The rearrangement of this equation gives:

$$\log C_i = (E - E^*)/S$$

or

$$C_i = \text{antilog}[(E - E^*)/S]$$
$$= [\text{antilog}(-E^*/S)][\text{antilog}(E/S)]$$

The first antilog term is a constant and therefore:

$$C_i = \text{const} . [\text{antilog} (E/S)]$$

If the species i is disappearing during the course of the titration, then it will do it linearly. The antilog term reduces linearly, and a plot of antilog (E/S) against volume of reagent added should give a straight line whose intercept with the volume axis will be the equivalence point, as shown in Fig. 11.

Applications

Precipitation and complex-formation titrations

The indicator electrode for a precipitation titration is often the metal from which the reacting cation is derived. Membrane electrodes that are sensitive to one of the ions involved in the titration process may be used. For example, fluoride-sensitive membrane electrode is used in the determination of the fluoride content of toothpastes. Lanthanum(III) solution is used as a precipitant.

Silver nitrate is the most commonly used reagent for precipitation titration, including potentiometric determination of endpoint. Argentometric methods exist for the determination of halides, halogenoids, mercaptans, sulfides, phosphates, oxalates, and arsenates. A silver electrode serves as indicator for the potentiometric determination of these ions. If the concentration of reagent and analyte is 0.1 M or higher, then a calomel electrode can be used. In dilute solutions, the slight leakage of chloride ions from the salt bridge could be a source of significant error, but not in more concentrated solutions.

Mercury electrode can be used for the potentiometric determination of 29 divalent, trivalent, and tetravalent cations with EDTA (11, 12).

Neutralization titrations

Potentiometric acid–base titrations are particularly useful for the analysis of mixtures of acids or polyprotic acids (or bases) because often, discrimination between the endpoints can be made. An approximate numerical value for the dissociation constant of a weak acid or base can be estimated from potentiometric titration curves. In theory, this quantity can be obtained from any point along the curve, but it is most easily derived from the pH at the point of half-neutralization.

In the case of weak acid HA, it can be assumed that at the midpoint, [HA] = [A⁻], and thus:

$$Ka = [H^+][A^-]/[HA] = [H^+]$$

which gives

$$pKa = pH$$

It must be noted that this constant is not correct because activities should be used in calculations:

$$Ka = [A^-]f_A/[HA]f_{HA}$$

and because

[HA] and [A⁻] are equal $Ka = f_A/f_{HA}$

Oxidation–reduction titrations

In oxidation–reduction titrations, an electrode potential related to the concentration ratio between the oxidized and reduced forms of either of the reactants is determined as a function of the titrant volume. The indicator electrode must be responsive to at least one of the couples involved in the reaction. Indicator electrodes for oxidation–reduction titrations are generally constructed from platinum, gold, mercury, or palladium. The metal chosen must be unreactive with respect to the components of the reaction. The indicator metal is merely a medium for electron transfer.

Automatic Titrators

An entire titration can be performed automatically by titrators equipped with microcomputers and analog-to-digital converters and using dedicated software (13). The most widely used apparatus for automatic reagent addition consists of a calibrated syringe that is activated by a motor-driven micrometer screw. The volume is determined from the number of turns the screw makes during the titration.

Another method uses a preset equivalence point potential applied across the electrodes by means of a calibrated potentiometer. A difference between this potential and that of the electrodes causes an "error" signal, which is amplified. This causes the electronic switch to close, permitting a flow of electricity through the solenoid-operated valve of the burette. As the signal approaches zero, the flow of titrant ceases as the current to the solenoid is switched off.

Second-derivative titrators have the advantage that no preknowledge of the equivalence point potential is required. The signal processor calculates the second derivative of the electrode potential of the indicator electrode. Change in the sign of the second derivative causes a switching device to turn off the flow of the titrant.

A fully automated unit accepts a series of samples placed on a turntable. After each titration, the turntable rotates, indexes the next sample beneath the electrode assembly, and starts the titration.

CONDUCTOMETRIC TITRATIONS

Theory

Conduction of an electric current through an electrolyte solution involves migration of positively charged species toward the cathode and negatively charged species toward the anode. The conductance of a solution is a measure of the current flow that results with application of a given electrical force. It is directly dependent on the number of charged species the solution contains (14). The conductance L of a solution is also the reciprocal of the electrical resistance and has the units of ohm:

$$L = 1/R$$

where R is the resistance in ohms.

The conductance is directly proportional to the length (l) of a uniform conductor. Thus:

$$L = kA/l$$

where k is a proportionality constant called the specific conductance, and A is the surface area.

The equivalent conductance, Λ, is defined as the conductance of a 1-g equivalent of solute contained between electrodes spaced 1 cm apart. It is equal to L when 1-g equivalent of solute is contained between electrodes spaced 1 cm apart. The volume V of solution(cm^3) that will contain 1 gram equivalent solute is given by:

$$V = 1000/C$$

where C is the concentration in equivalents per liter.

Volume can also be expressed in terms of the dimensions of the cell:

$$V = lA$$

when l is 1 cm

$$V = A = 1000/C$$

when $L = kA/l$,

when $L = kA/l$
and $\Lambda = L$, then $\Lambda = 1000k/C$

A conductometric titration involves measurement of the conductance of the sample after successive additions of reagent. The endpoint is determined from a plot of either the conductance or the specific conductance as a function of the volume of added titrant. Throughout a titration, the volume of the solution is always increasing. Unless the conductance is corrected for this effect, nonlinear titration curves result. The titrant should be at least 10 times as concentrated as the solution being titrated to keep the volume change small. Some temperature control is ordinarily required during a conductometric titration because the temperature coefficient for conductance measurements is approximately 2% per °C.

Titration Curves

Titration curves for conductometric titrations take a variety of shapes, depending on the chemical system under investigation. In general, they are characterized by straight line portions with dissimilar slopes on either side of the equivalence point, as shown previously in Fig. 3. To establish a conductometric endpoint, after correcting for volume changes, the conductance data are plotted as a function of titrant volume. The two linear portions are then extrapolated, and the point of intersection is taken as the equivalence point. Frequently, reactions fail to proceed to absolute completion, and the conductometric titration curves invariably show departures from strict linearity in the region of the equivalence point.

An advantage of the conductometric titration is that it can be used for titrations based on relatively unfavorable equilibria.

Applications

Acid–base titrations

Neutralization titrations are particularly well-adapted to the conductometric titration because of the very high conductance of the hydronium and hydroxide ions compared with the conductance of the reaction products. In neutralization of strong acids, hydronium ions are being replaced by an equivalent number of less mobile sodium ions, and the conductance decreases as a result of this substitution. At the equivalence point, the concentration of hydronium and hydroxide ions are at a minimum, and the solution exhibits its lowest conductance. After the endpoint, a reversal of slope occurs as the sodium ion and the hydroxide ion concentration from the excess base increase. There is an excellent linearity between conductance and the volume base added, except at very near equivalence point region. Very dilute solutions can be analyzed accurately.

In conductometric titrations, a change in conductance is caused after the endpoint owing to the increase in concentration of the mobile hydroxide ion. Very weak acids (such as boric acid) and moderately weak acids (such as acetic acid) can be titrated using conductometric titration.

If the titrant is a weak electrolyte (such as ammonia), the curve is essentially horizontal past the equivalence point, which causes less uncertainty to the extrapolation of a curve. In titration of a weak base, such as acetate ion, with a strong acid, a salt and undissociated acetic acid are formed. After the endpoint is passed, a sharp rise in conductance attends the addition of excess hydronium

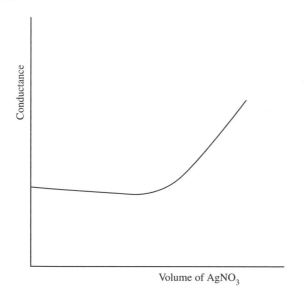

Fig. 12 Titration of chloride ion with silver nitrate.

ions. Salts whose acidic or basic character is too weak to give satisfactory endpoints with indicator are conveniently titrated with the conductometric method. The conductometric titration of a mixture of two acids that differ in degree of dissociation is frequently more accurate than a potentiometric titration.

Precipitation and complex-formation titrations

Figure 12 illustrates the titration of sodium chloride with silver nitrate. After all chloride is precipitated, the addition of excess silver nitrate causes a rapid increase in conductivity. The slope of the initial portion of the curve may be either downward or upward, depending on the relative conductance of the ion being determined and the ion of like charge in the reagent that replaces it. Slow reactions and coprecipitation are sources of difficulty with precipitation and complex-formation titrations.

COULOMETRIC TITRATIONS

Theory

A coulometric titration uses an electrolytically generated titrant for reaction with the analyte. In some analyses, the active electrode process involves only generation of the reagent. In other titrations, the analyte may also be directly involved at the generator electrode (15). The current in a coulometric titration is carefully maintained at a constant and accurately known level. The product of this current and the time required to reach the equivalence point for the reaction yield the number of coulombs and thus the number of equivalents involved in the electrolysis. The coulomb (C) is the quantity of electricity that is transported in 1 by a constant current of 1 ampere. The Faraday constant (F) is the quantity of electricity that produces one equivalent of chemical change at an electrode (16).

The so-called primary titration technique is attempted only with electrodes of silver metal, silver–silver halide, or mercury amalgams, which are the source of the electrogenerated species. The substance to be determined reacts directly at the electrode or with a reactant electrogenerated from the working electrode. This class of titrations is limited generally to nondiffusible reactants such as mercury amalgams, silver ions generated by anodization of silver metal, and halides liberated by reduction of the appropriate silver–silver halide electrode.

In secondary coulometric titrations, an oxidation–reduction buffer serves as the titrant precursor. An active intermediate from the titrant precursor must first be generated with 100% efficiency by the electrode process. The intermediate must react rapidly and completely with the substance being analyzed.

The endpoint may be detected by addition of colored indicators, provided the indicator itself is not electroactive. Potentiometric and spectrophotometric indication is used in acid–base and oxidation–reduction titrations. Amperometric procedures are applicable to oxidation–reduction and ion-combination reactions especially for dilute solutions.

The most obvious advantage of coulometric titration is the elimination of problems associated with the preparation, standardization, and storage of standard solutions. This is particularly important for labile reagent substance such as chlorine or bromine. Another advantage is the requirement of a small quantity of reagent. Instrumentation is simple; a single constant-current source can be used to generate precipitation, oxidation–reduction, or neutralization reagents. Furthermore, coulometric titration is easily automated.

Typical sources of error in coulometric titrations are variation in the current during electrolysis and errors in measurement of current and time. Departure of the process from 100% current efficiency is the primary error source. In some cases, the equivalence point is not the endpoint of the titration.

Applications

Neutralization titrations

Both weak and strong acids can be titrated with a high degree of accuracy using electrogenerated hydroxide ions.

Table 4 Coulorimetric titrations of oxidation–reduction reactions

Reagent	Substance determined
Br_2	As^{3+}, Sb^{3+}, U^{5+}, NH_3, N_2H_4, NH_2OH, phenol, aniline
Cl_2	As^{3+}, I^-
I_2	As^{3+}, Sb^{3+}, $S_2O_3^{2-}$, H_2S
Ce^{4+}	Fe^{2+}, Ti^{3+}, U^{4+}, As^{3+}, I^-, $Fe(CN)_6^{3-}$
Fe^{2+}	Cr^{6+}, Mn^{7+}, V^{3+}, Ce^{4+}
Ti^{3+}	Fe^{3+}, V^{5+}, Ce^{4+}, U^{6+}
$C_2Cl_3^{2-}$	V^{5+}, Cr^{6+}, IO_3^-

In this application, the platinum anode must be isolated by some sort of diaphragm to eliminate potential interference from the hydrogen ions produced. Alternatively, chloride or bromide ions can be added to the solution, and a silver wire used as an anode. The reaction at this electrode is:

$$Ag^+ + Br^- \leftrightarrow AgBr + e$$

Thus, this anode product does not interfere with the neutralization reaction.

Strong and weak bases can be titrated with hydrogen ions generated at a platinum anode.

Here also the cathode must be isolated from the solution to prevent interference from the hydroxide ions produced at that electrode.

Precipitation and complex-formation titrations

Anodically generated silver ions can be used for precipitation titrations of various substances. A cell constructed from a piece of heavy silver wire can be used. Substances precipitated include Cl^-, Br^-, I^-, and mercaptans. Similar applications using mercury(I) ion formed at a mercury anode have been used for the determination of Cl^-, Br^-, and I^-.

The complexing ability of ethylenediaminetetra-acetic acid (EDTA, H4Y) has been exploited in the coulometric titration of metal ions. The method depends on the reduction of the mercury(II) or cadmium chelate of EDTA and on the titration of the metal ion (for example, magnesium) to be determined by the anion of EDTA that is released.

Oxidation–reduction titrations

Applications of coulometric titrations involving oxidation–reduction reactions are shown in Table 4. Electrogenerated oxidizing agents such as bromine have proved to be useful, especially in organic analysis.

AMPEROMETRIC TITRATIONS

Theory

Polarographic methods can be used to estimate the equivalence point of a reaction, provided that at least one of the participants or products of the titration is oxidized or reduced at the microelectrode. When the potential applied across the two electrodes is maintained at some constant value, the current may be measured and plotted against the volume of the titrant, thus, the term amperometric titration. In the case of working electrode-reference electrode pair, the potential of the indicator electrode is maintained at a constant value with respect to a reference electrode, measuring a limiting current, which is proportional to the concentration of one or more of the reactants or products of the titration.

Amperometric titration is easily automated. The titrator can be programmed to shut off when a specified current level is reached. Titrant is run into a blank solution until a specified current is reached, the sample is added, and the titrant is again added until the specified current level is reached.

A correction for dilution is necessary to attain a linear relationship between current and volume of titrant. By working with a reagent that is 10-fold more concentrated than the solution being titrated, this correction becomes negligible. Amperometric and conductometric titrations are similar in the respect that the data for each are collected well away from the equivalence point. Therefore, reactions that are relatively incomplete can be used.

Titration Curves

Typical forms of amperometric titration curves are shown in Fig. 13. A titration in which the substance being analyzed reacts (is reduced) at the electrode while the reagent does not is shown in Fig. 13a. A sufficiently high potential is applied to give a diffusion current for

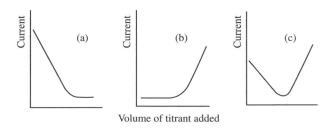

Fig. 13 Amperometric titration curves: (a) analyte is reduced, reagent is not; (b) reagent is reduced, analyte is not; (c) both reagent and analyte are reduced.

the substance, and a linear decrease in current is observed as substance ions are removed from the solution by precipitation. The curvature near the equivalence point reflects the incompleteness of the analytical reaction in this region. The endpoint is obtained by extrapolation of the linear portions. Nearly a mirror image curve is obtained for a titration in which the reagent reacts (is reduced) at the microelectrode, and the substance being analyzed does not (Fig. 13b). The third common curvature for amperometric titrations is obtained when both reagent and subtance analyzed react (are reduced) at the electrode Fig. 13c.

Amperometric Titrations with Two Polarized Microelectrodes

A modification of amperometric method involves the use of two stationary microelectrodes immersed in a well-stirred solution of a sample (17). A small potential is applied between these electrodes, and such current that flows is followed as a function of the volume of reagent added.

Oxidation–reduction titrations

Twin polarized platinum microelectrodes are conveniently used for endpoint detection for oxidation–reduction titrations. Consider a titration curve for oxidation–reduction titration where both reactants behave reversibly at the electrodes. An example of this kind of titration is titration of iron(II) with cerium(IV) (Fig. 14a). At the starting point of the titration, no current is observed because no suitable cathode reactant is available. With addition of cerium(IV), a mixture of iron(II) and iron(III) is produced, which permits the passage of current. Beyond the midpoint in the titration, iron(III) becomes in excess, and the current is then regulated by decreasing iron(II) concentration. At the equivalence point, the current approaches zero because iron(III) are present, and the applied potential is not great enough to cause these to react at the electrode. Beyond the equivalence point, the current

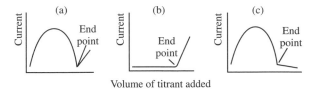

Fig. 14 Amperometric titration curves with twin polarized electrodes: (a) both reactants behave reversibly at the electrode; (b) only reagent behaves reversibly; (c) only analyte titrated behaves reversibly.

rises again because both cerium(III) and cerium(IV) are present to react at the electrodes.

In cases where only reagent behaves reversibly, a different form for titration curve is obtained. Although the reagent added can serve as an anode reactant, no cathode reactant is available because of the slow rate at which the substance analyzed is reduced at a platinum surface. Therefore, no current is observed. Beyond the equivalence point, depolarization of the cell can occur, and the current is dependent on the concentration of the reagent (Fig. 14b). In cases where only the species titrated behave reversibly, before equivalence point, a current is observed that depends on the concentration of the species present in lesser amount. At equivalence point, a zero current is reached, and beyond the equivalence point, no current is observed because the reagent does not behave reversibly at the electrodes (Fig. 14c).

Precipitation titrations

Twin silver microelectrodes permit observation of the endpoint for various titrations using silver nitrate as precipitation reagent (Table 5). Short of the equivalence point, essentially no current exists when a small potential is applied between two such electrodes during a titration of substance analyzed with silver ions because no easily reduced species is present in the solution. After equivalence, the cathode becomes depolarized owing to the presence of a significant amount of silver ions that can react to give silver. Current is permitted as a result of this half-reaction and the corresponding oxidation of silver at the anode. The magnitude of the current is directly proportional to the concentration of the excess reagent.

PHOTOMETRIC TITRATIONS

The change in absorbance of a solution may be used to follow the change in concentration of a radiation-absorbing

Table 5 Applications of amperometric titrations with precipitation products

Reagent	Substance determined
AgNO$_3$	Cl$^-$, Br$^-$, I$^-$, CN$^-$, RSH
Cupferron	Cu^{2+}, Fe^{3+}
Dimethylglyoxime	Ni^{2+}
Pb(NO$_3$)$_2$	SO$_4^{2+}$, MoO$_4^{2+}$, F$^-$, Cl$^-$
8-Hydroxyquinoline	Mg^{2+}, Cu^{2+}, Zn^{2+}, Cd^{2+}, Al^{3+}, Bi^{3+}, Fe^{3+},
K$_2$CrO$_4$	Pb^{2+}, Ba^{2+},

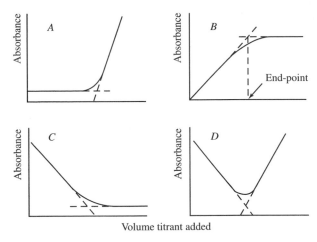

Fig. 15 Different shapes of photometric titration curves.

constituent during a titration (18). The absorbance is directly proportional to the concentration of the absorbing constituents. A plot of absorbance versus titrant consists, if the reaction is complete, of two straight lines that intersect at the endpoint. If the reaction is appreciably incomplete, extrapolation of the two linear segments of the titration curve establishes the intersection and endpoint volume.

Photometric titrations have several advantages over a direct photometric determination. The presence of other absorbing species at the analytical wavelength does not necessarily cause interference because only the change in absorbance is significant. However, if the absorbance of nontitratable components is intense, the absorbance readings are shifted to the undesirable upper end of the absorbance scale. Ideally, only a single absorber is present among the reactant, titrant, and products.

The analytical wavelength is selected to avoid the interference caused by other absorbing substances. Also, there is a need for a molar absorbtivity that causes the change in absorbance during the titration to fall within a convenient range. Often, the chosen wavelength lies well apart from an absorption maximum.

Titration Curves

Volume change, caused by addition of titrant, is seldom negligible, and straight lines for titration curve are obtained only if there is correction for dilution.

If correction is not made, the lines are curved downward toward the volume axis, and erroneous intersections are obtained. Use of a microsyringe and a relatively concentrated titrant is desirable.

Possible shapes of photometric titration curves are shown in Fig. 15. Curve A is typical of the titration where the titrant alone absorbs and where the absorbance readings are taken at the wavelength of the titrant. Curve B is characteristic of systems where the product of the reaction absorbs, and curve C is typical for reactions where the analyte is converted to a nonabsorbing product. When a colored analyte is converted to a colorless product by a colored titrant, curves similar to D are obtained.

Applications

Areas of particular applicability are for solutions so dilute that the indicator blank is excessive or when the color change is not sharp perhaps because titration reactions that are incomplete in the vicinity of the equivalence point or when extraneous colored materials are present in the sample. Titrations in solutions of high or low ionic strength and even in nonaqueous solution are easily performed. Sensitivity of the measurement can be changed easily by simply changing the wavelength or the length of the cell path, a feature that also makes photometric titration attractive. Indicators can be used in titrations where self-indicating systems are lacking.

REFERENCES

1. Grant, J. *Sutton's Volymetric Analysis*, 13th Ed.; Butterworth's Scientific Publications: London, 1955; 28–29.
2. Skoog, D.A.; West, D.M. *Fundamentals of Analytical Chemistry*, 2nd Ed.; Holt, Rinehart, Wilston: London, 1972; 225.
3. Skoog, D.A.; West, D.M. *Fundamentals of Analytical Chemistry*, 2nd Ed.; Holt, Rinehart, Winston: London, 1972; 226–227.
4. Laitinen, H.A. *Chemical Analysis*; McGraw-Hill: New York, 1960; 37.
5. Grant, J. *Sutton's Volymetric Analysis*, 13th Ed.; Butterworth's Scientific Pulications: London, 1955; 140.
6. Mitchell, J. Anal. Chem. **1951**, *23*, 1069.
7. Meites, L. *Handbook of Analytical Chemistry*; McGraw-Hill: New York, 1963; 3–226.
8. Reilley, C.N.; Barnard, A.J., Jr. *Handbook of Analytical Chemistry*; McGraw-Hill: New York, 1963; 3–166 to 3–200.
9. Gran, G. Acta Chem. Scand. **1950**, *4*, 559.
10. Gran, G. Analyst **1952**, *77*, 661.
11. Reilley, C.N.; Schmid, R.W. Anal. Chem. **1958**, *30*, 947.
12. Reilley, C.N.; Schmid, R.W.; Lamson, D.W. Anal. Chem. **1958**, *30*, 953.
13. Foreman, J.K.; Stockwell, P. *Automatic Chemical Analysis*; Wiley: New York, 1975; 42–62.

14. Shadlovsky, T.; Weisserger, A. *Physical Methods of Organic Chemistry*, 3rd Ed.; Interscience: New York, 1960; 1, 3011–3048.

15. Clem, R.G. Ind. Research **1973**, (September), 50.

16. Skoog, D.A.; West, D.M. *Fundamentals of Analytical Chemistry*, 4th Ed.; Holt, Rinehart, Winston: Hong Kong, 1986; 443–444.

17. Lingane, J.J. *Electroanalytical Chemistry*; Interscience: New York, 1958; 280–294.

18. Goddu, R.F.; Hume, D.N. Anal. Chem. **1954**, *26*, 1679.

19. Headridge, J.B. *Photometric Titrations*; Pergamon Press: New York, 1961.

20. Laitinen, H.A.; Harris, W.E. *Chemical Analysis*, 2nd Ed.; McGraw-Hill: New York, 1975.

21. Lingane, J.J. *Electroanalytical Chemistry*; Interscience: New York, 1958.

22. Ma, T.S.; Hassan, S.S.M. *Organic Analysis Using Ion-Selective Electrodes*; Academic Press: London, 1982; 1, 2.

23. Rechnitz, G.A. Bioanalysis with Potentiometric Membrane Electrodes. Anal. Chem. **1982**, *54*, 1194A.

24. Serjeant, E.P. *Potentiometry and Potentiometic Titrations*; John Wiley: New York, 1984.

25. Svehla, G. *Automatic Potentiometric Titrators*; Pergamon Press: New York, 1978.

TONICITY

Jaymin C. Shah
Pfizer Inc., Groton, Connecticut

INTRODUCTION

Parenteral formulations, both large and small volume, have been discussed in depth in Volume 11 of the Encyclopedia of Pharmaceutical Technology (V 11, pp. 201–217, 217–237). However, no discussion of parenteral formulations is complete without an adequate description of tonicity. Tonicity is an important factor in the formulation of products intended for application to sensitive mucous membranes of organs such as eye, ear, and nose. In this article, an attempt is made to first introduce tonicity with respect to its physiological significance, followed by a discussion of the physico-chemical basis for tonicity and colligative properties. Then, a brief review of methods of measuring and/or calculating tonicity is given, followed by the established methods of adjusting tonicity and the examples illustrating each of the methods. Tables listing the established values necessary to do the calculations are provided at the end of the article. Excellent comprehensive reviews dealing with various aspects of tonicity are available in the literature in the form of chapters in various textbooks for pharmacy students (Remington's Pharmaceutical Sciences, Physical Pharmacy by Martin, etc.). A list of such reading material is provided at the end of the article in the Bibliography.

Dosage forms are drug-delivery systems designed to deliver drug to the systemic circulation or to a localized region of the human body. These dosage forms should ideally be free of any undesired adverse effects from the drug and from the formulation components. Reasonable risks associated with the drug substance are sometimes tolerated with an objective of realizing significant therapeutic advantages, as in the case of cancer chemotherapeutic agents. However, any untoward side effect, even as minor as irritation, resulting from an excipient or the finished dosage form cannot be accepted and should not be tolerated. This concern is particularly important to parenteral formulations that breach the normal defensive barriers of the human body to deliver the drug. Therefore, any formulation that comes in contact with sensitive mucous membranes of organs such as the eye should not result in tissue irritation and pain attributable to the formulation itself. One of the

physicochemical means by which a formulation may result in pain and tissue irritation is caused by the nonphysiological concentration of dissolved solutes coming in contact with sensitive tissues. Tonicity is a formulation property that has a direct influence on the ability of the formulation to result in tissue irritation, as described by the following example.

If a small quantity of blood defibrinated to prevent clotting is mixed with a solution containing 0.9% w/v of NaCl, the red blood cells remain intact and retain their normal size and shape. The NaCl solution is considered to be isotonic and has essentially the same salt concentration as does the red blood cell. In contrast, if the blood is mixed with 1.8% w/v NaCl solution, erythrocytes shrink and become wrinkled or crenated as if the cell content has been sucked out. The salt solution that causes this is considered hypertonic with respect to the red blood cell contents. It is because the red blood cell contains a lower salt concentration than the surrounding 1.8% w/v salt solution and as if the water from the erythrocytes passes through the cell membrane to dilute the surrounding salt solution to equalize the two salt concentrations across the membrane. The opposite phenomenon occurs if blood is mixed with 0.45% w/v NaCl solution. Water from the surrounding salt solution enters the erythrocytes, causing them to swell and finally burst, with the liberation of hemoglobin. The 0.45% w/v salt solution is considered hypotonic, and the phenomenon is known as hemolysis. The physiological significance of hemolysis was reconfirmed recently by the report of 10 episodes of hemolysis among patients who received hypotonic 25% human albumin because of dilution with sterile water instead of isotonic sodium chloride (1). Two of these 10 recipients exhibited significant hemolysis and adverse pathological conditions, with one resulting in death (1). Also, it has been observed that hypertonic and hypotonic salt solutions tend to irritate sensitive mucous membranes of the eye, the nose, and the muscle when applied. However, an isotonic solution causes no tissue irritation when it comes in contact with the tissue. The crenation and the hemolysis of red blood cells in hypertonic and hypotonic salt solution, respectively, can be explained by the movement of water across the cell membrane. A membrane is defined as semipermeable if it allows only the movement of solvent molecules across it. The process of diffusion of a solvent through a semipermeable membrane from a less-concentrated solution to a more-concentrated solution is known as osmosis. The pressure that must be applied to the concentrated solution side of the membrane to prevent the flow of pure solvent across the membrane from the diluted solution is known as the osmotic pressure. In crenation, water diffuses from the inside of the erythrocyte across the membrane into the exterior hypertonic salt solution. Hemolysis occurs when water diffuses from the exterior hypotonic solution into the erythrocyte, causing it to swell and burst. An isotonic solution is an aqueous solution that generates the same "tone," or osmotic pressure, as the body fluids across biological membranes and thus prevents water flow in either direction and hence is nonirritating when injected, instilled, perfused, or brought into contact with sensitive mucous membranes. When a solution is hypertonic or hypotonic, osmotic water flow occurs and tone of the membrane is affected. Thus, formulators need to adjust the tone, or tonicity, of the solution to be isotonic with physiological fluids. To be able to adjust the tonicity of a formulation to the isotonic state, one has to understand the principles behind the generation of the osmotic pressure resulting from the dissolved solutes and how it can be altered to that of the physiological fluids.

Osmotic pressure is a colligative property unlike the additive and constitutive properties of solution. Simply stated, the colligative properties of a solution are dependent solely on the number of nonsolvent (solute) particles (molecule/ions) dissolved or in a true solution form in a given solvent and are independent of the specific physicochemical characteristics of the nonsolvent dissolved substance(s). For example, two nonelectrolyte solutes A and B when prepared as $0.1M$ solutions will exhibit the same osmotic pressure irrespective of the chemical nature of A and B. Experimentally, it has been found over the years that the colligative properties are indeed independent of the solute nature and dependent solely on the number of independent particles in dilute solutions for a wide variety of solutes, provided the number of particles is properly assessed. An implicit assumption in the statement above is that the solute is nonvolatile relative to the solvent and the reasoning will be clear from the discussion that follows. The colligative properties of solution are vapor pressure lowering, boiling-point elevation, freezing-point depression, and osmotic pressure. These four properties are effects of solute on the solvent, in that it reduces the escaping tendency of the solvent, and all of them can be related to vapor pressure lowering of the solution. Osmotic pressure is of primary importance from the formulation standpoint; however, it is

cumbersome to measure, and therefore other colligative properties are determined because they are all interrelated. The theory of the colligative properties has been well-established and reviewed in depth in the various textbooks and in the pharmaceutical literature (see the Bibliography). And because the focus of this *Encyclopedia* is on pharmaceutical technology rather than on the theoretical foundation, we briefly overview the theory of colligative properties as needed to understand the concepts used in methods to adjust tonicity of parenteral and ophthalmic formulations.

RAOULT'S AND HENRY'S LAWS AS BASIS FOR COLLIGATIVE PROPERTIES

Raoult's law states that in an ideal solution, the partial vapor pressure of each volatile constituent is equal to the vapor pressure of the pure component multiplied by its mole fraction in the solution. Thus, for two constituents A and B in solution:

$$P_B = P_B^o X_B \qquad (1)$$

$$P_A = P_A^o X_A \qquad (2)$$

where P_A and P_B are the partial vapor pressures of constituents A and B over their solution when the fractional molar concentrations are X_A and X_B, and the vapor pressure of the pure constituents are P_A^o and P_B^o. Therefore, it can be inferred that the vapor pressure of B above the solution by dilution with A is reduced relative to its vapor pressure in pure state and vice versa for A. This diminishes the escaping tendencies of each component, leading to a reduction in the rate of escape of the molecules of A and B from the surface of the solution. This law is valid only in ideal solutions in which there are no intermolecular interactions between components A and B (adhesive interactions) or in which interactions between the two components A and B are identical to the interactions of the pure components A and pure B (cohesive interactions between A and A and between B and B). In essence, the molecule of each component sees an environment identical to its molecular environment in the pure state. This refers to an infinitely dilute solution in which a component's thermodynamic activity is equal to its concentration. However, in the real solutions, the assumption noted above may not apply, and negative deviation from Raoult's law may occur when adhesive attractions between A and B are greater than cohesive attraction within pure A or pure B molecules; i.e., the vapor pressure of the solution or the partial vapor pressure of each component is lower than that expected based on Raoult's law applied to ideal solution. Similarly, positive deviations from Raoult's law can occur when interactions between A and B are less than the cohesive interactions of pure A or pure B, resulting in vapor pressures higher than that expected based on Raoult's law applied to ideal solution. In general, Raoult's law states that when a component A is diluted with another component B, the partial vapor pressure of A is reduced; in essence, a dilution effect.

Raoult's law does not apply over the entire concentration range in a nonideal, real solution. However, when one component is in a large enough excess to be considered a solvent, Raoult's law may be expressed as:

$$P_{\text{solvent}} = P^o_{\text{solvent}} X_{\text{solvent}} \qquad (3)$$

in such a dilute solution and is valid only for the solvent component of a nonideal solution that is sufficiently dilute for the other component, i.e., the solute in a dilute nonideal solution. In such a dilute solution, the solute molecule is completely surrounded by solvent molecules such that the solute molecule can interact only with the solvent molecules because there are very few solute molecules. Further dilution beyond this point does not alter a solute molecule's environment and, even if the solute molecule interacts with the solvent molecule, the solute's partial vapor pressure or the thermodynamic activity becomes proportional to its fractional molar composition as:

$$P_{\text{solute}} = K_{\text{solute}} X_{\text{solute}} \qquad (4)$$

Eq. 4 is known as Henry's law, and K_{solute} is the Henry's law constant, which is less than P^o_{solute}. Therefore, Henry's law applies to the solute in dilute solutions, and Raoult's law applies to solvent in dilute nonideal solutions. Note the similarities between Eqs. 1 and 2 and between Eqs. 3 and 4 for the nonideal dilute solution case. When the solution is ideal, Henry's law becomes identical to Raoult's law, and K_{solute} becomes identical to P^o_{solute}. When the partial pressures of the solute and the solvent are directly proportional to their mole fractions over the entire range, the solution is ideal. In a nonideal solution, Raoult's law will apply to the solvent over the entire concentration range, whereas Henry's law will apply to the solute in a limited concentration range in which it is in a sufficiently diluted form.

When a nonvolatile solute is dissolved in a solvent, the partial vapor pressure of the solvent above the solution is equal to the vapor pressure of the solution. And because

the mole fraction of the solvent is $X_{\text{solvent}} = 1 - X_{\text{solute}}$, Eq. 3 can be rewritten as:

$$P_{\text{solution}} - P_{\text{solvent}} = P^o_{\text{solvent}}(1 - X_{\text{solute}}) \qquad (5)$$

for the dilute solution of a nonvolatile solute of mole fraction X_{solute}. Therefore, the important conclusion from Raoult's and Henry's laws is that the thermodynamic activity of a solvent as measured by its vapor pressure is proportional solely on the mole fractional composition of the solute, irrespective of the physical and chemical nature of the dissolved species. The vapor pressure of the solvent above the solution thus depends solely on the number of particles (molecules/ions) of the dissolved solute and not on the weight concentration of the solute in solution. Therefore, the vapor pressure of a solvent above a dilute solution that obeys Henry's law is a colligative property of the solution. Henry's law has been found to be applicable to nonelectrolyte-type solute mole fractional concentrations of 0.1; however, the range is much smaller for electrolyte type solutes owing to the long-range nature of interionic interactions as noted above. Its impact is evaluated later below.

COLLIGATIVE PROPERTIES

Raoult's law forms the basis for the colligative properties, and Henry's law sets the limits of the applicability of Raoult's law to colligative properties of a solution as increasing amounts of solute are added to solution. As noted above, colligative properties are a consequence of the number of dissolved particles in solution and are all related to the escaping tendency of the solvent from solution.

The four colligative properties that are of importance are: 1) the vapor pressure lowering, 2) the elevation of boiling point, 3) the freezing-point depression, and 4) the osmotic pressure. An attempt is made below to describe qualitatively and quantitatively each colligative property of solutions, with an emphasis on their interrelationship and their application later in measurement and adjustment of the tonicity of solutions, with particular reference to parenteral formulations. Although theoretical derivations based on thermodynamics can be used to show how each of the colligative properties of solution arises and relate to each other, textbooks on physical chemistry for theoretical derivations are recommended.

Lowering of Vapor Pressure

The addition of a nonvolatile solute to a solvent leads to a reduction in the vapor pressure of the solvent because of a reduction in thermodynamic activity of the solvent. Also, because the solute is nonvolatile, the vapor pressure of the solvent is the vapor pressure of the solution, as seen from Eq. 5. Qualitatively, one can imagine that fewer numbers of solvent molecules are escaping per unit surface area of the solution than from the pure solvent because fewer solvent molecules are present per unit surface area of the solution owing to displacement by solute molecules. However, these solute molecules will not affect the condensation of solvent molecules with insufficient kinetic energy present in the vapor phase. The result is a net reduction in escaping tendency of solvent molecules on the surface, causing a lowering of vapor pressure and, consequently, the rate of vaporization. The resulting vapor pressure lowering ($P^o_{solvent} - P_{solution}$) and the relative vapor pressure lowering as a function of mole fractional concentration of solute can be obtained by rearranging Eq. 5 to Eq. 6:

$$\frac{P^o_{solvent} - P_{solution}}{P^o_{solvent}} = \frac{\Delta P}{P^o_{solvent}} = X_{solute} \qquad (6)$$

The left term is the relative vapor pressure lowering, which is solely dependent on the mole fraction concentration of a single solute or the sum of mole fraction of each solute dissolved in the solution. Thus, the relative vapor pressure lowering is a direct measure of the total number of dissolved solute particles, irrespective of their physico-chemical nature. The mole fractions can be converted into molality (m moles of solute per 1000 g of solvent) to result in the following equation for water as the solvent:

$$\frac{\Delta P}{P^o_{solvent}} = X_{solute} \cong \frac{m M_{solvent}}{1000}$$

$$\cong 0.018 \, m \text{ for Aq. solutions} \qquad (7)$$

where m is the concentration of solute expressed in molality, and $M_{solvent}$ is the molecular weight of the solvent in grams. For water, $M = 18$, and because the density of water is close to 1, for dilute aqueous solutions, the molality and molarity (moles/liter) can be used interchangeably, and Eq. 7 can be used to calculate the relative vapor pressure lowering from the molar concentration of the nonelectrolyte solute.

Elevation of the Boiling Point

The boiling point of a liquid is the temperature at which the vapor pressure of the liquid becomes equal to the external pressure acting on the liquid, which is 760 mm Hg at one atmospheric pressure. Therefore, the boiling point of a solution of nonvolatile solute will be higher than that of the pure solvent owing to the solute reducing the vapor

pressure of the solvent above the solution according to Raoult's law. The solution has to be heated to a higher temperature to achieve the same vapor pressure to result in boiling of the solvent. The elevation of the boiling point ($T_{solution} - T^o_b$) is directly proportional to the relative vapor pressure lowering based on the Clausius–Clapeyron equation, resulting in an equation relating it to molality as follows:

$$(T_{solution} - T^o_b) = \delta T_b = \Delta T_b = K \Delta P = K_b m \qquad (8)$$

where in K_b is called the molal elevation constant or the ebullioscopic constant, a characteristic constant for each solvent, and is the boiling point elevation of an ideal 1-molal solution of a nonvolatile solute. K_b can be obtained by measuring the $\delta T_b/m$ of several molal concentrations of solute in solutions and extrapolating the $\delta T_b/m$ versus molality curve to zero solute concentration. The value of K_b for water is 0.515° kg/mole. By measuring the boiling point elevation of a solvent in a solution and knowing the K_b for that solvent, one can calculate the molal concentration of a solute in the solution. From Eq. 8, it is evident that the elevation of boiling point is a colligative property like vapor pressure lowering because it is strictly dependent on the molal concentration of the solute: the number of particles in solute and, thus, independent of the physicochemical nature of the solute.

Freezing-Point Depression

The freezing point of a liquid or the melting point of a solid phase of a pure compound is the temperature at which the solid and liquid phases are in equilibrium at a pressure of 1 atm. The freezing point of a pure compound is described by a unique point in the phase diagram of the compound, and, at that point, the solid and liquid phases are in equilibrium, and the vapor pressure of the liquid phase coincides with the vapor pressure of the pure solid phase. Because in a solution, the vapor pressure of the solvent is lowered relative to the pure solvent, no freezing (or crystallization) takes place at the equilibrium temperature of the liquid and solid phases of the pure solvent; i.e., the freezing point. The phase with the lower vapor pressure is the more stable phase thermodynamically. Therefore, cooling of the solution below the freezing point of the pure solvent results in a greater reduction in vapor pressure of the pure solid phase than the solution phase, and when the vapor pressure of the two phases eventually coincides, freezing (crystallization) of the pure liquid solvent occurs. The dissolved solute reduces the escaping tendency of the solvent molecules to crystallize, and thus the temperature must be reduced to reestablish equilibrium between the solid and liquid phases and hence the depression of freezing point. It must be noted that the dissolved solute only affects the freezing of the liquid phase and does not alter the tendency of the molecules to leave the solid phase, although both processes are occurring in equilibrium at the freezing point. Also, the solvent should form a pure solid; if the solute cocrystallizes with the solvent, the phenomenon is complex and cannot be described as a colligative property. The more concentrated the solution, the greater the freezing-point depression, and using thermodynamic principles, Raoult's law, and Clausius–Clapeyron equation, the freezing-point depression can be related to solute concentration expressed in molality as follows:

$$(T_{solution} - T_f^o) = \delta T_f = \Delta T_f = K\Delta P = K_f m \tag{9}$$

where in K_f is called the molal depression constant or the cryoscopic constant, a characteristic constant for each solvent dependent on the physicochemical nature of the solvent, and is the freezing-point depression of an ideal 1-molal solution of a nonvolatile solute. K_f can be obtained experimentally by measuring the $\delta T_f/m$ of several molal concentrations of solute in solutions and extrapolating the $\delta T_f/m$ versus molality curve to zero solute concentration. The value of K_f for water is 1.86° kg/mole. By measuring the freezing-point depression of a solvent in a solution and knowing the K_f for that solvent, one can calculate the molal concentration of a solute in the solution. Freezing-point depression is a colligative property as seen from Eq. 9, because it is proportional to molal concentration of solute: the number of particles in solution, and not on the physicochemical characteristics of the solute.

Osmotic Pressure

As described in the Introduction, the process of diffusion of a solvent through a semipermeable membrane from a less-concentrated solution into a more-concentrated solution is osmosis. This results in the development of a hydrostatic pressure head on the more-concentrated solution side of the membrane. Alternatively, pressure may be applied to the more-concentrated solution side of the semipermeable membrane to prevent the diffusion of solvent. This applied pressure on the concentrated solution is identical to the hydrostatic pressure head that may develop owing to osmosis. It is known as the osmotic pressure and is directly proportional to the solute concentration in an ideal solution. A semipermeable membrane is one that allows the movement of only solvent molecules, and if the membrane is not semipermeable,

osmosis may not be observed because the solute will diffuse quickly through the membrane to equalize the concentration on two sides of the membrane.

Osmosis tends to equalize the escaping tendencies of the solvent on both sides of the semipermeable membrane. Escaping tendency can be measured in terms of partial vapor pressure of solvent above the solution. Alternatively, one can see that at the beginning, the solution and pure solvents have different thermodynamic activities for the solvent because they have different vapor pressures. For the solution and pure solvent on two sides of the semipermeable membrane to be in equilibrium, they should have identical escaping tendency or identical vapor pressure and, thus identical thermodynamic activity. The equilibrium is therefore established by the generation of the osmotic pressure that compensates for the difference in solvent concentration on the two sides of the membrane, which is responsible for the different vapor pressures, escaping tendencies, and thermodynamic activity. Therefore, osmosis is a process to reach equilibrium state whereby solvent spontaneously flows from the high-free-energy (low-vapor-pressure) side of the membrane to the low-free-energy (high-vapor-pressure) side of the membrane, until the solvent's free energies on both sides of the membrane are equal and identical. Obviously, the solute will not be able to attain equilibrium because it cannot diffuse through the semipermeable membrane. Because osmotic pressure is attributable to the difference in vapor pressure of the solvent above solution, it is also a colligative property as explained below.

Using thermodynamics and considering free energy of the solvent as a function of vapor pressure, the osmotic pressure (π) that develops when a solution is separated from pure solvent by semipermeable membrane can be related to vapor pressures as shown below:

$$\Pi = \frac{RT}{V_{solvent}^M} \ln \frac{P_{solvent}^o}{P_{solution}} \tag{10}$$

where in R is the gas constant, T is temperature, $V_{solvent}^M$ is the partial molar volume, (the volume occupied by 1 mole of solvent), and π is the developed osmotic pressure when a solution with vapor pressure $P_{solution}$ is separated from a solvent with vapor pressure $P_{solvent}^o$ by a semipermeable membrane. Applying Raoult's law and substituting mole fractions for the vapor pressures from Eq. 5 into Eq. 10 results in the following:

$$\Pi = \frac{-RT}{V_{solvent}^M} \ln(1 - X_{solute}) \cong \frac{RT}{V_{solvent}^M} X_{solute} \tag{11}$$

$$\text{since } \ln(1 - X_{solute}) \cong -X_{solute}$$

In a dilute solution, X_{solute} is approximately equal to the molar ratio $n_{solute}/n_{solvent}$, and Eq. 11 becomes:

$$\Pi = \frac{n_{solute}}{n_{solvent}V_{solvent}^M}RT = \frac{n_{solute}}{V_{solution}}RT = mRT \qquad (12)$$

in which the number of moles of solvent multiplied by the partial molal volume is equal to the volume of the solvent in solution. In a dilute solution, the volume of solvent can be approximated to the volume of solution, which results in the above equation relating osmotic pressure to molar or molal concentration of a solute in solution. Eq. 12 is known as Morse's expression and demonstrates how osmotic pressure is a colligative property directly proportional only on the number of particles dissolved in the solvent irrespective of the nature of the solute. Van't Hoff had recognized early on that there is a direct proportionality among osmotic pressure and concentration of solute and temperature, and suggested a relationship that was similar to the equation for an ideal gas as follows:

$$\Pi V_{solution} = n_{solute}RT \qquad (13)$$

Eq. 13 is analogous to the ideal gas equation, and van't Hoff concluded that osmotic pressure of a dilute solution was a pressure that the solute would exert if it behaved like a gas occupying that volume. Eq. 13 can also be expressed as:

$$\Pi = \frac{n_{solute}}{V_{solution}}RT = cRT \qquad (14)$$

which shows that osmotic pressure is directly proportional to the concentration of solute expressed in molarity. This equation is similar to Morse's expression, Eq. 12; however, it has been shown theoretically and experimentally that more accurate results can be obtained when solute concentration is expressed in molality rather than in molarity. Although the resemblance of Eq. 13 to the ideal gas equation is striking, osmotic pressure is a result of differences in the escaping tendencies of the solvent on two sides of the membrane rather than of the behavior of a solute such as a gas.

From Eqs. 12–14, one finds that 1-molar solution of any solute will generate an incredibly high osmotic pressure of approximately 24 atm at room temperature, which has been verified experimentally. Although this estimate is based on the assumption that the solution is dilute and behaving ideally, at high concentrations of solute, the theory overestimates the experimental findings. The discussion above deals primarily with the thermodynamic basis for the generation of osmotic pressure; however, it does not address the issue of how fast the equilibrium is attained or how fast the osmotic pressure will be generated. The rate of generation of osmotic pressure is a kinetic process and depends to a great extent on the characteristics of the semipermeable membrane. Red blood cell membrane or the mucous membrane in the eye are very thin and moist, and water can diffuse very rapidly through the membrane to generate the enormous osmotic pressure. However, the osmotic pressure may develop very slowly across synthetic and semisynthetic polymeric membranes, across which the diffusion is very slow.

COLLIGATIVE PROPERTIES OF ELECTROLYTES AS COMPARED WITH NONELECTROLYTE SOLUTES

The colligative properties, by definition, should be independent of the nature of the solute. Therefore, 0.1-molal solutions of sucrose and NaCl should exhibit similar colligative properties. It was observed by van't Hoff that colligative properties of dilute solutions of nonelectrolytes such as sucrose were expressed satisfactorily by the equations above. However, solutions of strong electrolytes such as salts gave osmotic pressure twice or three times as large as would be expected based on Eq. 14, depending on the electrolyte investigated. To account for this anomaly, van't Hoff proposed the following modification of Eq. 14 as shown below:

$$\Pi = icRT \qquad (15)$$

in which i can be considered to be a factor to account for the deviation of concentrated solutions of electrolytes and also nonelectrolytes from Raoult's law as applied to ideal solutions. After Arrhennius developed the theory of ionization or dissociation of salts into ions, van't Hoff and others recognized that the value of i approached or equaled the number of ions into which the electrolyte or the molecule dissociated as the solution was made more dilute. For example, a dilute 0.1-M solution of NaCl would be twice as active osmotically as a 0.1-M solution of sucrose, and i for NaCl was two. Similarly, 0.1-M solutions of $CaCl_2$ and $MgCl_2$ would generate three times the osmotic pressure of 0.1-M sucrose solution, and i for both is equal to three. Therefore, it was realized that i reflected the number of ions the electrolytes dissociated into and, thus, electrolytes at equimolar concentrations were more effective in generating osmotic pressure based on the number of ions they produced on dissociation. However, it was also observed that at moderate concentrations of electrolytes, osmotic pressures were less than that expected based on complete dissociation. In fact, this led the scientific community to suggest partial dissociation for even strong electrolytes and to use colligative properties as a measure of degree of dissociation. However, we know now that strong electrolytes do dissociate completely even in concentrated solutions from other measurements such as conductivity techniques. The lower-than-expected values of osmotic pressure in moderate concentrations of electrolytes is attributable to the influence of long-range ionic interactions that come into play as the solution gets increasingly concentrated. The basic assumption in Raoult law was that there was no interaction between solute particles and, even if there was any, it should equal that between the solute and the solvent. However, the strong attractive forces between ions of opposite charges do predominate in increasingly concentrated solutions of electrolytes, and their thermodynamic activity is reduced relative to that in an infinitely dilute solution. Also, the effect of ionic strength of a solution has been shown to influence the activity of electrolytes, and thus, it is the interionic forces rather than the partial dissociation that seems to influence the colligative properties of electrolytes being lower than expected based on complete dissociation.

All the colligative properties of all solutes with the modification by the van't Hoff factor i can be expressed as:

$$\Delta P = i P^o_{\text{solvent}} m; \quad \Pi = i RT m;$$
$$\Delta T_f = i K_f m; \quad \Delta T_b = i K_b m \qquad (16)$$

where in i for nonelectrolyte should be 1 and for strong electrolytes equal the number of ions formed on dissociation. For example, i should be 2 for NaCl, 3 for $CaCl_2$, and 4 for $FeCl_3$. However, in reality, i is less than that calculated, based on the number of ions produced in concentrated solutions, but will approach the theoretical number in infinitely dilute ideal solutions. When the i value is calculated, for a number of solutions with increasing concentration of the solute and then extrapolated to zero concentration of the solute, one can obtain the theoretical i value. The van't Hoff factor has also been considered the ratio of any colligative property of a real solution to that of an ideal solution of a nonelectrolyte.

PHYSIOLOGICAL AND CLINICAL SIGNIFICANCE OF TONICITY

Osmotic pressure becomes important from a physiological standpoint because a majority of biological membranes are semipermeable, and body fluids such as blood and tears exhibit significant osmotic pressure owing to a

number of solutes dissolved in them. As noted above in the Introduction, if a small quantity of blood is mixed with a solution containing 0.9% w/v NaCl, the red blood cells remain intact and retain their normal size and shape. The NaCl solution is considered to be isotonic because it maintained the tone of the membrane of the red blood cell. In contrast, if the blood is mixed with the hypertonic 1.8% w/v NaCl solution, cells shrink and become wrinkled or crenated owing to its content being sucked out. It is because the red blood cell content exerts a lower osmotic pressure than does the surrounding hypertonic 1.8% w/v salt solution, and the water inside the cells diffuses through the cell membrane to dilute the surrounding salt solution to equalize the osmotic pressure across the membrane. The exact opposite phenomenon occurs if blood is mixed with hypotonic 0.45% w/v NaCl solution. Water from the surrounding salt solution enters the cells, causing them to swell and finally burst with the liberation of hemoglobin, and the phenomenon is known as hemolysis. The crenation and hemolysis of red blood cells in hypertonic and hypotonic salt solution, respectively, are explained by the movement of water across the cell membrane owing to the osmotic pressure differential. However, it is well-known that the different physiological membranes are different with respect to their permeability characteristics. The red blood cell membrane has been found to be permeable to small polar and semipolar solutes such as alcohol, boric acid, and urea, etc. Thus, the erythrocyte membrane is not truly semipermeable, and although 2% boric acid solution is iso-osmotic with erythrocyte cell contents, it causes hemolysis because boric acid moves freely across the membrane and its solution being hypotonic acts like pure water in its effect on erythrocytes. However, the same 2% boric acid solution is both iso-osmotic and isotonic with eye secretions and causes no irritation when instilled in the eye because the mucous membrane of the eye is a true semipermeable membrane. To resolve the confusion created by different permeability characteristics of biological membranes, the word isotonicity was created. The word isotonic refers to solutions that are iso-osmotic with the cell contents, across a specific membrane, and in addition, maintains the tone of the membrane, i.e., no solvent movement across the membrane. Thus, 2% boric acid solution is iso-osmotic with blood but it behaves like a hypotonic solution with erythrocytes while it is both iso-osmotic and isotonic with respect to the mucous membrane of the eye.

It has been also observed that hypertonic and hypotonic salt solutions tend to irritate sensitive tissue and cause pain when applied to mucous membranes of the eye, ear, and nose, etc., whereas isotonic solution causes no tissue irritation when it comes in contact with the tissue. Obviously, the tonicity of formulations that come in to direct contact with blood, muscle, eye, nose, and delicate tissues is critical. Therefore, the issue of tonicity is important in small- and large-volume injectables, ophthalmic products, and products intended for tissue irrigation. The degree of tissue irritation or hemolysis or crenation observed depends on the degree of deviation from isotonicity, the volume injected, the speed of injection, the concentration of the solutes in the injection, and the nature of the membrane. The parenteral and ophthalmic formulations are therefore adjusted to isotonicity if possible. Hypotonic solutions can be easily adjusted to isotonicity by adding solutes such as dextrose or sodium chloride, commonly used for this purpose. However, at times, the formulation may be hypertonic and may have to be diluted with water to maintain isotonicity. This dilution of the hypertonic solution may be precluded owing to other limitations such as poor aqueous solubility of the drug. In such a case, the hypertonic solution can be administered slowly in small volumes into a large vein such as the subclavian vein in which the formulation will be diluted and distributed rapidly, minimizing chances of crenation of erythrocytes, pain, and tissue irritation on injection. It has also been observed that minor deviations such as 10% from isotonicity may result in no effect or only temporary effects at the site of injection. However, the effects of deviation from isotonicity of large-volume parenterals can be fairly severe and, thus, parenteral nutrient solutions and infusions of large volume need to be adjusted to isotonicity. Large-volume infusion of hypotonic solutions has been observed to cause effects ranging from hemolysis to water-retention problems such as convulsions and pulmonary edema. This was exemplified by the recent report of 10 episodes of hemolysis, with two patients exhibiting significant hemolysis and renal insufficiency resulting in one death. These severe episodes of hemolysis occurred because of the large volume infusion of 25% human albumin diluted with sterile water instead of with isotonic sodium chloride for therapeutic plasma exchange (1). In contrast, large-volume infusion of hypertonic solutions can result in severe conditions such as intracellular dehydration, osmotic diuresis, hyperglycemia, glycosuria, dehydration from loss of water, and coma. Also, hypertonic solution infusion should be terminated gradually to avoid sudden changes in osmotic pressure. In summary, any formulation that comes in to contact with sensitive tissues of the human body needs to be adjusted to isotonicity to minimize any adverse effects. To be able to adjust the formulation to isotonicity, a method to measure the tonicity and/or the osmotic pressure of the formulations has to be used. The methods to measure tonicity or osmotic pressure of solutions are reviewed briefly as below.

MEASUREMENT OF TONICITY OF SOLUTIONS

The most direct method for measurement of tonicity obviously would be to observe changes in erythrocytes on mixing solution with blood. If hemolysis or crenation or a marked change in the appearance of erythrocytes occurs, the solution is not isotonic. If the cells retain their normal size and shape, the solution is isotonic. Grosicki and Husa used this method early on; however, one has to be mindful of the fact that solutions may be iso-osmotic with erythrocyte contents, yet may cause hemolysis because solutes such as boric acid are permeable through erythrocyte membrane and, thus, solution is not isotonic (2). Therefore, Grosicki and Husa recommended that the word isotonic should be used with reference to solutions having equal osmotic pressures with respect to a particular membrane (2). Because hemolysis due to hypotonic solution results in release of oxyhemoglobin directly proportional to the number of cells hemolyzed, a quantitative method has been developed to calculate osmotic pressure and the van't Hoff i factor noted above. A limitation of observing changes in erythrocytes as a measure of tonicity is the fact that the specific chemical interaction of the solute with the cell, pH of the solution, presence of solvents, lipid solubility of the solute, and denaturant activity of solute may have influences on the cell membrane and, thus, osmotic pressure differences alone are not responsible for hemolysis. Furthermore, it was shown recently that hemolysis is related to the contact time in addition to hypotonicity of the formulation (3). To overcome this limitation, some investigators have used measurements of erythrocyte cell volumes as a function of tonicity of solution, which influence solvent (water) uptake or loss from erythrocytes. This method is more sensitive, objective, and reliable than observation of hemolysis. Recently, a method using fluorescence anisotropy for fluidity of erythrocyte membranes demonstrated differences between hypotonic and isotonic solutions (4). However, the method is involving, and more data need to be obtained to correlate tonicity with fluidity of the membrane to be reliable.

An alternative approach is based on the theoretical foundation described earlier for the colligative properties. If the solution is isotonic with blood, its osmotic pressure, vapor pressure, boiling-point elevation, and freezing-point depression should also be identical to those of blood. Thus, to measure isotonicity, one has to measure the osmotic pressure of the solution and compare it with the known value for blood. However, the accurate measurement of osmotic pressure is difficult and cumbersome. If a solution is separated from blood by a true semipermeable membrane, the resulting pressure due to solvent flow (the head) is accurately measurable, but the solvent flow dilutes the solution, thus not allowing one to know the concentration of the dissolved solute. An alternative is to apply pressure to the solution side of the membrane to prevent osmotic solvent flow. In 1877, Pfeffer used this method to measure osmotic pressure of sugar solutions. With the advances in the technology, sensitive pressure transducers, and synthetic polymer membranes, this method can be improved. However, results of the search for a true semipermeable membrane are still elusive, and this method is still cumbersome and inconvenient. The measurement of osmotic pressure using this method has been applied successfully to colloidal solution of proteins to measure their molecular weight because they are of relatively large molecular weight and are impermeable across number of membranes. Numerous instruments, known as osmometers, are commercially available to measure osmotic pressure (5,6). Only the Knauer membrane osmometer and colloid osmometer are true osmometers using a semipermeable membrane (5). Vapor pressure osmometers such as the Wescor osmometer, using the principle of vapor pressure lowering should not be called osmometers. These types of instruments measure the vapor pressure using the isopiestic method, or the thermoelectric method, or the measurement of the dew point of unknown solution in comparison with a standard, and then calculate osmotic pressure and osmolality using the theory of colligative properties. These instruments require a few microliters, and the method is fairly precise, simple, and totally automated. The presence of a volatile solvent such as ethanol will create problem with this method because the inherent assumption is that only water is present in the vapor phase. This can be a serious limitation because many parenteral and, ophthalmic formulations contain organic solvents for the purposes of drug solubility and, sometimes of stability. Commercial osmometers of this type have been found to measure osmolalities in the range of 100–3000 mmol/kg reliably.

Boiling-point elevation can also be used to measure osmotic pressure and tonicity of a solution using just a reflux condenser and a thermometer. The commercially available instrument is the Cottrell boiling-point apparatus. However, this method is affected by the ambient barometric pressure and the presence of volatile solvents in the solution.

Osmometers based on the freezing-point depression are the most commonly and widely used instruments for measurements of tonicity because of the simplicity, reliability, and ease of use. Freezing-point depression of solutions of a number of drugs at various concentrations has already been determined, and thus, an extensive database is available for adjustment of tonicity of solutions of these drugs, as addressed below. The freezing-point depression of a solution can be simply measured using a salt–ice bath, Dewars flask, and Beckmann's thermometer. Numerous commercial instruments requiring small quantities of solution such as Osmette from Precision Systems that use the principle of Beckmann's freezing-point method are now available. One of the problems with this method is the disengagement of ice and the need for determination of the actual equilibrium freezing point. The latter limitation can be overcome by use of the equilibrium method, in which solid solvent (ice) is placed in contact with solution (aq.) and the freezing point measured and compared with that of the pure solvent (water) in contact with the solid solvent (ice). Also, one has to consider the presence of other solvents in influencing the freezing-point depression. The freezing-point depression method is precise to the extent that the differences in freezing points of two systems within $\pm 0.0002°C$ can be measured. Freezing-point osmometry can be used for all samples with osmolalities less than 550 mmol/kg, including those that contain volatile solutes (6). Once the freezing point of the solution is known, inert solute such as sodium chloride is added to match the freezing point of solution with that of blood and lacrimal fluids. After considerable debate and experimentation, it is now well-established that $-0.52°C$ is the freezing point of blood and lacrimal fluids, following the work of Lund et al. (7). This is also the freezing point of 0.9% sodium chloride solution, which is therefore considered to be isotonic with both blood and lacrimal secretions. Therefore, to determine the tonicity of a solution, one has to measure its freezing-point depression and compare it with that of blood ($-0.52°C$). The freezing-point depressions of a number of drugs are listed in Table 1. A more comprehensive list of the freezing-point depressions of various concentrations of drugs can be found in The Merck Index, Remington's Pharmaceutical Sciences, and other literature sources listed in the Bibliography. An important consideration when using this method is that although all the solutes present in solution contribute to its freezing-point depression, those that permeate the biological membrane will not maintain the tone, for example, boric acid. In addition, association of solute molecules by processes such as complexation and micellar association, which are temperature-dependent, may have to be considered. The viscosity and presence of suspended particles can also affect the freezing point by altering the crystallization of the solvent. Nevertheless, freezing-point

Table 1 Freezing point depressions ($T_f^{1\%}$), L_{iso} values and sodium chloride equivalents (E) for drugs and excipients for adjusting their solutions to isotonicity[a]

Substance	MW[b]	$T_f^{1\%c}$	L_{iso}[d]	E[e]	V[f]
Alcohol, dehydrated	46.07	0.41	1.9	0.70	23.3
Aminophylline	456.46	0.10	4.6	0.17	5.7
Amphetamine sulfate	368.49	0.13	4.8	0.22	7.3
Antipyrine	188.22	0.10	1.9	0.17	5.7
Antazoline (Antistine) hydrochloride	301.81	0.11	3.2	0.18	6.0
Apomorphine hydrochloride	312.79	0.08	2.6	0.14	4.7
Ascorbic acid	176.12	0.11	1.9	0.18	6.0
Atropine sulfate	694.82	0.07	5.3	0.13	4.3
Aureomycin hydrochloride	544	0.06	3.5	0.11	3.7
Barbital sodium	206.18	0.29	3.5	0.29	10.0
Benadryl hydrochloride (diphenhydramine hydrochloride)	291.81	0.34	3.4	0.20	6.6
Boric Acid	61.84	0.29	1.8	0.50	16.7
Butacaine sulfate	710.95	0.12	8.4	0.20	6.7
Caffeine	194.19	0.05	0.9	0.08	2.7
Calcium gluconate	448.39	0.09	4.2	0.16	5.3
Calcium lactate	308.30	0.14	4.2	0.23	7.7
Camphor	152.23	0.12	1.8	0.20	6.7
Chloramphenicol (chloromycetin)	323.14	0.06	1.9	0.10	3.3
Chlorobutanol (chloretone)	177.47	0.14	2.5	0.24	8.0
Cocaine hydrochloride	339.81	0.09	3.2	0.16	5.3
Dextrose−H_2O	198.17	0.09	1.9	0.16	5.3
Dibucaine hydrochloride	379.92	0.08	2.9	0.13	4.3
Ephedrine hydrochloride	201.69	0.18	3.6	0.30	10.0
Ephedrine sulfate	428.54	0.14	5.8	0.23	7.7
Epinephrine bitartrate	333.29	0.11	3.5	0.18	6.0
Epinephrine hydrochloride	219.66	0.17	3.7	0.29	9.7
Fluorescein sodium	376	0.18	6.9	0.31	10.3
Glycerin	92.09	0.20	1.8	0.34	11.3
Homatropine hydrobromide	356.26	0.10	3.6	0.17	5.7
Lactose	360.31	0.04	1.7	0.07	2.3
Magnesium sulfate · $7H_2O$	246.50	0.10	2.5	0.17	5.7
Menthol	156.26	0.12	1.8	0.20	6.7
Meperidine hydrochloride	283.79	0.12	3.7	0.22	7.3
Methamphetamine hydrochloride	185.69	0.22	4.0	0.37	12.3
Morphine hydrochloride	375.84	0.09	3.3	0.15	5.0
Morphine sulfate	758.82	0.08	6.2	0.14	4.8
Naphazoline hydrochloride	246.73	0.16	3.3	0.27	7.7
Neomycin sulfate	−	0.06	−	0.11	3.7
Neostigmine bromide	303.20	0.11	3.2	0.22	6.0
Nicotinamide	122.13	0.15	1.9	0.26	8.7
Penicillin G potassium	372.47	0.11	3.9	0.18	6.0
Penicillin G Procaine	588.71	0.06	3.5	0.10	3.3
Penicillin G sodium	356.38	0.11	3.8	0.18	6.0
Phenacaine hydrochloride	352.85	0.11	3.3	0.20	5.3
Phenobarbital sodium	254.22	0.14	3.6	0.24	8.0
Phenol	94.11	0.20	1.9	0.35	11.7
Phenylephrine hydrochloride	203.67	0.18	3.5	0.32	9.7
Physostigmine salicylate	413.46	0.09	3.9	0.16	5.3
Physostigmine sulfate	648.45	0.08	5.0	0.13	4.3
Pilocarpine nitrate	271.27	0.14	3.7	0.23	7.7

(*Continued*)

Table 1 Freezing point depressions ($T_f^{1\%}$), L_{iso} values and sodium chloride equivalents (E) for drugs and excipients for adjusting their solutions to isotonicity[a] (*Continued*)

Substance	MW^b	$T_f^{1\%c}$	L_{iso}^d	E^e	V^f
Potassium acid phosphate (KH$_2$PO$_4$)	136.13	0.25	3.4	0.43	14.2
Potassium chloride	74.55	0.45	3.3	0.76	25.3
Potassium iodide	166.02	0.20	3.3	0.34	11.3
Procaine hydrochloride	272.77	0.12	3.4	0.21	7.0
Quinine hydrochloride	396.91	0.08	3.3	0.14	4.7
Scopolamine hydrobromide	438.32	0.07	3.1	0.12	4.0
Silver nitrate	169.89	0.19	3.3	0.33	11.0
Sodium acid phosphate (NaH$_2$PO$_4$.H$_2$O)	138.00	0.24	3.2	0.40	13.3
Sodium benzoate	144.11	0.24	3.4	0.40	13.3
Sodium bicarbonate	84.00	0.38	3.2	0.65	21.7
Sodium bisulfite	104.07	0.36	3.7	0.61	20.3
Sodium borate · 10H$_2$0	381.43	0.25	9.4	0.42	14.0
Sodium chloride	58.45	0.58	3.4	1.00	33.3
Sodium iodide	149.92	0.23	3.4	0.39	13.0
Sodium nitrate	85.01	0.39	3.4	0.68	22.7
Sodium phosphate, anhydrous	141.98	0.31	4.4	0.53	17.7
Sodium phosphate · 2H$_2$0	178.05	0.25	4.4	0.42	14.0
Sodium phosphate · 7H$_2$O	268.08	0.17	4.6	0.29	9.7
Sodium phosphate · 12H$_2$O	358.21	0.13	4.6	0.22	7.3
Sodium propionate	96.07	0.36	3.4	0.61	20.3
Sodium sulfite, exsiccated	126.06	0.38	4.8	0.65	21.7
Streptomycin sulfate	1457.44	0.04	6.0	0.07	2.3
Strong silver protein	—	0.0	—	0.08	2.7
Sucrose	342.30	0.05	1.6	0.08	2.7
Sulfacetamide sodium	254.25	0.14	3.4	0.23	7.7
Sulfadiazine sodium	272.27	0.14	3.8	0.24	8.0
Sulfamerazine sodium	286.29	0.14	3.9	0.23	7.7
Sulfanilamide	172.21	0.13	2.2	0.22	7.3
Sulfathiazole sodium	304.33	0.13	3.9	0.22	7.3
Tetracaine hydrochloride	300.82	0.11	3.2	0.18	6.0
Tetracycline hydrochloride	480.92	0.08	4.0	0.14	4.7
Tripelennamine hydrochloride	291.83	0.17	3.8	0.30	7.3
Urea	60.06	0.35	2.1	0.59	19.7
Zinc chloride	139.29	0.37	5.1	0.62	20.3
Zinc Sulfate·7H$_2$O	287.56	0.09	2.5	0.15	5.0

[a]Values vary somewhat with concentration, and those in the table are for 1 to 3% solutions of the drugs in most instances. A more comprehensive table of E and T_f, values is found in Ref. 8.

[b]MW is the molecular weight of the drug.

[c]$T_f^{1\%}$ is the freezing point depression of a 1% solution of the drug.

[d]L_{iso} is the molar freezing point depression of the drug at a concentration approximately isotonic with blood and lacrimal fluid.

[e]E is the sodium chloride equivalent of the drug.

[f]V is the volume in milliliters of isotonic solution that can be prepared by adding water to 0.3 g of the drug (the weight of drug in one fluid ounce of a 1% solution).

(Adapted with modifications from Ref. 9.)

depression has become popular because of its simplicity, reliability, and availability of commercial instruments. The methods of osmometry, the technology, and the limitations inherent in each method have been reviewed recently (5, 6) and should be consulted for more details.

Based on the theory of colligative properties and the principles of osmometry, it is understood that osmometer will read osmolalities and not osmolarities because colligative properties are directly proportional to the total solute concentration expressed in molality (see Eqs. 1–16).

The relationship between osmolality and osmolarity and its significance can be found in the Remington's Pharmaceutical Sciences and in a review article by Deardorff (10). However, it is more convenient to use osmolarity because it is based on weight/volume rather than on weight/weight as in osmolality. The U.S. Pharmacopeia also recommends that the labeling of parenteral and ophthalmic formulation should list osmolarity while the experimentally determined quantity is osmolality. Methods to convert osmolality to osmolarity using determinations of solution density and solute content (11, 12) or using partial molal volume of solute and solvent have been described (13, 14).

THEORETICAL METHOD TO CALCULATE TONICITY USING L_{ISO} VALUE

In the discussion above of colligative properties of electrolytes, the equations were modified by introduction of the van't Hoff i factor as shown in Eq. 16. Because the freezing-point depressions of strong and weak electrolytes are always greater than those calculated from Eq. 9, because of different degrees of ionization and interionic interaction, a new factor, $L = iK_f$, is introduced. The L value obtained from freezing-point depression of a solution of a particular type of electrolyte at a molar concentration (c) that is isotonic with blood is defined as L_{iso} ($L_{iso} = 0.52°/c$). For example, the L_{iso} value for an isotonic sodium chloride solution (0.9%w/v) is 3.4, and its freezing-point depression is 0.52°C. Because the colligative properties are independent of the chemical nature of the electrolyte and the interionic interactions in dilute solutions are similar, all electrolytes of the same type will have identical L_{iso} values. Therefore, all nonelectrolytes have $L_{iso} = 1.9$, whereas uni-univalent electrolyte's $L_{iso} = 3.4$ and triunivalent electrolyte's $L_{iso} = 6.0$. Thus, if the ionic nature of the solute and its molecular weight are known, using the appropriate L_{iso} value, freezing-point depression can be calculated for a solution of a given concentration. The average L_{iso} values for all types of solutes are available in the literature (9). This method is simple and does not require experimentation, but it is only approximate, with potential for some error. Also, one has to know the ionic nature of the solute, which can be difficult to determine for a new drug compound with a complex structure.

METHODS OF ADJUSTING TONICITY

From the theoretical background presented above, one can easily devise his or her own methods to adjust tonicity of solutions using the principles of colligative properties. However, in the practice of pharmacy, a number of simple methods to adjust tonicity of formulation in a prescription order on an extemporaneous basis were developed to help the pharmacist. The methods of adjusting tonicity could be classified into two types. In class I methods, some inert substance such as sodium chloride or dextrose is added to the solution to lower its freezing point to match that of blood ($-0.52°C$) i.e., made isotonic by the addition of inert excipient. In class II methods, a calculated quantity of water is added to the total solute content (drug) of the prescription to make it isotonic, which is then diluted with sufficient isotonic diluting solution to bring it to the final volume. These methods are explained below, followed by a simple example illustrating the method. However, the assumptions inherent in all the methods need to be considered carefully. The first assumption is that colligative properties are additive for mixture of solutes and that they are related linearly to their concentration expressed in molarity, molality, or in percentages. This assumption is true in dilute solutions of nonelectrolytes and electrolytes. However, when dealing with concentrated solutions, this assumption may not be valid. In cases of chemical interaction, association, complexation, or micellar interaction among solutes in solution, the colligative properties of solutes may not be additive. The second assumption is that they consider all solutes present in solution to be contributing to its tonicity. However, it is known from the discussion above that all biological membranes are not truly semipermeable, and thus, some solutes will not contribute to the tonicity of the solution across that membrane, for example, boric acid across erythrocytes membrane. Nevertheless, the errors introduced are small, and slight deviations from isotonicity on either side do not result in significant adverse effects. In the literature, one may also find methods known as the L value method or the L_{iso} method, which are identical to the theoretical method described above for solutes, for which one can calculate the freezing-point depression based on molecular weight and ionic nature. By knowing the freezing-point depression, any of the class I or class II methods can then be used to adjust their solution to isotonicity.

Class I Methods

Freezing-point depression method (cryoscopic method)

The freezing-point depression of a number of drugs and excipients, either experimentally determined by the method described above or calculated theoretically using the L_{iso} method, is available in the literature (8, 9, 15). Table 1 (adapted from Ref. 9.) lists the freezing point depression of 1% solution of various drugs. Basically, from the percentage of drug present in solution, the freezing point of the solution is calculated. This number is then subtracted from the freezing point of blood ($-0.52°C$) to obtain the freezing-point depression to be achieved by the addition of sodium chloride. Knowing that 0.9% sodium chloride is isotonic and freezes at $-0.52°C$, the amount of sodium chloride to be added is calculated as shown in the example below.

Example 1: Calculate the amount of sodium chloride needed to prepare 100 ml of 2% isotonic physostigmine salicylate solution.

Freezing-point depression of 2% physostigmine salicylate $= 2 \times 0.09°C = 0.18°C$ (Table 1). Therefore, the freezing-point depression to be achieved by adding sodium chloride $= 0.52° - 0.18°C = 0.34°C$. Sodium chloride (0.9%) produces a freezing-point depression of $-0.52°C$; therefore, the percentage of sodium chloride needed $= (0.34°C/0.52°C) \times 0.9\% = 0.59\% = 0.59$ g/100 ml.

Sodium chloride equivalent (E) method

The sodium chloride equivalent (E) is the amount of sodium chloride equivalent to 1 g of the drug in exerting the same osmotic effect. The E value for a new drug can be calculated from its L_{iso} value or from the freezing-point depression as shown below.

The freezing-point depression of a 1 g/L-solution of a new drug can be expressed as:

$$\Delta T_f = L_{iso} \frac{1\,g}{MW} \tag{17}$$

By definition, E gram of sodium chloride ($MW = 58.45$ and $L_{iso} = 3.4$) in 1 L will have similar freezing-point depression as shown below:

$$\Delta T_f = 3.4 \frac{E\,g}{58.45} \tag{18}$$

Therefore, equating Eqs. 17 and 18, results in the following equation for E:

$$E = 17 \frac{L_{iso}}{MW} \tag{19}$$

Wells developed a nomogram based on the above equation to readily calculate E values from the MW and L_{iso} value of the drug (16). Thus, the E value for physostigmine salicylate ($MW = 413.46$) calculated using $L_{iso} = 3.4$ for a uni-univalent electrolyte is equal to 0.14, which is close to 0.16 (E value) in Table 1. This small deviation is attributable to the difference between the experimentally determined L_{iso} (3.9) of physostigmine salicylate and the theoretical value of 3.4 for a uni-univalent

electrolyte. By knowing the E value, the solution can be adjusted to isotonicity as shown below.

Example 2: Calculate the amount of sodium chloride needed to prepare 100 ml of 2% isotonic physostigmine salicylate solution.

Physostigmine salicylate (2 g/100 ml) is equivalent to 2×0.16 (E) $= 0.32$ g/100 ml of sodium chloride. Therefore, 0.58 g (0.9–0.32 g) of sodium chloride has to be added to 100 ml of this solution to make it isotonic.

Note that the answers given by the two methods are not identical, but very close.

Class II Methods

The class II methods involve the calculation of a quantity of water needed to make an isotonic solution for a given amount of drug, followed by dilution with an isotonic solution to make up the volume. These methods were developed to enable pharmacists to prepare parenteral and ophthalmic formulations with simplicity and ease.

The White-Vincent method

In this method, the weight of the drug (w) is first multiplied by its sodium chloride (E) to obtain the quantity of sodium chloride osmotically equivalent to weight per gram of drug (17). Because 0.9 g of sodium chloride dissolved in 100 ml results in an isotonic solution, the volume of isotonic solution that can be prepared from weight per gram of drug is given by the following equation:

$$V = wE \frac{100}{0.9} = 111.1\,w\,E \tag{20}$$

Thus, dissolving weight per gram of drug in V ml of water will result in an isotonic solution that can be further diluted with isotonic solutions such as 0.9% sodium chloride or isotonic dextrose solution to make up the volume. The method can be illustrated by the following example.

Example 3: Prepare 100 ml of 2% physostigmine salicylate solution isotonic with blood.

Using Eq. 20 and E of physostigmine salicylate $= 0.16$ from Table 1, the volume of water needed to prepare isotonic solution, $V = 2$ g $\times 0.16 \times 111.1$ ml/g $= 35.55$ ml. This solution can be diluted with 64.45 ml of any isotonic diluting solution to obtain 100 ml of 2% isotonic physostigmine salicylate solution. To verify the results, if we assume that we dilute the above solution with 64.45 ml of isotonic sodium chloride solution, the equivalent amount of sodium chloride added is 0.58 g, which matches with results obtained using the class I methods.

The Sprowls method

In the early days of pharmacy practice, many prescriptions were written to prepare one fluid ounce of a 1% drug solution, thus, the amount of drug ($w = 0.3$ g) and the final volume were fixed (one fluid ounce or 30 ml). Sprowls, recognizing this fact, suggested a modification of the White–Vincent method to further simplify the calculations for the practicing pharmacist (18). In this method, the amount of drug is fixed at 0.3 g (30 ml of 1% solution), and the volume of water required to prepare the isotonic solution is calculated using Eq. 20 and listed in a table such as column 4 in Table 1 for all drugs that are commonly used in parenteral and ophthalmic formulations and for which sodium chloride equivalents are known. The pharmacist then makes up the volume of the preparation to 30 ml with an isotonic diluting solution to fill the prescription. For example, if one fluid ounce of 1% physostigmine salicylate solution is to be prepared, from Table 1, column 4, we recognize that 5.3 ml of water is required for 0.3 g of physostigmine salicylate to prepare an isotonic solution. After the preparation of this 5.3-ml solution, it can be diluted with any isotonic diluting solution to make up the volume to one fluid ounce. If one needed to prepare 100 ml of a 1% solution, the volume of water (V) should be multiplied by 3.33 to obtain the amount of water necessary to make it isotonic.

FUTURE DIRECTIONS

The theory of colligative properties is well-understood and successfully applied to parenteral formulations for making them isotonic and, thus, safe and acceptable. The techniques of osmometry have been refined, and now instruments that can estimate freezing-point depression, vapor pressure, or osmotic pressure from microliter quantities of samples in a few minutes are commercially available. At the same time, very few pharmacists are required to compound prescriptions requiring the knowledge of the various methods of adjustments of tonicity. Because of ever-increasing complexities in the structure of new drug entities, there is an increasing problem of their inadequate aqueous solubility, exemplified by drugs such as Cyclosporine and Taxol. A number of organic solvents and new classes of surfactants are being developed and used to aid in solubilization and, thus, in the formulation of these drugs for parenteral administration. The issue of tonicity needs to be addressed from this perspective because organic solvents and the surfactants behave differently in solution than do the traditional solutes whose characteristics in solution are well-understood. Also, dispersed systems such as nanocapsules, liposomes, and microemulsions are being developed as parenteral formulations. The colligative properties of these systems need to be investigated too. There is an increasing concern regarding tissue irritation and muscle injury at the site of injection resulting from formulations. With the advent of biotechnology, more peptide and protein drugs are in clinical trials than before, and, also, gene therapy is being considered for few diseases. The parenteral formulations of these newer drugs are more complex to maintain the integrity of their higher-order structure. Therefore, the issue of tonicity needs to be revisited with a newer approach and from a different perspective.

REFERENCES

1. Morbidity & Mortality Weekly Report **1999**, *48* (8), 157–159.
2. Grosicki, T.S.; Husa, W.J. J. Am. Pharm. Assoc., Sci. Ed. **1954**, *43*, 632–636.
3. Krzyzaniak, J.E.; Raymond, D.M.; Yalkowsky, S.H. PDA J. Pharm. Sci. Tech. **1996**, *50* (4), 223–226.
4. Au, K.S. Biochem. Mol. Bio. Int. **1994**, *32*, 49–53.
5. Bevan, D.R. Anesthesia **1978**, *33*, 794–800.
6. Sweeney, T.E.; Beuchat, C.A. Am. J. Physio. **1993**, *264*, R469–480.
7. Lund, C.G.; Nielsen, P.; Pedersen-Bjergaard, K. *The Preparation of Solutions Iso-Osmotic with Blood, Tears, and Tissue*; Danish Pharmacopeia Commission: Einar Munksgaard Copenhagen, 1947; 2.
8. Budavari, S., O'Neil, M.J., Smith, A., Heckelman, P.E., Kinneary, J.F., Eds. *The Merck Index: An Encyclopedia of Chemicals, Drugs and Biologicals*, 12th Ed.; Merck & Co. Inc.: Whitehouse Station NJ, 1996; 47–57, MISC.
9. Martin, A.; Bustamante, P.; Chun, A.H.C. Physical Pharmacy: Physical Chemical Principles. *The Pharmaceutical Sciences*; Lea & Febiger: Philadelphia, 1993; 101, 142, 169–189.
10. Deardorff, D.L. Am. J. Hosp. Pharm. **1980**, *37*, 504–509.
11. Murty, S.R.; Kapoor, J.N.; DeLuca, P.P. Am. J. Hosp. Pharm. **1976**, *33*, 546–551.
12. Gatlin, L.; Kulkarni, P.; Hussain, A.; DeLuca, P.P. Am. J. Hosp. Pharm. **1979**, *36*, 1357–1361.
13. Streng, W.H.; Huber, H.E.; Carstensen, J.T. J. Pharm. Sci. **1978**, *67*, 384–386.
14. Huber, H.E.; Streng, W.H.; Tan, H.G.H. J. Pharm. Sci. **1979**, *68*, 1028–1032.
15. Siegel, F.P. Tonicity, Osmoticity, Osmolality and Osmolarity. *Remington's Pharmaceutical Sciences*; Gennaro, A.R., Chase, G.D., Marderosian, A.D., Harvey, S.C., Hussar, D.A., Medwick, T., Rippie, E.G., Schwartz, J.B., Zink, G.L., Eds.; Mack Printing Co.: Easton Pennsylvania, 1990; 1481–1498.
16. Wells, J.M. J. Am. Pharm. Assoc. Prac. Ed. **1944**, *5*, 99–106.
17. White, A.I.; Vincent, H.C. J. Am. Pharm. Assoc. Prac. Ed. **1947**, *8*, 406–411.
18. Sprowls, J.B. J. Am. Pharm. Assoc., Prac. Ed. **1949**, *10*, 348–352.

BIBLIOGRAPHY

Flynn, G.L. J. Parenteral Drug Assoc. **1979**, *33*, 292–314.
Hadzija, B.W. Am. J. Pharm. Ed. **1995**, *59*, 191–195.

TRANSDERMAL DELIVERY: SONOPHORESIS

Samir S. Mitragotri
University of California, Santa Barbara, California

Hua Tang
Daniel Blankschtein
Robert Langer
Massachusetts Institute of Technology, Cambridge, Massachusetts

TRANSDERMAL DRUG DELIVERY

Systemic as well as topical delivery of drugs via the transdermal route is limited by the low skin permeability which is attributed to the stratum corneum (SC), the outermost layer of the skin (1). The SC consists of disk-like dead cells (keratinocytes) containing keratin fibers and water, surrounded by densely-packed lipid bilayers. The highly-ordered structure of the lipid bilayers confers a highly impermeable character to the SC. A variety of approaches have been suggested to enhance transdermal drug transport. These include: 1) use of chemicals to either modify the skin structure or to increase the drug concentration in the transdermal patch (2, 3); 2) applications of electric fields to create transient transport pathways [electroporation] (4, 5) or to increase the mobility of charged drugs through the skin [iontophoresis] (6); and 3) application of ultrasound [sonophoresis] (7–56).

Sonophoresis was shown to enhance transdermal drug transport about half a century ago by Fellinger et al. (16) who showed that application of ultrasound increases transport of hydrocortisone across the skin. Following this study, attempts were made to enhance transdermal transport of more than 15 drugs including steroidal anti-inflammatory drugs such as hydrocortisone, dexamethasone; non-steroidal anti-inflammatory drugs such as salicylates and ibuprofen; anesthetic agents such as lidocaine; and proteins such as insulin. This chapter provides a review of these studies with emphasis on associated techniques, mechanistic studies, and safety.

GENERATION AND APPLICATION OF ULTRASOUND FOR SONOPHORESIS

Generation of Ultrasound

Ultrasound is a sound wave possessing frequencies above 20 kHz (57, 58). These waves are characterized by two main parameters: frequency and amplitude. Amplitude of ultrasound waves can be represented in terms of peak wave pressure (in Pascals) or in terms of intensity (in the units of W/cm^2). Ultrasound can be applied either continuously or in a pulsed manner. In the latter case, an additional parameter, duty cycle, is required to characterize ultrasound application. Duty cycle is the fraction of time for which ultrasound is ON.

Ultrasound is generated using a device referred to as a sonicator. It consists of an electrical signal generator which generates an electrical AC signal at the desired frequency and amplitude. This signal is applied across a piezo-electric crystal (transducer) to generate ultrasound. The thickness of the piezo-electric crystal is selected so that it resonates at the operating frequency. Sonicators operating at various frequencies in the range of 20 kHz to 3 MHz are available commercially and can be used for sonophoresis.

If a sonicator operating at the desired frequency is not available commercially, it is possible to assemble one using commercially available signal generators, amplifiers, and transducers. Such sonicators operating at frequencies of 10 MHz and 16 MHz have been assembled by Bommannan et al. (11). (For a discussion of the relevant methods for making a custom sonicator, see Ref. 11.)

For sonophoretic delivery, the desired drug is dissolved in a solvent and applied on the skin. Ultrasound is applied by contacting the transducer with the skin (see Fig. 1A–C) through a coupling medium to ensure a proper contact between the transducer and the skin. This medium can be the same as the solvent used to dissolve the drug or it can be a commercially available ultrasound coupling gel (for example, Aquasonic, Polar, NJ).

Transmission of Ultrasound from the Transducer to the Skin

Transmission through the medium

Ultrasound requires a coupling medium for transmission from the transducer to the desired tissue. The coupling

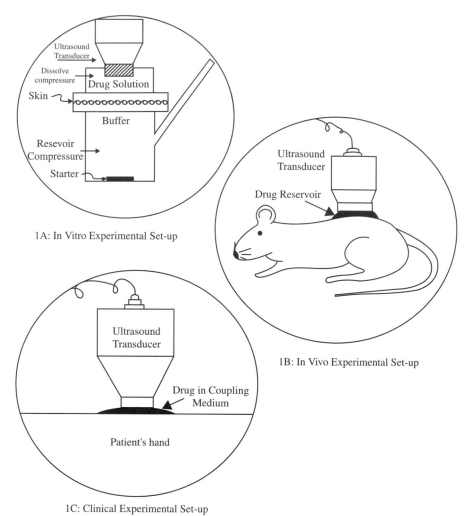

1A: In Vitro Experimental Set-up

1B: In Vivo Experimental Set-up

1C: Clinical Experimental Set-up

Fig. 1 Experimental set-up for sonophoresis delivery.

medium should result in proper transmission of ultrasound from the transducer to the skin. The transmittive properties of a medium are indicated by its acoustic impedance (Z). A coupling medium is appropriate for sonophoresis if its acoustic impedance (Z) is comparable to that of skin (1.6×10^6 kg/m^2/s). Z-values for various materials can be found in (57, 58). For example, water has a Z-value of 1×10^6 kg/m^2/s and is a reasonable coupling agent. Z-values for several media are listed in Table 1.

Absorption of ultrasound

Every medium absorbs ultrasound to a certain extent. The ability of a medium to absorb ultrasound is indicated by the absorption coefficient (α). The extent of absorption is given by the following equation.

$$f(\tau) = 1 - \exp(-\alpha\tau)$$

where $f(\tau)$ is the fraction of ultrasound intensity absorbed as the ultrasound beam propagates in a medium with absorption coefficient α and thickness τ. An estimation of α-values for various materials at various ultrasound frequencies may be found in Refs. (57, 58). In the case of water, the α-value is 0.0006 at an ultrasound frequency of 1 MHz, suggesting that a 1 cm thick column of water absorbs less than 0.1% of ultrasound (1 MHz) intensity, i.e, water is a reasonable coupling medium. Absorption coefficients for several media are listed in Table 1.

Ultrasound reflection

Ultrasound is reflected at the boundary of two media possessing different acoustic impedances. 99.99% of ultrasound is reflected at the air-water boundary when an ultrasound beam is incident upon it from either side. Hence occurrence of air bubbles should be minimized in

Table 1 Acoustic impedances and absorption coefficients of materials

Material	Acoustic impedance, Z (kg/m^2/s)	Absorption coefficient (α) at 1 MHz (cm^{-1})
Water	1.5×10^6	0.0006
Blood	1.6×10^6	0.028
Bone	6.3×10^6	3.22
Skin	1.6×10^6	0.62
Fatty tissue	1.54×10^6	0.14
Muscle	1.6×10^6	0.76
Air	0.0004×10^6	2.76

(From Hoogland, R., *Ultrasound Therapy*; Ernaf Nonius: Delft, Holland, 1986.)

the coupling medium in order to avoid ultrasound reflection. The reflection coefficient for various interfaces may be estimated from the acoustic impedances of two media forming the interface using equations described in (57, 58).

Selection of Ultrasound Parameters

Proper selection of ultrasound parameters is required to ensure safe and efficacious sonophoresis. Ultrasound parameters such as frequency, intensity, duty cycle, and distance of transducer from the skin influence the efficiency of sonophoresis. Below we present a general discussion of the role played by various ultrasound parameters in sonophoresis. Note that the objective of this discussion is not to point out the exact values of ultrasound parameters to be selected, but rather to present information regarding the dependence of sonophoretic enhancement on each parameter.

Ultrasound frequency

Ultrasound at various frequencies in the range of 20 kHz to 16 MHz has been used for sonophoresis. These studies of sonophoresis can be classified into three categories based on the ultrasound frequency used, i.e., therapeutic, high-frequency, and low-frequency ultrasound.

Therapeutic frequency ultrasound (1–3 MHz): This is the most commonly used ultrasound frequency range for sonophoresis. Specifically, over 90% of the previous studies of sonophoresis have been conducted using therapeutic ultrasound. A summary of these studies is provided in Table 2. Interestingly, in the therapeutic frequency range of 1–3 MHz, frequencies closer to 1 MHz

have been preferably used for sonophoresis. No reason has been given by investigators for the use of this particular frequency. Mitragotri et al. (36) reported that the sonophoretic enhancement in the therapeutic frequency range varies inversely with ultrasound frequency. They found that while 1 MHz ultrasound enhances transdermal transport of estradiol across human cadaver skin in vitro by 13-fold, 3 MHz ultrasound at the same intensity induces an enhancement of only 1.5-fold. They further hypothesized that the observed inverse dependence of sonophoretic enhancement on ultrasound frequency occurs since cavitational effects, which are primarily responsible for sonophoresis, vary inversely with ultrasound frequency (37, 59).

High-frequency ultrasound (above 3 MHz): Bommanan et al. (11, 12) performed sonophoresis of salicylic acid and lanthanum tracers across hairless rat skin in vivo using high-frequency ultrasound ($f = 2$, 10, and 16 MHz) (Table 3). They investigated the dependence of sonophoresis on ultrasound frequency in the high-frequency region and found that 10 MHz ultrasound is more effective in enhancing transdermal transport of salicylic acid than that at 16 MHz, which in turn, is more effective than that at 2 MHz. They proposed that the sonophoretic enhancement in the high-frequency region should vary directly with ultrasound frequency, though the anomolusly high efficiency of sonophoresis at 10 MHz was due to higher efficiency of the transducer operating at that frequency.

Low-frequency ultrasound (below 1 MHz): Tachibana et al. (52, 53) have reported use of low-frequency ultrasound (48 kHz) to enhance transdermal transport of lidocaine and insulin across hairless mice skin. Very low-frequency ultrasound has also been used by Mitragotri et al. (37, 38) to enhance transport of various low-molecular weight drugs including salicylic acid, corticosterone as well as high-molecular weight proteins including insulin, γ-interferon, and erythropoeitin across human cadaver skin in vitro. They investigated the dependence of sonophoretic enhancement in low-frequency region using two ultrasound frequencies, 20 and 40 kHz, and found that the sonophoretic enhancement of transdermal salicylic acid flux induced by 20 kHz ultrasound is up to 7-fold higher than that induced by 40 kHz ultrasound at the same intensity. The inverse dependence of sonophoretic enhancement on ultrasound frequency was hypothesized to occur due to inverse dependence of cavitational effects on ultrasound frequency (59).

Ultrasound intensity

Various ultrasound intensities in the range of 0.1–2 W/cm^2 have been used for sonophoresis. In most

Table 2 Literature reports of therapeutic sonophoresis

Drug	Molecular weight (Da)	Experimental system	Ultrasound conditions	Experimental conclusions[a]	Ref.
Caffeine	194	Human skin in vitro	1 MHz, 2 W/cm^2	0.2 ± 0.4	(37)
		Hairless rat in vitro	1 MHz, 2 W/cm^2	1	(33)
Corticosterone	346	Human skin in vitro	1 MHz, 2 W/cm^2	3 ± 0.6	(37)
Dexomethasone	392	Swine	1 MHz, 1.5 W/cm^2	Significant enhancement	(37)
Estradiol	272	Human skin in vitro	1 MHz, 2 W/cm^2	12 ± 1.5	(37)
Fluocinolone acetonide	452	Human skin in vivo	1 MHz, 2 W/cm^2	Significant enhancement	(35)
		Dogs	1 MHz, 0.3–1 W/cm^2	Significant enhancement	(42)
		Human skin in vivo	1 MHz, up to 2 W/cm^2	Significant enhancement	(42)
Hydrocortisone	362	Human skin in vivo	1 MHz, up to 3 W/cm^2	Significant enhancement	(42)
		Human skin in vivo	1 MHz, 1.5 W/cm^2	Significant enhancement	(42)
		Swine	1 MHz, 1.5 W/cm^2	Significant enhancement	(42)
		Pigs	1 MHz, up to 3 W/cm^2	Significant enhancement	(42)
Indomethacin	357	Rats	1 MHz, 0.75 W/cm^2	Significant enhancement	(40)
		Human skin in vitro	1 MHz, 2 W/cm^2	0.1 ± 0.6	b
Lidocaine	234	Human skin in vivo	1 MHz, 0.25 W/cm^2	No enhancement	(8)
		Human skin in vivo	1–3 MHz, 1.5 W/cm^2	No enhancement	(53)
Phenylbutazone	308	Human skin in vivo	1 MHz, 2 W/cm^2	Significant enhancement	(13)
Physostigmine	275	Hairless rats in vivo	1 MHz, 3 W/cm^2	Significant enhancement	(32)
Progesterone	274	Human skin in vitro	1 MHz, 2 W/cm^2	0.1 ± 0.5	(37)
Salicylate	138	Human skin in vivo	1 MHz, 1.5 W/cm^2	No significant enhancement	(15)
		Human skin in vivo	1 MHz, 1.5 W/cm^2	No significant enhancement	(14)
Testosterone	288	Human skin in vitro	1 MHz, 2 W/cm^2	4 ± 1.1	(37)

[a] The experimental conclusions are reported either as statistically significant or insignificant enhancement or in terms of a quantitative ratio of sonophoretic and passive skin permeability.
[b] Unpublished data by J. Kost and R. Langer.

cases, use of higher ultrasound intensities is limited by thermal effects. Several investigations have been performed to assess the dependence of sonophoretic enhancement on ultrasound intensity. Miyazaki et al. (41) found a relationship between the plasma concentrations of indomethacin transported across the hairless rat skin by sonophoresis (therapeutic conditions) and the ultrasound intensity used for this purpose. Specifically, the plasma indomethacin concentration at the end of three hours after sonophoresis ($0.25 \, W/cm^2$) was about 3-fold higher than controls at the same time. However, increasing intensity by 3-fold (to $0.75 \, W/cm^2$) further increased sonophoretic enhancement only by 33%. Mortimer et al. (42) found that application of ultrasound at $1 \, W/cm^2$ increased transdermal oxygen transport by 40% while that at $1.5 \, W/cm^2$ and $2 \, W/cm^2$ induced an enhancement by 50% and 55%, respectively.

In the very low-frequency ultrasound region (20 kHz), Mitragotri et al. (37) have reported that permeability of human skin in vitro to insulin increased by more than 100-fold as the ultrasound intensity increased from 12.5 to $125 \, mW/cm^2$. This variation of sonophoretic skin permeability with ultrasound intensity is quite different from that observed in therapeutic frequency region described above.

Pulse length

Ultrasound can be applied either in a continuous or a pulsed mode. A pulsed mode of ultrasound application is used many times because it reduces the severity of adverse side effects of ultrasound, such as thermal effects. However, pulsed application of ultrasound may have a significant effect on the efficacy of sonophoresis. As will be discussed later, cavitational effects, which play a crucial role in sonophoresis, vary significantly with the pulse length. For example, the cavitation threshold in an aqueous solution at 1 MHz changes from approximately $0.3 \, W/cm^2$ (60) to $33 \, W/cm^2$ (61) as the mode of ultrasound application changes from continuous to pulsed, with a pulse length of 1 ms applied every 10 ms. This is because under pulsed ultrasound, during the intervals between pulses, gas nuclei formed during the previous pulse have time to dissolve back into solution, and therefore, making it more difficult to cavitate the solution (62). Mitragotri et al. (36) reported that while a continuous application of therapeutic ultrasound (1 MHz, $2 \, W/cm^2$) increased human skin permeability to estradiol by 13-fold, a pulsed application (2 ms pulses applied every 10 ms) did not significantly enhance transdermal estradiol flux. In very low-frequency ultrasound region, Kost et al. (28) reported that urea permeability of cuprophane membranes

increased from 6 to 56% as the ultrasound (20 kHz) pulse length increased from 100 to 400 ms (applied every second).

Distance of the transducer from the skin

The ultrasound pressure (or intensity) field around a transducer is quite complex. The intensity of the ultrasound passes through a series of maxima and minima in a region near the transducer and beyond a certain distance, decreases monotonically with distance. The region in which the ultrasound intensity passes through the series of minima and maxima is referred to as the near field, and the region beyond the near field is referred to as the far field. The length of the near field of a transducer having an area of $1 \, cm^2$ operating at 1 MHz is 1.66 cm (57). In most of the experiments reported in the literature, for which ultrasound frequencies of 1 MHz or above have been used, the distance of the skin from the transducer was probably less than 1.66 cm. As a result, in most reported experiments, the skin was in the near-field region. In very low-frequency ultrasound region, Julian et al. (23) studied the effect of transducer distance on the sonophoretic permeability of benzoic acid through a polydimethylsiloxane membrane under low-frequency conditions. They observed that the effect of 20 kHz ultrasound on the permeability of the membrane is insensitive to the distance of the transducer from the membrane. This probably occurs because of the successive reflections of ultrasound waves in the diffusion cell which prevents any systematic pressure pattern form forming in the diffusion cell.

Ultrasound energy dose

In a recent systematic study of the dependence of 20 kHz sonophoresis on ultrasound parameters, Mitragotri et al. showed that the enhancement of skin permeability varies linearly with ultrasound intensity and ultrasound on-time (for pulsed ultrasound, ultrasound on-time equals the product of total ultrasound application time and duty cycle), while is independent of the ultrasound duty cycle. Based on those findings, the authors reported that there is a threshold energy dose for ultrasound induced transdermal drug transport. Once the threshold value is crossed, the enhancement of skin permeability varies linearly with the ultrasound energy dose (J/cm^2), which is calculated as the product of ultrasound intensity and ultrasound on-time. This result indicates that ultrasound energy dose can be used as a predictor of the effect of 20 kHz sonophoresis. The authors also indicated that it is important to determine the threshold energy dose for each individual sonophoresis system, for example, the

Table 3 Literature reports of high frequency sonophoresis

Drug	Molecular weight (Da)	Experimental system	Ultrasound conditions	Experimental conclusions[a]	Ref.
Salicylic acid	138	Hairless rat in vivo	2, 10, and 16 MHz 200 mW/cm^2	2–4 fold enhancement	(11)
Lanthanum tracers	—	Hairless rat in vivo	10 and 16 MHz 200 mW/cm^2	Significant enhancement	(12)

[a]The experimental conclusions are reported as statistically significant or insignificant enhancement.

real in vivo situation, because it may vary from system to system. Specifically, it may vary between different skin models, as well as with the ultrasound frequency and the distance of the transducer from the skin surface, etc.

PREVIOUS STUDIES OF SONOPHORESIS

Numerous attempts of sonophoresis have been performed over the last 40 years. As described earlier, these attempts can be classified into three categories: therapeutic frequency, high-frequency and low-frequency ultrasound.

Therapeutic Frequency Sonophoresis

The therapeutic ultrasound conditions correspond to a frequency in the range of 1–3 MHz and an intensity in the range of 0–2 W/cm^2. Therapeutic ultrasound has been attempted to enhance transdermal transport of more than 15 drugs (7–10, 14, 15, 18–22, 25, 22, 27, 28, 30–33, 36, 33, 42–45, 47–50, 55, 56, 63), a summary of which is provided in Table 2.

Historically, the transdermal route of drug administration has been considered for topical rather than systemic delivery of drugs. Accordingly, most of the sonophoresis experiments reported in Table 2 were intended for topical delivery of various drugs. Among all the drugs that have been used for sonophoresis, much attention has been focused on anti-inflammatory drugs. These include steroidal drugs such as hydrocortisone and dexamethasone and non-steroidal drugs such as indomethacin and salicylate. Sonophoresis of anti-inflammatory drugs offers an advantage over their passive topical delivery in that ultrasound may deliver drugs deeper into tissues. This is especially advantageous in the case of delivery of anti-inflammatory drugs to muscles which lie deeper into the body. Griffin et al. (18) reported that application of

ultrasound (1 MHz, 2 W/cm^2) delivered hydrocortisone about 5 cm deep into pig tissues. This characteristic property of sonophoresis has been used effectively by these investigators to deliver hydrocortisone to joints for the treatment of rheumatoid arthritis.

The most commonly used technique of sonophoresis in these studies was to apply hydrocortisone in the form of an ointment on the skin and then apply ultrasound by keeping the transducer in contact with the ointment. In some cases, the transducer was moved in circular patterns to avoid a continuous exposure of a certain part of the skin to ultrasound. Although these studies were performed using different animal models, application techniques, hydrocortisone concentrations in the ointment, and exposure time, a measurable enhancement of hydrocortisone transport was reported in almost all cases. In contrast, most of the attempts to enhance transdermal transport of lidocaine and salicylates have been less successful. In the case of lidocaine, the sonophoretic enhancement was measured in terms of reduction of onset time for anesthesia or prolonging duration of anesthesia. In most cases, no significant effect of ultrasound application on either induction time or duration of anesthesia has been reported (55). Similarly sonophoresis of salicylates from ointments has not been found to induce any significant increase in plasma salicylate levels (14).

Literature data reported in Table 2 indicate that except in the case of steroids including hydrocortisone, dexamethasone, testosterone, estradiol, and corticosterone, application of therapeutic ultrasound results in either minor or no enhancement of transdermal drug transport. Mitragotri et al. (36) presented a hypothesis for this variation of sonophoretic enhancement from drug to drug based on their mechanistic conclusion that ultrasound induces disorganization of the SC lipid bilayers, thus increasing drug diffusivity and hence permeability of the SC. This mechanism suggests that drugs such as steroids which possess low passive diffusion coefficients through the SC bilayers (36) compared to those through the disordered SC bilayers should be significantly

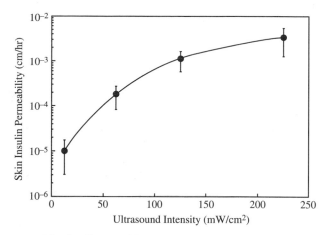

Fig. 2 Human skin permeability to insulin (37).

transport. Bommanan et al. (11) found that transdermally delivered salicylic acid appears much sooner in the urine if driven by sonophoresis than by passive permeation. These researchers also found that an electron dense tracer, such as lanthanum, was driven deep into the dermis by a 5 min. application of high-frequency ultrasound in hairless mouse in vivo.

MECHANISMS OF SONOPHORESIS

In order to understand the mechanisms of sonophoresis, it is important to identify various effects of ultrasound exposure on the human tissue since one or more of these effects may contribute to the mechanism of sonophoresis.

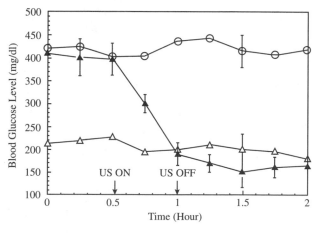

Fig. 3 Blood glucose levels of rats; ○ – diabetic hairless rats; △ – normal rats, ▲ – diabetic rats treated by sonophoresis and insulin for 30 min (37)

A brief description of the various biological effects of ultrasound is provided below.

Exposure Effects

Thermal effects

Absorption of ultrasound results in a temperature increase of the medium. Materials which posses higher ultrasound absorption coefficients, such as bones, experience severe thermal effects as compared to muscle tissues which have a lower absorption coefficient (α). α-values for several biological tissues can be found in (60, 66) (Table 1). The absorption coefficient of a medium increases proportionally with the ultrasound frequency indicating that, the thermal effects of ultrasound are proportional to the ultrasound frequency. The increase in the temperature of a medium upon ultrasound exposure at a given frequency varies proportionally with the ultrasound intensity and exposure time. The thermal effects can be substantially decreased by pulsed application. For a detailed discussion of the thermal effects of ultrasound (60).

Acoustic streaming

Acoustic streaming, by definition, is the development of time independent large fluid velocities in a medium under the influence of an ultrasound wave. The primary causes of acoustic streaming are the reflections and other distortions of the wave propagation. Oscillations of cavitation bubbles may also contribute to acoustic streaming. The shear stresses developed by streaming velocities may affect the neighboring structures (67).

Cavitational effects

Cavitation is the formation of gaseous cavities in a medium upon ultrasound exposure. The primary cause of cavitation is the ultrasound-induced pressure variations in the medium. Cavitation involves either rapid growth and collapse of a bubble (transient cavitation) or slow oscillatory motion of a bubble in ultrasound field (stable cavitation). Cavitation affects tissues in several ways. Specifically, collapse of cavitation bubbles releases a shock wave which can cause a structural alterations in its surroundings. Biological tissues contain numerous air pockets trapped in the fibrous structures which act as nuclei for cavitation upon ultrasound exposure. Accordingly, a significant cavitation activity is known to occur in biological tissues upon ultrasound exposure (60). The cavitational effects vary inversely with ultrasound frequency and directly with ultrasound intensity. Significant attention has been devoted to explore which of the above mentioned phenomena plays an important role in sonophoresis.

Mechanisms of Therapeutic Sonophoresis

Mortimer et al. (42) performed sonophoresis of oxygen across frog skin in vitro. They found that the sonophoretic enhancement of transdermal oxygen transport depends on ultrasound intensity, rather than pressure amplitude. Based on this observation, they hypothesized that cavitation cannot be responsible for sonophoresis. They hypothesized that the observed enhancement occurs due to acoustic streaming in the solution around the skin (42). Levy et al. (30) performed an in vitro investigation of the roles played by thermal effects, cavitation, and mixing in sonophoretic enhancement of urea transport across polymer membranes. They found that the observed enhancement can not be explained by the thermal effects or mixing. In an attempt to elucidate the role played by cavitation, they performed sonophoresis experiments using degassed solutions. Since degassing a solution decreases the cavitation activity in the solution, they hypothesized that if a decrease in the sonophoretic enhancement is observed upon degassing, it would indicate the importance of cavitation. Indeed, they found that degassing procedure reduced the sonophoretic enhancement of urea permeation by 2-fold suggesting that cavitation may play a role in sonophoresis.

Cavitation occurs in a variety of mammalian tissues, including muscle, abdominal tissues, brain, cardiovascular tissues, and liver upon exposure to ultrasound at a variety of conditions (60). As explained earlier, the occurrence of cavitation in biological tissues is attributed to the existence of a large number of gas nuclei. These nuclei are gas pockets trapped in either intracellular or intercellular structures. Simonin et al. (68) hypothesized that cavitation occurs in the follicles of the skin upon ultrasound exposure and enhances transdermal permeation by convective velocities through follicles. However, no evidence was presented to support this hypothesis. Mitragotri et al. (36) presnted results of the experiments indicating that cavitation inside the skin plays an important role in sonophoresis performed using therapeutic ultrasound.

In the first set of experiments, the known effect of static pressure on cavitation was utilized. It is known that cavitation in fluids and porous media (21) can be suppressed at high pressures. This effect is believed to occur due to the dissolution or collapse of the gaseous nuclei under the influence of pressure. Sonophoresis experiments were performed using skin compressed at 30 atm (between two smooth glass plates soaked in water placed in a compression press for two hours prior to sonophoresis experiments). They found that while application of ultrasound (1 MHz, 2 W/cm^2, continuous) enhances estradiol permeability of the normal human epidermis by 13-fold, the corresponding enhancement for compressed skin is only about 1.75-fold.

In the second set of experiments, the heat-stripped human cadaver skin was degassed (under a pressure of 0.05 mm Hg) prior to the permeability experiments. The authors hypothesized that when a skin piece soaked in buffer is subjected to high vacuum, the resulting low pressures should reduce the dissolved gas concentration in the buffer thereby forcing small gaseous nuclei in the skin to dissolve. When the degassed skin was exposed to ultrasound, once again, the effect of ultrasound on the estradiol permeability was minimal (1.5-fold), compared to 13-fold across the normal skin. Based on these two results, the authors concluded that cavitation inside the skin plays a major role in enhancing transdermal transport upon therapeutic ultrasound exposure. They provided the following hypothesis for the mechanism of sonophoresis performed using therapeutic ultrasound.

Ultrasound exposure in the therapeutic range causes cavitation in the keratinocytes of the stratum corneum. Oscillations of the ultrasound-induced cavitation bubbles near the keratinocyte-lipid bilayer interfaces may, in turn, cause oscillations in the lipid bilayers, thereby causing structural disorder of the SC lipids (Fig. 4). Shock waves generated by the collapse of cavitation bubbles at the interfaces may also contribute to the structure-disordering effect.

Since diffusion of permeants through a disordered bilayer phase can be significantly higher than that through a normal bilayer, transdermal transport in the presence of ultrasound is expected to be higher than passive transport.

Mechanisms of Low-Frequency Sonophoresis

Since cavitational effects in fluids vary inversely with ultrasound frequency (59), it is likely that cavitational effects should play an even more important role in low-frequency sonophoresis. Tachibana et al. (53) hypohesized that application of low-frequency ultrasound results into acoustic streaming in the hair follicles and sweat ducts of the skin, thus leading to enhanced transdermal transport. Mitragotri et al. (38) hypohesized that transdermal transport during low-frequency sonophoresis occurs across the keratinocytes rather than hair follicles. They provided

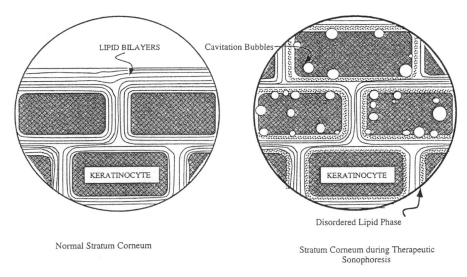

LIPID BILAYERS Cavitation Bubbles

KERATINOCYTE

KERATINOCYTE

Disordered Lipid Phase

Normal Stratum Corneum

Stratum Corneum during Therapeutic
Sonophoresis

Fig. 4 Ultrasound-induced cavitation bubbles in stratum corneum.

the following hypothesis for the higher efficacy of low-frequency sonophoresis.

Cavitation induced by low-frequency ultrasound may cause disordering of the SC lipids. In addition, oscillations of cavitation bubbles may result in significant water penetration into the disordered lipid regions. This may cause the formation of aqueous channels through the intercellular lipids of the SC through which permeants may transport (Fig. 5). The occurrence of transdermal transport through aqueous channels across the disordered lipid regions may enhance transdermal transport as compared to passive transport because i) the diffusion coefficients of permeants through water, which is likely to primarily occupy the channels generated by ultrasound, are up to 1000-fold higher than those through the ordered lipid bilayers (38), and ii) the transport path length of these aqueous channels may be much shorter (by a factor up to 25 (69)) than that though the tortuous intercellular lipids in the case of passive transport.

This hypothesis also explains why low-frequency ultrasound can induce transdermal transport of drugs which exhibit very low passive transport. Drugs possessing low passive permeabilities are either i) hydrophilic, which makes their partitioning into the SC bilayers difficult, or ii) large in molecular size (for example, proteins), which reduces their diffusion coefficients in the SC. Low-frequency ultrasound may overcome both of these limitations by providing aqueous transport channels across the skin. Since these channels are filled with saline, hydrophilic drugs can easily partition into the SC. In addition, diffusion of drugs through water is much faster

than that through ordered lipid bilayer regions, thus allowing drugs to transport across the skin at a faster rate. Therefore, molecules such as hydrophilic drugs or proteins, may permeate skin with relative ease in the presence of low-frequency ultrasound.

Mechanisms of High-Frequency Sonophoresis

Bommanan et al. (12) perfored sonophoresis of lanthanum tracers across hairless mice skin at an ultrasound frequency of 16 MHz in order to understand the transport pathways during high-frequency sonophoresis. They observed the skin under the electron microscope after sonophoresis and found that 5 min. of sonophoresis results in penetration of lanthanum tracers to dermal levels of the skin. They further reported that the tracer was patchily distributed within the intercellular lipid bilayers of the SC. They provided the following hypothesis for the mechanism of high-frequency sonophoresis. The micronuclei (air-pockets) present in the SC oscillate in response to oscillating pressure fields of ultrasound and eventually collapse. The oscillations of these bubbles result in enhanced skin permeation. They also hypothesized that the patchy distribution of the lanthanum tracer revealed in the micrographs corresponds to the location of oscillating air pockets in the SC. In a later report, Menon et al. (35) presented additional microscopic studies of the hairless mice skin after undergoing sonophoresis of lanthanum tracer. They reported the presence of long confluent channels in the intercellular lipids filled with lanthanum tracers in the hairless rat skin exposed to ultrasound. They

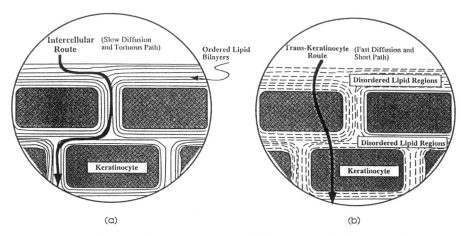

Fig. 5 Transdermal transport through the stratum corneum. (a) Passive and (b) during low-frequency sonophoresis.

presented the following hypothesis for the mechanism of sonophoresis: application of ultrasound opens and expands gas-filled cavities in the SC much like pumping air through a collapsed rubber tubing. Enhanced transport of drugs may then occur through these confluent channels across the SC.

SAFETY

The safety aspects of sonophoresis involve the reversibility of the skin barrier properties after turning ultrasound off, and the effect of ultrasound on the living parts of the skin and underlying tissues. Many reports exist in literature describing preliminary assessments of sonophoresis with respect to these two issues.

Recovery of the Skin Barrier Properties after Sonophoresis

Numerous reports exist to suggest that application of therapeutic ultrasound (1–3 MHz, 0–2 W/cm²) does not induce any irreversible change in the skin permeability to drugs in vivo. Quantitative measurements of estradiol transport across human skin (in vitro) have also shown that application of therapeutic ultrasound (1 MHz, 2 W/cm²) does not induce any statistically significant irreversible change in skin barrier properties (36). Similar studies have also been performed using very low-frequency ultrasound (20 kHz, 125 mW/cm², 100 ms pulses applied every second) to assess whether application of low-frequency ultrasound results in any permanent loss of the barrier properties of skin measured in terms of water permeability (38). It has been found that in the case of a 1 h long

ultrasound exposure, the skin permeability to water measured within 2 h post-exposure was comparable to the passive skin permeability to water. In the case of a 5-h long ultrasound exposure, the skin permeability 2 h post-exposure was about 6 times higher than the passive permeability to water. However, this value continued to decrease, and was within a factor of 2 of the passive skin water permeability 12 h post-exposure. Studies have also been performed (35) to assess whether application of high-frequency ultrasound induces any irreversible damage to the barrier properties of the skin measured in terms of trans-epidermal water loss (TEWL) across hairless mice skin exposed to high-frequency ultrasound (16 MHz). No significant difference in TEWL values of the skin exposed to ultrasound and that not exposed to ultrasound was found (35).

Biological Effects of Low-Frequency Ultrasound

Ultrasound over a wide frequency range has been used in medicine over last century. For example, therapeutic ultrasound (1–3 MHz) has been used for massage, low-frequency ultrasound has been used in dentistry (23–40 kHz) (70, 71), and high-frequency ultrasound (3–10 MHz) has been used for diagnostic purposes (66). In view of this, significant attention has been dedicated to investigate the effects of ultrasound on biological tissues. However, no conclusions have been reached regarding the limiting ultrasound conditions required to ensure safe exposure.

As described earlier, ultrasound affects biological tissues via three main effects, thermal effects, cavitational effects, and acoustic streaming. Conditions under which these effects become critical are given below (60).

Thermal effects may be important when

1. The tissue has a high protein content.
2. A high intensity continuous wave ultrasound is used.
3. Bone is included in the heated volume.
4. Vascularization is poor.

Cavitation may be important when

1. Low-frequency ultrasound is used.
2. Gassy fluids are exposed.
3. Small gas-filled spaces are exposed.
4. The tissue temperature is higher than normal.

Streaming may be important when

1. The medium has an acoustic impedance different from its surroundings.
2. The fluid in the biological medium is free to move.
3. Continuous wave application is used.

Numerous investigators have performed histological studies of animal and human skin exposed to ultrasound under various conditions in order to assess the effect of ultrasound on living skin cells. Levy et al. (30) exposed in vivo hairless rat skin to therapeutic ultrasound (1 MHz, 1.5 W/cm^2 continuous wave or 3 W/cm^2 pulsed wave, 3–5 min) and reported no damage to the skin. Nevertheless, Machet et al. (72) reported both epidermal and dermal alteration of human and hairless mouse skin when exposed to therapeutic ultrasound in vitro (3.3 MHz, 3 W/cm^2, 10 min). The authors proposed that a combined cavitation and thermal effect could explain these cellular lesions. Due to the higher likelihood of occurrence of cavitation under low-frequency ultrasound, the effect of low-frequency ultrasound on skin histology has drawn the most attention in the recent years. Tachibana et al. (52) exposed rabbit skin to 105 kHz ultrasound (5000 Pa, 5-s pulses applied at 5-s intervals, for 90 min) and reported no inflammation or destruction of skin. Mitragotri et al. (37) performed histological studies of hairless rat skin exposed to 20 kHz ultrasound (125 mW/cm^2, 100-ms pulses applied every second, for 1 h) and found no damage to the epidermis and underlying living tissues. In a more recent studies on skin microscopy, Yamashita et al. (54) exposed both human skin in vitro and hairless mouse skin in vivo to 48 kHz ultrasound at 0.5 W/cm^2 for 5 min, and reported that there was slight and complete removal of keratinocytes from human skin and hairless mouse skin, respectively. From the above reports, we can deduce that the effect of ultrasound, especially in the low-frequency range, on living skin cells strongly depends on the ultrasound parameters, i.e., frequency, intensity, exposure time and duty cycle. Further research focusing on safety

issues is required to evaluate limiting ultrasound parameters for safe exposure.

CONCLUSIONS

Application of ultrasound enhances transdermal drug transport, a phenomenon referred to as sonophoresis. Proper choice of ultrasound parameters including ultrasound energy dose, frequency, intensity, pulse length, and distance of transducer from the skin is critical for efficient sonophoresis. The numerous attempts made over the last 50 years can be classified into three categories: therapeutic frequency, high-frequency and low-frequency ultrasound; the first represents the most commonly used ultrasound condition for sonophoresis, although recently, attention has been more focused on low- and high-frequency conditions. Mechanistic experiments performed by several investigators suggest that cavitation plays a major role. It has been suggested that cavitation disorganizes the lipid bilayers of the skin through which enhanced transport of drugs may occur. Various studies have indicated that application of ultrasound under conditions used for sonophoresis does not cause any permanent damage to the skin or underlying tissues, although more work is required before arriving at definite conclusions regarding the safety of ultrasound exposure.

REFERENCES

1. Jarrett, A. *The Physiology and Pathology of the Skin*; Ed.; Academic Press: London, 1978.
2. Walters, K.A. Penetration Enhancers and Their Use in Transdermal Therapeutic Systems. *Penetration Enhancers and their Use in Transdermal Therapeutic Systems*; Hadgraft, J., Guy, R.H., Eds.; Marcel Dekker, Inc.: New York, 1989, 197–233.
3. Junginger, H.E.; Bodde, H.E.; de Haan, F.H.N. Penetration. In *Visuallization of Drug Transport across Human Skin and the Influence of Penetration Enhancers*; Hsieh, D.S., Ed.; Marcel Dekker, Inc.: New York, 1994; 59–90.
4. Bommanon, D.; Tamada, J.; Leung, L.; Potts, R. Effects of Electroporation on Transdermal Iontophoretic Delivery of Leutinizing Hormone Releasing Hormone. Pharm. Res. **1994**, *11*, 1809–1814.
5. Prausnitz, M.R.; Bose, V.; Langer, R.; Weaver, J.C. Electroporation of Mammalian Skin: Mechanism to Enhance Transdermal Drug Delivery. Proc. Natl. Acad. Sci. **1993**, *90*, 10504–10508.
6. Burnette, R.R. Iontophoresis. In *Transdermal Drug Delivery: Development Issues and Research Initatives*; Hadgraft, J., Guy, R.H., Eds.; Marcel Dekker, Inc.: New York, 1989; 247–291.

7. Antich, T.J. Phonophoresis: The Principles of the Ultrasonic Driving Force and Efficacy in Treatment of Common Orthopedic Diagnoses. J. Orth. Sports Phys. Ther. **1982**, *4*, 99–102.

8. Benson, H.A.E.; McElnay, J.C.; Harland, R. Phonophoresis of Lingocaine and Prilocaine from Emla Cream. Int. J. Pharm. **1988**, *44*, 65–69.

9. Benson, H.A.E.; McElnay, J.C.R.H. Use of Ultrasound to Enhance Percutaneous Absorption of Benzydamine. Phys. Ther. **1989**, *69*, 113–118.

10. Benson, H.A.E.; McElnay, J.C.J.H. Influence of Ultrasound on the Percutaneous Absorption of Nicotinate Esters. Pharm. Res. **1991**, *9*, 1279–1283.

11. Bommannan, D.; Okuyama, H.; Stauffer, P.; Guy, R.H. Sonophoresis. I. The Use of High-Frequency Ultrasound to Enhance Transdermal Drug Delivery. Pharm. Res. **1992**, *9*, 559–564.

12. Bommannan, D.; Menon, G.K.; Okuyama, H.; Elias, P.M.; Guy, R.H. Sonophpresis. II. Examination of the Mechanism(s) of Ultrasound-Enhanced Transdermal Drug Delivery. Pharm. Res. **1992**, *9*, 1043–1047.

13. Brondolo, W. Arch. Orthop. **1960**, *73*, 532–540.

14. Ciccone, C.D.; Leggin, B.Q.; Callamaro, J.J. Effects of Ultrasound and Trolamine Salicylate Phonophoresis on Delayed-Onset Muscle Soreness. Phys. Ther. **1991**, *71*, 666–678.

15. Davick, J.P.; Martin, R.K.; Albright, J.P. Distribution and Deposition of Tritiated Cortisol Using Phonophoresis. Phys. Ther. **1988**, *68*, 1672–1675.

16. Fellinger, K.; Schmidt, J. Klinik und Therapie des Chronischen. Gelenkreumatismus, Maudrich, Vienna, Austria **1954**, ,549–554.

17. Fogler, S.; Lund, K. Acoustically Augmented Diffusional Transport. J. Acous. Soc. Am. **1973**, *53*, 59–64.

18. Griffin, J.E.; Touchstone, J. Ultrasonic Movement of Cortisol into Pig Tissue. Am. J. Phys. Med. **1965**, *44*, 20–25.

19. Griffin, J.E. Physiological Effects of Ultrasonic Energy as it is Used Clinically. J. Am. Phys. Ther. Assoc. **1966**, *46*, 18–26.

20. Griffin, J.E.; Echternach, J.L.; Proce, R.E.; Touchstone, J.C. Patients Treated with Ultrasonic Driven Hydrocortisone and with Ultrasound Alone. Phys. Ther. **1967**, *47*, 600–601.

21. Griffin, J.E.; Touchstone, J.C. Low-Intensity Phonophoresis of Cortisol in Swine. Phys. Ther. **1968**, *48*, 1136–1344.

22. Griffin, J.E.; Touchstone, J.C. Effects of Ultrasonic Frequency on Phonophoresis of Cortisol into Swine Tissues. Am. J. Phys. Med. **1972**, *51*, 62–78.

23. Julian, T.N.; Zentner, G. Ultrasonically Mediated Solute Permeation through Polymer Barriers. J. Pharm. Pharmacol. **1986**, *38*, 871–877.

24. Julian, T.N.; Zentener, G.M. Mechanim for Ultrasonically Enhanced Transmembrane Solute Permeation. J. Control. Rel. **1990**, *12*, 77–85.

25. Kleinkort, J.A.; Wood, F. Phonophoresis with 1 Percent Versus 10 Percent Hydrocortisone. Phys. Ther. **1975**, *55*, 1320–1324.

26. Kost, J.; Levy, D.; Langer, R. Ultrasound as a Transdermal Enhancer. *Percutaneous Absorption Mechanisms-Methodology-Drug Delivery*; Bronaugh, R., Maibach, H.I. Eds.; Marcel Dekker, Inc.: New York, 1989; 595–601.

27. Kost, J.; Langer, R. Ultrasound-Mediated Transdermal Drug Delivery. *Topical Drug Bioavailability, Bioequivalence, and Penetration*; Shah, V.P., Maibach, H.I., Eds.; Plennum: New York, 1993; 91–103.

28. Kost, J. Ultrasound for Controlled Delivery of Therapeutics. Clin. Mater. **1993**, *13*, 155–161.

29. Lenart, I.; Auslander, D. The Effects of Ultrasound on Diffusion through Membranes. Ultrasonics **September 1980**, 216–217.

30. Levy, D.; Kost, J.; Meshulam, Y.; Langer, R. Effect of Ultrasound on Transdermal Drug Delivery to Rats and Guinea Pigs. J. Clin. Invest. **1989**, *83*, 2974–2078.

31. Machluf, M.; Kost, J. Ultrasonically Enhanced Transdermal Drug Delivery. Experimental Approaches to Elucidate the Mechanism. J. Biomat. Sci. **1993**, *5*, 147–156.

32. McElnay, J.C.; Matthews, M.P.; Harland, R.; McCafferty, D.F. The Effect of Ultrasound on the Percutaneous Absorption of Lingocaine. Br. J. Clin. Pharmacol. **1985**, *20*, 421–424.

33. McElnay, J.C.; Kennedy, T.A.R.H. The Influence of Ultrasound on the Percutaneous Absorption of Fluocinolone Acetonide. Int. J. Pharm. **1987**, *40*, 105–110.

34. McEnlay, J.C.; Benson, H.A.E.; Harland, R.; Hadgraft, J. Phonophoresis of Methyl Nicotinate: A Preliminary Study to Elucidate the Mechanism. Pharm. Res. **1993**, *4*, 1726–1731.

35. Menon, G.; Bommanon, D.; Elias, P. High-Frequency Sonophoresis: Permeation Pathways and Structural Basis for Enhanced Permeability. Skin Pharmacol. **1994**, *7*, 130–139.

36. Mitragotri, S.; Edwards, D.; Blankschtein, D.; Langer, R. A Mechanistic Study of Ultrasonically Enhanced Transdermal Drug Delivery. J. Pharm. Sci. **1995**, *84*, 697–706.

37. Mitragotri, S.; Blankschtein, D.; Langer, R. Ultrasound-Mediated Transdermal Protein Delivery. Science **1995**, *269*, 850–853.

38. Mitragotri, S.; Blankschtein, D.; Langer, R. Transdermal Drug Delivery Using Low-Frequency Sonophoresis. Pharm. Res. **1996**, *13*, 411–420.

39. Mitragotri, S.; Blankschtein, D.; Langer, R. An Explanation for the Variation of the Sonophoretic Transdermal Transport Enhancement from Drug to Drug. J. Pharm. Sci. **1997**, *86*, 1190–1192.

40. Mitragotri, S.; Farrell, J.; Tang, H.; Terahara, T.; Kost, J.; Langer, R. Determination of Thresholds Energy Dose for Ultrasound-Induced Transdermal Drug Transport. J. Control. Rel. **2000**, *63*, 41–52.

41. Miyzaki, S.; Mizuoka, O.; Takada, M. External Control of Drug Release and Penetration: Enhancement of the Transdermal Absorption of Indomethacin by Ultrasound Irradiation. J. Pharm. Pharmacol. **1990**, *43*, 115–116.

42. Mortimer, A.J.; Trollope, B.J.; Roy, O.Z. Ultrasound-Enhanced Diffusion through Isolated Frog Skin. Ultrasonics **1988**, *26*, 348–351.

43. Newman, J.T.; Nellermo, M.D.; Crnett, J.L. Hydrocortisone Phonophoresis: A Literature Review. J. Am. Pod. Med. Assoc. **1992**, *82*, 432–435.

44. Novak, E.J. Experimental Transmission of Lidocaine through Intact Skin by Ultrasound. Arch. Phys. Med. Rehab. **May 1964**, ,231–232.

45. Oziomek, R.S.; Perrin, D.H.; Herold, D.A.; Denegar, C.R. Effect of Phonophoresis on Serum Salicylate Levels. Med. Sci. in Sports and Exer. **1990**, *23*, 397–401.

46. Policoff, L.D. Effective Use of Physical Modalities. Orthopedic Clinics of North America **1982**, *13*, 579–586.

47. Pottenger, J.F.; Karalfa, L.B. Utilization of Hydrocortisone Phonophoresis in United States Army Physical Therapy Clinics. Milit. Med. **1989**, *154*, 355–358.

48. Pratzel, H.; Ditrich, P.; Kukovetz, W. Spontaneous and Forced Cutaneous Absorption of Indomethacin in Pigs and Humans. J. Rheumat. **1986**, *13*, 1122–1125.

49. Quillen, W.S. Phonophoresis: A Review of the Literature and Technique. Athelet. Train. **1980**, *15*, 109–110.

50. Skauen, D.M.; Zentner, G.M. Phonophoresis. Int. J. Pharm. **1984**, *20*, 235–245.

51. Tachibana, K.; Tachibana, S. Transdermal Delivery of Insulin by Ultrasonic Vibration. J. Pharm. Pharmacol. **1991**, *43*, 270–271.

52. Tachibana, K. Transdermal Delivery of Insulin to Alloxan-Diabetic Rabbits by Ultrasound Exposure. Pharm. Res. **1992**, *9*, 952–954.

53. Tachibana, K.; Tachibana, S. Use of Ultrasound to Enhance the Local Anesthetic Effect of Topically Applied Aqueous Lidocaine. Anestheiology **1993**, *78*, 1091–1096.

54. Yamashita, N.; Tachibana, K.; Ogawa, K. Scanning Electron Microscopy Evaluation of the Skin Surface after Ultrasound Exposure. Anat. Rec. **1997**, *247*, 455–461.

55. Williams, A.R. Phonophoresis: An In Vivo Evaluation Using Three Topical Anaesthetic Preparations. Ultrasonics **1990**, *28*, 137–141.

56. Wing, M. Phonophoresis with Hydrocortisone in the Treatment of Temporomandibular Joint Dysfunction. Phys. Ther. **1981**, *62*, 32–33.

57. Kinsler, L.W.; Frey, A.R.; Coppens, A.B.; Sandes, J.V. *Fundamentals of Acoustics*; John Wiley & Sons: New York, 1982.

58. Hueter, T.F.; Bolt, R.H. *Sonics: Techniques for the Use of Sound and Ultrasound in Engineering and Science*; John Wiley & Sons: New York, 1962.

59. Gaertner, W. Frequency Dependence of Acoustic Cavitation. J. Acoust. Soc. Am. **1954**, *26*, 977–80.

60. Suslick, K.S. *Ultrasound: Its Chemical, Physical and Biological Effects*; VCH Publishers: New York, 1989.

61. Crum, L.A.; Folwlkes, J.B. Acoustic Cavitation Generated by Microsecond Pulses of Ultrasound. Nature **1986**, *52*, 319.

62. Ciaravino, V.; Flynn, H.G.; Miller, M.W. Pulsed Enhancement of Acoustic Cavitation: A Postulated Model. Ultrasound Med. Biol. **1981**, *7*, 159–166.

63. Tyle, P.; Agrawala, P. Drug Delivery by Phonophoresis. Pharm. Res. **1989**, *6*, 355–360.

64. Hanch, C.; Leo, A. *Substituent Constants for Correlation Analysis in Chemistry and Biological Sciences*; Wiley: New York, 1979.

65. Flynn, G.L. Physiochemical Determinants of Skin Absorption. *Physiochemical Determinants of Skin Absorption*; Gerrity, T.R., Henry, C.J., Eds.; Elsevier: New York, 1990; 93–127.

66. Wells, P.N.T. *Biomedical Applications of Ultrasound*; Plenum Press: New York, 1977.

67. Nyborg, W.L. Acoustic Streaming. *Acoustic Streaming*; Mason, W.P., Ed.; Academic Press: New York, 1965; II B, 265–331.

68. Simonin, J.P. On the Mechanisms of In Vitro and In Vivo Phonophoresis. J. Control. Rel. **1995**, *33*, 125–141.

69. Edwards, D.; Langer, R. A Linear Theory of Transdermal Transport Phenomena. J. Pharm. Sci. **1994**, *83*, 1315–1334.

70. Walmsley, A.D. Applications of Ultrasound in Dentistry. Ultrasound Med. Biol. **1988**, *14*, 7–14.

71. Walmsley, A.D. Potential Hazards of the Dental Ultrasonic Descaler. Ultrasound Med. Biol. **1988**, *14*, 15–20.

72. Machet, L.; Pinton, J.; Patat, F.; Arbeille, B.; Pourcelot, L.; Vaillant, L. In Vitro Phonophoresis of Digoxin across Hairless Mice and Human Skin: Thermal Effect of Ultrasound. Int. J. Pharm. **1996**, *133*, 39–45.

ULTRASONIC NEBULIZERS

Kevin M.G. Taylor

University of London, London, United Kingdom

Orla McCallion

Vandsons Research, Islington, London, United Kingdom

INTRODUCTION

Ultrasonic nebulizers use ultrasonic energy to convert liquid, usually an aqueous solution, into an aerosol for inhalation. They are used to deliver β_2-agonists, corticosteroids, antiallergics, anticholinergics, and antiviral and mucolytic agents to the respiratory tract (1). Recent innovations have increased the popularity of nebulizers, both ultrasonic and air-jet, and new devices with improved portability, compared with traditional models, are capable of generating aerosols with high respirable fractions (deep lung delivery) with a high drug output. Nebulized drugs may be inhaled during normal tidal breathing through a mouthpiece or face mask, permitting their use for patients, such as the hospitalized, the elderly, children, and patients with arthritis, who experience difficulties with other devices. Nebulizers represent ideal delivery systems for drugs that cannot be conveniently formulated into pressurized metered-dose inhalers (pMDIs) or dry powder inhalers (DPIs) or when the therapeutic dose is too large for delivery with these systems.

Ultrasonic nebulizers were first developed in the 1960s and were initially used for air humidification in respiratory care units (2). Generally, ultrasonic nebulizers have higher mass outputs than do air-jet nebulizers, in which compressed gas is used as a means of generating the aerosol. However, this is achieved at the expense of a large aerosol droplet size (3–7). Consequently, the majority of ultrasonically generated aerosols have a mean droplet size considered unsuitable for efficient targeting of a drug to the alveolar region of the lung. However, the size distribution of droplets within aerosols produced by ultrasonic nebulization is generally less than that from air-jet nebulizers. Nevertheless, the generated aerosols are polydisperse in nature, and as with air-jet nebulizers, they require baffles to remove the larger droplets from the emitted aerosol. Because ultrasonic nebulizers have a high mass output, with increased droplet concentration, which is independent of the airflow, the duration of nebulization is shorter than with air-jet nebulizers. This, together with their quieter mode of operation, may make them particularly attractive to patients. Ultrasonic nebulizers are reported to produce bronchodilator responses comparable with those of air-jet nebulizers and pMDIs (8).

MECHANISM OF AEROSOL GENERATION

The energy required to atomize a liquid is produced by a piezoelectric crystal transducer, usually a synthetic ceramic material, vibrating at a high frequency (1–3 MHz). When an alternating electric current is applied, the crystal shrinks and expands and the resultant vibrations are transmitted to the nebulized fluid, either directly or via a coupling liquid, usually water. A fountain of liquid is produce at the liquid surface, with large droplets being emitted from its apex and a "fog" of small droplets being produced from the lower part.

Fig. 1 illustrates the two mechanisms proposed for the processes of liquid disintegration and aerosol generation within ultrasonic nebulizers (9). The capillary-wave theory relates to the production of capillary waves in the bulk liquid. These waves constructively interfere to form peaks and a central geyser. When the amplitude of the applied energy is sufficiently high, the crests of the capillary waves break off, and droplets are formed. The rate of generation of capillary waves is dependent on both the physicochemical properties of the nebulized fluid and the intensity of the ultrasonic vibration. Mercer (3) used Eq. 1 to calculate the threshold amplitude for the generation of capillary waves:

$$A = 4\frac{v}{f\lambda} \tag{1}$$

where A is the threshold amplitude, v is the kinematic viscosity of the liquid, f is the acoustic frequency, and λ the capillary wavelength. When the amplitude exceeds the threshold value by a factor of approximately four, droplets are formed. Lang (10) noted that the mean droplet size generated from thin liquid layers was proportional to

Encyclopedia of Pharmaceutical Technology

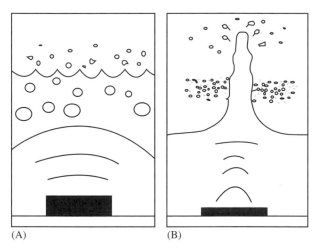

Fig. 1 Proposed ultrasonic nebulizer aerosolization mechanisms. (A) Cavitation bubble formation at low frequency; (B) capillary-wave formation at high frequency. (From Ref. 9.)

the capillary wavelength on the liquid surface. Using an experimentally determined factor of 0.34, the droplet diameter D is given by Eq. 2;

$$D = 0.34\lambda \qquad (2)$$

where D is the number median diameter and λ is the capillary wavelength. Lobdell (11) concurred with these findings and calculated a theoretical value of 0.36 for the proportionality constant. The capillary wavelength can be calculated from Kelvin's equation, as in Eq. 3:

$$\lambda = (8\pi y / \rho f^2)^{1/3} \qquad (3)$$

where γ is the surface tension, ρ is the density, and f the acoustic frequency. When γ is in mN/m (dyne/cm), ρ is in g/cm^3, and f is in megacycles/s, then D is given in micrometers. Good correlation exists between calculated and experimentally derived values (12).

The second mechanism proposed for aerosol generation is based on the piezoelectric crystal operating at low frequency and imparting vibrations to the bulk liquid. This results in the formation of cavitation bubbles, which move to the air–liquid interface (13). The internal pressure within the bubbles equilibrates with that of the atmosphere, causing their implosion. When this occurs at the liquid surface, portions of the liquid break free from the turbulent bulk liquid, resulting in droplet formation. The dependence of atomization on cavitation phenomena has been demonstrated for frequencies between 0.5 and 2.0 MHz (14, 15). Boguslavskii and Eknadiosyants (16) combined these theories with their proposal that droplet formation resulted from capillary waves initiated and driven by cavitation bubbles.

NEBULIZER DESIGN

Ultrasonic nebulizers exist in a number of basic designs that differ in the configuration of the piezoelectric crystal transducer, nebulizer chamber, baffles, and auxiliary airflow systems (Fig. 2) (9). Once the aerosol cloud is generated from the nebulizer fluid, it is transferred from the chamber and made available to the patient. Ultrasonic nebulizers produce a large number of droplets per unit volume, which tend to aggregate and settle in the absence of air circulating through the device. Larger droplets impact on the baffles or internal surfaces to return to the reservoir surface for recirculation under the influence of gravity. Smaller droplets leave the device aided by an internal fan (e.g., Medix Electronic®, Easimist®) or by entrainment into the inspiratory flow of the patient (e.g., DeVilbiss Pulmosonic®). Air velocity over the reservoir surface may be modified by fan speed (and flow constrictors), thereby influencing both droplet size and aerosol output rate. For instance, changing the fan speed

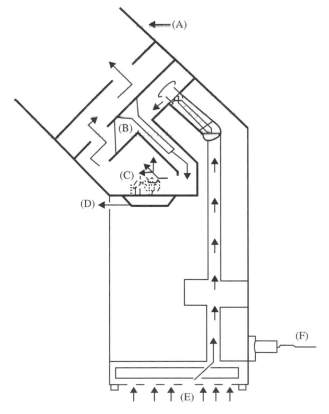

Fig. 2 Schematic diagram of a typical ultrasonic nebulizer. (A) Face mask or mouthpiece; (B) baffles; (C) geyser of respiratory solution or suspension; (D) piezoelectric crystal; (E) internal fan; (F) battery or electrical source. (From Ref. 9.)

Table 1 Design features of ultrasonic nebulizers determining particle size distribution and mass output

Design features	Nebulizer characteristics
Piezoelectric crystal	
	Frequency of vibration
	Amplitude of vibration
	Surface morphology (flat or curved)
	Coupling between crystal and fluid
Fluid reservoir	
	Size
	Shape
	Baffles
Auxiliary air flow	
	Velocity

(Modified from Ref. 7.)

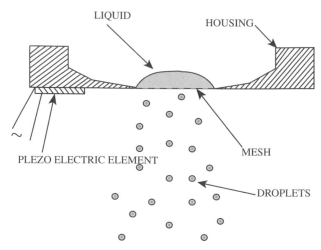

Fig. 3 Schematic diagram of the sprayhead of the Bespak Piezo Electric Actuator. (Reproduced courtesy of Bespak plc, UK.)

setting of the Sonix 2000® (Medix) ultrasonic nebulizer can vary flow output between 1 ml per min and 1 ml per 6 min. The important design features influencing mass output and the particle size of the generated aerosols are summarized in Table 1.

Whereas air-jet nebulizers are usually disposable or sterilizable, ultrasonic nebulizers are too expensive to be produced as disposable units and are thus used repeatedly (17), running the risk of bacterial contamination (18). Cleaning nebulizers and connecting tubing is difficult, and the transfer of Gram-negative bacteria between nebulization equipment and patients has been reported (19).

Although most ultrasonic devices share a basic design, some novel devices have been developed. The Respimat® (Boehringer Ingelheim) offered direct delivery of a metered dose from a valve similar to that used in pMDIs to the surface of a vibrating crystal (2.5 MHz). Although the mass median aerodynamic diameter (MMAD) of the aerosol generated was closed to 10 μm, generally considered too large for effective inhalation therapy, equivalence to an equivalent pMDI formulation was claimed (20).

The Bespak Piezo Electric Actuator® is a novel aerosol delivery system based on a piezoelectric crystal combined with an electroformed mesh (Fig. 3). It produces droplets of "adjustable" size from a single metered drop or fluid reservoir (21). The mesh hole dimension (as small as 3 μm) determines the size of the droplets produced, whereas the size and density of the holes control the rate of fluid delivery. These can be varied according to the formulation. Although solutions are more readily nebulized, suspensions can be aerosolized if the particle size of the

suspended particles is two to three times smaller than the mesh size.

More recently, The Technology Partnership has created several new forms of a perforated mesh atomizer known as TouchSpray® (22). TouchSpray devices deliver suspensions without requiring these to be formulated with small suspended particles. Furthermore, they can produce small droplets from large mesh holes. For example, TouchSpray devices can deliver 5 μm droplets of suspensions containing normally micronized drug suspensions, which typically include particles of 3 μm or larger. These droplets can be produced by devices having mesh hole sizes of 15 μm. TouchSpray allows small droplets to be produced from solutions. A review of the development of perforated mesh devices is given in Humberstone et al. (23). An inhalation droplet spray plume produced by the TouchSpray is shown in Fig. 4.

Future devices are likely to be hybrids of ultrasonic nebulizer technology and pMDI or DPI technology. Vibrating transducer or grids, incorporated into pMDIs, could break down large propellant droplets that would otherwise be wasted into a more respirable size range. Alternatively, the dependence of DPIs on patient-generated turbulent airstreams could be minimized by deaggregating powder by vibrational elements within the inhalation device or by generating aerosols electrostatically (Spiros®, Dura).

AEROSOL DROPLET SIZE

The efficacy of a therapeutic inhalation aerosol depends on its ability to penetrate the respiratory tract. This is

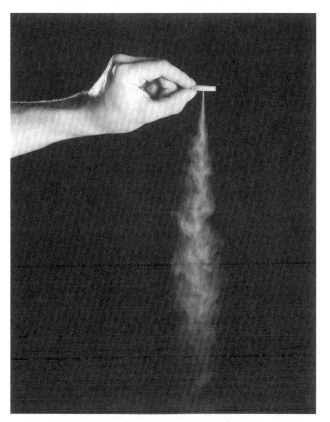

Fig. 4 Inhalation droplet spray plume produced by TouchSpray device. (Reproduced courtesy of The Technology Partnership plc, UK.)

primarily dependent on the particle size of the particles or droplets. To penetrate to the peripheral (respiratory) airways, aerosols generally require a size less than approximately 5–6 μm, with a size less than 2 μm being optimal for alveolar deposition (24, 25).

Clinical performance is often predicted from in vitro measurements of the droplet size of an aerosol. Nebulized aerosols are usually assessed by a multistage liquid impinger (MSLI), cascade impactor, or laser diffraction methods. The MSLI and cascade impactors comprise a series of progressively finer jets and collection plates, permitting fractionation of aerosols according to their MMADs (26). Problems associated with the cascade impactors for the assessment of nebulized aerosols are that the high flow rates involved (typically 28–90 L/min) give rise to rapid solvent evaporation and droplet entrainment. Additionally, these inertial impaction techniques are invasive, laborious, and time-consuming. Alternatively, nebulized aerosols may be sized by passing the spray through a beam of a laser diffraction analyzer. The volume or mass median diameter is then calculated from the generated diffraction pattern. Provided the liquid density is known, the MMAD can be calculated.

Numerous investigators have compared the aerosol droplet size of nebulized aerosols from ultrasonic and air-jet devices (3, 4, 6, 27–31). Because droplet size is inversely proportional to the acoustic frequency, smaller droplets are generated from ultrasonic devices with higher frequencies. Ultrasonic nebulizers with high operating frequencies (2–3 MHz) are capable of generating droplets of sizes comparable to arrow air-jet devices. However, devices with low frequencies (<0.5 MHz) tend to generate droplets outside the respirable range (4, 32). Most commercially available ultrasonic nebulizers have an operating frequency between 1 and 2 MHz. Although these produce aerosol droplets, which are significantly larger than those produced by air-jet nebulizers (3, 4), the size distributions are generally less polydisperse (3, 33).

NEBULIZATION TIME, DRUG OUTPUT, AND RESIDUAL VOLUME

Patient compliance with prescribed nebulization regimes is primarily determined by the duration of the therapy. Nebulizer fluids may be atomized for a set period, or more usually, a measured volume of therapeutic liquid is nebulized to "dryness." The time taken to achieve this is directly related to the volume to be delivered. However, not all the fluid in the nebulizer can be atomized, and some fluid remains associated with the baffles, internal structures, and walls of the nebulizer as the "dead" or "residual" volume (34). The proportion of fluid remaining as the residual volume and thus unavailable to patients is higher for smaller fill volumes.

Ultrasonic devices typically produce a much larger fluid output per unit of time than do jet nebulizers. Although Sterk et al. (4) suggested that high airflow through these devices resulted in lower droplet concentrations per unit volume than for air-jet nebulizers, more recent findings indicate that the reduced volume of dilution air in modern ultrasonic devices gives a more concentrated aerosol cloud. Ultrasonic nebulizers may retain a higher residual volume than do comparable air-jet nebulizers (35), but they show less tendency to increase the solute concentration within the nebulizer chamber during operation (27, 29).

In comparing DeVilbiss ultrasonic and jet devices, Newman et al. (29) reported shorter nebulization times for the ultrasonic devices with higher fluid outputs. Furthermore, the air-jet devices tended to increase the concentration of drug in the nebulizer chamber more than did the ultrasonic counterparts. The output from nebulizers comprises droplets of drug solutions and suspensions and solvent vapor, which saturates the outgoing air, causing solute concentration to increase during nebulization. Because ultrasonic nebulizers generally have higher fluid outputs and larger droplet sizes than do air-jet nebulizers, there is more solvent available within the dense aerosol cloud to saturate the outgoing air. Thus, the changes in solute concentration within the dead volume are much smaller than for air-jet devices.

THERMAL EFFECTS

Excess energy within the nebulizer is converted to heat, causing the temperature of the liquid in the reservoir to increase until the input energy balances the energy removed by evaporation and by conduction to the surroundings and circulating air (12). The temperature of a liquid in an ultrasonic nebulizer may thus increase by as much as 20°C above ambient temperature during use (6, 36). This results in changes in the properties of the fluid, including surface tension and viscosity. Although such changes may affect the aerosol particle size characteristics and overall drug output, little variation was seen during prolonged operation of Medix Electronic or Easimist nebulizers (37) or when the temperature in a DeVilbiss Aerosonic nebulizer was increased using a heating coil (38).

Warming may have a beneficial effect. For instance, the temperature of fluids atomized in air-jet nebulizers decreases by approximately 10–15°C during use (34, 39), resulting in bronchoconstriction in some asthma suffers (40). Bronchoconstriction, which is most marked at 5°C, disappears at 37°C and thus may be minimized by using an ultrasonic device. Furthermore, when solutions of drugs with low solubility are to be nebulized, ultrasonic nebulizers, which warm the solutions, may be preferable (36) to air-jet devices, which cool them and may cause precipitation (39). However, the heat generated may harm heat-labile materials such as diethylenetriaminepentoacetic acid (^{99}mTc-/DTPA) (41), proteins (31), and some antibiotic solutions (42). Thus, ultrasonic nebulizers are specifically prohibited for aerosolization of recombinant human deoxyribonuclease (rhDNase) (1).

FORMULATION OF NEBULIZER FLUIDS

Respiratory solutions are the mainstay of nebulized inhalation therapy. These typically contain drug dissolved in aqueous, isotonic solvent systems, with the inclusion of cosolvents (e.g., ethanol) if necessary. Suspensions are less common for nebulization, although corticosteroid preparations such as budesonide are available. Antioxidant and antimicrobial preservatives may be included in the formulations; however, some (e.g., sodium metabisulfate, benzalkonium chloride, EDTA) may have paradoxical effects and cause coughing and bronchoconstriction (43). To prevent this, "preservative-free" unit dose products are marketed. Isotonicity is generally achieved using sodium chloride. Although iso-osmotic solutions of pH 3–8.5 are usually employed, the osmolarity and pH may change during use, resulting in bronchospasm (44).

The size and output characteristics of aerosols generated from such liquids depend on their physico-chemical properties (density, surface tension, viscosity) in conjunction with the nebulizer design and operating conditions. Empirical and semiempirical formulas predict that the droplet size of the aerosols is proportional to surface tension and inversely related to viscosity, whereas the effect of density, over the concentration range normally encountered, is negligible. The filtering effects of the baffles and solvent evaporation may modify the secondary aerosol produced, but studies (32, 37, 45, 46) have found viscosity to be a major determinant of aerosol size and output characteristics. High-viscosity fluids offer greater resistance to the integral fountain-disintegration process, thereby producing not only lower output but also larger droplets. Gershenzon and Eknadiosyants (14) noted higher droplet outputs with lower viscosity fluids, whereas Boucher and Kreuter (32) reported that it was difficult to ultrasonically aerosolize fluids with viscosities exceeding 10 cP. Gershenzon and Eknadiosyants (14) stated that the atomization rate for a wide range of fluids (except water) is given by the proportionality of A^2 to $\pi\rho/\eta\sigma$, where A is the atomization rate, ρ is the liquid vapor pressure, η is the viscosity, and σ is the surface tension.

Il'in and Eknadiosyants (15) suggested that the dynamic viscosity coefficient was the most important property determining the nebulization rate. The rate of nebulization for solutions of tyloxapol or N-acetyl-L-cysteine decreased progressively as the solution viscosity increased. When certain oily and viscous liquids (e.g., Lipiodal®; a radio-opaque diagnostic agent) were nebulized, a fountain of liquid was generated, although this did not disintegrate to produce an aerosol. Similar results were reported by McCallion et al. (37), who compared a range of different model fluids, finding that ultrasonic nebulizers could not efficiently atomize the more viscous liquids and tended to produce poor total fluid outputs. Furthermore, when the fluid viscosity increased, larger droplets were generated.

Surface tension is also important because it represents the force resisting the formation of new surfaces. These forces tend to impair atomization by opposing any distortion or irregularity on the liquid surface, thereby delaying the onset of fountain formation. In suspension formulations, surfactants may be present as suspending agents. Reduction in liquid surface tension, through the addition of these agents, may decrease nebulization rate. This may be attributed to reduction in capillary wavelength, causing an increase in threshold amplitude (45) or through their influence on the diffusion of gas into cavitation bubbles (47). When a range of pharmaceutically relevant surfactant systems was nebulized, an inverse relationship was found between droplet size and surface tension over the entire concentration range investigated or to a peak value (33). There was no relationship between this peak value and a specific surface tension or the critical micelle concentration. In most cases, the total fluid output was unchanged.

Most nebulizer formulations are solutions, but a few corticosteroid suspension formulations have been marketed. In general, ultrasonic nebulizers are less efficient and more variable in delivering suspensions than are air-jet nebulizers. Although soluble radiopharmaceuticals may be more appropriate for delivery from ultrasonic nebulizers (48), Lin et al. (49) successfully used an ultrasonic nebulizer to deliver radiolabeled sulfur and tin colloids for lung imaging. McCallion et al. (50) nebulized a range of latex sphere suspensions in air-jet and ultrasonic nebulizers. No correlation was found between the size of the suspended spheres and the size distribution of the nebulized droplets. Higher outputs of smaller spheres were reported, with a concentrating effect occurring in the residual volume. The ultrasonic nebulizer studied was less efficient than the jet nebulizers, degrading some of the larger spheres and being unable to atomize suspended spheres of a specific size range.

Nebulizers, particularly air-jet devices, have been studied extensively for the delivery of liposomes to the lung (e.g., 51, 52). Because in ultrasonic nebulizers, the temperature of fluid in the reservoir is raised during use, they have generally been avoided for delivering liposomes, which exhibit temperature-dependent drug release. Barber and Shek (53) reported that egg phosphatidylcholine (egg PC) liposomes with a mean size of 281 nm or smaller were stable to nebulization in a DeVilbiss Ultra-Neb 99® ultrasonic nebulizer. However, dipalmitoylphosphatidylcholine liposomes of 499 nm increased in size within the nebulizer reservoir, suggesting fusion of vesicles, which could result in loss of entrapped hydrophilic materials. A later study (54) showed that the size of large multilamellar egg PC liposomes remaining in a Medix Electronic nebulizer decreased markedly during nebulization, suggesting vesicle disruption, which was reduced by including cholesterol in the formulations.

Ultrasonic nebulizers are less suitable than jet nebulizers for delivery of proteins to the airways because of their thermal sensitivity. In a comparison of eight air-jet and two ultrasonic nebulizers, all air-jet nebulizers maintained the enzymatic activity of rhDNase in both the collected aerosol and the residual volume (31). With the ultrasonic nebulizers, some thermal denaturation of the enzyme was evident toward the end of the nebulization period when the liquid volume was minimal and its temperature highest. The maximum temperature of the rhDNase solution was 58°C, which was near the thermal transition temperature (approximately 65°C) of the enzyme (31).

Ip et al. (55) investigated DeVilbiss Aerosonic®, Mountain Medical Microstat®, and Medix Electronic® ultrasonic nebulizers for the delivery of recombinant consensus α-interferon. The extent of protein aggregation was governed by the type of nebulizer used with, the Easimist causing the least and Microstat the most aggregation. This was related to the increase in temperature and could be minimized by cooling the nebulizer solution during use. The Aerosonic® nebulizer completely inactivated lactate dehydrogenase after 20 min (38). The profile of inactivation differed from that of an air-jet nebulizer and was associated both with the temperature increase of the nebulizer fluid and the aerosol production. The activity of the enzyme was almost completely retained if Tween 80 or PEG 8000 was included in the nebulizer fluid.

GUIDELINES AND STANDARDIZATION FOR THE USE OF NEBULIZERS

The British Thoracic Society Nebulizer Project Group published a set of guidelines for nebulizer treatment (18). Their findings relating to ultrasonic devices are summarized as follows.

1. The aim of treatment is to deliver a therapeutic dose of the drug as an aerosol in the form of respirable particles within 5–10 min.
2. Nebulizers are useful when large doses of drug are to be inhaled by patients too ill to use alternative devices and when drugs are not available for delivery from pMDIs and DPIs.
3. Nebulizers are generally used to treat acute exacerbations of asthma or chronic obstructive pulmonary

disease. Other indications include long-term bronchodilator treatment of chronic airflow obstruction;
prophylactic treatment for asthma; antimicrobial
drugs for cystic fibrosis, bronchiectasis, and
HIV/AIDS; and symptomatic relief in palliative care.
4. When drugs other than bronchodilators are being
    nebulized, equipment known to provide a suitable
    output should be used, and specific instructions should
    be given to patients. Such treatment should be
    supervised by hospital specialists.
5. Nebulization times for bronchodilators should be less
    than 10 min. Nebulization times and correct operation
    of devices should be familiar to the patients.

Convenience and patient preference determine whether
a mouthpiece or face mask is used.

Currently, there are no *U.S. Pharmacopeia* or *European
Pharmacopoeia* standard tests for characterizing the
output of respiratory solutions or suspensions generated
by air-jet or ultrasonic nebulizers. If nebulizers are to truly
compete with pMDIs and DPIs, standardization of
methods to measure dead volume, quantity of aerosol
emitted from the device, nebulization times, and the
size distribution of nebulized clouds is a logical and
fundamental requirement.

REFERENCES

1. British National Formulary 38, British Medical Association
    and Royal Pharmaceutical Society of Great Britain:
    London, 2000.
2. Tovell, R.M.; D'Ambruoso, D.C. Humidity in Inhalation
    Therapy. Anesthesiology **1962**, *23*, 452–459.
3. Mercer, T.T. Output Characteristics of Three Ultrasonic
    Nebulizers. Chest **1981**, *80*, 813–817.
4. Sterk, P.J.; Plomp, A.; Van der Vate, J.F.; Quanjer, P.H.
    Physical Properties of Aerosols Produced by Several Jet
    and Ultrasonic Nebulizers. Bull. Eur. Physiopathol. Respir.
    1984, *20*, 65–72.
5. Matthys, H.; Kohler, D. Pulmonary Deposition of Aerosols
    by Different Mechanical Devices. Respiration **1985**, *48*,
    269–276.
6. Phipps, P.R.; Gonda, I. Droplets Produced by Medical
    Nebulizers: Some Factors Affecting Their Size and Solute
    Concentration. Chest **1990**, *97*, 1327–1332.
7. Hardy, J.G.; Newman, S.P.; Knoch, M. Lung Deposition
    from Four Nebulizers. Respir. Med. **1993**, *87*, 461–465.
8. Ballard, R.D.; Bogin, R.M.; Pak, J. Assessment of
    Bronchodilator Response to a β-Adrenergic Delivered
    from an Ultrasonic Nebulizer. Chest **1991**, *100*, 410–415.
9. Dalby, R.N.; Hickey, A.J.; Tiano, S.L. Medical Devices for
    the Delivery of Therapeutic Aerosols to the Lungs.
    *Inhalation Aerosols: Physical and Biological Basis for
    Therapy*; Hickey, A.J., Ed.; Marcel Dekker, Inc.: New
    York, 1996; 441–473.
10. Lang, R.J. Ultrasonic Atomization of Liquids. J. Acoust.
    Soc. Am. **1962**, *36*, 6–8.
11. Lobdell, D.D. Particle Size-Amplitude Reactions for the
    Ultrasonic Atomizer. J. Acoust. Soc. Am. **1968**, *43*,
    229–231.
12. Mercer, T.T.; Goddard, R.F.; Flores, R.L. Output
    Characteristics of Three Ultrasonic Nebulizers. Ann.
    Allergy **1968**, *26*, 18–27.
13. Sollner, K. The Mechanism of the Formation of Fogs
    By Ultrasonic Waves. Trans. Faraday Soc. **1936**, *32*,
    1532–1536.
14. Gershenzon, E.L.; Eknadiosyants, O.K. The Nature of
    Liquid Atomization in an Ultrasonic Fountain. Sov. Phys.
    Acoust. **1964**, *10*, 156–162.
15. Il'in, B.I.; Eknadiosyants, O.K. Nature of Liquid Atomiza-
    tion in an Ultrasonic Fountain. Sov. Phys. Acoust. **1966**, *12*,
    310–318.
16. Boguslavskii, Y.Y.; Eknadiosyants, O.K. Physical Mech-
    anism of the Acoustic Atomization of a Liquid. Sov. Phys.
    Acoust. **1969**, *15*, 14–21.
17. Greenspan, B.J. Ultrasonic and Electrodynamic Methods of
    Aerosol Generation. *Inhalation Aerosols: Physical and
    Biological Basis for Therapy*; Hickey, A.J., Ed.; Marcel
    Dekker, Inc.: New York, 1996; 313–335.
18. The Nebuliser Project Group of the British Society
    Standards of Care Committee. Current Best Practice for
    Nebuliser Treatment. Thorax **1997**, *52* (Suppl. 2),
    S1–S106.
19. Rhoades, E.R.; Ringrose, R.; Mohr, J.A.; Brooks, L.;
    McKown, B.A.; Felton, F. Contamination of Ultrasonic
    Nebulization Equipment with Gram Negative Bacteria.
    Arch. Intern. Med. **1971**, *127*, 228–232.
20. Zierenberg, B.J. The Respimat, a New Inhalation System
    Based on the Piezoelectric Effect. Biopharmaceut. Sci.
    1992, *3*, 85–90.
21. Baker, P.G.; Stimpson, P.G. Electronically Controlled Drug
    Delivery Systems Based on the Piezo Electric Crystal.
    Respir. Drug Del. **1994**, *4*, 273–285.
22. Humberstone, V.C.; Newcombe, G.C.F.; Sant, A.J.;
    Palmer, M.R. Fluid Droplet Production Apparatus and
    Method. EP-615-470: 1994.
23. Humberstone, V.C.; Sant, A.J.; van Rensburg, R.J.
    Piezoelectric Aerosol Inhalers: Technology to Product.
    Conference Proceedings of New Horizons in Pulmonary
    Drug Delivery, Management Forum: London, October
    1–2, 1996.
24. Stahlhofen, W.; Gebhart, J.; Heyder, J. Experimental
    Determination of the Regional Deposition of Aerosol
    Particles in the Human Respiratory Tract. Am. Ind. Hyg.
    Assoc. J. **1980**, *41*, 385–398.
25. Newman, S.P.; Clarke, S.W. Therapeutic Aerosols. I.
    Physical and Practical Considerations. Thorax **1983**, *38*,
    881–886.
26. Hallworth, G.W.; Andrews, H.G. Size Analysis of
    Suspension Inhalation Aerosols by Inertial Separation
    Methods. J. Pharm. Pharmacol. **1976**, *28*, 898–907.
27. Ferron, G.A.; Kerrebijn, K.F.; Weber, J. Properties of
    Aerosols Produced with Three Nebulizers. Am. Rev.
    Respir. Dis. **1976**, *114*, 899–908.
28. Ryan, G.; Dolovich, M.B.; Obminski, G.; Cockroft, D.W.;
    Juniper, E.; Hargreave, F.E.; Newhouse, M.T. Standardi
    zation of Inhalation Provocation Tests: Influence of

Nebulizer Output, Particle Size and Method of Inhalation. J. Allergy Clin. Immunol. **1981**, *67*, 156–161.

29. Newman, S.P.; Pellow, P.G.D.; Clarke, S.W. In Vitro Comparison of DeVilbiss Jet and Ultrasonic Nebulizers. Chest **1987**, *92*, 991–994.

30. Smalldone, G.C.; Perry, R.J.; Deutsch, D.G. Characteristics of Nebulizers Used in the Treatment of AIDS-Related *Pneumocystis Carinii* Pneumonia. J. Aerosol Med. **1988**, *1*, 113–126.

31. Cipolla, D.C.; Clarke, A.R.; Chan, H.-K.; Gonda, I.; Shire, S.J. Assessment of Aerosol Delivery Systems for Recombinant Human Deoxyribonuclease. STP Pharm. Sci. **1994**, *4*, 50–62.

32. Boucher, R.M.G.; Kreuter, J. The Fundamentals of the Ultrasonic Atomization of Medicated Solutions. Ann. Allergy **1968**, *26*, 591–600.

33. McCallion, O.N.M.; Taylor, K.M.G.; Thomas, M.; Taylor, A.J. The Influence of Surface Tension on Aerosols Produced by Medical Nebulisers. Int. J. Pharm **1996**, *129*, 123–136.

34. Clay, M.M.; Pavia, D.; Newman, S.P.; Lennard-Jones, T.; Clarke, S.W. Assessment of Jet Nebulisers for Lung Aerosol Therapy. Lancet **1983**, *2*, 592–594.

35. Flament, M.-P.; Leterme, P.; Gayot, A.T. Factors Influencing Nebulizing Efficiency. Drug Dev. Ind. Pharm. **1995**, *21*, 2263–2285.

36. Taylor, K.M.G.; Hoare, C. Ultrasonic Nebulisation of Pentamidine Isethionate. Int. J. Pharm. **1993**, *98*, 45–49.

37. McCallion, O.N.M.; Taylor, K.M.G.; Thomas, M.; Taylor, A.J. Nebulization of Fluids of Different Physicochemical Properties with Air-Jet and Ultrasonic Nebulizers. Pharm. Res. **1995**, *12*, 1682–1688.

38. Niven, R.W.; Ip, A.Y.; Mittelman, S.; Prestrelski, S.J.; Arakawa, T. Some Factors Associated with the Ultrasonic Nebulization of Proteins. Pharm. Res. **1995**, *12*, 53–59.

39. Taylor, K.M.G.; Venthoye, G.; Chawla, A. Pentamidine Isethionate Delivery from Jet Nebulisers. Int. J. Pharm. **1992**, *85*, 203–208.

40. Lewis, R.A. Nebulisers for Lung Aerosol Therapy. Lancet **1983**, *2*, 849.

41. Waldman, D.L.; Weber, D.A.; Oberdörster, G.; Drago, S.R.; Utell, M.J.; Hyde, R.W.; Morrow, P.E. Chemical Breakdown of Technetium-99m DTPA During Nebulization. J. Nucl. Med. **1987**, *28*, 378–382.

42. Dennis, J.H.; Hendrick, D.J. Design Characteristics for Drug Nebulizers. J. Med. Eng. Technol. **1992**, *16*, 63–68.

43. Beasley, R.; Rafferty, P.; Holgate, S.T. Adverse Reactions to the Non-Drug Constituents of Nebuliser Solutions. Br. J. Clin. Pharmacol. **1988**, *25*, 283–287.

44. Schöni, M.H.; Kraemer, R. Osmolarity Changes in Nebulizer Solutions. Eur. Respir. J. **1989**, *2*, 887–892.

45. Davis, S.S. Physico-Chemical Studies on Aerosol Solutions for Drug Delivery I. Water-Propylene Glycol Systems. Int. J. Pharm. **1978**, *1*, 71–83.

46. Newman, S.P.; Pellow, P.G.D.; Clarke, S.W. Dropsizes from Medical Atomisers (Nebulisers) for Drug Solutions with Different Viscosities and Surface Tensions. Atom. Spray Tech. **1987**, *3*, 1–11.

47. Kapustina, O.A. Effect of Surface Active Substances on Bubble Growth Kinetics in a Sound Field. Sov. Phys. Acoust. **1969**, *15*, 110–111.

48. Istiman, A.T.; Manoli, R.; Schmidt, G.H.; Holmes, R.A. An Assessment of Alveolar Deposition and Pulmonary Clearance of Radiopharmaceuticals After Nebulization. Am. J. Roentgenol. **1974**, *120*, 776–781.

49. Lin, M.S.; Hayes, T.M.; Goodwin, D.A.; Kruse, S.L. Distal Penetration in Radioaerosol Inhalation with an Ultrasonic Nebulizer. Radiology **1974**, *112*, 443–447.

50. McCallion, O.N.M.; Taylor, K.M.G.; Thomas, M.; Taylor, A.J. Nebulisation of Monodisperse Latex Sphere Suspensions in Air-Jet and Ultrasonic Nebulisers. Int. J. Pharm. **1996**, *133*, 203–214.

51. Farr, S.J.; Kellaway, I.W.; Parry-Jones, D.R.; Woolfrey, S.G. 99m-Technetium as a Marker of Liposomal Deposition and Clearance in the Human Lung. Int. J. Pharm. **1985**, *26*, 303–316.

52. Taylor, K.M.G.; Taylor, G.; Kellaway, I.W.; Stevens, J. The Influence of Liposomal Encapsulation on Sodium Cromoglycate Pharmacokinetics in Man. Pharm. Res. **1989**, *6*, 633–636.

53. Barber, R.F.; Shek, P.N. Liposome Stability during Ultrasonic Nebulization. Proceedings of the 33rd Harden Conference, The Biochemical Society: Ashford, UK, 1989; 53.

54. Leung, K.K.M.; Bridges, P.A.; Taylor, K.M.G. The Stability of Liposomes to Ultrasonic Nebulisation. Int. J. Pharm. **1996**, *145*, 95–102.

55. Ip, A.Y.; Arakawa, T.; Silvers, H.; Ransone, C.M.; Niven, R.W. Stability or Recombinant Consensus Interferon to Air-Jet and Ultrasonic Nebulization. J. Pharm. Sci. **1995**, *84*, 1210–1214.

UNIT PROCESSES IN PHARMACY: FUNDAMENTALS

Anthony J. Hickey

The University of North Carolina at Chapel Hill, Chapel Hill, North Carolina

David Ganderton

Vectora Ltd., Bath, United Kingdom

INTRODUCTION

Pharmaceutical manufacturing can be divided into a number of unit process on the basis of a few fundamental principles. The following monograph describes briefly fluid flow and heat and mass transfer.

FLUID FLOW

Fluids (liquids and gases) are a form of matter that cannot achieve equilibrium under an applied shear stress but deform continuously, or flow, as long as shear stress is applied.

Streamlines are hypothetical lines without width drawn parallel to all points to the motion of the fluid. As velocity increases, pressure decreases. Pressure field around an object is the reverse of velocity field. This may appear to contradict common experience. However, it follows from the principle of conservation of energy and finds expression in Bernoulli's theorem.

Bernoulli's Theorem

At any point in system through which a fluid is flowing, the total mechanical energy can be expressed in terms of potential energy, pressure energy, and kinetic energy.

Potential energy of a body is its capacity to do work by reason of its position relative to some center of attraction. For unit mass of fluid at a height z above some reference level, the potential energy is zg.

Pressure energy or flow energy is an energy form peculiar to the flow of fluids. The work done and the energy acquired in transferring the fluid is the product of the pressure P and the volume.

Volume of unit mass of the fluid is the reciprocal of the density ρ. For an incompressible fluid, the density is not dependent on the pressure, so for unit mass of fluid the pressure energy is P/ρ.

Kinetic energy is a form of energy possessed by a body by reason of its movement. If the mass of the body is m and

its velocity u, the kinetic energy is $1/2\, mu^2$, and for unit mass of fluid the kinetic energy is $u^2/2$.

The total mechanical energy of unit mass of fluid is therefore

$$\frac{u^2}{2} + \frac{P}{\rho} + zg$$

and proved no energy is lost or gained by the system, the mechanical energy at two points A and B is the same as that expressed by Eq. 1.

$$\frac{u_A^2}{2} + \frac{P_A}{\rho} + z_A g = \frac{u_B^2}{2} + \frac{P_B}{\rho} + z_B g \tag{1}$$

This relationship neglects the frictional degradation of mechanical energy that occurs in real systems. A fraction of the total energy is dissipated in overcoming shear stresses induced by velocity gradients in the fluid. Energy E lost during flow between A and B must be considered. The dimensions of each component are $L^2 T^{-2}$, $\text{Length}^2\,\text{Time}^{-2}$. In practice, each term is divided by g (LT^{-2}) to give the dimension of length. The terms are then referred to as velocity head, pressure head, potential head, and friction head, the sum giving the total head of the fluid as shown in Eq. 2.

$$\frac{u_A^2}{2g} + \frac{P_A}{\rho g} + z_A = \frac{u_B^2}{2g} + \frac{P_B}{\rho g} + z_B + \frac{E}{g} \tag{2}$$

The evaluation of the kinetic energy term requires consideration of the variation in velocity found in the direction normal to flow. The kinetic energy, given by the term $u_{\text{mean}}^2/2$, differs from the true kinetic energy found by summation across the flow direction. The former can be retained, however, if a correction factor a is introduced. Then

$$\text{velocity head} = \frac{u_{\text{mean}}^2}{2ga},$$

where a has a value of 0.5 in laminar flow and approaches unity in fully turbulent flow. Mechanical energy is added to the system at some point by means of a pump. The work W done, in absolute units, on a unit mass of fluid at A is given by Eq. 3.

$$\frac{W}{g} + \frac{u_A^2}{2g} + \frac{P_A}{pg} + z_A = \frac{u_B^2}{2g} + \frac{P_B}{\rho g + z_B} + \frac{E}{g} \qquad (3)$$

The power required through a system at a certain rate may be calculated using Eq. 3 to drive a liquid. The sum of heads, ΔH, being the total head against which the pump must work is therefore

$$\frac{W}{g} + H$$

If the work performed and energy acquired by unit mass of fluid is ΔHg, the power required to transfer mass m in time t is given by

$$\text{Power} = \frac{Hgm}{t}$$

As the volume flowing in unit time Q is $m/\rho t$, the power is given by Eq. 4.

$$\text{Power} = QHg\rho \qquad (4)$$

Flow Measurement

The Bernoulli theorem can also be applied to the measurement of flow rate. The passage of an incompressible fluid through a constriction results in an increase in velocity from u_1 to u_2, which is associated with a decrease in pressure from P_1 to P_2, which can be measured directly. The volumetric flow rate $Q = u_1 a_1 = u_2 a_2$ by algebraic rearrangement (which is not shown). The final linear velocity u_2 can be described by Eq. 5.

$$\frac{u_2^2}{2} - \frac{u_1^2}{2} = \frac{P_1 - P_2}{p} \qquad (5)$$

The volumetric flow rate can be described by Eq. 6.

$$Q = a_2 \sqrt{\frac{2(P_1 - P_2)}{p\left(1 - a_2^2/a_1^2\right)}} \qquad (6)$$

This derivation neglects the correction of kinetic energy loss due to nonuniformity of flow in both cross sections and the frictional degradation of energy during passage through the constriction. This is corrected by the introduction of a numerical coefficient, C_D, known as the coefficient of discharge, as shown in Eq. 6.

$$Q = C_D a_2 \sqrt{\frac{2(P_1 - P_2)}{p\left(1 - a_2^2/a_1^2\right)}}$$

The value of C_D depends on conditions of flow and shape of the constriction. For a well-shaped constriction (notably circular cross section), it would vary between 0.95 and 0.99 for turbulent flow. The value is much lower in laminar flow because the kinetic energy correction is larger. The return of the fluid to the original velocity by means of a diverging section forms a flow-measuring device known as a Venturi meter.

The Venturi meter is shown in Fig. 1(a). The converging cone leads to the narrowest cross section known as the throat. The change in pressure is measured across this part of the meter and the volumetric flow rate found by substitution into Eq. 6. Values of the coefficient of discharge are given previously. The diverging section or diffuser is designed to induce a gradual return to the original velocity. This minimizes eddy formation in the diffuser and permits the recovery of a large proportion of the increased kinetic energy as pressure energy. The permanent loss of head due to friction in both converging and diverging sections is small. The meter is therefore efficient.

When the minimization of energy degradation is less important, the gradual economic return to the original velocity may be abandoned, compensation for loss of efficiency being found in a device that is simpler, cheaper, and more adaptable than the Venturi meter. The orifice meter, to which this statement applies, consists simply of a plate with an orifice. A representation of flow through the meter is depicted in Fig. 1(b), indicating convergence of the fluid stream after passage through the orifice to give across section of minimum area called the *vena contracta*. The downstream pressure tapping is made at this cross section. The volumetric flow rate is given by Eq. 6 in which a_2 is the jet area at the *vena contracta*. The measurement of this dimension is inconvenient. It is therefore related to the area of the orifice, a_0, which can be accurately measured by the coefficient of contraction C_c by the relation $C_c = a_2/a_0$.

The coefficient of contraction, frictional losses between the tapping points, and kinetic energy corrections are absorbed in the coefficient of discharge. The volumetric flow rate is then given by Eq. 7.

$$Q = C_D a_0 \sqrt{\frac{2(P_1 - P_2)}{p\left(1 - a_0^2/a_1^2\right)}} \qquad (7)$$

If the orifice is small compared with the pipe cross section, the term $(1 - (a_0^2/a_1^2))$ approaches unity. As $P_1 - P_2 = \Delta h\rho g$, Δh being the difference in head developed by the orifice, Eq. 7 reduces to Eq. 8.

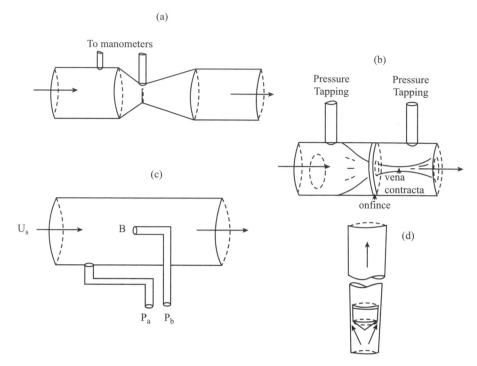

Fig. 1 (a) Venturi meter; (b) orifice meter; (c) Pitot tube; (d) rotameter.

$$Q = C_D a_0 (h\rho g)^{1/2} \qquad (8)$$

The value of C_D for the orifice meter is about 0.6, varying with construction, the ratio a_0/a_1, and flow conditions within the meter. Due to its complexity, it cannot be calculated.

After passage through the orifice, flow disturbance during retardation causes the dissipation of most of the excess kinetic energy as heat. The permanent loss of head is therefore high, increasing as the ratio of a_0/a_1 falls, ultimately reaching the differential head produced within the meter.

The Bernoulli theorem may be used to determine the change in pressure caused by retardation of fluid at the upstream side of a body immersed in a fluid stream. This principle is applied in the Pitot tube, shown in Fig. 1(c). The fluid velocity is reduced from u_a, the velocity of the fluid filament in alignment with the tube, to zero at B, an position known as the stagnation point. The pressure, P_b, is measured at this point by the method shown in Fig. 1(c). The undisturbed pressure, P_a, is measured in this example with a tapping point in the wall connected to a manometer. As the velocity at B is zero, Eq. 10 reduces to

$$\frac{u_a^2}{2} = \frac{p_b - P_a}{\rho}$$

and u_2 can be calculated. As only a local velocity is measured, variation of velocity in a section can be studied by altering the position of the tube. This procedure must be used if the flow rate in a pipe is to be measured. The mean velocity is derived from velocities measured at different distances from the wall. This derivation and the low pressure differential developed render the Pitot tube less accurate than either the venturi tube or the orifice meter for flow measurement. Hence, the tube is small in comparison with the pipe diameter and, therefore, produces no appreciable loss of head.

The rotameter (a variable area meter), shown in Fig. 1(d), is commonly used, giving a direct flow rate reading by the position of a small float in a vertical, calibrated glass tube through which the fluid is flowing. The tube is internally tapered toward the lower end so that the annulus between float and wall varies with the position of the float. Acceleration of the fluid through the annulus produces a pressure differential across the position of the float and an upward force upon it. At the equilibrium position, which may be stabilized by a slow rotation of the float, this upward force is balanced by the weight force acting on the float. If the equilibrium is disturbed by increasing the flow rate, the balance of weight force and the pressure differential are produced by movement of the float upward to a position at which the area of the annulus is bigger. For accurate measurement, the rotameter is calibrated with the fluid to be metered. Its use is, however, restricted to that fluid.

Laminar and Turbulent Flow

The nature of flow may be examined by introducing a dye into the axis of the tube. At low speeds, the dye forms a coherent thread, which grows very little in thickness with distance down the tube. However, with progressive increase in speed, the line of dye begin to waver and then break up. Secondary motions crossing and recrossing the general flow direction occur. Finally, at very high speeds, no filament of dye is detected and mixing is instantaneous. In this experiment, flow changes from laminar to turbulent, the change occurring at a critical speed. Generalizing, in laminar flow, the instantaneous velocity at a point is always the same as the mean velocity in both magnitude and direction. In turbulent flow, order is lost and irregular motions are imposed upon the main steady motion of the fluid. At any instant of time, the fluid velocity at a point varies in both magnitude and direction, having components perpendicular as well as parallel to the direction of net flow. Over a period of time, these fluctuations even out to give the net velocity in the direction of flow.

In turbulent flow, rapidly fluctuating velocities produce high velocity gradients within the fluid. Proportionately large shear stresses are developed, and to overcome them, mechanical energy is degraded and dissipated in the form of heat. The degradation of energy in laminar flow is much smaller.

The turbulent mechanism that carries motion, heat, or matter from one part of the fluid to another is absent in laminar flow. The agency of momentum transfer is the shear stress arising from the variations in velocity, that is, the viscosity. Similarly, heat and matter can only be transferred across streamlines on a molecular scale, heat by conduction and matter by diffusion. These mechanisms that are present but less important in turbulent flow are comparatively slow. Velocity, temperature, and concentration gradients are, therefore, much higher than in turbulent flow.

The Flow of Liquids in Pipes

The many pharmaceutical processes that involve the transfer of a liquid confer great importance on the study of flow in pipes. This study permits the evaluation of pressure loss due to friction in a simple pipe and assesses the additional effects of pipe roughness, changes in diameter, bends, exists, and entrances. When the total pressure drop due to friction is known for the system, the equivalent head

can be derived and the power requirement for driving a liquid through the system can be calculated from Eq. 9.

Streamline flow in a tube

The mathematical analysis of streamline flow in a simple tube results in the expression known as Poiseuille's law, one form of which is Eq. 9.

$$Q = \frac{P\pi d^4}{128\eta l} \tag{9}$$

where Q is the volumetric flow rate or discharge, ΔP is the pressure drop across the tube, d and l are the diameter and length of the tube, respectively, and η is the viscosity of the fluid.

Where flow in the tube is streamline or turbulent, an infinitesimally thin stationary layer is found at the wall. The velocity increases from zero at this point to a maximum at the axis of the tube. The velocity profile of streamline flow is shown in Fig. 9(a). The velocity gradient du/dr varies from a maximum at the wall to zero at the axis. In flow through a tube, the rate of shear is equal to the velocity gradient, and Eq. 1 dictates the same variation of shear stress.

To derive Poiseuille's law, the form of the velocity profile must first be established. For a fluid contained within a radius r flowing in a tube of radius R, the pressure drop across length l is ΔP; therefore, the pressure force driving this section is $\Delta P \pi r^2$. If the flow is steady, this force can only be balanced by opposing viscous forces acting on the "wall" of the section. This force is

$$\tau = \frac{Pr}{2l}$$

Substituting for Eq. 1 gives

$$-\frac{du}{dr} = \frac{Pr}{2\eta l}$$

The velocity gradient is negative because u decreases as r increases. If $r = R$, then $u = 0$. Integration gives

$$\int_0^u du = \frac{P}{2\eta l} \int_R^r r \, dr$$

Therefore, Eq. 10 can be written as

$$u = \frac{P}{2\eta l} \left(\frac{R^2 - r^2}{2} \right) \tag{10}$$

This relation shows that the velocity distribution across the tube is parabolic. For such a distribution, the maximum velocity is twice the mean velocity.

The volumetric flow rate across an annular section between *r and (r + dr)* is given by

$$Q = 2\pi r \, dr \, r.$$

Substituting for *u* for Eq. 10 gives

$$Q = \frac{P\pi}{2\eta l}(R^2 r - r^2) r \, dr$$

The total volumetric flow rate is the integral between the limits *r = R* and *r = 0*:

$$Q = \frac{P\pi}{2\eta l}\int_0^R (R^2 r - r^3)dr = \frac{P\pi}{2\eta l}R^2\left(\frac{r^2}{\frac{2-r^4}{4}}\right)_o^R$$

Therefore Eq. 9 is valid:

$$Q = \frac{P\pi R^4}{8\eta l} = \frac{P\pi d^4}{128\eta l}$$

where *d* is the diameter of the tube.

As $Q = u_{mean}\pi(d2/4)$, substitution and rearrangement gives Eq. 11.

$$P = \frac{32 u_{mean}\eta l}{d^2} \tag{11}$$

The Significance of Reynolds Number *Re*

The Reynolds number describes the ratio of the inertia and viscous or frictional forces. Higher the Reynolds number, greater is the relative contribution of inertial effects. At very low *Re*, viscous effects predominate and the contribution of inertial forces can be ignored.

Calculation of the Pressure Drop in a Pipe Due to Friction

If the volumetric flow rate of a liquid of density ρ and viscosity η through a pipe of diameter *d* is *Q*, the derivation of the mean velocity *u* from the flow rate and pipe area completes the data required for calculating *Re*. If the pipe roughness factor is known, the equivalent value of $R/\rho u^2$ can be read from Fig. 2, and the shear stress at the pipe wall calculated. The total frictional force opposing motion is the product of *R* and the surface area of the pipe, π*dl*, where *l* is the length of the pipe. If the unknown pressure drop across the pipe is Δ*P*, the force driving through the pipe is Δ*P*· π*d²*/4. Equating pressure force and frictional force,

$$P = \frac{\pi d^2}{4} = R\pi dl$$

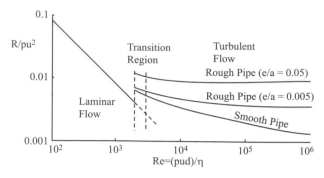

Fig. 2 Pipe friction chart $R/\rho u^2$ versus *Re*.

Therefore, Eq. 12 follows.

$$P = \frac{4Rl^2}{d} \tag{12}$$

Division by ρg gives the pressure loss as a friction head.

Flow in Tubes of Noncircular Cross Section

The foregoing arguments may be applied to turbulent flow in noncircular ducts by introducing a dimension equivalent to the diameter of a circular pipe. This is known as the mean hydraulic diameter, d_m, which is defined as four times the cross-sectional area divided by the wetted perimeter. The following examples are given:

For a square channel of side *b*,

$$d_m = \frac{4b^2}{4b} = b.$$

For an annulus of outer radius r_1 and inner radius r_2,

$$\frac{4(\pi r_2^1 - \pi r_2^2)}{2\pi r_1 + 2\pi r_2} = 2(r_1 - r_2)$$

This simple modification does not apply to laminar flow in noncircular ducts.

Frictional Losses at Pipe Fittings

In addition to the friction losses at the wall of a straight pipe, losses occur at the various fittings and valves used in practical systems. In general, these losses are derived from sudden changes in the magnitude or direction of flow induced by changes in geometry. They can be classified as losses due to a sudden contraction of enlargement, losses at entrance or exit, and losses due to pipe curvature. Losses can be conveniently expressed as a length of straight pipe offering the same resistance. This is usually in the form of a number of pipe diameters. For example, the loss at a right-angled elbow is equivalent to the length of a straight pipe equal to 40 diameters. The sum of the equivalent lengths of all fittings and vales is then added to the actual pipe length and the total frictional loss estimated by Eq. 20.

Motion of Bodies in a Fluid

Viscous and inertial forces operate to determine the flow pattern and drag force on a body moving relative to a fluid. The Reynolds number, which expresses their ratio, is used as a parameter to predict flow behavior. The relation between the drag force and its controlling variables is presented in a manner similar to that employed for flow in a pipe. Considering a sphere moving relative to a fluid, the projected area normal to flow is $\pi d^2/4$, where d is the diameter of the sphere. The drag force acting on the unit projected area R' is determined by the velocity u, the viscosity η, and the density ρ of the fluid and the diameter of the sphere d. Dimensional analysis yields Eq. 13.

$$\frac{R}{\rho u^2} = f(Re) = f\left(\frac{ud\rho}{\eta}\right) \tag{13}$$

This form of Reynolds number, Re', employs the diameter of the sphere as the linear dimensions.

With the exception of an analysis at very low Re. values, the form of this function is established by experiment. Results are presented on logarithmic coordinates in Fig. 3. When Re' is less than about 0.2,

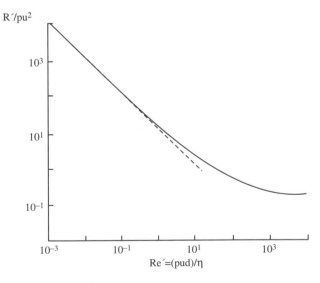

R´/pu²

10^3

10^1

10^{-1}

10^{-3} 10^{-1} 10^1 10^3

Re´=(pud)/η

Fig. 3 $R'/\rho u^2$ versus Re' number for a smooth sphere.

viscous forces are solely responsible for drag on the sphere and Eq. 13 becomes

$$\frac{R}{\rho u^2} = \frac{12}{Re}$$

Therefore,

$$\text{Total drag force} = R\frac{\pi d^2}{4} = \rho u_2 \frac{12}{Re}\frac{\pi d^2}{4} = 3\pi\eta du \tag{14}$$

This is the normal form of Stokes law.

At larger Re' values, the experimental curve progressively diverges from this relation, ultimately becoming independent of Re' and giving a value of $R/\rho u^2$ equal to about 0.22. As Re' increases, the form drag increases, ultimately becoming solely responsible for the force opposing motion.

For nonspherical particles, the analysis employs the diameter of a sphere of equivalent volume. A correction factor, which depends upon the shape of the body and its orientation in the fluid, must be applied.

An important application of this analysis is the estimation of the speed at which particles settle in a fluid. Under the action of gravity, the particle accelerates until the weight force mg is exactly balanced by the opposing drag. The body then falls at a constant terminal velocity u. Equating weight and drag forces gives Eq. 15.

$$mg = \frac{\pi}{6}d^3(\rho_s - \rho)g = R\frac{\pi d^2}{4} \tag{15}$$

where ρ is the density of the particle.

For a sphere falling under streamline conditions (Re' 0.2), $R' = \rho u^2 (12/Re')$. Substituting in Eq. 15 gives Eq. 16.

$$u = \frac{d^2(\rho_s - \rho)g}{18\eta} \tag{16}$$

This expression follows more simply from the equation $mg - 3\pi d\eta u$.

Flow of Fluids Through Packed Beds

The analysis of the flow of fluids through a permeable bed of solids is widely applied in filtration, leaching, and several other processes. A first approach may be made by assuming that the interstices of the bed correspond to a large number of discrete, parallel capillaries. If the flow is streamline, the volumetric flow rate Q is given for a single capillary by Eq. 14:

$$Q = \frac{P\pi d^4}{128\eta l}$$

where l is the length of the capillary and d its diameter, ΔP is the pressure drop across the capillary, and η is the viscosity of the fluid. The length of the capillary exceeds the depth of the bed by a value that depends upon its tortuosity. The depth of bed, L, is however, proportional to the capillary length l so that

$$Q = \frac{Pd^4}{k\eta L},$$

where k is a constant for a particular bed. If the area of the bed is A and it contains n capillaries per unit area, the total flow rate is given by

$$Q = \frac{Pd^4 nA}{k\eta L}$$

Both n and d are not normally known. However, they have certain values for a given bed, expressed by Eq. 17.

$$Q = KA \frac{P}{\eta L} \qquad (17)$$

where $K = d^4 n/k$. This constant is a permeability coefficient and its reciprocal, $1/K$, is the specific resistance. Its value characterizes a particular bed.

The postulate of discrete capillaries precludes valid comment on the factors that determine the permeability coefficient. Channels are not discrete but are interconnected in a random manner. Nevertheless, the resistance to the passage of fluid must depend on the number and dimensions of the channels. These can be expressed in terms of the fraction of the bed which is void, that is, the porosity, and the manner in which the void fraction is distributed. Illustrating this reference to a specific example, water would flow more easily through a bed with a porosity of 40% than through a bed of the same material with a porosity of 25%. It would also flow more quickly through a bed of coarse particles than through a bed of fine particles packed to the void fraction or porosity. The latter effect can be expressed in terms of the surface area offered to the fluid by the bed. This property is inversely proportional to the size of the particles forming the bed. Permeability increases as the porosity increases and the total surface of the bed decreases and these factors may be combined to give the hydraulic diameter d' of an equivalent channel. This is defined by:

$$d = \frac{\text{Volume of voids}}{\text{Total surface of material forming bed}}$$

The volume of voids is the porosity, and the volume of solids is $(1 - \varepsilon)$. If the specific surface area, that is, the surface area of unit volume of solids, is S_0, the total surface presented by unit volume of the bed is $S_0(1 - \varepsilon)$.

Therefore, Eq. 18 applies.

$$d = \frac{\varepsilon}{S_0(1 - \varepsilon)} \qquad (18)$$

Under streamline conditions, the rate at which a fluid flows through this equivalent channel is given by Poiseuille's Eq. 14.

The velocity u' in the channel is derived by dividing the volumetric flow rate by the area of the channel, $k'd'^2$. Combining the constants,

$$u = \frac{Q}{kd^2} = \frac{Pd^2}{k\eta L}$$

This velocity, when averaged over the entire area of the bed, solids, and voids, gives the lower value u. These velocities are related by

$$u = u\varepsilon$$

Therefore:

$$\frac{u}{\varepsilon} = \frac{Pd^2}{k\eta L}$$

Substituting for d' by means of Eq. 18 gives

$$\frac{u}{\varepsilon} = \frac{P}{k\eta L} \frac{\varepsilon^2}{(1 - \varepsilon)^2 S_0^2}$$

and Eq. 19.

$$u = \frac{P}{-k\eta L} \frac{\varepsilon^3}{(1 - \varepsilon)^2 S_0^2} \qquad (19)$$

In this equation, known after its originator as Kozeny's equation, the constant k'' has a value of 5 ± 0.5. As $Q = uA$, where A is the area of the bed, Eq. 19 can be transformed to Eq. 20.

$$Q = \frac{PA}{\eta L} \cdot \frac{\varepsilon^3}{5(1 - \varepsilon)^2 S_0^2} \qquad (20)$$

This analysis shows that permeability is a complex function of porosity and surface area, the latter being determined by the size distribution and shape of the particles. The appearance of specific surface in Eq. 20 offers a method for its measurement and provides the basis of fluid permeation methods of size analysis. This equation also applies in the studies of filtration.

Pumps

Eqs. 8 and 9 examine the power requirement for driving a liquid through a system against an opposing head. This energy is normally generated by a pump. In different processes, the quantities to be delivered, the opposing head, and the nature of the fluid vary widely, and many pumps are made to meet these differing requirements. Basically, however, pumps can be divided into positive-displacement pumps, which may be reciprocating or rotary, and impeller pumps. Positive-displacement pumps seek to displace a fixed volume of fluid with each stroke or revolution; impeller pumps, on the other hand, impart high kinetic energy to the fluid which is subsequently converted to pressure energy. The volume discharged depends upon the opposing head.

The equipment for pumping gases and liquids is essentially similar. Machines delivering gases are commonly called compressors or blowers; compressors discharge at relatively high pressures and blowers at relatively low pressures. The lower density and viscosity of gases results in higher operating speeds and, to minimize leakage, smaller clearance between moving parts.

HEAT TRANSFER

Heat transfer in process vessels has been described previously in this encyclopedia (1). The following is a more complete review of heat transfer as a unit operation in pharmacy. Heat energy can only be transferred from a region of higher to a region of lower temperature. Understanding heat transfer requires the study of the mechanism and rate of this process.

Heat is transferred by three mechanisms: conduction, convection, and radiation. It is unusual for the transfer to take place by one mechanism only.

Conduction is the most widely understood mechanism of heat transfer and the main method in solids. The flow of heat depends upon the transfer of vibrational energy from one molecule to another and, in the case of metals, the movement of free electrons. Radiation is rare in solids but examples are found among glasses and plastics. Convection by definition, is not possible under these conditions. Conduction in the bulk of fluids is normally overshadowed by convection, but it assumes great importance at fluid boundaries.

Heat is transferred from or to a region by the motion of fluids and the phenomenon of convection. In natural convection, the movement is caused by buoyancy forces induced by variations in the density of the fluid; these variations are caused by differences in temperature. In forced convection, movement is created by an external agency such as a pump.

All bodies with a temperature above absolute zero radiate heat in the form of electromagnetic waves.

The radiation may be transmitted, reflected, or absorbed by matter, the fraction absorbed being transformed into heat. Radiation is of great importance at very high or very low temperatures and under circumstances in which the other modes of heat transmission are suppressed. Although the heat losses can, in some cases, equal the losses by natural convection, the mechanism is, from the standpoint of pharmaceutical processing, least important and needs only brief consideration.

Heat transfer in many systems occurs as a steady-state process, and the temperature at any point in the system does not vary with time. In other important processes, temperatures in the system do vary with time. This situation, which is common among the small-scale, batch-operated processes of the pharmaceutical and fine chemical industry, is known as unsteady heat transfer and, as warming or cooling occurs, the thermal capacity (i.e., the size and specific heat), of the system becomes important. Analysis of unsteady heat transfer is complex.

Heat Transfer Through a Wall

Heat transfer by conduction through walls follows the basic relation given by Fourier's equation (Eg. 21), which states that the rate of heat flow, Q, is proportional to the temperature gradient, dT/dx, and to the area normal to the heat flow, A.

$$Q = -kA\frac{dT}{dx} \tag{21}$$

As the distance x increases, the temperature T decreases. Hence, measuring in the x direction, the temperature gradient, dT/dx, is algebraically negative. The proportionality constant k is the thermal conductivity. Its numerical value depends on the material of which the body is made and on its temperature.

Metals exhibit high conductivity, although values vary widely. Nonmetallic solids normally have lower conductivities than do metals. For the porous materials of this group, the overall conductivity lies between that of the homogeneous solid and the air that permeates the structure. Low resultant values lead to wide use as heat insulators. Carbon is an exception among nonmetals. Its relatively high conductivity and chemical inertness permit its wide use in heat exchangers.

Steady nondirectional heat transfer through a plane wall of thickness x and area A is represented in Fig. 4(a). Assuming that thermal conductivity does not change with temperature, the temperature gradient is linear and equal to $(T_1 - T_2)/x$, where T_1 is the temperature of the hot face and

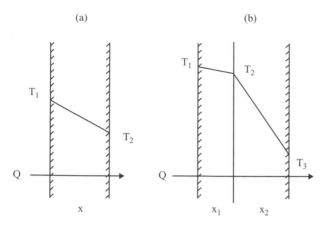

Fig. 4 Conduction of heat through (a) a plane wall and (b) a composite wall.

T_2 the temperature of the cool face. Eq. 21 then becomes Eq. 22

$$Q = kA \frac{T_1 - T_2}{x} \qquad (22)$$

This may be rearranged to Eq. 23

$$Q = A \frac{T_1 - T_2}{x/k} \qquad (23)$$

where x/k is the thermal resistance. Thus, for a given heat flow, a large temperature drop must be created if the wall or layer has a high thermal resistance.

Conversely, the heat flow promoted by a given temperature difference is reduced if the thermal resistance is increased. This is the principle of insulation by lagging, and it is illustrated by a composite wall, as shown in Fig. 4(b). If steady-state heat transfer exists, the rate of heat transfer is the same for both materials. Therefore,

$$Q = \frac{k_1 A (T_1 - T_2)}{x_1} = \frac{k_2 A (T_2 - T_3)}{x_2}$$

The major temperature drop occurs across the distance x_2, indicating that this material provides the major thermal resistance. (In the case of heavily lagged, thin metal walls, the temperature drop and thermal resistance of the metal are so small that they can be ignored). Rearrangement of this equation and the elimination of the junction temperature gives Eq. 24.

$$Q = A \frac{(T_1 - T_2)}{(x_1/k_1 + x_2/k_2)} \qquad (24)$$

Equations of this form can be applied to any number of layers.

Heat Transfer in Pipes and Tubes

Pipes and tubes are common as barriers over which heat exchange takes place. Conduction is complicated in this case by the changes in the area over which heat is transferred. If Eq. 21 is to be retained, some value of A must be derived from the length of the pipe, l, and the internal and external radii, r_1 and r_2, respectively. If the pipe is thin-walled and the ratio r_2/r_1 is less than approximately 1.5, the heat transfer area can be based on an arithmetic mean of the two radii, and Eq. 21 becomes Eq. 25.

$$Q = k 2\pi \frac{r_2 + r_1}{2} l \frac{T_1 - T_2}{r_2 - r_1} \qquad (25)$$

This equation is inaccurate for thick-walled pipes, where the heat transfer area must be based on a logarithmic mean radius r_m. Heat transfer is then expressed by Eq. 26

$$Q = k 2\pi r_{ml} \frac{T_1 - T_2}{r_2 - r_1} \qquad (26)$$

where

$$r_m \frac{r_2 - r_1}{\log_e \frac{r_2}{r_1}}$$

Heat Exchange Between a Fluid and a Solid Boundary

Conduction and convection contribute to the transfer of heat from a fluid to a boundary. The distribution of temperatures at a plane barrier separating two fluids may be considered. If the fluids are turbulent motion, temperature gradients are confined to a relatively narrow region adjacent to the wall. Outside this region, turbulent mixing, the mechanism of which has been explained earlier, is very effective in the transfer of heat. Temperature gradients are quickly destroyed and equalization at values T_1 and T_2 occurs. Within the region, there exists a laminar sublayer across which heat is transferred by conduction only. The temperature gradients produced by a given heat flow are correspondingly high. Outside the laminar layer, eddies contribute to the transfer of heat by moving fluid from the turbulent bulk to the edge of the sublayer, where heat can be lost or gained, and by corresponding movements in the opposite direction. The temperature gradients in this region, where both convection and conduction contribute to heat transfer, are smaller than in the sublayer.

The major resistance to the flow of heat resides in the laminar sublayer. Its thickness, therefore, is of critical importance in determining the rate of heat transfer from the fluid to the boundary. It depends on the physical properties of the fluid, the flow conditions, and the nature of the surface. Increase in flow velocity, for example, decreases the thickness of the layer and, therefore, its resistance to heat flow.

To evaluate the rate of heat transfer at a boundary, a film, transmitting heat only by conduction is postulated. This fictitious film presents the same resistance to heat transfer as the complex turbulent and laminar regions near the wall. If on the hot side of the wall the fictitious layer had a thickness x_1, the equation of heat transfer to the wall would be

$$Q = kA\frac{T_1 - T_{1\,\text{wall}}}{x_1}$$

where k is the thermal conductivity of the fluid. A similar equation applies to heat transfer at the cold side of the wall. The thickness of the layer is determined by the same factors that control the extent of the laminar sublayer. In general the layer thickness is not known and the above equation is rewritten as Eq. 27.

$$Q = h_1 A(T_1 - T_{1\,\text{wall}}) \tag{27}$$

where h_1 is the heat-transfer coefficient for the film under discussion. It corresponds to the ratio k/x_1 and is the Btu/ft^2 · h · °F. It is a convenient numerical expression of heat flow by conduction and convection at a boundary. The approximate evaluation of these coefficients is discussed later.

The film coefficient h_2 may be used to characterize heat transfer from the barrier to the colder fluid.

$$T_1 - T_{1\,\text{wall}} = \frac{Q}{h_1 A} \qquad T_{1\,\text{wall}} - T_{2\,\text{wall}} = \frac{Qx_{\text{w}}}{h_{\text{w}}A}$$

where k_{w} is the thermal conductivity of the wall, and

$$T_{2\,\text{wall}} - T_2 = \frac{Q}{h_2 A}$$

Addition and rearrangement of these equations gives Eq. 28.

$$Q = \frac{A}{(1/h_1 + x_{\text{w}}/k_{\text{w}} + 1/h_2)}(T_1 - T_2) \tag{28}$$

The quantity

$$\frac{1}{(1/h_1 + x_{\text{w}}/k_{\text{w}} + 1/h_2)}$$

is called the overall heat-transfer coefficient U. A general expression of the rate of heat transfer then becomes Eq. 29.

$$Q = UAT \tag{29}$$

or

$$\frac{ql}{Tk} = \text{constant}\left(\frac{l^3 Tag\rho^2}{\eta^2}\right)\left(\frac{C_p\eta}{k}\right)^q \tag{30}$$

Heat transfer by free convection can thus be presented as a relation between three dimensionless groups: $C_p\eta/K$ is known as the Prandtl number, the combination $l_3\Delta Tag\rho^2/\eta^2$ as the Grashof number, and $ql/\Delta T$, the Nusselt number may also be written hl/k.

The specific relation in which these groups stand is established for a particular system experimentally.

The fluid properties, C_p, k, η, and ρ are themselves temperature dependent. In establishing a correlation, the temperature at which these properties are to be measured must be chosen. This is usually the temperature of the main body of the fluid or the mean of this temperature and the temperature of the surface.

The exponents r and q are usually found experimentally to be equal to 0.25 in streamline flow and 0.33 in turbulent flow. The constant varies with the configuration. As an example, the heat transfer to gases and liquids from a large horizontal pipe by free convection is described by Eq. 31.

$$\frac{qd}{kT} = 0.47\left(\frac{d^3 Tag\rho^2}{\eta^2}\right)\left(\frac{C_p\eta}{k}\right)^{0.25} \tag{31}$$

The linear dimension in this correlation is the pipe diameter d. The fluid properties are to be measured at the mean of the wall and bulk fluid temperatures.

In forced convection, the fluid is moved over the surface by a pump or blower neglecting natural convection are usually neglected. The study of forced convection is of great practical importance and vast amount of data have been amassed for streamline and turbulent flow in pipes, across and parallel to tubes, across plane surfaces, and in other important configurations such as jackets and coils.

In forced convection, the heat transferred per unit area per unit time q, is determined by a linear dimension which characterizes the surface l, the temperature difference between the surface and the fluid, ΔT, the viscosity η, the density ρ, and the velocity u, of the fluid, its conductivity k, and its specific heat C_p. Dimensional analysis yields Eq. 32

$$\frac{qd}{kT} = \text{constant}\left(\frac{C_p\eta}{k}\right)^x\left(\frac{u l\rho}{\eta}\right)^y \tag{32}$$

where ql/kT is the Nusselt number, Nu, $C_p\eta/k$ is the Prandtl number, Pr, and $ul\rho/\eta$ is the Reynolds number, Re, a parameter discussed previously. The values of the indices, x and y and of the constant are established for a particular system experimentally. In the case of turbulent flow in pipes, the correlation for fluids of low viscosity is given by Eq. 33.

$$Nu = 0.023 \, Pr^x Re^{0.8} \qquad (33)$$

where x has the value 0.4 for heating and 0.3 for cooling. The linear dimension used to calculate Re or Nu is the pipe diameter, and the physical properties of the fluid are to be measured at the bulk fluid temperature. This relation shows that in a given system, the film coefficient varies as the fluid velocity$^{0.8}$. If the flow velocity is doubled, the film coefficient increases by a factor of 1.7.

Heat Transfer to Boiling Liquids

Heat transfer to boiling liquids occurs in a number of operations, for example, distillation and evaporation. Heat is transferred by both conduction and convection in a process further complicated by the phase change that occurs at the heating boundary. When boiling is induced by a heater in contact with a pool of liquid, the process is known as pool boiling. Liquid movement is derived only from heating effects. In other systems, the boiling liquid may be driven through or over heaters, a process referred to as boiling with forced circulation.

Pool boiling

If a horizontal heating surface is in contact with a boiling liquid, a sequence of events occurs as the temperature difference between the surface and the liquid increases.

When ΔT is small, the degree of superheating of the liquid layers adjacent to the surface is low and bubble formation (growth and disengagement), if present, is slow. Liquid disturbance is small and heat transfer can be estimated from expressions for natural convection given, for example, in Eq. 29.

Vapor formation becomes more vigorous and bubble chains rise from points that progressively increase in number and finally merge. This movement increases liquid circulation. This phase is called nucleate boiling and is the practically important regime. A peak flux occurs and a maximum heat-transfer coefficient is obtained. At this point, ΔT is known as the critical temperature drop. For water, the value lies between 40 and 50°F (4–10°C). The critical temperature drop for organic liquids is somewhat higher. Beyond the critical temperature, vapor formation is so rapid that escape is inadequate and a progressively larger fraction of the heating surface becomes covered with a vapor film. This represents a transition from nucleate boiling to film boiling. When this transition is complete, the vapor entirely covers the surface, film boiling is fully established, and the heat flux rises again.

The low heat-transfer coefficient renders film boiling undesirable and equipment is designed for and operated at temperature differences which are less than the critical temperature drop. If a constant temperature heat source such as steam or hot liquid is employed, exceeding the critical temperature drop results simply in a drop in heat flux and process efficiency. If, however, a constant heat-input source is used, as in electrical heating, decreasing heat flux as the transition region is entered causes a sudden and possibly damaging increase in the temperature of the heating element; such damage is known as boiling burn-out.

Boiling heat-transfer coefficients depend upon both the physical character of the liquid and the nature of the heating surface. Through the agencies of wetting, roughness, and contamination, the latter greatly influences the formation, growth, and disengagement of bubbles in the nucleate boiling regime. There is, at present, no reliable method of estimating the boiling coefficients of heat transfer from the physical properties of the system.

Boiling inside a vertical tube

Heat transfer to liquids boiling in vertical tubes is common in evaporators. If a long tube of suitable diameter in which liquid lies at a low level is heated, the pattern of boiling is established Fig. 5. At low levels, boiling may be suppressed by the imposed head [Fig. 5(a)]. Higher in the tube, bubbles are produced, which rise and coalesce [Fig. 5(b)]. Slug formation due to bubble coagulation occurs [Fig. 5(c) and 5(d)]. The slugs finally break down [Fig. 5(e)]. Escape is hindered and both liquid and vapor move upward at an increasing speed. Draining leads to separation of the phases, giving an annular film of liquid dragged upward by a core of high velocity vapor [Fig. 5(f)]. In long tubes, the main heat transfer takes place in this region by either forced convection or nucleate boiling. At low temperature differences between wall and film, heat transfer occurs quietly as in forced convection. This is the normal regime in a climbing film evaporator and heat flux can be calculated from correlations of the type given in Eq. 40. At high temperatures differences, nucleate boiling takes place in the film and the vigorous movement leads to an increase in heat transfer coefficient.

Boiling with forced circulation

In many systems, movements other than those caused by boiling are imposed. For example, boiling in agitated vessels is common in many batch processes. The boiling heat-transfer coefficients depend upon the properties of the liquid, the nature of the surface, and the agitation. The coefficients obtained are slightly higher than those of pool boiling. Inside the tubes, the pattern of forced circulation

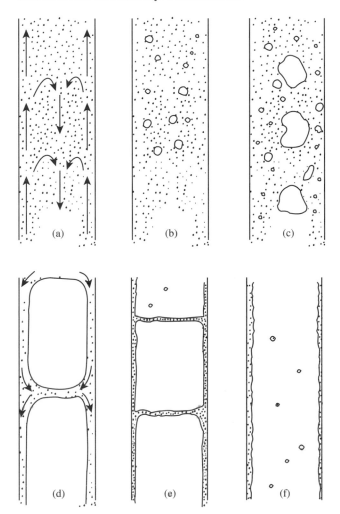

Fig. 5 Boiling in a narrow vertical tube. (a) Boiling suppressed by head, natural convection is shown; (b) bubble formation; (c) slug formation due to bubble coagulation; (d) fully developed slug flow; (e) breakdown of slugs at high vapor rates; (f) annular-flow-climbing film.

boiling is similar to that described in the previous section. Coefficients, however, are higher because the velocities attained are higher.

Heat Transfer from Condensing Vapors

When a saturated vapor is brought into contact with a cool surface, heat is transferred to the surface and a liquid condenses. The vapor may consists of a single substance or a mixture, some components of which may be noncondensable.

The process is described by the following sequence. The vapor diffuses to the boundary where actual condensation takes place. In most cases, the condensate

forms a continuous layer over the cooling surface, draining under the influence of gravity. This is known as film condensation. The latent heat liberated is transferred through the film to the surface by conduction. Although this film offers considerable resistance to heat flow, film coefficients are usually high.

Dropwise condensation

Under some surface conditions, the condensate does not form a continuous film. Droplets are formed which grow, coalesce, and then run from the surface. As a fraction of the surface is always directly exposed to the vapor, film resistance is absent, and heat-transfer coefficients, which may be ten times those of film condensation, are obtained. This process is known as dropwise condensation. Although highly desirable, its occurrence, which depends upon the wettability of the surface, is not predictable and cannot be used as a basis for design.

Condensation of a pure vapor

For film condensation, a theoretical analysis of the laminar flow of a liquid film down an inclined surface and the progressive increase in thickness due to condensation yields Eq. 34 for the mean-transfer coefficient h_m

$$h_m = \text{constant} \left(\frac{\rho^2 k^3 \lambda g}{T \eta x} \right)^{0.25} \tag{34}$$

where λ is the latent heat of vaporization; ρ, k, and η are the density, thermal conductivity, and viscosity of the liquid, respectively; ΔT is the difference in temperature between the surface and vapor. Experimentally determined coefficients confirm the validity of Eq. 34. In practice, however, the coefficients are somewhat higher due to disturbance of the film arising from a number of actors. As the condensation rate rises, the thickness of the condensate layer increases and the film coefficient falls. However, a point may be reached in long vertical tubes at which flow in the layer becomes turbulent. Under these conditions, the coefficient rises again and Eq. 34 is not valid. Coefficients may also be increased if high vapor velocities induce ripples in the film.

Condensation of mixed vapors

If a mixture of condensable and noncondensable gases is cooled below its dew point at a surface, the former condenses, leaving the adjacent layers richer in the latter, thus creating an added thermal resistance. The condensable fraction must diffuse through this layer to reach the film of condensate and heat-transfer coefficients are normally very much lower than the corresponding value for the pure vapor. For example, the presence of 0.5% of air has been found to reduce the heat transfer by condensation of steam by as much as 50%.

Heat Transfer by Radiation

Of the radiation that falls on a body, a fraction a is absorbed, a fraction r is reflected, and a fraction t is transmitted. These fractions are called absorptivity, reflectivity, and transitivity, respectively. Most industrial solids are opaque such that the transmissivity is zero and Eq. 35 holds.

$$a + r = 1 \tag{35}$$

Reflectivity, and therefore, absorptivity depend greatly on the nature of the surface. The limiting case, that of a body which absorbs all and reflects none of the incident radiation, is called a black body.

Exchange of radiation

The exchange of radiation is based upon two laws. The first, known as Kirchoff's law, states that the ratio of the emissive power to the absorptivity is same for all bodies in thermal equilibrium. The emissive power of a body, E, is the radiant energy emitted from unit area in unit time. A body of area A_1 and emissivity E_1, therefore, emits energy at a rate $E_1 A_1$. If the radiation falling on unit area of the body is E_b, the rate of energy absorption is $E_b a_1 A_1$, where a_1 is the absorptivity. At thermal equilibrium, $E_b a_1 A_1$. For another body in the same environment, $E_b a_1 A_2 = E_2 A_2$, leading to Eq. 36

$$E_b = \frac{E_1}{a_1} = \frac{E_2}{a_2} \tag{36}$$

For a black body, $a = 1$. The emissive power is therefore E_b. The black body is a perfect radiator and is used as the comparative standard for other surfaces. The emissivity e of a surface is defined as the ratio of the emissive power E of the surface to the emissive power of a black body at the same temperature E_b, as shown by Eq. 37.

$$e = \frac{E}{E_b} \tag{37}$$

Emissivity is numerically equal to absorptivity. As emissive power varies with wavelength, the ratio should be quoted at a particular wavelength for many materials. However, the emissive power is a constant fraction of the black body radiation, that is, the emissivity is constant. These materials are known as gray bodies.

The second fundamental law of radiation, known as the Stefan–Boltzmann law, states that the rate of energy emission from a black body is proportional to the fourth power of the absolute temperature T, as shown by Eq. 38

$$E = \sigma T^4 \tag{38}$$

where E is the total emissive power and σ is the Stefan–Boltzmann constant. It is sufficiently accurate to say that the heat emitted in unit time Q from a black body of area A is given by

$$Q = \sigma A T^4$$

and for a body that is not perfectly black by Eq. 39

$$Q = \sigma e A T^4 \tag{39}$$

where e is the emissivity.

The net energy gained or lost by a body can be estimated by these laws. The simplest case is that of a gray body in black surroundings. These conditions, in which none of the energy emitted by the body is reflected back, are approximately those of a body radiating to atmosphere. If the absolute temperature of the body is T_1, the rate of heat loss is $\sigma e A T_4^1$ (Eq. 40), where A is the area of the body and e its emissivity. Surroundings at a temperature T_2 emit radiation proportional to σT_4^2, and a fraction, determined by area and absorptivity a, is absorbed by the body; this heat is $\sigma a A T_4^2$, and as absorptivity and emissivity are equal, Eq. 40 is valid.

$$\text{Net heat-transfer rate} = \sigma e A (T_1^4 - T_2^4) \tag{40}$$

If part of the energy emitted by a surface is reflected back by another surface, the calculation of radiation exchange is more complex. Equations for various surface configurations take the following general form:

$$Q = F_1 F_2 \sigma A (T_A^4 - T_B^4)$$

where F_1 and F_2 are factors determined by the configuration and emissivity of surfaces at temperatures T_A and T_B.

MASS TRANSFER

Mass transfer in unit operations has been described in detail previously in this encyclopedia (2). the following is a brief review to complete the overview of unit processes in pharmacy.

In mass transfer operations, two immiscible phases are normally present, one or both of which are fluid. In general, these phases are in relative movement and the rate at which a component is transferred from one phase to the other is greatly influenced by the bulk movement imposed upon the fluids. In most drying processes, for example, water vapor diffuses from a saturated layer in contact with the drying surface into a turbulent air stream. The boundary layer, as described earlier, consists of a sublayer in which flow is laminar and an outer region in which flow is turbulent. The mechanism of diffusion differs in these regimes. In the laminar layer, movement of water vapor molecules across streamlines can occur only by molecular diffusion. In the turbulent region, the movement of relatively large units of gas, called eddies, from one region to another causes mixing of the components of the gas. This is called eddy diffusion. Eddy diffusion is a more rapid process and although molecular diffusion is still present, its contribution to the overall movement of material is small. In still air, eddy diffusion is virtually absent and evaporation occurs by molecular diffusion.

Molecular Diffusion of Gases

Transport of material in stagnant fluids or across streamlines of a fluid in laminar flow occurs by molecular diffusion. Two adjacent compartments, separated by a partition containing pure gases A or B may be envisaged. Random movement of all molecules occurs so that after a period tome, molecules are found quite remote from their original positions. If the partition is removed, some molecules of A move toward the region occupied by B, their number depending on the number of molecules at the point considered. Concurrently, molecules of B diffuse toward regimes formerly occupied by pure A.

Ultimately, complete mixing occurs. Before this point in time, a gradual variation in the concentration of A occurs along an axis, designated x, which joins the original compartments. This variation, expressed mathematically, is $-dC_A/dx$, where C_A is the concentration of A. The negative sign arises because the concentration of A decreases as the distance x increases. Similarly, the variation in the concentration of gas B is $-dC_B/dx$. The rate of diffusion of A, N_A, depends on the concentration gradient and the average velocity with which the molecules of A move in the x direction. This relationship is expressed by Fick's law, given by Eq. 41

$$N_A = -D_{AB} \frac{d/C_A}{dx} \tag{41}$$

where D is the diffusivity of A in B, a property proportional to the average molecular velocity and, therefore, dependent on the temperature and pressure of the gases. The rate of diffusion N_A is usually expressed as the number of moles diffusing across unit area in unit time. As

with the basic equations of heat transfer, Eq. 41 indicates that the rate of a process is directly proportional to a driving force, which, in this context, is a concentration gradient.

This basic equation can be applied to a number of situations. Restricting discussion exclusively to steady-state conditions, in which neither dC_A/dx or dC_B/dx change with time, equimolecular counterdiffusion is considered first.

Equimolecular counterdiffusion

If no bulk flow occurs in an element of length dx, the rates of diffusion of the two gases A and B must be equal and opposite, that is, $N_A = -N_B$.

The partial pressure of A changes by dP_A over the distance dx. Similarly, the partial pressure of B changes dP_B. As there is no difference in total pressure across the element (no bulk flow), dP_A/dx must equal $-dP_B/dx$. for an ideal gas, the partial pressure is related to the molar concentration by the relation

$$P_A V = n_A R T$$

where n_A is the number of moles of gas A in a volume V. As the molar concentration C_A is equal to n_A/V, therefore

$$P_A = C_A R T$$

Consequently, for gas A, Eq. 40 can be written as in Eq. 42,

$$N_A = -\frac{D_{AB}}{RT} \frac{dP_A}{dx} \tag{42}$$

where D_{AB} is the diffusivity of A in B. Similarly,

$$N_B = -\frac{D_{BA}}{RT} \frac{dP_B}{dx} = \frac{D_{AB}}{RT} \frac{dP_A}{dx}$$

It, therefore, allows that $D_{AB} = D_{BA} = D$. If the partial pressure of A at x_1 is P_{A_1} and at x_2 is P_{A2}, integration of Eq. 42 gives Eq. 43.

$$N_A = -\frac{D}{RT} \left(\frac{P_{A_2} - P_{A_1}}{x_2 - x_1} \right) \tag{43}$$

A similar equation may be derived for the counter-diffusion of gas B.

Diffusion through a stationary, nondiffusing gas

An important practical case arises when a gas A diffuses through a gas B, there being no overall transport of gas B. It arises, for example, when a vapor formed at a drying surface diffuses into a surrounding gas. At the liquid surface, the partial pressure of A is dictated by the temperature. For water, it would be 12.8 mm Hg (1.7 kPa) at 15°C. Some distance away the partial pressure is lower, and the concentration gradient causes diffusion of A away from the surface. Similarly, a concentration gradient for B must exist, the concentration being lowest at the surface. Diffusion of this component takes place toward the surface. There is, however, no overall transport B so that diffusional movement must be balanced by bulk flow away from the surface. The total flow of A is, therefore, the diffusional flow of A plus the transfer of A associated with this bulk movement.

Molecular Diffusion in Liquids

Equations describing molecular diffusion in liquids are similar to those applied to gases. The rate of diffusion of material A in a liquid is given by Eq. 40.

$$N_A = D\frac{dC_A}{dx}$$

Fick's law for steady-state equimolal counterdiffusion is then expression by Eq. 44

$$N_A = -D\frac{C_{A_2} - C_{A_1}}{x_2 - x_1} \qquad (44)$$

where C_{A2} and C_{A1} are the molar concentrations at points x_2 and x_1 respectively.

Equations for diffusion through a layer of stagnant liquid can also be developed. The applicability of these equations is, however, limited because diffusivity in a liquid varies with concentration. In addition, unless the solutions are very dilute, the total molar concentration varies from point to point. These complications do not arise with diffusion in gases.

Diffusivities in liquids are very much lower than diffusivities in gases, commonly by a factor of 10^4.

Mass Transfer in Turbulent and Laminar Flow

As already explained, movement of molecules across the streamlines of a fluid in laminar flow can occur only by molecular diffusion. If the concentration of a component A varies in a direction normal to the streamlines, the molar rate of diffusion is given by Eq. 44.

When a fluid flows over a surface, the surface retards the adjacent fluid region, forming a boundary layer, If the flow throughout the fluid is laminar, the equation for molecular diffusion may be used to evaluate the mass transferred across the boundary layer. In most important cases, however, the flow in the bulk of the fluid is turbulent. The boundary layer is then considered to consist of three distinct flow regimes. In the region of the boundary layer most distant from the surface, flow is

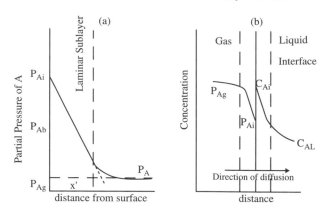

Fig. 6 Mass transfer at (a) a boundary and (b) an interface.

turbulent, and mass transfer is the result of the interchange of large portions of the fluid. Mass interchange is rapid and concentration gradients are low. As the surface is approached, a transition from turbulent to laminar flow occurs in the transition or buffer region. In this region, mass transfer by eddy diffusion and molecular diffusion are of comparable magnitude. In a fluid layer at the surface, a fraction of a millimeter thick, laminar flow conditions persist. This laminar sublayer, in which transfer occurs by molecular diffusion only, offers the main resistance to mass transfer as shown in Fig. 6(a). As flow becomes more turbulent, the thickness of the laminar sublayer and its resistance to mass transfer decrease.

An approach to the evaluation of the rate of mass transfer under these conditions lies in the postulation of a film, the thickness of which offers the same resistance to mass transfer as the combined laminar, buffer, and turbulent regions. The analogy with heat transfer by conduction and convection is exact and quantitative relations between heat and mass transfer can be developed for some situations. This, however, is not attempted here. The postulate of an effective film is explained by Fig. 6(b). As a gas flows over a surface, equimolecular counterdiffusion of components A and B occurs, A away from the surface and B toward the surface. The variation in partial pressure of A with distance from the surface is shown in Fig. 6a. At the surface, the value of P_{Ai}, a linear fall to P_{Ab} occurs over the laminar sublayer. Beyond this, the partial pressure falls less steeply to the value P_A at the edge of the boundary layer. A value slightly higher than this is P_{Ag}, the average partial pressure of A in the entire system. In general, the gas content of the laminar layer is so small that P_A and P_{Ag} are virtually equal. If the molecular diffusion were solely responsible for diffusion, the partial pressure P_{Ag} would be reached at some fictitious distance x' from the surface, over which the concentration gradient $(P_{Ai} - P_{Ag})/x'$ exists. The molar rate of mass transfer would then be

$$N_A = \frac{D}{RT} \cdot \frac{P_{Ai} - P_{Ag}}{x}$$

However, x' is not known, and Eq. 45 may be written as

$$N_A = -\frac{k_g}{RT}(P_{Ai} - P_{Ag}) \qquad (45)$$

where k_g, is a mass transfer coefficient, the units of which are cm sec^{-1}. As $C_A = P_A/RT$, it can also be written as

$$N_A = k_g(C_{Ai} - C_{Ag})$$

where C_{Ai} and C_{Ag} are the gas concentrations at either side of the film. Similar equations describe the diffusion of B in the opposite direction.

Diffusion across a liquid film is described by Eq. 46

$$N_A = k_1(C_{Ai} - C_{A1}) \qquad (46)$$

where C_{Ai} is the concentration of component A at the interface and C_{A1} is its concentration in the bulk of the phase.

In all cases, the mass-transfer coefficient depends upon the diffusivity of the transferred material and the thickness of the effective film. The latter is largely determined by the Reynolds number of the moving fluid, that is, its average velocity, density, and viscosity, and some linear dimension of the system. Dimensional analysis gives the following relation:

$$\frac{kd}{D} = \mathrm{const}(Re)^q \left(\frac{\eta}{\rho D}\right)^r$$

where Re is the Reynolds number, k the mass transfer coefficient, D the diffusivity, and d a dimension characterizing the geometry of the system.

This relation is analogous to the expression for the heat transfer by forced convection given earlier. The dimensionless group kd/D corresponds to the Nusselt group in heat transfer. The parameter $\eta/\rho D$ is known as the Schmidt number and is the mass-transfer counterpart of the Prandtl number. For example, the evaporation of a thin liquid film at the wall of a pipe into a turbulent gas is described by the equation

$$\frac{kd}{D} = 0.023 \, Re^{0.8} Sc^{0.33}$$

where Sc is the Schmidt number. Although this equation expresses experimental data, comparison with Eq. 41

again demonstrates the fundamental relation of heat and mass transfer.

Similar relations have been developed empirically for other situations. The flow of gases normal to and parallel to liquid surfaces can be applied to drying processes, and the agitation of solids in liquids can provide information for crystallization or dissolution.

Interfacial Mass Transfer

On a macroscopic scale, the interface can be regarded as a discrete boundary. On the molecular scale, however, the change from one place to another takes place over several molecular diameters. Due to movement of molecules, this region is in a state of violent change, the whole surface layer changing many times a second. Transfer of molecules at the actual interface is, therefore, virtually instantaneous and the two phases are, at this point in equilibrium.

As the interface offers no resistance, mass transfer between phases can be regarded as the transfer of a component from one bulk phase to another through two films in contact, each characterized by a mass-transfer coefficient. This is the two-film theory and the simplest of the theories of interfacial mass transfer. For the transfer of a component from a gas to a liquid, the theory is described in Fig. 6b. Across the gas film, the concentration, expressed as partial pressure, falls from a bulk concentration P_{Ag} to an interfacial concentration P_{Ai}. In the liquid, the concentration falls from an interfacial value C_{Ai} to bulk value C_{A1}.

At the interface, equilibrium conditions exist. The break in the curve is due to the different affinity of component A for the two phases and the different units expressing concentration. The bulk phases are not, of course, at equilibrium and it is the degree of displacement from equilibrium conditions that provides the driving force for mass transfer. If these conditions are known, an overall mass-transfer coefficient can be calculated and used to estimate the mass-transfer rate.

Transfer of a component from one mixed phase to another, as described above, occurs in several processes. Liquid–liquid extraction, leaching, gas absorption, and distillation are examples. In other processes such as drying, crystallization, and dissolution, one phase may consist of only one component. Concentration gradients are set up in one phase only, with the concentration at the interface given by the relevant equilibrium conditions. In drying, for example, a layer of air in equilibrium (i.e., saturated) with the liquid is postulated at the liquid surface and mass transfer to a turbulent air stream is described by Eq. 44, the interfacial concentration being the saturation concentration. The rate of solution is determined by the difference between the interfacial concentration and the concentration in the bulk solution, and the mass-transfer coefficient.

REFERENCES

1. Markovitz, R.E. Heat Transfer in Process Vessels. *Encyclopedia of Pharmaceutical Technology*; Swarbrick, J., Boylan, J.C., Eds.; Marcel Dekker, Inc.: New York, 2001.
2. Graham Nairn, J. Mass Transfer in Unit Operations. *Encyclopedia of Pharmaceutical Technology*; Swarbrick, J., Boylan, J.C., Eds.; Marcel Dekker, Inc.: New York, 2001.

BIBLIOGRAPHY

Beard, J. *Dynamics of Fluids in Porous Media*; Dover Publications, Inc.: Mineola, NY, 1972.

Bird, R.B.; Stewart, W.E.; Lightfoot, E.N. *Transport Phenomena*; John Wiley & Sons: New York, 1960.

Chhabra, R.P. *Bubbles, Drops and Particles in Non-Newtonian Fluids*; CRC Press: Boca Raton, FL, 1993.

Cheremisinoff, N.P. *Practical Fluid Mechanics for Engineers and Scientists*; Technomic Publishing Co., Inc.: Lancaster, PA, 1990.

Cho, Y.I.; Hartnett, J.P. Non-Newtonian Fluids in Circular Pipe Flow. Adv. Heat Transfer **1982**, *15*, 59–141.

Coulson, J.M.; Richardson, J.R. *Chemical Engineering*; Pergamon Press: New York, 1977; 1.

The Mathematics of Diffusion; Crank, J. Ed.; reprinted 1992 Oxford University Clarendon Press: Oxford, 1975.

Cussler, E.L. *Diffusion Mass Transfer in Fluid Systems*; Cambridge University Press: New York, 1984.

Fayed, M.E.; Otten, L. *Handbook of Powder Science and Technology*; Van Nostrand Reinhold, Co. New York, 1984.

Hartnett, J.P.; Kostic, M. Heat Transfer to Newtonian and Non-Newtonian Fluids in Rectangular Ducts. Adv. Heat Transfer **1989**, *19*, 24–356.

McCabe, W.L.; Smith, J.C.; Harriott, P. *Unit Operations of Chemical Engineering*; McGraw Hill, Inc.: New York, 1993.

Meyer, R.E. *Introduction to Mathematical Fluids Dynamics*; Dover Publications, Inc.: Mineola, NY, 1982.

Neumann, B.S. The Flow Properties. In *Advances in Pharmaceutical Sciences*; Bean, H.S., Beckett, A.H., Carless, J.E. Eds.; Academic Press: New York, 1967; 2, 181–221.

Orr, C. *Particulate Technology*; Macmillan: New York, 1966.

Ozisik, M.N. *Boundary Value Problems of Heat Conduction*; Dover Publications, Inc.: Mineola, NY, 1968.

Prandtl, L.; Tietjens, O.G. *Fundamentals of Hydro- an Aeromechanics*; Dover Publications, Inc.: Mineola, NY, 1957.

Perry, R.H.; Chilton, C.H. *Chemical Engineer's Handbook*; McGraw Hill: New York, 1973.

Taylor, R.; Krishna, R. *Multicomponent Mass Transfer*; John Wiley & Sons: New York, 1993.

UNIT PROCESSES IN PHARMACY— THE OPERATIONS

Anthony J. Hickey
University of North Carolina at Chapel Hill, Chapel Hill, North Carolina

David Ganderton
Vectura Ltd., Bath, United Kingdom

INTRODUCTION

The fundamentals of unit processes have been described elsewhere (1, 2). The following is a summary of the major operations. Although it is broad in scope, the abbreviated form of this article has resulted in selected omissions. References are given, wherever possible, to make up for this deficiency.

EVAPORATION AND DISTILLATION

Evaporation

The term evaporation, in the pharmaceutical industry, is primarily associated with the removal of water and other solvents by boiling in batch processes.

Heat transfer to boiling liquids in an evaporator

The heat required to boil a liquid in an evaporator is usually transferred from a heating fluid, such as steam or hot water, across the wall of a jacket or tube in or around which the liquid boils. A qualitative discussion of the methods used to secure high rates of heat flow can be used on Equation (1),

$$Q = UA \, \Delta T \tag{1}$$

where Q is the rate of heat flow, U is the overall heat transfer coefficient, A is the area over which heat is transferred, and ΔT is the difference in temperature between the fluids.

Other factors described by Eq. 1 are the area of the heat transfer surfaces, which should be as large as possible, and the temperature difference between the heating surface and the boiling liquid. As long as the critical heat flux is not exceeded, the latter also should be large.

The physical properties of solution and liquids

A number of physical factors, which are inter-related, are relevant to the study of evaporation. For a given heating fluid, the temperature difference across the wall of an evaporator is determined by the boiling temperature, a variable controlled by the external pressure and the concentration of the solute in the solution. The boiling temperature and the solute concentration both influence the viscosity of the solution, a factor which greatly affects the heat transfer coefficient. The boiling temperature also determines the solubility of dissolved constituents and the degree of concentration which can be carried out without separation of solids.

The effect of heat on the active constituents of a solution: The thermal stability of components of a solution may determine the type of evaporator to be used and the conditions of its operation. If a simple solution contains a hydrolyzable material and the rate of its degradation during evaporation depends on its concentration at any time, an exponential relation between the remaining fraction, F, and the time, t, characteristic of a first-order reaction, is obtained, as shown in Eq. 2.

$$F = e^{-kt} \tag{2}$$

The dependence of the reaction velocity constant, k, on the absolute temperature, T, is expressed by Eq. 3,

$$k = Ae^{-B/T} \tag{3}$$

where A and B are constants characteristic of the reaction. Thus, at temperatures T_1, T_2, and T_3, where $T_1 > T_2 > T_3$, the relation between the remaining fraction and the time of heating becomes clear, as shown in Fig. 1. This indicates the importance of the temperature and time of heating. If the latter can be shortened, the temperature of evaporation can be increased greatly without increasing the fraction which is degraded. If, therefore, the effect of temperature on the rate of evaporation is known, it is possible to define the conditions of time and temperature at which decomposition is minimum.

In practice, the kinetics of degradation and the relation of evaporation rate and temperature are usually not known. This is particularly true when the criteria by which the product is judged are color, taste, or smell. In addition, this

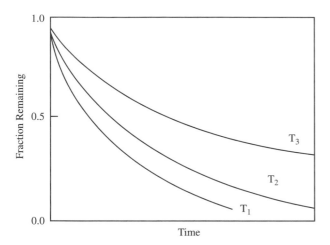

Fig. 1 The effect of time and temperature of degradation.

analysis neglects the temperature variation in the evaporating liquid and the degradation in boundary films where temperatures are higher. Therefore, experiments are often necessary to determine the suitability of an evaporation process.

In batch processes, the time of exposure to heat is well defined. This is also true of continuous processes in which the liquid to be evaporated is passed only once through the heater. In continuous processes, is where the liquid is recirculated through the heater, the average residence time, a, is given by the ratio.

The volumetric discharge is only an indication of the damage that may be caused by prolonged heating. If perfect mixing occurs in the evaporator, the fraction, f, which is in the unit for time t or less, is given by Eq. 4.

$$f = 1 - e^{-t/a} \tag{4}$$

This relation shows that an evaporator, for example, with an average residence time of 1 h holds 13.5% of active principles for 2 h and about 2% for 4 h.

Evaporators

It is convenient to classify evaporators into natural circulation evaporators, forced-circulation evaporators, and film evaporators.

Natural circulation evaporators

Small-scale evaporators consist of a simple pan heated by a jacket or a coil, or both. Admission of the heating fluid to the jacket induces the liquid in the vessel to boil. Very small evaporators may be open, the vapor escaping to atmosphere or into a vented hood. Larger pan evaporators are closed, the vapor escaping through a pipe. Small

jacketed pans are efficient and easy to clean and may be fitted for the vacuum evaporation of thermolabile materials. Their size, however, is limited because the ratio of heating area to volume decreases as the capacity increases. Larger vessels must employ a heating coil which increases their evaporating capacity but it also makes cleaning more difficult.

Forced-circulation evaporators

On the smallest scale, forced-circulation evaporators are similar to the pan evaporators described previously, modified only by the inclusion of an agitator. Vigorous agitation increases the boiling film coefficient, the degree of which depends on the type and speed of the agitator. An agitator should be used for the evaporation of viscous materials to prevent degradation of material at the heated surfaces. Some large-scale continuous units are similar to the natural circulation evaporators already described.

Film evaporators

In the short tubes of the calandria, an intimate mixture of vapor and liquid is discharged at the top as shown in Fig. 2a. If the length of the tube is greatly increased, progressive phase separation occurs until a high velocity core of vapor is formed which propels an annular film of liquid along the tube. This phenomenon, which is one stage of flow when a liquid and a gas pass in the same direction along a tube, is employed in film evaporators. The turbulence of the film gives very high heat transfer coefficients, and the bubbles and vapor evolved are rapidly swept into the vapor stream. Although recirculation may be adopted, it is possible with the high evaporation is found in long tubes to sufficiently concentrate the liquid in a single pass. Because a very short residence time is obtained, very thermolabile materials may be concentrated at relatively high temperatures. Film evaporators are also

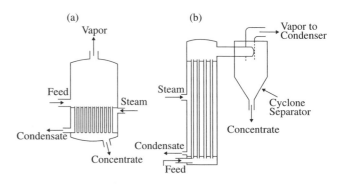

Fig. 2 (a) Evaporator with calandria; (b) climbing film evaporator.

suitable for materials which foam strongly. Various types have been developed, but all are essentially continuous in operation and their capacity starts from a few liters per hour upward.

The climbing film evaporator, which is the most common film evaporator, consists of tubes 15 to 30 feet (4.5–13.6 m) long and 1 to 2 in. (2.5–5 cm) in diameter mounted in a steam chest (Fig. 2b). The feed liquid enters the bottom of the tubes and flows upward for a short distance before boiling begins. The length of this section, which is characterized by low heat transfer coefficients, may be minimized by preheating the feed to its boiling point. The pattern of boiling and phase separation follows and a mixture of liquid and vapor emerges from the top of the tube to be separated by baffles or by a cyclone separator. Climbing film evaporators are not suitable for the evaporation of viscous liquids.

In the falling film evaporator, the liquid is fed to the top of a number of long heated tubes. Because the gravity assists the flow down the tube, this arrangement is better suited to the evaporation of moderately viscous liquids. The vapor evolved is usually carried downward and the mixture of liquid and vapor emerges from the bottom for separation. Even distribution of liquid must be secured during feeding. The tendency to channel in some tubes leads to drying in others.

The rising-falling film evaporator concentrates a liquid in a climbing film section and leads the emerging liquid and vapor into a second tube section which forms a falling film evaporator. Good distribution of liquid is claimed in the falling film section and this type is particularly suitable for liquids which greatly increase in viscosity during evaporation.

In mechanically aided film evaporators, a thin film of material is maintained on the heat transfer surface irrespective of the viscosity. This is usually achieved by means of a rotor, concentric with the tube, which carries blades that either scrape the tube or ride with low clearance in the film. Mechanical agitation permits the evaporation of highly viscous materials or those that have a low thermal conductivity. Because the temperature variations in the film are reduced and residence times are shortened, the vacuum evaporation of viscous thermolabile materials becomes possible.

Evaporation without boiling

During heating, some evaporation takes place at the surface of a batch of liquid before boiling begins. Similarly, liquids that are very viscous or excessively froth may be concentrated without boiling. The diffusion of vapor from the surface is described by Eq. 5,

$$N_A = k_g RT(P_{Ai} - P_{Ag}) \tag{5}$$

where N_A is the number of moles evaporating from unit area in unit time, k_g is the mass transfer coefficient across the boundary layer, R is the gas constant, T is the absolute temperature, P_{Ai} is vapor pressure of the liquid, and P_{Ag} is the partial pressure of the vapor in the gas stream; k_g is proportional to the gas velocity.

Distillation

Distillation is a process in which a liquid mixture is separated into its component parts by vaporization. The vapor evolved from a boiling liquid mixture is normally richer in the more volatile components than the liquid with which it is in equilibrium. Distillation rests upon this fact. Although multicomponent mixtures are most common in distillation processes, an understanding of the operation can be based on the vapor pressure characteristics of two-component or binary mixtures.

Binary mixtures of immiscible liquids: steam distillation

If the components of a binary mixture are immiscible, the vapor pressure of the mixture is the sum of the vapor pressures of the two components, each exerted independently and not as a function of their relative concentrations in the liquid. This property is employed in steam distillation, a process particularly applicable to the separation of high boiling substances from nonvolatile impurities. The steam forms a cheap and inert carrier. The principles of the process also apply to other immiscible systems.

The composition of the distillate is calculated in the following way. For two components, A and B, the total vapor pressure, P, is the sum of the vapor pressures of the components, P_A and P_B. Since the partial pressure of a component in a gaseous mixture is proportional to its molar concentration, the composition of the vapor is given by Eq. 6,

$$\frac{n_A}{n_B} = \frac{P_A}{P_B} \tag{6}$$

where n_A and nB are the number of moles of A and B in the vapor, respectively. If W_A and W_B are the weights of A and B in the vapor, Eq. 7 holds,

$$\frac{W_A}{M_A} = \frac{M_B}{W_B} = \frac{P_A}{P_B} \tag{7}$$

where M_A and M_B are the respective molecular weights. The distillate obtained from the vapor is $W_A + W_B$, and the percentage of A in the distillate is expressed by Eq. 8.

$$\frac{W_A}{M_A + W_B} \times 100 = \frac{P_A M_A}{P_A M_A + P_B W_B} \times 100 \qquad (8)$$

The ratio of immiscible organic liquid to water in the distillate is increased if the former has a high molecular weight or a high vapor pressure. Steam distillation under vacuum may be employed when the thermal stability of the material prohibits temperatures of approximately 100°C.

The relation of vapor pressure and mixture composition: In a binary mixture of two completely miscible components, the vapor pressure is a function of the mixture composition as well as of the vapor pressures of the two pure components. If the liquids are ideal, the relation of vapor pressure and composition is given by Raoult's law. At a constant temperature, the partial vapor pressure of a constituent of an ideal mixture is proportional to its mole fraction in the liquid. Thus, for a mixture of A and B, the partial vapor pressure of A is given by Eq. 9,

$$P_A = P_A^0 \cdot x_A \qquad (9)$$

where P_A^0 is the vapor pressure of pure A and x_A is its mole fraction. Similarly, the partial vapor pressure of B is expressed by Eq. 10.

$$P_B = P_B^0 \cdot x_B \qquad (10)$$

The total pressure of the system, P, is simply $P_A + P_B$.

Very few liquid mixtures rigidly obey Raoult's law. Consequently, the vapor pressure data must be determined experimentally. Mixtures that deviate positively from this law give a total vapor pressure curve which lies above the theoretical straight line. Negative deviations fall below the line. In extreme cases, deviations are so large that a range of mixtures exhibits a higher or lower vapor pressure than either of the pure components.

Returning to ideal systems, the partial pressure of a component in the vapor is proportional to its mole fraction, as shown in Eq. 11 for component A,

$$P_A = y_A P \cdot \qquad (11)$$

where P_A is the partial pressure of A in the vapor and y_A is its mole fraction. Because, $P_A = P_A^0 \cdot x_A$, Eqs. 12 and 13 can be written as:

$$y_A = \frac{x_A P_B^0}{P} \qquad (12)$$

similarly,

$$y_B = \frac{x_B P_B^0}{P} \qquad (13)$$

If A is the more volatile component, P_A^0 is greater than P. Therefore y_A is greater than x_A, that is, the vapor is richer in the more volatile component than the liquid with which it is in equilibrium.

Systems that form minimum boiling mixtures are common. Ethyl alcohol and water provide an example, the azeotrope containing 4.5% by weight of water. The boiling point at atmospheric pressure is 78.15°C that is 0.25°C lower than the boiling point of pure alcohol. Maximum boiling mixtures are less common. The most familiar example is hydrochloric acid which forms an azeotrope boiling at 108.6°C containing 20.2% by weight of hydrochloric acid. Mixtures that form azeotropes cannot be separated into the pure components by normal distillation methods. However, separation into the azeotrope and one pure component is possible.

Simple or differential distillation

In simple or differential distillation, the vapor evolved from the boiling mixture is immediately removed and condensed. Unless the boiling points of the two pure components differ widely, a reasonable degree of separation is not possible. This method may be used to remove low boiling solvents from aqueous solutions.

Rectification or fractionation

In simple distillation, vapor enrichment is small. In fractionation, a term synonymous with rectification, the vapor leaving the boiling liquid is led up a column to meet a liquid stream or reflux which originates higher in the column as part of the condensate. In a series of partial condensations and vaporizations, the rising vapor becomes richer in the more volatile component at the expense of the falling liquid and high degrees of separation become possible. The columns, called fractionating columns, are of two basic types: packed columns and plate columns.

Packed columns: These are used for laboratory and small-scale industrial distillation and are usually operated as a batch process. The column consists of a vertical, hollow, cylindrical shell containing a packing designed to offer a large interfacial contact area between liquid and vapor. The form of the packing varies but Raschig rings, which consist of small metallic or ceramic cylinders, are the most commonly used. In general, packed columns operate under widely varying conditions without serious loss of efficiency.

Plate columns: A plate column consists of a series of plates or trays on which the liquid is retained for some period during its movement down the column. The rising vapor is bubbled through this liquid, providing intimate contact between the phases. Liquid in reflux moves downward between plates and is usually carried by a downcomer. Contact between the vapor and liquid takes place in stages.

Plate columns operate efficiently over a limited range of conditions. They are mainly used in large-scale continuous installations in which the conditions of distillation can be closely maintained.

Molecular distillation

Molecular distillation is carried out without boiling at very low pressures of the order 0.001 mm Hg (0.133 Pa). At these pressures, collision of molecules in the evolving vapor and reflection back to the liquid surface is greatly decreased and the mean free path of the molecules is of the same order as the distance between the evaporating surface and a condenser placed a short distance away. It then becomes possible to distil liquids of very high boiling point although the degree of separation cannot exceed one theoretical plate. The process therefore is used primarily to concentrate nonvolatile components in a high boiling medium. The vitamins in cod liver oil can be concentrated this way. For the separation of liquids of comparable volatility, several separate distillation stages are necessary.

Because agitation due to boiling is absent, an alternative method of maintaining the more volatile component at the evaporating surface must be adopted. In the industrial molecular still shown in Fig. 3, the feed is introduced at the bottom of a heated conical rotor and flows upward as a thin liquid layer under the action of centrifugal force. The residue is caught in a gutter at the top. The vapor is condensed on a concentric, water-cooled condenser a short distance away and discharged.

AIR CONDITIONING AND HUMIDIFICATION

General principles of the supply of air in pharmaceutical processes are similar to conventional air conditioning. The control of its quality, however, may be more stringent. In areas where sterile materials are made and handled, for example, the cleaning process must remove bacteria. In other situations, it may be necessary to remove water vapor. The flow of powders is a sensitive function of moisture content, and the equilibrium moisture content of a material is determined by the humidity. Some tableting processes break down if the humidity is too high. In such processes, the scale of the air conditioning varies. It may be necessary to supply a whole room with air of a certain quality. Alternatively, conditioning may be restricted to a small area surrounding a particular piece of equipment.

Vapor and Gas Mixtures

The study of the properties of the air–water vapor mixture is called psychometry, and data are presented in various forms of psychrometric charts presenting various data. In Fig. 4, humidity is plotted as ordinate and temperatures as abscissa. Percentage of relative humidity is plotted as curves running across the chart. The use of this simplified chart is demonstrated later.

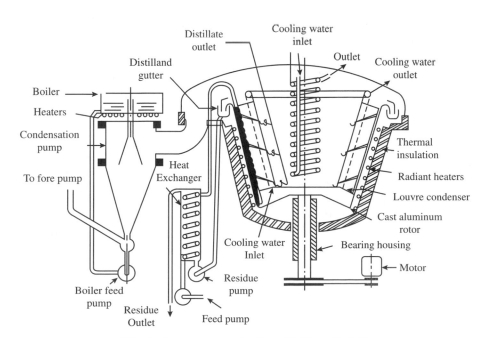

Fig. 3 Large-scale molecular still. (From Ref. 3)

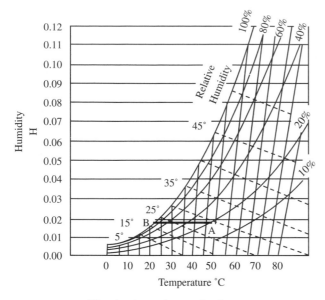

Fig. 4 A psychrometric chart.

Hygrometry, the Measurement of Humidity

The accurate determination of the humidity of air is carried out gravimetrically. The water vapor present in a known volume of air is chemically absorbed with a suitable reagent and weighed. In less laborious methods, the humidity is derived from the dew point or the wet-bulb depression of a water–vapor mixture.

The dew point is the temperature at which a vapor condenses when cooled at constant pressure. If air of the condition denoted by point A in Fig. 4 is cooled, the relative humidity increases until the mixture is fully saturated. This condition is given by point B; the temperature coordinator is the dew point, which can be measured rapidly by evaporating ether in a silvered bulb. The temperature at which dew deposits from the surrounding air is noted and the humidity is read directly from a psychrometric chart.

The derivation of the humidity from the wet-bulb depression requires a preliminary study of the transfer of mass and heat at a boundary between air and water. The difference between the air temperature and the wet-bulb temperature is the wet-bulb depression. If these temperatures are denoted by T_a and T_{wb}, the rate of heat transfer, Q, is given by Eq. 14,

$$Q = hA(T_a - T_{wb}) \tag{14}$$

$$Q = \rho k_g A(H_i - H_a) \tag{15}$$

Equating Eqs. 14 and 15 gives Eq. 16.

$$H_i - H_a = \frac{h}{\rho k_g \lambda}(T_a - T_{wb}) \tag{16}$$

Both the heat and mass transfer coefficients are functions of air velocity. However, at air speeds greater than about 15 ft/s (4.5 m/s), the ratio $h{:}k_g$ is approximately constant. The wet-bulb depression is directly proportional to the difference between the humidity at the surface and the humidity in the bulk of the air. In the wet- and dry-bulb hygrometer, the wet-bulb depression is measured by two thermometers, one of which is fitted with a fabric sleeve wetted with water. These thermometers are mounted side by side and shielded from radiation, an effect neglected in the derivation above. Air is drawn over the thermometers by means of a small fan. The derivation of the humidity from the wet-bulb depression and a psychrometric chart are discussed later.

Many wet- and dry-bulb hygrometers operate without any form of induced air velocity at the wet bulb. This may be explained by examining another air–water system. If a limited quantity of air and water is allowed to equilibrate under conditions in which heat is neither gained nor lost by the system, the air becomes saturated and the latent heat required for evaporation is drawn from both fluids which cool to the same temperature. This temperature is the adiabatic saturation temperature, T_∞. It is a peculiarity of the air–water system that the adiabatic saturation temperature and the wet-bulb temperature are the same. If water at this temperature is recycled in a system through which air is passing, the incoming air is cooled till it reaches the adiabatic saturation temperature at which point it is saturated. The temperature of the water, on the other hand, remains constant and all the latent heat required for evaporation is drawn from the sensible heat of the air. Equilibrium is expressed by Eq. 17,

$$(T_a - T_\infty)S = (H_\infty - H_a)\lambda \tag{17}$$

where T_a is the temperature of the incoming air and S is its specific heat, H_a and H_∞ are the humidities of the incoming air and the saturated air, and λ is the latent heat of evaporation for water.

When both wet- and dry-bulb temperatures have been found, the humidity is read from the psychrometric chart in the following way. The point on the saturation curve corresponding to the wet-bulb temperature is found first. An adiabatic cooling line is then interpolated and followed until the coordinate corresponding to the dry-bulb temperature is reached. The humidity is read from the other axis.

Humidification and Dehumidification

Most commonly, air is humidified by passage through a spray of water. Small quantities of air are easily dehumidified by adsorbing the water vapor with alumina or silica gel arranged in columns. These are mounted in pairs so that one can be regenerated while the other is in use. Alternatively, the air can be cooled below the dew point. Excess water vapor condenses and the cold saturated air is reheated.

CRYSTALLIZATION

The term crystallization describes the production of a solid, single-component, crystalline phase from a multi-component fluid phase. The importance of crystallization lies primarily in the purification achieved during the process and in the physical properties of the product. A crystalline powder is easily handled, stable, and often possesses good flow properties and an attractive appearance.

Crystallization from a vapor, which occurs naturally, e.g., in the formation of hoar frost, is employed in sublimation processes and for the condensation of water vapor during freeze-drying.

Crystallization in Melts

A melt may be defined as the liquid form of a single material or the homogeneous liquid form of two or more materials which solidify on cooling. Crystallization in such a system passes through the following stages: supercooling, nuclei formation, and crystal growth.

If a single-component liquid is cooled, some degree, often high, of supercooling must be established before crystal nuclei form and growth begins. A metastable liquid region exists below the melting point which only can be entered by cooling. In this metastable, supercooled region, the absence of nucleation precludes the formation and growth of crystals. If, however, a crystal seed is added, growth occurs. The deliberate seeding of a metastable system is commonly employed in industrial crystallization. With further cooling, spontaneous nucleation usually takes place and the released heat of crystallization raises the temperature of the melt to its true melting point.

Nucleation

In certain single-component systems, such as piperine, nucleation and crystal growth are independent and can be separately studied. The rate of nucleation as a function of supercooling is studied by maintaining the melt for a certain time at the given temperature and then quickly raising the temperature to the metastable region where further nucleation is negligible but the already formed nuclei can grow.

Spontaneous nucleation occurs when sufficient molecules of low kinetic energy come together in such a way that the attraction between them is sufficient to overcome their momentum.

Crystal Growth

If nucleation and crystal growth are independent, the latter can be studied by seeding a melt with small crystals under conditions of little or no natural nucleation. The rate of growth can then be measured. The form of the crystal growth curve is again explained by the kinetics of the molecules. At temperatures just below the melting point, molecules have too much energy to remain in the crystal lattice. As the temperature falls, more molecules are retained and the growth rate increases. Ultimately, however, diffusion to and orientation at the crystal surface is depressed.

For crystal growth in a single component melt, the molecules at the crystal surface must reach the correct position at the lattice and become suitably orientated, losing kinetic energy. These energy changes appear as heat of crystallization, which must be transferred from the surface to the bulk of the melt. The rate of crystal growth is influenced by the rate of heat transfer and the changes taking place at the surface. Agitation of the system increases heat transfer by reducing the thermal resistance of the liquid layers adjacent to the crystal until the changes at the crystal face become the controlling effect.

In multicomponent melts and solutions, deposition of material at the crystal face depletes the adjacent liquid layers and a concentration gradient is set up with saturation at the face and supersaturation in the liquid. Diffusion of molecules to the crystal face is discussed in the next section.

Crystallization from Solutions

During crystal growth, a high degree of supersaturation promotes a high growth rate. A reaction at the surface, in which, solute molecules become correctly orientated in the crystal lattice, provides a second resistance to the growth of the crystal. Simultaneously, the heat of crystallization must be conducted away.

For given conditions of temperature and saturation, agitation modifies the rate of crystal growth. Initially, agitation quickly increases the growth rate by decreasing the thickness of the boundary layer and the diffusional resistance. However, as agitation is intensified, a limiting value is reached which is determined by the kinetics of the surface reaction.

As with melts, soluble impurities may increase or reduce nucleation rate. Insoluble materials may act as nuclei and promote crystallization. Impurities may also affect crystal form and, in some cases, are deliberately added to secure a product with good appearance, absence of caking, or suitable flow properties.

Crystallizers

Although other methods may be adopted, crystallizers can be classified conveniently in the same way, a solution is supersaturated. This leads to the self-explanatory terms, cooling crystallizer and evaporate crystallizer. In vacuum crystallizers, evaporation and cooling both take place.

FILTRATION

Filtration may be defined as the removal of solids suspended in a liquid or gas by passage through a pervious medium on which the solids are retained. The pervious medium or septum is normally supported on a base and these, together with a suitable housing providing free access of fluid to and from the septum, comprise the filter.

Methods

Clarification

Clarification of parenteral solutions eliminates unwanted solids normally present in very small concentrations. This may be carried out with the help of thick media, which allow the penetration and arrest of particles by entrapment, impingement, and electrostatic effects. This procedure leads to the concept of depth filtration in which particles, perhaps a hundred times smaller than the dimensions of the passages through the medium, are removed. Such filters are not absolute and must be designed with sufficient depth so that the probability of the smallest particle under consideration passing right through the filter is extremely small.

Depth filtration fundamentally differs from the use of media in which pore size determines the size of particle retained. Such filters may be said to be "absolute" at a particle diameter closely related to the size of the pore, so that there is a relatively sharp division between particles which pass the filter and those that are retained. An analogy

with sieving may be drawn for this mechanism. The life of such filters depends on the number of pores available for the passage of fluid. Once a particle is trapped at the entrance to the pore, the contribution of the latter to the overall flow of liquid is very much reduced. Coarse straining with a wire mesh and membrane filter employ this mechanism. Sterilization of liquids by filtration could be regarded as an extreme application of clarification in which the complete removal of particles as small as 0.3 μm must be ensured.

Cake filtration

The most common industrial application is the filtration of slurries containing a relatively large amount of suspended solids, usually 3 to 20%. The septum acts only as a support in this operation, the actual filtration being carried out by the solids deposited as a cake. In such cases, solids may completely penetrate the septum until the deposition of an effective cake occurs. Until this time, cloudy filtrate may be recycled. The physical properties of the cake largely determine the method employed. Washing and partial drying or dewatering are often integral parts of the process. Effective discharge of the cake completes the process. The solids, the filtrate, or both may be wanted.

The Theories of Filtration

Filtration theory has two important aspects. The first describes the flow of fluids through porous media and is applicable to both clarification and cake filtration. The second, which is of primary importance only in clarification, is the retention of particles on a depth filter.

Flow of fluids through porous media

The concept of a channel with a hydraulic diameter equivalent to the complex interstitial network which exists in a powder bed leads to Eq. 18,

$$Q = \frac{KA\ \Delta P}{\eta L} \qquad (18)$$

where Q is the volumetric flow rate, A is the area of the bed and L its thickness, ΔP is the pressure difference, and η is the viscosity of the fluid. The permeability coefficient, K, is given by

$$\frac{\varepsilon^3}{5(1-\varepsilon)^2 S_0^2}$$

where ε is the porosity of the bed and S_0 its specific surface area (cm^2/cm^3).

In clarification, high permeability and filtration rate oppose good particle retention. In the formation of clarifying media from sintered or loose articles, accurate control of particle size, specific surface and porosity is possible, and, a medium can be designed which offers the best compromise between permeability and particle retention. The analysis of permeability given above can be accurately applied to these systems. Because of extremes of shape, this is not so with the fibrous media used for clarification. Here it is possible to develop a material of high permeability and high retentive capacity. Such a material is, however, intrinsically weak and must be adequately supported.

A mathematical account of the theories of clarification with depth filters is found in the work of Ives (4, 5) and Maroudas and Eisenklam (6).

Filters

The method by which the filtrate is driven through the filter medium and cake, if present may be used to classify filters into:

- Gravity filters
- Vacuum filters
- Pressure filters

Each group may be further subdivided into filters employed in continuous or batch processes although, due to technical difficulties, continuous pressure filters are uncommon and expensive. Centrifugation is another means of removing filtrate. Extensive surveys can be found in the literature (7, 8).

Many small-scale filters simply consist of a fixed, rigid medium, robust enough to withstand limited pressures, mounted in a suitable housing. These filters, which are also vacuum operated, are used to clarify by depth filtration. Media are composed of sintered metals, ceramics, plastics, or glass. Filters prepared from closely graded and sintered chemical powders are suitable for the sterilization of solutions by filtration on a manufacturing scale.

Filter Media

In cake filtration, the medium must oppose excessive penetration and promote the formation of a junction with the cake, to high permeability. The medium should also give free discharge of cake after washing and dewatering.

Rigid media

Rigid media may be loose or fixed. The former is exemplified by the deposition of a filter aid on a suitable support. Filtration characteristics are governed mainly by particle size, size distribution, and shape in a manner described earlier. These factors may be varied for different filtering requirements.

Fixed media vary from perforated metals used for coarse straining for the removal of very fine particles with a sintered aggregate of metal, ceramic, plastic, or glass powder. The size, size distribution, and shape of the powder particles together with the sintering conditions control the size and distribution of the pores in the final product. The permeability may be expressed in terms of the coefficient given in Eq. 18. Alternatively, the medium may be characterized by air permeability. The maximum pore size, which is important in the selection of filters for sterilization, may be determined by measuring the pressure difference required to blow a bubble of air through the medium while it supports a column of liquid with a known surface tension.

Flexible media

Flexible media may be woven or unwoven. Filter media, woven from cotton, wool, synthetic and regenerated fibers, and glass and metal fibers, are used as septa in cake filtration. Cotton is the most widely used natural fiber, nylon is predominant among synthetic fibers. Terylene is a useful medium for acid filtration. Penetration and cake discharge are influenced by twisting and plying of fibers and by the adoption of various weaves such as duck and twill. The choice of a particular cloth often depends on the chemical nature of the slurry.

Nonwoven media in the form of felts and compressed cellulose pulps, are used for clarification by depth filtration. Unless carefully prepared, they have the disadvantage of losing fibrous material from the downstream side of the filter. The application of sheet media has been discussed earlier. High wet strength is conferred on paper sheets by resin impregnation. An alternative technique employs asbestos fibers supported in a cellulose framework.

Mechanism of air filtration

A theoretical foundation for the filtration of air by passage through fibrous media was laid in the early 1930s by studies of the flow of suspended particles around various obstacles. In studies of the filtration of smokes (9, 10) it has been shown that the following factors operate simultaneously in the arrest of a particle during its passage through a filter, although their relative importance varies with the type of filter and the conditions under which it is operated.

- Diffusion effects due to Brownian movement
- Electrostatic attraction between particles and fibers
- Direct interception of a particle by a fiber
- Interception as a result of inertial effects acting on a particle and causing it to collide with a fiber
- Settling and gravitational effects

Air filters operate under conditions of streamline flow as indicated by the streamlines drawn around a cylindrical fiber. It was assumed that capture of a particle takes place if any contact is made during its movement around the fiber. Once captured, the particle is not re-entrained in the air stream and deposited deeper in the bed. Support for this assumption has been found by using an atomized suspension of *Staphylococcus albus* and spores of *Bacillus subtilis* (11). Nevertheless, some fiber filters are treated with viscous oils, presumably to make capture more positive and to reduce re-entrainment.

Deviation of particles from streamlines can occur in a number of ways (10, 12). The chance of capture increases if Brownian movement causes appreciable migration across streamlines, an effect only important for small particles (less than 0.5 μm) and low air speeds, when the time span spent in the vicinity of a fiber is relatively long. These conditions also apply to capture which is the result of electrostatic attraction.

Sampling efficiency has been demonstrated for bacterial aerosols (13) in a study of the efficiency with which a glass fiber mat collected *B. subtilis* spores atomized as particles just over a micrometer in radius. A theoretical approach to the removal of industrial dusts has been developed (14–16).

Design, operation, and testing of air filters

Granular beds, fibrous media, and "absolute filters" prepared from cellulose and asbestos are used for high-efficiency air filtration. With fibrous and granular filters, the fractional reduction in particle content is assumed to be the same through successive incremental thicknesses of the filter, expressed by Eq. 19,

$$\frac{dC}{dx} = -kC \tag{19}$$

where C represents the number of particles entering a section of thickness dx. The constant, k, is a measure of the filter's ability to retain a particle. It is a complex function of fiber diameter, interfiber distance, and the operational air velocity. Integration between inlet and outlet conditions gives Eq. 20.

$$\log \frac{C_{out}}{C_{in}} = -kC \tag{20}$$

The use of this log penetration effect in filter design has been described elsewhere (17). If a certain filter thickness is capable of retaining 90% of the entering particles and 10^6 particles enter, 10^5 penetrate. If six thicknesses are used, Eq. 21 predicts that only one particle penetrates. The

log-penetration effect has been confirmed for fibrous filters (13) and granular beds (18).

Centrifugal Operations

An object moving in a circular path is subjected to an outward centrifugal force which balances the centripetal force moving the object toward the center of rotation. This principle is used in the mechanical separations called centrifugal filtration and centrifugal sedimentation. In the former, a material is placed in a rotating perforated basket which is lined by a filter cloth used to separate a solid, which is retained at the cloth, from a liquid. It is essentially a filtration process in which the driving force is of centrifugal origin. This does not depend upon a difference in the density of the two phases.

In centrifugal sedimentation, the separation is due to the difference in the density of two or more phases. This is the more important process, where both solid–liquid mixtures and liquid–liquid mixtures can be completely: separated. If, however, the separation is incomplete, there is a gradient in the size of the dispersed phase within the centrifuge due to the faster radial velocity of the larger particles. Operated in this way, the centrifuge becomes a classifier.

Centrifugal sedimentation

The motion of a particle in a liquid is described by Stokes' equation. If its diameter is d, the rate u at which it settles by gravity in a liquid of viscosity η and density ρ is given by Eq. 21

$$u \quad \frac{1}{18} \ d^2 \ \frac{\rho_s - \rho}{\eta} g \tag{21}$$

where g is the acceleration due to gravity, and ρ_s is the density of the particle. In the centrifuge, the gravitational force causing separation is replaced by a centrifugal force. If the particle has a mass m and moves at an angular velocity ω in a circle of radius r, the centrifugal force is $\omega^2 r \cdot (m - m_1)$, where m_1, is the mass of the displaced ligand. The expression

$$\frac{\omega^2 r}{g}$$

is, therefore, the ratio of the centrifugal and gravitational forces in the example described previously. Its value can exceed 10,000. The separation is quicker, more complete, and effective in systems containing very fine particles which do not settle by gravity because of Brownian movement.

Expressing the mass of the particle in terms of its volume and effective density, the centrifugal force can be written as in Eq. 22.

$$\frac{\pi}{6} d^2 (\rho_s - \rho)\omega^2 r \tag{22}$$

In streamline conditions, the opposing viscous force is $3\pi\, d\eta u$, where u is the terminal velocity of the particle. Equating these expressions gives Eq. 23.

$$u = \frac{1}{18} d^2 \frac{(\rho_s - \rho)}{\eta}\omega^2 r \tag{23}$$

The rate of sedimentation is proportional to the radius of the basket and the square of the speed at which it rotates. Centrifugal sedimentors can be divided into a number of types. For operations at very high speeds, the centrifuge bowl is tubular with a length/diameter ratio from 4 to 8. The solids are periodically discharged by scraping the walls of the centrifuge tube. Uses include the cleaning of fats and waxes, the fractionation of blood, and the recovery of viruses.

DRYING

Drying may be defined as the vaporization and removal of water or other liquid from a solution, suspension, or other solid–liquid mixture to form a dry solid. The change of phase from liquid to vapor distinguishes drying from the mechanical methods of separating solids from liquids such as filtration. The latter often precede drying because they offer a cheaper method for removing a large part of the liquid, where applicable.

Adjustment and control of moisture levels by drying, is important in the manufacture and development of pharmaceutical products. Apart from the obvious requirement of dry solids for many operations, drying may be carried out in order to:

- Improve handling characteristics, as in bulk powder filling and other operations involving powder flow, and
- Stabilize moisture-sensitive materials, such as aspirin and ascorbic acid.

Theory

The following terms are employed in discussing drying: humidity and humidity of saturated air, relative humidity, wet-bulb temperature, and adiabatic cooling line. Other terms may be defined as:

- Moisture Content. It is usually expressed as weight per unit weight of dry solids.
- Equilibrium Moisture Content. If a material is exposed to air at a given temperature and humidity, it will gain or lose moisture until equilibrium is reached. The moisture present at this point is defined as the equilibrium moisture content for the given exposure conditions. At a given temperature, it will vary with the partial pressure of the water vapor in the surrounding atmosphere.

Equilibrium moisture content curves vary greatly with the type of material examined. Insoluble, nonporous materials, such as talc or zinc oxide, have equilibrium moisture contents of almost zero over a wide humidity range. A moisture content between 10 and 15% may be expected for cotton fabrics under; normal atmospheric conditions. Drying below the equilibrium moisture content for room conditions may be deliberately undertaken, particularly if the material is unstable in the presence of moisture; subsequent storage becomes important.

The effects of storage after drying also may be assessed from the equilibrium moisture content curves. Storage conditions are not critical for the lactose granulation (19, 20). If the antacid formulation is stored at a relative humidity of only 65% it would, given sufficient time, absorb moisture until the content was 91%. This could be associated with poor flow characteristics and its attendant difficulties during compression.

Evaporation of Water into an Air Stream

The evaporation of moisture into a warm air stream, with the latter providing the latent heat of evaporation, is a common drying mechanism although it is not easily adapted to the recovery of the liquid. In the evaporation from a liquid surface which, with the passage of air, falls to the wet bulb temperature corresponding to the temperature and humidity of the air, the rate at which water vapor is transferred from the saturated layer at the surface to the drying stream is described by Eq. 15,

$$N = \frac{k_g}{RT}(P_{\text{wi}} - P_{\text{wa}})$$

where P_{wi} is the partial pressure of the water vapor at the surface, P_{wa} is the partial pressure of water vapor in the air, k_g is a mass transfer coefficient, and N the number of moles vapor transferred from unit area in unit time. Rewriting this in terms of the total mass, W, transferred in unit time from the entire drying surface A gives Eq. 6,

$$W = \frac{M_w A}{RT} k_g (P_{\text{wi}} - P_{\text{wa}})$$

where M_w is the molecular weight of water vapor, R is the gas constant, and T the absolute temperature. The mass transfer coefficient, k_g, is a function of the temperature, the air velocity, and the angle of air incidence. A high velocity or angle of incidence diminishes the thickness of the stationary air layer in contact with the liquid surface and therefore lowers the diffusional resistance.

The rate of evaporation may also be expressed in terms of the heat transferred across the laminar film from the drying gases to the surface, as shown in Eq. 9,

$$Q = hA(T_a - T_s)$$

where Q is the rate of heat transfer, A is the area of the surface, T_a and T_s, are the temperatures of the drying air and the surface, respectively, and h is the heat transfer coefficient. The last is also a function of air velocity and the angle of impingement. If the latent heat of evaporation is λ, this affords a mass transfer rate, W, which is given by Eq. 24.

$$W = \frac{hA}{\lambda}(T_a - T_s) \tag{24}$$

When these conditions pertain to drying, the surface temperature, T_s, which is the wet bulb temperature, is normally much lower than the temperature of the drying gases. This is of great importance in the drying of thermolabile materials. If solids are present in the surface, the rate of evaporation is modified, the overall effect depending on the structure of the solids and the moisture content.

Static Beds of Nonporous Solids

The drying of wet granular beds containing nonporous particles, which are insoluble in the wetting liquid, has been extensively studied. The operation is presented as the relation of moisture content and time of drying in Fig. 5a.

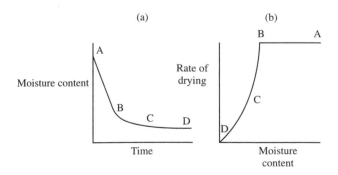

Fig. 5 (a) Relation of moisture content and time of drying; (b) rate of drying and moisture content.

It should be noted that the equilibrium moisture content is approached slowly. A protracted period may be required for the removal of water just above the equilibrium value. This is not justified if a small amount of water can be tolerated in further procession establishing realistic drying requirements.

The data have been converted to a curve relating the rate of drying to moisture content in Fig. 5b. The initial heating period during which equilibrium is established is short and has been omitted from both figures. Assuming that sufficient moisture is initially present, the drying-rate curve exhibits three sections limited by the points A, B, C, and D. In section A-B, called the constant-rate period, moisture is evaporating from a saturated surface at a rate governed by the stationary air film in contact with it. An analogy with evaporation from a plain water surface can therefore be drawn and Equations (11) and (13) apply. The rate of drying during this period depends upon the air temperature, humidity, and speed, which in turn determine the temperature of the saturated surface. Assuming that these are constant, all variables in the drying equations given earlier are fixed, and a constant rate of drying is established which is largely independent of the material being dried. The drying rate is somewhat lower than for a free-water surface and to some extent depends on the particle size of the solids. During the constant-rate period, liquid must be transported to the surface at a rate sufficiently high to maintain saturation. The mechanism of transport is discussed later.

At the end of the constant-rate period B, a break in the drying curve occurs. This point is called the critical moisture content, and a linear fall in the drying rate occurs with further drying. Because section, B-C, is called the first falling-rate period. At and below the critical moisture content, the movement of moisture from the interior is no longer sufficient to saturate the surface. As drying proceeds, moisture reaches the surface at a decreasing rate and the mechanism which controls its transfer influences the rate of drying. Because the surface is no longer saturated, it tends to rise above the wet bulb temperature.

For any material, the critical moisture content decreases as the particle size decreases. Eventually, moisture ceases to reach the surface which becomes dry. The plane of evaporation recedes into the solid, the vapor reaching the surface by diffusion through the pores of the bed. This section is called the second falling-rate period and is controlled by vapor diffusion, a factor which is largely independent of the conditions outside the bed but markedly affected by the particle size due to its influence on the dimensions of pores and channels. During this period, the surface temperature approaches the temperature of the drying air.

Considerable migration of liquid occurs during the constant-rate and first falling-rate periods. Associated with the liquid is any soluble constituent which forms a concentrating solution in the surface layers as drying proceeds. Deposition of these materials takes place when the surface dries. Considerable segregation of soluble elements in the cake can occur, therefore, during drying. These effects have been fully investigated (21).

The Internal Mechanism of Drying

Capillary forces offer a coherent explanation for the drying periods of many materials. If a tapered capillary is filled with water and exposed to a current of air, the meniscus at the smaller end remains stationary while the tube empties from the wider end. A similar situation exists in a wet particulate bed and the phenomenon is explained by the concept of suction potential. A negative pressure exists below the meniscus of a curved liquid surface which is proportional to the surface tension, λ, and inversely proportional to the radius of curvature, r. (The meniscus is assumed to be a part of a hemisphere.) This negative pressure or suction potential may be expressed as the height of liquid, expressed by Eq. 25,

$$h = \frac{2\lambda}{\rho g r} \tag{25}$$

where ρ is the density of the liquid.

The suction potential, h_x, acting at a depth x below the meniscus is given by Eq. 26.

$$h_x = h - x \tag{26}$$

The particles of the bed enclose spaces called pores connected by passages, the narrowest part of which is called the waist. The dimensions of the latter are determined by the size of the surrounding particles and the manner in which they are packed. In a randomly packed bed, pores and waists of varying sizes are found. Thus, the radius of a capillary running through the bed varies continuously. The depletion of water in this network is controlled by the waists because the radii of curvature are smaller and the suction potentials are greater than for the pores. The application of this mechanism has been described fully elsewhere (22, 23).

Through Air-Circulation Drying

If the particles are in a suitable granular form, it is often possible to pass the air stream downward through the bed of solids. Drying follows the pattern described previously, except that each particle or agglomerate behaves as a drying bed. The surface area exposed to the drying gases is greatly increased, and the drying rates are 10 to 20 times higher than those encountered when air is passed over a free surface.

Methods Involving Movement of the Solid

As an extension of drying by passing the air stream through a static bed of solids, it is possible to project air upward through the bed at a velocity high enough to fluidize the particles. Alternatively, the material may be mechanically subdivided and introduced into the drying stream. Both methods give high drying rates due to high interfacial contact between the drying surfaces and the air stream. Fluidized bed driers and spray driers, respectively, are based on these principles.

Solids Moving Over a Hot Surface

Conditions in which the solids move over a heated surface are employed in tumbling and agitated driers. Drying rates are higher than those obtained in static beds because fresh solids are continually exposed to the hot surface. The heat treatment received by the solid is more uniform.

Batch Driers

Hot air ovens

Ovens operating by passing hot air over the surface of a wet solid which is spread over trays arranged in racks, provide the simplest and cheapest drier. In small installations, the air is passed over electrically heated elements and once through the oven. Larger units may employ steam-heated, finned tubes, and thermal efficiency is improved by recirculating the air. This is controlled by manually set dampers, and a common operating position gives 90% recirculation and 10% bleed-off. The heater blank is placed in such a position that the solids do not receive radiant heat and incoming air may be filtered.

The chief advantage of the hot air oven, apart from its low initial cost, is its versatility. With the exception of dusty solids, materials of almost any physical form may be dried. Thermostatically controlled air temperatures between 40 and 120°C permit heat-sensitive materials to be dried. For small batches this may be the equipment of choice. However, the following characteristics have led to development of other small driers:

- A large floor space is required for the oven and tray loading facilities.

- Labor costs for loading and unloading the oven are high.
- Long drying times, usually of the order of 24 h, are necessary.
- Solvents can be recovered from the air only with difficulty.
- Unless carefully designed, nonuniform distribution of air over the trays results in variations in temperature and drying times within the oven. Variations of ±7°C in temperature have been found from location to location during the drying of tablet granules (19). Poor air circulation may permit local saturation and the cessation of drying.

An extensive analysis of tray drying and the effect of operational variables has been given by Shepherd et al. (24).

If the material is of suitable granular form, drying times may be reduced to 1 h or less by passing the air downward through the material laid on mesh trays. The oven in this form is called a batch through-circulation drier.

Vacuum tray driers

Vacuum tray driers offer an alternative method for drying small quantities of material. When scaled up, construction becomes massive to withstand the applied vacuum and cost is further increased by the associated vacuum equipment. Vacuum tray driers are, therefore, only used when a definite advantage over the hot air oven is secured, such as low temperature drying of thermolabile materials or the recovery of solvents from the bed. The exclusion of oxygen may also be advantageous or necessary in some operations.

Heat is usually supplied by passing steam or hot water through hollow shelves. Radiation from the shelf above may cause a significant increase in temperature at the surface of the material if high drying temperatures are used. Drying times are long, usually of the order of 12 to 48 h.

Tumbling driers

The limitations of ovens, particularly with respect to the long drying times, has, where possible, promoted the design and application of other batch driers. The simplest of these is the tumbler drier. Its most common shape is the double cone (19). Operating under vacuum, it provides controlled low temperature drying, the possibility of solvent recovery, and increased drying rates. Heat is supplied to the tumbling charge by contact with the heated shell and heat transfer through the vapor.

A normal charge would be about 60% of the total volume and, for driers 2–7 ft (0.6–2 m) in diameter, drying times of 2–12 h may be expected. In studying the

application of tumbler driers to drying tablet granules, periods of 2–3.5 h were sufficient instead of 18 h required by hot air ovens (25). The mixing and granulating capacity of the tumbling action has suggested that these operations could precede drying in the same apparatus.

Fluid-bed driers

The term "fluidization" is applied to processes in which a loose, porous bed of solids is converted to a fluid system, having the properties of surface leveling, flow, and pressure-depth relationships, by passing the fluid up through the bed.

Fluidized-bed techniques, employing air as the fluidizing medium, have been successfully applied to the drying of solids of the suitable physical form. The high interfacial contact between drying air and solids gives drying rates 10 to 20 times higher than those obtained during tray drying.

Fluidized-bed driers are particularly suitable for granulated materials and are being increasingly used for tablet granulations, providing that product changeover is not too frequent. Machines vary in size, handling up to 250 kg. Drying times, maximum, minimum, and optimum air velocities, air temperature, and the tendency to cake and channel are established experimentally as those cannot be predicted accurately at present.

Agitated batch driers

Agitated batch driers consist of a jacketed cylindrical vessel with agitator blades designed to scrape the bottom and walls. They may operate at atmospheric pressure or under vacuum. Pasty materials that could not be handled in tumbling or fluidized-bed driers, may be successfully dried at rates higher than can be achieved in an oven.

Freeze drying

Freeze drying is an extreme form of vacuum drying in which the solid is frozen and drying takes place by subliming the solid phase (26–30) at low temperatures and pressures. Establishing and maintaining these conditions, together with the low drying rates obtained, constitutes the most expensive method of drying which is only used on a large scale when other methods are inadequate.

Freeze drying is extensively used when rapid decomposition occurs during normal drying. Another application concerns substances that can be dried at high temperatures but are thereby changed in some way.

Freeze drying is theoretically a simple technique. Pure ice exhibits an equilibrium vapor pressure of 4.6 mm Hg (611 Pa) at 0°C and 0.1 mm Hg (13.3 Pa) at −40°C. The vapor pressure of ice containing dissolved substances is, of course, lower. If, however, the pressure above the frozen solution is less than its equilibrium vapor pressure, the ice sublimes, eventually leaving the solute as a sponge-like residue equal in apparent volume to the original solid.

Continuous Driers

Although many types of continuous driers are available, the scale of the operation for which they are designed is rarely appropriate to pharmaceutical manufacture. As with most continuous operations, the cost is disproportionately high for small units. Spray and drum driers provide an exception, because residence times in the driers are short and thermal degradation is minimized. Under some conditions, freeze drying may be the only practicable alternative.

Spray driers

The solution or suspension to be dried is sprayed into a hot air stream and circulated through a chamber. The dried product may be carried out to cyclone or bag separators or may fall to the bottom of the drying chamber and be expelled through a valve. The chambers are normally cylindrical with a conical bottom although proportions vary widely. The process can be divided into four sections: atomization of the fluid, mixing of the droplets, drying, and finally removal and collection of the dry particles.

In vertical spray driers, the flow of the drying gas may be concurrent or counter-current with respect of the movement of droplets. The movement of the gas is, however, complex and highly turbulent. Good mixing of droplets and gas occurs, and the heat and mass transfer rates are high. In conjunction with the large interfacial area conferred by atomization, these factors give very high evaporation rates. The residence time of a droplet in the drier is only a few seconds (5–30 s). Since the material is at wet bulb temperature for much of this time, high gas temperatures of 150–200°C may be used even with thermolabile materials. Although the temperature of the material rises above the wet-bulb temperature at the end of the process, the drying gas is cooler and the material is almost dry, a condition in which many materials are thermally less sensitive.

Drying is considered to take place by simple evaporation rather than by boiling and it has been observed that a droplet reaches a terminal velocity within about one foot of the atomizer. Beyond this, there is no relative velocity between the droplet and the drying gas unless the former is very large. The droplets may dry to form a solid, spherical particle. If, however, the emerging solids form a skin, internal pressure may inflate the particle and the final dry form will consist of hollow spheres which may or may not have a blow hole. These xenospheres may also fragment, resulting in a final product of agglomerates of finely divided solids.

The capital and running costs of spray driers are high, but if the scale is sufficiently large, it may provide the cheapest method. When thermolabile materials are dried on a small scale, costs will be 10 to 20 times higher than for oven drying. Air used to dry fine chemicals or food products is heated indirectly, thus reducing thermal efficiency and increasing costs. In some other installations, hot gases from combustion may be used directly.

Drum driers

The drum drier consists of one or two slowly rotating, steam-heated cylinders. These are coated with solution or slurry by means of a dip feed in which the lower portion of the drum is immersed in an agitated trough of feed material or, in the case of some double-drum driers, by feeding the liquor into the gap between the cylinders. Spray and splash feeds are also used. In dip feeding, the hot drum must not boil the liquid in the trough. Drying takes place by simple evaporation rather than by boiling. The dried material is scraped from the drum by a knife at a suitable point.

Drying capacity is influenced by the speed of the drum and the temperature of the feed, which may be preheated. With the double-drum drier, the gap between the cylinders determines the thickness of the film.

Drum driers, like spray driers, are relatively expensive in small sizes and their use in the pharmaceutical industry is largely confined to drying thermolabile materials where the short contact time is advantageous. Drums are normally fabricated from stainless or chrome-plated steel to reduce contamination. The heat treatment to which the solid is subjected is more intense than in spray drying and the physical form of the produce is often less attractive during drying, the liquid approaches its boiling point and the dry solids attain the temperature of the drum surface.

SIZE REDUCTION AND CLASSIFICATION

The theoretical strength of crystalline materials can be calculated from interatomic attractive and repulsive forces. The strength of real materials, however, is found to be many times smaller than the theoretical value. The discrepancy is explained in terms of flaws of various kinds, such as minute fissures or irregularities of lattice structure known as dislocations. These have the capacity to concentrate the stress in the vicinity of the flaw. Failure may occur at a much lower overall stress than is predicted from the theoretical considerations. Failure occurs with the development of a crack tip which propagates rapidly through the material, penetrating other flaws which may, in turn, produce secondary cracks. The strength of the material depends therefore on the random distribution of flaws and is a statistical quantity varying within fairly side limits. This concept explains why a material becomes progressively more difficult to grind. Since the probability of containing an effective flaw decreases as the particle size decreases, the strength increases until, with the achievement of faultless domains, the strength of the material equals the theoretical strength. This position is not realized in practice due to complicating factors such as aggregation.

The strength of most materials is greater in compression than in tension. It is therefore unfortunate that technical difficulties prevent the direct application of tensile stresses. The compressive stresses commonly used in comminution equipment do not cause failure directly but generate by distortion sufficient tensile or shear stress to form a crack tip in a region away from the point of primary stress application. This is an inefficient but unavoidable mechanism. Impact and attrition are the other basic modes of stress application. The distinction between impact and compression is referred to later. Attrition, which is commonly employed, is difficult to classify but is probably primarily a shear mechanism.

The deformation and subsequent failure of a brittle material is not only a function of stress but also of the rate at which the stress is applied. Different results may be obtained from slow compressive breaking and impact breaking at the same energy level. Particle shape, size, and size distribution may be affected. In impact breaking, the rate of stress application is so high that the limiting strain energy may be exceeded several times by the suddenness of the operation. The reason is that fracture is time dependent, a lag occurring between the application of maximum stress and failure.

Stress application is further complicated by "free crushing" and "packed crushing" mechanisms. In free crushing, the stress is applied to an unconstrained particle and released when failure occurs. In packed crushing, the application of stress continues on the crushed bed of particles. Although further size reduction occurs, the process is less efficient due to vitiation of energy by the effects of interparticulate friction and stress transmission via particles which do not themselves fracture. This is easily demonstrated when a crystalline material is ground in a pestle and mortar. The fine powder initially produced protects coarser particles. If the material is sieved and

oversize particles are returned, the operation may be completed with far less effort.

Various hypotheses relate the net grinding energy applied to a process and the size reduction achieved. The first, proposed by Karl von Rittinger in 1867, states in Eq. 27 that the energy necessary for size reduction is directly proportional to the increase in surface area,

$$E = k(S_p - S_f) \qquad (27)$$

where E is the energy consumed, and S_p and S_f are the surface area of the product and feed materials, respectively. The constant, k, depends on the grinding unit employed and represents the energy consumed in enlarging the surface area by one unit. The relation between surface area and particle size has already been derived, and Eq. 28 may therefore be written,

$$E = k\left(\frac{1}{d_p} - \frac{1}{d_f}\right) \qquad (28)$$

where d_f and d_p are the particle sizes of feed and product particles, respectively.

The hypothesis indicates that energy consumption per unit area of new surface produced increases faster than the linear ratio of feed and product dimensions, a phenomenon already noted and explained. The proportionality of net energy input and new surface produced has been confirmed in some grinding operations.

Conversion of grinding energy to surface energy is neglected in Kick's law, promulgated in 1885. It is based on the deformation and brittle failure of elastic bodies and states that the energy required to produce analogous changes of configuration of geometrically similar bodies is proportional to the weight or volume of those bodies. The energy requirements are independent of the initial particle size and depend only on the size reduction ratio. Kick's law predicts lower energies than the relation proposed by Rittinger. The theory, however, demands that the resistance to crushing does not change with particle size. The role of flaws present in real materials is not considered, with the result that the energy required for fine grinding, when the apparent strength may have greatly risen, is underestimated.

A third theory of comminution gives results intermediate between the predictions of the laws of Kick and Rittinger (31). It rests upon three principles: the first states that any divided material must have a positive energy register. This can only be zero when the particle size becomes infinite. The input energy, E, for any size reduction process then equals the product energy register minus the feed energy register. The energy associated with a powder increases as the particle size decreases, and it may be assumed that the energy register is inversely proportional to the particle size to an exponent, n. Hence, Eq. 29 is valid.

$$E = E_p - E_f = \frac{K}{d_p^n} - \frac{K}{d_f^n} \qquad (29)$$

The second principle of this theory (31) assigns to n a value of i, stating that "the total work useful in breaking, which has been applied to a stated weight of an homogeneous material, is inversely proportional to the square root of the diameter of the product particles."

The third principle states that breakage of the material is determined by the flaw structure. This aspect of size reduction has already been discussed.

A modification to Kick's law, sometimes known as the fourth law of comminution, has also been proposed (32). For its discussion, the reader is referred to the original paper.

An empirical, but realistic approach to mill efficiency is gained through experiments in which the energy consumed and size reduction achieved are compared with values obtained in a laboratory test operating under free crushing conditions. All energy supplied in the latter is available for crushing and the test is assumed to be 100% efficient. Both slow crushing and impact tests are used. A large number of single particles may be simultaneously crushed and the work done is measured (33). The latter is related to the size reduction. Similar measurements can be made during practical milling, expressing the efficiency of the process as a percentage of the free crushing value. On this basis, the approximate efficiency of the roll crusher is 80%, of the swing hammer mill 40%, of the ball mill 10%, and of the fluid energy mill only 1%.

The Operation of Mills

Heywood (34) has stated that any type of crushing or grinding machine exhibits optimal comminution conditions for which the ratio of the energy to new surface is minimal. If finer grinding is attempted in such a machine, the; ratio is increased. Mills may thus become grossly inefficient if called upon to grind at a size for which they were not designed. A limited size reduction ratio is imposed upon a single operation, larger ratios being obtained by the adoption of several stages, each employing a suitable mill. The fluid energy mill, which presents a size reduction ratio of up to 400, is exceptional.

A low retention time is inherent in free crushing machines. Little overgrinding takes place and the production of excessive undersize material or fines is avoided. Protracted milling times are found with many low-speed mills, with the result that considerable overgrinding takes place. Accumulation of product particles within the mill reduces the effectiveness of breaking stresses and the efficiency of milling progressively decreases.

Dry and wet grinding

Between the approximate limits of 5 and 50% moisture, materials cake and do not flow. Both factors oppose effective grinding. Dry grinding is carried out at low moisture contents, the upper limit depending on the nature of the material. Although 5% or more moisture may be permissible for vegetable drugs, it would prove excessive during the milling of a coarse, impervious solid.

Wet grinding is a common procedure when a fluid suspension is required and drying, which would provide a significant drawback, is unnecessary. An excellent dispersion can be produced simultaneously, which in some operations provides the primary objective, size reduction being of secondary importance. Wet grinding also may be adopted when the size reduction achieved during dry grinding is prematurely linked by aggregation.

Certain general advantages are secured during wet grinding, including increased mill capacity, a lower energy consumption, the elimination of hazards from dust, and easier handling of materials. The principal disadvantage, apart from the possible inclusion of a drying stage, is the increased wear of the grinding medium.

Temperature sensitivity

Care must be exercised during the milling of temperature-sensitive materials, especially for a very fine product; caking results if the softening point is exceeded. Materials may be chilled before grinding or facilities provided for cooling the mill during grinding. Waxy solids can be successfully ground with dry ice, the low temperatures conferring brittle characteristics on the material. Chemical degradation may occur at high grinding temperatures. Oxidative changes can be prevented by grinding in an inert atmosphere such as nitrogen.

Structural changes

Several examples of change of physical structure during very fine grinding have been reported, for example, changes in the crystal form of calcium carbonate after ball milling (35), distortion of the kaolinite lattice (36), and formation of various barbiturate polymorphs (37). Changes such as these could affect solubility and other physical characteristics which, in turn, might influence formulation and therapeutic value.

Dust hazards

Hazards from dust may become acute during dry grinding. Extremely potent materials require dust proofing of machines and dust-proof clothing and masks for operators. Danger may also arise from the explosive nature of many dusts.

Grinding Equipment

The following equipment are in regular use for dry-grinding pharmaceutical materials: edge- and end-runner mills, hammer mills, pin mills, ball mills, vibratory mills, fluid energy mills, colloid mills, and roller mills.

Classification or Size Separation

Although a number of particle properties can be used to classify a powder, only two are important. The first is based on the ability of a particle to pass through an aperture. This is sieving or screening. The second employs the drag forces on a particle moving through a fluid. The term "classification" is sometimes restricted to this method of separation but here the terms "elutriation" and "sedimentation" are used. In general, screening is applied to the separation of coarse particles and sedimentation to the separation of fine particles.

Sieving and screening

Sieves and screens are widely used for the classification of relatively coarse materials. For very large particles (>0.5 in.) a robust plate perforated with holes is used. However, the pharmaceutical applications of screening are for much smaller particles and screens are in the form of woven meshes. Unless special methods are used to prevent clogging and powder aggregation, the lower useful limit is in a cloth woven with 200 mesh/in. (70–80 μm). Fine screens of this type are extremely fragile and must be used with great care.

As the scale of the operation increases it becomes, in general, less precise. For continuous screening, the feed material is made to move across the screen to a point of discharge. The residence time on the screen is usually short and many undersize particles traverse it without falling through. With an increase of sieving area, the meshes become more fragile and the finest meshes must be supported with a coarser wire. An example of a large-scale separator utilizes a circular screen, up to 5 ft (1.5 m) in diameter, vibrated in a horizontal plane, the gyratory movement being imparted by an out-of-balance fly wheel connected to the assembly. In other machines, the mesh is rectangular and inclined at a shallow angle (5–30°).

A gyratory movement is developed and the material to be classified is fed to the top. These machines may bear more than one deck, thus allowing the separation of the powder into several fractions at one time.

Elutriation and sedimentation

The simplest classifier is a rising current of fluid in which the particles are suspended. In this case, the force opposing the upward drag is gravitational. If the opposition develops a terminal velocity higher than the current speed, the particle falls. This is the principle of elutriation; the particle size d at which the separation is made follows from a rearrangement of Eq. 29 for conditions in which Stokes' law is valid; it is given by Eq. 30,

$$d = \sqrt{\frac{18\eta\mu}{(\rho_s - \rho)g}} \tag{30}$$

where $\rho_s - \rho$ is the density difference between solid and fluid, η is the viscosity of the fluid, and μ is the speed of the upward current.

In practice, fluctuations in flow conditions due to natural convection and a violation of the conditions for which Stokes' law is valid, blur the point of separation.

The centrifuge is normally operated to completely separate two phases. If, however, the rate at which the feed passes through does not allow all particles to settle, the action of a classifier is developed. This is illustrated by a solid-bowl centrifuge which consists of a steel shell in the form of a frustum mounted horizontally. It contains a conveying screw at the wall which rotates at a slightly higher speed than the shell. Particles that settle at the wall are conveyed to the narrow end of the shell and discharged. Fine particles are entrained with the overflow to the other end. Further details of this and other centrifugal classifiers have been given by Treasure (38).

MIXING

Mixing has been defined (39) as an operation in which two or more ingredients in separate or roughly mixed condition are treated so that each particle of any one ingredient is adjacent to a particle of each of the other ingredients, as nearly as possible. The term "blending" is synonymous and "segregation" or "demixing" is the opposite.

Mixing has been classified (40) as follows:

- *Positive mixing* which applies to systems that, given time, would spontaneously and completely mix. Examples are provided by two gases or two miscible liquids; mixing apparatus is used on such systems to accelerate mixing.

- *Negative mixing* is demonstrated by suspensions of solids in liquids. Any two-phase system in which the phases differ in density separates unless continuously agitated.
- *Neutral mixing* occurs when neither mixing nor demixing takes place unless the system is acted upon by a system of forces. Examples are found in the mixing of solids and of solids with liquids when the concentration of the former is high.

Theoretical knowledge is, however, insufficient to predict the performance of mixers. More commonly, choice is based upon broad empirical principles which are supported by practical tests.

Mixing of Solids

The mixing of all systems of matter involves a relative displacement of the particles, whether they are molecules, globules, or small crystals, until a state of maximum disorder is created and a completely random arrangement is achieved.

In 1953, Lacey (41) showed that the variation in the composition of samples drawn from a random mixture of two materials could be expressed by Eq. 31,

$$s = \sqrt{\frac{p(1-p)}{n}} \tag{31}$$

where s is the standard deviation of the samples, p is the proportion of one component, and n is the number of particles in the sample. The relation requires that the two components are alike in particle size, shape, and density and only can be distinguished by some neutral property, such as color. If very many samples are withdrawn from a mixture of equal parts of two materials, each containing a given number of particles, the results of analysis can be presented in the form of a frequency curve in which the samples are normally distributed around the mean content of the mixture, and 99.7% of the samples will fall within the limits $p = 0.5 + 3\sigma$. The standard deviation of the samples is inversely proportional to the square root of the number of particles in a sample. If the particle size is reduced to the extent that the same weight of sample contains four times as many particles, the standard deviation is halved.

In a critical examination of pharmaceutical mixing, Train (42) showed that samples of a random mixture of equal parts A and B must contain at least 800 particles if 997 out of every 1000 samples were to lie between ±10% of the stated composition, that is, the proportion, p, of

A = 0.5 ± 0.05, where σ = 0.05/3. If limits of ±1% were substituted, 90,000 particles must be present in each sample. The true standard deviation is given by σ. The standard deviation estimated by the withdrawal of a number of samples is denoted as s.

If, instead of equal parts A and B, the proportion of an active ingredient, A, in the mixture was 0.1 (10%), imposition of limits of ±10% (in 997 cases out of 1000) requires that each sample shall contain over 8000 particles. If the proportion of active constituent is 0.01, or 1%, a figure of 90,000 particles per sample is obtained, and if the limits are reduced to +1%, the active constituent is 0.01, or 1% a figure of 90,000 particles per sample is obtained, and if the limits are reduced to ±1%, the figure is 9×10^6.

The theoretical derivation of these results is based on component particles which vary in size, shape, and density. This condition is not encountered in the practical mixing of solids and, as described later, any of these factors may prevent the formation of a random mixture. The value of the number of particles per sample derived in any example must therefore be raised if the limits given are to be maintained.

As already shown, a series of samples drawn from a random mix exhibits a standard deviation of s_r. An index of mixing, M, suggested by Lacey (43) is given by Eq. 32,

$$M = \frac{s_r}{s} \tag{32}$$

where s is the standard deviation of samples drawn from the mixture under examination. This approaches unity as mixing is completed. Eq. 33 has been suggested,

$$M = \frac{s_0 - s}{s_0^2 - s_r} \tag{33}$$

where s_0 is the standard deviation of samples drawn from the unmixed materials. It is equal to $p(1-p)$, where p is the proportion of the component in the mix. It has been modified (43) to Eq. 34, using the variance of the samples,

$$M = \frac{s^2 - s_r^2}{s_0^2 - s_r^2} \tag{34}$$

This is a fundamental equation for expressing the state of the mixture, the index M varying from zero to one.

The binomial and Poisson distributions have also been used to examine the state of a mixture. If the proportion of black particles in a random mixture of black and white particles is p, the probability, $P(x)$, of obtaining x black particles in a sample of n particles is given by Eq. 35.

$$P(x) = \binom{n}{x} p^x (1-p)^{n-x} \tag{35}$$

If p is small (<0.15) and n is large, the Poisson distribution can be used, applying Eq. 36,

$$P(x) = e^{-m} \frac{m^x}{x!} \qquad (36)$$

where $m = np$, the mean number of black particles in the samples of n particles. This relation may be used in an assessment of dry mixing equipment (44). If m is greater than 20 and more than 10 samples are taken, then:

- About 10 of the samples have the number of black particle's outside the limits $m \pm 1.7\sqrt{m}$,
- About 5% of the samples have the number of black particles outside the limits $m \pm 2.0\sqrt{m}$, and,
- About 1% of the samples has the number of black particles outside the limits $m \pm 2.6\sqrt{m}$.

Mechanism of mixing and demixing

The randomization of particles by relative movement, one to another, is achieved by the following mechanisms:

- *Convective mixing*, where groups of adjacent particles are transferred from one location in the mass to another.
- *Diffusive mixing*, where the particles are distributed over a freshly developing surface, and
- *Shear mixing*, where slip planes are set up within the mass.

Convective mixing predominates in machines utilizing a mixing element moving in a stationary container, for example, the horizontal ribbon mixer. Groups of adjacent particles are moved from one position to another, steadily decreasing the scale of segregation.

Diffusive mixing predominates in tumbler mixers. The material is tumbled as it is lifted past its angle of repose. Mixing occurs when a particle changes its path of circulation through a collision or by being trapped in voids presented by another layer of particles.

Shear mixing occurs when forces acting on the particles induce the formation of a slip place, resulting in relative displacement of two regions. Shear mixing occurs, for example, in the rearrangement of shapes as the main charge falls from end to end in a double cone mixer. Train (42) has stressed the importance of expansion or dilation of the material so that shear forces may be effective. A practical corollary is that efficiency will be reduced if the machine is overfilled.

As long as one type of particle is not preferentially caught, random mixing eventually occurs in the radial plane. If, however, one component is smaller, denser, or has certain shape characteristics, it is preferentially trapped and moves into the lower layers of the mixing zone until it finally concentrates as a central core running

the length of the mixer. Similar effects occur in axial mixing, and the final shape of the segregated zone formed under the influence of axial and radial movement depends on the flow properties of the material. Similar effects have been reported with a double-cone blender (44). Segregation also occurs with materials dumped from the mixer.

Mixing rate

Because mixing is a process of achieving uniform randomness, the rate of mixing is proportional to the amount of mixing still to be done. If, at the start a particle changes its path of circulation, it is most likely to find itself in a different environment. The mixing rate is therefore high. At the end of the process, the particle is less likely to find a different environment, and such a change gives no useful mixing. Fewer mixing events take place, and the mixing rate finally reaches zero. It can be represented for any mixing mechanism by Eq. 37,

$$\frac{dM}{dt} = k(1 - M) \qquad (37)$$

where M, the index of mixing, has already been defined. Integration of Equation (37) gives Eq. 38.

$$M = I - e^{-kt} \qquad (38)$$

The rate constant, k, depends on the physical nature of the materials being mixed and on the geometry and operation of the mixer.

Mixing Machines

Trough and ribbon mixers

A simple trough mixer consists of a semicircular trough in which an impeller, such as a number of paddles mounted at diverse angles on a shaft running the length of the trough, rotates, lifting and distributing the material in an irregular manner. Convective and shear mixing occurs, as well as some fine-scale diffusive mixing when the impeller lifts material clear of the main charge.

The ribbon mixer employs a ribbon-like conveying scroll. The helix, which may be continuous or interrupted, is rotated in a semicircular trough and mixing again occurs through convection and shear, giving rapid coarse-scale dispersion. Two ribbons set to convey material in opposite directions are frequently fitted to the shaft. Although little axial mixing in the vicinity of the shaft occurs, mixtures with high homogeneity can be produced by prolonged mixing, even when components differ in particle size, shape, or density or tend to aggregate.

Tumbler mixers

Tumbler mixers operate primarily by a diffusive mechanism; their use is confined to freeflowing and granular materials. The mild forces are employed, which preclude the mixing of materials that aggregate strongly, allow friable materials to be handled satisfactorily. The more elaborate geometrical forms are most commonly used because movement of material in all planes, which is necessary for rapid overall mixing, is induced. Internal baffles and lifter blades may also be incorporated. For example, axial movement of material along the length of a simple drum mixer is slow and can be enhanced by these methods.

Mixing of Liquids

Miscible liquids are most commonly mixed by impellers rotating in tanks, including paddles, propellers, and turbines. All the material should pass through the impeller zone at frequent intervals of time, the design of the mixer preventing the formation of "dead" zones. The turbulent, high velocity flow of liquid from the impeller causes mixing by projecting eddies into, and entraining liquid from, the neighboring zones. The thin ribbons of one component in another rapidly become diffuse and finally disappear through molecular diffusion.

The flow pattern may be analyzed in terms of its three components of motion:

- Radial flow, in a direction perpendicular to the impeller shaft.
- Longitudinal or axial flow, in a direction parallel to the shaft, and
- Tangential flow, in which the liquid follows a circular path around the shaft.

A satisfactory flow pattern depends on the correct balance of these components. In a cylindrical tank, radial flow gives rise to axial flow by reaction at the wall of the tank. Tangential flow receives no such modification. Its predominance as laminar flow circulation supports stratification at various levels. Furthermore, a vortex is created at the surface of the liquid which may penetrate to the impeller, causing air to be dispersed in the liquid. In general, tangential flow should be minimized by moving the impeller to an off-center position, thus destroying the symmetry of the mixer, or by modification of the flow pattern by means of baffles. Tanks with vertical agitators may be baffled by one, two, or more strips mounted vertically on or just away from the vessel wall. These reduce but do not eliminate tangential flow, whereas little modification of radial and axial flow occurs. Baffles produce additional turbulence.

Paddle mixers

For a simple paddle, with upper and lower blades, suitable for mixing miscible liquids of low viscosity a tangential flow pattern predominates with zones of turbulence to the rear of the blades (10–100 rpm). The gate paddle is suitable for mixing liquids of higher viscosity and the anchor paddle with low clearance between pan and blade is useful for working across a heat transfer surface. Stationary paddles intermeshing with the moving element suppress swirling in the mixer. In other examples, baffles are also necessary. Unless paddle blades are pitched, poor axial turnover of the liquid occurs. Paddles are therefore not suitable for mixtures that separate.

Propeller mixers

Propellers are commonly used for mixing miscible and immiscible liquids of low viscosity. The marine propeller is typical of the group. High speed rotation (400–1500 rpm) of the relatively small element provides high shear rates in the vicinity of the impeller and a flow pattern with mainly axial and tangential components. They may be used in unbaffled tanks when mounted in an off-center position or inclined from the vertical. In large-scale operations, horizontal mounting in the side of the vessel is frequently used.

Turbines

Turbine designs are intermediate between paddles and propellers. Turbines are effective mixers over a wide viscosity range and provide a very versatile mixing tool. The ratio of radial to tangential flow, the predominating parameters with this impeller, increases as the operating speed increases. Pitched-blade turbines are sometimes used to increase axial flow. Baffles must be used to limit swirling unless the turbine is shrouded. This impeller produces a discharge with no tangential component.

STERILIZATION

Sterilization processes do not result in a product that can be described as absolutely sterile or nonsterile inasmuch as the process is a statistical phenomenon. A variety of techniques are available (45), including heat, radiation, ethylene oxide sterilization, and sterile filtration.

Thermal Sterilization

The amount of heat required to sterilize depends upon the magnitude (T), duration (t), and amount of moisture present, t 1/T. For example, heat coagulates protein in the living cell. The temperature required for this phenomenon to occur is inversely proportional to the moisture present.

Dry heat

Relatively stable substances that resist degradation at high temperatures (>140°C) are suitable candidates for dry heat sterilization. A 2-h exposure at 180°C or 45 min at 260°C kills spores as well as vegetative forms of micro-organisms. These exposure periods do not include the lag time from loading of the oven until sterilization temperature is reached. The lag time depends on the geometry and operating features of the oven and the characteristics of the load.

Both natural and forced-convection oven types can be employed; they have been described in the section on drying. The forced-convection oven offers the advantages of uniformity of heat distribution and reduction in lag time in comparison with the natural-convection system. The dry-heat method is reserved almost exclusively for glass or metal as other materials char (cellulose), oxidize (rubber), or melt (plastic) at these temperatures.

Moist heat

Moist heat offers the advantage of greater effectiveness at low temperatures. The thermal capacity of steam is much greater than that of hot air. Spores and vegetative forms of bacteria may be effectively destroyed in an autoclave employing steam (121°C) under pressure (15 psig) for 20 min or (27 psig at 132°C), for 3 min. The lag time to complete exposure of the material to be sterilized is important.

Radiation

Ultraviolet light is frequently employed to reduce airborne microbial contamination. Surface sterilization is usually achieved by employing a mercury vapor lamp with an emitted light of 253.7 run.

Radiation sterilization includes the use of the ionizing radiation of x-rays and gamma-rays. The former are derived from bombardment of a heavy metal target with electrons. Gamma-rays are obtained from atomic nucleus decay from excited to ground state.

The energy evolved from radiation can be equated to photon behavior where E hv and $v = $ C/λ, (E and v are the energy and frequency of a photon, respectively), h is Planck's constant, and C and λ are the speed and wavelength of light, respectively. The energy absorbed from the radiation sources equates to the dose.

$$1\tilde{~}\text{rad} = 100\,\text{erg/g of material absorbing}$$
$$= 6.24 \times 10^{13}\,\text{eV/g}$$
$$= 2.4 \times 10^{-6}\,\text{cal/g}(10 \times 10^{-6}\,\text{J/g})$$

There are a variety of radiation sources. ^{60}Cobalt decays to ^{59}Co in the core of a nuclear reactor to emit two photons (1.17 and 1.33 MeV) and an electron (0.31 MeV). The half-time for decay is 5.3 years. ^{137}Cesium decays emitting one photon (0.661 MeV). Cesium has a 33-year half-life. An electron beam can be accelerated to an energy equivalent of 5–10 MeV. At energies below 5 MeV, penetration is insufficient for sterilization. Depth of penetration can be correlated with energy levels; for example, materials with density equivalent to water ($\rho = 1$ g/cm^3) are penetrated 0.5 cm/MeV. ^{60}Cobalt gives rise to radiation that penetrates 30 cm through water. Accelerating electrons have a high dose rate and exposure is only required for seconds. ^{60}Cobalt has a lower dose rate, and an exposure for hours is required.

Ionizing radiation arises from the photoelectric effect, the Compton effect, or ion pair production. Gamma radiation causes local and intense damage and may break chemical bonds. The primary target is the deoxyribonucleic acid (DNA) of the micro-organism. In addition, free radicals may be formed, such as peroxides that result in intracellular and extracellular peroxides by a chain reaction that causes damage.

Resistance to damage

Damage depends on the amount of energy absorbed relative to the number and resistance of the micro-organisms being irradiated. Unicellular organisms have greater resistance than multicellular ones. Gram-positive bacteria have greater resistance than gram-negative bacteria. Finally, bacterial spores have greater resistance than vegetative forms. Viruses are more resistant than bacteria. The energy required to reduce the population of viruses by 90% (D value), is 0.5 Mrg i d (5 mGy). Fungi are equivalent to bacterial spores in their resistance.

In order to evaluate the dose, a number of parameters must be known. What magnitude of source (e.g., ^{60}Co) is available? A typical source ranges from 500,000 to 2×10^6 Curies (Ci) where 1 Ci is 3.7×10^{10} disintegrations per second. The product geometry and the speed of the conveyor carrying it to the source must be known. The dose can be evaluated by a variety of dosimetric techniques. In bulk or ampoules containing liquids, ferric ammonium sulfate and ceric sulfate can be used and the absorbance change evaluated by UV spectroplidtometry; however, this is only accurate for ^{60}CO and ^{137}CS.

Radiochromic solids can be utilized and evaluated by visible spectrophotometry. Amber and red polymethyl methacrylate are used to evaluate 0.1–1.0 Mrad and 0.5–5.0 Mrad, respectively. Nylon film is examined for opacity following exposure and may be used to evaluate exposures of 0.1–5.0 Mrad.

Validation requires the determination of the bioburden and the *D* value. These represent the dose required to achieve sterilization and the estimated dose. If low *D* values are obtained, the dose may be regarded as overkill. Bocillus pumulis exhibits inherently high resistance to gamma-ionization radiation (*D* values 0.15–0.22 Mrad). The FDA prefers a 12-log reduction in microorganisms. The dose required is approximately 2.6 Mrad.

Ethylene Oxide

Ethylene oxide (bp, 10.8°C) is a gaseous alkylating agent. It alkylates proteins and ribonucleic and deoxyribonucleic acid in micro-organisms. It replaces labile hydrogen with hydroxyethyl groups. Ethylene oxide is utilized as a surface sterilant. Bulk crystalline materials can occlude vegetative bacterial cells or spores with crystals. Consequently, ethylene oxide does not reach them. The final step prior to sterilization is an aseptic recrystallization step.

Ethylene oxide is a colorless gas with an aromatic odor. The threshold limit for the odor is 700 ppm. The OSHA specification for worker exposure is 10 ppm. The toxicity of ethylene oxide is similar to that of ammonia. It causes conjunctival and respiratory irritation, dizziness, headaches, and vomiting. It is known to be mutagenic and may be carcinogenic. By-products include ethylene glycol (bp, 198.9°C) and ethylene chlorhydrin (bp, 128.4°C). Pure ethylene oxide is flammable and explosive. It is generally mixed with propellant (88:12) or carbon dioxide (90:10). Ethylene oxide polymerizes in the liquid state in 90–120 days. In this form it may plug lines or deposit polymerized sludge.

Ethylene oxide inactivates all micro-organisms. The sterilizing rate depends upon its concentration, the temperature, the duration of exposure, and the water content of the micro-organism. Inactivation follows classical first-order kinetics and is irreversible. Relative humidity is synergistic, at 30–60% the micro-organism hydrates. The water acts as a vehicle to transport the gas through polyethylene and polypropylene. Polystyrene traps ethylene oxide and dissipates it over years and thus is not appropriate for ethylene oxide sterilization. Temperatures of 40–60°C are suitable for heat-sensitive articles. Cycle times are longer at low temperatures, relative humidities, or ethylene oxide concentrations.

Generally, concentrations of 350–700 mg/ml are employed; cycle times vary from 4 to 12 h.

Following sterilization the load is degassed by a dynamic process wherein filtered air is passed over the product for 12–72 h. Degassing usually takes place in the treatment chamber but may be moved to a sterile facility. The process is monitored using *Bacillus subtilis var. niger* as a biological indicator, commercially available as spore strips (10^6 spores per strip). In addition, the load is probed with thermocouples during validation. The gaseous mixture is sampled at different points in the sterilizer for gas chromatographic analysis.

Sterile Filtration

Several filter geometries are available for sterile filtration. They consist of flat membranes in a stainless steel press (<293 mm), pleated membranes housed in stainless steel cartridges, and stacked plates in the form of flat segments of membrane filters.

Matrix filters consist of fibers with pores having a depth up to 120 μm. Cellulose nitrate may be dissolved in a highly volatile solvent, such as amyl acetate, ether, or dioxane. A gel-forming solvent, acetone, ethanol, or propanol, may be added. The mixture is poured on a flat plate and placed in a controlled-temperature environment to dry. Pore size is dependent on the concentration of the gel-forming solvent. A number of other substances may be used as filter material, including cellulose, acetate and butyrate, polyamides (nylon), polysulfones, fluorocarbons (Durapore membranes), polyvinylidene difluoride (hydrophobic), or surfaces modified with organic amides (hydrophilic), acrylic polymers, or polyvinyl chloride. To make some membranes hydrophilic, surfactants may be added including Tween 80, Triton X-100, hydroxypropyl cellulose, or glycerol. Sieve filters are made of polycarbonate (Nucleopore, 10 μm thick). Collimated uranium fission products form nucleation tracks in film. Exposure to chemical etching determines the pore size.

Adsorption and screening

Most membrane filters, when wetted, have a negative charge. Bacteria have a similar negative charge and do not necessarily remain on the filter. Filters with other characteri stics can be selected under these circumstances. Positively charged (AMF Zeta Plus Membrane) or protein- and peptide-adsorbing (Pall Posidyne Nylon 66) filters can be selected.

Ionic strength, pH, pressure, and flow rate affect particle adsorption. The flow rate through a filter is expressed by Eq. 39,

$$Q = \frac{C_i A P}{V} \qquad (39)$$

where C_i is the inherent resistance of the filter to flow (a function of void volumes), A is the surface area, P is the pressure, and V is the viscosity. Filters are rated according to nominal pore size and absolute pore size (the largest pore in the filter); this recognizes that a pore size distribution exists.

Filter integrity

The filter integrity can be evaluated by a number of techniques. The destructive test involves filtering a suspension of bacterial cells (*Pseudomonas diminuta*, 0.3×1 μm, through a 0.2 μm-filter. If 6 L of suspension containing 1×10^7 organisms per mL are passed through a 1-μm filter, there should be no microorganism and an 8-log reduction would have occurred. The bubble-point test assumes that pores can be characterized as capillaries. When totally wetted, all the capillaries should be full of water or solution. The pore length is generally much greater than the diameter. Pressure is applied to the wetted filter. The bubble-point pressure, P, may be described by Eq. 40,

$$P = \frac{4\gamma \cos \Theta}{D} \qquad (40)$$

where γ is the surface tension (72 dynes/cm^2 or 7.2 Pa), θ is the contact angle, and D is the diameter of capillary. The bubble-point test is performed before and after sterile filtration.

A specified area of filter must be soaked in a specified volume of product for a designated time. The accelerated stability of active ingredients at 40–60°C for 60 days must be established prior to the selection of a filter for a particular purpose. The extent of damage, and the nature and quantity of extractables and their potency have to be evaluated.

EXTRACTION AND LEACHING

Leaching or solid–liquid extraction are terms that describe the extraction of soluble constituents from a solid or semisolid by means of suitable solvents. The process, which is used whenever tea or coffee is made, is an important stage in the production of many fine chemicals found naturally in animal and vegetable tissue. Examples are found in the extraction of fixed oils from seeds, in the preparation of alkaloids, such as strychnine from *Nux vomica* beans or quinine from Cinchona bark; and in the isolation of enzymes, such as rennin, and hormones, such as

insulin, from animal sources. In the past, a wider importance attended the process because the products of simple extraction procedures, known as galenicals, formed the major part of the ingredients used to fulfill a doctor's prescription.

Whatever the scale of the extraction, leaching is performed in one of two ways. In the first, the raw material is placed in a vessel, forming a permeable bed through which the solvent or menstrum percolates. The wanted constituents are dissolved, and the solution issues from the bottom of the bed. This liquid is sometimes called the miscella and the exhausted solids, the marc. The process is called leaching by percolation. The second process employs immersion and consists of immersing the solid in the solvent and stirring. After a suitable period of time, solid and liquid are separated.

Percolation

Coarsely ground material is placed in the body of the extractor which may be jacketed for control of the extraction temperature. The packing must be even or the solvent flows preferentially through a limited volume of the bed and leaching is inefficient. In large extractors, channeling is prevented or reduced by horizontal, perforated plates placed at intervals in the bed; these redistribute the percolating liquid.

Solvent inhibition swells dried materials and reduces the permeability of the bed. This is most marked with aqueous solvents. If swelling occurs, it is necessary to moisten the material with water or with the solvent before it is packed into the extractor.

Immersion

In pharmaceutical processes, leaching by immersion is carried out in simple tanks which may be agitated by a turbine or paddle. If the solids are adequately suspended, intimate contact between the phases promotes efficient extraction. Incomplete extraction due to channeling is avoided and difficulties due to swelling do not arise. Problems arise, however, in the subsequent separation of the phases. The materials to which leaching by immersion is applied are normally either finely divided or coarse and compressible. When agitation ceases, the solids settle and the leach liquid can be siphoned or pumped off by lines suitably placed in the tank. The sediment, however, contains a large volume of the leach liquid which must be recovered by resuspending the solids in fresh solvent, allowing the solids to sediment and decanting the supernatant liquid. Cake filtration provides an alternative method of separation. The leach liquid remaining in the cake is displaced by passing a wash liquid. In some cases, a filter press may be used for both extraction and separation.

Solvent

The ideal solvent is cheap, nontoxic, and nonflammable. It is highly selective, dissolving only the wanted constituents of the solid. It should have a low viscosity, allowing easy movement through a bed of solids, and, if the resulting solution is to be concentrated by evaporation, have a high vapor pressure. Water and alcohol, and mixtures of the two, are widely used. Both, however, are nonselective, leaching varying proportions of gums, mucilages, and other unwanted components. Most of the tinctures and liquid extracts used in pharmacy are simple, impure extracts made with, water or mixtures of water and alcohol. Acidified or alkaline mixtures of water and alcohol are used to extract insulin from comminuted pancreas. A more selective extraction is given by petroleum solvents, benzene, and related solvents. In the preparation of many pure alkaloids, the powdered material is moistened with an alkaline solution, packed into a bed, and leached with petroleum. Subsequent purification by fractional crystallization is facilitated by the absence of gums. Acetone and chlorinated hydrocarbons also find applications in leaching. In some cases, specific properties of the wanted constituents may suggest a particular solvent. Eugenol, for example, can be readily extracted from cloves with a solution of potassium hydroxide.

Leaching Rate

Whatever method is adopted, leaching consists of a number of consecutive diffusional or mass transfer processes. The solvent first penetrates the raw material and dissolves the soluble elements. These diffuse in the opposite direction to the surface of the solid matrix and through the liquid layers at its surface to reach the bulk solution. These processes are under the influence of an overall concentration gradient, the concentration being lowest in the bulk solution. Any of these processes may be responsible for limiting the rate at which leaching proceeds. In pharmaceutical leaching, however, the solid matrix is usually cellular, a structure which normally offers the highest diffusional resistance. The complexity of such structures does not permit a strict analysis of the processes of mass transfer. Nevertheless, the simple diffusional concepts expressed in Fick's law suggest that the following factors influence the leaching rate:

- The size distribution of the leached particles,
- The temperature of leaching,
- The physical properties of solvent, and
- The relative movement imposed upon the solids and the liquid.

Size and Size Distribution of the Solid Particles

The particle size of the solids determines the distance which solvent and solute must diffuse within the solid matrix. Since this distance offers the major diffusional resistance, its reduction by comminution raises the rate of leaching, the concentration gradient being effectively increased. In addition, the inverse relationship between particle size and surface area requires an increase in the area of contact between the matrix and the surrounding liquid. Transfer of solute at this boundary is therefore facilitated. In leaching by immersion, a further advantage conferred by size reduction is the ease with which finer particles are suspended. Finally, extensive cell rupture occurs during grinding, allowing more direct contact between solvent and solute and more rapid dissolution and diffusion.

Other factors, however, operate against size reduction. Leaching by percolation demands the formation of a permeable bed. Low permeability gives low flow rates and low extraction rates. Permeability is a complex function of both particle size and porosity, the former determining how a given void space is to be disposed within the bed. The disposition of the void space consists of few channels of relatively large diameter, that is, a bed of high permeability, if the particle size is large. In leaching by immersion, the difficulties of separating solid and liquid increase as the particle size decreases.

The opposition of the factors suggests an optimum particle size for any particular extraction. This is determined to some extent by the physical nature of the solids. A dense, woody structure would be extracted as a fine powder. An example is given by the root of Ipecacuanha. A leafy structure, on the other hand, would be more satisfactorily leached as a coarse powder.

Both porosity and permeability are influenced by the particle size distribution. A high porosity is secured if the distribution is narrow. Small particles may otherwise fill the interstices created by the contact of larger particles. After grinding it is often necessary, therefore, to classify the product and remove undersize material. This material would then be bulked with the fines from other batches and extracted separately. A further advantage arising from a narrow size distribution is even packing and the creation of a regular system of pores and waists. This promotes even movement of solvent and solution through the bed.

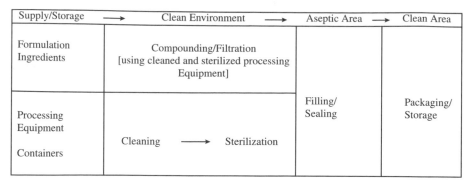

Fig. 6 Flow diagram illustrating the various processes in sterile parenterals production.

Temperature

Within the limits imposed by the thermal stability of the wanted constituents, a high extraction temperature appears desirable. The solubility of most materials increases with increasing temperature, allowing higher solute concentrations and higher concentration gradients. Both this and the increased diffusivity result in higher extraction rates. In many cases, however, materials are susceptible to heat degradation and cold extraction must be used. In addition, the selectivity of a solvent may be impaired at high temperatures. An example of the use of moderately high temperatures is the extraction of Rauwolfia alkaloids with boiling methanol.

The Relative Movement Imposed Upon the Solids and the Liquid

The major and controlling resistance to the diffusion of the solute to the bulk solution is normally found in the cell matrix. Increase in the rate of movement of the solution past the surface does not, therefore, greatly affect the rate of extraction. This is in marked contrast to the processes of dissolution and crystallization. Nevertheless, movement is imposed upon the solvent in both general methods described above.

In the percolation of a liquid through a bed of solids, mass transfer of the solute from the surfaces of the solid to the liquid in the interstices of the bed takes place by molecular diffusion and by natural convection arising from the density changes created by dissolution. Although these processes are slow, they are much faster than mass transfer in the matrix under the same concentration differences. Concentration gradients in the liquid outside the particles are, therefore, very low. At any point in the bed, the introduction of dilute solution from above and the loss of concentrated solution to below decrease the interstitial concentration by dilution or displacement. This effect can be considered simply to reduce the solute concentration at the junction of solid and solution, thus imposing a favorable concentration gradient within the matrix.

APPLICATIONS

The processes described here are integrated in order to facilitate the production of pharmaceutical dosage forms. The following examples are intended to illustrate the application of the processes in the dominant pharmaceutical settings. They have been selected to demonstrate the broad application of unit operations in pharmaceutical manufacturing. Unique processes are associated with each dosage form. This is no less the case for dermatologics, intranasal and inhalation products, and the range of alternative pharmaceuticals than for the examples given. Nevertheless, the majority of processes and their underlying principles (11) are similar from one dosage form to the next.

Parenteral Products

Parenteral products are intended for injection into a variety of subdermal and submucosal locations (46). Their manufacture can be defined as a sequence of operations intended to be performed in certain environments or under specific conditions. Fig. 6 illustrates the sequence in which these processes may be combined. This flow diagram shows the relationship of the unit operations to the underlying physical-organic chemistry of compounding and the subsequent processes pertaining to packaging.

Solid Dosage Forms

The majority of solid dosage forms are intended for oral ingestion. The drug released from the dosage form is available at the site of absorption or action within the gastrointestinal tract.

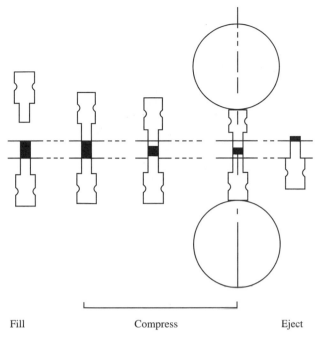

Fill   Compress   Eject

Fig. 7   Sequence of events in tablet press operation.

Additional processes are required for the production of tablets beyond those described previously. As these processes are not ubiquitous in pharmaceutical manufacturing they are dealt with only briefly here.

Granulation

Following particle size reduction and blending the formulation may be granulated (47), which provides

homogeneity of drug distribution in the blend. In addition, it may help flow properties and compression characteristics of the powder. Large granules can be prepared from primary particles by drying from a slurry (with techniques described above) or spraying with granulating solution. Fig. 7 shows a top-spray granulator. An alternative method (Fig. 7) employs an auger to force the blend between rollers, thereby forming a compressed solid which disintegrates into large aggregates (48).

The steps involved in granulation begin with transferring powders to a mixer and blending the product. The granulation solution can be added and coarse milling or wet granulation begun. Finally, the product is dried and milled to an appropriate size.

Compression

Compressed solids, tablets, or caplets, are prepared by placing the blend of component additives in a cylinder or die, above a moveable piston or punch. An upper punch is brought into the top of the piston, and pressure applied to the distal ends of the punches forces the powder into a compact (Fig. 7). The quality of the product depends upon the cohesive forces acting on the powder upon compression. These cohesive forces are influenced by the selection of additives in the dosage formulation. One method of evaluating tablet manufacture considers the effect of the applied pressure on porosity of a compressed powder (49). Data may be plotted as the negative natural logarithm of porosity against applied pressure in the form of a Heckel plot (50). The slope of this plot is proportional to the yield value (ϕ, elastic limit) with a value of $1/3\phi$).

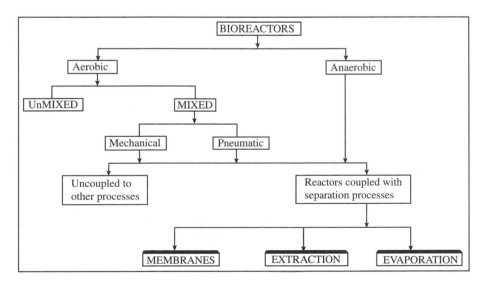

Fig. 8   Schematic of types of bioreactors.

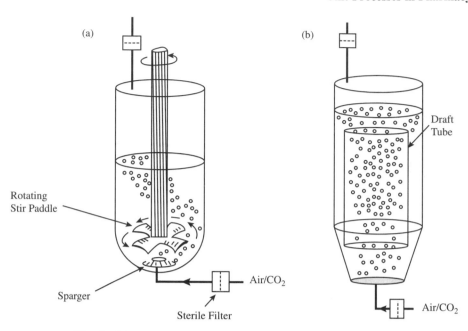

Fig. 9   Bioreactors: (a) stirred tank reactor; (b) airlift fermentor.

Bioprocessing

The use of biotechnology in the manufacture of pharmaceuticals is of increasing interest Consequently these techniques require attention in the planning of unit processes. Bioprocessing can be considered in terms of small-scale bioreactors, or fermenters, and the translation of such processes into large-scale economically viable production operations (51, 52).

Bioprocessing is by no means a new field. The topicality of this subject is due to the increased interest in the use of isolated cells and microorganisms as manufacturing tools. It might well be argued that this technology was developed millennia ago for the purposes of wine and beer production. More recently, the use of attenuated microorganisms or isolated antigenic materials for vaccination resulted in further developments. In the last decade, the interest in genetic engineering and manipulation of the genetic code of certain microorganisms has produced a revolution in the manufacturing of pharmaceuticals.

Bioreactors

The major difference between a biotechnological process and other pharmaceutical manufacturing operations is the need for a bioreactor (Fig. 8). These bioreactors may be required to produce expressed proteins utilizing bacteria, yeast, insect, or mammalian cells. It would be difficult to describe the various bioreactor elements and their permutations. Some of simplest examples of bioreactors are shown in Fig. 9.

CONCLUSION

Pharmaceutical manufacturing entails the combination of a number of unit processes. The major processes have been described in this article. Brief outlines of the applications of these processes to parenteral, solid dosage form, and biological materials production are given.

The efficiency, quality, and economy of manufacturing depends upon an understanding of the individual operations involved in processing. In many cases, unlike in other industrial processing, safety and efficacy of a therapeutic agent may be affected. A guide or introduction to the practical aspects of unit processes in pharmacy is provided here.

REFERENCES

1.   Ganderton, D.; Hickey, A.J. Unit Process in Pharmacy: Fundamentals. *Encyclopedia of Pharmaceutical Technology*; Swarbrick, J., Boylan, J.C., Eds.; 1st Ed.; Marcel Dekker, Inc.: New York, 1996; 15, 341–398.
2.   McCabe, W.L.; Smith, J.C.; Harriott, P. *Unit Operations in Chemical Engineering*; 5th Ed.; Ind. McGraw-Hill, Inc.: New York, 1993.

3. Hickman, K.C.D. Commercial Molecular Distillation. Eng. Chem. **1947**, *39*, 686.
4. Ives, K.J. Proc. Inst. Civ. Engrs. **1963**, *25*, 345.
5. Ives, K.J. Symposium: Interaction Between Fluids and Particles. Inst. Chem. Engr. **1962**, ,260.
6. Maroudas, A.; Eisenklam, P. Clarification of Suspensions: A Study of Particle Deposition in Granular Media. Chem. Eng. Sci. **1965**, *20*, 867.
7. Salter, K.C.; Hosking, A.P. Chem. Eng. Pract. **1958**, *6*, 487.
8. Dickey, G.D. *Filtration*; Reinhold: New York, 1961.
9. Suits, C.G. *The Collected Works of Irving Langmuir*; Pergamon: New York, 1961; 10, 394.
10. Hinds, W.C. *Aerosols Technology, Properties, Behavior and Measurement of Airborne Particles*; John Wiley and Sons: New York, 1982; 164–186.
11. Terjsen, S.G.; Cherry, C.B. Trans. Inst. Chem. Engrs. **1947**, *25*, 89.
12. Reist, P.C. *Aerosol Science and Technology*; 2nd Ed.; McGraw-Hill, Inc.: New York, 1992.
13. Gaden, E.L.; Humphrey, A.E. Fibrous Fitters for Air Sterilization. Design Procedure. Ind. Eng. Chem. **1956**, *48*, 2172.
14. Stairmand, C.J. Trans. Inst. Chem. Engrs. **1950**, *28*, 130.
15. Hesketh, H.E.; EI-Shobokshy, M.S. *Predicting and Measuring Fugitive Dust*; Technomic Publishing Co., Inc.: Lancaster, PA, 1985, 1–33.
16. Fuchs, N.A. *The Mechanics of Aerosols*; Dover Publications, Inc.: New York, 1964.
17. Humphrey, A.E.; Gaden, E.L. Air Sterilization by Fibrous Media. Industr. Eng. Chem. **1955**, *47*, 924.
18. Cherry, G.B.; McCann, E.P.; Parker, A. The Removal of Bacteria from Air by Filtration: Application to Industrial-Scale Fermentations. J. Appl. Chem. **1951**, I,S103.
19. Scott, M.W.; Lieberman, H.A.; Chow, F.S.; Rankell, A.S.; Johnston, G.W. Drying as a Unit Operation in the Pharmaceutical Industry. I. J. Pharm. Sci. **1963**, *52*, 284.
20. Scott, M.W.; Lieberman, H.A.; Chow, F.S. Pharmaceutical Applications of the Concept of Equilibrium Moisture Contents. J. Pharm. Sci. **1963**, *52*, 994.
21. Newitt, D.M.; Na Nagara, P.; Papadopoulos, A.L. Trans Inst. Chem. Engrs. **1960**, *38*, 273.
22. Ceaglske, N.H.; Hougen, O.A. Drying Granular Solids. Indust. Eng. Chem. **1937**, *29*, 805.
23. Pearse, J.F.; Oliver, T.R.; Newitt, D.M. Trans. Inst, Chem. Engrs. **1949**, *27*, 1.
24. Shepherd, C.B.; Hadlock, C.; Brewer, R.C. Drying Materials in Trays. Evaporation of Surface Moisture. Industr. Eng. Chem. **1938**, *30*, 388.
25. Cooper, J.; Swartz, C.J.; Suydam, W. Drying of Tablet Granulations. J. Pharm. Sci. **1961**, *50*, 67.
26. Pikal, M.J.; Roy, M.L.; Shah, S. Mass and Heat Transfer in Vial Freeze-Drying of Pharmaceuticals: Role of the Vial. J. Pharm. Sci. **1984**, *73*, 1224–1237.
27. Nail, S.N. The Effect of Chamber Measure on Heat Transfer in the Freeze Drying of Parenteral Solutions. J. Parent. Drug Assoc. **1980**, *34*, 358–368.
28. Jennings, T.A. Discussion of Primary Drying During Lyophilization. J. Parent. Sci. Techn. **1988**, *42*, 118–121.
29. Dushman, S.; Lafferty, J.M. *Scientific Foundations of Vacuum Technique*; 2nd Ed.; John Wiley and Sons: New York, 1962; 48.
30. Ho, N.F.H.; Roseman, T.J. Lyophilization of Pharmaceutical Injections: Theoretical Physical Model. J. Pharm. Sci. **1979**, *68*, 1170–1174.
31. Bond, F.C. The Third Theory of Comminution. Trans. Amer. Inst. Min. Metall. Engrs. **1952**, *193*, 484.
32. Holmes, J.A. Trans. Inst. Chem. Engrs. **1957**, *3S*, 125.
33. Carey, W.F.; Stairmand, C.J. Recent Advances in Mineral Dressing. Inst. Min. Metall. **1953**, 117.
34. Heywood, H. Chem. Eng. Pract. **1957**, *3*, 8.
35. Gammage, R.B.; Glasson, D.R. Crystal Changes in Vateritic Calcium Carbonate During Ball Milling. Chem. Ind. **1963**, 1466.
36. Gregg, S.J. Trans. Br. Ceram. Soc. **1955**, *54*, 257.
37. Cleverley, B.; Williams, P.P. Polymorphysm and Changes of Infrared Spectra of Barbiturates During Sample Preparation. Chem. Ind. **1959**, 49.
38. Treasure, C.R. G. Trans. Inst. Chem. Engrs. **1965**, *43*, T199.
39. Perry, R.H.; Chilton, C.H. *Chemical Engineer's Handbook*; 5th Ed.; McGraw-Hill: New York, 1973.
40. Dankwerts, P.V. The Theory of Mixtures and Mixing. Research **1953**, *6*, 355.
41. Lacey, P.M.C. Trans. Inst. Chem. Engrs. **1953**, *21*, 53.
42. Train, D. Pharmaceutical Aspects of Mixing Solids. Pharm. J. **1960**, *185*, 129.
43. Lacey, P.M.C. Developments in the Theory of Particle Mixing. J. Appl. Chem. **1954**, *4*, 257.
44. Adams, J.F.E.; Baker, A.G. Trans. Inst. Chem. Engrs. **1956**, *34*, 91.
45. Avis, K.E.; Akers, M.J. Sterilization. *The Theory and Practice of Industrial Pharmacy*, 3rd Ed.; Lachman, L., Lieberman, H.A., Kanig, J.L. Eds.; Lea & Feblger: Philadelphia, 1986; 619–638.
46. Boylan, J.C.; Fites, A.L. *Modern Pharmaceutics*; 2nd Ed. Marcel Dekker, Inc.: New York, 1990, 491–538.
47. Carstensen, J.T. Heterogenous Systems. *Theory of Pharmaceutical Systems*; Academic Press: New York, 1973; 2, 223.
48. Doelker, E. Assessment If Powder Compaction. *Powder Technology and Pharmaceutical Processes*; Chulia, D., Deleuil, M., Pourcelot, Y., Eds.; Elsevier: Amsterdam, 1994; 403–471.
49. Carstensen, J.T. *Pharmaceutical Principles of Solid Dosage Form*; Technomic Publishing Company: Lancaster PA, 1993; 73.
50. Heckel, R.W. Density Pressure Relationships in Powder Compaction. Trans. Metal. Soc. AIME **1961**, *221*, 671.
51. Propkop, A.; Bajpai, R.K. *Recombinant DNA Technology and Applications*; Prokop, A., Bajpai, R.K., Ho, C., Eds.; McGraw-Hill, Co.: New York, 1991; 415–459.
52. Hofmann, F.K. Scaleup of Production and Purification of Cell Expressed Proteins. *Pharmaceutical Biotechnology, Fundamentals and Essentials*; Klegerman, M.E., Groves, M.J., Eds.; Interpharm Press: Buffalo Grove IL, 1992;, 138–164.

BIBLIOGRAPHY

Allen, T. *Particle Size Measurement*, 4th Ed.; Chapman and Hall: New York, 1990.

Andrews, G.A.; Kniseley, R.M.; Wagner, H.N. *Radioactive Pharmaceuticals*; US Atomic Energy Commission: Washington, 1966.

Ansel, H.C.; Popovich, N.G.; Allen, L. *Pharmaceutical Dosage Forms and Drug Delivery Systems*, 6th Ed.; Williams and Wilkins: Malvern, PA, 1995.

Avis, K.E. *Process Engineering Applications* Interpharm Press, Inc.: Buffalo Grove, IL, 1995.

Banker, G.S.; Rhodes, C.T. *Modem Pharmaceutics*, 2nd Ed.; Marcel Dekker, Inc.: New York, 1990.

Carey, V.P. *Liquid-Vapor Phase-Change Phenomena* Hemisphere Publishing Corporation: New York, 1992.

Carstensen, J.Y. *Pharmaceutical Principles of Solid Dosage Forms;* Technomic Publishing Co.: Lancaster, PA, 1993.

Cheremisinoff, P.N. *Air/Particulate Instrumentation and Analysis;* Ann Arbor Science: Ann Arbor, 1981.

Chulia, D.; Deleuil, M.; Pourcelot, Y. *Powder Technology and Pharmaceutical Processes;* Elsevier Science B.V.: Amsterdam, 1994.

Groves, M.J. *Parenteral Technology Manual*, 2nd Ed.; Interpharm Press: Buffalo Grove, IL, 1988.

Groves, M.J.; Olson, W-P.; Anisfeld, M.H. *Sterile Pharmaceutical Manufacturing*; Interpharm Press: Buffalo Grove IL, 1991.

Hesketh, H.E.; EI-Shobokshy, M.S. *Predicting and Measuring Fugitive Dust*; Technomic Publishing Company: Lancaster, 1985.

Hyman, D. Mixing and Agitation. *Advances in Chemical Engineering*; Academic Press: New York, 1962; 3.

Klegerman, M.E.; Groves, M.J. *Pharmaceutical Biotechnology Fundamentals and Essentials*; Interpharm Press: Buffalo Grove, IL, 1992.

Lachman, L.; Lieberman, H.A.; Kanig, J.L. *The Theory and Practice of Industrial Pharmacy*; 3rd Ed.; Lea & Febiger: Philadelphia, 1986.

Lefebvre, A.H. *Atomization and Sprays*; Hemisphere Publishing Corporation: New York, 1989.

Little, A.; Mitchell, K.A. *Tablet Making*, 2nd Ed.; The Northern Publishing Co., Ltd. Liverpool, 1963.

Masters, K. *Spray Drying Handbook*, 5th Ed.; Longman Scientific and Technical and John Wiley and Sons, Inc.: New York, 1991.

Mullin, J.W. *Crystallization*, 3rd Ed.; Butterworth-Heinemann: London, 1993.

Wert, C.A.; Thomson, R.M. *Physics of Solids* 2nd Ed. McGraw-Hill, Inc.: New York, 1970.

Mullin, J.W. *Crystallization*; Butterworth: London, 1961.

Pietsch, W. *Size Enlargement by Agglomeration*; John Wiley and Sons: New York, 1991.

Prokop, A.; Bajpai, R.K.; Ho, C. *Recombinant DNA Technology and Applications*; McGraw-Hill, Inc.: New York, 1991.

Tien, C. *Granulator Filtration of Aerosols and Hydrosols* Butterworths: Boston, 1989.

Van-Hook, A. *Crystallization: Theory and Practice*; A.C.S. Monograph No. 152 Chapman and Hall: London, 1961.

Weidenbaum, S.S. Mixing of Solids. *Advances in Chemical Engineering*; Academic Press: New York, 1958; 2.

VACCINES AND OTHER IMMUNOLOGICAL PRODUCTS

Suresh K. Mittal
Harm HogenEsch
Kinam Park
Purdue University, West Lafayette, Indiana

VACCINES

Introduction

The concept of vaccination was introduced in the late 18th century by Edward Jenner when he used cowpox virus as a vaccine to protect humans against smallpox virus infections. This led to the development of vaccines over the next 2 centuries to provide protection against various bacterial and viral pathogens. Undoubtedly, the effective vaccination against infectious diseases is the best method of reducing suffering of human and animals caused by viral, bacterial, and parasitic infections. Over the last 200 years, the technology of vaccine development and production has not changed significantly. This usually involves the use of either a killed pathogen combined with an adjuvant or a live pathogen with reduced virulence. Apart from the tremendous success of killed and attenuated virus vaccines over the years, many of such vaccines do not provide satisfactory protection, and there are a number of other disadvantages associated with these vaccines. Additionally, there are important pathogens against which attempts to develop effective vaccines using traditional approaches were unsuccessful. Various protective viral antigens (envelope and/or capsid proteins or glycoproteins and other viral proteins) and bacterial antigens (surface, internal, or fimbria proteins; bacterial polysaccharides; bacterial toxins; and other proteins involved in bacterial metabolism) have been identified as potential vaccine candidates. These protective antigens are used by various means to develop effective vaccines. The field of vaccine technology is not limited to infectious diseases but has shown potential in other areas, such as cancer treatment, reproduction, and modulation of animal productivity. An overview of vaccine strategies is depicted in Fig. 1.

Conventional Vaccines

Inactivated vaccines

Inactivated (killed) pathogenic organisms can be used in vaccines. This is the simplest way to produce vaccines,

provided the organisms can be cultured easily. Therefore, this method is often first tested to develop a potential-vaccine. As with any other technique of vaccine production, this procedure is only good for some organisms. There are a number of methods of inactivating pathogenic organisms; the most common are treatment with chemicals (formalin, formaldehyde, or propiolactate), heat, or γ-irradiation. In some instances, the procedure of inactivation may enhance antigenicity of some antigens important in protection. Inactivated vaccines usually result in good humoral immune response after multiple inoculations. Because inactivated vaccines in general fail to elicit effective mucosal and cell-mediated immune responses, they may provide limited protection against mucosal and intracellular pathogens. Failure to inactivate the pathogenic organisms completely could result in disease instead of protection. During the 1950s, some lots of poliovirus vaccine were not inactivated completely (1, 2). Now, the methods used to detect residual infectivity are more stringent, therefore, inactivated vaccines are considered safe with extremely low or no chance of infection.

There have been instances in which inactivated vaccines led to atypical disease or enhanced disease severity. For example, in the 1960s, formalin-inactivated respiratory syncytial virus (RSV) vaccine actually enhanced the disease symptoms when vaccinated children were naturally exposed to RSV (3, 4). It was later discovered that a change in the antigenicity of RSV F and G glycoproteins (5) resulted not only in alteration in humoral immune response but also in the Th1 and Th2 components of the CD4+ T-cell response to RSV (6).

Live attenuated vaccines

Mostly attenuated organisms are being used as live virus vaccines; however, in some instances, even virulent organisms could be used, provided they are not administered via the natural route of infection. For example, human adenovirus types 4 and 7 may cause acute respiratory infections in humans when administered via the oronasal route but provide protection when given orally in enteric-coated capsules (7).

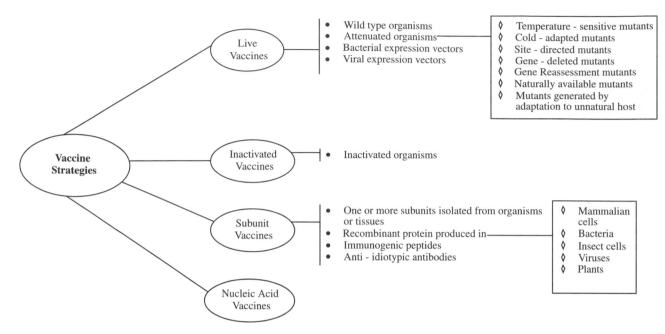

Fig. 1 Overview of vaccine strategies.

There are different ways to attenuate pathogens for vaccine production. Attenuation of organisms can be achieved by growing them under abnormal conditions, which include cultivation in unnatural hosts or cell lines. Some organisms are attenuated when they replicate at different pH levels and/or temperatures. In cells infected with multiple viruses with a segmented genome (e.g., influenza virus, reovirus), genome segments are randomly recombined in the progeny. This process of recombination is known as reassortment and is also useful in generating attenuated viruses. A natural pathogen of one host may be attenuated for another host, e.g., vaccinia virus worked as an attenuated vaccine for small poxvirus eradication program during the 1960s and 1970s, and turkey herpesvirus works as an attenuated vaccine for Marek's disease virus (a chicken herpesvirus). In an inoculated host, the attenuated organism replicates without causing disease symptoms, thereby leading to induction of immune response somewhat similar to the natural infection with the disease-causing organism. The Bacille Camet–Guerin (BCG) strain of *Mycobacterium tuberculosis* was attenuated after more than 200 passages on media containing increasing amounts of bile. The Sabin poliovirus vaccine was attenuated by a number of passages in monkeys and in monkey kidney epithelial cells (8). Measles virus was initially adapted to monkey kidney cells and subsequently attenuated in duck embryo and human tissue culture cell lines (9–11).

Temperature-sensitive (*ts*) mutants have proven to be the most useful type of mutants for a number of viruses and bacteria because of their conditional-lethal phenotype. The (*ts*) mutants are produced by alteration in the nucleotide sequence of a gene so that the resulting protein product of the gene is unable to assume or maintain its functional configuration at the nonpermissive (37–39°C) temperature. The protein, however, is able to assume a functional configuration at the permissive temperature (32–34°C), e.g., herpesviruses, adenoviruses, and influenza viruses. Thus, these mutants can replicate in mucosal sites with a lower temperature, e.g., the nasal cavity, but are unable to cause systemic infections and disease.

A number of advantages associated with live vaccines are that: 1) they are cheap to produce because the inoculum dose is relatively less, 2) they require fewer inoculations, 3) they do not require adjuvants, 4) they elicit both humoral and cell-mediated immune responses, and 5) they can be inoculated by the natural route of infection. Some of the disadvantages associated with live vaccines are that 1) they are usually less stable than inactivated vaccines and may require refrigeration for storage, 2) some of these vaccines under certain situations may revert to virulent form in the host and thereby lead to clinical disease, 3) they may not be recommended for immunosuppressed, immature, older, or pregnant hosts, 4) they may have a low level of residual virulence, and 5) they may be contaminated with other adventitious organisms.

Recombinant Vaccines

Recombinant vector vaccines

Viral vectors: For the development of an effective vaccine strategy for protection against mucosal pathogens such as respiratory and enteric viruses, a vaccine-delivery system that can induce a protective mucosal immunity in the form of secretory IgA antibody, in addition to a systemic immune response, is extremely important. The route of vaccine delivery also plays an important role in determining the type of resultant immunity induced. A number of viruses, such as adenoviruses, poxviruses, herpesviruses, picornaviruses, togaviruses, orthomyxoviruses, paramyxoviruses, and others, have demonstrated considerable potential as vectors for antigen delivery at mucosal surfaces (12). Immunogenic foreign epitopes can be expressed on the virus surface by modifying the viral capsid or envelope protein (13). A wide variety of foreign viral antigens has been expressed in viral vectors, and vaccination-challenge studies in experimental animals have demonstrated moderate to complete protection. Immunization with such vectors leads to the foreign viral antigen expression similar to that of natural infection without causing disease. Antigenic peptides are expressed along with major histocompatibility (MHC) class I and class II antigens and, thus, result in both humoral and cytotoxic T-cell responses.
Both adenovirus-and poxvirus-based vectors have a number of common advantages including that 1) vector construction is easy, ii) relatively high levels of foreign protein expression are easily attained, 3) relative thermostability, 4) they have a large capacity for foreign DNA insertion, 5) vector derivatives are nonpathogenic, and 6) they have a wide host range. More than one foreign antigen can be expressed in the same vector to provide protection against a number of diseases by inoculation with a single vector.

Vaccinia virus expressing rabies glycoprotein has been licensed for use to control rabies in the wildlife population, especially raccoons, foxes, skunks, and coyotes (14). Baits containing a live vaccinia-rabies glycoprotein recombinant virus vaccine are distributed in the rabies endemic area with the intention that rabies-susceptible wild animals that eat these baits will become immunized against rabies virus (15), and this approach has demonstrated satisfactory results. Vaccinia virus expressing the F and H gene of rinderpest virus has shown potential for its use to control rinderpest in developing countries (16, 17).

To increase the safety of viral vectors for immuno-compromised hosts and to control their indiscriminate spread, replication defective viral vectors have been developed. These vectors can be grown to high titers in vitro, but they are defective for in vivo replication. Replication-defective vectors undergo an abortive infection in an inoculated host that leads to foreign antigen expression similar to replication-competent vectors. Replication-defective adenovirus vectors are generated by deleting the early region 1 (E1) genes (18,19). E1-deleted vectors can be grown in an E1-complementing cell line, and animals immunized with such vectors elicit a protective immune response (20). Avian poxviruses grow normally in avian cells but would result in an abortive infection in mammalian hosts. Dogs and cats immunized with an avipox-rabies glycoprotein recombinant are protected against rabies virus infection (21).

Bacterial vectors: Similar to viral expression vectors, attenuated bacteria can be developed as vectors for foreign gene expression and delivery for the purpose of multivalent vaccines. Immungenic foreign epitopes can be expressed on bacteria surfaces by modifying cell surface proteins, fimbria, or flagella. It has been demonstrated that *M. bovis* BCG strain induces both strong humoral and cell-mediated immunity, therefore, it has been developed as a delivery vector with the assumption that foreign proteins expressed by *M. bovis* in inoculated individuals will also raise a strong protective immune response (22). Because *Salmonella* and *Vibrio* colonize in the intestinal tract, attenuated strains of these bacteria were developed as vectors for mucosal delivery (23–26).

Various bacterial vectors have been used to express a number of bacterial (*B. pertussis, S. pneumoniae, Y. pestis,* and *L. monocytogenes*), viral (herpesvirus, influenza virus, human immunodeficiency virus, simian immunodeficiency virus, and hepatitis B virus), and parasitic (*S. mansoni,* and *L. major*) antigens (26). Significant improvements in attenuation of bacteria, and the stability, localization, and expression levels of heterologous antigens are required to market the bacterial vector-based vaccines for use in humans or animals.

To enhance foreign gene expression, "balanced lethal," plasmid-based expression vehicles have been developed (27). A foreign antigen may form inclusion bodies or localize in intracellular compartment of the vector thereby affecting the type, levels, and duration of immune response elicited against the antigen. The *Escherichia coli* α-hemolysin secretion system (HSS) that includes HlyB, HlyD, and TolC is involved in exporting the HlyA-fused foreign antigens to extracellular compartment (28). Using the HSS system for attenuated *Shigella dysenteriae,* the expression and secretion of Shiga toxin-B subunit were obtained (29).

Gene-deleted vaccines

Many attenuated vaccines are derived after introduction of random mutations in the genomes of various pathogens. In situations in which these random mutations may be point mutations, attenuated organisms may regain virulence owing to back mutations. Because of our increased understanding of virulence of various pathogens at the molecular level, one or more genes responsible for virulence has been identified in many pathogens. The genes associated with virulence may be genes involved with nucleic acid replication and other nonstructural and structural components of the organism. This has made it possible to delete one or more of these genes involved in virulence—another strategy to produce safer attenuated vaccines.

Pseudorabies virus has been attenuated by deleting genes associated with viral virulence. These genes include the thymidine kinase gene (nonstructural protein) involved in viral DNA replication and the gC, gG, and gE genes (nonessential glycoproteins) involved in virus assembly (30, 31). A gene-deleted vaccine of pseudorabies virus has proved highly effective in controlling this viral infection under field conditions. It has been demonstrated that *Salmonella typhimurium* aroA, aroB, and aroC deletion mutants fail to grow in its host because of the absence of aromatic amino acid production. These genes have been targeted to reduce the virulence of the bacterium. *S. typhimurium* gene-deleted mutants are capable of replication at least for a short period in its host, thus raising a protective immune response (32). Vaccination with gene-deleted vaccines also allows eradication of wild-type pathogens from the population. Because antibodies against the deleted gene product will only be developed in infected animals, it is feasible to differentiate between vaccinated and naturally infected animals (33, 34). The process of gene deletion not only attenuates the pathogen but also offers a unique opportunity to insert foreign genes for developing viral or bacterial-vectored vaccines.

Subunit vaccines

A subunit vaccine consists of one or more immunogenic epitopes, proteins, or other components of a pathogenic organism. Immunogenic epitopes can be chemically synthesized and are known as peptide vaccines, e.g., peptide vaccine candidates for foot-and-mouth disease virus (35, 36). The pathogen could be disrupted, and one or more immunogenic proteins such as bacterial cell wall proteins; flagella or pili; and viral envelope, capsid, or nucleoproteins can be purified. The isolation of such components in purified form is sometimes cumbersome and expensive. However, bacterial exotoxins can be easily purified, inactivated, and used as toxoid vaccines.

A number of expression systems including bacteria, yeasts, mammalian cells, insect cells, and plants are now available for foreign protein expression. High amounts of a foreign protein can be produced in a bacterial-expression system at a low cost. Because scale-up and downstream processing have been well worked out for bacterial-expression systems, they are usually first tested for subunit vaccine production. Many of the immunogenic proteins, especially of viral origin, require secondary modifications that are important for their antigenicity. A bacterial-expression system may produce proteins of altered immunogenicity because the bacterial system lacks many posttranslational processes. However, some viral glycoproteins expressed in bacteria induce protective immunity, e.g., the gp 70 gene of feline leukemia virus (37). A yeast-expressed hepatitis B virus surface antigen (HbsAg)-based subunit vaccine is currently in use for humans and has demonstrated excellent protection against hepatitis B virus infection (38). This vaccine is an excellent example of the potential of recombinant subunit vaccines for providing protection against many viral and bacterial infections.

Because mammalian cells are known to process viral glycoproteins to their functional form by secondary modifications, they are considered one of the means to produce viral antigens for subunit vaccine production. However, the expression of such proteins in mammalian cells is usually too low. It was demonstrated that the stable expression of the transmembrane anchor-deleted form of many viral glycoproteins in mammalian cells results in the secretion of truncated products in the medium in large quantities that could be used as a subunit vaccine without further purification. However, the removal of transmembrane anchor may potentially alter antigenicity of the secreted protein. A number of viral glycoproteins that were expressed either in mammalian or in insect cells and secreted in form of proteins were suitable for providing protective immune response include F and G genes of respiratory syncytial virus (39), the HN and F genes of parainfluenza virus (40), and the gD gene of bovine herpesvirus type 1 (41).

Immunogenic antigen production in plants: In the past decade, significant progress has been made in the stable integration and expression of a wide variety of genes in plant cells, resulting in the creation of novel plants for agricultural and industrial use. The inserted genes confer resistance to insect pathogen and herbicides; enhanced tolerance to drought, salt, and frost; and improved agricultural production. Undoubtedly, improvements in plant attributes by genetic engineering will have a great impact on agriculture production. However, it has been estimated that the major economic (over 90%) gain of plant biotechnology will result from the use of plants as bioreactors to produce high-valued products such as vaccines, industrial enzymes, and other pharmaceuticals.

Production of subunit vaccines in mammalian cells is usually expensive because of the low level of foreign gene expression and high processing cost. High levels of foreign gene expression can be obtained in bacteria and yeast, but many animal viral or mammalian proteins expressed in these systems fail to undergo proper secondary modifications such as glycosylation, phosphorylation, sulfation, etc. Therefore, these recombinant proteins may have altered antigenicity. Because most mechanisms regulating secondary modifications of proteins are present in plants, transgenic plants offer an attractive alternative to produce functional viral, bacterial, or parasitic proteins in large quantities at a very low cost for subunit vaccine production (42). Similarly, the production of functional multimeric antibody molecules in plants has made it possible to manufacture antibodies in bulk amounts for passive immunization (43).

Two major strategies have been devised to produce foreign proteins in plants. These are: 1) the stable integration of chimeric gene into the plant genome under a suitable constitutive or inducible plant promoters (44, 45), and 2) manipulation of plant pathogenic viruses (46). Foreign protein expression in plants usually range from 0.01 to 1% of the total plant protein.

The hepatitis B virus (HBV) surface antigen HBsAg produced in transgenic tobacco elicits an immune response when injected In mice (47). Mice fed transgenic potato tuber expressing B subunit of heat-labile enterotoxin (LT-B) of enterotoxigenic E. coli developed antibodies to LT-B, particularly IgA antibodies (44). Dalsgaard et al. (46) demonstrated that immunization of mink with the VP2 capsid protein of mink enteritis virus, expressed in cowpea after infection with modified cowpea mosaic virus, elicited a protective immune response. Protection against challenge with virulent foot-and-mouth disease virus (FMDV) in mice inoculated with the structural protein VP1 of FMDV produced in transgenic Arabidopsis has been shown (45). It has been hypothesized that transgenic plants could serve as "edible vaccine," thereby providing a very inexpensive mean of oral immunization (48).

Anti-idiotypic vaccines

Another approach to provide protective immune response is the use of anti-idiotype antibodies as vaccines. Antibodies have unique sequences in the variable (V) region in their binding site known as "idiotypic determinants". Some of the idiotypic determinants make up the antigen-binding site (paratope) of the antibody. The part of the antibody that binds to the antigen is called a paratope. Antibodies to a specific paratope of an idiotype mimic the epitope of immunizing antigen and are known as anti-idiotypic antibodies. Thus, anti-idiotype antibodies are mirror images of

antigens and can be used instead of immunogens to elicit a protective immune response. Monoclonal anti-idiotypic antibodies could serve as a source of antigen. Anti-idiotype vaccines are useful in cases in which actual antigen is poorly immunogenic or similar to host antigens. Some of the pathogens against which anti-idiotype vaccines have been tested include Listeria monocytogenes, Streptococcus pneumoniae, hepatitis B virus, Semliki forest virus, and Sendai virus (49, 50). This type of vaccine is still in the developmental stage.

DNA Vaccines

Immunization of mammalian hosts with a plasmid DNA containing a gene under control of a heterologous promoter has introduced a new approach in the area of recombinant vaccine design. The introduced DNA is taken up by cells, and the gene of interest is expressed. The cells expressing the foreign antigen are recognized by the host immune system, leading to humoral and cell-mediated immune responses. DNA vaccines can also be called polynucleotide vaccines or nucleic acid (NA) vaccines. Such vaccines appear to have the primary advantages of both attenuated and inactivated vaccines but without their known limitations. NA vaccines elicit an immune response similar to that obtained with live attenuated vaccines. They also provide safety similar to that of inactivated vaccines, however, without the obvious side effects of adjuvants or animal-derived proteins.

The concept of NA vaccine evolved from initial studies in experimental animals in which the inoculation with naked plasmid DNA resulted in a protective immune response (51). After inoculation into a muscle, the efficiency of cellular uptake of the naked DNA is poor, and a large portion of the DNA is degraded before it reaches the nucleus for transcription. To increase the efficiency of DNA uptake by host cells and to reduce DNA degradation within the cell, a number of delivery systems,

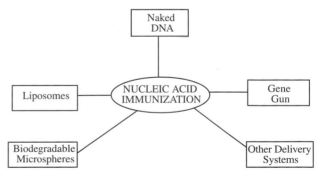

Fig. 2 Methods of nucleic acid delivery.

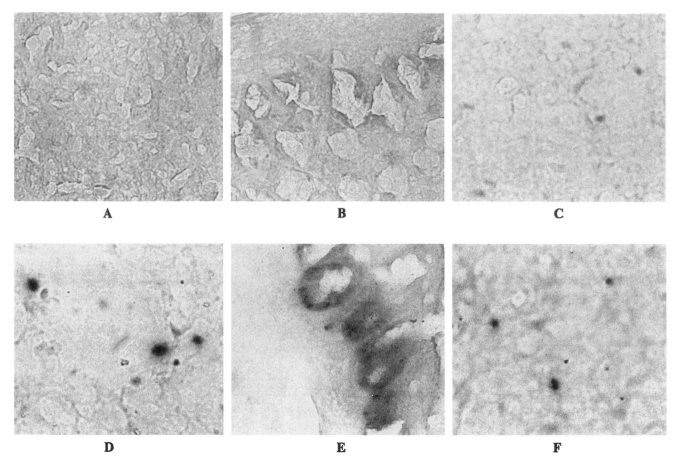

Fig. 3 β-Galactosidase expression in tissues of mice inoculated orally with alginate microspheres containing plasmid DNA: (A) liver, (B) intestine, and (C) spleen sections from the animal inoculated with microspheres containing bovine adenovirus type 3 (BAd3). (D) Liver, (E) intestine, and (F) spleen sections from the animal inoculated with microspheres containing LacZ plasmid +, BAd3. (From Ref. 57.)

such as bombardment with gold microparticles coated with NA (52, 53), incorporation of NA into liposomes and other polycationic lipids (54, 55), biological erodable polymers (56), and others, have been developed (Fig. 2). Recently, it has been demonstrated that alginate microspheres can be used for the encapsulation, delivery, and expression of plasmid DNA (57) (Fig. 3). Inoculation of mice with microspheres containing both plasmid DNA and bovine adenovirus type 3 (BAd3) resulted in a significant increase in transgene expression compared with those inoculated with microspheres containing only the plasmid DNA. As with other delivery systems, alginate microspheres led to a stronger mucosal or systemic immune response, depending on route of inoculation (58). Because alginate microspheres are most likely taken up by macrophages and dendritic cells, it may have a positive effect on the type of immune response elicited.

A number of factors that have an impact on the level and type of immune response produced by an NA vaccine include the type of immunogen, the dosage and number of inoculations, the heterologous regulatory sequences, the delivery system, the route of inoculation, and the presence or absence of immunomodulatory molecules. A variety of immunogenic antigens including HIV-1, SIV, HTLV-1, influenza virus, hepatitis B virus, hepatitis C virus, herpesvirus, M. tuberculosis, *Leishmania,* malaria, and many more have been expressed by NA vaccines and have demonstrated encouraging results (59–63).

Adjuvants

Adjuvants are compounds that, when administered in combination with antigens, enhance the immune response to those antigens. This enhanced immunogenicity can be measured as an increase of antigen-specific antibody levels in serum and/or mucosal secretions, a response against an increased number of epitopes, an increase of cell-mediated immune responses, or a combination thereof. Adjuvants are particularly important for the induction of protective immune responses against weak immunogens such as subunit vaccines. The mechanisms by which adjuvants enhance the immunogenicity of antigens are not completely understood, but they include immunostimulation, altered processing of antigens, and sustained release of antigens (depot effect). A different type of immune response is obtained by administration of antigens via the oral route, and this has different delivery requirements.

Many compounds can act as adjuvants. Their classification is made difficult by the variety in chemical composition and the overlapping, often poorly understood, mechanisms of action. Only aluminum adjuvants are approved by the FDA for use in human vaccines. Quil A is a saponin that is commonly used as an adjuvant in veterinary vaccines and is also a component of immune-stimulating complexes (ISCOM). These adjuvants are addressed in some detail below. A detailed discussion of other types of adjuvants can be found in recent books (64–66) and reviews (67) on this subject.

Immunostimulation

The immune system can be divided into the adaptive immune system, comprising of B and T lymphocytes, and the innate immune system, which includes neutrophils, macrophages, dendritic cells, and soluble factors such as the complement system. The innate immune system plays a critical role in the activation of the adaptive immune system. Dendritic cells are antigen-presenting cells that integrate the signals from the innate immune system and activate T-cells and possibly B-cells. T-cells have antigen-specific receptors that recognize peptides displayed by MHC I molecules (CD8$^+$ cytotoxic T-cells) and MHC II molecules (CD4$^+$ T helper cells). Engagement of the antigen-specific T-cell receptor is not sufficient, and T-cells also need to receive costimulatory signals delivered via CD28 and CD40-ligand. Dendritic cells express both MHC I and MHC II and, on activation, increase the expression of the costimulatory molecules CD80 and CD86 (ligands for CD28) and CD40. The signals that activate dendritic cells include microbial molecules. The innate immune system is equipped with receptors (called pattern-recognition receptors) that can recognize molecules that are expressed by pathogens, but not by mammalian cells, and alert the innate immune system on infection. These molecules, pathogen-associated molecular patterns, include lipopolysaccharides (LPS), mannose, and bacterial DNA with unmethylated CpG motifs. In addition, dendritic cells are stimulated by host cell components that are expressed and/or released by cells when they undergo stress and pathologic cell death (necrosis). The identity of these components, called danger signals, is uncertain but

may include heat shock proteins. The microbial molecules and danger signals can directly activate dendritic cells, or they can activate other components of the innate immune system resulting in the secretion of cytokines and other mediators that activate dendritic cells. The activated dendritic cells, in turn, activate T- and B-cells.

Immune responses can be divided into type 1 and type 2, based on the pattern of cytokine secretion and functional outcome of the immune response. Type 1 immune responses are characterized by secretion of IFN-gamma, production of IgG2a in mice, and activation of macrophages, NK cells, and cytotoxic T-cells. Type 2 responses are characterized by secretion of IL-4, IL-5, and IL-13 and by IgG1 and IgE production. The responses are reciprocally regulated. How the polarization of the immune response toward type 1 or type 2 is determined is not exactly understood. IL-12 is an important factor that drives the type 1 response, and IL-4 is implicated in the type 2 response. Microbial products such as LPS and bacterial DNA stimulate the secretion of IL-12 by dendritic cells and preferentially induce type 1 immune responses.

It is likely that the primary mechanism by which adjuvants stimulate the immune response is by direct or indirect signaling through pattern-recognition and danger signal receptors. Very strong adjuvants are often composed of or include microbial components such as LPS and mycobacteria or derivatives thereof. These type of adjuvants bind to pattern-recognition receptors to stimulate IL-12 production and a type 1 immune response. Coadministration of cytokines can directly activate and influence dendritic cells and the outcome of the immune response. This was clearly demonstrated with an experimental Leishmania vaccine using IL-12 as an adjuvant. Immunization of genetically susceptible BALB/c mice with a Leishmania antigen did not result in protection, but when IL-12 was injected with the antigen, the mice became markedly resistant to infection. The effect of IL-12 correlated with increased IFN-γ and decreased IL-4 secretion by antigen-specific T-cells in vitro.

Altered processing of antigens

Most T-cells that carry the $\alpha-\beta$-T-cell receptor do not recognize and react with intact proteins. Instead, the T-cells recognize small peptides that are derived from proteins and that are linked to MHC I and MHC II molecules. The MHC I-linked peptides are generated in the cytoplasm (endogenous pathway) and recognized by CD8$^+$ T-cells. Proteins in the cytoplasm are degraded by a complex of proteolytic enzymes, the proteasome, and the peptides are transported into the rough endoplasmic reticulum where they associate with MHC I molecules. Peptide binding stabilizes the MHC I molecules, and the complexes are transported to the cell surface. In contrast, proteins that enter cells by endocytosis are partially degraded into peptides in endosomal vesicles. The peptides bind MHC II molecules that have been transported from the endoplasmic reticulum to the endosomes. The MHC II–peptide complexes are then displayed on the cell surface and are available for recognition by $CD4^+$ T-cells.

Vaccines that contain single proteins or inactivated pathogens can readily activate $CD4^+$ T-cells because the antigens are endocytosed and processed by MHC II–positive antigen-presenting cells. Activation of the $CD4^+$ T-cells can result in a type 1 or a type 2 immune response, depending on the type of adjuvant included. However, such vaccines usually do not activate $CD8^+$ cytotoxic T-cells because activation of $CD8^+$ T-cells requires processing of antigen via the endogenous pathway. Certain adjuvant formulations such as liposomes, the saponin QS-21, and poly-(lactic-*co*-glycolic acid) (PLGA) are able to induce cytotoxic T-cell responses to protein antigens (68). These adjuvants appear to target some of the injected antigens into the cytosol of antigen-presenting cells for processing via the endogenous pathway. The mechanism by which this occurs is not known.

Sustained release of antigens

The slow and continued release of antigens has been postulated to induce a strong immune response through continued activation of the immune system. This may contribute to the adjuvant effect of aluminum-based adjuvants and mineral oils. Newer technologies may allow for the design of vaccines that release antigens from a depot at certain time intervals after a single injection. One example is the use of poly PLGA microspheres for encapsulation of antigens. By varying the polymer composition and size of the microspheres, the release of antigen can be varied. Pulsatile release of antigen can be attained by combining multiple variations of PLGA microspheres in a single dose of the vaccine (69). Relatively little is known about the desired pattern of antigen release to obtain a maximal response. It was recently suggested that continued release of antigen is not desirable for the induction of strong memory cell responses. Mathematical models may help design appropriate strategies for the release of antigens from depots after a single injection (70).

Aluminum

Aluminum adjuvants in human vaccines are either aluminum hydroxyphosphate (commonly referred to as aluminum phosphate) or aluminum oxyhydroxide (aluminum hydroxide) (71). Aluminum-based vaccines are prepared by adsorption of antigen to commercial aluminum hydroxide or aluminum phosphate gels or by mixing antigen with alum (potassium aluminum sulfate), resulting in precipitation. The alum-precipitated adjuvants resemble aluminum phosphate in their chemical and physical properties (71). The surface charge and morphology of the aluminum adjuvants affect their adsorptive capacity. The rate and degree of adsorption are further dependent on the pH, ionic strength of the antigen solution, and isoelectric point of the antigen.

Aluminum adjuvants are universally used in diptheria–tetanus–pertussis (DTP) vaccines and in most hepatitis B vaccines and have an excellent safety record. They are not ideal adjuvants, however, because the enhancement of the immune response is relatively weak, they are not effective with all antigens, and, most important, they only enhance the humoral (type 2) immune response and have little effect on the cell-mediated (type 1) immune response.

The mechanism by which aluminum enhances the immune response is not clear. Early studies suggested that aluminum adjuvants slowly release the adsorbed antigen over time (depot effect). However, recent experiments demonstrated that antigens are rapidly desorbed after injection in animals. Moreover, aluminum phosphate enhanced the immune response to DNA-encoded antigen after DNA immunization, clearly indicating that adsorption may not be critical to the adjuvant effect of aluminum compounds. These data indicate that aluminum enhances the immune response via other mechanisms. A satisfactory explanation of the adjuvant effect of aluminum also needs to take into account its selective mode of enhancing the immune response, i.e., a predominant type 2 immune response. Aluminum adjuvants induced differentiation toward type 2 immune responses, even in the absence of IL-4 or IL-13. Aluminum stimulated a type 1 and type 2 immune response in genetically engineered mice with a defective IL-4 and IL-13 response, suggesting that aluminum-induced IL-4 and/or IL-13 secretion suppresse the type 1 response but are dispensable for a type 2 response in intact animals (72). The lack of a type 1 immune response is a drawback for the use of aluminum in vaccines for intracellular pathogens and tumors. A recent study demonstrated that aluminum adjuvant with adsorbed IL-12 induces a strong type 1 response, indicating that it is possible to overcome the aluminum-induced suppression of type 1 responses (73).

Saponins

The saponins of the bark of the *Quillaja saponaria* Molina tree have long been known to have immunostimulatory activity. A partially purified fraction, Quil A, has reduced toxicity and more potent adjuvant activity and is used in veterinary vaccines. Quil A can be further fractionated into fractions that have different degrees of toxicity. QS-21 is a less toxic component with strong adjuvant activity. Saponins probably act by direct stimulation of the immune system (74). They stimulate both the humoral (primarily IgG2a antibodies in the mouse) and cell-mediated immune responses. QS-21 causes protein antigens to be processed and presented via the MHC I pathway, resulting in cytotoxic T-cell responses. Cytokine analysis indicates that QS-21 stimulates type 1 cytokine production.

Immune-stimulating complexes (ISCOMs) are 30–40 nm particles consisting of Quil A, cholesterol, antigen, and phospolipids (74). They are used in a commercial vaccine for equine influenza. ISCOM-adjuvanted vaccines stimulate a strong humoral and cell-mediated immune response caused by the immunostimulatory actions of Quil A and targeting of the particles to macrophages. As with Quil A, ISCOMs target antigens for processing via the MHC I pathway, resulting in induction of cytotoxic T-cell responses.

Delivery of Vaccines

Parenteral versus mucosal route

The success of vaccination depends primarily on the method of presenting the antigen to the host immune system. Antigens have usually been delivered by parenteral (such as intravenous, intramuscular, intraperitoneal, intradermal, and subcutaneous) administration, but recent studies have shown that other routes of delivery such as intranasal, oral, and transdermal delivery have also been effective. In some cases, vaccination through mucosal routes resulted in better responses in IgA production. Because nonparenteral vaccine delivery presents many obvious advantages, numerous attempts have been made on the development of nonparenteral delivery of vaccines.

Parenteral route: Parenteral vaccination remains the immunization method of choice for most antigens because it provides more effective immune response than do any other routes of vaccination in most cases. Every years millions of people receive inactivated influenza vaccine by parenteral administration. Subcutaneous vaccination with inactivated influenza vaccine is known to induce simultaneous immune responses in the blood and upper respiratory tract of subjects. The immune response, i.e., the increase in the number of influenza virus-specific antibody-secreting cells in peripheral blood and tonsils, increased rapidly to reach a peak within 1 week after vaccination (75). Parenteral vaccination of a DNA vaccine encoding glycoprotein D of herpes simplex virus type 2

resulted in systemic cellular and humoral responses. The mucosal humoral responses generated by intramuscular and intradermal vaccination were comparable with those obtained by mucosal vaccination. The DNA vaccine was able to stimulate a response in the Peyer's patches, a major inductive site for mucosal responses (76). For many other antigens, however, the usefulness of parenteral vaccination is limited by the insufficient induction of mucosal immune responses.

Parenteral vaccination is difficult for those living in the developing countries where medical care is not well-established. Vaccination of a large number of subjects using hypodermic needles, which is a highly labor-intensive procedure requiring healthcare personnel, is not practical. The problem becomes even more significant for vaccination of millions of animals. For example, vaccination for routine control of Newcastle disease in chickens by intramuscular injection requiring individual handling of the birds is not practical (77). Recent advances in needleless injectable systems have made the parenteral vaccination easier, but it still requires individual handling. Examples of needleless injection systems are Powder-Ject®, Medi-Jector®, Biojector®, Vitajet®, Bio-Set®, and Intraject®. They all use high pressure released in a very short period to deliver drugs through the skin. A jet-immunization technique was used for intraoral administration of DNA in the cheek, resulting in high IgA mucosal responses (78). The intraoral jet-injection technique for DNA vaccine delivery has the advantages of being a simple and rapid way to administer the DNA in solution and to provoke specific mucosal IgA after administration in the mucosal-associated lymphoid tissue.

The results of parenteral vaccination depend on the route of administration. For plasmid DNA vaccines, the highest levels of antibodies were induced by intramuscular and intravenous injections, although significant titers were also obtained with sublingual and intradermal delivery. Delivery to the skin by the gene gun induced exclusively IgG1 antibodies (Th2-like) at 4 weeks and only very low IgG2a levels at later times. Other routes, such as intraperitoneal, intraperineal, subcutaneous, intranasal inhalation, intranasal instillation, intrarectal, intravaginal, ocular, and oral, did not result in significant immune responses (79).

Dual-chamber syringe. For delivery of two established vaccines (e.g., polyribosyl ribitol phosphate conjugated to tetanus toxoid and diphtheria–tetanus–whole cell pertussis and inactivated poliovirus vaccine) at the same time, a dual-chamber syringe delivery system can be used. The proximal chamber may contain a vaccine in the freeze-dried solid state, and the distal chamber contains a vaccine in the liquid formulation that allows reconstitution of the vaccine in the proximal chamber. The immune response by the dual-chamber delivery of vaccination was equivalent to that by the separate-injection method of vaccination. The dual-chamber syringe can be used for safe and effective delivery of two different vaccines that are not yet available as a single formulation for pediatric applications (80). The primary advantage of the dual-chamber syringe is that it reduces the cost of vaccine delivery and, at the same time, increases the vaccine acceptability and coverage rate of vaccines (81).

Mucosal route: Vaccination through mucosal routes provides new avenues of vaccination with a unique advantage of mucosal immunity, that may not be obtained, through parenteral vaccination. Mucosal immunization presents a realistic alternative to parenteral administration for inducing protective immune responses. Vaccination by mucosal route provides a number of advantages over parenteral vaccination. First, mucosal vaccination does not involve hypodermic needles, which are not user-friendly. Second, the total surface area of the mucosal surfaces in the gastrointestinal, respiratory, and urogenital tracts where many infectious pathogens come into contact with the host is huge. Thus, preventing infections at the mucosal surface

provides an immunological first line of defense against diseases (82). This makes priming of the mucosal-associated lymphoid tissue (MALT) by vaccination most desirable. Parenteral vaccination alone is quite often insufficient in inducing mucosal immune responses, because stimulation of the MALT usually requires direct contact between the immunogen and the mucosal surface (83). The mucosal tissues are protected by interconnected local immune system, which is essentially separated from systemic immunity (84). In a common mucosal-defense system, an antigen interacting with localized lymphoid tissue can stimulate IgA precursor cells that may then migrate to other mucosal surfaces to elicit immune reaction in other mucosal tissues. It is known that the mucosal immune system produces 70% of the body's antibodies (85). Fig. 4 shows a schematic description of the common mucosal-immunization system. Mucosal delivery of numerous antigens by a variety of routes (oral, nasal, tracheal, and rectal) has been shown to elicit immunity at mucosal surfaces mediated by secretory IgA. The presence of MALT indicates that mucosal vaccination at a certain site in the body can be achieved by mucosal immunization at the distal site of the body. Although the mucosal and

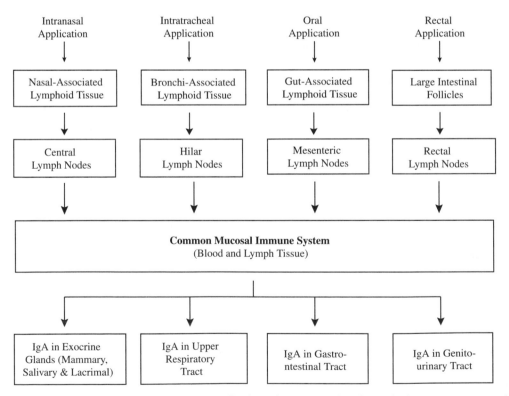

Fig. 4 Mucosal immunization and production of IgA antibodies in various mucosal surfaces via the common mucosal-simmunization system. Nasal and rectal vaccinations usually result in IgA production in upper respiratory tract and genitourinary tract, respectively, whereas effector sites by oral vaccination are expected to include many mucosal surfaces.

systemic humoral immune systems function essentially independent of each other, an antigen administered by one route can modify responsiveness to subsequent immunization by an alternate route (86).

Oral vaccination of the various mucosal routes, oral vaccination is the most preferable mode of vaccination because of its ease of use and low cost of manufacturing (87). Furthermore, the gastrointestinal (GI) tract provides the largest component of the mucosal immune system that has been well-characterized. Oral administration of vaccines has high acceptability, by avoidance of injection, to individuals of all ages. Fig. 5 shows the current understanding of oral vaccination. After oral vaccination, an antigen, which is typically loaded in microspheres, is taken up by M-cells in the Peyer's patch of the gut-associated lymphoid tissue. The antigen is then passed to the macrophages and B-cells (B). These cells in turn present the antigen to T helper lymphocytes. These cells migrate into the blood via the mesenteric lymph nodes (MLN) and the thoracic duct (TD). These cells subsequently localize in the effector sites, i.e., mucosal membranes of the GI tract, upper respiratory tract, genitourinary tract, and glandular tissue. At the effector sites, the migrating B-cells develop into plasma cells that produce IgA antibodies. Polymeric IgA is then released as secretory IgA (sIgA) through epithelial cells.

The maximal intestinal immunization can be achieved by intra-Peyer's patch immunization, and thus this method can be used to screen oral vaccine candidate antigens without the added complication of simultaneously testing

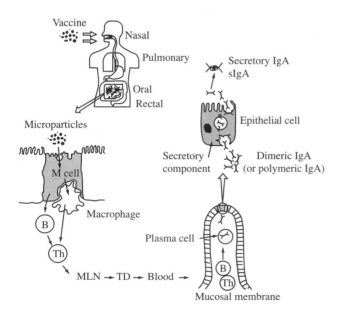

Fig. 5 Mucosal immunization by oral vaccination.

oral-delivery systems (88). Immunization of subjects against *Helicobacter pylori* by intra-Peyer's patch resulted in an 84–91% reduction in *H. pylori* infection compared with unimmunized controls. The therapeutic efficacy of the recombinant *H. pylori* urease vaccine in mice was shown to be comparable with that achieved with the combined antibiotic/antacid treatment in humans. The oral vaccination is preferred to conventional treatment of ulcers because it is a very simple and quick procedure compared with long-term conventional treatment. In addition, vaccines use the defense mechanisms of the body to establish long-lasting immunity (89).

One of the limitations of oral vaccination is that it does not always induce sufficient immunity. There are a few good reasons for this. First, the GI tract is designed to digest proteins by acidic and enzymatic degradation for absorption. Because most antigens are proteins in nature, they may be degraded by enzymes in the GI tract as well as by acids in the stomach. This is why soluble antigens administered orally are not effective. Thus, prevention of the antigen degradation is the first step toward successful oral vaccination. Adding protease inhibitors before oral vaccination may induce complete immunity, but this approach is not practical. There are many different enzymes that may not be inhibited by a particular protease inhibitor, and, more important the action of protease inhibitors may not occur at the same time that the antigens are present in the GI tract. Second, the systemic uptake of antigens from the GI tract is very poor. Even after oral intake of gram quantities of antigen, only a nanogram range of antigenic material was found to pass the intestinal barrier (90). It is also possible that for certain antigens, oral vaccination may simply be less effective than parenteral vaccination in induction of systemic immunity (91). The protection resulting from oral vaccination is known to last for a relatively short period, ranging from a few months to 1 year. To obtain the desirable immunity equivalent to systemic immunization, oral vaccination requires much higher and more frequent oral doses. The use of highly effective adjuvants in oral vaccine formulation may result in strong and long-lasting immunity in mucosal tissues.

The issues of degradation of antigens in the GI tract and the poor systemic uptake of antigens from the GI tract have led to encapsulation of antigens in microparticles (also called microcapsules or microspheres). Antigens that are encapsulated in microparticles are protected from degradation, and the microparticulate nature allows better uptake by the M-cells in the Peyer's patches. A large number of studies have shown that antigens orally delivered in microparticles resulted in good mucosal immunity. It is noted here that virus itself can be regarded as a particulate vaccine-delivery system. Many viruses are highly effective in inducing immunization after oral vaccination. Norwalk virus, which is a major cause of epidemic gastroenteritis, was immunogenic in healthy human adults even when administered without adjuvants (92). Influenza virus can also elicit immune response after oral administration. Successful oral vaccination relies on targeting of microparticles to the Peyer's patches. It is known that the surface chemistry of microparticles affects the targeting to and uptake by M-cells in the Peyer's patches (93). The exact relationships between the surface chemistry and the uptake by Peyer's patches, however, have not been fully understood. Development of better oral vaccines requires understanding of such relationships.

Intranasal vaccination route has received growing interest for noninvasive immunization. Intranasal immunization has been quite effective for various vaccine-delivery systems. Both solution and microsphere formulations tend to show good immune responses after intranasal administration. Immunization of mice with tetanus toxoid, in solution and microsphere-encapsulated formulations, resulted in high levels of specific IgG and IgA antibodies (94). Nasal vaccine delivery is known to be superior to oral delivery in inducing specific IgA and IgG antibody responses in the upper respiratory tract (95). Nasal immunization is also known to be preferable to the oral route for distant mucosal vaccination that might be used to prevent adhesion of pathogens to the urogenital tract (95). It is interesting to note that the volume of the nasally instilled vaccine is important (94). The larger-volume (e.g., 50 μL) of microsphere suspension resulted in the higher percentage of particles entering the lungs than did the lower, volume (e.g., 10 μL) instillation.

It is generally believed that microspheres that adhere to the nasal mucus elicit better immune response, and for this reason, many microspheres made of mucoadhesive polymers, such as chitosan, have been used extensively in the preparation of nasal vaccine formulations.

Transdermal vaccination or transcutaneous immunization, is attractive, because it does not require specially trained personnel necessary for needle injections. Topical application of antigens to intact skin has shown promising results for the administration of DNA-based vaccines. Noninvasive gene delivery by pipetting adenovirus- or liposome-complexed plasmid DNA onto the outer layer of skin was able to achieve localized transgene expression within a restricted subset of skin in mice. It also elicited an immune response against the protein encoded by the DNA (96).

For improved results, transdermal electroporation was also tried to explore the feasibility of nonadjuvant, needle-free skin immunization (97). The transdermal electroporation route elicited higher responses to a myristylated peptide than did intradermal immunization. For diphtheria toxoid, however, the result was the opposite. It appears that transdermal electroporation is a promising technique for nonadjuvant skin immunization, especially with low-molecular-weight, weakly immunogenic antigens. Topical application of antigen and cholera toxin or bacterial exotoxin to the skin surface resulted in detectable antigen-specific IgG in plasma and mucosal secretions (98, 99). It appears that transcutaneous immunization can induce potent, protective immune responses to both systemic and mucosal challenge (100).

Pulmonary vaccination is especially useful in mass vaccination campaigns. A conventional method of pulmonary delivery of drugs using metered-dose, propellant-driven, small-particle aerosols was used to deliver killed whole bacterium vaccines. The results showed good stimulation of mucosal immunity against respiratory infections in animals (101). Recent advances in powder inhaler devices have made it possible to deliver vaccines via the pulmonary route using dry powder inhalation technologies (102). Dry powder vaccine in the size range from 1 to 5 μm in diameter is used for the maximum alveolar (deep lung) deposition (101).

Direct gene transfer into the respiratory system can be carried out for either therapeutic or immunization purposes. Cells in the lung can take up and express plasmid DNA whether it is administered in naked form or formulated with cationic liposomes. For a given dose of DNA, the results can be improved when the DNA is mixed with the minimum amount of lipid that can complex it completely (103). Such a complex formation can be considered a formation of microparticles that can enhance cellular uptake and subsequent immune responses.

Parenteral and mucosal combination vaccination: The combination of mucosal and systemic immunization routes (e.g., parenteral immunization followed by oral immunization or vice versa) generally induces mucosal immune responses that are superior to immunization by either route alone (91). Pigs showed some protection after intramuscular inoculation with formalin-inactivated *M. hyopneumoniae* vaccine in incomplete Freund's adjuvant and a booster inoculation with the same vaccine in microspheres onto the mucosal surface of Peyer's patches by a surgical operation (104).

Antigen delivery systems

The primary goal of antigen-delivery systems is to maintain a stable dosage form during storage and, when administered to present antigens to elicit a vigorous immune response in vivo. It is necessary to develop vaccine formulations that would preserve the antigen and deliver it to a specific target organ over a desired period. Continuous release or multiple pulsatile release during the desired period would eliminate the inconvenience of multiple vaccine administration for obtaining satisfactory immune responses. The antigen-delivery system plays one of the most crucial roles in the outcome of the immunization. The way that antigens are delivered affects the immune response significantly. Currently, antigen-delivery systems are classified into two systems: live attenuated microorganisms and nonliving microparticulate systems.

Live attenuated organisms: Live attenuated bacteria and viruses have been used not only as vaccines but also as a delivery system that elicits humoral, mucosal, and cellular immune responses against exogenous antigens. Since the success with live attenuated oral vaccines against tuberculosis and polio more than 3 decades ago, a number of live attenuated microorganisms have been used as antigen-delivery systems. Live vaccines are relatively easy and cheap to manufacture, because they do not require purification of antigens or formulation with adjuvants (82). Attenuated strains of microorganisms can be formed spontaneously or induced by heat, chemical, or UV mutagenesis. Another advantage of the attenuated live vaccines is that they can be administered by the natural route of infection. Recently, pathogenic microorganisms have been attenuated by genetic engineering, i.e., mutating specific genes or removing some toxic genes. Because much of the infection occurs through the mucosal surfaces, live attenuated vaccines are best suited for protection against pathogens that access the body through the mucosal surfaces. Live attenuated oral vaccines are expected to provide the most convenient and effective means of vaccinating against enteric disease (105). Orally administered attenuated *Salmonella* are known to interact with the MALT (82). Other examples of live attenuated microorganism vaccines are BCG (bacilli Calmette–Guérin), adenovirus, and poliovirus.

Some viruses and bacteria are inherently quite stable. For example, polio virus can be formulated as a frozen liquid. A live poliovirus vector expressing a foreign antigen generates both antibody and cytotoxic T-lymphocyte responses in mice (106). Most live bacteria and viruses, however, are usually stored as powders after freeze-drying or lyophilization. Preserving the live state through freeze-drying often requires the presence of a stabilizer, which is selected primarily through trial and error. The most widely used nonspecific stabilizers are sugars, amino acids, polyols, and neutral salts which are known to act as bound water substitutes for maintaining the conformational integrity of proteins. An example of lyophilized vaccine products is *S. typhi* bacteria lyophilized to a powder that is encapsulated into gelatin for oral administration (107).

One of the drawbacks of using live microorganisms is that attenuated pathogens may invoke the very disease they are designed to prevent if they are insufficiently attenuated. Even if they are sufficiently attenuated, they still may cause severe infections in immunocompromised individuals. In addition, they always have a potential to revert to full virulence if lesions causing attenuation are not fully characterized (82). If pathogens are over-attenuated, they fail to trigger an appropriate immune response. Thus, it is highly important to attain the right balance between minimal virulence and maximal immunogenicity. This balance can be achieved in a normal population but may not be the same in a population with even minor defects in immune competence (108) Another aspect to notice in using live vaccines is that the distribution of live vaccines requires a cold chain that may not be readily accessible in many developing countries, and this may offset advantages of using live-vectored vaccines (109).

Nonliving microparticulate delivery systems: Nonliving immunogens generally result in immune responses of lesser magnitude and of shorter duration than do those by living immunogens (82). Nonliving immunogens are usually made of microparticulate forms to protect antigens and to improve cellular uptake. Nonliving microparticulates that can be used as antigen-delivery systems include polymeric microparticles, liposomes, virus-like particles, neosomes, and cross-linked protein crystals. The definition of microparticles should be broad enough to include all other forms, such as protein aggregates. The size of microparticles used in the vaccine area is usually less than 50 μm (110). It is common, however, to call any particles less than a few hundred micrometers microparticles. For this reason, it is important to specify the average size of microparticles for particular applications, because the size of microparticles often affect the outcome.

Polymeric microparticles and liposomes have been used extensively as controlled-release dosage forms for many drugs including antigens. They have been quite useful in oral delivery of antigens because encapsulation in microparticles can protect antigens from acidic and enzymatic degradation in the GI tract, and thus serve as a stable vaccine vehicle with extended shelf life. Delivery of antigens by microparticulate-delivery systems has the potential benefits of reducing the number of inoculations, enhancing the immune response via both parenteral and oral vaccination routes, and reducing the total antigen dose required to achieve immune protection (111). Microparticulate vaccine-delivery systems show improved immune responses because of the protection of the loaded antigens from degradation and the slow release of the antigens. For this reason, microparticulate-delivery systems are often considered adjuvants (66).

Polymer microparticles, a large number of polymers, such as poly(methyl methacrylate), poly(butyl cyanoacrylate), poly(lactide-*co*-glycolide), polyarcylstarch, dextran, albumin, and alginic acid, have been used for making microparticles for vaccine delivery. All the polymers that have been used for controlled drug delivery can be used for vaccine delivery (112). Preparation of microparticles from water-insoluble polymers [e.g., poly(methyl methacrylate), poly(butyl cyanoacrylate), and poly(lactide-*co*-glycolide)] requires use of organic solvents or high temperature, both of which may not be good for maintaining tertiary structures of antigens. Preparation from water-soluble polymers frequently requires cross-linking reaction to make the polymers remain insoluble. It is possible that cross-linking agents cross-link not only polymer chains but also antigen molecules. Absorption of water into hydrophilic polymers results in swelling of the network, i.e., formation of hydrogels, or aquagels. Preparation of microparticles from hydrophilic polymers is preferred because it does not require organic solvents or high temperature. Polymers that have been used in the immunization vary depending on the route of administration.

For parenteral vaccination, biodegradable polymeric microparticles made of poly(lactide-*co*-glycolide) are commonly used as vaccine carriers. Poly(lactide-*co*-glycolide) has been well-characterized and known to be highly biocompatible. The size of microparticles can be easily controlled, and microparticles of less than 100 μm in diameter can be easily administered by injection through standard-sized needles (22 gauge or smaller). Because of the slow degradation of the polymer, antigens are slowly released from the microparticles for long term in much the same way as do alum adjuvants, and this results in enhanced immune responses. Other polymers, such as chitosan, have been used for preparation of vaccine formulations. Because one of the important roles that microparticles play in immunization is the slow release of antigens, a number of approaches have been tried to achieve antigen release at desired rates. The surface of microparticles can be modified to alter the adsorption and desorption kinetics of antigens. Alternatively, the pore size can be varied to control the release of antigens from microparticles.

The size of microparticles is known to play a critical role in oral immunization. In addition to protecting antigens from acidic and enzymatic degradation in the GI tract, microparticulates are known to enhance uptake by M-cells in the Peyer's patches, and the effectiveness of the uptake depends on the size of microparticles. It is generally thought that microparticles smaller than 10 μm

are preferentially absorbed by M-cells, and the smaller the size, the better the absorption. One study using microparticles of different sizes showed that the efficiency of uptake of 100-nm particles by the intestinal tissue was 15- to 250-fold higher than that of larger size microparticles (113). In addition to the small size, microparticles with more hydrophobic surface property are absorbed better than those with more hydrophilic surface property. There are, however, no definite studies confirming or supporting these assumptions. Once microparticles are placed in the GI tract, adsorption of numerous proteins and polysaccharides present in the GI tract would alter the surface chemistry drastically, and it is difficult to correlate a particular surface chemistry of the native microparticles with the absorption ability.

Virus-like particles (VLPs) consist of one or more viral-coat proteins. They are very immunogenic molecules that allow for covalent coupling of the epitopes of interest (114). Recently, parvovirus-like particles have been engineered to express foreign polypeptides in certain positions, resulting in the production of large quantities of highly immunogenic peptides, and to induce strong antibody, helper T-cell, and cytotoxic T-lymphocyte responses (114). Parenteral administration of recombinant VLPs of papillomavirus induced VLP-specific humoral and cellular immune responses (115). Immunization of VLPs without adjuvant via mucosal route is also known to elicit specific antibody at mucosal surfaces and also systemic VLP epitope-specific T-cell responses (115).

Liposomes are vesicles composed of naturally occurring or synthetic phopholipids. The bilayer structure can be single- or multicompartment. The size can also vary from smaller than 1 μm to larger than 10 μm. When negatively charged lipid molecules, which form liposomes, interact with divalent cations, a solid, multilayered, crystallaine structure called cochleate is formed. Because liposomes and cochleates can protect antigens from the GI tract and deliver them to the Peyer's patches, they have been exploited as an effective delivery system for oral vaccination.

Liposomes, like other vaccine-delivery systems, can exert immunoadjuvant effects. The surface charge of liposomes is known to affect the immune responses. Positively charged liposomes containing soluble antigens were reported to function as a more potent inducer of antigen-specific, cytotoxic T-lymphocyte responses and delayed-type hypersensitivity responses than negatively charged and neutral liposomes containing the same concentrations of antigens (116). Studies showed that the positively charged liposomes delivered proteinaceous antigens efficiently into the cytoplasm of the macrophages/antigen-presenting cells where the antigens are processed to be presented by class I MHC molecules to induce the cell-mediated immune response (116).

Liposomes containing highly immunogenic glycoproteins of the Sendai virus on their surface, which are called fusogenic liposomes, showed enhanced antigen-specific humoral immunity in mice. The levels of antiovalbumin antibody were markedly increased in serum from mice immunized with OVA encapsulated in fusogenic liposomes. It appears that the fusogenic liposomes function as an immunoadjuvant in inducing antigen-specific antibody production (117).

Virosomes are liposomes containing viral fusion proteins that allow efficient entering into cells fusion with endosome membranes. Viral fusion proteins become activated in the low pH environment in the endosome to release its contents into the cytosol (118). Hepatitis A and influenza vaccines constructed on virosomes elicited fewer local adverse reactions than did their classic counterparts and displayed enhanced immunogenicity. Virosome-formulated influenza vaccine has also been shown to be safe and immunogenic when administered by the intranasal route (119). Other studies have suggested that immunopotentiating reconstituted influenza virosomes can be a suitable delivery system for synthetic peptide vaccines. The virosomes have a great potential for the design of combined vaccines targeted against multiple antigens and multiple pathogens (120).

Micelles are aggregates of detergent molecules in aqueous solution. Detergents are water-soluble, surface-active agents composed of a hydrophilic head group and a hydrophobic or lipophilic tail group. They can also align at aqueous/nonaquous interfaces, reducing surface tension, increasing miscibility, and stabilizing emulsions. Polymeric micelles made of block copolymers, such as poly(ethylene oxide)-poly(propylene oxide)-poly(ethylene oxide), have been used as a delivery system for hydrophobic drugs. They can also encapsulate antigens for vaccination.

Niosomes are nonionic surfactant vesicles. They have been used to develop a vaccine-delivery system by peroral and oral routes. Ovalbumin was encapsulated in various lyophilized niosome preparations consisting of sucrose esters, cholesterol, and dicetyl phosphate. Encapsulation of ovalbumin into niosomes consisting of 70% stearate sucrose ester and 30% palmitate sucrose ester (40% mono-, 60% di/triester) resulted in a significant increase in antibody titers in serum, saliva, and intestinal washings (121).

Cross-linked protein crystals have been used as antigens. The immunogenicity of cross-linked protein crystals of human serum albumin was 6- to 30-fold higher in antibody titer than that of the soluble protein over an almost 6-month study (122). It is likely that the cross-linked protein crystals release antigen in a slow-release manner, and in this sense, the cross-linked protein crystals function as a depot. The cross-linked protein crystals present high stability, purity, biodegradability, and ease of manufacturing, all of which are highly attractive features for vaccine formulation (122). Because the cross-linked protein crystals are microparticulates, they can also be used for vaccination through various routes.

IMMUNOMODULATION

Immunomodulation refers to treatments that alter immune responsiveness in a nonantigen-specific manner. Enhancement of the immune response is desired in the treatment of chronic infectious diseases and neoplastic diseases, whereas suppression is needed in cases of inappropriate or exaggerated immune response, including allergies and autoimmune diseases. There are numerous treatments that affect the activity of the immune system. The effect of currently available immunosuppressive drugs is very broad, giving these drugs undesirable side effects. The aim of the research in this area is to design treatments that selectively enhance or suppress immune responses. Some of the newer treatment options are those that target costimulatory molecules, and the use of CpG DNA, and cytokines.

Costimulation

Activation of T-cells requires two signals. The first signal is provided by recognition of MHC/peptide complex by the T-cell receptor. This does not result in proliferation and differentiation of the T-cell unless the T-cell receives a second, costimulatory signal. Several costimulatory signals have been identified, but the major costimulatory signal appears to result from the binding of CD28 on T-cells to B7 molecules on antigen-presenting cells. There are at least two B7 molecules, B7-1 (CD80) and B7-2 (CD86). Activation of antigen-presenting cells results in increased expression of B7-2, followed by B7-1. A second T-cell ligand of the B7 molecules is cytotoxic T lymphocyte antigen-4 (CTLA-4 or CD152) that, other than its name implies, is rapidly expressed on both CD4[+] and CD8[+] T-cells after binding of the T-cell receptor to the MHC/peptide complex on antigen-presenting cells. However, in contrast to the positive signal provided by CD28, CTLA-4 downregulates T-cell responses (123). CTLA-4 has a higher affinity for the B7-molecules than does CD28 and may prevent the activation of T-cells when B7 expression by dendritic cells is low and terminate the immune response when its expression is strongly increased. A soluble chimeric protein, CTLA4Ig, blocks the binding of both CD28 and CTLA-4 to the B7 molecules and, thus, may prevent T-cell activation. Administration of this protein to patients with psoriasis vulgaris, an immune-mediated skin disease, in a phase I clinical trial resulted in significant improvement in approximately 50% of the patients (124). Selective inhibition of CTLA-4 with specific antibodies may boost the immune system. The combination of surgery and anti-CTLA-4 antibody therapy was highly effective in the prevention of metastatic recurrence in a mouse prostatic carcinoma model (125).

Other CD28 and B7 homologs continue to be identified and appear to play a role in costimulation (126). These molecules may provide additional targets for immunomodulation and suggest that it may be possible to fine-tune the immune response through pharmacologic intervention.

CpG DNA

Bacterial DNA has a higher content of the CpG dinucleotide than does vertebrate DNA, and, in contrast to vertebrate DNA, the CpG is not preferentially methylated. The unmethylated CpG DNA sequences provides a strong stimulus for the immune system (127). CpG DNA stimulates the secretion of IL-12 by macrophages and dendritic cells and thus provides a potent stimulus for type 1 immune responses. It also directly stimulates B cells to proliferate and differentiate into immunoglobulin secreting cells. A cellular receptor for CpG DNA has not been identified. The DNA appears to enter the cell via endocytosis, and some of the DNA escapes the endosomes into the cytoplasm of the cell where it activates various signaling pathways.

Applications for oligonucleotides containing unmethylated CpG sequences (CpG–ODN) are being explored in various areas of immunotherapy. Administration of CpG–ODN to mice protected against subsequent challenge with the intracellular bacteria *Listeria monocytogenes* and the intracellular protozoa *Leishmania major*. In addition, the CpG–ODN cured established *L. major* infections. The strong type 1 immunostimulatory property of CpG–ODN makes this compound a good candidate for vaccine adjuvants. Indeed, coadministration of CpG–ODN with antigen markedly boosts the humoral and cell-mediated immune responses. Allergic diseases such as asthma and atopic dermatitis are caused by type 2 immune responses directed against otherwise innocuous antigens. Treatment with CpG–ODN cleared established disease in a mouse model of airway hyper-reactivity, suggesting a CpG-induced reversal to type 1 immune

responses. CpG DNA may also have a place in immunotherapy of cancer because of its ability to activate NK cells through the induction of IL-12. Administration of CpG–ODN in combination with monoclonal antibodies directed against tumor antigens greatly enhanced the survival of mice that had been inoculated with tumor cells.

Cytokines

Cytokines play a critical role in the regulation of the immune and inflammatory response, and they are potential targets for therapy. Important limitations, however, are the pleiotropy and redundancy in the cytokine system and the short half-life and short action range of most cytokines. In spite of these limitations, considerable effort is spent on developing reagents that either block or enhance the activity of a specific cytokine.

Two remarkable successes of cytokine therapy are the treatment of multiple sclerosis with interferon-β and the treatment of rheumatoid arthritis and inflammatory bowel disease with tumor necrosis factor-α inhibitors.

Interferon-β

Clinical trials have demonstrated that subcutaneous injections of recombinant or natural interferon-β reduces the rate of exacerbation of relapsing-remitting multiple sclerosis (128, 129). The mode of action of interferon-β has not been determined. Interferon-β reduces the production of tumor necrosis factor-α and increases the secretion of IL-10 in vitro. TNF-α is a proinflammatory cytokine that may contribute to demyelination in multiple sclerosis. IL-10 suppresses macrophage function and the production of TNF-α. In addition, interferon-β may reduce the entry of leukocytes into the central nervous system, a critical component in the inflammation that causes the lesions in multiple sclerosis.

Tumor necrosis factor-α inhibitors

Tumor necrosis factor-α (TNF-α) is a cytokine with multiple biological effects. It is produced as a transmembrane precursor molecule by various cells in the body. It is cleaved by the TNF-α-converting enzyme and forms trimeric aggregates that bind to either the TNF-receptor (TNFR) I or the TNFR II that are expressed on many different types of cells. The extracellular domains of the TNFR can be cleaved by enzymes and can inhibit TNF-α activity by preventing binding of TNF-α to cell-bound receptors. Recent studies have demonstrated that inhibition of TNF-α activity resulted in significant improvement of the clinical condition of many patients with rheumatoid arthritis and inflammatory bowel disease (130, 131). These studies clearly demonstrate an important role of TNF-α in rheumatoid arthritis and inflammatory bowel disease, although the precise mechanisms remain to be determined. The inhibition of TNF-α activity is achieved by treatment with anti-TNF-α monoclonal antibodies or with soluble TNFR-fusion protein. To reduce the induction of antibodies against the mouse monoclonal antibodies, the monoclonal antibodies are chimeric (i.e., the constant portion is derived from human immunoglobulins and the TNF-α-specific variable portion is derived from mice) or humanized (all of the immunoglobulin is human except for the complementarity determining regions that fold into the TNF-α-binding region). The TNFR-fusion protein is constructed from the extracellular domain of TNFRII and the Fc portion of human immunoglobulins. This construct has a much longer half-life than does the naturally occurring soluble TNFR.

CHALLENGES IN FUTURE VACCINE FORMULATIONS

Recent advancements in microbial pathogenesis, immunology, genetic engineering, plant genetics, and expression vector technology have formed the foundation for a new generation of vaccines and other pharmaceutical products. New developments in the delivery system have provided us with novel ways to enhance the immunogenicity of subunit antigens or nucleic acids by their controlled release and reduced degradation.

For more convenient and more effective immunization, current vaccine-delivery technologies need to be improved. Currently, vaccination of many inactivated or subunit antigens requires booster doses because of the lack of inherent immunogenicity found in the natural organism. Thus, reducing the number of doses is one of the primary goals in vaccination. Theoretically, various controlled-release technologies can be used to release antigens over time in a sustained or pulsatile manner and to direct antigens to specific antigen-presenting cells for increased vaccine efficacy. In addition to controlled-release technology, the single-shot vaccination requires development of better adjuvants. The mechanism of action of such adjuvants should be known so that reproducible results can be obtained in a mass vaccination program. The requirements and problems of immunizing immunocompromised, immature, older, or pregnant hosts need to be addressed effectively. Further improvement in our understanding of how to modulate Th1 and Th2 responses effectively would certainly help us design better vaccines. Another means of improvement is to combine a number of vaccines into multivalent vaccines. This will improve the immunization compliance in people living in developed or developing countries. Because the majority of pathogens enter their hosts via mucosal routes, the new-generation vaccines should have the advantage of providing effective protection at the mucosal sites. An ideal vaccine would be one that provides life-long protection with a single inoculation. The new-generation vaccine formulations should also have high stability, thus avoiding the problems commonly observed during storage.

REFERENCES

1. Peterson, L.J.; Benson, W.W.; Graeber, F.O. Vaccination Induced Poliomyelitis in Idaho. J. A. Med. Assoc. **1955**, *159*, 241–244.
2. Nathanson, N.; Langmuir, A.D. The Cutter Incident. Poliomyelitis Following Formaldehyde-Inactivated Poliovirus Vaccination in the United States During the Spring of 1955. I. Background. Am. J. Hygiene **1963**, *78*, 16–28.
3. Kapikian,, A.Z.; Mitchell, R.H.; Chanock, R.M.; Shvedoff, R.A.; Stewart, C.E. An Epidemiologic Study of Altered Clinical Reactivity to Respiratory Syncytial (RS) Virus Infection in Children Previously Vaccinated with an Inactivated RS Virus Vaccine. Am. J. Epidemiol. **1969**, *89*, 405–421.
4. Kim, H.W.; Canchola, J.G.; Brandt, C.D.; Pyles, G.; Chanock, R.M.; Jensen, K.; Parrott, R.H. Respiratory Syncytial Virus Disease in Infants Despite Prior Administration of Antigenic Inactivated Vaccine. Am. J. Epidemiol. **1969**, *89*, 422–434.
5. Murphy, B.R.; Prince, G.A.; Walsh, E.E.; Kim, H.W.; Parrott, R.H.; Hemming, V.G.; Rodriguez, W.J.; Chanock, R.M. Dissociation Between Serum Neutralizing and Glycoprotein Antibody Responses of Infants and Children Who Received Inactivated Respiratory Syncytial Virus Vaccine. J. Clin. Microbiol. **1986**, *24*, 197–202.
6. Connors, M.; Kulkarni, A.B.; Firestone, C.Y.; Holmes, K.L.; Morse, H.C., III; Sotnikov, A.V.; Murphy, B.R. Pulmonary Histopathology Induced by Respiratory Syncytial Virus (RSV) Challenge of Formalin-Inactivated RSV-Immunized BALB/c Mice is Abrogated by Depletion of CD4+ T Cells. J. Virol. **1992**, *66*, 7444–7451.
7. Top, F.H., Jr.; Buescher, E.L.; Bancroft, W.H.; Russell, P.K. Immunization with Live Type 7 and Type 4 Adenovirus Vaccines. II Antibody Response and Protective Effect Against Acute Respiratory Disease Due to Adenovirus Type 7. J. Infect. Dis. **1971**, *124*, 155–160.
8. Sabin, A.B.; Boulger, L. History of Sabin Attenuated Poliovirus Oral Live Vaccine Strains. J. Biol. Standardization **1973**, *1*, 115–118.
9. Parkman, P.D.; Meyer, H.M., Jr.; Kirschstein, R.L.; Hopps, H.E. Attenuated Rubella Virus. I. Development and Laboratory Characterization. New Engl. J. Med. **1966**, *275*, 569–574.
10. Plotkin, S.A.; Farquhar, J.; Katz, M.; Ingalls, T.H. A New Attenuated Rubella Virus Grown in Human Fibroblasts: Evidence for Reduced Nasopharyngeal Excretion. Am. J. Epidemiol. **1967**, *86*, 468–477.

11. Bunyak, E.B.; Hilleman, M.R.; Weiber, R.E.; Stokes, J., Jr. Live Attenuated Rubella Virus Vaccines Prepared in Duck Embryo Cell Culture. I. Development and Clinical Testing. J. Am. Med. Assoc. **1968**, *204*, 195–200.

12. Morrow, C.D.; Novak, M.J.; Ansardi, D.C.; Porter, D.C.; Moldoveanu, Z. Recombinant Viruses as Vectors for Mucosal Immunity, Defence of Mucosal Surfaces: Pathogenesis, Immunity and Vaccines. *Current Topics in Microbiology and Immunology*; Kraehenbuhl, J.P., Neutra, M.R., Eds.; Springer-Verlag: Berlin, 1999; 236, 255–273.

13. Muster, T.; Ferko, B.; Klima, A.; Purtscher, M.; Trkola, A.; Schulz, P.; Grassauer, A.; Engelhardt, O.G.; Garcia-Sastre, A.; Palese, P. et al. Mucosal Model of Immunization Against Human Immunodeficiency Virus Type 1 with a Chimeric Influenza Virus. J. Virol. **1995**, *69*, 6678–6686.

14. Pastoret, P.P.; Brochier, B.; Languet, B.; Thomas, I.; Paquot, A.; Bauduin, B.; Kieny, M.P.; Lecocq, J.P.; De Bruyn, J.; Costy, F. et al. First Field Trial of Fox Vaccination Against Rabies Using a Vaccinia-Rabies Recombinant Virus. Vet. Rec. **1988**, *123*, 481–483.

15. Robbins, A.H.; Borden, M.D.; Windmiller, B.S.; Niezgoda, M.; Marcus, L.C.; O'Brien, S.M.; Kreindel, S.M.; McGuill, M.W.; DeMaria, A., Jr.; Rupprecht, C.E.; Rowell, S. Prevention of the Spread of Rabies to Wildlife by Oral Vaccination of Raccoons in Massachusetts. J. Am. Vet. Med. Assoc. **1998**, *213*, 1407–1412.

16. Yilma, T.; Hsu, D.; Jones, L.; Owens, S.; Grubman, M.; Mebus, C.; Yamanaka, M.; Dale, B. Protection of Cattle Against Rinderpest with Vaccinia Virus Recombinants Expressing the HA or F Gene. Science **1988**, *242*, 1058–1061.

17. Yilma, T. Vaccinia Virus Recombinant Vaccines for Rinderpest. Dev. Biol. Standardization **1995**, *84*, 201–208.

18. Graham, F.L.; Prevec, L. Adenovirus Expression Vectors and Recombinant Vaccines. *In Vaccines; New Approaches to Immunological Problems*; Ellis, R.W., Ed.; Butterworth-Heinemann: Boston, 1992; 363–390.

19. Imler, J.-L. Adenovirus Vectors as Recombinant Viral Vaccines. Vaccine **1995**, *13*, 1143–1151.

20. Mittal, S.K.; Papp, Z.; Tikoo, S.K.; Baca-Estrada, M.; Yoo, D.; Benko, M.; Babiuk, L.A. Induction of Systemic and Mucosal Immune Responses in Cotton Rats Immunized with Human Adenovirus Type 5 Recombinants Expressing the Full and Secretory Forms of Bovine Herpesvirus Type 1 Glycoprotein gD. Virology **1996**, *222*, 299–309.

21. Taylor, J.; Paoletti, E. Pox Viruses as Eukaryotic Cloning and Expression Vectors: Future Medical and Veterinary Vaccines. Prog. Vet. Microbiol. Immunol. **1988**, *4*, 197–217.

22. Jacobs, W.R.; Snapper, S.B.; Lugosi, L.; Bloom, L.; Bloom, B.R. Development of BCG as a Recombinant Vaccine Vehicle. *T-Cell Paradigms in Parasitic and Bacterial Infections. Current Topics in Microbiology and Immunology*; Kaufmann, S.H.E., Ed.; Springer-Verlag: Berlin, 1990; 155, 153–160.

23. Ryan, E.T.; Crean, T.I.; John, M.; Butterton, J.R.; Clements, J.D.; Calderwood, S.B. Vivo Expression and Immunoadjuvancy of a Mutant of Heat-Labile Enterotoxin of *Escherichia coli* in Vaccine and Vector Strains Of *Vibrio cholerae*. Infect. Immun. **1999**, *67*, 1694–1701.

24. Cardenas, L.; Dasgupta, U.; Clements, J.D. Influence of Strain Viability and Antigen Dose on the Use of Attenuated Mutants of Salmonella as Vaccine Carriers. Vaccine **1994**, *12*, 833–840.

25. Cardenas, L.; Clements, J.D. Oral Immunization Using Live Attenuated Salmonella Spp. As Carriers of Foreign Antigens. Clin. Microbiol. Rev. **1992**, *5*, 328–342.

26. Killeen, K.; Spriggs, D.; Mekalanos, J. Bacterial Mucosal Vaccines: Vibrio Cholerae as a Live Attenuated Vaccine/Vector Paradigm, Defence of Mucosal Surfaces: Pathogenesis, Immunity and Vaccines. *Current Topics in Microbiology and Immunology*; Kraehenbuhl, J.P., Neutra, M.R., Eds.; Springer-Verlag: Berlin, 1999; 236, 237–254.

27. Nakayamma, K.; Kelly, S.M.; Curtiss, R., III Construction of an ASD+ Expression-Cloning Vector: Stable Maintenance and High Level Expression of Cloned Genes in a Salmonella Vaccine Strain. Biotechnology **1998**, *6*, 693–697.

28. Gentschev, I.; Hess, J.; Goebel, W. Change in the Cellular Localization of Alkaline Phosphatase by Alteration of Its Carboxy-Terminal Sequence. Mol. Gen. Genetics. **1990**, *222*, 211–216.

29. Tzschaschel, B.D.; Klee, S.R.; de Lorenzo, V.; Timmis, K.N.; Guzman, C.A. Towards a Vaccine Candidate Against Shigella Dysenteriae 1: Expression of the Shiga Toxin B-subunit in an Attenuated Shigella Flexneri AroD Carrier Strain. Microbial Pathogenesis **1996**, *21*, 277–288.

30. Kit, S.; Kit, M. Genetically Engineered Herpesvirus Vaccines. Accomplishments in Pigs and Prospects in Humans. Prog. Med. Virol. **1991**, *38*, 128–66.

31. Kit, S. Genetically Engineered Vaccines for Control of Aujeszky's Disease (Pseudorabies). Vaccine **1990**, *8*, 420–424.

32. Chatfield, S.N.; Roberts, M.; Dougan, G.; Hormaeche, C.; Khan, C.M.A. The Development of Oral Vaccines Against Parasitic Diseases Utilizing Live Attenuated Salmonella. Parasitology. **1995**, *110*, S17–S24.

33. Mettenleiter, T.C. New Developments in the Construction of Safer and More Versatile Pseudorabies Virus Vaccines. Dev. Biol. Standardization **1995**, *84*, 83–87.

34. Kimman, T.G.; Gielkens, A.L.J.; Glazenburg, K.; Jacobs, L.; de Jong, M.C.M.; Mulder, W.A.M.; Peeters, B.P.H. Characterization of Live Pseudorabies Virus Vaccines. Dev. Biol. Standardization **1995**, *84*, 89–96.

35. Briand, J.P.; Benkirane, N.; Guichard, G.; Newman, J.F.; Van Regenmortel, M.H.; Brown, F.; Muller, S. A Retro-Inverso Peptide Corresponding to the GH Loop of Foot-and-Mouth Disease Virus Elicits High Levels of Long-Lasting Protective Neutralizing Antibodies. Proceedings of the National Academy Science USA **1997**, *94*, 12545–12550.

36. Brown, F. Foot-and-Mouth Disease and Beyond: Vaccine Design, Past, Present and Future. Arch. Virol. (Suppl) **1999**, *15*, 179–188.

37. Marciani, D.J.; Kensil, C.R.; Beltz, G.A.; Hung, C.H.; Cronier, J.; Aubert, A. Genetically-Engineered Subunit Vaccine Against Feline Leukaemia Virus: Protective Immune Response in Cats. Vaccine **1991**, *9*, 89–96.

38. Valenzuela, P.; Medina, A.; Rutter, W.J.; Ammerer, G.; Hall, BD. Synthesis and Assembly of Hepatitis B Virus Surface Antigen Particles in Yeast. Nature **1982**, *298*, 347–350.

39. Brideau, R.J.; Walters, R.R.; Stier, M.A.; Wathen, M.W. Protection of Cotton Rats Against Human Respiratory Syncytial Virus by Vaccination with a Novel Chimeric FG Glycoprotein. J. Gen. Virol. **1989**, *70*, 2637–2644.

40. Brideau, R.J.; Oien, N.L.; Lehman, D.J.; Homa, F.L.; Wathen, M.W. Protection of Cotton Rats Against Human Parainfluenza Virus Type 3 by Vaccination with a Chimeric FHN Subunit Glycoprotein. J. Gen. Virol. **1993**, *74*, 471–477.

41. Kowalski, J.; Gilbert, S.A.; van Drunen-Littel-van den Hurk, S.; van den Hurk, J.; Babiuk, L.A.; Zamb, T.J. Heat-Shock Promoter-Driven Synthesis of Secreted Bovine Herpesvirus Glycoproteins in Transfected Cells. Vaccine **1993**, *11*, 1100–1107.

42. Ma, J.K.-C.; Vine, N.D. Plant Expression Systems for the Production of Vaccine, Defence of Mucosal Surfaces: Pathogenesis, Immunity and Vaccines. *Current Topics in Microbiology and Immunology*; Kraehenbuhl, J.P., Neutra, M.R., Eds.; Springer-Verlag: Berlin, 1999; 236, 275–292.

43. Ma, J.K.-C.; Hiatt, A.; Hein, M.; Vine, N.D.; Wang, F.; Stabila, P.; van Dolleweerd, C.; Mostov, K.; Lehner, T. Generation and Assembly of Secretary Antibodies in Plants. Science **1995**, *268*, 716–719.

44. Haq, T.A.; Mason, H.S.; Clements, J.D.; Arntzen, C.J. Oral Immunization with a Recombinant Bacterial Antigen Produced in Transgenic Plants. Science **1995**, *268*, 714–716.

45. Carrillo, C.; Wigdorovitz, A.; Oliveros, J.C.; Zamorano, P.I.; Sadir, A.M.; Gomez, N.; Salinas, J.; Escribano, J.M.; Borca, M.V. Protective Immune Responses to Foot-Mouth-Disease Virus with VP1 Expressed in Transgenic Plants. J. Virol. **1998**, *72*, 1688–1690.

46. Dalsgaard, K.; Uttenthal, A.; Jones, T.D.; Xu, F.; Merryweather, A.; Hamilton, W.D.O.; Langeveld, J.P.M.; Boshuizen, R.S.; Kamstrup, S.; Lomonossoff, G.P.; Porta, C.; Vela, C.; Casal, J.I.; Meloen, R.H.; Rodgers, P.B. Plant-Derived Vaccine Protects Target Animals Against a Viral Disease. Nature Biotechnol. **1997**, *15*, 248–252.

47. Thanavala, Y.; Yang, Y.-F.; Lyons, P.; Mason, H.S.; Arntzen, C. Immunogenicity of Transgenic Plant-Derived Hepatitis B Surface Antigen. Proceedings of the National Academy Science USA **1995**, *92*, 2258–3361.

48. Arntzen, C.J.; Mason, H.S.; Shi, J.; Haq, T.A.; Estes, M.K.; Clements, J.D. Production of Candidate Oral Vaccines in Edible Tissues of Transgenic Plants. *Vaccines '94: Modern Approaches to New Vaccines Including Prevention of AIDS*; Brown, F., Chanock, R.M., Ginsberg, H.S., Lerner, R.A., Eds.; Cold Spring Harbor Laboratory Press Cold Spring Harbor: New York, 1994; 339–344.

49. Zanetti, M.; Secarz, E.; Salk, J. The Immunology of New Generation Vaccines. Immunol. Today **1987**, *8*, 18–22.

50. Oosterlaken, T.A.; Harmsen, M.; Jhagjhoor-Singh, S.S.; Ekstijn, G.L.; Kraaijeveld, C.A.; Snippe, H.A. Protective Monoclonal Anti-Idiotypic Vaccine to Lethal Semliki Forest Virus Infection in BALB/c Mice. J. Virol. **1991**, *65*, 98–102.

51. Wolff, J.A.; Malone, R.W.; Williams, P.; Chong, W.; Acsadi, G.; Jani, A.; Felgner, P.L. Direct Gene Transfer into Mouse Muscle In Vivo. Science **1990**, *24*, 1465–1468.

52. Yang, N.S.; Burkholder, J.; Roberts, B.; Martinell, B.; McCabe, D. In Vivo and In Vitro Gene Transfer to Mammalian Somatic Cells by Particle Bombardment. Proceedings of the National Academy Science USA **1990**, *87*, 9568–9572.

53. Williams, R.S.; Johnston, S.A.; Riedy, M.; DeVit, M.J.; McElligott, S.G.; Sanford, J.C. Introduction of Foreign Genes into Tissues of Living Mice by DNA-Coated Microprojectiles. Proceedings of the National Academy Science USA **1991**, *88*, 2726–2730.

54. Felgner, P.L.; Ringold, G.M. Cationic Liposome-Mediated Transfection. Nature **1989**, *337*, 387–388.

55. Barthel, F.; Remy, J.S.; Loeffler, J.P.; Behr, J.P. Gene Transfer Optimization with Lipospermine-Coated DNA. DNA Cell. Biol. **1993**, *12*, 553–560.

56. Mathiowitz, E.; Jacob, J.S.; Jong, Y.S.; Carino, G.P.; Chickering, D.E.; Chaturvedi, P.; Santos, C.A.; Vijayaraghavan, K.; Montgomery, S.; Bassett, M.; Morrell, C. Biologically Erodable Microspheres as Potential Oral Drug Delivery Systems. Nature **1997**, *386*, 410–414.

57. Aggarwal, N.; HogenEsch, H.; Guo, P.; North, A.; Suckow, M.; Mittal, S.K. Biodegradable Alginate Microspheres as a Delivery System for Naked DNA. Can. J. Vet. Res. **1999**, *63*, 148–152.

58. Mittal, S.K.; Aggarwal, N.; Sailaja, G.; van Olphen, A.; HogenEsch, H.; North, A.; Hays, J.; Moffatt, S. Immunization with DNA, Adenovirus or Both in Biodegradable Alginate Microspheres: Effect of Route of Inoculation on Immune Response. Vaccine *,in press.*

59. Ulmer, J.B.; Donnelly, J.J.; Parker, S.E.; Rhodes, G.H.; Felgner, P.L.; Dwarki, V.J.; Gromkowski, S.H.; Deck, R.R.; DeWltt, C.M.; Friedman, A. Heterologous Protection Against Influenza by Injection of DNA Encoding a Viral Protein. Science **1993**, *259*, 1745–1749.

60. Donnelly, J.J.; Ulmer, J.B.; Liu, MA. DNA Vaccines. Life Sci. **1993**, *60*, 163–172.

61. Lowrie, D.B.; Silva, C.L.; Colston, M.J.; Ragno, S.; Tascon, R.E. Protection Against Tuberculosis by a Plasmid DNA Vaccine. Vaccine **1997**, *15*, 834–838.

62. Lowrie, D.B.; Tascon, R.E.; Bonato, V.L.; Lima, V.M.; Faccioli, L.H.; Stavropoulos, E.; Colston, M.J.; Hewinson, R.G.; Moelling, K.; Silva, C.L. Therapy of Tuberculosis in Mice by DNA Vaccination. Nature **1999**, *400*, 269–271.

63. Koprowski, H.; Weiner, D.B. *DNA Vaccination/Genetic Vaccination. Current Topics in Microbiology and Immunology*; Springer-Verlag: Berlin, 1998; 226.

64. Powell, M.F.; Newman, M.J. *Vaccine Design: The Subunit and Adjuvant Approach*; Plenum Press: San Diego, 1995.

65. Stewart-Tull, D.E.S. *The Theory and Practical Application of Adjuvants*; John Wiley & Sons: Chichester, UK, 1995.

66. O'Hagan, D.T. *Vaccine Adjuvants. Preparation Methods and Research Protocols*; Humana Press: Totowa, NJ, 2000; 342.

67. Singh, M.; O'Hagan, D. Advances in Vaccine Adjuvants. Nature Biotechnol. **1999**, *17*, 1075–1081.

68. Raychaudhuri, S.; Rock, K.L. Fully Mobilizing Host Defenses: Building Better Vaccines. Nature Biotechnol. **1998**, *16*, 1025–1031.

69. Cleland, J.L. Design and Production of Single-Immunization Vaccines Using Polylactide Polyglycolide Microsphere Systems. *Vaccine Design: The Subunit and Adjuvant Approach*; Powell, M.F., Newman, M.J., Eds.; Plenum Press: New York, 1995; 439–462.

70. Rundell, A.; DeCarlo, R.; HogenEsch, H.; Doerschuk, P. The Humoral Immune Response to Haemophilus Influenzae Type B: A Mathematical Model Based on T-Zone and Germinal Center B-Cell Dynamics. J. Theor. Biol. **1998**, *194*, 341–381.

71. Hem, S.L.; White, J.L. Structure and Properties of Aluminum-Containing Adjuvants. *Vaccine Design. The Subunit and Adjuvant Approach*; Powell, M.F., Newman, M.J., Eds.; Plenum Press: New York, 19951 249–276.

72. Brewer, J.M.; Conacher, M.; Hunter, C.A.; Mohrs, M.; Brombacher, F.; Alexander, J. Aluminium Hydroxide Adjuvant Initiates Strong Antigen-Specific Th2 Responses in the Absence of IL-4- or IL-13-Mediated Signaling. J. Immunol. **1999**, *163*, 6448–6454.

73. Jankovic, D.; Caspar, P.; Zweig, M.; Garcia-Moll, M.; Showalter, S.D.; Vogel, F.R.; Sher, A. Adsorption to Aluminum Hydroxide Promotes the Activity of IL-12 as an Adjuvant for Antibody as well as Type 1 Cytokine Responses to HIV-1 GP120. J. Immunol. **1997**, *159*, 2409–2417.

74. Barr, I.G.; Sjolander, A.; Cox, J.C. ISCOMs and Other Saponin Based Adjuvants. Adv. Drug Del. Rev. **1998**, *32*, 247–271.

75. Brokstad, K.A.; Cox, R.J.; Olofsson, J.; Jonsson, R.; Haaheim, L.R. Parenteral Influenza Vaccination Induces a Rapid Systemic and Local Immune Response. J. Infect. Dis. **1995**, *171*, 198–203.

76. Shroff, K.E.; Marcucci-Borges, L.A.; de Bruin, S.J.; Winter, L.A.; Tiberio, L.; Pachuk, C.; Snyder, L.A.; Satishchandran, C.; Ciccarelli, R.B.; Higgins, T.J. Induction of HSV-gD2 Specific CD4(+) Cells in Peyer's Patches and Mucosal Antibody Responses in Mice Following DNA Immunization by Both Parenteral and Mucosal Administration. Vaccine **1999**, *18*, 222–230.

77. Fontanilla, B.C.; Silvano, F.; Cumming, R. Oral Vaccination Against Newcastle Disease of Village Chickens in the Philippines. Prev. Vet. Med. **1994**, *19*, 39–44.

78. Lundholm, P.; Asakura, Y.; Hinkula, J.; Lucht, E.; Wahren, B. Induction of Mucosal IgA By a Novel Jet Delivery Technique for HIV-1 DNA. Vaccine **1999**, *17*, 2036–2042.

79. McCluskie, M.J.; Brazolot Millan, C.L.; Gramzinski, R.A.; Robinson, H.L.; Santoro, J.C.; Fuller, J.T.; Widera, G.; Haynes, J.R.; Purcell, R.H.; Davis, H.L. Route and Method of Delivery of DNA Vaccine Influence Immune Responses in Mice and Non-Human Primates. Mol. Med. **1999**, *5*, 287–300.

80. Langue, J.; Ethevenaux, C.; Champsaur, A.; Fritzell, B.; Begue, P.; Saliou, P. Safety and Immunogenicity of Haemophilus Influenzae Type B-Tetanus Toxoid Conjugate, Presented in a Dual-Chamber Syringe with Diphtheria–Tetanus-Pertussis and Inactivated Poliomyelitis Combination Vaccine. Eur. J. Pediatr. **1999**, *158*, 717–722.

81. Kanra, G.; Yurdakok, K.; Ceyhan, M.; Ozmert, E.; Turkay, F.; Pehlivan, T. Immunogenicity and Safety of Haemophilus Influenzae Type B Capsular Polysaccharide Tetanus Conjugate Vaccine (PRP-T) Presented in a Dual-Chamber Syringe with DTP. Acta Paediatr. Jpn. **1997**, *39*, 676–680.

82. Roberts, M.; Chatfield, S.N.; Dougan, G. *Salmonella as Carriers of Heterologous Antigens, In Novel Delivery Systems for Oral Vaccines*; O'Hagan, D.T.,Ed.; CRC Press Inc.: Ann Arbor MI, 1994; 27–58.

83. McGhee, J.R.; Mestecky, J.; Dertzbaugh, M.T.; Eldridge, J.H.; Hirasawa, M.; Kiyono, H. The Mucosal Immune System: From Fundamental Concepts to Vaccine Development. Vaccine **1992**, *10*, 75–88.

84. Hornquist, E.; Lycke, N.; Czerkinsky, C.; Holmgren, J. Cholera Toxin and Cholera B Subunit as Oral-Mucosal Adjuvant and Antigen Carrier Systems. *Novel Delivery Systems for Oral Vaccines*; O'Hagan, D.T. Ed.; CRC Press, Inc.: Ann Arbor MI, 1994; 157–173.

85. Service, R.F. Triggering the First Line of Defense. Science **1994**, *265*, 1552–1554.

86. Heritage, P.L.; Underdown, B.J.; Brook, M.A.; McDermott, M.R. Oral Administration of Polymer-Grafted Starch Microparticles Activates Gut-Associated Lymphocytes and Primes Mice for a Subsequent Systemic Antigen Challenge. Vaccine **1998**, *16*, 2010–2017.

87. Dale, J.W.; Dellagostin, O.A.; Norman, E.; Barrett, A.D.T.; McFadden, J. Multivalent BCG Vaccines. *Novel Delivery Systems for Oral Vaccines*; O'Hagan, D.T. Ed.; CRC Press, Inc.: Ann Arbor, MI, 1994; 87–109.

88. Dunkley, M.L.; Harris, S.J.; McCoy, R.J.; Musicka, M.J.; Eyers, F.M.; Beagley, L.G.; Lumley, P.J.; Beagley, K.W.; Clancy, R.L. Protection Against *Helicobacter pylori* Infection by Intestinal Immunisation with a 50/52-kDa Subunit Protein. FEMS Immunol. Med. Microbiol. **1999**, *24*, 221–225.

89. Corthesy-Theulaz, I.; Porta, N.; Glauser, M.; Saraga, E.; Vaney, A.C.; Haas, R.; Kraehenbuhl, J.P.; Blum, A.L.; Michetti, P. Oral Immunization with *Helicobacter pylori* Urease B Subunit as a Treatment Against Helicobacter Infection in Mice. Gastroenterology **1995**, *109*, 115–121.

90. Husby, S.; Jensenius, J.C.; Svehag, S.-E. Passage of Undegraded Dietary Antigen into the Blood of Healthy Adults. Further Characterization of the Kinetics of the Uptake and the Size Distribution of the Antigen. Scand. J. Immunol. **1986**, *24*, 447–455.

91. Eaton, K.A.; Krakowka, S. Chronic Active Gastritis Due to *Helicobacter pylori* in Immunized Gnotobiotic Piglets. Gastroenterology **1992**, *103*, 1580–1586.

92. Ball, J.M.; Graham, D.Y.; Opekun, A.R.; Gilger, M.A.; Guerrero, R.A.; Estes, M.K. Recombinant Norwalk Virus-Like Particles Given Orally to Volunteers: Phase I Study (see Comments). Gastroenterology **1999**, *117*, 40–48.

93. Foster, N.; Clark, M.A.; Jepson, M.A.; Hirst, B.H. Ulex Europaeus 1 Lectin Targets Microspheres to Mouse Peyer's Patch M-Cells In Vivo. Vaccine **1998**, *16*, 536–541.

94. Eyles, J.E.; Williamson, E.D.; Alpar, H.O. Immunological Responses to Nasal Delivery of Free and Encapsulated Tetanus Toxoid: Studies on the Effect of Vehicle Volume. Int. J. Pharm. **1999**, *189*, 75–79.

95. Rudin, A.; Riise, G.C.; Holmgren, J. Antibody Responses in the Lower Respiratory Tract and Male Urogenital Tract in Humans After Nasal and Oral Vaccination with Cholera Toxin B Subunit. Infect. Immun. **1999**, *67*, 2884–2890.

96. Shi, Z.; Curiel, D.T.; Tang, D.C. DNA-based Noninvasive Vaccination Onto the Skin. Vaccine **1999**, *17*, 2136–2141.

97. Misra, A.; Ganga, S.; Upadhyay, P. Needle-Free, Nonadjuvanted Skin Immunization by Electroporation-Enhanced Transdermal Delivery of Diphtheria Toxoid and a Candidate Peptide Vaccine Against Hepatitis B Virus. Vaccine **1999**, *18*, 517–523.

98. Scharton-Kersten, T.M.; Glenn, G.; Vassell, R.; Yu, J.; Walwender, D.; Alving, C.R. Principles of Transcutaneous Immunization Using Cholera Toxin as an Adjuvant. Vaccine, Suppl 17 **1999**, *2*, s37–43.

99. Glenn, G.M.; Scharton-Kersten, T.; Vassell, R.; Matyas, G.R.; Alving, C.R. Transcutaneous Immunization with Bacterial ADP-Ribosylating Exotoxins as Antigens and Adjuvants. Infect. Immun. **1999**, *67*, 1100–1106.

100. Glenn, G.M.; Scharton-Kersten, T.; Vassell, R.; Mallett, C.P.; Hale, T.L.; Alving, C.R. Transcutaneous Immunization with Cholera Toxin Protects Mice Against Lethal Mucosal Toxin Challenge. J. Immunol. **1998**, *161*, 3211–3214.

101. Brown, A.R.; George, D.W.; Matteson, D.K. Vaccinator Device for Delivering Propellant-Driven Aerosols of *Streptococcus suis* Bacterin into the Respiratory Tracts of Swine. Vaccine **1997**, *15*, 1165–1173.

102. LiCalsi, C.; Christensen, T.; Bennett, J.V.; Phillips, E.; Witham, C. Dry Powder Inhalation as a Potential Delivery Method for Vaccines. Vaccine **1999**, *17*, 1796–1803.

103. McCluskie, M.J.; Chu, Y.; Xia, J.L.; Jessee, J.; Gebyehu, G.; Davis, H.L. Direct Gene Transfer to the Respiratory Tract of Mice with Pure Plasmid and Lipid-Formulated DNA. Antisense Nucleic Acid Drug Dev. **1998**, *8*, 401–414.

104. Weng, C.N.; Tzan, Y.L.; Liu, S.D.; Lin, S.Y.; Lee, C.J. Protective Effects of an Oral Microencapsulated *Mycoplasma hyopneumoniae* Vaccine Against Experimental Infection in Pigs. Res. Vet. Sci. **1992**, *53*, 42–46.

105. Forrest, B.D. Clinical Evaluation of Attenuated *Salmonella typhi* Vaccines in Human Subjects. *Novel Delivery Systems for Oral Vaccines*; O'Hagan, D.T., Ed.; CRC Press, Inc.: Ann Arbor, MI, 1994; 59–85.

106. Crotty, S.; Lohman, B.L.; Lu, F.X.; Tang, S.; Miller, C.J.; Andino, R. Mucosal Immunization of Cynomolgus Macaques with Two Serotypes of Live Poliovirus Vectors Expressing Simian Immunodeficiency Virus Antigens: Stimulation of Humoral, Mucosal, and Cellular Immunity. J. Virol. **1999**, *73*, 9485–9495.

107. Aunins, J.G.; Lee, A.L.; Volkins, D.B. Vaccine Production. *The Biomedical Engineering Handbook*; Bronzino, J.D., Ed.; CRC Press: Boca Raton, FL, 1995; 1502–1517.

108. Bussiere, J.L.; McCormick, G.C.; Green, J.D. Preclinical Safety Assessment Considerations in Vaccine Development. *Vaccine Design: The Subunit and Adjuvant Approach*; Powell, M.F., Newman, M.J., Burdman, J.R., Eds.; Plenum Press: New York, 1995; 61–79.

109. Lawrence, D.N.; Goldenthal, K.L.; Boslego, J.W.; Chandler, D.K.F.; La Montagne, J.R. Public Health Implications of Emerging Vaccine Technologies. *Vaccine Design: The Subunit and Adjuvant Approach*; Powell, M.F., Newman, M.J., Burdman, J.R., Eds.; Plenum Press: New York, 1995; 43–60.

110. O'Hagan, D.T. Microparticles as Oral Vaccines. In *Novel Delivery Systems for Oral Vaccines*; CRC Press, Inc.: Ann Arbor, MI, 1994; 175–205.

111. Morris, W.; Steinhoff, M.C.; Russell, P.K. Potential of Polymer Microencapsulation Technology for Vaccine Innovation. Vaccine **1994**, *12*, 5–11.

112. Kuntz, R.M.; Saltzman, W.M. Polymeric Controlled Delivery for Immunization. Trends Biotechnol. **1997**, *15*, 364–369.

113. Desai, M.P.; Labhasetwar, V.; Amidon, G.L.; Levy, R.J. Gastrointestinal Uptake of Biodegradable Microparticles: Effect of Particle Size. Pharm. Res. **1996**, *13*, 1838–1845.

114. Casal, J.I.; Rueda, P.; Hurtado, A. Parvovirus-Like Particles as Vaccine Vectors. Methods **1999**, *19*, 174–186.

115. Liu, X.S.; Abdul-Jabbar, I.; Qi, Y.M.; Frazer, I.H.; Zhou, J. Mucosal Immunisation with Papillomavirus Virus-Like Particles Elicits Systemic and Mucosal Immunity in Mice. Virology **1998**, *252*, 39–45.

116. Nakanishi, T.; Kunisawa, J.; Hayashi, A.; Tsutsumi, Y.; Kubo, K.; Nakagawa, S.; Nakanishi, M.; Tanaka, K.; Mayumi, T. Positively Charged Liposome Functions as an Efficient Immunoadjuvant in Inducing Cell-Mediated Immune Response to Soluble Proteins. J. Controlled Rel. **1999**, *61*, 233–240.

117. Hayashi, A.; Nakanishi, T.; Kunisawa, J.; Kondoh, M.; Imazu, S.; Tsutsumi, Y.; Tanaka, K.; Fujiwara, H.; Hamaoka, T.; Mayumi, T. A Novel Vaccine Delivery System Using Immunopotentiating Fusogenic Liposomes. Biochem. Biophys. Res. Commun. **1999**, *261*, 824–828.

118. Lasic, D.D. *Liposomes in Gene Delivery*; CRC Press: Boca Raton, FL, 1997; 67–112.

119. Cryz, S.J. BERNA: A Century of Immunobiological Innovation. Vaccine **1999**, *17*, S1–S5.

120. Poltl-Frank, F.; Zurbriggen, R.; Helg, A.; Stuart, F.; Robinson, J.; Gluck, R.; Pluschke, G. Use of Reconstituted Influenza Virus Virosomes as an Immunopotentiating Delivery System for a Peptide-Based Vaccine. Clin. Exp. Immunol. **1999**, *117*, 496–503.

121. Rentel, C.O.; Bouwstra, J.A.; Naisbett, B.; Junginger, H.E. Niosomes as a Novel Peroral Vaccine Delivery System. Int. J. Pharm. **1999**, *186*, 161–167.

122. St Clair, N.; Shenoy, B.; Jacob, L.D.; Margolin, A.L. Cross-Linked Protein Crystals for Vaccine Delivery. Proc. Natl. Acad. Sc. USA **1999**, *96*, 9469–9474.

123. Thompson, C.B.; Allison, J.P. The Emerging Role of CTLA-4 as an Immune Attenuator. Immunity **1997**, *7*, 445–450.

124. Abrams, J.R.; Lebwohl, M.G.; Guzzo, C.A.; Jegasothy, B.V.; Goldfarb, M.T.; Goffe, B.S.; Menter, A.; Lowe, N.J.; Krueger, G.; Brown, M.J.; Weiner, R.S.; Birkhofer, M.J.; Warner, G.L.; Berry, K.K.; Linsley, P.S.; Krueger, J.G.; Ochs, H.D.; Kelley, S.L.; Kang, S.W. CTLA4Ig-Mediated Blockade of T-Cell Costimulation in Patients with Psoriasis Vulgaris. J. Clin.Invest. **1999**, *103*, 1243–1252.

125. Kwon, E.D.; Foster, B.A.; Hurwitz, A.A.; Madias, C.; Allison, J.P.; Greenberg, N.M.; Burg, M.B. Elimination of Residual Metastatic Prostate Cancer After Surgery and

Adjunctive Cytotxic T Lymphocyte-Associated Antigen 4 (CTLA-4) Blockade Immunotherapy. Proceedings of the National Academy Science USA **1999**, *96*, 15074–15079.

126. Abbas, A.K.; Sharpe, A.H. T-cell Stimulation: An Abundance of B7s. Nature Med. **1999**, *5*, 1345–1346.

127. Krieg, A.M.; Yi, A.-K.; Hartmann, G. Mechanisms and Therapeutic Applications of Immune Stimulatory CpG DNA. Pharmacol. Therapeutics **1999**, *84*, 113–120.

128. Hall, G.L.; Compston, A.; Scolding, N.J. Beta-Interferon and Multiple Sclerosis. Trends Neurosci. **1997**, *20*, 63–67.

129. Yong, V.W.; Chabot, S.; Williams, G. Interferon Beta in the Treatment of Multiple Sclerosis. Mechanisms of Action. Neurology **1998**, *51*, 682–689.

130. Moreland, L.W. Inhibitors of Tumor Necrosis Factor for Rheumatoid Arthritis. J. Rheumatol. **1999**, *57*, 7–15, Suppl. 26.

131. Sandborn, W.J.; Hanauer, S.B. Antitumor Necrosis Factor Therapy for Inflammatory Bowel Disease: A Review of Agents, Pharmacology, Clinical Results, and Safety. Inflamm. Bowel Dis. **1999**, *5*, 119–133.

VALIDATION OF PHARMACEUTICAL PROCESSES

Robert A. Nash
Consultant, Mahwah, New Jersey

INTRODUCTION

Process validation is a requirement of current Good Manufacturing Practices (GMPs) for finished pharmaceuticals (21 CFR 211) and of the GMP regulations for medical devices (21 CFR 820) and therefore applies to the manufacture of both drug products and medical devices.

According to the FDA Guidelines on General Principles of Process Validation (1), process validation is defined, "... as establishing documented evidence, which provides a high degree of assurance, that a specific process will consistently produce a product meeting its predetermined specifications and quality characteristics." The process for making a drug product consists of a series (flow diagram in logically defined steps) of unit operations (modules) that result in the manufacture of the finished pharmaceutical.

There is much confusion regarding the definition of process validation and what constitutes process validation documentation. The term validation is used here generically to cover the entire spectrum of current GMP concerns, essential most of which are: facility, equipment, component, method, and process qualification. Based upon the FDA process validation guidelines (1), the specific term should be reserved for the final stage(s) of the product and process development sequence. The essential or key steps or stages of a successfully completed development program are shown in Table 1.

The end of the development sequence, which should be assigned to formal (three-batch) process validation, derives from the fact that the specific exercise of process validation should never be designed to fail. Failure in carrying out the formal process validation assignment is often the result of incomplete or faulty understanding of the process capability, in other words, what the process can and cannot accomplish under a given set of operational requirements.

In a well-designed validation program, most of the effort should be spent on facilities, equipment, components, methods, and process qualification. In such a program, the formalized, final three-batch validation sequence provides only the necessary process validation documentation required by the FDA to show product reproducibility and a manufacturing process in a state of control. Such a strategy is consistent with the FDA preapproval inspection program directive (2).

PROCESS VALIDATION OPTIONS

The guidelines on general principles of process validation (1) mention three options: prospective process validation (also called premarket validation), retrospective process validation, and revalidation. Actually there are four, if concurrent process validation is included.

Prospective validation is carried out prior to the distribution of a new product or an existing product made under a revised manufacturing process where such revisions may affect product specifications or quality characteristics. The prospective approach features critical step analysis in which the unit operations are challenged during the process qualification stage to determine those critical process variables that may affect overall process performance, using either worst-case analysis or a fractional–factorial design. During formal, three-batch, prospective validation, critical process variables should be set within their operating ranges and should not exceed their upper and lower control limits during process operation. Output responses should be well within finished-product specifications.

Retrospective validation is recognized in both current GMPs [21 CFR 211.110(b)] and the FDA process validation guidelines (1). It involves accumulated in-process production and final product testing and control (numerical) data to establish that the product and its manufacturing process are in a state of control. Valid in-process results should be consistent with the final specifications of the drug product and shall be derived from previous acceptable process average and process variability estimates where possible and determined by the application of suitable statistical procedures (quality control charting) where appropriate.

The retrospective validation option is chosen for established products whose manufacturing processes are considered to be stable and when, on the basis of economic considerations and resource limitations, prospective qualification and validation experimentation cannot be justified.

Encyclopedia of Pharmaceutical Technology

Table 1 Development sequence with respect to process validation

Developmental stages	Batch size
Product design	1 X
Product characterization	
Product selection	
Process design	
Product optimization	10 X
Process characterization	
Process optimization	
Process qualification	
Process qualification	100 X
Process validation	
Process certification	
Process revalidation	100 X to 1000 X

Prior to undertaking either prospective or retrospective validation, the facilities, equipment, and subsystems used in connection with the manufacturing process must be qualified in conformance with cGMP requirements.

Concurrent validation studies are carried out under a protocol during the course of normal production. The first three production-scale batches must be monitored as comprehensively as possible. The evaluation of the results is used in establishing the acceptance criteria and specifications of subsequent in-process control and final product testing. Some form of concurrent validation, using statistical process control techniques (quality control charting) may be employed throughout the product manufacturing life cycle.

Revalidation is required to ensure that changes in the process and/or in the process environment, whether introduced intentionally or unintentionally, do not adversely affect product specifications and quality characteristics (2). There should be a quality assurance program (change control) in place which requires revalidation whenever there are significant changes in formulation, equipment, process, and packaging that may impact on product and manufacturing process performance (3). Furthermore, when a change is made in a raw material supplier, the drug manufacturer should be made aware of subtle, potentially adverse differences in raw material characteristics that may adversely affect product and manufacturing process performance.

It is recommended that every requested change be reviewed by the validation or CMC committee. Such a committee should judge if a change is significant for revalidation and decide on a course of action to be taken. The following conditions require revalidation study and documentation:

1. Change in a critical component (usually refers to active pharmaceutical ingredient, key excipients, or primary packaging);
2. Change or replacement in a critical piece of modular (capital) equipment;
3. Significant change in processing conditions that may affect subsequent unit operations and product quality;
4. Change in a facility and/or plant (usually location, site, or support systems);
5. Significant increase or decrease in batch size that affects the operation of modular equipment; and
6. Sequential batches that fail to meet product and process in-process specifications.

In some situations process performance requalification studies may be required prior to undertaking specific revalidation assignments. With the exception of sterile products manufacture, periodic revalidation is not required at the present time. The performance and state of control of the product and its manufacturing process can be adequately covered during the annual product and process review. The FDA has issued an interim guidance document that addresses what constitutes major and minor formulation and manufacturing changes for immediate-release solid dosage forms (4). Such documentation and others to follow should simplify manufacturing decisions about the need to revalidate.

VALIDATION PRIORITIES

There is a basic concept with respect to which pharmaceutical processes should be given a higher priority over others. All pharmaceutical manufacturing processes require process validation documentation, but there is an accepted logical approach to priority selection, in the following order:

Sterile products and their processes

- large volume parenterals (LVPs) infusions greater than 100 ml
- small volume parenterals (SVPs) single and multiple dose injections
- ophthalmics and sterile devices

Nonsterile products and their processes

- low dose high potency tablets and capsules
- drugs with inherent stability problems
- transdermal delivery (TDD) and inhalation products
- the rest of the oral solid dosage forms
- oral liquids and topical products

The best approach to assessing problems with respect to a terminal sterilization method (i.e., moist heat, dry heat, radiation, and chemical methods) is to first establish the qualification, validation and stability of the pharmaceutical process prior to conducting a given sterilization procedure.

THE VALIDATION COMMITTEE

In most companies, the validation or Chemistry, Manufacturing and Control (CMC) committee is charged with the responsibility of establishing and operating the complete validation program for the specific manufacturing site. In some companies the program is led by a validation manager whereas in others, quality assurance personnel have taken on expanded responsibilities in this regard.

Specific process validation assignments are carried out by those with the necessary training and experience. The specifics of how the committee is organized to conduct process validation assignments is beyond the scope of this article. The responsibilities that must be carried out and the traditional organizational structures best equipped to handle each of these assignments are outlined in Table 2. Other members may include Quality Control, Regularity affairs, etc.

VALIDATION MASTER PLAN

The creation of a master plan permits the development of a logical overview of the validation effort. It lays out in a logical sequence the activities or key elements or both to be performed in accordance with the approximate time schedule in a Gantt or PERT chart format. The master plan establishes the critical path through the chart against which progress can be monitored.

The validation program starts with the design and development of raw materials and components, followed by the IQ/OQ of facilities, equipment, and systems through performance and process qualification stages, and terminates in the protocol-driven, three-batch, formal process validation

program. Most of these activities move forward in series. However, by combining activities and elements and moving in parallel, where possible, on independent tracks with respect to active pharmaceutical ingredients (APIs) analytical methods development, facilities, equipment, support systems, and the drug product design and manufacturing process development, a great deal of time can be saved before the individual elements or grouping of activities are combined prior to the formal process validation program. A Process Validation progress chart is shown in Fig. 1.

Installation Qualification (IQ)

This includes procedures and documentation to show that all important aspects of the installation of the facility, support system, or piece of modular equipment, having been properly calibrated, meet its design specifications and that the vendor's recommendations had been suitably considered.

Operational Qualification (OQ)

Following IQ, procedures and documentation show that the facility, support system, or piece of modular equipment perform as intended throughout all anticipated operating ranges under a suitable load.

Performance Qualification (PQ)

Following IQ and OQ, actual demonstrations during the course of the validation program show that the facility, support system, or piece of modular equipment perform according to a predefined protocol and achieve process reproducibility and product acceptability.

VALIDATION PROTOCOL
AND REPORT

The following validation protocol and format for the completed validation report have been suggested in the WHO Guidelines on Validation of Manufacturing Processes (TRS 823) (5).

Table 2 Composition of the process validation committee

Representative of	Function
Engineering	Qualifies for plant, facilities, equipment, and support systems
Development	Qualifies for products and their specific manufacturing processes
Manufacturing	Operates plant, facilities, equipment, support systems and the various manufacturing processes
Quality assurance	Audits plant, facilities, equipment, support systems, the various manufacturing processes, and their products

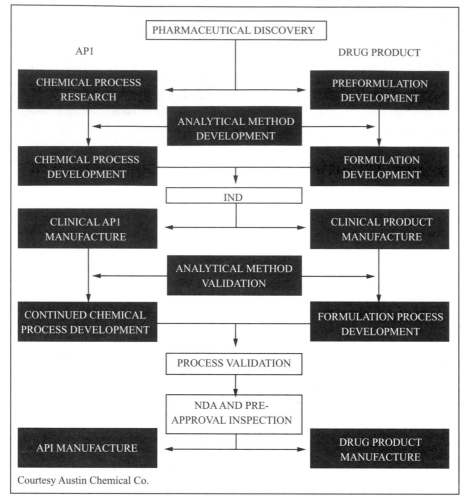

Fig. 1   Process validation progress chart.

1. Purpose (for the whole validation) and prerequisites
2. Presentation of the whole process and subprocesses including flow diagram and critical step analysis
3. Validation protocol approvals
4. Installation and operational qualifications, including blueprints or drawings
5. Qualification report(s)

- Subprocess 1
- Purpose
- Methods and procedures
- Sampling and testing procedures, release criteria
- Reporting function
- Calibration of test equipment
- Test data
- Summary of results
- Approval and requalification procedure
- Subprocess 2 (repeat)

6. Product qualification, test data from prevalidation batches
7. Product validation, test data from three formal validation batches
8. Evaluation and recommendations (include revalidation and requalification requirements)
9. Certification (approval)
10. Summary report with conclusions

The validation protocol and report may also include copies of the product stability report or its summary as well as validation documentation on cleaning and analytical methods.

PREAPPROVAL INSPECTION

The FDA Preapproval Inspection Program (2) is designed to provide a basis for determining the adequacy and accuracy of reported and factual information in New Drug Application (NDA) and Abbreviated New Drug Application (ANDA) submissions with respect to the suitability of cGMP product development, analytical laboratory, and manufacturing facilities.

A preapproval inspection checklist should include the following documentation which may be required prior to the formal inspection:

1. API development and validation report(s) including impurity profile and polymorphic forms;
2. Pharmaceutical (dosage form) development report;
3. Stability and clinical batch records and history, including phase-III program;
4. Data for API and key excipients used in the manufacture of clinical and biobatches;
5. Bioequivalency report;
6. Technical transfer report (development to manufacturing/QA/QC);
7. Copy of the CMC section of the NDA including information on suppliers and vendors;
8. Copy of proposed production monograph and master batch record;
9. Equipment validation report establishing IQ and OQ;
10. Cleaning validation report;
11. Analytical methods validation and computer systems validation reports;
12. Stability report establishing expiry dating; and
13. Process validation protocol for formal three-batch validation of production-size batches.

During preapproval inspection, the FDA accepts a process-validation protocol based on the company's commitment to complete successfully three production-size validation batches prior to product launch. In some situations a prevalidation (process demonstration qualification) production-size batch is completed before the entire formal three-batch program is carried out.

PILOT SCALE-UP AND TECHNOLOGY TRANSFER

The pilot-production program may be carried out as a shared responsibility between the development laboratories and their appropriate manufacturing counterpart or as a process demonstration by a separate, designated pilot-plant or process development department. Supporting technology transfer documentation applies to both the specific process and system being qualified and validated and the related testing standards and testing methods. The formal technology transfer is normally made from the development laboratories or the process development pilot-plant to pharmaceutical production function.

In actuality, a number of technology transfer points and documents are generated as prospective validation proceeds through the various stages of product development. These stages of technology transfer in terms of scale-up are illustrated in Fig. 2.

Solid pharmaceutical dosage forms (tablets and capsules) are used to illustrate the various stages of product and process development. These principles and practices also apply in a general way to the development of liquid and semisolid pharmaceutical dosage forms (not discussed here).

STAGES OF VALIDATION

Elements of the validation concept should be incorporated during each of the various stages of the product and process development continuum. These stages can be summarized as follows.

Stage Preformulation Studies: APIs plus rey excipients

Stage I Product design and development
Stage II Preparation of clinical and biobatches
Stage III Process scale-up and evaluation
Stage IV Formal process validation

Preformulation Studies: API

Preformulation testing of the specific API of interest and key excipients to be used in the product design stage, alone and in combinations with the API, should be included as a preliminary first step in the product and process development sequence. A simple check list of items

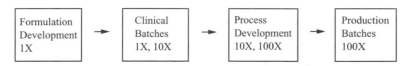

Fig. 2 Technology transfer stages.

worth consideration in preformulation studies with APIs and important or critical excipients is provided as follows:

API

- Key excipients

  Fillers and diluents
  Binders
  Disintegrants
  Glidants and lubricants

- Establish chemical and physical compatibility
- Minimize lot-to-lot variability in properties
- Worldwide availability from comparable suppliers
- Properties for possible evaluation

  Color, odor, taste, solubility;
  Particle morphology (DSC, TGA, x-ray diffraction);
  Particle size distribution and surface area;
  Crystal and bulk density, compaction index;
  Angle of repose and flowability index;
  Spectrophotometry (UV, FTIR, NMR, OR);
  Water content, LOD, moisture uptake;
  Microbial limits and heavy metals;
  HPLC assay and impurity profile.

Before preformulation studies are undertaken, two-way technical communication between the manufacturers of the API (laboratory and plant) and the pharmaceutical product development laboratories must be established (see Fig. 1). It should start early and be maintained through-out the product and process development program.

In addition to potency, purity, and stability considerations of the API, the product development department is especially interested in the chemical and physical form (free acid or base, salts, esters, amides, polymorphs, solvates, particle size and shape) of the API. Time spent early in the cycle in establishing these particular factors often aids and/or simplifies the subsequent product and process development program.

Not every subject shown above must be tested or addressed. However, aspect, particle morphology and size, compaction and flowability, water content, spectrophotometric and chromatographic data should be studied and monitored throughout the product and process development program (6, 7).

Because key excipients are well established in most new product and process development programs, the same degree of preformulation scrutiny is often not required. Compatibility studies with the API, however, should be performed to study possible untoward interactions between the active ingredients and the excipients. It should be kept in mind that small or minor changes in

physical and possibly chemical properties upon intimate contact in binary studies with key excipients should not automatically exclude a favored excipient without further critical testing.

Stage I: Product Design and Development

Following successful preformulation studies, the API is transferred to the formulations laboratory for preliminary product design and development studies. In most cases, the drug is mixed with an appropriate diluent or filler and glidant combination and filled into two-piece opaque hard-shell capsules for preliminary stability and subsequent phase I clinical studies versus matching placebo capsules (8). At or about the same time, initial studies of a prototype tablet formulation should be started. The key steps in the product design and development sequence are given below.

Stage I: Product Design: 1× Laboratory Scale (1–10 kg)

- Hard-shell capsule (phase I clinical trials) followed by prototype tablet dosage form

  Direct compression versus wet granulation
  Maximize chemical and physical stability
  Minimize product and process costs
  Product characterization
  Product selection
  Process design

- Excipients are selected among the following categories:

  Binder, diluents, and disintegrants including alginates, calcium phosphate, cellulose, dextrates, gelatin, povidones, starch and derivatives, sorbitol, sucrose, and derivatives. Glidants and lubricants including colloidal silicon dioxide, hydrogenated vegetable oil, mineral oil, PEG, silica gel, sodium lauryl sulfate, stearates, talc.

Although the work is conducted in the research or formulations laboratory using small-scale processing equipment, it is important to gain early experience with colorant systems that have been selected for the finished tablet product; color aids in blend-uniformity evaluation.

In addition to excipient screening and selection, it is important to gauge processing parameters that are more fully explored during the scale-up phases. These processing factors include flowability, compaction and compressibility of powders and granules, content uniformity of powder and granule blends and finished tablets, moisture uptake, in vitro dissolution release profiles, and subsequent full-scale stability testing.

Products used in human clinical trials must, of course, conform to good laboratory, good clinical, and good manufacturing practice requirements (1, 9).

Stage II: Process Development: Pilot Laboratory (Clinical)

After the (1X) "go" laboratory batch has been determined to be both physically and chemical stable, based upon accelerated, elevated temperature testing (1 month at 45°C or 3 month at 40°C and 80% relative humidity) the next step (stage II) is to scale the product and its process to (10X) pilot-laboratory size batch(es). This batch represents the first replicated scale-up of the designated formula. Its size usually ranges between 10 and 100 kg, 10 and 100 L, or 10,000 to 100,000 units. Often these pilot-laboratory batches are used in clinical trials and bioequivalency studies. According to the FDA, the minimum requirement for a biobatch is 100,000 units (10).

Pilot-laboratory batches are usually prepared in small pilot equipment within a designated current GMP approved facility. The number and size of these pilot-laboratory batches may vary, depending on one or more of the following factors:

- Equipment availability
- API availability
- Cost of raw materials
- Inventory requirements for both clinical and nonclinical studies

Process development (process qualification) or process capability studies are normally started in this important stage II of the scale-up sequence. The scope of stage-II process development consists essentially of product optimization and process characterization studies.

Product Optimization:

- Establish formula rationale and boundary conditions for API and excipients

Process Characterization:

- Define unit operations, process variables, and response parameters.
  - Define critical process variables and response parameters using simple experimental designs.
  - Establish provisional control limits for critical process variables and their response parameters based on process replication.
- Maintain product stability.

Unit operations for solid dosage-form development include:

- Granulation
- Drying
- Sizing
- Blending and mixing
- Encapsulation andar tablet compression
- Coating
- Filling and packaging

Unit operations are selected for the development of a tablet (coated or noncoated) or capsule (hard shell or softgel) process (11). Unit operations that are considered to be critical are determined through analysis of the process variables and their respective measured response for each unit operation (Table 3) (12–14).

In order to determine critical control parameters and their unit operations, constraint analysis techniques (15) followed by fractional factorial designs (Table 4) are used to challenge the tentative control limits (so-called worst-case analysis) established for the process at this intermediate stage. Time and effort spent to qualify the process at the 10X stage often simplifies the work that follows during stages III and IV.

Von Doehren et al. (13) and Chowhan (16) have described the various stages of solid dosage form process development as it relates to technology transfer and process validation. Their respective approaches to the topic have been integrated in this article.

Fahrner (17) raises the following issues regarding the new role for pilot plants in product development.

- Too much time is devoted to preliminary or applied research and not enough to the proper development of the process.
- Often a suitable manufacturing strategy is lacking during the early phases of the program, which results in poorly planned technology transfer and an inappropriate division of responsibility with respect to the overall program.
- Most laboratory processes are rarely scalable, since piloting is a scaled-down version of manufacturing not a scaled-up version of the laboratory batch.

Fahrner makes the case for a separate pilot facility (process development function) to bridge the communication gap between R & D and production.

Stage-III: Pilot Production

The technology transfer of the product and process from the traditional product development function to a separate process development (pilot plant) function or production

Table 3 Control parameters for solid-dosage-form development

Unit Operation	Process variables (X)[a]	Measured responses (Y)[b]
Granulation (Power type)	Load Speed (main chopper) Liquid addition rate Granulation time	Power consumption
Drying	Load Inlet temperature Air-flow rate Drying time	Moisture content Bulk density
Sizing (Screening)	Load Screen size Speed Feed rate	Particle size distr. Bulk density
Blending (Mixing)	Load Speed Mixing time	Blend uniformity
Encapsulation	Fill volume Tamper setting Speed Glidant (type, amount)	Capsule weight Moisture content Dissolution Content uniformity Potency
Tablet compression	Press speed Feed rate Precompression force Compression force	Tablet weight Moisture content Hardness/friability Thickness Dissolution/disintegration Content uniformity Potency
Coating (Film type)	Load Pan speed Spray rate Air flow	Weight gain

[a]7–23 possible variables.
[b]11–16 possible responses.

itself is normally carried out at the (100×) pilot-production batch stage (100–1000 kg):

- Full-scale production batch
- For possible future commercial or clinical use
- Evaluate critical process parameters; product and process are scaled to another order of magnitude (100×)
- Process optimization

  — Mixing and blending times
  — Drying times
  — Milling operations
  — Press speed, compression force
  — Encapsulation speed, tamping settings
  — Speed, air flow, spray settings, temperature

- Process qualification (prevalidation batches); determine process capability, challenge in-process control limits
- Maintain product stability

The creation of a separate pilot plant or process development unit has been favored in recent years because it is ideally suited to carry out key process qualification and/or process validation studies in a timely manner (18, 19).

The objective of the pilot-production batch is to scale the product and its process by another order of magnitude (100×). For most solid dosage forms it represents a full production scale batch, in standard equipment. The technology transfer documents should include the technical information normally required for preapproval inspection:

Table 4 Fractional factorial design for process development[a]

Trials	Key variables[b]							Sums
	X_1	X_2	X_3	X_4	X_5	X_6	X_7	
1	−	−	−	−	−	−	−	0/7
2	−	−	−	+	−	−	−	1/6
3	−	−	+	−	−	+	−	2/5
4	+	+	−	−	+	−	−	3/4
5	+	+	−	−	−	+	+	4/3
6	+	−	+	+	+	−	+	5/2
7	−	+	+	+	+	+	+	6/1
8	+	+	+	+	+	+	+	7/0
Sums	4/4	4/4	4/4	4/4	4/4	4/4	4/4	28/28

[a]Adapted from Hendrix, C. D., What every technologist should know about experimental design, *CHEMTECH* (March 1979).
[b]Key variables are randomly assigned an "X" value.

1. Preformulation information
2. Product development report
3. Product stability report
4. Analytical methods report
5. Proposed manufacturing formula, manufacturing instruction, in-process and final product specifications at the 100X-batch size

The objectives of prevalidation trials at stage III (100X pilot production) is to qualify and optimize the process in full-scale production equipment and their facilities.

Rushing through the first (100X) pilot-production batch in order to proceed with formal validation should be discouraged. Small problems that often arise during (100X) scale-up should be addressed immediately and not ignored. Such problems are often best addressed by returning to the laboratories (10X) for supplemental process characterization and qualification studies.

Many companies, however, proceed directly to three-batch formal validation without stage III prevalidation work and often complete formal trials prior to preapproval inspection. The downside of this alternative strategy is that finished production batches often remain in the warehouse beyond their approved expiry dating period.

When faced with a choice of strategies, there is no one ideal way of completing the pilot scale-up and validation sequence other than depending on prior experience with related products and their processes.

Stage-IV: Formal Process Validation

In the normal course of events and following a successfully completed preapproval inspection, formal, three-batch process validation is carried out in accordance with the protocol approved during the preapproval inspection. The primary objective of the formal process validation exercise is to establish process reproducibility and consistency. The program is not designed to challenge upper and lower control limits (so-called worst-case analysis) of critical process variables. Such upper and lower control limit challenging is normally conducted during the stage II (10X size) process characterization, optimization, and qualification program, using suitable and reasonable experimental designs (Table 4).

The documentation to be established before, during, and after formal process validation is shown below. The protocols and the subsequent formal validation studies are designed to establish uniformity among the three batches with respect to granulation, blending, finished tablet, and finished capsule stages (1, 2, 10).

100× production batches

- Complete product development program and report
- Prepare protocol for prospective process validation
- Complete preapproval inspection requirements; conduct three-batch formal process validation, establish reproducibility for mixing, blending, and compression or encapsulation operations
- Establish process documentation

  — Preformulation report
  — Analytical methods validation report
  — IQ/OQ and cleaning validation reports
  — Formula development report
  — Process feasibility report
  — Manufacturing bioequivalency report
  — Product development report
  — Process validation protocol
  — Process validation report
  — Product stability report

In that respect, the following test data and results are used to show process reproducibility and consistency among validation batches: particle or granule size distribution, bulk density, moisture content, hardness, thickness, friability, weight uniformity, potency uniformity, disintegration–dissolution profile, and product stability. Not every one of these categories have to be addressed nor followed both during in-process and final product testing. Nevertheless, testing must be sufficient to establish process reproducibility and demonstrate, with a high degree of certainly, that the product and process are in a state of control.

Whenever possible, formal validation studies should continue through packaging and labeling operations (whole or in-part), so that machinability and stability of the finished product can be established and documented in the primary container–closure system.

Recently the FDA, with the cooperation of the Pharmaceutical Industry has developed a series of guidance procedures to speed approval of post approval changes with or without process scale-up changes. At the present time the SUPAC (scale-up post approval change) program covers the following product categories:

- Immediate Release (IR) solid dosage forms
- Extended Release (ER) solid dosage forms
- Delayed Release (MR) solid dosage forms
- Semisolids (SS) dosage forms
- API changes presently called BACPAC
- Packaging changes called PACPAC
- Analytical Methods changes called AMPAC
- Sterile Aqueous Solutions called SUPAC-SAS

If the program is successful, other dosage form categories will be added later.

The following changes are covered:

- Components and Composition Changes
- Manufacturing Equipment and Process Changes
- Batch Size (scale-up) Changes
- Manufacturing Site Changes

The program consists of three levels:

- Level 1 or minor changes that are made without FDA approval and reported in the Annual Report (AR).
- Level 2 or intermediate changes that may be instituted by first filing a Change Being Effected (CBE) Supplement with the FDA and waiting 30 days for a reply before instituting the change.
- Level 3 or major change in which a prior approval supplement (PAS) is filed with the FDA and approval must be obtained from the FDA before proceeding with the change.

This new program is off to a good start and is intermittently involved with the need for adequate process validation studies and documentation to support the changes requested.

CHANGE CONTROL

Procedures with respect to establishing change control should be in place before, during, and after the completion of the formal validation program. A change control system maintains a sense of functionality as the process evolves and provides the necessary documentation trail that ensures that the process continues in a validated,

operational state, even when small noncritical adjustments and changes have been made. Such minor, noncritical changes in materials, methods, and machines should be reviewed by the validation commitee (development, engineering, production, and QA/QC) to ensure that process integrity and comparability have been maintained and documented before the specific change that has been requested can be approved by the head of the quality control unit.

The change control system, based upon an approved standard operating procedure(s) (SOPs), takes on added importance as the vehicle or instrument through which innovation and process improvements can be made more easily and more flexibly without prior formal review on the part of the NDA and ANDA reviewing function of the FDA. If more of the supplemental procedures with respect to the chemistry and manufacturing control sections of NDAs and ANDAs could be covered through annual review documentation procedures, with appropriate safeguards, process validation will become more innovative (20–22).

OUT-OF-SPECIFICATIONS

Probably the single most important technical issue facing the pharmaceutical industry at the present time is the question: what constitutes process or batch failure in terms of an out-of-specification (OOS) assay value? The concept of product and/or process failure appears twice in the cGMPs (3).

According to 21 CFR Sect. 211.165(f), "Drug products failing to meet established standards or specifications and other relevant quality control criteria shall be rejected." In CFR Sect. 211.192 it is stated:

> Any unexplained discrepancy (including a percentage of theoretical yield exceeding the maximum or minimum percentages established in master production and control records) or the failure of a batch or any of its components to meet any of its specifications shall be thoroughly investigated [regardless] whether the batch has already been distributed. The investigation shall extend to other batches of the same drug product and other drug products that may have been associated with the specific failure or discrepancy. A written record of the investigation shall be made and shall include the conclusions and follow-up.

The key to establishing product and/or process failure is to verify the accuracy, relevance, and reproducibility of deviant assay value(s), test result(s), and recorded number(s) that are reported (23). All companies should have SOPs in place that cover first the verification of deviant numbers in the quality control laboratories and, following that investigation and a report showing the test result to be deviant, a second set of SOPs covering follow-up actions taken as described in the following steps:

1. A written procedure for full investigation when there is not a verified laboratory error.
2. Scientific criteria for retesting and resampling during the formal investigation.
3. Description and results of the formal investigation into possible causes of the OOS result(s).
4. Results of all testing involved during the investigation.
5. A scientific basis and justification for discarding any OOS test result and accepting the batch in question.
6. Final determination of conformity to appropriate specifications and justification of the actions taken, and
7. Signature of individual(s) responsible for final decision(s) and the action(s) taken.

Even though the responsibility for batch acceptance or rejection lies with the head of the quality control unit, the help of the validation committee should prove useful in reviewing the process of OOS investigation and arriving at a recommendation for action taken.

CLEANING VALIDATION

According to 21 CFR Sect. 211.67, Equipment Cleaning and Maintenance of cGMP regulations (3), equipment and utensils should be cleaned, maintained, and sanitized at appropriate intervals to prevent malfunction or contamination that would alter the safety, identity, strength, quality, or purity of the drug product. Written procedures shall be established and followed for cleaning and maintenance of equipment. These procedures shall include, but are not limited to the assignment of responsibility for cleaning and maintaining equipment; maintenance, cleaning, and sanitizing schedules where appropriate; description in sufficient detail of methods, equipment, and materials used in cleaning and maintenance operations, and the methods of disassembling and reassembling equipment as necessary to assure proper cleaning and maintenance; removal or obliteration of previous batch identification, protection of clean equipment from contamination prior to use; and inspection of equipment for cleanliness immediately before use.

Records shall be kept of maintenance, cleaning, sanitizing, and inspection.

The objective of cleaning validation of equipment and utensils is to reduce the residues of one product below established limits so that the residue of the previous product does not affect the quality and safety of the subsequent product manufactured in the same equipment.

According to 21 CFR Sect. 211.63, Equipment Design, Size, and Location, of cGMP regulations (3), equipment used in the manufacture, processing, packing, or holding of a drug product shall be of appropriate design, adequate size, and suitably located to facilitate operations for its intended use and for its cleaning and maintenance. Some of the equipment design considerations include type of surface to be cleaned (stainless steel, glass, plastic), use of disposables or dedicated equipment and utensils (bags, filters, etc.), of stationary equipment (tanks, mixers, centrifuges, presses, etc.), of special features (clean-in-place systems, steam-in-place systems), and identifying the difficult-to-clean locations on the equipment (so-called hot spots or critical sites).

The specific cleaning procedure should define the amounts and the specific type of cleaning agents and/or solvents used. The cleaning procedure should give full details as to what is to be cleaned and how it is to be cleaned. The cleaning method should focus on worst-case conditions, such as highest-strength, least-soluble, most difficult to clean formulations. Cleaning procedures should identify the time between processing and cleaning, cleaning sequence, equipment dismantling procedure, need for visual inspection, and provisions for documentation.

The choice of a particular analytical method (HPLC, TLC, spectrophotometric, total organic carbon (TOC), pH, conductivity, gravimetric, etc.) and sampling technique chosen (direct surface by swabs and gauze, or by rinsing) depends on the residue limit to be established, based upon the sampling site, type of residue sought, and equipment configuration (critical sites vs. large surface area) considerations. The analytical and sampling methods should be challenged in terms of specificity, sensitivity, and recovery.

The established residue limits must be practical, achievable, verifiable, and assure safety. The potency of selected drug and presence of degradation products, cleaning agents, perticulates and microorganisms should be taken into consideration.

The following residue limits have been suggested: not more than (NMT) 10 ppm or NMT 0.001% of the dose of any product appears in the maximum daily dose of another product and no residue visible on the equipment after cleaning procedures have been performed.

PHARMACEUTICAL EXCIPIENTS

Pharmaceutical Excipients are components of finished drug products and site active components are recognized in the USP/NF. A list of key excipients for solid dosage forms is given:

Diluents, Fillers, and Binders:
    Calcium phosphate, dibasic
    Dextrates
    Dextrin
    Lactose (anhydrous, fast flow)
    Mannitol
    Starch (corn)
    Sugar, compressible

Tablet Disintegrants:
    Cellulose, microcrystalline
    Croscarmellose sodium
    Crospovidone
    Sodium starch glycolate
    Starch, pregelatinized

Tablet and Capsule Lubricants:
    Magnesium stearate
    Mineral oil, light
    Polyethylene glycol
    Sodium stearyl fumarate
    Stearic acid, purified
    Talc
    Vegetable oil, hydrogenated

Other Excipients:
    Carboxymethylcellulose sodium
    Cellulose acetate phthalate
    Ethylcellulose
    Hydroxypropyl cellulose
    Hydroxypropyl methylcellulose
    Hydroxypropyl methylcellulose pathalate
    Methacrylic acid copolymer
    Polysorbates
    Polyvinyl acetate phthalate
    Povidone
    Sodium lauryl sulfate

ACTIVE PHARMACEUTICAL INGREDIENTS (API)

A chemical is considered to be an API if it is intended for medicinal purposes. Regulatory agencies however, place greater emphasis and priority on the manufacture and validation of APIs than UPS/NF exciepients.

According to Sect. 501 (a)(2)(b) of the Food, Drug, and Cosmetic (FD&C) Act, all drugs must be manufactured, processed, packed, and held in accordance with cGMPs. No distinction is made between APIs and finished drug products.

Elements common to both APIs and finished drug products include facilities and equipment qualification (IQ/OQ, and PQ), cleaning validation, validation of water supplies, microbial limits for nonsterile material, manufacture of sterile and pyrogen-free material, in-process blending and mixing, analytical methods validation, laboratory controls and in-process testing, change control procedures and revalidation, reprocessing, packaging and labeling, and stability testing.

Process

There are four primary processes used in the manufacture of APIs. They are chemical synthesis, fermentation, extraction, and purification. A flow diagram (Fig. 3) and a description of the chemistry involved are helpful in defining the process. The process description should include appropriate parameters, such as charging quantities or volumes of reactants or solvents, reaction times, temperatures, pressures, etc. Critical processing steps and critical operating parameters should be maintained to ensure batch-to-batch consistency, product yield, and quality.

Where in the chain of unit operations (chemical process) does API validation start? As long as key intermediates are made in the plant, they and their reaction and processing steps should be subjected to an appropriate cGMP and process qualification-validation program. A key intermediate is defined as an intermediate in which an essential molecular characteristic, usually related to stereochemical configuration, is introduced into the final API structure (moeity).

Physical Characteristics

Besides purity (chemical potency), the physical characteristics and properties of the API are extremely important to the end user (drug product manufacturer). Characteristics such as crystal morphology, particle size and shape, bulk density, melting point, optical rotation, etc., have a profound effect upon the final drug product and its performance and stability. In addition to the reaction or extraction step, crystallization, milling, and blending unit operations must be subject to qualification and validation.

Impurity Profile

The USP permits up to 2% of ordinary nontoxic impurities. However, impurities above 0.1% should be

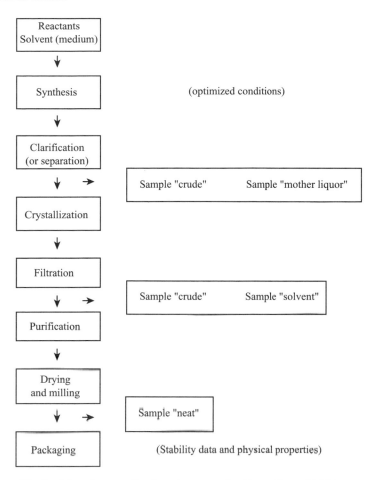

Fig. 3   Manufacture of active pharmaceutical ingredients (APIs).

fully characterized and quantified. Impurities may include starting materials, by-products, intermediates, degradation products, reagents, catalysts, heavy metals, electrolytes, filter aids, and residual solvents. Known toxic impurities must be held to a tighter standard, i.e., below 0.1%.

The ISO quality standards series

The ISO 9000 Series was developed in 1987 by the International Organization for Standardization (ISO) in Geneva, Switzerland. It is a comprehensive set of management standards governing the operation of quality assurance to help develop and document a quality system that is useful for individual companies.

The ISO 9000 Quality Management and Quality Assurance Standards, Guidelines for Selection and Use, provide basic definitions and concepts and explain how to use the rest of the series (9001, 9002, 9003, and 9004).

The ISO 9001 Quality System—Model for Quality Assurance in Design and Development provides for quality assurance in the areas of design, installation, servicing, development, and production. It is useful primarily for companies that design and develop their own products.

The ISO 9002 Quality System—Model for Quality Assurance in Production, Installation and Service applies to manufacturers, distributors, and service vendors whose products have been designed and serviced by a subcontractor. Such companies are exempt from design control requirements. Both ISO 9001 and ISO 9002 are directly applicable to cGMPs. The connection between the two independent systems is shown in Table 5. Except for language, shades of meaning, and stresses the documents are similar.

The ISO 9003 Quality Systems—Model for Quality Assurance in Inspection and Testing, designed for testing laboratories and equipment distributors only requires conformance to final inspection and testing procedures.

The ISO 9004 Quality Management and Quality Systems Elements—Guidelines provide standards and guidelines for quality management planning and implementation.

Table 5 Meeting quality standards

	ISO 9000 series	cGMPs
1.	Management responsibility	Organization and personnel
2.	Quality system	Organization and personnel, laboratory, controls, records, reports
3.	Contract review	Holding and distribution
4.	Design control	Production and process controls
5.	Document control	Records and reports
6.	Purchase products	Control of components, drug product containers, closures
7.	Supplied product	Holding and distribution
8.	Product identification, traceability	Packaging and labeling control
9.	Process control	Production and process control
10.	Procedures for inspection, testing	Laboratory controls
11.	Inspection, measuring, testing equipment	Laboratory controls production, and process controls
12.	Inspection, testing status	Laboratory controls
13.	Control of nonconforming products	Returned and salvaged drug products
14.	Corrective action	Records and reports
15.	Handling, storage, packaging, delivery	Packaging and labeling control holding, distribution
16.	Quality records	Records and reports
17.	Internal quality audits	Laboratory controls
18.	Training needs	Organization and personnel
19.	Servicing procedures	Equipment
20.	Statistical techniques	Building, facilities production and process controls

APPENDIX

Glossary of Terms Used in Process Validation

Acceptance activities
Acceptance criteria
Active Pharmaceutical
   Ingredient (API)
Analytical methods
   validation
Audit of suppliers
Calibration
Certification
Challenge testing
Change control
Chemistry and
   manufacturing
   control (CMC)
Cleaning validation
Component
Computer qualification
Concurrent validation
Critical processing
   variables
Design change
Design history
Design input

Design of experiments
Design output
Design review
Design transfer
Design validation
Design verification
Development report
Equipment suitability
Good manufacturing
   practices
In-process control
Installation
   qualification (IQ)
ISO 9000 series
Manufacturing process
Master plan
Master record
Methods validation
Module
Operating range
Operational
   qualification (OQ)
Out-of-specifications

Packaging validation
Performance
   qualification (PQ)
Policy
Preapproval inspection
Prequalification
Prevalidation
Process capability
Process characterization
Process flow diagram
Process optimization
Process optimization
Process parameters
Process performance
Process qualification
Process suitability
Process validation
Process
Product attribute
Product optimization
Product performance
Product qualification
Protocol
Proven acceptable range
Qualification
Qualified person
Quality assurance

Quality audit
Quality control
Quality policy
Quality system
Quality
Representative sample
Reprocessing
Requalification
Retrospective validation
Revalidation
Supac
Technical transfer
Time limitation
Total quality
   management
Traceability
Unit operation
Validation change control
Validation manager
Validation master plan
Validation protocol
Validation report
Validation committee,
   group, team
Validation
Verification
Worst-case

REFERENCES

1. Berry, I.R.; Harpaz, D. *Validation of Active Pharmaceutical Ingredients*; Interpharm Press, Inc.: Buffalo Grove, IL, 2001.
2. Validation of Pharmaceutical Processes, Sterile Products. Carleton, F.J., Agalloco, J.P., Eds.; Marcel Dekker, Inc.: New York, 1998.
3. Chow, S.-C., Liu, J.-P., Eds. *Validation, Process Controls and Stability, Statistical Design and Analysis in Pharmaceutical Science;* Marcel Dekker, Inc.: New York, 1995.
4. Gibson, W.; Powell-Evans, K. *Validation Fundamentals*; Interpharm Press, Inc.: Buffalo Grove, IL, 1998.
5. Sucker, H., Ed. *Validation in Practice;* Wissenchaftliche Verlagsgesellschaft GmbH: Stuttgart, 1983.
6. Validation of Manufacturing Processes Fourth European Seminar on Quality Control, Geneva, Sept. 25 1980.
7. FDA. Guideline on General Principles of Process Validation, FDA, Rockville, MD, May 11, 1987.
8. FDA. Pre-Approval Inspection/Investigations Guidance Manual, FDA, Rockville, MD, Oct. 1, 1990; 7346.832.
9. Fed. Reg. 43(190) Human and Veterinary Drugs, Current Good Manufacturing Practice in Manufacturing, Processing, Packing or Holding, Sept. 29 1978; 45,014–45,089.
10. Lucisano, L.J.; Franz, R.M. FDA Proposed Guidance for CMC Changes: A Review and Industrial Perspective. Pharm. Technol. **1995**, *19* (5), 30–40.
11. WHO. Good Manufacturing Practices for Pharmaceutical Products—Guidelines on the Validation of Manufacturing Processes, WHO, Geneva, 1993.
12. Skelly, J.P. Scale-Up of Immediate-Release Oral Solid Dosage. Forms. Pharm. Res. **1993**, *10*, 313–316.
13. Skelly, J.P. Scale-Up of Oral Extended-Release Dosage Forms. Pharm. Res. **1993**, *10*, 1800–1804.
14. Bolton, S. Process Validation for Hard Gelatin Capsules. Drug Cosm. Ind. **1984**, *134* (3), 42–48–85–87.
15. Avallone, H.L. Development and Scale-Up of Pharmaceuticals. Pharm. Eng. **1990**, *10* (4), 38–41.
16. FDA, Guide to Inspections of Oral Solid Dosage Forms Pre/Post Approval Issues for Development and Validation, FDA, Rockville, MD, Jan 1994.
17. Berry, I.R. Process Validation for Soft Gelatin Capsules. Drug Cosm. Ind. **1984**, *134* (4), 26–35.
18. Nash, R.A. Process Validation for Solid Dosage Forms. Pharm. Technol. **1979**, *3* (6), 105–107.
19. von Doehren, P.J.; St. John, Forbe F.; Shively, C.D. An Approach to the Characterization and Technology Transfer of Solid Dosage Form Processes. Pharm. Technol. **1982**, *6* (9), 139–156.
20. Sucker, H., Ed. *Validation in Practice;* Wissenschaftliche Verlagsgesellschaft GmbH: Stuttgart, 1983.
21. Berry, I.R., Nash, R.A., Eds. *Pharmaceutical Process Validation,* 2nd Ed.; Marcel Dekker, Inc.: New York, 1993; Revised and Expanded.
22. Chowhan, Z.T. Development of a New Drug Substance into a Compact Tablet. Pharm. Technol. **1992**, *16* (9), 58–67.
23. Fahrner, R. New Role for Pilot Plants in Product Development. Biopharm **1993**, *6* (3), 34–37.
24. Avallone, H.L.; D'Eramo, P. Scale-Up and Validation of ANDA/NDA Products. Pharm. Eng. **1992**, *12* (6), 36–39.
25. Bala, G. An Integrated Approach to Process Validation. Pharm. Eng. **1994**, *14* (3), 57–64.
26. Chapman, K.G. A History of Validation in the United States, Part I. Pharm. Technol. **1991**, *15* (10), 82–96.
27. Akers, J. Simplifying and Improving Process Validation. J. Parent. Sci. Technol. **1993**, *47*, 281–284.
28. Tomamichel, K. Pharmaceutical Quality Assurance: Basics of Validation. Swiss Pharma **1994**, *16* (3), 13–23.
29. Bolton, S. When is it Appropriate to Average and its Relationship to the Barr Decision. Clin. Res. Reg. Affairs **1994**, *11*, 171–179.

VETERINARY DOSAGE FORMS

J. Desmond Baggot
Monash University, Parkville, Victoria, Australia

INTRODUCTION

Veterinary dosage forms are drug preparations designed for use in, or topical application to, one or more species of domestic animal and/or other species of veterinary interest. Although the majority of veterinary dosage forms contain the same drugs as human dosage forms, some veterinary preparations contain drugs that are not widely used in humans. Examples include benzimidazole anthelmintics, macrolide endectocides, salicylanilide flukicides, synthetic pyrethroids, chloramphenicol derivatives, α_2-adrenoceptor agonists (sedative–analgesics), and antagonists. The converse applies to some classes of pharmacological agent (e.g., benzodiazepine derivatives, tricyclic antidepressants) because of limited clinical indications for use in animals. Veterinary pharmacology differs from human pharmacology both in the diversity of species of interest and in the emphasis placed on the various classes of drug. Some types of dosage forms are suitable for use in humans and certain animal species. They include parenteral solutions (although the concentration of the drug, the nature of the vehicle, and other constituents of the preparation must be considered); conventional tablets and capsules (amount of the drug relative to dosage requirement must be considered); oral solutions and suspensions (pediatric preparations are generally appropriate for administration to small animals, especially cats); and conventional ophthalmic preparations. Sustained-release tablets and controlled-release transdermal drug-delivery systems designed for use in humans could be used in medium to large breeds of dog. It is because of the unique physiological characteristics of each species, or closely related group of species, and the variation among species in the dose–effect relationship of pharmacological agents that veterinary dosage forms of drugs are required. Veterinary dosage forms designed specifically for use in certain animals species include long-acting parenteral dosage forms of antimicrobial agents for intramuscular injection, oral pastes containing antimicrobial agents or anthelmintics for horses, granules containing nonsteroidal anti-inflammatory drugs or anthelmintics for addition to the feed for horses or pigs, respectively, modified-release ruminal boluses containing anthelmintics for cattle or sheep, intramammary antimicrobial preparations for cows, preparations containing ectoparasiticides for topical application to various species, and darts containing sedative drugs for capture and restraint of exotic animal species. The avoidance of drug residues in tissues and animal products (milk and eggs) is a regulatory requirement of veterinary preparations administered to food-producing species.

VETERINARY DRUGS

Although the majority of drugs available as veterinary dosage forms were initially developed for use in humans, based on experimental findings in laboratory animals, some drugs have been developed specifically for veterinary use. Anthelmintics and ectoparasiticides/insecticides are primarily veterinary drugs. Some anthelmintics (e.g., ivermectin, mebendazole, albendazole, pyrantel, piperazine, levamisole, praziquantel, bithionol) have been adopted for the treatment of parasitic infections in humans. Most ectoparasiticides are exclusively veterinary drugs. Some antimicrobial agents within certain classes, which include sulfonamides, fluoroquinolones, macrolides, chloramphenicol derivatives, and carboxylic ionophores, are available only for use in animals. Relatively few pharmacological agents were initially developed as veterinary drugs, although some drugs have indications for use in animals that do not apply to humans (Table 1). Other pharmacological agents have largely become veterinary drugs by virtue of their clinical efficacy in animals and replacement by alternative drugs for use in humans. Examples include phenylbutazone, quinidine, phenobarbital, and thiopental.

Steroid (sex) hormones, gonadotrophins, gonadotrophin-releasing hormones (synthetic forms and GnRH analog), and synthetic prostaglandins ($F_{2\alpha}$ type or analog) are used in female animals (cows, ewes, sows, and mares) to regulate various stages of the estrous cycle, whereas synthetic prostaglandins may be used to induce parturition. Melatonin, a modified-release dosage form implanted subcutaneously behind the ear of ewes, is used to stimulate the onset of cyclical ovarian activity. Progestogens are used to synchronize estrus in groups of animals or to enable

Encyclopedia of Pharmaceutical Technology

Table 1 Some pharmacological agents that are used exclusively in animals

Drug	Classification	Clinical indications
Xylazine	α_2, (α_1)-adrenoceptor agonist	Sedation; analgesia preanesthetic medication
Yohimbine	α_2, (α_1)-adrenoceptor antagonist agonist	Xylazine reversal
Detomidine	α_2-adrenoceptor agonist	Preanesthetic medication
Atipamezole	α_2, (α_1)-adrenoceptor antagonist	Detomidine reversal
Acepromazine	Phenothiazine-derivative tranquilizer	Preanesthetic medication; sedation
Etorphine–Acepromazine	Potent opioid agonist-PTZ-derivative tranquilizer	Neuroleptanalgesia
Diprenorphine	Opioid antagonist	Etorphine reversal
Droperidol–Fentanyl	Butyrophenon μ-opioid agonist	Neuroleptanalgesia
Azeperone	Butyrophenone	Preanesthetic medication; Behavior modification (pigs)
Alfadolone–Alfaxalone	Steroid anaesthetic(contraindicated in dogs)	Anesthesia
Flunixin	Cyclo-oxygenase inhibitor	Anti-inflammatory; analgesia; antipyresis
Metamizole (Dipyrone)	Cyclo-oxygenase inhibitor	("Similar" to other NSAIDs)

prediction of the onset of estrus. On removal of the progestogen source (intravaginal device for cows and ewes; added to feed for sows and mares), the negative feedback effect on the pituitary and hypothalamus is terminated, and estrus is initiated. Progestogens (medroxyprogesterone, megestrol, proligestone), generally administered by subcutaneous injection, are used to suppress ovarian activity (estrus) in dogs and cats, whereas altrenogest (added to feed) is used to suppress estrus in cycling mares or to synchronize estrus in gilts and sows.

Monensin, a carboxylic ionophore antibiotic, is available as a premix (for addition to feed) used for the prevention of coccidiosis caused by *Eimeria* spp. in broiler chickens. Turkeys over 16 weeks of age, guinea fowl, and other game birds should not be given access to monensin-containing feed. Monensin is used as a production enhancer (improves feed conversion efficiency and growth rate) in beef cattle and dairy heifers up to the time of first service. It is available for use in cattle as a premix (sodium salt) for addition to the feed and as a modified-release ruminal bolus. The oral LD50 (mg/kg) of monensin differs among species: horses, 2–3; sheep, 12; pigs, 16; cattle, 22; and chickens, 200. Extreme care should be taken not to feed cattle, pig, or poultry rations or supplements to horses and to avoid accidental contamination in feedmills. Steroid hormone-growth promoters (bovine somatotropin, porcine somatotropin, bovine growth hormone-releasing factor) are available for use as production enhancers in some countries, whereas in others (European Union member states), their use is banned. The properties of somatotropins and the dosage forms that have been studied were comprehensively reviewed by Foster (1). The use of β_2-adrenoceptor agonists such as clenbuterol for production enhancement in cattle is illegal.

Some antidotal substances used in the treatment of plant or heavy metal toxicity in animals could be considered veterinary drugs. They include methylthioninium chloride (methylene blue), sodium nitrite, sodium thiosulfate, ammonium molybdate, and sodium calciumedetate. Phytomenadione (vitamin K_1) is indicated for the treatment of warfarin and coumarin poisoning in animals. The substances are present in sweet vernal grass *Anthoxanthum odoratum* and in spoiled sweet clover (*Melilotus officinalis* and *M. alba*) hay, and silage. Acetylcysteine and ascorbic acid are used concurrently in the treatment of acetaminophen (paracetamol) toxicity in cats. The acetylcysteine, which is administered by intravenous injection, serves as a precursor for glutathione replenishment, whereas ascorbic acid (administered intravenously or orally) reduces methemoglobin to hemoglobin. Feline hemoglobin is particularly susceptible to oxidative damage (methemoglobinemia). Atropine sulfate is widely used in animals for preanesthetic medication (although glycopyrronium is preferred in horses) and at a much higher dose (25 to 40 times the preanesthetic dose, 44 μg/kg), often in conjunction with a cholinesterase-reactivating agent (pralidoxime mesilate), in the treatment of organophosphate toxicity.

This overview of veterinary drugs shows applications of these drugs in animals and how some aspects of veterinary and human pharmacology differ in their orientation.

CATEGORIZATION OF SPECIES

Even though mammalian species differ in physical characteristics (notably body weight) and behavior, they possess the same body systems that perform generally similar physiological functions. There are, however, species-related adaptations that account for the uniqueness of each species. The character of the adaptations underlies the feasibility of extrapolating scientific information obtained in certain species (such as laboratory animals) to other species (domestic animals) and human beings. Because the pattern of quantifiable adaptations can be generally described mathematically, it is possible to make some predictions regarding interspecies extrapolation. The reliability of predictions on drug bioavailability and disposition depends on knowledge of both the anatomical and physiological similarities of and differences among the species of interest.

The anatomical arrangement of the gastrointestinal tract serves as a basis for broadly categorizing domestic animals as ruminant species (cattle, sheep, and goats) or monogastric species (horses, pigs, dogs, and cats). Consideration of dietary habit somewhat refines the categorization and enables the pattern of drug absorption to be explained as well as the potential interaction among commensal microbial flora in the digestive system and drugs, especially antimicrobial agents. Ruminant species are herbivores with a voluminous forestomach compartment in which microbial fermentation takes place continuously. Horses are monogastric herbivores with a small-capacity stomach and large-capacity colon where microbial digestion takes place. Dogs and cats are monogastric carnivores, whereas pigs are monogastric omnivores (similar to humans) fed a vegetable diet. Because the urinary pH reaction is determined primarily by the composition of the diet, the usual pH range differs among herbivorous species (pH 7.2–8.4) and carnivorous species (pH 5.5–7.0), whereas in omnivorous species, urinary pH can vary over a wide range (pH 4.5–8.2), but would be expected to be alkaline in pigs, whereas it is usually acidic in humans. Urinary pH influences the extent of reabsorption from the distal renal tubules and the half-life of weak organic acids and bases when a significant fraction (arbitrarily >20%) of the systemically available dose is eliminated by renal excretion.

The character of the female reproductive (estrous) cycle varies with the animal species in several respects, that include duration of cycle, length of estrus (sexual receptivity), and time of ovulation (Table 2) (2). In seasonal breeding species (mare, ewe, doe, and queen), the time of year during which estrous cycles occur is strongly influenced by the photoperiod. The mare and queen become anestrous in late autumn owing to decreasing daylight hours, and cycles are re-established with increasing daylight in early spring. The converse situation applies to ewes and does. The plane of nutrition can affect the onset of estrous cycles in seasonal breeding species. The queen is unique among domestic animal species in that ovulation is induced by coitus. Pharmacological intervention at any stage of the reproductive cycle, whether it be to induce ovulation in mares, ewes, or cows or to suppress estrus or prevent ovum implantation in bitches or queens, is based on changing the plasma concentrations of the reproductive hormones that influence the particular process. To be successful, knowledge of the temporal pattern of the various hormone concentrations in plasma is essential.

Because avian and mammalian species differ in many respects, these distinct classes of animal should be considered separately. Avian species that are "farmed" include chickens, turkeys, ducks, geese, ostriches, guinea fowl, quail, and pheasants. The term poultry refers to farmed domestic fowl that, in common usage, includes chickens, turkeys, ducks and geese, whereas other farmed avian species are considered game birds. Application of the collective term poultry overlooks species differences in dosage requirements and drug residues in tissues as well as differences in susceptibility to toxicity of some drugs.

Birds (and reptiles) have a well-developed renal portal system that drains blood from the caudal portion of the body. Consequently, drugs administered parenterally in the lower extremities (hind limbs) of those species pass through the kidneys before entering the systemic circulation. This feature of blood flow to the kidneys provides the opportunity for first-pass excretion of water-soluble ionized drugs (e.g., β-lactam and aminoglycoside antibiotics) to occur.

Fish, reptiles (which include crocodiles and alligators), and amphibians are poikilothermic, i.e., cold-blooded animals. In contrast to homeothermic animals, the disposition of drugs in poikilothermic animals is influenced by environmental temperature. When applied to fish, the rate of drug elimination varies with the temperature of the water to which the fish are acclimatized. Studies of drug disposition in fish should generally be carried out at more than one water temperature, and whether fresh water or sea water is contained in the tank depends on the species of fish. A complication arises in the case of salmon for example, because adult salmon live in sea water but spawn and grow as fingerlings in fresh water.

DOSAGE FORMS AND ROUTES OF ADMINISTRATION

The type of dosage form, the route of administration, and site of injection of parenteral preparations depend on the animal species or group of related species (such as

Table 2 Average length of various stages of reproductive cycles of domestic animals

Species	Duration of estrus cycle	Length of estrus	Time of ovulation	Time fertilized ova enter uterus (after conception)	Time of implantation (after conception)	Type of placenta	Length of pregnancy
Mare[a]	21 days	5–6 days	Last day of estrus	3–4 days	30–35 days	Epitheliochorial	345 days
Cow	21 days	18 h	12 h after end of estrus	3–4 days	30–35 days	Epitheliochorial	280 days
Ewe[a]	17 days	36 h	30 h after beginning of estrus	3–5 days	15–18 days	Syndesmochorial	147 days
Doe[a] (goat)	20 days	40 h	30–36 h after beginning of estrus	4 days	20–25 days	Syndesmochorial	147 days
Sow	21 days	45 h	36–40 h after beginning of estrus	3–4 days	14–20 days	Epitheliochorial	113 days
Bitch	In estrus at 7–8 month intervals depending on breed	Proestrus, 9 days; estrus, 7–9 days	First or second day of estrus	5–6 days	15 days	Endotheliochorial	64 days
Queen[a]	16 days (nonbred) (pseudopregnancy lasts 36 days)	5–6 days	Induced 24–32 h after coitus	4 days	13 days	Endotheliochorial	65 days

[a]Seasonally polyestrous.
(Modified from Ref. 2.)

ruminant animals or poultry). The greatest differences relate to oral dosage forms and topical preparations. Whether a veterinary dosage form is intended for individual animal treatment or for administration/application to a large group of animals (herd or flock medication) should be decided before the development of a dosage form. Convenience of administration and cost of the drug preparation are foremost considerations in determining the use of a veterinary dosage form by animal owners.

GASTROINTESTINAL ABSORPTION

The anatomical arrangement of the gastrointestinal tract and associated digestive physiology govern the pattern of drug absorption. In pigs, dogs, cats, and humans, the plasma concentration profile after the administration of an oral solution or conventional (immediate-release) dosage form is generally similar in that it shows a reasonably well-defined single peak. Because the rate of gastric emptying differs among monogastric species and the anterior (upper) portion of the small intestine is the principal site of absorption, the time at which the peak plasma concentration occurs may vary. An effective pH value of 5.3 in the microenvironment of the intestinal mucosal surface, rather than the reaction of intestinal contents (average pH 6.6), is consistent with observations on the absorption of drugs that are weak organic acids or bases. Under normal conditions, weak acids with pK_a values above 3.0 and bases with pK_a values below 7.8 are well-absorbed from the small intestine (3). An alteration in the pH of the stomach or small intestine contents can markedly change the degree of ionization of drugs that are weak organic electrolytes (acids or bases). At pH values below the pK_a, weak acids exist primarily in the nonionized form, which is the moiety that can readily be absorbed; the converse applies to weak bases. Lipid-soluble neutral molecules (digoxin, chloramphenicol) and fluoroquinolones (amphoteric compounds) are well-absorbed in dogs, although the systemic availability of norfloxacin is much lower than that of enrofloxacin/ciprofloxacin or marbofloxacin. Because of their polar nature, aminoglycoside antibiotics are poorly absorbed from the gastrointestinal tract and must be administered parenterally in the treatment of systemic bacterial infections.

After the administration of a sustained-release oral dosage form, the duration of drug availability for absorption is limited by the sum of the residence times of the dosage form in the stomach and small intestine. This has been estimated to be 9–12 h in dogs. In the development of a sustained-release dosage form for use in dogs, the aim is to provide an effective plasma concentration of the drug throughout the dosage interval (12 h) with an acceptable degree of fluctuation in steady-state concentrations. The latter is determined both by the half-life of the drug and the dosage interval (4). Suitable candidate drugs should have reasonably high oral bioavailability, which implies reliable absorption from the gastrointestinal tract and no more than partial inactivation by the first-pass effect unless active metabolites are formed, a half-life in the range of 4 to 6 h, and a relatively high potency but reasonably wide range of therapeutic plasma concentrations. Because of variation between dogs and humans in the oral bioavailability and the rate of elimination of most lipid-soluble drugs, those that would be suitable for formulating as sustained-release dosage forms often differ between the two species. Theophylline meets the criteria that make it suitable for formulating as a sustained-release oral preparation for administration to dogs. Of the sustained-release oral dosage forms that are commercially available, anhydrous theophylline in tablet form (200 and 300 mg) is preferred for use in dogs. This product has an oral bioavailability (theophylline) of 76%, and the dosage regimen (20 mg/kg administered at12-h intervals) has been predicted to maintain plasma concentrations within the therapeutic range (6–16 µg/ml) with less fluctuation in peak-to-trough theophylline concentrations than other sustained-release dosage forms (5). The dosage regimen for the conventional dosage form (aminophylline tablets) is 10 mg/kg administered at 8-h intervals to dogs.

Other drugs of veterinary interest that have been formulated as sustained-release oral dosage forms include morphine, propranolol, quinidine, procainaminde, and verapamil or diltiazem. Of these, sustained-release morphine sulfate (tablets, 15 mg) has the greatest potential for use in dogs over 10 kg body weight. The proposed dosage regimen, 1–2 mg/kg administered at 8- or 12-h dosage intervals, may be effective in the management of chronic pain (6). The sustained-release dosage form overcomes the shortcoming of conventional oral preparations of morphine, which is their short duration of action in dogs. Phenytoin is a likely candidate drug for formulating as a sustained-release dosage form because it would enable phenytoin to be used in dogs for the prevention/treatment of generalized tonic–clonic seizures (grand mal epilepsy). The average oral bioavailability of phenytoin administered as the conventional dosage form is 36%, the half-life in dogs is 3.5–4.5 h (dose-dependent), and the therapeutic range of plasma concentrations is 10–20 µg/ml. Oral bioavailability of phenytoin in humans is 90%, and the apparent half-life, which is dose-dependent, is 15–24 h. The slower elimination of phenytoin in humans obviates the need for the development of a sustained-release dosage form.

Even though the horse is a monogastric species, the stomach has a small capacity (8.5% of the gastrointestinal tract) compared with that of the pig (29%) and the dog (62%). Expressed on the basis of volume capacity, the stomach of the horse, pig, and dog can hold 7–14, 5.5–7, and 3–8 L, respectively. The average pH value of gastric contents in horses is less acidic (pH 5.5; range, 4.5–6.0) than in other monogastric species (pH 3–4), and a substantial portion of the stomach lining is composed of stratified squamous epithelium. Under natural conditions of management, horses feed continuously. The fibrous component of the feed is digested primarily in the large intestine, although horses digest fiber less efficiently than do ruminant species. Microbial digestion of fibrous carbohydrates to volatile fatty acids and break down of undigested dietary protein to peptides and amino acids takes place in the large intestine. The combined capacity of the caecum and colon occupies approximately 55% of the gastrointestinal tract, and the pH of large intestinal contents is 6.6–6.8. Two unrelated features of the digestive system are that horses do not possess a gall bladder (similarly camelids and giraffes) and are unable to vomit. The temporal relationship between feeding and oral dosing can greatly influence the pattern of drug absorption. Because the systemic availability of most antimicrobial agents administered orally (paste formulations) or by nasogastric tube (aqueous suspensions) to horses is significantly decreased by feeding shortly before dosing, food should be withheld for up to 2 h after administration of an antimicrobial agent. Feeding horses close to the time of administering phenylbutazone in various oral dosage forms changed the pattern without altering the extent of absorption of the nonsteroidal anti-inflammatory drug (7). The availability of a drug for absorption from the small intestine of the horse, particularly when administered in conjunction with or shortly after feeding, may be limited by adsorption to the ingested feed, especially hay. Under these circumstances, absorption may occur in two phases, initially (1–2 h after drug administration) from the small intestine and several (8–10) hours later from the large intestine (principal site) after microbial digestion of the fibrous material in feed (7, 8). The inadvertent contamination of horse feed with a feed additive premix approved for use as a production enhancer/growth promotant in cattle or pigs, may cause toxicity, even death, in horses.

The anatomical arrangement of the gastrointestinal tract distinguishes ruminant (cattle, sheep, and goats) from monogastric(horses, pigs, dogs, and cats) species (Table 3). The difference in digestive physiology between the two groups of species determines the types of oral dosage forms appropriate to administer and influences oral bioavailability of drugs. Susceptibility to ingested plant toxicity differs between ruminant and monogastric species. The volume capacity of the mature reticulorumen is 100–225 L in cattle and 10–25 L in sheep and goats and accounts for approximately 60% of the total capacity of the gastrointestinal tract. The forestomach contents vary from liquid to semisolid consistency, and the pH reaction is normally maintained within the range 5.5 to 6.5 owing to copious secretion of alkaline saliva (pH 8.2–8.4) particularly rich in bicarbonate and phosphate buffers but devoid of amylase. In addition to its buffering action, saliva has an antifoaming action that serves to prevent dietary bloat. Salivary secretion, at a daily rate of 100–190 L in cattle and 6–16 L in sheep, is essential for microbial digestion, which takes place continuously in the reticulorumen. Based on average values of saliva flow and volume of the rumen liquid pool, the turnover rate for reticuloruminal fluid was estimated to be 2.0/day for cattle and 1.1–2.2/day for sheep (9). Despite the stratified squamous nature of its epithelial lining, the rumen has considerable absorptive

Table 3 Relative capacity of components of digestive tract of domestic animal species

| | Relative capacity (%) | | | | Relative capacity (%) |
Component	Horse	Pig	Dog	Component	(Sheep and Goat)
Stomach	8.5	29.2	62.3	Rumen	52.9
Small intestine	30.2	33.5	23.3	Reticulum	4.5
Cecum	15.9	5.6	1.3	Omasum	2.0
Large colon	38.4			Abomasum	7.5
		31.7	13.1		
Small colon and rectum	7.0			Small intestine	20.4
				Cecum	2.3
				Colon and rectum	10.4

capacity (10, 11). Because absorption takes place by passive diffusion, lipid-soluble drugs, whether neutral molecules or the nonionized form of weak organic acids or bases, may be absorbed from the rumen. The theoretical equilibrium distribution, expressed as concentration ratio, of weak organic acids and bases of different pK_a values between saliva (pH 8.2) or ruminal contents (pH range 5.5–6.5) and plasma (pH 7.4) is presented graphically (Fig.1) (12).

Ruminal micro-organisms are capable of at least partially metabolizing some drugs (e.g., trimethoprim, chloramphenicol, nitroxynil, digitalis glycosides) either by hydrolysis or reduction, which would decrease the amount of drug available for absorption. Intraruminal biotransformation makes ruminant species susceptible to toxicity caused by ingestion of plants containing cyanogenetic glycosides (cyanide poisoning) or accumulated nitrate (nitrite poisoning). Overuse of nitrogenous fertilizers contributes to the incidence of nitrite poisoning. Antidotal substances that are used (injected intravenously) to treat these toxicities are sodium nitrite, followed by sodium thiosulfate for cyanide poisoning and methylthioninium chloride (methylene blue) for nitrite poisoning. In ruminant species, in which chemical compounds can be altered (activated or detoxified) by microbial action in the forestomach and in which the whole physiological tempo of the body is so dependent on ruminal activity, no pharmacological or toxicological investigation can be interpreted without full consideration of the basic diet and feeding regimen (13).

After comminution by rechewing and microbial digestion, the liquid component with suspended particles of reticuloruminal contents is "pumped" by the omasum (third compartment of the forestomach) into the abomasum (true stomach). During the two-stage transfer process, water and electrolytes are absorbed, and the size of particulate matter in the digesta is reduced. The abomasum, which accounts for approximately 4–5% of the capacity of the gastrointestinal tract in adult cattle and 7.5% of gastrointestinal capacity in sheep and goats, is the only compartment of the ruminant stomach that secretes digestive juices. Secretions from the fundic area of the abomasum contain hydrochloric acid, pepsin and, in suckling preruminant animals, rennin (a milk-coagulating enzyme). Mucus is produced by the columnar epithelial cells that line the abomasum. The pH reaction of abomasal contents does not vary much and is usually close to pH 3.0 (14).

Because of the large volume of reticuloruminal contents, a drug can attain only a low concentration in the reticulorumen, whether administered in solution, suspension, or solid dosage form. In dissolution of solid dosage forms, dilution in the large volume of fluid and binding to particulate matter would decrease the rate, but not necessarily the extent, of drug absorption. Lipid-soluble neutral molecules and the nonionized form of weak organic electrolytes, particularly organic acids, should normally be well-absorbed from the reticulorumen. When aspirin (pK_a 3.5) in a solid dosage form (60 g, which is equivalent to 3.9 g of oral bolus) was administered to cows, salicylate was slowly absorbed, and systemic availability was 50–70% (15). The 12-h dosage interval for aspirin in adult cattle is based on the rate of absorption rather than on the half-life of salicylate, which is 0.8 h.

Benzimidazole anthelmintics (albendazole, fenbendazole, oxfendazole, which is fenbendazole sulphoxide); probenzimidazoles (netobimin and febantel, which are metabolically converted to albendazole and fenbendazole, respectively); and salicylanilide flukicides (closantel, rafoxanide, oxyclozanide) are administered as oral suspensions to ruminant animals. For anthelmintic drugs oral suspensions have an advantage over oral solutions in that the delayed availability of drug for absorption extends the duration of action. Reducing the level of feed intake (for 36 h before and 36 h after dosing) delays the onward passage of ruminal fluid with suspended matter from the reticulorumen to the abomasum and small intestine and

Selection of Dosage Form

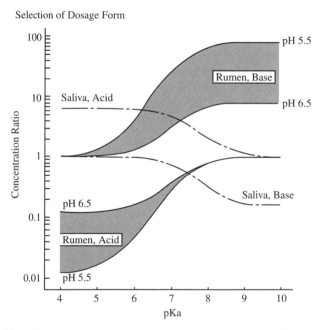

Fig. 1 Expected equilibrium distribution between saliva or rumen contents and plasma of acids and bases of differing pKa. Concentration ratio is the ratio of the salivary or ruminal concentration to concentration free in the plasma, calculated separately for acids and bases, for saliva of pH 8.2 and rumen contents over a range of pH5.5–6.5, assuming plasma is pH 7.4. (From Ref. 12.)

would allow more time for drug dissolution and absorption to occur. When the rate of onward passage of ruminal fluid was decreased, by temporarily reducing feed intake, in sheep, the systemic availability of oxfendazole was increased (16). The systemic availability of rafoxanide and triclabendazole, administered as oral suspensions, was higher in housed lambs fed hay and concentrates than in lambs grazing on pasture (17). The effect of dietary regimen/composition on systemic availability of the flukicides could be attributed to the time allowed for dissolution and absorption of the drugs.

Closure of the reticular groove would allow an oral solution to flow directly from the cardiac orifice of the rumen into the absomasum, bypassing the rumen. Spontaneous closure of the groove occurs reflexly in some animals although at least partial closure can be chemically induced. Should rapid absorption of a drug (such as a nonsteroidal anti-inflammatory drug) from the gastrointenstinal tract be desired, an oral solution of the drug could be administered immediately after inducing closure of the reticular groove. This can be achieved generally in cattle by administering orally a solution containing sodium bicarbonate and in sheep by administering orally a copper sulfate solution or injecting intravenously a dose (0.3 U/kg) of lysine–vasopressin. Closure of the reticular groove would be unwanted in the case of an oral liquid, such as dimeticone emulsion or poloxaline, used to treat frothy bloat in cattle. In young ruminant animals, reflex closure of the reticular groove, induced by suckling, allows milk to flow directly to the abomasum.

Advantage can be taken of the anatomical arrangement of the forestomach of ruminant animals by administering a modified-release ruminal bolus that will remain lodged in the reticulorumen for a prolonged period. Slow-release ruminal boluses containing trace elements (cobalt oxide, copper oxide, cobalt and copper in sodium phosphate glass matrix, and selenium as sodium selenate) are commercially available for administration to cattle or sheep, and the compound ruminal bolus can be administered to farmed adult deer. Controlled-release ruminal boluses containing certain anthelmintic drugs (ivermectin, fenbendazole, oxfendazole, morantel) or the production enhancer monensin are available for oral administration, using a specialized delivery device, to beef cattle within a specified range of body weight (100–400 kg). These systems are designed either to continuously release the drug into ruminal fluid for a prolonged period (generally 120–140 days) or to intermittently release pulse doses (oxfendazole bolus) at a predetermined interval (approximately 3 weeks). This interval generally coincides with the prepatent period of the major gastrointestinal tristrongylids of cattle (18). Controlled-release ruminal boluses that continuously release ivermectin, fenbendazole, or morantel into ruminal fluid are available for use in beef cattle, whereas controlled-release boluses that deliver albendazole or ivermectin over a period of 100 days are available for use in sheep (35–65 kg in body weight). The delivery systems are retained in the reticulorumen at least throughout the entire period of drug release. The retention of oral controlled-release drug delivery systems designed for use in humans is limited by gastric emptying time, which can be up to 12 h (19).

FIRST-PASS EFFECT

Having traversed the gastrointestinal mucosal barrier, drug molecules are conveyed in hepatic portal blood to the liver, where they are subjected to the first-pass effect before entering the systemic circulation. The first-pass effect applies to all animal species and, owing to the generally higher capacity of the liver of herbivorous species (ruminant animals and horses) to metabolize lipid-soluble drugs by microsomal oxidative reactions, is likely to decrease the systemic availability of these drugs to a greater extent in herbivorous than in nonherbivorous species(dogs, cats, pigs, humans). In ruminant species (cattle, sheep, goats) and *Equidae* (horses, ponies, donkeys), triclabendazole, administered as an oral suspension, is converted by hepatic first-pass metabolism to triclabendazole sulfoxide (active metabolite), which is subsequently converted to the sulfone (inactive) metabolite. In many species, the first-pass effect can substantially reduce the systemic availability of orally administered lipid-soluble drugs that undergo extensive biotransformation in the liver (e.g., diazepam, propranolol, verapamil). Although presystemic metabolism occurs primarily in the liver, it can also take place in the small intestinal mucosa during the absorption process. Some drugs that show incomplete systemic availability after oral administration to dogs are listed in Table 4. Presystemic metabolism in the liver is responsible for incomplete systemic availability of the majority of these drugs. The oral bioavailability of digoxin was enhanced in humans when the drug was administered as an aqueous alcoholic solution in gelatin capsules rather than in tablet form, even though the tablets had a satisfactory dissolution rate (20–22). In a similar manner, increased relative bioavailability, based on comparison of areas under the plasma concentration–time curves of flufenamic acid, was achieved in dogs when the drug was administered in soft rather than hard gelatin capsules; the average increase was 34% (23). In both instances, the higher oral bioavailability was attributed to physicochemical factors brought into play by adjuvants in the soft gelatin capsules. The influence that

Table 4 Systemic availability of some orally administered drugs in dogs

Drugs (dosage form)	Dose (mg/kg)	Systemic availability (%)	Site of metabolism/ other factor
Phenobarbitone (tablet)	10	86–96	Liver
Valproic acid(tablet)	40	78	Liver
Phenytoin (tablet)	15	36[a]	Liver
Salicylate (aspirin tablet)	250 mg total	45	Liver
Ibuprofen (gelatin capsule)	5	60–86	Liver
Naproxen[b](gelatin capsule)	5	68–100	—
Theophylline (conventional aminophylline tablet)	10	91	Liver
Diazepam (tablet)	2	1–3 86[c]	Liver + (intestinal mucosa)
Lidocaine (solution)	10	15	Liver
Procainamide (tablet)	25	85[a,d]	
Propranolol (conventional tablet)	80 mg total	2–17	Liver
Verapamil	0.5	15	Liver
Digoxin (Lanoxin tablet)	1 mg total	80	Dissolution
Cephalexin monohydrate(capsule)	20	57	Dissolution
Norfloxacin (tablet)	5	35[a]	Dissolution + liver
Enrofloxacin (tablet)	5	100[e]	—
Allopurinol (tablet)	15	70[f]	Intestine + liver (xanthine oxidase)

[a]Average oral bioavailability; wide individual dog variation.
[b]Naproxen has an unusually long half-life in dogs.
[c]Total active benzodiazepine.
[d]Dogs do not form N-acetylprocainamide (active metabolite).
[e]Total antimicrobial active fluoroquinolone.
[f]Average oral bioavailability is 14% in the horse.

formulation, or rather dosage form, can have on the systemic availability of an orally administered drug was shown in horses given racemic ketoprofen (2.2 mg/kg). The systemic availability of the S(+)- and R(−)-enantiomers was 54.2 and 50.5%, respectively, after administration of micronized racemic ketoprofen powder in hard gelatin capsules to horses with restricted access to feed. When ketoprofen powder from the same batch was administered as an oil-based paste, systemic availability of the S(+)- and R(−)-enantiomers was 5.75 and 2.7%, respectively, regardless of the feeding schedule (24). To avoid hepatic first-pass metabolism, glyceryl trinitrate (nitroglycerin) is formulated in a variety of dosage forms, which include parenteral solution, spray for sublingual application, sustained-release tablet, and transdermal therapeutic systems, for use in humans, and as an ointment for topical application to dogs (cardiogenic pulmonary edema) or horses (acute laminitis). Sublingual administration avoids the first-pass effect, but it is not feasible to administer solid dosage forms by this route to animals.

Although the first-pass effect is a major source of species variation in systemic availability of orally administered drugs that undergo extensive hepatic metabolism, another important source of variation is metabolism by ruminal microorganisms. Some drugs (nitroxynil, chloramphenicol, digitalis glycosides) are metabolized in the rumen to such an extent that parenteral administration is required for clinical efficacy.

An advantage of rectal over oral administration of lipid-soluble drugs is partial avoidance of the first-pass effect. The extent to which the first-pass effect is avoided appears to be less in dogs than in humans. Because venous drainage of the rectum of the horse, unlike in the humans and dog, appears to be substantially into the hepatic portal vein, minimal avoidance of hepatic first-pass metabolism of drugs absorbed from the rectum could be anticipated in horses.

ORAL DOSAGE FORMS

The oral route of drug administration is safer than parenteral routes and avoids tissue irritation at injection sites. However, wide variation, both inter- and intraspecies, in systemic availability is a feature of orally administered drugs. The convenience of oral drug administration depends on the species of animal and the dosage form of the drug. To facilitate drug administration and take into account the anatomy and physiology of the digestive system and the average body weight of the various animal species, the requirements of oral dosage forms differ among species. Consideration must be given to size of the total dose (amount of drug) to be administered and oral bioavailability in the animal species.

Oral dosage forms available for administration to animals include oral solutions, liquids, suspensions, gels, pastes, capsules, tablets, ruminal boluses, powders and granules for addition to feed, soluble powders for addition to drinking water or fish medicating baths, and premixes for addition to feed for livestock or poultry. The type of dosage form is determined by the solubility and physicochemical properties of the drug, the species of animal for which the dosage form is intended, and whether a reasonably rapid onset or a prolonged duration of effect is required. Liquid dosage forms (oral solutions and liquids) provide readily available drug for absorption, particularly in monogastric species. Oral liquids, such as dimeticone emulsion and poloxaline (anionic surfactant), are used for the treatment of frothy bloat in cattle. An oral liquid containing propylene glycol (glucose precursor) for addition to drinking water or for preparation of an oral solution is indicated for adjunctive treatment of ketosis in cattle and sheep. Aqueous suspensions are administered by nasogastric tube to horses, by mouth (as a drench) to ruminant animals and by mouth (sometimes with the aid of an oral syringe) to dogs and cats. Oral pastes and gels are semisolid dosage forms supplied in preloaded calibrated syringes designed for convenience of drug administration to horses by their owners. The formulation of a paste must be such that it is syringeable over a wide range of ambient temperatures, is moderately tenacious so that it will adhere to the tongue, and is tasteless or suitably flavored (mint or apple flavor appears to be preferred by horses). Classes of drugs that could be formulated as oral pastes or gels for administration to horses include anthelmintics, nonsteroidal anti-inflammatory drugs, and some antimicrobial agents. Application of an anthelmintic paste, at the appropriate dose of the drug, to the distal forelimbs of cats is a convenient alternative to oral administration of a tablet or capsule. Solid dosage forms must undergo disintegration and dissolution in the stomach before absorption of the drug can occur. Drug release from solid dosage forms delays the rate of absorption compared with that from an oral solution. With regard to the quality of solid dosage forms, capsules offer an advantage over tablets in that the particle size and distribution of the active ingredient are rarely altered by the capsule-filling process, whereas

physical stresses (compression and heat) are imposed in the manufacturing process of tablets. In addition, capsules provide more rapid dissolution than do conventional tables of the same active ingredient. The pattern of release of coated pellets or granules is more predictable when packed in capsules than compressed into tablets. Capsules, however, are generally more expensive than tablets containing the same drug. Because of the higher manufacturing cost, soft gelatin capsules should probably be used in preference to hard gelatin capsules only when the fill is liquid or bioavailability of the drug is significantly superior. An encapsulated active ingredient, until released, would be protected against metabolism by ruminal micro-organisms and/or chemical degradation in the ruminal environment. Encapsulation of insect development inhibitors (e.g., diflubenzuron) or insect growth regulators (e.g., methoprene) has potential application in cattle. These substances interfere with the metamorphosis and reproductive capacity of arthropod parasites, many of which breed in cattle dung. Dichlorvos, an organophosphorus compound with activity against gastrointestinal nematodes including whipworms (*Trichuris* spp.), is incorporated into polyvinyl chloride resin pellets (plasticization) for addition to the feed for pigs or canned food for dogs. This dosage form protects dichlorvos from hydrolytic degradation and provides slow release into the gastrointestinal tract, which greatly increases the margin of safety of the drug.

A sustained-release dosage form provides an initial amount of drug sufficient to provide a desired therapeutic concentration and continuously releases the drug at a constant (zero-order) rate for an extended period. The margin of safety of the drug is an important consideration, because sustained-release dosage forms contain a large amount of drug and the potential exists for "dose-dumping" with resultant toxicity. For drugs with half-lives in the range of 4 to 6 h, sustained-release dosage forms could provide a dosage interval of 12 h in dogs or 24 h in horses. Very few sustained-release preparations have been developed for use in either species. This type of dosage form has to be swallowed intact.

Controlled-release ruminal boluses are designed either to continuously release drug (an anthelmintic or production enhancer) at a constant rate for a prolonged specified period or to intermittently deliver pulse (usually five) doses at predetermined intervals. Each product is designed for use in either cattle or sheep within a specified range of body weight. Retention of orally administered controlled-release systems in the reticulorumen is dependent on either density or geometry of the system. The ivermectin (Ivomec) ruminal bolus, designed for use in cattle between 100 and 400 kg body weight, contains 1.72 g of ivermectin that is continuously released into ruminal fluid at a constant rate (12.5 mg/day) over a period of 135 days. The bolus is a cylindrical device that consists of an outer semipermeable membrane enclosing a metal density element at one end, an osmotic energy source at the other end, and a formulation containing the drug in the center. The osmotic energy source is composed of a tablet containing a polymeric salt mixture. Absorption of water through the semipermeable membrane causes expansion of the tablet, which drives the ivermectin wax formulation through the exit port (channel) in the density element (25) (Fig. 2a). The

Dosage Formulations

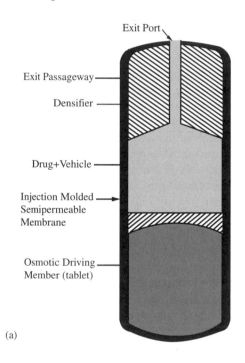

(a)

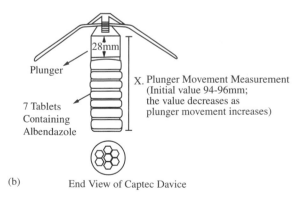

(b)   End View of Captec Davice

Fig. 2   (a) IVOMEC schematic; (b) captec schematic.

fenbendazole ruminal bolus (Panacur), designed for use in cattle between 100 and 300 kg body weight, contains 12 g of the anthelmintic which, is continuously released into ruminal fluid over a period of up to 140 days. Release of fenbendazole is controlled by the erosion of two magnesium alloy tubes; each tube contains five tight-fitting cylindrical tablets (6 g of fenbendazole). The magnesium alloy tubes are protected from the ruminal contents by a series of close-fitting rigid plastic rings; the central ring connects both tubes. The bolus is completely biodegradable and leaves no residual device in the forestomach (26). The morantel tartrate (Paratect Flex) ruminal bolus, designed for use in cattle over 100 kg body weight, contains 11.8 g of morantel base. The bolus consists of a drug-impregnated polymer packaged in a cylindrical trilaminate cartridge. Release of the drug (approximately 150 mg/day) takes place by diffusion through the semipermeable membrane into ruminal fluid over a period of at least 90 days. There is no withdrawal period associated with the use of the morantel tartrate trilaminate bolus because the combination of poor absorption and first-pass hepatic metabolism makes systemic availability of morantel exceedingly low. The Captec, also known as the Laby (27), device is a controlled-release ruminal capsule designed for use in sheep within a specified range of body weight that continuously releases the anthelmintic contained within, either albendazole (32.5 mg/day) or ivermectin (1.6 mg/day), over a period of 100 days. The device consists of a polypropylene barrel with a spring-loaded plunger at the closed (top) end and an orifice(series of perforations) at the base (Fig. 2b). A pair of polypropylene wings attached to the top of the barrel is secured in a folded position (compressed configuration) by water-soluble tape to enable oral administration. The barrel is loaded with tablets containing the anthelmintic, either albendazole (3.85 g) or ivermectin (160 mg). After administration of the ruminal capsule, the tape securing the pair of wings dissolves, and the wings open to a predetermined angle(expanded configuration) that prevents both regurgitation and reticulo-omasal passage. The rate of drug release is determined by a combination of factors that include the formulation of the tablets, the diameter of the orifice, and the pressure exerted on the tablets by the plunger. The ruminal fluid bathing the orifice of the device brings about dissolution of the tablets.

The modified-release ruminal bolus containing oxfendazole, designed for use in cattle in the body weight range of 200 to 400 kg, delivers pulse doses (1.25 g) at 3-week intervals over a period of 105 days (18). The bolus containing five tablets (Autoworm 5) releases the first dose at 21 days after administration whereas the bolus containing six tablets (Autoworm 6) releases the first dose on the day of administration.

Drugs in powder form or prepared granules can be added to the feed for pigs. Shortcomings associated with this method of administration include uncertainty as to the amount of drug (dose) ingested and interanimal variation in oral bioavailability. The drug must have a wide margin of safety and be palatable in the feed and, importantly, the animal must be feeding. Inappetence or indifference to feeding is a usual feature of illness in animals. Addition to feed, often referred to as top dressing of feed, is generally an unreliable method of drug administration to horses. However, the packaging of powders or granules in unit dose sachets provides convenience of drug administration for owners when the number of animals to be dosed is small. Unit dose sachets must be prepared on an individual species basis because the dose level (mg/kg) may differ among species, and the average body weight range of domestic animal species differs by approximately 200-fold. Soluble salts of drugs in prepared solutions or powder form can be administered to poultry and other farmed avian species by addition to drinking water or to fish by addition to the water in a medicating bath of known volume capacity. Sachets containing various trace elements (cobalt, copper, iodine, selenium) for addition to drinking water delivered by dispenser are available for the correction of mineral deficiencies in cattle. The mineral content of each sachet suffices for 25 cattle for a period of 7 days. Several factors to consider in the design of premix formulations and to ensure their satisfactory mixing in bulk feed are addressed in detail by Klink et al. (28). Premixes must always be diluted to the approved use level, usually parts per million (ppm) [g/tonne (feed) or mg/L(water)], for the animal species.

INTRAMUSCULAR INJECTION

Intramuscular injection is a commonly used route for drug administration in animals. This route offers convenience in that it is easy to apply and, because a sizeable proportion of veterinary parenteral preparations are formulated as long-acting dosage forms, either a single dose may suffice or a long dosage interval can be used. There are, however, a number of factors to consider before choosing this route of administration. They include the purpose for administering the drug, the acceptable time interval between drug administration and onset of the desired effect, the suitability of available parenteral preparations for use in the particular animal species, the withdrawal period(s) in food-producing animals, and the cost of the drug preparation

for the anticipated course of treatment. The suitability of a parenteral preparation for use in a particular species primarily depends on the formulation of the preparation. Significant formulation variables include the concentration of drug in a preparation, which determines the volume to be injected, the nature of the vehicle and other ingredients(solubilizers, preservatives), and the likelihood of causing irritation at the injection site. The horse is the least tolerant of domestic animal species to injection-site irritation, and drugs in oily vehicles should never be administered by injection to horses.

Whereas the formulation of a preparation determines the pattern of absorption and influences systemic availability of the drug, the volume of the preparation deposited in muscle and the vascularity of the injection site determines the rate of absorption. The barrier to absorption is the capillary endothelium, which most drugs readily penetrate by passive diffusion, although small water-soluble molecules may enter capillaries by bulk flow through intercellular "pores" in the endothelial membrane. Aqueous channels(pores) in the capillary endothelium are approximately 10-fold larger in diameter (40–80 Å) than those in the intestinal epithelium. Polar drugs such as aminoglycoside antibiotics are rapidly and completely absorbed from intramuscular injection sites, whereas they are very poorly absorbed from the gastrointenstinal tract when the epithelial membrane is intact. Drug absorption from intramuscular injection sites is generally assumed to be a first-order process. However, this assumption may not be entirely valid, particularly during the initial stage when absorption may obey zero-order (nonlinear) kinetics. Local and systemic factors that influence the rate of absorption seldom remain constant throughout the absorption process. Increased blood flow to skeletal muscle at the site of injection promotes absorption, whereas the administration of a drug that causes local vasoconstriction or the presence of a disease state that decreases skeletal muscle perfusion delays absorption. Deposition of the injected preparation between muscle masses (intermuscular) or in adipose tissue and the injection of a preparation that causes tissue irritation or precipitation of the drug at the injection site produce an erratic pattern of absorption that is reflected in the plasma concentration profile of the drug.

The site of intramuscular injection can affect the plasma concentration profile and bioavailability of a drug, particularly when a long-acting preparation is administered. The variation in the pattern of absorption can be attributed to regional differences in blood flow to skeletal muscles and in absorptive surface area. In cattle and goats, intramuscular injection in the lateral neck provides superior absorption to injection in the buttock

(*M. semitendineus*) and thigh muscle (*M. quadriceps femoris*), respectively, or subcutaneous injection in the lateral neck. In pigs, the lateral neck should always be used as the site for intramuscular injection of parenteral preparations. The reasons for selecting this site include better absorption than in other sites, less residual drug at the injection site, and avoidance of damage to the carcass. In dogs and cats, the quadriceps muscle mass is the preferred site for intramuscular injection, which should be performed slowly, of parenteral preparations. After the injection of procaine penicillin G (20,000 IU/kg) at various intramuscular sites and subcutaneously in the cranial part of the pectoral area in horses, the peak plasma concentration and systemic availability of penicillin G were highest when the long-acting preparation was injected i.m. in the neck region (*M. serratus ventralis cervicis*). This was followed, in descending order of injection site, by *M. biceps* > *M. pectoralis* > *M. gluteus*, or subcutaneously (Fig. 3) (29). The intramuscular injection technique must ensure that inadvertent intravenous administration does not occur.

Potential disadvantages of intramuscular injection are the deposition of the preparation in adipose tissue or intermuscular fascial planes and the production of tissue damage with persistence of drug residue at the site of injection (30–32). Tissue damage is more likely to be caused by constituents of the formulation than the drug substance *per se*. Useful antemortem methods of assessing the extent of tissue irritation and the rate of resolution at an intramuscular injection site include the echographical examination of the muscle tissue in the immediate vicinity of the injection site (33) and the monitoring of plasma creatine kinase (CK) activity (34, 35). These methods have

the distinct advantage of being applicable to the live animal. Should moderate to severe tissue damage be evident, the extent of the damage and precise nature of the lesion can be described on postmortem examination. The use of some tissue-damaging parenteral preparations in food-producing animals is unavoidable, and the specified withdrawal period(s) must be applied. The withdrawal period for a drug varies with the formulation of the dosage form (preparation), which should be administered only by the recommended route and may differ between animal species. Fish are ectothermic and their basal metabolic rate, which markedly influences the rate of elimination of drugs, varies with the temperature of the water to which they are acclimatized. It follows that withdrawal periods, stated in degree days, for drugs used in "farmed" fish (primarily by addition to feed or bath water) will vary with ambient water temperature.

In cats, puppies, and piglets, particular attention should be given to the drug concentration in parenteral preparations and, when giving an intramuscular injection in the thigh (particularly of cats), to avoid causing damage to the sciatic nerve. Because avian and reptilian species have a well-developed renal portal system, first-pass renal excretion may decrease the systemic availability of drugs that are primarily eliminated by the kidneys (e.g., β-lactam and aminoglycoside antibiotics) when injected intramuscularly in the thigh of birds or caudal half of the body of reptiles.

SUBCUTANEOUS INJECTION

Subcutaneous injection is an alternative route to intramuscular injection for administration of parenteral preparations to domestic animals. This route of administration is used most often in dogs and cats and only occasionally in horses. Most of the factors that influence drug absorption from skeletal muscle also apply to subcutaneous sites. They include the concentration of drug in the parenteral preparation, the nature of the vehicle and other components of the formulation, the total volume of the preparation administered, blood supply to subcutaneous tissue and area of the absorptive surface, tissue irritation, precipation of drug at the site of injection, and persistence of drug residues. Absorption from subcutaneous sites is often slower and more erratic than from intramuscular sites because of the limited and more variable blood flow to subcutaneous tissue. However, the absorptive area may be larger and can be expanded by massaging the skin covering the region of the injection site. The degree of tissue irritation caused by some parenteral preparations appears to be greater after subcutaneous than intramuscular

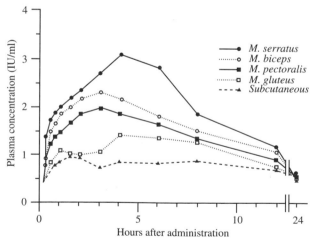

Fig. 3 Mean plasma penicillin concentration–time curves after 20,000 IU of procaine penicillin g/kg was administered to 5 animals (4 horses, 1 pony) at 5 different sites. (From Ref. 29.)

injection(36, 37). Because the damaged tissue surrounding a subcutaneous injection site can be trimmed from the carcass of a slaughtered animal, the likelihood of violative drug residues in the meat is reduced. Subcutaneous injection is the preferred route of administration for some poorly soluble suspensions. When formulating sustained-release parenteral preparations, a compromise may have to be made between the rate of drug release and the degree of tissue irritation caused by the preparation. Various modified-release devices for subcutaneous implantation have been developed as an alternative to injection of sustained-release oily suspensions. Devices developed include an implantable osmotic pump that delivers growth hormone-releasing factor over a period of 7 days in steers and wethers (38). Another subdermal implant is a diffusion polymeric matrix system that releases estradiol at an approximately zero-order rate. A modified-release melatonin implant designed to advance the time of onset of cyclical ovarian activity in ewes is commercially available. Although great efforts have been made toward technological development of modified-release devices for subcutaneous implantation in cattle and sheep, the use of implants in food-producing animals does not appear to have gained wide acceptance over the past decade.

INTRAVENOUS INJECTION

When a parenteral drug solution is administered intravenously, it is assumed that the total dose of the drug is completely available systemically. This assumption overlooks the fact that an intravenously administered drug passes through the lungs, which constitute an organ of biotransformation, before being distributed throughout the body. Intravenous injection produces a prompt pharmacological response and overcomes the variability in absorption associated with other routes of drug administration. Parenterals, excluding long-acting preparations, that are too irritant to be injected by other routes may be cautiously administered intravenously. It must be ensured that perivascular leakage at the site of injection does not occur. Intravenous injection of irritant solutions can cause thrombophlebitis. Once a drug has entered the systemic circulation, its removal from the body is entirely dependent on the elimination(biotransformation and excretion) processes. Pharmacokinetic parameters that describe the disposition(distribution and elimination) of drugs are based on the plasma concentration profiles after intravenous injection of single doses. Assumptions made in the estimation of absolute bioavailability, which is based on comparison of total areas under the plasma concentration–

time curves after extravascular and intravenous administration of the drug, are that the intravenously administered dose is completely available systemically and that the clearance of the drug is not changed by the route of administration.

The vein commonly used for injecting drugs intravenously varies with the species of animal. In horses, cattle, sheep, and goats, the jugular vein is used, whereas in dogs and cats, either the cephalic (usually) or the jugular vein is used, and in pigs, an ear vein is often used. In anesthetized dogs and cats, the jugular vein is convenient to use for administering supplemental doses of intravenous anesthetics, whereas in dogs, the sublingual vein may be used in emergency situations for injecting drug solutions of small volume. In pharmacokinetic studies of drug bioavailability and disposition, blood samples are collected from the jugular vein of all species apart from pigs, in which the anterior vena cava is generally used. It is very unlikely that the vein used for collection of blood samples, with the exception of the vein used for injection of the drug, would influence the results obtained in a pharmacokinetic study involving the measurement of plasma drug concentrations over an extended period.

Because of practical considerations, intravenous infusion is used far less widely for drug administration to animals than to humans. Intravenous administration, especially constant-rate infusion, has two important advantages over other routes. It provides complete systemic availability of the drug and allows greater control over the intensity (magnitude) of the effects produced. The relatively short dosage interval associated with multiple dosing is the principal disadvantage of the use of intravenous injection in animals. Long-acting preparations administered by intramuscular injection constitute the parenteral dosage form most widely used in farm animals.

Intraosseous administration is a feasible alternative to intravenous injection of some antimicrobial agents (sodium ampicillin or amoxicillin, cefotaxime, gentamicin or amikacin sulfate) in neonatal foals (less than 7 days of age). This particularly applies in the treatment of septicemia in neonatal foals that are in a state of septic shock or dehydration or both. The plasma concentration profiles for amikacin administered intraosseously and intravenously to neonatal foals are similar (Fig. 4) (39).

PARENTERAL DOSAGE FORMS

Parenteral dosage forms for use in animals include aqueous, aqueous organic and oily solutions, emulsions,

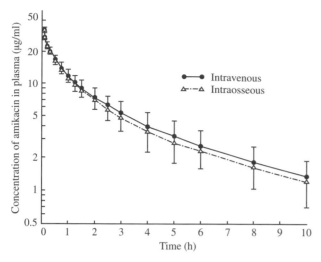

Fig. 4 Concentrations (mean ± S.D.) of amikacin in plasma after i.v. and i.o. administration of amikacin sulphate (7 mg/kg body weight) to 6 foals at 3 to 5 days of age.

aqueous and oily suspensions for injection, and modified-release devices for subcutaneous implantation. Parenteral preparations must be sterile and pyrogen-free; liquid formulations should, if possible, be buffered close to physiological pH and preferably be isotonic with body fluids. The advantages and disadvantages associated with the various types of parenteral dosage forms have been addressed elsewhere (40).

The formulation of an extravascularly injected parenteral preparation primarily determines the plasma concentration profile of the drug. A drug is immediately available for absorption only when administered as an aqueous solution and when neither precipitation nor tissue irritation occurs at the injection site. Gentamicin sulfate (50 mg/ml aqueous solution) is rapidly and completely absorbed in that the peak plasma concentration is attained within 30–60 min, and systemic availability exceeds 90% from intramuscular injection sites in horses, dogs, and cats. After intravenous, intramuscular, and subcutaneous injection of gentamicin (3 mg/kg) in dogs, the peak plasma concentration (10.7 μg/ml i.m.; 10.2 μg/ml s.c.) and absolute bioavailability (96% i.m.; 94.3% s.c.) of the antibiotic provided by the intramuscular and subcutaneous routes were similar (41). Administration of amikacin sulfate (50 mg/ml aqueous solution) by subcutaneous injection at three dose levels (5, 10, and 20 mg/kg) to dogs showed that area under the curve, which reflects the extent of absorption, was proportional to the dose administered (42). After intramuscular injection of ceftiofur sodium(as reconstituted aqueous solution) at dose levels of 1.1 and 2.2 mg of ceftiofur free acid

equivalents per kilogram of body weight to sheep, the peak plasma concentrations(C_{max}) of ceftiofur and metabolites (measured as desfuroylceftiofur acetamide by HPLC) were 4.33 and 7.13 μg/ml, the apparent half-lives were 6.5 and 7.65 h, respectively, and the area under the curve (from time zero to the limit of quantification of the assay) was proportional to the dose administered (43). The drug was rapidly(t_{max}, 0.5–1 h) and completely absorbed from the intramuscular injection site. Ketamine hydrochloride (100 mg/ml aqueous solution) is rapidly absorbed from the intramuscular injection site in cats, but pain may be evident before onset of the anesthetic effect. In horses, dogs and cats, ketamine administration is preceded by sedative premedication with an α_2-adrenoceptor agonist (detomidine, medetomidine, or xylazine). Parenteral solutions of an irritant nature (thiopental sodium, ticarcillin sodium-clavulanate potassium combination, cefuroxime, cefotaxime, ceftriaxone, flunixin meglumine) and digoxin injection should be administered only by the intravenous route. Formulations containing sparingly soluble drugs in a water-miscible solvent, such as propylene glycol, may cause precipitation of drug at the intramuscular injection site. This makes these preparations unsuitable for intramuscular administration (e.g., diazepam, phenytoin). Diazepam injection (5 mg/ml solution or emulsion) may be administered to dogs and cats by intravenous injection and, after appropriate dilution, by intravenous infusion.

In parenteral preparations containing a poorly soluble salt of a drug, availability of the drug for absorption, which is dependent on dissolution rather than on the absorption process per se, generally controls the rate of absorption, the peak plasma concentration, and the length of time over which effective plasma concentrations are maintained. Long-acting parenteral preparations are formulated in a nonaqueous vehicle (such as an oil), or a poorly soluble salt of the drug is used (usually an aqueous suspension). These preparations provide slow absorption of the drug over an extended period owing to its gradual or staged availability for absorption (44). Avermectins and milbemycins (macrocyclic lactones) are highly lipophilic substances that determine the extent of their distribution and deposition in body fat, whereas the formulation of parenteral dosage forms (for subcutaneous injection in cattle or sheep, but not horses) influences the plasma concentration profile after the administration of a single dose (200 μg/kg). The commercially available preparations differ in formulation; ivermectin is a nonaqueous preparation (60% propylene glycol/40% glycerol formal), doramectin is an oil-based preparation containing sesame oil/ethyl oleate (90/10), and moxidectin is an aqueous-based solution. The pharmacokinetic parameters describing the rates of absorption and elimination of these

Table 5 Pharmacokinetic parameters describing the rate of absorption and elimination of ivermectin (IVM), doramectin (DRM), and moxidectin (MXD) after subcutaneous injection (shoulder region) of single doses (200 μg/kg) of the commercially available preparations to 10-month-old hereford calves (180–210 kg body weight)

Kinetic parameter	IVM	DRM	MXD
C_{max}(ng/ml)	42.8 ± 3.8	37.5 ± 3.9	39.4 ± 3.4
t_{max} (days)	4.00 ± 3.94^{a}	6.00 ± 1.35	0.32 ± 0.0^{c}
$t_{1/2}$ (days)	17.2 ± 4.26^{b}	6.25 ± 0.16	14.5 ± 1.20^{c}
Cl_{B}/F(ml/day·kg)	457 ± 52.5^{a}	322 ± 164	938 ± 62.5^{c}

[a]Mean kinetic parameters for IVM are significantly different from those obtained for MXD at $P < 0.05$.
[b]Mean kinetic parameters for IVM are significantly different from those obtained for DRM at $P < 0.05$.
[c]Mean kinetic parameters for MXD are significantly different from those obtained for DRM (c) at $P < 0.05$.
Results are expressed as mean $\pm$ sem ($n = 4$).

endectocides after administration by subcutaneous injection (shoulder region) in 10-month-old Hereford calves are compared in Table 5 (45). Because the systemic availability (F) of the drugs was not determined in this study, the term clearance/systemic availability (CL_{B}/F) is used. Comparison of three commercially available parenteral preparations (one conventional and two long-acting) of oxytetracycline (20 mg/kg) injected intramuscularly in the lateral neck of pigs showed statistically significant differences between the preparations in peak plasma concentration (C_{max}), time of peak concentration (t_{max}), and mean residence time (MRT), whereas area under the curve (AUC) did not significantly differ among the preparations (Table 6) (46). The results indicate that a 24-h dosage interval should be used for the conventional preparation, whereas a 48-h interval would be appropriate for either of the long-acting preparations. A single intramuscular dose (20 mg/kg) of a long-acting preparation of oxytetracycline provides plasma concentrations above 0.5 μg/ml for 48 h in pigs, ruminant calves, cattle, goats, red deer (*Cervus elaphus*), fallow deer (*Dama dama*), and camels (*Camelus dromedarius*). The commercially available long-acting preparations of oxytetracycline should not be administered to *Equidae* (horses, ponies, and donkeys). When comparing parenteral preparations of an antimicrobial agent on the basis of potential clinical efficacy, it is generally useful to compare the areas under the inhibitory plasma concentration–time curves (AUIC = AUC/MIC_{90}) for the duration of the recommended dosage interval because this term indicates the degree of exposure of susceptible micro-organisms to the drug.

The plasma concentration profiles can vary widely among different parenteral preparations of the same drug administered by intramuscular injection, even when the same injection site is used. Comparison of the plasma concentration profiles obtained after intramuscular injec-

Table 6 Pharmacokinetic parameters describing the absorption and disposition of three oxytetracycline formulations administered intramuscularly (lateral neck) to pigs ($n = 8$) at a dose of 20 mg/kg body weight

Pharmacokinetic term	Product A	Product B	Product C
C_{max} (μg/ml)	6.27 ± 1.47	5.77 ± 1.0	4.68 ± 0.61
t_{max} (h)	3.0 $(2.0–4.0)$	0.5 $(0.083–2.0)$	0.5 $(0.083–2.0)$
AUC (μg h/ml)	79.22 ± 25.02	91.53 ± 20.84	86.64 ± 14.21
MRT (h)	11.48 ± 2.01	25.27 ± 9.22	37.66 ± 15.62
$C_{p(24\ h)}$ (μg/ml)	0.81 ± 0.34	1.01 ± 0.26	0.97 ± 0.29
$C_{p(48\ h)}$ (μg/ml)	$< LOQ$	0.40 ± 0.17	0.50 ± 0.09

LOQ = limit of quantification (0.1 μg/ml).
Product A, Engemycine 10% in polyvinylpyrrolidone.
Product B, Oxyter LA 20% in dimethylacetamide.
Product C, Terramycin LA 20% in pyrrolidone-2 and polyvinylpyrrolidone.
Results are expressed as mean $\pm$ S.D.

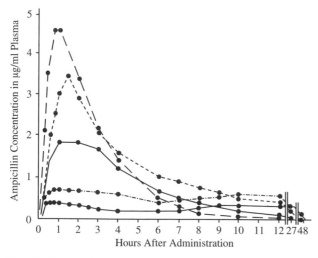

Fig. 5 Mean plasma ampicillin concentrations after i.m. injection of 5 different parenteral ampicillin formulations at similar dose levels (7.7 ± 1.0 mg/kg) to 5 calves. (From Ref. 47.)

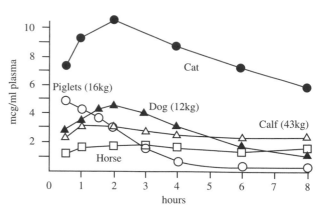

Fig. 6 Effect of species and weight on the bioavailability of amoxicillin after i.m. injection of amoxicillin trihydrate aqueous suspension (100 mg/ml) at the same dose (7 mg/kg) in the various species except cats (10–12 mg/kg).

tion in the lateral neck of ruminant calves of five different parenteral preparations of ampicillin at a similar dose level (7.7 ± 1.0 mg/kg) serves to illustrate the variation that can exist among preparations (Fig. 5) (47). Estimation of the bioavailability of each preparation relative to a reference preparation is useful. A crossover design incorporating an appropriate washout period between the phases of the bioavailability study should be used whenever feasible.

The drug concentration in a parenteral suspension can influence the plasma concentration profile. When different concentrations of amoxicillin (100 and 200 mg/ml) in aqueous suspensions of amoxicillin trihydrate were administered intramuscularly at the same site and same dose level (10 mg/kg) to horses, the preparation of lower concentration (10%) provided relatively better absorption and a more consistent plasma concentration profile. Intramuscular injection of amoxicillin trihydrate (15% in a mixed oil base) in the neck (10 cm behind the ear) of pigs produced two peaks, 1.7 and 0.8 μg/ml at 1.3 and 6.6 h, respectively, rather than a single peak in the plasma concentration profile and an eight-fold longer mean residence time of the antibiotic than a preparation of the same concentration in oil (48). The two peaks in the plasma concentration profile could be ascribed to the mixture of oil vehicles releasing amoxicillin at different rates.

Age and body weight (45, 55, and 62, kg) of calves was shown to influence the systemic availability of amoxicillin administered intramuscularly as amoxicillin trihydrate (10% aqueous suspension). When the same preparation was administered intramuscularly to different animal species, the trend was for smaller animals (piglets, dogs, cats) to show an early high peak concentration followed by

a rapid decline, whereas larger animals (calves, horses) show a lower and relatively constant plasma concentration of amoxicillin over at least an 8-h period (Fig. 6) (49).

BOVINE MAMMARY GLAND

Antimicrobial agents, as with other drugs, cross the blood–milk barrier, which is a somewhat restrictive functional rather than anatomical barrier, primarily by passive diffusion. Both nonpolar lipid-soluble compounds and polar substances with sufficient lipid solubility passively diffuse through the predominantly lipoidal blood–milk barrier (50). At a moderate level of milk production, the ratio of the volume of blood circulating through the mammary gland to the volume of milk produced has been estimated to be 670:1; this provides ample opportunity for drugs to diffuse passively from the systemic circulation into milk. The composition (g/dL) of milk varies among breeds of cow in protein, from 3.1 (Holstein) to 3.9. (Jersey, Zebu, and buffalo) and fat, from 3.5 (Holstein) to 5.5 (Jersey, Zebu, and buffalo) content.

The milk-to-plasma equilibrium concentration ratio of total (nonionized plus ionized) drug is determined by the degree of ionization of the drug, which is pK_a/pH-dependent, in blood and milk, the charge on the ionized moiety, and the extent of binding to plasma proteins and milk macromolecules. It has been shown that only the lipid-soluble, nonionized moiety of a weak organic acid or base that is free (not bound to proteins) in the plasma can diffuse through cellular barriers and enter the milk (51). In normal lactating cows (milk pH range 6.5–6.8), weak organic acids attain milk ultrafiltrate-to-plasma ultrafiltrate equilibrium concentration ratios less than 1; oxytetracycline and rifampin, amphoteric drugs with moderate and high lipid solubility, attain equilibrium concentration ratios of 0.75 and approximately 1, respectively; weak organic bases, apart from aninoglycosides, spectinomycin, and polymyxin B (drugs with low solubility in lipid) attain milk ultrafiltrate-to-plasma ultrafiltrate concentration ratios greater than 1 (Table 7) (52). The high concentration ratios attained by lipophilic organic bases (macrolides, lincosamides, trimethoprim) are attributed to the ion-trapping effect in acidic milk. Enrofloxacin and its active metabolite ciprofloxacin, formed by *N*-deethylation (a microsomal-mediated oxidative reaction in the liver), would be expected to attain concentrations in milk that would be effective against susceptible Gram-negative aerobic bacteria, in particular *Escherichia coli*.

In the presence of mastitis, the pH of milk increases to within the range of 6.9 to 7.2. As a consequence, the ion-trapping effect on lipophilic organic bases is reduced, whereas the concentrations attained by weak organic acids are somewhat increased. The higher pH of milk does not change the concentrations attained by amphoteric drugs (fluoroquinolones, tetracyclines, rifampin); however, antimicrobial activity of these drugs is often lower in milk than in extracellular fluid or in vitro determination would predict.

Antimicrobial therapy is generally applied in the treatment of clinical mastitis during lactation and in treating subclinical mastitis at the end of lactation, whereas the implementation of preventive measures is essential for decreasing the incidence of mastitic infection in the dairy herd. The common causative pathogenic microorganisms of clinical mastitis are *Streptococcus uberis*, coliforms (*E. coli*, *Klebsiella* spp.), *S. aureus*, *S. dysgalactiae*, and *S. agalactiae*. It is usual to treat clinical mastitis both systemically using a parenteral antimicrobial preparation and locally with a quick-release intramammary prep-

Table 7 Comparison of calculated and experimentally obtained milk: plasma concentration ratios for antimicrobial agents under equilibrium conditions

Drug	Lipid solubility	pK$_a$	Milk pH	Concentration ratio (Milk ultrafiltrate: plasma ultrafiltrate) Theoretical	Experimental
Acids					
Penicillin G	Low	2.7	6.8	0.25	0.13–0.26
Cloxacillin	Low	2.7	6.8	0.25	0.25–0.30
Ampicillin	Low	2.7, 7.2	6.8		0.24–0.30
Cephaloridine	Low	3.4	6.8	0.25	0.24–0.28
Cephaloglycin	Low	4.9	6.8	0.25	0.33
Sulfadimethoxine	Moderate	6.0	6.6	0.20	0.23
Sulfadiazine	Moderate	6.4	6.6	0.23	0.21
Sulfamethazine	Moderate	7.4	6.6	0.58	0.59
Rifampin[a]	Moderate/high	7.9	6.8	0.82	0.90–1.28
Bases					
Tylosin	High	7.1	6.8	2.00	3.5
Lincomycin	High	7.6	6.8	2.83	3.1
Spiramycin	High	8.2	6.8	3.57	4.6
Erythromycin	Very high	8.8	6.8	3.87	8.7
Trimethoprim	High	7.3	6.8	2.32	2.9
Aminoglycosides	Low	7.8[b]	6.8	3.13	0.5
Spectinomycin	Low	8.8	6.8	3.87	0.6
Polymyxin B	Very low	10.0	6.8	3.97	0.3
Amphoteric					
Oxytetracycline	Moderate	—	6.5–6.8	—	0.75
Doxycycline	Moderate/high	—	6.5–6.8	—	1.53

[a]Rifampin is an amphoteric drug substance; theoretical concentration ratio was based on its behavior as an organic acid.
[b]pK$_a$ value given for aminoglycosides is unconfirmed.

aration. The infusion via the teat canal of an intramammary preparation alone would be inadequate for the treatment of moderate to severe infection because of the decreased ability of an infused drug to ascend partially occluded milk ducts and the requirement, particularly in coliform mastitis, for frequent milkout (stripping) of the infected quarter of the mammary gland. In mild cases of mastitis diagnosed at an early stage of infection, the infusion of a quick-release intramammary preparation may suffice without concurrent systemic treatment. Slow-release intramammary preparations are used at the end of lactation (after the last milking) to treat subclinical mastitis and to prevent the establishment of new infections, including summer mastitis commonly caused by *Actinomyces pyogenes* during the nonlactating (dry) period. Because *S. aureus* is the principal causative microorganism of subclincial mastitis, the slow-release intramammary preparation selected for treatment should contain an antimicrobial effective against all strains of the bacterium.

PARENTERAL PREPARATIONS

An "ideal" antimicrobial agent for systemic therapy of bovine mastitis should possess the following properties (53):

1. low minimum inhibitory concentration (MIC) for the majority of mastitis-causing pathogenic microorganisms;
2. high systemic availability after intramuscular injection;
3. lipid-soluble and predominantly nonionized in the blood and have a low degree of binding to plasma proteins;
4. long apparent half-life to ensure that concentrations above (preferably severalfold) the MIC are maintained at the site of infection in the mammary gland throughout the recommended dosage interval (12 h is desirable);
5. minimal adverse effects in cows treated at effective dosage; and
6. short withdrawal periods (milk and slaughter).

Parenteral preparations with antimicrobial activity, which depends on the causative pathogenic microorganism, and pharmacokinetic properties that meet most of these criteria include procaine penicillin G (aqueous suspension), amoxicillin trihydrate–clavulanate potassium combination (aqueous suspension), and enrofloxacin (solution). Enrofloxacin is not approved for use in cows producing milk for human consumption. To attain effective concentrations in the mammary gland, oxytetracycline

hydrochloride (conventional preparation) has to be administered by slow intravenous injection. Even though macrolide antibiotics attain high concentrations in milk, they also diffuse passively into ruminal fluid (pH 5.5–6.5) where the ion-trapping effect applies. This feature of their distribution may be undesirable. Moreover, slow intravenous injection is the preferred manner of administration because the available parenteral preparations cause tissue irritation at intramuscular injection sites. Because spiramycin binds avidly to tissue components, long withdrawal periods would be associated with the use of this antimicrobial agent.

INTRAMAMMARY PREPARATIONS

Intramammary preparations are formulated to provide either quick release of the antimicrobial agent or slow release of the antimicrobial over an extended period. A requirement of all intramammary preparations is that they be reasonably nonirritating to the parenchyma (epithelial tissue) of the udder. Quick-release preparations are used primarily in lactating cows for the treatment, often in conjunction with systemic therapy, of clinical mastitis. They should have short withdrawal periods. The vehicle used and viscosity of the formulation should allow rapid release of the antimicrobial while ensuring that effective concentrations will be maintained throughout the recommended dosage interval. Access of the released antimicrobial to the site of infection is determined by its uptake and distribution in mammary tissue, which are governed by the chemical nature and physiochemical properties (in particular, lipid solubility) of the drug. Binding to milk proteins or components of mammary tissue limits distribution and extends the withdrawal periods. The transfer of an antimicrobial agent from treated to untreated quarters of the udder takes place via the bloodstream and involves passive diffusion in both directions across the blood–milk barrier. Examples of intramammary preparations formulated as suspensions and having a recommended dosage interval of 12 h include cloxacillin sodium, ampicillin sodium–cloxacillin sodium combination, trimethoprim–sulfadiazine combination, and oxytetracycline hydrochloride (oily suspension), whereas erythromycin is formulated as an intramammary solution. Cefuroxime sodium and cefoperazone sodium (third-generation cephalosporins) are formulated as an oily paste and oily suspension, respectively. Quick-release intramammary preparations have short withdrawal periods, typically slaughter, 7 days and milk-withholding, 3.5 days, or either may be shorter depending on the preparation.

Slow-release intramammary preparations may be infused at the end of lactation (after the last milking) and into the teat canal of nonlactating cows to treat subclinical mastitis and to prevent the establishment of new infections during the nonlactating period. Either a poorly soluble salt of an antimicrobial agent may be used or the formulation of the preparation be such that the rate of antimicrobial release is relatively constant, approaching zero-order. The antimicrobial must remain active (be stable) throughout the extended duration in the udder, and the preparation should not cause tissue irritation. Antimicrobial binding to mammary tissue components is not of particular concern because slow-release preparations are not used in lactating cows. However, the ability to penetrate cell membranes is important because, in chronic staphylococcal mastitis, the pathogenic bacteria often reside within epithelial cells, neutrophils, and macrophages (54). Examples of slow-release intramammary preparations include cloxacillin (benzathine salt) with aluminium monostearate (suspension), ampicillin (trihydrate) and cloxacillin (benzathine) with aluminium monostearate (suspension) or formulated without aluminium monostearate as an oily suspension, procaine penicillin G (oily paste), dihydrostreptomycin sulfate and procaine penicillin G (oily paste). Penicillins and especially aminoglycosides have limited ability to penetrate cell membranes, whereas fluroquinolones, rifampin, and macrolides have this capacity.

Compound preparations containing one or more antimicrobial agents and a corticosteroid (hydrocortisone or prednisolone) are available for intramammary infusion in lactating cows. The reduction in inflammation of the mammary gland is desirable; however, the immunosuppressant effect and decrease in phagocyte function produced by glucocorticoids are undesirable. Amoxicillin trihydrate–clavulanate potassium combination with prednisolone is an example of a compound preparation (oily suspension) that can be administered by intramammary infusion at 12-h intervals and has short withdrawal periods (slaughter, 7 days; milk, 2 days). Unlike glucocorticoids, the nonsteroidal anti-inflammatory drugs do not cause immunosuppression. Flunixin meglumine (2.2 mg/kg) administered by intravenous injection at 24-h dosage intervals may have a place in the treatment of acute *E. coli* (endotoxin) mastitis. The significance of the antipyretic, anti-inflammatory, and analgesic effects produced by the drug is primarily dependent on the stage of the inflammatory process at which treatment is begun. Early diagnosis of coliform mastitis and prompt initiation of treatment with flunixin greatly increase the beneficial effect of the drug. The half-life of flunixin in cows is 8.1 h and the withdrawal periods are short (slaughter, 7 days; milk, 12 h). Flunixin does not interfere with the activity of concurrently administered antimicrobial agents, should antimicrobial therapy be applied. There is no evidence to support the contention that systemic antimicrobial therapy causes a massive release of endotoxin in cows with coliform mastitis. Frequent stripping of the infected quarter(s) to remove bacteria and cellular debris is important, perhaps essential, in coliform mastitis (55). The slow intravenous injection of oxytocin, 5–10 U of diluted solution (10 U/ml), facilitates the completeness of stripping (milkout).

THERAPEUTIC CONCENTRATIONS

The principal pharmacological effects produced are generally associated with the same range of therapeutic plasma concentrations in domestic animals as in humans (Table 8). The mechanisms of action of drugs appear to be the same in mammalian species. The calculation of a dosage regimen (dose and dosage interval) for a drug preparation is based on a knowledge of the therapeutic concentration range and the pharmacokinetic parameters

Table 8 Principal pharmacological effect and range of therapeutic plasma concentrations of some drugs

Drug	Pharmacological effect	Therapeutic concentrations
Quinidine	Antiarrhythmic	0–6 μg/ml
Procainamide	Antiarrhythmic	6–14 μg/ml
Lignocaine	Antiarrhythmic	1.5–5.0 μg/ml
Propranolol	Antihypertensive	20–80 ng/ml
Digoxin	Positive inotropic	0.6–2.4 ng/ml
Phenobarbitone	Anticonvulsant	10–25 μg/ml
Pethidine	Analgesic	0.4–0.7 μg/ml
Theophylline	Bronchodilator	6–16 μg/ml

that describe bioavailability and disposition of the drug. Complete systemic availability can be assumed only when a drug is administered intravenously. Species differences in the dosage regimen for a drug preparation administered by a particular route can generally, but not always, be attributed to variation among species in pharmacokinetic behavior of the drug. Species differences in susceptibility (dosage requirement) to certain drugs (morphine, xylazine) appear to be attributable to pharmacodynamic variation (affinity and/or efficacy).

Dosage of anthelmintics, which usually refers to a single dose, is based on semiquantitative assessment of clinical efficacy, although, when appropriate, bioavailability and the plasma concentration profile of the active moiety (parent drug and/or active metabolite) are considered in the development of anthelmintic dosage forms and selection of their routes of administration for various animal species (56). Because anthelmintics are administered in different dosage forms to ruminant species (cattle, sheep, and goats), pigs, horses, and small animals (dogs and cats), a wide variety of preparations are commercially available for use in animals.

DRUG DISPOSITION

Species variations in the disposition of a drug may be attributed to differences in the extent of distribution and/or the rate of elimination of the drug. Variations are usual between ruminant and monogastric species and between herbivorous and nonherbivorous species, depending on the classification system used for mammalian species. The rate of elimination of drugs differs widely between homeothermic and poikilothermic species. Little is known regarding drug distribution in poikilothermic species (fish and reptiles).

EXTENT OF DISTRIBUTION

Significant differences in the extent of distribution of drugs, particularly lipid-soluble organic bases, are usual between ruminant and monogastric species. After parenteral administration, lipophilic bases diffuse passively from the systemic circulation into ruminal fluid (pH 5.5–6.5), where they become "trapped" by ionization. These drugs are slowly reabsorbed or, if they possess functional groups suitable for metabolism by hydrolysis or reduction, they may be partially inactivated by ruminal micro-organisms.

The volume of distribution at steady state ($V_{d(ss)}$) is useful for determining the significance of changes in the extent of distribution of a drug in the presence of disease states or by plasma protein binding displacement (drug interaction) and for comparing the extent of drug distribution in neonatal and adult animals of the same species. The volume of distribution at steady state, unlike $V_{d(area)}$, is at least theoretically independent of changes in the rate of drug elimination (57).

PLASMA PROTEIN BINDING

Although the extent of plasma protein binding of a drug varies among domestic animal species, the range of binding is reasonably narrow in the collective species, and the difference among individual species is often not of clinical significance. Species variation in the binding of acidic drugs could be attributed to differences in the conformation of plasma albumin; the lower concentration of plasma albumin in birds than in mammals may generally account for the lower binding of acidic drugs in birds.

ELIMINATION PROCESSES

In domestic animal species, the liver constitutes 1.25–2.5% of live body weight, and hepatic arterial blood flow represents 26–29% of cardiac output. The hepatic portal vein contributes additionally to liver blood flow. The kidneys constitute 0.25–0.6% of live body weight and receive 22–24% of cardiac output. In avian species and reptiles, the renal portal system contributes to blood flow to the kidneys. In proportion to organ weight (mass), the kidneys are more richly perfused with blood than is the liver.

The liver metabolizes drugs, other foreign chemical compounds (xenobiotics), and certain endogenous substances (e.g., steroid hormones, bilirubin) by a variety of pathways. They include hepatic microsomal-mediated oxidative reactions, reductive and hydrolytic reactions (phase I), and conjugation (synthetic) reactions with various endogenous substances (phase II) (58, 59). Phase I metabolic reactions occur ubiquitously and are qualitatively similar in mammals, birds, and fish, but differ widely and unpredictably among species in the rates at which they take place. Although molecular structure is the primary determinant of the phase I reaction that will most likely occur, at least a moderate degree of lipid solubility is required for microsomal oxidation. The situation is

Table 9 Domestic animal species with defects in certain conjugation reactions

Species	Conjugation reaction	Major target groups	State of synthetic reaction
Cat	Glucuronide synthesis	$-OH, -COOH, -NH_2, =NH, -SH$	Present, slow rate
Dog	Acetylation	$Ar-NH_2$	Absent
Pig	Sulfate conjugation	$Ar-OH, Ar-NH_2$	Present, low extent

(From Ref. 50.)

different with regard to phase II metabolic reactions because some of these are either defective or absent in certain species, which makes the final pathways of metabolism somewhat predictable (Table 9) (50). Requirements of phase II reactions include the presence in a drug molecule (either parent drug or phase I metabolite) of a functional group that is suitable for undergoing conjugation, an endogenous reacting substance (conjugating agent), and a transferring enzyme. The major transferring enzymes are UDP-glucuronyltransferase, sulfotransferase, N-acetyltransferase, GSH-S-transferase, and methyltransferase. Conjugates of drugs are polar, less lipid-soluble, and consequently less widely distributed extravascularly than the parent drug or phase I metabolite, and the vast majority are pharmacologically inactive. Apart from a few exceptions (e.g., the N^4-acetyl derivative of most sulfonamides), drug conjugates are more water-soluble than the parent drug. Glucoronide conjugates are especially suitable for carrier-mediated active excretion in urine or bile or both. Species variations in conjugate formation could be attributed to the availability of the conjugating agent, the ability to form the "activated" nucleolide, or the activity of the transferring enzyme (60). Fish may have a low capacity to form the activated nucleolide uridine–diphosphate–glucuronic acid, which would limit glucuronide synthesis. Prodrugs belong to a different category of drug, in that prodrugs per se are devoid of activity but are metabolically converted by phase I, usually hydrolytic reactions to the active parent drug. Examples of orally administered prodrugs include enalapril (enalaprilat), pivampicillin (ampicillin), netobimin (albendazole), and febantel (fenbendazole). Metabolic conversion (activation) of these prodrugs occurs presystemically in that it is brought about by ruminal micro-organisms or takes place during passage through the intestinal mucosa or the liver (first-pass metabolism).

Ruminal microorganisms are capable of at least partially inactivating orally administered drugs (chloramphenicol, trimethoprim, nitroxynil, digoxin) by hydrolytic and reductive reactions. The susceptibility of ruminant animals to toxicity caused by ingestion of plants containing cyanogenetic glycosides (e.g., *Prunus* spp., *Acacia* spp.,

Eucalyptus cladocalyx) is attributed to ruminal hydrolysis of the glycosides with liberation of hydrogen cyanide. Intestinal micro-organisms containing β-glucuronidase can reactivate (by hydrolysis) glucuronide conjugates of drugs excreted in bile. Renal excretion is the principal process for elimination of drugs that are predominantly ionized in the plasma, polar drugs, and drug metabolites. Extensive (>80%) binding to plasma proteins limits the availability of drugs for glomerular filtration but does not hinder carrier-mediated active tubular secretion. Although a drug may enter tubular fluid both by glomerular filtration and by proximal tubular secretion, its renal clearance may nonetheless be low when substantial reabsorption occurs in the distal nephron. Because reabsorption takes place by passive diffusion, it is influenced by the concentration of drug and its degree of ionization in distal tubular fluid and by the rate of passage of glomerular filtrate through the distal nephron. The degree of ionization is determined by the pK_a value of the drug and the urinary pH reaction. The usual urinary reaction in carnivorous species is acidic (pH 5.5–7.0), whereas in herbivorous species it is alkaline (pH 7.2–8.4). The excretion of weak organic acids is enhanced under alkaline and decreased under acidic urinary conditions; the converse applies to weak organic bases. Species variations in the rate of elimination of renally excreted drugs (penicillins, most cephalosporins, aminoglycosides, most diuretics, nondepolarizing neuromuscular blocking drugs) are primarily attributable to differences in the glomerular filtration rate (GFR). Based on inulin clearance, mean values of GFR (ml/min × kg) are 3.96 in dogs; 2.94 in cats; 2.80 in pigs; 2.26, 2.25, and 2.20 in goats, cattle, and sheep, respectively; and 1.65 in horses; the estimated value of GFR in humans is 1.84 ml/min × kg. Urinary pH influences the rate of elimination of drugs that are moderately lipid-soluble and undergo elimination both by hepatic metabolism and by renal excretion (amphetamine, trimethoprim, phenobarbital, sulfonamides).

The rate of hepatocyte secretion of bile in domestic animal species is 12–24 ml/kg per day; the lower end of the range applies to the dog and cat, and the upper end applies to the horse (a species that does not have a gall bladder). Compounds excreted in bile have molecular weights exceeding 300 and a degree of polarity that enables them to be transported by a carrier-mediated process from hepatic parenchymal cells into bile. Drugs and drug metabolites (primarily conjugates) excreted in bile enter the duodenum, from which some (depending on their lipid solubility) may be reabsorbed by passive diffusion.

RATE OF ELIMINATION

Half-life is the pharmacokinetic parameter used to measure the overall rate of drug elimination. The half-life of most drugs that are primarily eliminated by hepatic biotransformation varies widely among species (Table 10). The usual trend is that half-life is shorter in cattle and horses (herbivorous species) than in dogs and cats (carnivorous species), whereas the half-life of several drugs is longer in humans than in domestic animals. There are, however, notable exceptions to this trend, such as the methylxanthines (caffeine and theophylline) in horses and phenylbutazone in cattle. The half-life of phenylbutazone in cattle varies from 42 to 66 h and, unlike in horses, dogs, and humans, does not appear to be dose-dependent. Because of differences in the rate of hepatic elimination (presumably by biotransformation), the half-life of various drugs (sulfamethazine, trimethoprim, ceftiofur/desfuroylceftiofur, closantel, clorsulon) is shorter in goats (especially dwarf goats) than in sheep, whereas the half-life of some drugs (phenylbutazone, norfloxacin) is shorter in donkeys than in horses and ponies.

Because phenytoin, valproate, carbamazepine and clonazepam have a much shorter half-life in dogs than in humans (Table 11), the dosage intervals that would be required for anticonvulsant effectiveness in dogs make conventional dosage forms of these drugs impractical for therapeutic use (61). The half-life of phenobarbital and naproxen is 2-fold longer in mongrel (mixed-breed) dogs than in Beagles. The long half-life of naproxen in dogs (74 h in mongrels, 35 h in Beagles) is unusual for a nonsteroidal anti-inflammatory drug. Naproxen half-life is 13.9 h in humans, 8.3 h in horses, 4.8 h in minipigs, and 1.9 h in Rhesus monkeys.

The half-life of salicylate, which is primarily eliminated by glucuronide conjugation, is 25–35 h and dose-dependent in cats, compared with 10–15 h in humans, 8.6 h in dogs, 1 h in horses, and 0.8 h in cattle. A relative deficiency of hepatic microsomal glucuronyl-transferase activity appears to be characteristic of *Felidae*, because it applies not only to the domestic cat (*Felis catus*) but also to the lion (*Panthera leo*), African civet (*Viverra civetta*), and forest genet (*Genetta pardina*) (62). Even though dogs and foxes (*Canidae*) are unable to acetylate aromatic ($ArNH_2$) and hyrazine ($RNHNH_2$ or $ArNHNH_2$) amino groups, the absence of this metabolic pathway does not appear to delay the elimination of drugs with these functional groups (sulfonamides, procainamide). Either a larger fraction of the systemically available dose is excreted as parent drug in the urine or an alternative metabolic pathway compensates for the absence of acetylation of these amino groups. Amino acid conju-

Table 10 Species variations in the half-life of some drugs that are primarily eliminated by hepatic metabolism

Drug	Cattle	Horse	Dog	Human
Pentobarbitone	0.8	1.5	4.5	22.3
Thiopentone	3.3	2.5	8.3	11.5
Salicylate	0.8	1.0	8.6	12.0
Phenylbutazone	42–66	4.1–4.7[a]	2.5–6.0[a]	72.0[a]
Flunixin	6.9	1.9	3.7	—
Morphine	—	1.0	0.95	1.9
Ketamine	0.9	0.7	1.0	2.5
Caffeine	3.8	18.2	4.25	4.9
Theophylline	6.9	14.8	5.7	9.0
Norfloxacin	2.4	6.4	3.6	5.0
Enrofloxacin	1.7	5.0	3.4	—
Chloramphenicol	3.6	0.9	4.2	4.6
Metronidazole	2.8	3.9	4.5	8.5
Trimethoprim[b]	1.25	3.2	4.6	10.6
Sulphadiazine[b]	2.5	3.6	5.6	9.9
Sulphadimethoxine[b]	12.5	11.3	13.2	40

[a]Half-life is dose-dependent.
[b]Half-life may be influenced by urinary pH reaction.

Table 11 Comparison of the average half-life (h) after intravenous administration (apart from carbamazepine) of a single dose of anticonvulsant drugs in dogs and humans

Drug	Dog	Human	Therapeutic range of plasma concentrations (μg/ml)
Phenobarbitone	64	96	10–25
Phenytoin	3.5–4.5[a]	15–24[a]	10–20
Sodium valproate	2	14	40–100
Carbamazepine (PO)	1.5	15	4–10
Clonazepam	1.5–2.5[a]	24–36[a]	0.01–0.08
Diazepam	7.6[b]	32.9[b]	>0.15

[a]Half-life is dose-dependent.
[b]Parent drug and active metabolites.

gation in domestic animal species often involves glycine as the endogenous reacting substance. Glycine conjugation takes place in both the liver and the kidneys of domestic animals other than the dog, in which it occurs only in the kidneys. The transferring enzyme, which is located in mitochondria, is acyl-CoA glycinetransferase. Glycine is replaced by ornithine as the conjugating agent in birds classified as anseriformes (ducks, geese) and galliformes (chickens, turkeys) but not in columbiformes (pigeons, doves) (59).

Even though exceptions exist, which is inevitable in view of the variety of metabolic pathways, the half-life of the majority of drugs that undergo extensive hepatic biotransformation is shorter in laboratory animal species (mice, rats, guinea pigs, rabbits) and Rhesus monkeys than in domestic animal species and humans. Consistent with this trend is that the average half-life of antipyrine, a marker substance used to indicate hepatic microsomal oxidative activity, is shorter in laboratory animals (0.2–1.4 h) and Rhesus monkeys (1.2 h) than in domestic animals (1.75–3.25 h) and especially humans (10.3–12.7 h). It has been hypothesized (63) that the lesser capacity of humans to metabolize drugs by hepatic microsomal oxidation may be correlated with their enhanced longevity, expressed as maximum lifespan potential. Based on an equation using brain weight and body weight, maximum lifespan potential is estimated to be 93 y in humans, 39 y in horses, 20 y in dogs, 14 y in cats and, for comparative purposes, 77 y in African elephants.

As with the situation in mammals, wide variations exist among avian species in the half-life of drugs that are primarily eliminated by hepatic biotransformation (64). The half-life of antimicrobial agents is prolonged in poikilothermic species (fish and reptiles), which is consistent with their much lower metabolic turnover rate (65), and is influenced by ambient (in the case of fish, water) temperature (Table 12). The rate of drug elimination

increases (i.e., half-life decreases) with increase in ambient temperature and varies among fish species.

Species variations in the half-life of drugs that are eliminated by renal excretion is less pronounced than for lipid-soluble drugs that undergo extensive hepatic biotransformation. The half-life of gentamicin, which is eliminated solely by glomerular filtration, is 0.5–1 h in laboratory animals, 1.25–2.5 h in domestic animals, 2.75 h in humans, 1.25–3.4 h in various avian species, and 12 h in channel catfish (*Ictalurus punctatus*) acclimatazed at 22°C. In mammalian species, the half-life of gentamicin reflects the relative (not actual) rate of glomerular filtration and is unrelated to urinary pH reaction. The volume of distribution of gentamicin is similar (250–300 ml/kg) in the various species.

The half-life of drugs that undergo a high degree of enterohepatic circulation may vary widely among species and may be relatively more prolonged in fish. The half-life of oxytetracycline is 80.3 h in African catfish (*Clarias gariepinus*) acclimatazed at 25°C and 89.5 h in rainbow trout (*Salmo gairdneri*) at 12°C (66) compared with half-life of 9 h in humans, 3.4–9.6 h in domestic animals, and 1.3 h in rabbits. A combination of variables, which include the extent of distribution and the degree of enterohepatic circulation, contributes to species variation in the half-life of digoxin, which ranges from 7.8 h in cattle to 35 h in cats.

CLEARANCE

The systemic clearance of propofol, based on measurement of blood concentrations, in humans (31 ml/min × kg) and dogs (59 ml/min × kg) exceeds liver blood flow, which is 24 and 42 ml/min per kilogram of body weight in humans and dogs, respectively. It can be concluded that another organ (the lungs) or extrahepatic tissue contrib-

Table 12 Half-life of some antimicrobial agents in various species of fish

Antimicrobial agent	Fish species	Acclimatization temperature (°C)	Half-life (h)
Trimethoprim	Carp	10	40.7
	(*Cyprinus carpio* L.)	24	20.0
Sulphadiazine	Carp	10	47.0
	(*Cyprinus carpio* L.)	24	33.0
Sulphadimidine	Carp	10	50.3
	(*Cyprinus carpio* L.)	20	25.6
	Rainbow trout	10	20.6
	(*Salmo gairdneri*)	20	14.7
Ciprofloxacin	Rainbow trout	12	11.2
	(*Salmo gairdneri*)		
	Carp	20	14.5
	(*Cyprinus carpio*)		
	African catfish	25	14.2
	(*Clarias gariepinus*)		
Florfenicol	Atlantic salmon	10.8 ± 1.5	12.2
	(*Salmo salar*)	(Sea water)	
Oxytetracycline	Rainbow trout	12	89.5
	(*Salmo gairdneri*)		
	African catfish	25	80.3
	(*Clarias gariepinus*)		
Gentamicin	Channel catfish	22	12.0
	(*Ictalurus punctatus*)		

utes to the elimination (metabolism) of propofol. The blood propofol concentration at which dogs return to the sternal position and human beings regain consciousness appears to be the same (1 µg/ml).

When applied to conventional (immediate-release) aminophylline tablets, the dosing rates that would provide an average steady-state plasma theophylline concentration of 10 ug/ml and produce a sustained bronchodilator effect are 10 mg/kg administered at 8-h dosage intervals to dogs and 5 mg/kg administered at 12-h intervals to horses or cats. The systemic clearance of theophylline is 2.5 times higher in dogs (100 ml/h × kg) than in horses and cats (40 ml/h × kg), whereas systemic availability of the drug from the oral dosage form is similar (90–100%).

INTERSPECIES SCALING

The basic assumption in interspecies scaling is that physiological variables and biochemical processes are related to the body weight of mammalian species. The use of clearance, a physiologically based parameter, may be more appropriate than half-life (a hybrid parameter) for interspecies allometric scaling of drug elimination. A double logarithmic plot of the pharmacokinetic parameter of interest versus body weight of the animal species is used to verify the linearity of the allometric relationship.

The systemic clearance of structurally unrelated drugs that undergo elimination by various processes shows a high degree of correlation with the body weight of several animal species (Table 13). Inulin (marker substance) and gentamicin are eliminated by glomerular filtration and ampicillin by glomerular filtration and proximal tubular secretion, whereas oxytetracycline undergoes enterohepatic circulation and consequently is slowly excreted by glomerular filtration. Enrofloxacin, theophylline, and antipyrine are poorly extracted by the liver, which implies that their clearance may be influenced both by the unbound fraction in blood and by the metabolic capacity of the liver and are eliminated by phase I hepatic metabolism. Enrofloxacin and theophylline are eliminated primarily by microsomal-mediated oxidative reactions, whereas antipyrine (marker substance) is eliminated entirely by microsomal oxidation. Interspecies scaling of antipyrine clearance identifies the human as a nonconforming species, which is attributed to the substantially lower microsomal oxidative capacity of humans relative to the 10 other species studied. Because of species variations in

Table 13 Allometric relationship between the clearance (ml/min) of some drugs and body weight (kg) of various mammalian species

Drug	Elimination process	No. of species	Allometric Coefficient	Exponent	Correlation coefficient
Inulin	E (r)	8[a]	4.13	0.86	0.989
Gentamicin	E (r)	8[a]	2.60	0.86	0.970
Ampicillin	E (r)	8[b]	5.47	0.94	0.959
Oxytetracycline	E (r)	8[c]	7.96	0.73	0.978
Enrofloxacin	M (h)	8[d]	12.53	0.93	0.984
Theophylline	M (h)	9[c]	1.98	0.83	0.978
Antipyrine	M (h)	10[f]	8.16	0.85	0.989

[a] Cat, dog, goat, sheep, pig, human, cattle, horse.
[b] Rabbit, dog, sheep, pig, human, donkey, cattle, horse.
[c] Rabbit, dog, goat, sheep, pig, donkey, cattle, horse.
[d] Rabbit, cat, dog, sheep, pig, ilama, horse, cow.
[e] Rat, guinea pig, rabbit, cat, dog, pig, human, cattle, horse.
[f] Mouse, rat, guinea pig, rabbit, monkey, dog, goat, sheep, pig, cattle (human is a nonconforming species).
For each drug, the level of significance is $P < 0.001$.

binding to plasma proteins, the use of hepatic intrinsic clearance of unbound drug, rather than systemic clearance, would represent a refinement of the allometric scaling technique. This refinement has been applied to interspecies scaling of antipyrine (67) and theophylline (68). Additional correction could be made for maximum lifespan potential (63). Because the clearance of highly extracted drugs that undergo extensive phase I hepatic metabolism is primarily determined by a single physiological variable (liver blood flow), interspecies allometric scaling should be feasible for drugs in this category. The index of drug elimination (half-life, systemic clearance, organ clearance of unbound drug) to use depends on the level of refinement required.

With regard to organ (liver, kidney, heart) weights, physiological variables (liver blood flow, renal function, cardiac output, basal oxygen consumption), and the pharmacokinetic parameters systemic clearance and volume of distribution, the numerical value of the allometric exponent is generally in the range of 0.67 to 1. For physiological periods(heartbeat time, duration of respiratory cycle), turnover times (serum albumin, total body water, blood circulation), and drug half-life, the allometric exponent is often close to 0.25, which represents that for energy expenditure in mammalian species (69) and the turnover time of endogenous processes (63).

The reliability of predictions based on interspecies allometric scaling of drug disposition depends on the use of a sensitive and precise analytical method for quantification of the drug (and active metabolite) in blood or plasma, a knowledge of the principal elimination

process for the drug, the use of at least four animal species representing a wide range of body weight (based on log body weight ratio), and the identification, for possible exclusion, of any nonconforming species. Because of the uniqueness of each animal species, application of the technique for predictive purposes should be limited to the preclinical stage of drug development.

IMPLICATIONS OF STEREOISOMERISM

Stereoisomerism has implications in the formulating of dosage forms and because a chiral environment exists within the body, in determining both the degree of activity and the disposition of racemates. The enantioselective behavior of drugs used in domestic animals was comprehensively reviewed by Landoni et al. (70).

Because stereoselective processes are species-related, the enantiomeric ratios of plasma concentrations at various times and areas under the plasma concentration-time curves may differ among animal species after the administration of a drug racemate. Chiral inversion, which occurs to a variable extent in different species, can be equivocally established only by administering individual enantiomers to the animal species of interest and measuring, using a sensitive stereospecific analytical method, the enantiomer administered and the optical antipode in biological fluids and tissues. The pharmacokinetic parameters based on plasma concentration−time data for each of the enantiomers can be statistically compared.

The 2-arylpropionic acid ("profen") nonsteroidal anti-inflammatory drugs, each of which contains a single chiral center, are formulated as racemic (50:50) mixtures of the S(+)- and R(−)- enantiomers, with the exception of naproxen, which is formulated as the S(+)-enantiomer. Based on inhibition of cyclo-oxygenase activity, the S(+)-enantiomer is the eutomer (more potent enantiomer). These drugs differ markedly in both pharmacodynamic activity and pharmacokinetic behavior and, in addition, enantiomer pharmacokinetics of each drug varies among animal species. After intravenous administration of racemic ketoprofen to horses, sheep, and 20-week-old calves and measurement of individual enantiomers in plasma, significant differences between the enantiomers were found in systemic clearance in horses and in both systemic clearance and volume of distribution in sheep (Table 14), whereas values of the pharmacokinetic parameters in calves did not differ between the enantiomers (71–73). The S(+)- to R(−) ratio of area under the curve was 1.35:1 in horses, 0.54:1 in sheep, and 1.05:1 in calves. The predominant enantiomer in plasma was S(+) in horses, R(−) in sheep, and both enantiomers were present in equal concentrations in calves. After the administration of each enantiomer separately to these species, the extent of chiral inversion from the R(−)- to S(+)-enantiomer was estimated to be 49% in horses, 5.9% in sheep, and 31% in calves (72, 74, 75). Unidirectional chiral inversion was estimated to be 49% in Cynomolgus monkeys (*Macaca*) (76), 9% in humans (77), and varied from 27 to 66% in laboratory animal species (78). The oral bioavailability of the S(+)-enantiomer of ketoprofen in Beagle dogs is not affected by the proportion of the R(−)-enantiomer in the oral dosage form, even though considerable (73%) metabolic inversion from the R(−) to the S(+)-enantiomer occurs in dogs (79).

It is usual in humans for the S(+)-enantiomer of 2-arylpropionic acids to predominate in plasma and for the S(+)- to R(−)-enantiomeric ratio of plasma concentrations to increase with time after administration of the racemate, which is often attributed to metabolic inversion of the chiral center of the R(−)-enantiomers to their S(+)-antipodes (80). In humans, the S(+)-enantiomer is generally eliminated more slowly than is the R(−)-enantiomer. The extent of chiral inversion of fenoprofen, which has been attributed to the differential rate of formation of the CoA-thioester by hepatic microsomes (81, 82), varies widely among species. It has been estimated to be 90% in dogs (83), 80% in sheep (81), 73% in rabbits (84), 60% in humans (85), 42% in rats (86), and 38% in horses (83).

Carprofen, a weak inhibitor of cyclo-oxygenase but which produces a significant antioedematous effect in dogs (87) and horses (88) and has potent antiplatelet-aggregating properties, does not appear to undergo chiral inversion in either direction in horses, calves, dogs, cats, and humans. After intravenous or oral administration of racemic carprofen, which contains a 50:50 mixture of the enantiomers, to horses (i.v.), 8- to 10-week-old calves (i.v.), cats (i.v.), and dogs (p.o.), the R(−)-enantiomer predominated in the plasma and the R(−)- to S(+)-enantiomeric ratio of plasma concentrations increased with time after administration of the racemate. The increasing R(−):S(+) enantiomeric ratio of plasma concentrations with time can be attributed to stereoselective hepatic metabolism, although stereoselective binding to plasma albumin could contribute. A contrasting situation to that which occurs in domestic animals was found in rats and humans, in that the S(+)-enantiomer predominated in plasma and the R(−):S(+) enantiomeric ratio of plasma concentrations decreased (although only slightly in humans) with time after administration of the racemate (89, 90). The R(−)- to- S(+) ratio of area under

Table 14 Pharmacokinetic parameters describing disposition of S(+)- and R(−)-enantiomers after intravenous administration of racemic ketoprofen (KTP) to horses($n = 6$) and sheep ($n = 6$)

Pharmacokinetic parameter	Horses		Sheep	
	S(+)-KTP	R(−)-KPT	S(+)-KTP	R(−)-KTP
$t_{1/2(\alpha)}$ (h)	0.13 ± 0.03	0.10 ± 0.02	0.14 ± 0.01	0.13 ± 0.03
$t_{1/2(\beta)}$ (h)	1.51 ± 0.45	1.09 ± 0.19	0.86 ± 0.08	0.87 ± 0.10
V_d (ml/kg)	491 ± 206	472 ± 146	256 ± 21	168 ± 15[a]
CL_B (ml/h × kg)	202 ± 22	277 ± 35[a]	351 ± 50	196 ± 32[a]
MRT (h)	2.23 ± 0.15	2.63 ± 0.33	0.79 ± 0.11	0.95 ± 0.13
AUC (μg × h/ml)	5.67 ± 0.47	4.19 ± 0.37[a]	4.74 ± 0.71	8.73 ± 1.22[a]

[a]$P<0.05$.
Values are expressed as mean ± S.E.M.
(From Refs. 71 and 72)

the plasma concentration–time curve (AUC) was 4.5:1 in horses (91), 2.0:1 in cats (92), 1.8:1 in dogs (87), and 1.4:1 in calves (93), after administration of the racemate. Area under the curve enantiomeric ratios in rats and humans were not determined.

Ketamine, which is present in the commercially available preparation as a 50:50 mixture of the S(+)- and R(−)-enantiomers, is metabolized by hepatic microsomal N-demethylation to the corresponding norketamine (metabolite I) enantiomers. Based on the reported eudismic ratio of S(+):R(−) for ketamine enantiomers of 2.9:1 and the observed duration of unconsciousness in dogs and the plasma concentrations in humans at time of emergence from anesthesia which are 0.5 [S(+)] and 1.7 [R(−)] μg/ml, it can be concluded that the S(+)-enantiomer is three times more active than is the R(−)-enantiomer (94, 95). After intravenous injection of racemic ketamine, the S(+)-enantiomer of norketamine predominated in the plasma of horses (96) and dogs (97). This could be attributed to enantioselective N-demethylation. Systemic clearances of racemic ketamine are 15, 28, and 29 ml/min ×kg in humans, horses, and dogs, respectively. Because the disposition of the individual enantiomers administered separately has not been studied, comment cannot be made regarding the extent of chiral inversion.

Whether a racemate or an enantiomer of a chiral drug should be used in formulating dosage forms depends on the relative pharmacodynamic activity and the potential toxicity (or side effects) of the individual enantiomers, their pharmacokinetic profiles, and, importantly, the proportions formed over time in the target animal species. Binding to plasma and tissue proteins, hepatic microsomal oxidative reactions, and probably glucuronide conjugation and carrier-mediated excretion processes are stereoselective and vary among animal species. First-pass metabolism may influence oral bioavailability of the enantiomers of chiral drugs that are highly extracted by the liver and administered as racemic mixtures. When both enantiomers of a drug with a single chiral center show distinct and desirable effects (e.g., most opioids, dobutamine, bupivacaine), even though they differ in pharmacodynamic activity or when their action and the effects produced are not stereoselective, the formulating of racemic mixtures may be entirely justifiable (98). Nonetheless, because of species variation, pharmacokinetic profiles of the individual enantiomers should be determined using stereospecific analytical methods (99–102) to calculate optimum dosage for the various animal species. Use of the more active enantiomer (eutomer) in formulating dosage forms should be considered when the enantiomers differ widely in pharmacodynamic activity [e.g., S(−)-propranolol, the S(+)-enantiomer of the 2-arylpropionic acid nonsteroidal

anti-inflammatory drugs, d-propoxyphene] or toxic potential (levamisole is the l-isomer of racemic tetramisole, which can produce many side effects). To selectively produce a certain effect, a distomer (less potent enantiomer) could be formulated as a particular dosage form, e.g., R(+)-timolol as eyedrops to reduce intraocular pressure (glaucoma), R(+)-verapamil as a parenteral or oral dosage form for the treatment of angina (103). The use of an enantiomer, a single chemical entity, would increase selectivity of action, reduce total exposure to the racemate, and simplify dose–response relationships. When an enantiomer is used in formulating dosage forms, it must be optically pure. Bioequivalence assessment of a generic drug preparation requires that the generic preparation contain the racemic drug or the enantiomer corresponding to whichever is present in the innovator (reference) dosage form.

PERCUTANEOUS ABSORPTION

The skin accounts for approximately 10% of live body weight in cattle, goats, and dogs; 7.5% in horses; and 3.7% in humans. Although skin receives approximately 6% of cardiac output, cutaneous blood flow rate to various regions differs among species (104). In humans and pigs, the cutaneous circulation supplies blood (in musculocutaneous arteries) to both the skin and the underlying musculature, whereas in dogs and cats (loose-skin species), blood is supplied directly to the skin.

ABSORPTION PROCESS

The absorption process for a topically applied drug essentially involves the following stages: dissolution of the drug in and release from the vehicle, drug penetration (by diffusion) through the *stratum*, and permeation through the "living" layers of the epidermis to the underlying dermis where absorption into the systemic circulation takes place. Although the initial stage is formulation-dependent in that it relates to the form of the drug and the nature of the vehicle, the translocation stages are primarily governed by the molecular structure and physiocochemical properties of the drug. Penetration of the stratum corneum is generally the rate-limiting step in the absorption process (105). Only lipid-soluble drugs can diffuse through the dead, compacted, keratinized cells (corneocytes) of the stratum corneum. However, passive diffusion through the epidermis, including the stratum corneum, can take place by one, or more, of the following routes:

transcellular through the corneocytes, intercellular through the lipid matrix (a tortuous path), or along the sweat gland ducts and hair follicles (appendageal path). Even though lipophilic substances may penetrate the stratum corneum by transcellular diffusion, some degree of water solubility is required for passage through the "living" layers of the epidermis. Polar drugs have a low capacity to penetrate the stratum corneum but may gain access to the "living" epidermal layers by shunt diffusion along the appendageal path. Additional factors that influence percutaneous absorption include the nature of the vehicle, the state of hydration of the stratum corneum, drug persistence in the stratum corneum or other strata of the epidermis, biotransformation in the epidermis, and species differences in histological structure of skin. In aquatic mammals, the stratum corneum is very thick, and the corneocytes are solidly apposed, whereas the epidermis is devoid of a stratum granulosum regardless of whether the skin is glabrous (as in whales) or hairy (as in seals) (106).

The average thickness of the stratum corneum in laboratory and domestic animals and humans is in the range of 10 to 35 μm. The thickness of this epidermal layer might not influence the penetration of chemical substances, whereas the density of appendages per unit surface area, which differs among animal species, does influence passage through the epidermis. Human skin contains an average of 40–70 hair follicles and 200–250 sweat glands per square centimeter, whereas cattle skin contains approximately 2000 hair follicles, with associated sweat and sebaceous glands, per square centimeter (107). The mean follicle density in 10 British breeds of sheep varies from 1000 to 2000 per square centimeter of skin, with a secondary-to-primary follicle ratio of 2.4:1–5.9:1 (108). The ratio of secondary to primary follicles appears to be higher in Merino sheep skin in wool-growing regions. The sebaceous glands of cattle and sheep exude large quantities of lipoid material (lanolin in the case of sheep) that serve to protect their skin. The emulsifying properties of exocrine secretions may enhance dissolution and thus facilitate percutaneous absorption of topically applied compounds in cattle and sheep. Seasonal changes in the composition of secretions may cause variations in absorption of moderately lipid-soluble drugs (e.g., levamisole applied by "pour on") at different times of the year (109). Because of the larger number of skin appendages per unit of surface area, the appendageal path will likely contribute more to percutaneous absorption of hydrophilic substances in cattle and sheep than in other species. Horses and humans have highly effective sweat glands, whereas cattle, sheep, pigs, dogs, and cats are unable to sweat profusely. Changes in ambient temperature appear to affect animal skin temperature to a higher degree than human skin temperature, which suggests that skin plays a greater role in thermoregulation in humans than in animals.

The state of hydration of the stratum corneum, which is normally maintained at 10–15%, affects the rate of penetration of chemical substances. By increasing the state of hydration to 50%, the rate of permeation of some chemical substances through the epidermis can be increased up to 10-fold (110). Occlusion has been shown to enhance the pharmacological effect of topically applied hydrocortisone and fluocinolone acetonide (111); however, percutaneous absorption of drugs is not necessarily increased. The degree of occlusion-induced absorption enhancement appears to increase with increasing lipophilicity of drug substances.

Formulations containing an absorption-promoting substance, such as propylene glycol or sodium lauryl sulfate, may increase the permeability of the stratum corneum to water-soluble drugs. Propylene glycol is a commonly used vehicle in topical corticosteroid preparations for veterinary use. Various aprotic solvents, which include dimethylacetamide, dimethylformamide, dimethylsulfoxide, tetrahydrofurfuryl alcohol, and 2-pyrrolidone, serve as penetration enhancers of polar drugs (112). Dimethylsulfoxide (DMSO) is used in formulating some topical veterinary preparations. The penetration-enhancing property of DMSO is markedly concentration-dependent. At concentrations below 50% DMSO is water, the penetration rate of many drugs differs little than from aqueous solutions. The penetration rate of levamisole through skin of cattle and sheep was somewhat slower from a formulation containing DMSO (concentration not specified) than from an aqueous solution of the drug (107). Plasma and gastrointestinal fluid concentrations of levamisole were lower after pour-on application to cattle than after oral administration or subcutaenous injection of the drug (109). Parathion penetrated the skin of pigs more rapidly when formulated in DMSO than in other vehicles (glycerol–formal/isopropranol mixture, octanol, macrogol 400) (Table 15) (113). The formation of a stable 2:1 water hydrate at a concentration of 67% v/v DMSO may explain its dehydrating and penetration-enhancing effects when present at high concentration (114). These effects are accompanied by, or perhaps attributable to, epidermal tissue damage. Mineral oil may be used in formulating long-acting, water-based topical preparations of synthetic pyrethroids (permethrin, cypermethrin) for application to ruminant animals. This type of preparation would not be washed off by rain and could provide protection against flies for an extended period. Water-insoluble substances can be formulated as emulsifiable concentrates. The emulsifiable concentrate contains one or more surfactants and produces an emulsion or micellar solution with the

Table 15 Pharmacokinetic parameters for parathion (50 mg/kg) applied topically in various vehicles to pigs

Pharmacokinetic parameter	Vehicles			
	GFI[a]	DMSO	Octanol	Macrogol 400
AUC (μg × h/L)	1460–1795	1630–3050	2010–3310	595–600
MRT (h)	57–106	9.7–14.5	22–31	54–60
MAT (h)	55–104	7.5–12.5	20–29	52–58
Bioavailability (%)	16–20	19–28	15–29	3.9–54

[a]GFI = glycerol–formal/isopropanol mixture.
Bioavailability (absolute) was based on $AUC_{topical}/AUC_{IV}$, with correction for dose.
(From Ref. 113.)

water-insoluble drug in the nonaqueous phase when mixed with water (107).

SPECIES VARIATIONS

The barrier properties of skin vary with the species of animal and within a species may differ between regions of the body. Based on limited data obtained from in vitro studies of skin permeability, it could be speculated that species can, in general, be ranked in the following order: rabbits > rats > guinea pigs > cats > dogs > pigs and Rhesus monkeys > humans (least permeable skin). Because of a lack of data, horses, cattle, sheep, and goats are not included in the comparison of skin permeability. The emulsifying property and occlusive effect of sebum and the high density of appendages per unit of surface area would be expected to facilitate percutaneous absorption of substances in ruminant species.

The maximal rate of penetration of an organophosphorus compound through skin sections excised from the dorsal thorax of various species generally supports the skin permeability ranking of species vide supra (Table 16) (115). The compound rapidly penetrated the skin of rabbits and rats, whereas penetration through pig skin occurred more slowly than through skin of the other species. Even though pig skin and human skin are similar in many respects (116), percutaneous absorption of a variety of compounds in the pig was found to range from zero to four times that in humans in vivo (117). Advantage can be taken of the often similar permeability characteristics of pig and human skins with avoidance of the systemic/fat distribution difference in vivo by using the isolated perfused porcine skin flap in vitro model (118, 119). The diffusion of chemical substances through skin and

metabolism within the skin can be determined by assay of the perfusate. The sum of the amount of compound that diffused into the perfusate and the residual amount in the skin preparation at the end of the exposure period to the drug provide an estimation of percutaneous absorption.

Regional variations in percutaneous absorption contribute to differences in the systemic availability of a drug depending on the site of topical application. The Rhesus monkey (*Macaca mulatta*) could probably serve as an animal model for human skin regional variation (120).

The absolute bioavailability of a topically applied drug can be determined only by measurement of plasma concentrations and comparing total areas under the curves or, less reliably, the amounts excreted in urine over a period of at least six half-lives after topical application and intravenous injection of the drug. An appropriate washout period must be allowed to elapse between the phases of a crossover study, which is the experimental design that should be used whenever feasible. Because of species

Table 16 Maximal penetration of radiolabeled organophosphorus compound through excised skin from dorsal thorax of various species

Species	Rate (μg/cm^2/min)
Pig	0.3
Dog	2.7
Monkey	4.2
Goat	4.4
Cat	4.4
Guinea pig	6.0
Rabbit	9.3
Rat	9.3

(From Ref. 115.)

variations in ultrastructure of skin, cutaneous blood supply, density of appendages per unit of surface area, and activity of biotransformation pathways, the percutaneous absorption (rate and extent) of a drug is best determined by performing the study in the species of interest.

CUTANEOUS BIOTRANSFORMATION

Epidermal cytochrome P450 and hydrolytic enzymes in the lipid matrix of the stratum corneum as well as in the stratum granulosum may be involved in conversion reactions of topically applied steroids (121). In pigs, epidermal cytochrome P450 has been shown to convert parathion to paraoxon by oxidative desulfuration (122). The oxygen analog formed is rapidly hydrolyzed to inactive metabolites. The significant difference between mammals and insects in the rate at which the hydrolytic reaction takes place accounts for the selective toxicity of thiophosphate insecticides. The extent to which the ultrastructural difference in the epidermis of aquatic and terrestrial mammals affects the activity of drug-metabolizing enzymes in skin is not known. Fish appear to be unable to detoxify thiophosphate insecticides.

Benzoyl peroxide, the active ingredient in some shampoos for dogs, is almost completely metabolized to benzoic acid in the epidermis. Benzoic acid undergoes conjugation with glycine, primarily in the liver, and is excreted in urine as hippuric acid. Methylation of norepinephrine to epinephrine, an *N*-transferase-mediated conjugation reaction, in human and animal skin preparations has been reported (123).

Biotransformation of propranolol, which involves microsomal-mediated oxidative reactions and glucuronide conjugation, is stereoselective in both the liver and the skin. Based on in vitro studies, using intact human skin and microsomal preparations, of percutaneous absorption and metabolism of racemic propranolol, it was concluded that the S(−)-enantiomer (eutomer) is metabolized more efficiently by skin than is the R(+)-enantiomer (124). The converse applies to hepatocytes, which metabolize the R(+)-enantiomer more efficiently (125). The cytochrome P450 mono-oxygenase enzymes in skin, as in the liver, can be induced (by dexamethasone, for example) or inhibited (chloramphenicol, imidazole antifungal agents). The clinical significance of altered microsomal enzyme activity in the epidermis has not been established. Metronidazole, which is available as a topical gel, inhibits acetaldehyde dehydrogenase (a nonmicrosomal enzyme); however, whether the enzyme is present in skin does not appear to be known.

TOPICAL PREPARATIONS

There is a wide variety of veterinary drug preparations available for topical application to the skin. Although most of these preparations are intended to produce local effects, some are formulated to distribute via the systemic circulation to skin covering all regions of the body or to produce systemic effects. Because of the prevalence of ectoparasites, several ectoparasiticidal preparations are available for topical application by various methods depending on the animal species (Table 17). Liquid concentrates, which must be appropriately diluted before use, and prepared solutions are convenient to apply and, depending on susceptibility of the ectoparasite and persistence of the drug in skin, may provide effective treatment and protection against reinfestation for an extended period. The usual method of application of prepared solutions is by pour on to cattle, sheep, pigs, and horses, whereas "spot on" is preferred for dogs and cats. The active ingredient in preparations for pour-on application must be sufficiently lipid-soluble for percutaneous absorption to occur, and the preparation should provide residual activity in the stratum corneum and stratum germinativum and not be removed from the skin by environmental conditions (such as rain) or by rubbing. Diluted liquid concentrates are applied by spray to cattle, horses, pigs, and poultry and by either dip or spray to sheep. Because of the large quantity of drug required for dipping sheep and the difficulty of safe disposal of dip, application of diluted liquid (dip) concentrate as a spray, but at a higher

Table 17 Dosage forms and methods of application of topical ectoparasiticide preparations to individual species

Animal species	Dosage form	Method of application
Cattle	Solution	Pour on
	Liquid concentrate[a]	Spray
	Ear tag	Attach to ears
Sheep	Liquid concentrate[a]	Dip, spray
	Solution	Spot on, pour on
Pigs	Solution	Pour on, spot on
	Liquid concentrate[a]	Spray
Horses	Solution	Pour on
	Liquid concentrate[a]	Spray, shampoo
	Lotion	Dab on
Dogs and cats	Solution	Spot on, spray (dogs)
	Collar	Surrounding neck
	Dusting power	Apply to coat
	Liquid concentrate[a]	Sponge on (dogs)
	Shampoo	Wash (dogs)

[a]Liquid concentrates must be appropriately diluted before use on animals.

Table 18 Dosage forms of preparations containing synthetic pyrethroids and the methods of topical application to various species

Dosage form	Animal species	Method of application
Solution	Cattle, sheep, horses, pigs, dogs, cats	Pour on
		Spot on, spray (dogs)
Liquid concentrate	Cattle, sheep, horses, poultry	spray, dip (sheep)
Dusting powder	Dogs, cats	Apply to coat
Shampoo	Dogs	Wash
Collar	Dogs, cats	Surrounding neck
Ear tag	Cattle	Attach to ears

Synthetic pyrethroids: cypermethrin, deltamethrin, fenvalerate, flumethrin, permethrin.

concentration than that used in the dip bath, is becoming a popular method of ectoparasiticide application by sheep farmers. The relative effectiveness of spraying versus dipping sheep for the treatment and prevention of ectoparasite infestation is open to question. When choosing between an organophosphorus compound (dimpylate, propetamphos) and a synthetic pyrethroid (flumethrin, cypermethrin) for dipping sheep, a consideration (in addition to residual protection) that could be of practical relevance is that there is no withdrawal period associated with the use of synthetic pyrethroids. The low toxicity of pyrethroids in mammals is primarily attributed to the rapid biotransformation by ester hydrolysis and/or hydroxylation (phase I metabolic reactions). Unlike mammals, fish are extremely sensitive to pyrethroid toxicity.

Synthetic pyrethroids (cypermethrin, deltamethrin, fenvalerate, flumethrin, permethrin) are available in a variety of dosage forms for topical application to domestic animals (Table 18). The appropriate dosage form of a pyrethroid is primarily determined by the animal species, whereas due consideration is given to the ectoparasites and insects that affect the species. Aerosol sprays are more suitable for application to dogs than to cats, because cats resent (fearful response) being sprayed and lick the applied preparation from their coat. The combination preparation containing fenvalerate (0.09%), a synthetic pyrethroid, and diethyltoluamide (9.5%), a cutaneous penetration-enhancing substance, has been reported to cause acute toxicity in cats and occasionally in dogs (126, 127).

Macrolide endectocides (avermectins and milbemycins) have activity at low concentrations against both internal (nematode) and external (arthropod) parasites. Veterinary preparations of avermectins include parenteral solutions (for subcutaneous injection), various oral dosage forms, and topical solutions (Table 19). The different preparations are specifically designed for use in certain animal species. The topical solution of ivermectin or doramectin is applied to cattle by pouron, whereas the

Table 19 Dosage forms and routes of administration of avermectins to various animal species

Dosage form	Avermectin	Animal species	Route of administration
Parenteral			
Solution	Ivermectin, doramectin	Cattle, sheep	S.C. injection
	Ivermectin	pigs, (cats)	S.C. injection
Oral			
Solution	Ivermectin	Sheep, goats	Drench
Controlled-release ruminal bolus	Ivermectin	Cattle	P.O.
Controlled-release ruminal capsule	Ivermectin	Sheep	P.O.
Premix	Ivermectin	Pigs	Addition to feed
Paste	Ivermectin	Horses	P.O.
Tablet	Ivermectin	Dogs	P.O.
Topical			
Solution	Ivermectin, doramectin	Cattle	Pour on
Solution	Selamectin	Dogs, cats	Spot on

topical solution of selamectin is applied to dogs and cats by spot-on. Preparations for spot-on application contain concentrated solutions of ectoparasiticides and should be applied directly to the skin at one (cats) or two (dogs) locations where the animal is unable to ingest the drug by licking. The back of the neck is one such site. The total dose of drug to apply will vary with the animal species (lower dose for cats) and with the range of body weight (dogs). Selamectin solution, for example, is commercially available in six dose sizes (from 15 to 240 mg).

The classes of ectoparasiticide and the dosage forms used in cattle, an arbitrarily selected species, are shown in Table 20. Even though different classes of drug may have activity against a similar range of ectoparasites, the drugs that belong to the various classes differ in clinical effectiveness. Quantitative differences in clinical effectiveness could be attributed to parasite susceptibility, which would be decreased by the development of resistance, and to the combined effect of drug access to the site where the parasite is located and persistence of the drug in skin. Both access and persistence are influenced by the physicochemical properties of the drug, the formulation of the preparation, and the method of application to the animal.

Dermatological preparations containing antibacterial agents include aerosol sprays (oxytetracycline hydrochloride, neomycin sulfate in propylene glycol), gels (metronidazole, fusidic acid), creams (gentamicin sulfate, neomycin sulfate and zinc bacitracin, silver sulfadiazine), ointments (chlortetracycline hydrochloride, sodium fusidate, framycetin sulfate and gramicidin, neomycin sulfate, zinc bacitracin, polymyxin B sulfate), and dusting powders (chlortetracycline hydrochloride and benzocaine). The type of preparation influences the stability and release of the active ingredients. Gels and creams are generally easier to apply to animals but are less occlusive than ointments. Ointments provide a longer duration of drug action, and the occlusive effect may enhance preparation of the active ingredient(s) to the site of infection.

The selection of an antibacterial agent should be based on the clinical diagnosis and, whenever feasible, in vitro culture and susceptibility testing (when considered necessary) of the micro-organisms(s) isolated. In the treatment of superficial skin infections, a topically applied antibacterial preparation may suffice. However in severe and deep-seated skin infections, both local and systemic therapy should be applied. The avoidance of antagonism requires that due consideration be given to the mechanisms of action of drugs selected for concurrent use.

Cutaneous mycotic infections caused by filamentous or dermatophytic fungi can be treated either topically or systemically, depending on the location and severity of the skin lesions. Topical antifungal preparations should be

Table 20 Representative ectoparasiticides for application to cattle

Ectoparasiticide class (representative drugs)	Spectrum of activity	Dosage forms (methods of application)
Organophosphate:		
(Phosmet)	Mites, lice Warble-fly larvae	Solution (pour on)
Pyrethroid:		
(Cypermethrin)	Lice, flies	Solution (pour on)
(Deltamethrin)		Solution (spot on)
(Fenvalerate)		Liquid concentrate (spray)[a]
(Permethrin)		Ear tag
Amidine:		
(Amitraz)	Lice, mites, ticks	Liquid concentrate (spray)
Avermectin:		
(Ivermectin)	Mites, lice,	Solution (pour on)
(Doramectin)	Horn fly,	Parenteral solution
(Abamectin)	Warble-fly larvae	(S.C. injection);
(Eprinomectin)		Controlled-release ruminal bolus (ivermectin)
Milbemycin:		
(Moxidectin)	Similar to avermectins	Solution (pour on); parenteral solution (S.C. injection)

[a]Liquid concentrates must be appropriately diluted before use.

formulated to promote penetration and persistence of the drug at the site of infection. Drugs that may be applied topically include various imidazole derivatives (clotrimazole, enilconazole, ketoconazole, miconazole), natamycin, nystatin, and tolnaftate, whereas orally administered drugs include ketoconazole, fluconazole, itraconazole, nystatin, and griseofulvin. Superficial infections caused by *Candida* spp. may be treated locally by applying an imidazole derivative or nystatin.

In domestic animals and humans, the common fungal organisms that cause skin infections are *Trichophyton mentagrophytes* (the usual cause of ringworm in calves between 2 and 7 months of age), *Microsporum gypseum*, and *T. verrucosum* (in species other than dogs and cats). Superficial mycotic skin infections are also caused by *T. equinum* (horses, cattle, humans), *M. nanum* (pigs, cattle, humans), and *M. canis* (dogs and cats). Filamentous fungal keratitis in horses is usually caused by *Fusarium* spp. Yeasts, primarily *Candida* spp., can cause mastitis in cows and metritis in mares and occasionally inhabit the skin, primarily at mucocutaneous junctions, in dogs.

For topical application, individual imidazoles and nystatin are formulated as creams, whereas tolnaftate and nystatin are available as ointments. Enilconazole is formulated as a liquid concentrate, that must be diluted before topical application by wash to horses and dogs or by spray to cattle. Topically applied enilconazole may be used in conjunction with systemic (oral) treatment with griseofulvin. Ketoconazole alone and miconazole nitrate combined with chlorhexidine gluconate are commercially available as shampoos for dogs. After topical applciation, imidazoles attain effective concentrations and persist in the outer layers of the epidermis, and percutaneous absorption appears to be minimal. Natamycin is commercially available as a suspension, to be diluted before application by spray to horses or cattle. In addition to spraying horses affected with ringworm, all grooming utensils and tackle must be thoroughly cleansed and immersed in the natamycin suspension, which should be diluted in plastic or galvanized containers. Natamycin (5% aqueous suspension) is effective in the treatment of filamentous fungal keratitis, particularly when caused by *Fusarium* spp. in horses.

The selectivity of action of antifungal azoles is attributed to their greater affinity for fungal than for mammalian cytochrome P450 enzymes. Because imidazole derivatives (clotrimazole, enilconazole, ketoconazole, miconazole) are less selective in their action than are triazoles (itraconazole, fluconazole), the former subgroup would be expected to cause greater interference with the biosynthesis of endogenous steroid hormones and to show a higher incidence of pharmacokinetic interactions with other drugs that undergo microsomal-mediated biotransformation.

The therapeutic effectiveness of topically applied corticosteroids is attributed primarily to their anti-inflammatory activity. The relative efficacy of topical corticosteroids appears to be in the following order: hydrocortisone, prednisolone, betamethasone < hydrocortisone valerate or butyrate, betamethasone valerate, triamcinolone acetonide, flucinolone acetonide < betamethasone dipropionate, fluocinonide. In addition to the nature of the corticosteroid, its solubility, and, to a lesser extent, the concentration used, clinical efficacy is influenced by the formulation of the preparation. Glucocorticoids appear to have greater efficacy when formulated in ointment bases than in cream or lotion vehicles. This could be attributed to the occlusive effect provided by ointments. The application of an occlusive dressing further enhances penetration and persistence of the steroid (reservoir effect) in the stratum corneum (112, 128).

TRANSDERMAL THERAPEUTIC SYSTEMS

A transdermal therapeutic system is a rate-controlled drug-delivery system that, applied to the surface of the skin, continuously releases the drug at a rate that will provide a desired steady-state plasma concentration for a specified duration.

The transdermal therapeutic system containing fentanyl [μ (primarily)-opioid agonist], which was designed to release the drug at a constant rate for 72 h, may have application in dogs for the control of postoperative (surgical) pain. Secure placement of the transdermal system that releases 50 μg of fentanyl/h on the dorsal aspect of the thorax of Beagle dogs (11.4–16.5 kg body weight) provided an average steady-state plasma fentanyl concentration of 1.6 ng/ml, which is within the range of plasma concentrations (1–2 ng/ml) considered to provide analgesia without producing other significant effects (129, 130). A steady-state concentration of fentanyl in plasma was reached at approximately 24 h after placement of the transdermal system, as would be expected because the half-life of fentanyl in Beagles is 6 h and was maintained until removal of the system at 72 h. Because the dosing rate (3.7 μg/h × kg) exceeded the systemic clearance (2.7 μg/h × kg) and the transdermal bioavailability of fentanyl is 64%, a fraction of the released drug either persists in the stratum corneum or is metabolized in the epidermis before absorption into the systemic circulation, or both may contribute to incomplete systemic availability of the drug. Because of the 24 h delay in achieving plasma concentrations within the analgesia-producing range, either an intravenous dose (approximately 30 μg/kg) could be administered at the time of placement of the transdermal system or the system could be securely placed on the animal 12 h before performing the surgery.

Whenever a drug-delivery device such as an insecticidal collar or a transdermal system is securely placed on an animal, the increased potential for drug interaction must be kept in mind at the time of selecting another drug for administration by any route and throughout the course of therapy.

REFERENCES

1. Foster, T.P. Protein/Peptide Veterinary Formulations. *Development and Formulation of Veterinary Dosage Forms*; Hardee, G.E., Baggot, J.D., Eds.; Marcel Dekker, Inc.: New York, 1998; 231–282.
2. Hansel, W.; McEntee, K. Female Reproductive Processes. *Duke's Physiology of Domestic Animals*; Swenson, M.J., Ed.; Comstock Publishing Associates (Cornell University Press): Ithaca, NY, 1977; 772–800.
3. Hogben, C.A.M.; Tocco, D.J.; Brodie, B.B.; Schanker, L.S. On the Mechanism of Intestinal Absorption of Drugs. J. Pharmacol. Exp. Ther. **1959**, *125*, 275–282.
4. Theeuwes, F.; Bayne, W. Dosage Form Index: An Objective Criterion for Evaluation of Controlled-Release Drug Delivery Systems. J. Pharm. Sci. **1977**, *66*, 1388–1392.
5. Koritz, G.D.; McKiernan, B.C.; Neff-Davis, C.A.; Munsiff, I.J. Bioavailability of Four Slow-Release Theophylline Formulations in the Beagle Dog. J. Vet. Pharmacol. Ther. **1986**, *9*, 293–302.
6. Dohoo, S. Steady-State Pharmacokinetics of Oral Sustained-Release Morphine Sulphate in Dogs. J. Vet. Pharmacol. Ther. **1997**, *20*, 129–133.
7. Maitho, T.E.; Lees, P.; Taylor, J.B. Absorption and Pharmacokinetics of Phenylbutazone in Welsh Mountain Ponies. J. Vet. Pharmacol. Ther. **1986**, *9*, 26–39.
8. van Duijkeren, E.; Vulto, A.G.; Sloet van Oldruitenborgh-Oosterbann, M.M.; Kessels, B.G.F.; van Miert, A.S.J.P.A.M.; Breukink, H.J. Pharmacokinetics of Trimethoprim-Sulphaclorpyridazine in Horses after Oral, Nasogastric and Intravenous Administration. J. Vet. Pharmacol. Ther. **1995**, *18*, 47–53.
9. Hungate, R.E. *The Rumen and its Microbes*; Academic Press: New York, 1966; 218.
10. Phillipson, A.T.; McAnally, R.A. Studies on the Fate of Carbohydrates in the Rumen of the Sheep. J. Exp. Biol. **1942**, *19*, 199–214.
11. Masson, M.J.; Phillipson, A.T. The Absorption of Acetate, Propionate and Butyrate from the Rumen of Sheep. J. Physiol. (Lond) **1951**, *113*, 189–206.
12. Dobson, A. Physiological Peculiarities of the Ruminant Relevant to Drug Distribution. Federation Proceedings **1967**, *26*, 994–1000.
13. Clark, R.; Wessels, J.J. The Influences of the Nature of the Diet and of Starvation on the Concentration Curve of Sulphanilamide in the Blood of Sheep After Oral Dosing. Onderstepoort J. Vet. Res. **1952**, *25*, 75–83.
14. Masson, M.J.; Phillipson, A.T. The Composition of the Digesta Leaving the Abomasum of Sheep. J. Physiol. (Lond) **1952**, *116*, 98–111.
15. Gingerich, D.A.; Baggot, J.D.; Yeary, R.A. Pharmacokinetics and Dosage of Aspirin in Cattle. J. Am. Vet. Med. Assoc. **1975**, *167*, 945–948.
16. Ali, D.N.; Hennessy, D.R. The Effect of Temporarily Reduced Feed Intake on the Efficacy of Oxfendazole in Sheep. Int. J. Parasitol. **1995**, *25*, 71–74.
17. Taylor, S.M.; Malton, T.R.; Blanchflower, J.; Kennedy, D.G.; Hewitt, S.A. Effects of Dietary Variations on Plasma Concentrations of Oral Flukicides in Sheep. J. Vet. Pharmacol. Ther. **1993**, *16*, 48–54.
18. Rowlands, D.ap T.; Shepherd, M.T.; Collins, K.R. The Oxfendazole Pulse Release Bolus. J. Vet. Pharmacol. Ther. **1988**, *11*, 405–408.
19. Singh, B.N.; Kim, K.H. Floating Drug Delivery Systems: An Approach to Oral Controlled Drug Delivery Via Gastric Retention. J. Controlled. Release **2000**, *63*, 235–259.
20. Mallis, G.I.; Schmidt, D.H.; Lindenbaum, J. Superior Bioavailability of Digoxin Solution in Capsules. Clin. Pharmacol. Ther. **1975**, *18*, 761–768.
21. Johnson, B.F.; Bye, C.; Jones, G.; Sabey, G.A. A Completely Absorbed Oral Preparation of Digoxin. Clin. Pharmacol. Ther. **1976**, *19*, 746–751.
22. Lindenbaum, J. Greater Bioavailability of Digoxin Solution in Capsules: Studies in the Postprandial State. Clin. Pharmacol. Ther. **1977**, *21*, 278–282.
23. Angelucci, L.; Petrangeli, B.; Celletti, P.; Favilli, S. Bioavailability of Flufenamic Acid in Hard and Soft Gelatin Capsules. J. Pharm. Sci. **1976**, *65*, 455–456.
24. Landoni, M.F.; Lees, P. Influence of Formulation on the Pharmacokinetics and Bioavailability of Racemic Ketoprofen in Horses. J. Vet. Pharmacol. Ther. **1995c**, *18*, 446–450.
25. Baggott, D.G.; Ross, D.B.; Preston, J.M.; Gross, S.J. Nematode Burdens and Productivity of Grazing Cattle Treated with a Prototype Sustained-Release Bolus Containing Ivermectin. Vet. Rec. **1994**, *135*, 503–506.
26. Berghen, P.; Hilderson, H.; Vercruysse, J.; Claerebout, E.; Dorny, P. Field Evaluation of the Efficacy of the Fenbendazole Slow-Release Bolus in the Control of Gastrointestinal Nematodes of First-Season Grazing Cattle. Vet. Q. **1994**, *16*, 161–164.
27. Laby, R.H. US Patent 3, 844, 284, 1974
28. Klink, P.R.; Ferguson, T.H.; Magruder, J.A. Formulation of Veterinary Dosage Forms. *Development and Formulation of Veterinary Dosage Forms*; Hardee, G.E., Baggot, J.D., Eds.; Marcel Dekker, Inc.: New York, 1998; 145–229.
29. Firth, E.C.; Nouws, J.F.M.; Driessens, F.; Schmaetz, P.; Peperkamp, K.; Klein, W.R. Effect of the Injection Site on the Pharmacokinetics of Procaine Penicillin G in Horses. Am. J. Vet. Res. **1986**, *47*, 2380–2384.
30. Rasmussen, F. Tissue Damage at the Injection Site after Intramuscular Injection of Drugs in Food-Producing Animals. *Trends in Veterinary Pharmacology and Toxicology*; van Miert, A.S.J.P.A.M., Frens, J., van der Kreek, F.W., Eds.; Elsevier: Amsterdam, 1980; 27–33.

31. Nouws, J.F.M. Irritation, Bioavailability and Residue Aspects of Ten Oxytetracycline Formulations Administered Intramuscularly to Pigs. Vet Q **1984**, *6*, 80–84.

32. Nouws, J.F.M. Injection Sites and Withdrawal Times. Annal. de. Rech. Vet. **1990**, *21* (Suppl 1), 145S–150S.

33. Banting, A.deL; Tranquart, F. Echography as a Tool in Clinical Pharmacology. Acta. Vet. Scand. Suppl. **1991**, *87*, 215–216.

34. Aktas, M.; Lefebvre, H.P.; Toutain, P.-L.; Braun, J.P. Disposition of Creatine Kinase Activity in Dog Plasma Following Intravenous and Intramuscular Injection of Skeletal Muscle Homogenates. J. Vet. Pharmacol. Ther. **1995**, *18*, 1–6.

35. Toutain, P.-L.; Lassourd, V.; Costes, G.; Alvinerie, M.; Bret, L.; Lefebvre, H.P.; Braun, J.P. A Non-Invasive and Quantitative Method for the Study of Tissue Injury Caused by Intramuscular Injection of Drugs in Horses. J. Vet. Pharmacol. Ther. **1995**, *18*, 226–235.

36. Nouws, J.F.M.; Vree, T.B. Effect of Injection Site on the Bioavailability of an Oxytetracycline Formulation in Ruminant Calves. Vet. Q. **1983**, *5*, 165–170.

37. Korsrud, G.O.; Boison, J.O.; Papich, M.G.; Yates, W.D.G.; MacNeil, J.D.; Janzen, E.D.; Cohen, R.D.H.; Landry, D.A.; Lambert, G.; Yong, M.S.; Messier, J.R. Depletion of Intramuscularly and Subcutaneously Injected Procaine Penicillin G from Tissues and Plasma of Yearling Beef Steers. Can. J. Vet. Res. **1993**, *57*, 223–230.

38. Wheaton, J.E.; Al-Raheem, S.N.; Godfredson, J.A.; Dorn, J.M.; Wong, E.A.; Vale, W.W.; Rivier, J.; Mowles, T.F.; Heimer, E.P.; Felix, A.M. Use of Osmotic Pumps for Subcutaneous Infusion of Growth Hormone-Releasing Factors in Steers and Wethers. J. Anim. Sci. **1988**, *66*, 2876–2885.

39. Golenz, M.R.; Wilson, W.D.; Carlson, G.P.; Craychee, T.J.; Mihalyi, J.E.; Vinox, L. Effect of Route of Administration and Age on the Pharmacokinetics of Amikacin Administered by the Intravenous and Intraosseous Routes to 3- and 5-Day-Old Foals. Equine. Vet. J. **1994**, *26*, 367–373.

40. Baggot, J.D.; Brown, S.A. Basis for Selection of the Dosage Form. *Development and Formulation of Veterinary Dosage Forms*; Hardee, G.E., Baggot, J.D., Eds.; Marcel Dekker, Inc.: New York, 1998; 7–143.

41. Wilson, R.C.; Duran, S.H.; Horton, C.R., Jr.; Wright, L.C. Bioavailability of Gentamicin in Dogs after Intramuscular or Subcutaneous Injections. Am. J. Vet. Res. **1989**, *50*, 1748–1750.

42. Baggot, J.D.; Ling, G.V.; Chatfield, R.C. Clinical Pharmacokinetics of Amikacin in Dogs. Am. J. Vet. Res. **1985**, *46*, 1793–1796.

43. Craigmill, A.L.; Brown, S.A.; Wetzlich, S.E.; Gustafson, C.R.; Arndt, T.S. Pharmacokinetics of Ceftiofur and Metabolites After Single Intravenous and Intramuscular Administration and Multiple Intramuscular Administration of Ceftiofur Sodium to Sheep. J. Vet. Pharmacol. Ther. **1997**, *20*, 139–144.

44. Rasmussen, F.; Svendsen, O. Tissue Damage and Concentration at the Injection Site After Intramuscular Injection of Chemotherapeutics and Vehicles in Pigs. Res. Vet. Sci. **1976**, *20*, 55–60.

45. Lanusse, C.; Lifschitz, A.; Virkel, G.; Alvarez, L.; Sanchez, S.; Sutra, J.F.; Galtier, P.; Alvinerie, M. Comparative Plasma Disposition Kinetics of Ivermectin, Moxidectin and Doramectin in Cattle. J. Vet. Pharmacol. Ther. **1997**, *20*, 91–99.

46. Banting, A.deL; Baggot, J.D. Comparison of the Pharmacokinetics and Local Tolerance of Three Injectable Oxytetracycline Formulations in Pigs. J. Vet. Pharmacol. Ther. **1996**, *19*, 50–55.

47. Nouws, J.F.M.; van Ginneken, C.A.M.; Hekman, P.; Ziv, G. Comparative Plasma Ampicillin Levels and Bioavailability of Five Parenteral Ampicillin Formulations in Ruminant Calves. Vet. Q. **1982**, *4*, 62–71.

48. Agerso, H.; Friis, C. Bioavailability of Amoxycillin in Pigs. J. Vet. Pharmacol. Ther. **1998**, *21*, 41–46.

49. Marshall, A.B.; Palmer, G.H. Injection Sites and Drug Bioavailability. In *Trends in Veterinary Pharmacology and Toxicology*; van Miert, A.S.J.P.A.M., Frens, J., van der Kreek, F.W. Eds.; Elsevier: Amersterdam, 1980, 54–60.

50. Baggot, J.D. *Principles of Drug Disposition in Domestic Animals: The Basis of Veterinary Clinical Pharmacology*; WB Saunders: Philadelphia, 1977, 10–13, 73–112.

51. Rasmussen, F. *Studies on the Mammary Excretion and Absorption of Drugs*; Carl Fr. Mortensen: Copenhagen, 1966.

52. Prescott, J.F.; Baggot, J.D. Principles of Antimicrobial Drug Disposition; Antimicrobial Drug Use in Bovine Mastitis. *Antimicrobial Therapy in Veterinary Medicine*, 2nd Ed., Iowa State University Press: Ames Iowa, 1993; 37–60, 553–561.

53. Ziv, G. Drug Selection and Use in Mastitis: Systemic Vs Local Drug Therapy. J. Am. Vet. Med. Assoc. **1980**, *176*, 1109–1115.

54. Pyorala, S. Staphylococcal and Streptococcal Mastitis. *The Bovine Udder and Mastitis*; Sandholm, M., Honkanen-Buzalski, T., Kaartinen, L., Pyorala, S., Eds.; University of Helsinki, Faculty of Veterinary Medicine: Helsinki, 1995; 143–148.

55. Sandholm, M.; Pyorala, S. Coliform Mastitis. *The Bovine Udder and Mastitis*; Sandholm, M., Honkanen-Buzalski, T., Kaartinen, L., Pyorala, S., Eds.; University of Helsinki, Faculty of Veterinary Medicine: Helsinki, 1995; 149–160.

56. Baggot, J.D.; McKellar, Q.A. The Absorption, Distribution and Elimination of Anthelmintic Drugs: The Role of Pharmacokinetics. J. Vet. Pharmacol. Ther. **1994**, *17*, 409–419.

57. Benet, L.Z. Pharmacokinetic Parameters: Which are Necessary to Define a Drug Substance? Eur. J. Resp. Dis. **1984**, *65* (Suppl. 134), 45–61.

58. Williams, R.T. *Detoxication Mechanisms*; Chapman & Hall: London, 1959, 1–22, 732–740.

59. Williams, R.T. Comparative Patterns of Drug Metabolism. Fed. Proc. **1967**, *26*, 1029–1039.

60. Williams, R.T. Species Variations in Drug Biotransformations. *Fundamentals of Drug Metabolism and Drug Disposition*; LaDu, B.N., Mandel, H.G., Way, E.L., Eds.; Williams & Wilkins: Baltimore, 1971; 187–205.

61. Frey, H.-H.; Loscher, W. Pharmacokinetics of Anti-Epileptic Drugs in the Dog: A Review. J. Vet. Pharmacol. Ther. **1985**, *8*, 219–233.

62. French, M.R.; Bababunmi, E.A.; Golding, R.R.; Bassir, O.; Caldwell, J.; Smith, R.L.; Williams, R.T. The Conjugation of Phenol, Benzoic Acid, I-Naphthylacetic Acid and Sulphadimethoxine in the Lion, Civet and Genet. FEBS Letters **1974**, *46*, 134–137.

63. Boxenbaum, H. Interspecies Scaling, Allometry, Physiological Time, and the Ground Plan of Pharmacokinetics. J. Pharmacokinet. Biopharm. **1982**, *10*, 201–227.

64. Dorrestein, G.M.; van Miert, A.S.J.P.A.M. Pharmacotherapeutic Aspects of Medication of Birds. J. Vet. Pharmacol. Ther. **1988**, *11*, 33–44.

65. Calder, W.A., III *Size, Function and Life History*; Harvard University Press: Cambridge, MA, 1984.

66. Grondel, J.L.; Nouws, J.F.M.; Schutte, A.R.; Driessens, F. Comparative Pharmacokinetics of Oxytetracycline in Rainbow Trout (*Salmo gairdneri*) and African Catfish (*Clarias Gariepinus*). J. Vet. Pharmacol. Ther. **1989**, *12*, 157–162.

67. Boxenbaum, H. Interspecies Variation in Liver Weight, Hepatic Blood Flow, and Antipyrine Intrinsic Clearance: Extrapolation of Data to Benzodiazepines and Phenytoin. J. Pharmacokinet. Biopharm. **1980**, *8*, 165–176.

68. Gaspari, F.; Bonati, M. Interspecies Metabolism and Pharmacokinetic Scaling of Theophylline Disposition. Drug. Metab. Rev. **1990**, *22*, 179–207.

69. Kleiber, M. Metabolic Turnover Rate: A Physiological Meaning of the Metabolic Rate Per Unit Body Weight. J. Theoret. Biol. **1975**, *53*, 199–204.

70. Landoni, M.F.; Soraci, A.L.; Delatour, P.; Lees, P. Enantioselective Behaviour of Drugs Used in Domestic Animals: A Review. J. Vet. Pharmacol. Ther. **1997**, *20*, 1–16.

71. Landoni, M.F.; Lees, P. Comparison of the Anti-Inflammatory Actions of Flunixin and Ketoprofen in Horses Applying PK/PD Modelling. Equine. Vet. J. **1995**, *27*, 247–256.

72. Landoni, M.F.; Comas, W.; Mucci, N.; Anglarilla, G.; Bidall, D.; Lees, P. Enantiospecific Pharmacokinetics and Pharmacodynamics of Ketoprofen in Sheep. J. Vet. Pharmacol. Ther. **1999**, *22*, 349–359.

73. Landoni, M.F.; Cunningham, F.M.; Lees, P. Pharmacokinetics and Pharmacodynamics of Ketoprofen in Calves Applying PK/PD Modelling. J. Vet. Pharmacol. Ther. **1995**, *18*, 315–324.

74. Landoni, M.F.; Lees, P. Pharmacokinetics and Pharmacodynamics of Ketoprofen Enantiomers in the Horse. J. Vet. Pharmacol. Ther. **1996**, *19*, 466–474.

75. Landoni, M.F.; Lees, P. Pharmacokinetics and Pharmacodynamics of Ketoprofen Enantiomers in Calves. Chirality **1995**, *7*, 586–597.

76. Mauleon, D.; Mis, R.; Ginesta, J.; Ortega, E.; Vilageliu, J.; Basi, N.; Carganico, G. Pharmacokinetics of Ketoprofen Enantiomers in Monkeys Following Single and Multiple Oral Administration. Chirality **1994**, *6*, 537–542.

77. Rudy, A.C.; Liu, Y.; Brater, D.C.; Hall, S.D. Steieoselective Pharmacokinetics and Inversion of (R)-ketoprofen in Healthy Volunteers. J. Clin. Pharmacol. **1998**, *38*, 3S–10S.

78. Aberg, G.; Ciofalo, V.B.; Pendleton, R.G.; Ray, G.; Weddle, D. Inversion of (R)- to (S)-Ketoprofen in Eight Animal Species. Chirality **1995**, *7*, 383–387.

79. Garcia, M.L.; Tost, D.; Vitageliu, J.; Lopez, S.; Carganico, G.; Mauleon, D. Bioavailability of S(+)-Ketoprofen After Oral Administration of Different Mixtures of Ketoprofen Enantiomers to Dogs. J. Clin. Pharmacol. **1998**, *38*, 22S–26S.

80. Hutt, A.J.; Caldwell, J. The Importance of Stereochemistry in the Clinical Pharmacokinetics of the 2-Arylpropionic Acid Non-Steroidal Anti-Inflammatory Drugs. Clin. Pharmacokinet. **1984**, *9*, 371–373.

81. Soraci, A.L.; Benoit, E.; Olivier, L.; Delatour, P. Comparative Metabolism of R(−)-Fenoprofen in Rats and Sheep. J. Vet. Pharmacol. Ther. **1995**, *18*, 167–171.

82. Soraci, A.L.; Benoit, E. In Vitro Fenoprophenyl-Coenzyme A Thioester Formation: Interspecies Variations. Chirality **1996**, *7*, 534–540.

83. Benoit, E.; Soraci, A.; Delatour, P. *Chiral Inversion as a Parameter for Interspecies and Intercompound Discrepancies in Enantiospecific Pharmacokinetics*, 6th International Congress European Association for Veterinary Pharmacology and Toxicology, Blackwell Scientific Publications: Edinburgh, 1994; S5/7, 07

84. Hayball, P.J.; Meffin, P.J. Enantioselective Disposition of 2-arylpropionic Acid Nonsteroidal Anti-Inflammatory Drugs. III. Fenoprofen Disposition. J. Pharmacol. Exp. Ther. **1987**, *240*, 631–636.

85. Rubin, A.; Knadler, M.P.; Ho, P.P.K.; Bechtol, L.D.; Wolen, R.L. Stereoselective Inversion of (R)-Fenoprofen to (S)-Fenoprofen in Humans. J. Pharm. Sci. **1985**, *74*, 82–84.

86. Berry, B.W.; Jamali, F. Presystemic and Systemic Chiral Inversion of R(−)-Fenoprofen in the Rat. J. Pharmacol. Exp. Ther. **1991**, *258*, 695–701.

87. McKellar, Q.A.; Delatour, P.; Lees, P. Stereospecific Pharmacodynamics and Pharmacokinetics of Carprofen in the Dog. J. Vet. Pharmacol. Ther. **1994**, *17*, 447–454.

88. Lees, P.; McKellar, Q.A.; May, S.A.; Ludwig, B.M. Pharmacodynamics and Pharmacokinetics of Carprofen in the Horse. Equine Vet. J. **1994**, *26*, 203–208.

89. Kemmerer, J.M.; Rubio, F.A.; McClain, R.M.; Koechlin, B.A. Stereospecific Assay and Stereospecific Disposition of Racemic Carprofen in Rats. J. Pharm. Sci. **1979**, *68*, 1274–1280.

90. Stoltenberg, J.K.; Puglisi, C.V.; Rubio, F.; Vane, F.M. High-Performance Liquid Chromatographic Determination of Stereoselective Disposition of Carprofen in Humans. J. Pharm. Sci. **1981**, *70*, 1207–1212.

91. Lees, P.; Delatour, P.; Benoit, E.; Foster, A.P. Pharmacokinetics of Carprofen Enantiomers in the Horse. Acta. Vet. Scand. Suppl. **1991**, *87*, 249–251.

92. Taylor, P.M.; Delatour, P.; Landoni, M.F.; Deal, C.; Pickett, C.; Shojaee, AliabadiF.; Foot, R.; Lees, P. Pharmacodynamics and Enantioselective Pharmacokinetics of Carprofen in the Cat. Res. Vet. Sci. **1996**, *60*, 144–151.

93. Delatour, P.; Foot, R.; Foster, A.P.; Baggot, D.; Lees, P. Pharamacodynamics and Chiral Pharmacokinetics of Carprofen in Calves. Br. Vet. J. **1996**, *152*, 183–198.

94. Muir, W.W.; Hubbell, J.A. Cardiopulmonary and Anesthetic Effects of Ketamine and Its Enantiomers in Dogs. Am. J. Vet. Res. **1988**, *49*, 530–534.

95.   White, P.F.; Ham, J.; Way, W.L.; Trevor, A.J. Pharmacology of Ketamine Isomers in Surgical Patients. Anesthesiology **1980**, *52*, 231–239.

96.   Delatour, P.; Jaussaud, P.; Courtot, D.; Fau, D. Enantioselective N-demethylation of Ketamine in the Horse. J. Vet. Pharmacol. Ther. **1991**, *14*, 209–212.

97.   Deleforge, J.; Davot, J.L.; Boisrame, B.; Delatour, P. Enantioselectivity in the Anaesthetic Effect of Ketamine in Dogs. J. Vet. Pharmacol. Ther. **1991**, *14*, 418–420.

98.   Caldwell, J. The Importance of Stereochemistry in Drug Action and Disposition. J. Clin. Pharmacol. **1992**, *32*, 925–929.

99.   Foster, R.T.; Jamali, F. High-Performance Liquid Chromatographic Assay of Ketoprofen Enantiomers in Human Plasma and Urine. J. Chromatogr. **1987**, *416*, 388–393.

100. Delatour, P.; Garnier, F.; Benoit, E.; Claude, I. Chiral Behaviour of the Metabolite Albendazole Sulphoxide in Sheep, Goats and Cattle. Res. Vet. Sci. **1991**, *50*, 134–138.

101. Pasutto, F.M. Mirror Images: The Analysis of Pharmaceutical Enantiomers. J. Clin. Pharmacol. **1992**, *32*, 917–924.

102. Carr, R.A.; Foster, R.T.; Lewanczuk, R.Z.; Hamilton, P.G. Pharmacokinetics of Sotalol Enantiomers in Humans. J. Clin. Pharmacol. **1992**, *32*, 1105–1109.

103. Drayer, D.E. Pharmacodynamic and Pharmacokinetic Differences between Drug Enantiomers in Humans: An Overview. Clin. Pharmacol. Ther. **1986**, *40*, 125–133.

104. Monteiro-Riviere, N.A.; Bristol, D.G.; Manning, T.O.; Rogers, R.A.; Riviere, J.E. Interspecies and Interregional Analysis of the Comparative Histologic Thickness and Laser Doppler Blood Flow Measurements at Five Cutaneous Sites in Nine Species. J. Invest. Dermatol. **1990**, *95*, 582–586.

105. Riegelman, S. Pharmacokinetics: Pharmacokinetic Factors Affecting Epidermal Penetration and Percutaneous Absorption. Clin. Pharmacol. Ther. **1974**, *16*, 873–883.

106. Montagna, W. Comparative Anatomy and Physiology of the Skin. Arch. Dermatol. **1967**, *96*, 357–363.

107. Pitman, I.H.; Rostas, S.J. Topical Drug Delivery to Cattle and Sheep. J. Pharm. Sci. **1981**, *70*, 1181–1193.

108. Ryder, M.L. A Survey of the Follicle Populations in a Range of British Breeds of Sheep. J. Agric. Sci. **1957**, *49*, 275–284.

109. Forsyth, B.A.; Gibbon, A.J.; Pryor, D.E. Seasonal Variations in Anthelmintic Response by Cattle to Dermally Applied Levamisole. Aust. Vet. J. **1983**, *60*, 141–146.

110. Idson, B. Vehicle Effects on Percutaneous Absorption. Drug Metab. Rev. **1983**, *14*, 207–222.

111. McKenzie, A.W. Percutaneous Absorption of Steroids. Arch. Dermatol. **1962**, *86*, 91–94.

112. Barry, B.W. Properties that Influence Percutaneous Absorption. *Dermatological Formulations: Percutaneous Absorption*; Marcel Dekker, Inc. New York, 1983, 127–233.

113. Gyrd-Hansen, N.; Brimer, L.; Rasmussen, R. Percutaneous Absorption and Recovery of Parathion in Pigs. Acta Vet. Scand. Suppl. **1991**, *87*, 410–412.

114. Scheuplein, R.J. Site Variations in Diffusion and Permeability. In *The Physiology and Pathophysiology of the Skin*; Jarrett, A., Ed.; Academic Press: New York, 1978; 5, 1731–1752.

115. McCreesh, A.H. Percutaneous Toxicity. Toxicol. Appl. Pharmacol. **1965**, *7* (Suppl. 2), 20–26.

116. Monteiro-Riviere, N.A.; Stromberg, M.W. Ultrastructure of the Integument of the Domestic Pig (*Sus scrofa*) from one through Fourteen Weeks of Age. Zbl Vet Med [Reihe C] **1985**, *14*, 97–115.

117. Bartek, M.J.; LaBudde, J.A.; Maibach, H.I. Skin Permeability *In Vivo*: Comparison in Rat, Rabbit, Pig and Man. J. Invest. Dermatol. **1972**, *58*, 114–123.

118. Riviere, J.E.; Monteiro-Riviere, N.A. The Isolated Perfused Porcine Skin Flap as an In Vitro Model for Percutaneous Absorption and Cutaneous Toxicology. Crit. Rev. Toxicol. **1991**, *21*, 329–344.

119. Riviere, J.E.; Monteiro-Riviere, N.A.; Williams, P.L. The Isolated Perfused Porcine Skin Flap as an In Vitro Model for Predicting Transdermal Pharmacokinetics. Eur. J. Pharmac. Biopharm. **1995**, *41*, 152–162.

120. Wester, R.C.; Maibach, H.I. Regional Variation in Percutaneous Absorption. *Percutaneous Absorption*; Bronaugh, R.L., Maibach, H.I., Eds.; Marcel Dekker, Inc.: New York, 1999; 107–116.

121. Behrendt, H.; Korting, H.Ch.; Braun-Falco, O. Zum Metabolismus von Pharmaka in der Haut. Hautarzt **1989**, *40*, 8–13.

122. Riviere, J.E.; Chang, S.K. Transdermal Penetration and Metabolism of Organophosphate Insecticides. In *Organophosphates: Chemistry, Fate and Effects*; Academic Press: New York, 1992.

123. Kao, J.; Carver, M.P. Cutaneous Metabolism of Xenobiotics. Drug Metab. Rev. **1990**, *22*, 363–410.

124. Ademola, J.I.; Chow, C.A.; Wester, R.C.; Maibach, H.I. Metabolism of Propranolol During Percutaneous Absorption in Human Skin. J. Pharm. Sci. **1991**, *82*, 767–770.

125. Ward, S.; Walle, T.; Walle, K.; Wilkinson, G.R.; Branch, R.A. Propranolol's Metabolism is Determined by Both Mephenytoin and Debrisoquin Hydroxylase. Clin. Pharmacol. Ther. **1989**, *45*, 72–78.

126. Dorman, D.C.; Buck, W.B.; Trammel, H.L.; Jones, R.D.; Beasley, V.R. Fenvalerate/ *N*, N-Diethyl-*m*-Toluamide (DEET) Toxicosis in Two Cats. J. Am. Vet. Med. Assoc. **1990**, *196*, 100–102.

127. Mount, M.E.; Moller, G.; Cook, J.; Holstege, D.M.; Richardson, E.R.; Ardans, A. Clinical Illness Associated with a Commercial Tick and Flea Product in Dogs and Cats. Vet. Human. Toxicol. **1991**, *33*, 19–27.

128. Munro, D.D.; Stoughton, R.B. Dimethylacetamide (DMAC) and Dimethylformamide (DMFA): Effect on Percutaneous Absorption. Arch. Dermatol. **1965**, *92*, 585–586.

129. Kyles, A.E.; Papich, M.; Hardie, E.M. Disposition of Transdermally Administered Fentanyl in Dogs. Am. J. Vet. Res. **1996**, *57*, 715–719.

130. Holley, F.O.; van Steennis, C. Postoperative Analgesia with Fentanyl: Pharmacokinetics and Pharmacodynamics of Constant-Rate IV and Transdermal Delivery. Br. J. Anaesthesia. **1988**, *60*, 608–613.

WATER SORPTION OF DRUGS AND DOSAGE FORMS[a]

Mark J. Kontny

Pharmacia, Kalamazoo, Michigan

James J. Conners

Dura Pharmaceuticals, San Diego, California

INTRODUCTION

The physical, chemical, and mechanical properties of pharmaceutical drugs and dosage forms are critically dependent on the presence of moisture. Pharmaceutical scientists can cite numerous examples of desirable and undesirable properties that result from varied levels of moisture associated with a particular solid or formulation consisting of mixtures of solids. Flow, compaction, caking, disintegration, dissolution, hardness, and chemical stability are just some of the properties influenced by moisture. Because water is present in bulk liquid form or as a vapor at some relative humidity in virtually all stages of solid manufacture (active ingredient and excipients), storage, processing into formulations, and final product packaging, a fundamental understanding of the role of water in affecting solid properties (and vice versa) is necessary.

Although the properties of individual solids and the performance of solid dosage forms are dependent on moisture, characterization of the underlying water–solid interaction is often nebulous. For example, many solids are described as "hygroscopic" without further reference to whether and how this relates to the rate and amount of moisture uptake as a function of relative humidity and temperature (1). To illustrate this ambiguity, consider that water-soluble, nonhydrating crystalline substances such as sodium chloride sorb very low levels of moisture (e.g., less than 0.1%) below their critical relative humidities, where the solid actually dissolves in the sorbed moisture. On the other hand, some typical excipient materials used in solid dosage forms, such as starches, celluloses, and gelatin capsules, sorb significant quantities of moisture (e.g., 25–50%), and even though they do not dissolve, they do undergo significant morphological change at high relative humidities (i.e., swelling). Moisture uptake rate

for a material depends on both the relative humidity of the environment and the time-dependent moisture content of the solid. For situations in which the environmental relative humidity is significantly different from the relative humidity at which the excipient (gelatin, for example) was previously equilibrated, the initial moisture uptake/loss rate will be significant, but it will approach zero over time. On the other hand, a water-soluble, nonhydrating crystalline substance such as sodium chloride will have a very low moisture uptake/loss rate that will decrease to zero if the environmental relative humidity is kept below its critical relative humidity. However, the uptake rate will be relatively large and continuous, until all the solid has dissolved, if the relative humidity is above the critical value. Obviously, very different mechanisms of water sorption/desorption occur for the different samples. In this light, describing sodium chloride and/or starch as "hygroscopic" offers very little toward understanding the water–solid interactions that might affect their physico-chemical properties. These examples illustrate the need to understand the underlying mechanism(s) of uptake for a particular solid. In this regard, therefore, addressing the following questions provides a basis for studying the various mechanisms of water–solid interaction:

1. How much water is present and what is the corresponding water activity (approximated by relative pressure or percent relative humidity/100)?
2. What are the kinetics of moisture uptake or loss, and is the rate constant or changing over time?
3. Where is the water located (i.e., adsorbed to the external surface of crystals, absorbed into crystals as specific or nonspecific water of hydration, absorbed into amorphous regions, condensed into pores, etc.)?
4. What is the state of the moisture associated with the solid (i.e., bulk water, water of hydration, physisorbed water, etc.)?
5. What form of the solid is present (i.e., particle size and morphology, polymorphic species, degree of crystallinity, state of hydration) and is this form

---

[a]This work was taken in part from a chapter entitled "Sorption of Water by Solids," in *Physical Characterization of Pharmaceutical Solids*, H. Brittain, Ed., Marcel Dekker, Inc.: New York, 1995.

thermodynamically stable over the temperature and relative humidity range that the solid is expected to encounter?

It is the objective of this chapter to highlight the various mechanisms whereby water can interact with solid substances, present methodologies that can be used to obtain the necessary data, and then discuss moisture uptake for nonhydrating and hydrating crystalline solids below and above their critical relative humdities for amorphous solids and for pharmaceutically processed substances. Finally transfer of moisture from one substance to another will be discussed.

THE WATER SORPTION ISOTHERM

The most fundamental manner of demonstrating the relationship between sorbed water vapor and a solid is the water sorption–desorption isotherm. The water sorption–desorption isotherm describes the relationship between the equilibrium amount of water vapor sorbed to a solid (usually expressed as amount per unit mass or per unit surface area of solid) and the thermodynamic quantity, water activity (a_w), at constant temperature and pressure. At equilibrium the chemical potential of water sorbed to the solid must equal the chemical potential of water in the vapor phase. Water activity in the vapor phase is related to chemical potential by

$$\mu = \mu^0 + RT \ln a_w \tag{1}$$

where μ is the chemical potential of water in the system at equilibrium, μ^0 is the standard chemical potential of water at a specific reference temperature and pressure, R is the gas constant, and T is the absolute temperature. Lewis et al. (2) defined the relative activity of any pure substance or component (such as water) as a ratio of fugacities:

$$a_w = \frac{f_w}{f_w^0} \tag{2}$$

where f_w is the fugacity of water in the system at equilibrium and f_w^0 is the fugacity of pure water at a standard temperature and pressure. For all practical purposes, the fugacity (or "escaping tendency") of water vapor can be approximated by the water vapor pressure in the system. This assumption is valid as long as the water vapor behaves as an ideal gas. For the water vapor pressure range of relevance for pharmaceutical systems at temperatures less than 50°C, this approximation is excellent (<0.2% relative error) (3). Thus, the relative

pressure of water vapor, P/P^0, is usually employed as an estimate of the relative water activity in the system:

$$a_w = \frac{P}{P^0} \tag{3}$$

where P is the water vapor pressure in the system and P^0 is the vapor pressure above pure water at the temperature of interest. Relative humidity (RH) is defined as the relative pressure expressed on a percentage basis:

$$RH = 100 \frac{P}{P^0} \tag{4}$$

The sorption branch of the isotherm is obtained experimentally by measuring the equilibrium amount of water sorbed to a solid at known relative pressure, beginning with a known mass of absolutely dry solid and then progressively increasing the relative pressure in the system. Drying the solid sample under heat, possibly using vacuum to facilitate the removal of desorbed water vapor, is usually necessary to eliminate residual moisture. One must be aware, however, of the effects of such conditions on the chemical and physical stability of the solid. The desorption portion of the isotherm is obtained by progressively decreasing the relative pressure in the system from a relative pressure of approximately unity, again monitoring the equilibrium amount of moisture sorbed at each relative pressure. Remember that the moisture sorption isotherm is an equilibrium measurement of the interaction of water with a solid. In theory, information regarding the kinetics of moisture uptake is not explicitly derived from this experiment. This distinction is an important one that will be explored in more depth later.

Generation of water sorption–desorption isotherms for a particular solid can lend considerable insight into the nature of the water–solid interaction, as well as the surface characteristics of the solid. This information is readily obtained from the amount of moisture sorbed at lower relative humidities in comparison with the specific surface area of the sample, from the general shape of the isotherm, from whether or not water uptake is a completely reversible process (i.e., whether hysteresis is observed between sorption and desorption), and from the shape of the hysteresis loop if it is present. With knowledge of the aforementioned, one can usually obtain an indication of the mechanism of moisture sorption for the material of interest. For example, a material that exhibits sorption at lower relative humidities in much greater amounts than one might expect based on the specific surface area of the sample, and that exhibits hysteresis over the complete range of relative humidities, is most likely absorbing water into its internal structure. On the other hand, a material exhibiting a closed hysteresis loop over the higher relative humidity range while sorbing moisture over the lower relative humidity range similar to what might be expected based on its specific surface area, is probably quite porous in nature and is most likely sorbing water via capillary condensation over the higher relative humidity range.

MODELS DESCRIBING VAPOR ADSORPTION

Brunauer, Emmett, and Teller Equation

The model most commonly referred to in the literature describing vapor adsorption onto solid surfaces was put forth in 1938 by Brunauer, Emmett, and Teller (4). The so-called BET model was originally derived using kinetic arguments in a manner very similar to those used by Langmuir (5). The BET model has since also been derived using statistical mechanics (6–8). The BET model assumes that vapor molecules, behaving as an ideal gas, exist in a state of equilibrium with a solid that consists of identical, homogeneous adsorption sites. The first vapor molecule adsorbed to an adsorption site on the solid is proposed to be bound, whereas molecules adsorbing beyond the first layer are assumed to have the properties of the bulk liquid. Furthermore, adsorption is proposed to occur such that the adsorbed molecules do not interact laterally. The linear form of the BET equation is

$$\frac{1}{W\left[\dfrac{P^0}{P-1}\right]} = \frac{(C_b - 1) * \dfrac{P}{P^0}}{W_m C_b} + \frac{1}{W_m C_b} \tag{5}$$

where W is the mass of vapor adsorbed per gram of solid at a particular relative pressure, P/P^0; W_m is the theoretical quantity of vapor adsorbed when each adsorption site has one vapor molecule adsorbed to it; and

$$C_b = k \exp\left(\frac{H_1 - H_L}{RT}\right) \tag{6}$$

where H_1 is the heat of adsorption of the first vapor molecule adsorbed to a site, H_L is the heat of condensation of the bulk adsorbate, R is the universal gas constant, T is the absolute temperature, and k is a constant, usually assumed to be close to unity. The two BET constants, W_m and C_b, can easily be obtained from the linear plotting form of the BET equation given in Eq. 5. Plotting the quantity $1/[W(P^0/P - 1)]$ versus P/P^0 gives a slope equal

to $(C_b - 1)/W_m C_b$ and an intercept equal to $1/W_m C_b$. Algebraic manipulation gives

$$W_m = \frac{1}{\text{slope} + \text{intercept}} \tag{7}$$

and

$$C_b = 1 + \frac{\text{slope}}{\text{intercept}} \tag{8}$$

In general, the BET equation fits adsorption data quite well over the relative pressure range 0.05–0.35, but predicts considerably more adsorption at higher relative pressures than is experimentally observed. This is consistent with an assumption built into the BET derivation that an infinite number of layers are adsorbed at a relative pressure of unity. Application of the BET equation to nonpolar gas adsorption results is carried out quite frequently to obtain estimates of the specific surface area of solid samples. By assuming a cross-sectional area for the adsorbate molecule, one can use W_m to calculate specific surface area by the following relationship:

$$S = \frac{W_m X N_{av}}{M \Sigma} \tag{9}$$

where S is the specific surface area in m^2/g; W_m is the mass of adsorbate adsorbed at monolayer coverage; X is the cross-sectional area of an adsorbed adsorbate molecule (assumed to be 19.5 Å^2 for krypton, 16.2 Å^2 for nitrogen, 12.5 Å^2 for water (9, 10)); N_{av} is Avogadro's number; M is the molecular weight of adsorbate; and Σ is the mass of the sample. Obviously, calculating surface areas from moisture uptake data that does not lead to monolayer coverage at W_m [either incomplete coverage (see the section on "Water Sorption onto Nonhydrates" below) or absorption into the solid (see the section on "The Meaning of Specific Surface Areas Calculated from Water Absorption Studies")] will result in incorrect values that have no physical meaning. Therefore, comparison of the surface area measured by nonpolar gas adsorption to that calculated from a moisture sorption isotherm can lend insight into the fundamental interactions between the water and the solid. This will be explored in some depth later.

Guggenheim and deBoer Equation

Many attempts to modify the BET adsorption theory have been made since its original derivation. Its simplicity and ability to fit adsorption data extremely well at lower relative pressures, however, have made it the model of choice for estimating surface areas from nonpolar gas adsorption. Most modifications of the BET model, developed to analyze data over the entire range of relative pressures, usually add at least one fitting parameter to the equation. This makes computer fitting a necessity, because only two measurable parameters, W and P/P^0, are available. From a modeling perspective, additional fitting parameters of unknown or undefined physical meaning that arise from such approaches are often a deterrent to the use of multiparameter models because of the consequent difficulty in interpreting results. In this regard, therefore, only a single modification of the BET model, which has been shown to extend the relative pressure range over which vapor adsorption data can be fit, will be considered here. This extension of the BET model, independently derived by Guggenheim (11) and deBoer (12), accounts for the adsorption of an intermediate state of vapor between the tightly bound first molecule adsorbing to an adsorption site and the condensed molecules adsorbed at very high relative pressures. Molecules adsorbed in the intermediate range can be considered to interact with the solid, but the interaction is assumed to be considerably less than that of the first molecule sorbed at an adsorption site. Obviously, this addition of a "third state" of interaction is an approximation. In all likelihood, there is a continuum of interaction states. However, from a computational point of view, the existence of three or more states is indistinguishable. The equation for the three-state interaction model is given as

$$W = \frac{W_m C_G K \frac{P}{P^0}}{\left[1 - K \frac{P}{P^0}\right]\left[1 - K \frac{P}{P^0} + C_G K \frac{P}{P^0}\right]} \tag{10}$$

where P, P^0, H_L, W, and W_m are identical to the parameters used in the BET equation, and

$$K = B \exp\left(\frac{H_L - H_m}{RT}\right) \tag{11}$$

where B is a constant and H_m is the heat of adsorption of vapor adsorbed in the intermediate layer. The constant C_G is defined as

$$C_G = D \exp(H_1 - H_m RT) \tag{12}$$

where D is a constant, H_1 is the heat of adsorption of the first molecule adsorbed at a site, and H_m is the heat of adsorption of the intermediately bound molecule.

Water Vapor Absorption by Amorphous Solids

The process of water vapor interaction with amorphous solids has been likened to the production of a solid solution in which the water is dissolved in the solid matrix. As more

water is absorbed, the fundamental properties of this solid matrix (e.g., viscosity) can undergo significant change that can then result in visually apparent changes in physical properties (e.g., collapse, recrystallization) (13–17). This will be discussed in further detail later.

Although water vapor is absorbed into amorphous solids and not simply adsorbed on the surface, it still has been found that such sorption isotherms can be fit to the BET equation up to a P/P^0 of about 0.40 as with vapor adsorption, and over the entire range of P/P^0 using its extension, Eq. 10. Because this was first reported by Anderson (18) to be the case for water absorption, Eq. 10, when applied to water vapor sorption, is often called the GAB equation for Guggenheim, Anderson, and deBoer (19). Because the theoretical process for the derivation of the original equation does not translate directly to the absorption process, which involves dissolution of water in the amorphous solid, the significance of fit to the GAB equation is somewhat limited. It is, however, a very useful equation because it does allow one to describe the entire isotherm and to draw out some useful parameters (to be discussed in what follows).

Since water vapor dissolves in the solid during absorption, several models based on solution theory, proposing that the sorbate is taken up into the solid as a solid solution, have been derived and used to describe water sorption on polymers [e.g., Flory-Huggins (20), Hallwood-Horrobin (21)]. More recently, Vrentas et al. (22, 23) developed a solution-based model that accounts for the plasticizing effect of water on a polymer that has been shown to describe the entire moisture uptake isotherm for the polymer (24). While these sorption theories and the many modifications of the BET adsorption model are based on meaningful physicochemical principles, further work is still required to elucidate the molecular mechanisms underlying moisture uptake into polymeric systems. From this perspective, other models based on entirely different theoretical concepts will not be considered further in this chapter. For further reference, the reader is directed to several excellent literature reviews of the many sorption theories that have been proposed (25, 26).

Capillary Condensation

Vapor sorption onto porous solids differs from vapor uptake onto the surfaces of flat materials in that a vapor (in this case, water) will condense to a liquid in a pore structure at a vapor pressure, P_r, below the vapor pressure, P^0, where condensation occurs on flat surfaces. This is generally attributed to the increased attractive forces between adsorbate molecules that occur as surfaces become highly curved, such as in a pore or capillary. This phenomenon is referred to as capillary condensation and is described by the Kelvin equation (27):

$$\ln\left(\frac{P_r}{P^0}\right) = -2\gamma V_m rRT \tag{13}$$

where γ is the surface tension of the adsorbed film (assumed equal to that of the bulk liquid), V_m is the molar volume of the liquid, r is the pore radius, R is the gas constant, and T is the temperature. The Kelvin equation has been shown to be applicable to pore radii as low as 5 nm for water adsorption onto mica (28, 29). As mentioned in the section on The Water Sorption Isotherm, capillary condensation will result in a closed hysteresis loop in the adsorption/desorption isotherm of a porous material. Calculating P_r/P^0 by assuming a surface tension of water of 72.8 ergs/cm^2 and a density of 0.998 g/cm^3 at 293 K [this is an assumption for the purposes of this calculation as it has been shown that the density of water is lower in a pore than the bulk value (30)] shows that condensation is predicted at relative pressures of 0.998, 0.989, 0.898, and 0.340 for pore radii of 1000, 100, 10, and 1 nm, respectively. In this regard, it is clear that capillary condensation need only be considered for very small pore dimensions. In practical terms, one should be concerned about this mechanism of water uptake for microporous pharmaceutical powders that exhibit a relatively large specific surface area (i.e., >100 m^2/g), as determined from nonpolar gas adsorption studies.

METHODOLOGY

Control of Relative Humidity

Maintenance of constant relative humidity environments is essential for studying water–solid interactions. There are primarily four techniques that are frequently employed to maintain constant relative humidity:

1. Colligative solutions.
2. Temperature modification of an aqueous solution.
3. Control of total pressure over the solid.
4. Mixing wet and dry air streams.

Saturated salt solutions and sulfuric acid solutions establish relative humidity by reducing the vapor pressure above an aqueous solution (a colligative effect). Saturated salt solutions at controlled temperature maintain a constant relative humidity as long as excess salt and bulk solution are present. As water is added or removed from the solution,

moisture from the headspace will either condense or evaporate (as appropriate), with subsequent dissolution or precipitation of salt to maintain the equilibrium vapor pressure. Because the degree of vapor pressure depression is dependent on the number of species in solution and, further, since the solubility of most salts is somewhat dependent on temperature, the relative humidity generated is also temperature dependent. Hence, use of the same salt at different temperatures can result in different relative humidities. Refs. 31–35 can be consulted for specific saturated salt solutions that result in defined relative humidities as a function of temperature. Because relative humidity is dependent on the number of dissolved species, it is essential that saturation be attained prior to beginning experimentation. In this regard, preparing the salt solutions several days before beginning a sorption study is recommended. Sulfuric acid solutions of varying concentration (35) are also used to establish relative humidity. Addition or removal of water from the solution by desorption or sorption of water to the solid, however, will alter the concentration of sulfuric acid (and water) in solution, and thus change the relative humidity of the headspace. This technique for controlling relative humidity in the headspace is practically more useful when small amounts of water are sorbed/desorbed from the solid.

Temperature modification of an aqueous solution can also be used to maintain constant relative humidity in the headspace (19). This technique maintains the solid at one temperature and an aqueous solution connected to the system at another temperature. Due to strong vapor pressure dependence on temperature, very tight temperature control of the aqueous solution and the solid are required to maintain constant relative humidity in the vicinity of the solid by this technique.

Control of the vapor pressure in the headspace over a solid can also be used to maintain a relative humidity over a solid. As shown in Eq. 4, the relative humidity is directly correlated to the partial pressure of water in the vapor phase. To utilize this technique for relative humidity control, the headspace above the sample must be completely evacuated prior to analysis. Pure water vapor can then be carefully admitted to the vapor phase. Because only water vapor is present, the pressure measured over the system is directly related to the relative humidity over the sample (36).

Mixing dry and water vapor saturated air in defined proportions also can be used to generate constant relative humidity. Control of flow rates and the water vapor content of the dry and saturated air are essential to ensure accurate, reproducible relative humidity production (37, 38).

Measurement of Relative Humidity

Measurement of relative humidity depends on the system used. Systems employing vacuum are usually evacuated prior to introduction of water vapor (36, 39). For cases in which a gas-forming reaction is not occurring, measurement of total pressure in the system can be used as a measure of water vapor pressure. Systems in which air is not evacuated require specific measurement of water vapor pressure. (For the latter type of system, caution should be taken to assure that the relative humidity source is in close proximity to the solid, since the diffusion of water vapor through air to the solid is required to maintain a constant relative humidity in the immediate vicinity of the solid.) A wide variety of pressure measuring instrumentation is commercially available with varying accuracy, precision, and cost.

Measurement of the Critical Relative Humidity, RH_0

The relative humidity at which a solid begins to deliquesce, RH_0, can be determined in three ways: 1) directly, by measuring the relative humidity above a saturated solution of the substance; 2) by determining the relative humidity at which significant moisture uptake and simultaneous dissolution occurs, or; 3) indirectly, by measuring the steady state moisture uptake rate at relative humidities above RH_0 and then extrapolating to the relative humidity at which the moisture uptake rate is zero (1, 40, 41).

Although other techniques can be used to measure the relative humidity above a saturated solution, one relatively simple procedure is to evacuate the headspace (to remove air by vapor phase expansions) and then, with the vacuum pumps isolated and the saturated solution maintained at a constant temperature, to measure water vapor pressure. Water vapor pressure can then be converted to relative humidity by dividing by P^0, the vapor pressure above pure water at the temperature of interest (42).

Measurement of Moisture Uptake (Kinetics of Deliquescence)

The rate of moisture uptake above RH_0 requires maintenance and measurement of a range of relative humidities, and the capability of measuring the moisture content of the solid over time. Use of a vacuum system can minimize vapor diffusion through the headspace, thus maintaining constant relative humidity in the vicinity of the sample. Also, because the most reliable estimate of the steady-state moisture uptake rate is when the integrity of the solid is intact and the film of sorbed moisture is thin

(and saturation most likely), it is advisable to determine the moisture uptake rate at early time periods. In this regard, it is also helpful to be able to view the solid during the experiment to verify that integrity is maintained and excess solid remains (41, 43).

Measurement of Equilibrium Moisture Sorption

Generation of water sorption/desorption isotherms in a controlled relative humidity environment can be carried out either gravimetrically or volumetrically. Gravimetric methods require

1. A dry sample weight,
2. Constant temperature of the sample,
3. Maintaining predetermined constant relative humidities in the headspace, and
4. Attaining and measuring an equilibrium weight of sorbed water vapor. Gravimetric measurement of moisture uptake can occur continuously or discontinuously. Continuous measurement usually involves placing a sample on a balance in a temperature- and relative humidity-controlled environment. Microbalances in closed systems have been used successfully for this purpose (37–39, 44), and commercial systems are now available that can accurately and precisely control relative humidity and simultaneously monitor sample weight.

Volumetric methods require

1. A dry sample weight,
2. Constant temperature of the sample,
3. Water vapor pressure measurement in a dosing volume and, later, in the headspace above the equilibrated sample, and
4. Measuring dead volumes of the individual chambers, including the sample chamber. In essence, volumetric methods equilibrate a known headspace dosing volume at a given (measured) water vapor pressure, followed by exposure of the pre-equilibrated sample to this water, with subsequent measurement of the water vapor pressure after equilibration. The mass of water sorbed, Δn (in moles), at the final pressure in the system, P_f, is obtained from the difference, ΔP, between P_f^{calc}, the calculated water vapor pressure at equilibrium, and P_f^{meas}, the final measured water vapor pressure:

$$\Delta n = \frac{\Delta P V}{RT} \tag{14}$$

where V is the final volume, R is the gas constant, and T is the absolute temperature (39).

WATER SORPTION BY CRYSTALLINE SOLIDS

General Model

Fig. 1 schematically describes the important steps in the uptake of water vapor by crystalline water-soluble solids. At low relative humidities, water is adsorbed to the surface of a nonhydrate-forming solid. As the relative humidity is increased, some tendency for multilayer sorption is expected. At some relative humidity (characteristic for a given substance), the solid will begin to dissolve in the sorbed film of water. A saturated solution of solute will most likely exist, and this will cause the vapor pressure over the sorbed film of water to be depressed relative to pure water and to be constant and equal to that above a saturated solution of the substance. This vapor pressure may be expressed as the critical relative humidity, RH_0. If the relative humidity in the atmosphere is greater than that over the saturated solution (RH_0), water will spontaneously condense on the aqueous film. This will dilute the film allowing more solid to dissolve, which, in turn, will maintain the pressure gradient. The process of water vapor uptake will continue until all the solid has dissolved and further solution dilution has occurred. Only when the relative humidity above the solution is elevated to that of the atmosphere will this process terminate. This phenomenon is called deliquescence. Although hydrates undergo solid state transitions in transforming from the anhydrate to hydrate, as well as from one hydrate species to another, behavior similar to that previously described for nonhydrates is also noted at and above RH_0 for hydrates. In pharmaceutical systems, water-soluble species are frequently encountered in dosage forms. Thus, it is important to understand the conditions responsible for deliquescence and the molecular events occurring at relative humidities below the deliquescence point.

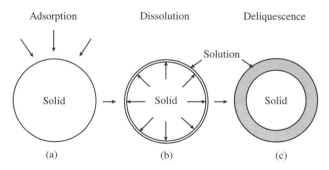

Fig. 1 Water vapor adsorption and deliquescence of a water-soluble solid at (a) atmospheric relative humidity, $RH_i < RH_0$; (b) $RH_i = RH_0$; (c) $RH_i > RH_0$.

Water Sorption onto Nonhydrates below RH_0

The sorption of water vapor onto nonhydrating crystalline solids below RH_0 will depend on the polarity of the surface(s) and will be proportional to surface area. For example, water exhibits little tendency to sorb to nonpolar solids like carbon or polytetrafluoroethylene (Teflon) (29), but it sorbs to a greater extent to more polar materials such as alkali halides (45–48) and organic salts like sodium salicylate (48). Because water is only sorbed to the external surface of these substances, relatively small amounts (i.e., typically less than 1 mg/g) of water are sorbed compared with hydrates and amorphous materials that absorb water into their internal structures.

Unfortunately, the literature is relatively sparse with examples showing the water uptake profile onto crystalline, nonhydrating substances below RH_0. This is most likely due to the difficulty in accurately measuring the small amounts of water that are sorbed. Alkali halides are an exception, however, likely due to their well-characterized particle morphologies (45–48). Figure 2 shows a water uptake isotherm onto recrystallized sodium chloride (48). Note that the amount of water sorbed as a function of relative humidity is normalized to the specific surface area of the sample. Because water is sorbed only to the external surface of this material, this allows comparison of water uptake data from different lots of material, whereas plotting this data on a "per gram" basis would have little or no meaning. For the sodium chloride sample in Fig. 2 (specific surface area = 0.0875 m^2/g from krypton adsorption studies), only 5×10^{-4} g water/m^2 of sodium chloride is sorbed, even up to 70% relative humidity. Also, note the apparent step-like nature of the isotherm. From BET analysis of the sorption data at the lower relative humidities, a W_m value of 7.6×10^{-5} g/m^2 is obtained. This value is only about 0.32 that of the predicted value for monolayer coverage assuming an area per water molecule of 12.5 Å^2. This suggests that it is quite meaningless to refer to the number of layers of sorbed water as multiples of W_m, except as a point of reference. Interestingly, the second step plateau in Fig. 2 occurs at about three times the moisture content corresponding to W_m, suggesting that for sodium chloride, the monolayer is actually completed during the second step of the isotherm. Isosteric heat of sorption results for sodium chloride from Barraclough and Hall (45) suggest that the heat of sorption of water up to W_m is invariant, whereas the heat of sorption decreases and becomes constant at about two times W_m. Considering the experimental error involved in obtaining W_m and the isosteric heats of sorption, this suggests that

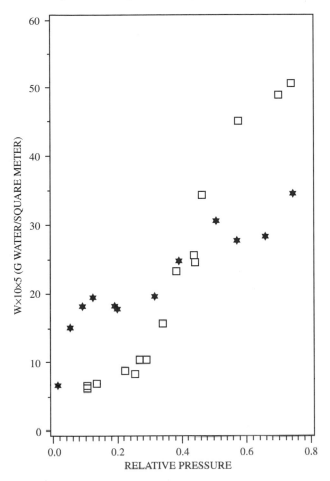

Fig. 2 Water vapor sorption for recrystallized (□) and ground (*) sodium chloride at 20°C. (From Ref. 48.)

Water Sorption onto Hydrates below RH_0

Many drugs and excipients (cephalexin monohydrate, quinidine sulfate dihydrate, ampicillin trihydrate, codeine sulfate trihydrate, morphine sulfate dihydrate, dicalcium phosphate trihydrate, raffinose pentahydrate, lactose monohydrate) utilize water as an integral part of their crystal structure. Solids that form specific crystal hydrates tend to sorb relatively small amounts of water to their external surface below a characteristic relative humidity, when initially dried to an anhydrous state. Below this characteristic relative humidity, these materials behave similarly to nonhydrates. Once the characteristic relative humidity is attained, addition of more water to the system will not result in a further increase in relative humidity. Rather, this water will be sorbed so that the anhydrate crystal will be converted to the hydrate. The strength of the water–solid interaction depends on the level of hydrogen bonding possible within the lattice (29, 49). In some hydrates (e.g., caffeine and theophylline) where hydrogen bonding is relatively weak, water molecules can aid in hydrate stabilization primarily due to their space-filling role (29, 49, 50).

Since water molecules occupy regular positions within the lattice of a hydrate with a specific stoichiometry (e.g., 1:1 monohydrate, 2:1 dihydrate, 5:1 pentahydrate) to the solid, relatively large quantities of water are sorbed. Fig. 3 shows a moisture uptake isotherm for ipratropium bromide (51). This substance undergoes an apparent hydration of the crystal between 63% and 75% relative humidity. Above 75% relative humidity, approximately 4.6% water is sorbed (theoretical monohydrate is 4.4%). Interestingly, as anhydrous ipratropium bromide is equilibrated for extended time periods (e.g., 2 and 5 months respectively, as shown in Fig. 3), hydration of the crystal appears to occur at 53% and 63% relative humidity. This example clearly shows that a time period of many months may be required to attain a reliable estimate of the equilibrium uptake at select relative humidities. Characteristic of many hydrates, ipratropium bromide exhibits significant hysteresis between the sorption and desorption isotherms. This is attributed to the degree of binding and the physical fit of water in the hydrated lattice.

Nonspecific hydration, or hydration of the lattice without a first-order phase transition, also must be considered. Cox et al. (52) reported the moisture uptake profile of cromolyn sodium, and the related effects on the physical properties of this substance. Although up to nine molecules of water per molecule of cromolyn sodium are sorbed into the crystalline lattice at 90% relative humidity,

water is sorbed with a homogeneous binding energy up to W_m and then interacts to a lesser extent until the monolayer is complete.

As shown in Fig. 2 (48) and also in the work of Barraclough and Hall (45), moisture uptake onto sodium chloride as a function of relative humidity is reversible as long as RH_0 is not attained. This is evidence that actual dissolution of water-soluble crystalline substances does not occur below RH_0. This is consistent with the thermodynamic rationale that dissolution below RH_0 would require a supersaturated solution (i.e., an increased number of species in solution would be necessary to induce dissolution at a relative humidity below that of the saturated solution, RH_0). In this regard, one should only need to consider the solid state properties of a purely crystalline material below RH_0. As will be described, other considerations may be warranted for a substance that exists in multiple polymorphic forms or contains amorphous material.

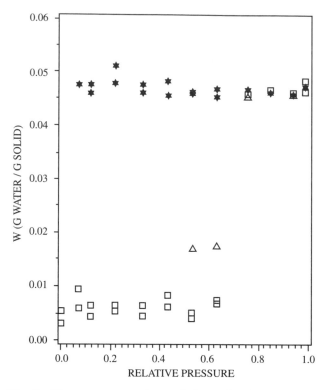

Fig. 3 Water vapor sorption and desorption isotherms for ipratropium bromide at 20°C. (□) 2- month sorption results; (△) 5- month sorption results; (*) 2- and 5- month desorption results. (Note: All 2- month sorption results, except at 53% and 63% relative humidity, were verified at 5 months.)

the sorption profile does not show any sharp plateaus corresponding to fixed hydrates. Rather, the uptake profile exhibits a gradual increase in moisture content as relative humidity increases, which results in marked changes in X-ray diffraction patterns, density, and other physical properties. For this example, moisture uptake onto cromolyn sodium was correlated with expansion of the lattice in the b crystallographic direction, which was shown to be reversible on dehydration.

A thorough understanding of the hydration profile for a solid forming a crystal hydrate is important for several reasons. First, because an anhydrate and hydrate(s) are distinct thermodynamic species, they will have different physicochemical properties (e.g., solubility) that may affect dissolution or bioavailability. Second, a desired hydrate species can be formed and used (and retained) simply by controlling the established environmental conditions. Third, because significant quantities of water can be sorbed/liberated as a hydrate becomes hydrated/dehydrated, the physicochemical properties of the immediate system (including other nearby solids) can be markedly affected.

The Critical Relative Humidity, RH_0

Knowledge of RH_0 for each component in a formulation, and for the entire system, is extremely important for predicting relative humidities where gross physical changes of the system are expected due to dissolution of water-soluble components. The value of RH_0, as a colligative property, is significantly influenced by the number of species in solution. As a rule of thumb, two general comments can be made. First, compounds exhibiting poor water solubility typically have RH_0 values well above 95% relative humidity. Second, as solubility increases, RH_0 decreases. Since nonidealities are introduced as solutions become more and more concentrated, it is not usually possible to use dilute solution models (e.g., Raoult's law) to predict the expected RH_0 for a solute of significant aqueous solubility. Hence, RH_0 should be measured for individual solids. Examples of RH_0 values for single component systems are shown in Table 1.

Values of RH_0 for mixtures, on the other hand, can be calculated from the RH_0 values of single components using an equation developed by Ross (54):

$$\frac{(RH_0)_{mix}}{100} = \left(\frac{(RH_0)_1}{100}\right) * \left(\frac{(RH_0)_2}{100}\right) * \left(\frac{(RH_0)_3}{100}\right) \cdots$$

(15)

Table 1 RH_0 values for single component systems at 25°C

Compound	RH_0	Reference
Potassium chloride	84	(41)
Potassium bromide	81	(41)
Potassium iodide	68	(41)
Sodium chloride	75	(41)
Choline iodide	72	(41)
Choline bromide	41	(41)
Choline chloride	23	(41)
Tetrabutylammonium bromide	61	(41)
Potassium acetate	23	(31)
Potassium carbonate	43	(31)
Sucrose	84	(41)
Fructose	64	(41)
Glucose	87	(41)
Sodium salicylate	79	(39)
Sodium benzoate	88	(39)
Salicylic acid	>99	(53)
Benzoic acid	>99	(53)
Malic acid	78	(53)
Tartaric acid	93	(53)
Fumaric acid	98	(53)
Succinic acid	95	(53)

Table 2 RH$_0$ values for single component systems at 25°C

Mixture	RH$_0$ calculated	Experiment
Sodium cloride–potassium bromide	61	64
Potassium chloride–sodium chloride	64	67
Potassium chloride–potassium bromide	68	73
Sucrose–potassium bromide	68	66
Sucrose–dextrose monohydrate	69	68
Sucrose–sodium chloride–potassium bromide	51	57
Choline bromide–potassium bromide	33	40
Tetrabutylammonium bromide–potassium bromide	49	57
Tetrabutylammonium bromide–choline bromide	25	34

where $(RH_0)_{mix}$ is the relative humidity above a saturated solution of the mixture and $(RH_0)_i$ represents the relative humidities of the individual saturated salt solutions. The Ross equation was derived assuming dilute solutions and negligible interaction between the components in solution. The results presented in Table 2 compare RH$_0$ values obtained by calculating RH$_0$ values for mixtures from the Ross equation and those obtained experimentally. Agreement is very good, especially considering the high levels of dissolved solute(s) that are attained (i.e., estimated as high as 50 molal for the choline bromide/tetrabutylammonium bromide system) (43).

The Kinetics of Deliquescence above RH$_0$

Initial work by Edgar and Swan (55), Adams and Merz (56), Prideaux (57), Morkowitz and Boryta (58), and Carstensen (1) suggested that the rate of moisture uptake onto water-soluble solids above RH$_0$ should depend on the difference between the partial pressure of water in the environment and that of the partial pressure of water above a saturated solution of the water-soluble substance, the temperature, the exposed surface area of the solid, the velocity of movement of the moist air, and a specific reaction constant that is characteristic of the individual solid.

Van Campen et al. (41) developed models describing the rate of moisture uptake above RH$_0$ that consider both the mass transport of water to the solid substance and the heat transfer away from the surface. For the special case of an environment consisting of pure water (i.e., initial vacuum conditions), the Van Campen et al. model is greatly simplified because vapor diffusion need not be considered. Here, only the rate at which heat is transported away from the surface is assumed to

be an important factor in limiting the sorption rate, W'. For this special case, an expression was derived to express the rate of moisture uptake solely as a function of RH$_I$, the relative humidity of the environment, and RH$_0$.

This model was shown to be applicable for describing moisture uptake kinetics (in vacuum) above RH$_0$ for single component systems of alkali halides, sugars, and choline salts (41). The model later was extended to consider the moisture uptake kinetics above RH$_0$ for multicomponent systems of these substances (43).

WATER SORPTION BY AMORPHOUS SOLIDS

Isotherm Analyses at Ambient Temperatures

The amount of moisture sorbed by amorphous solids is typically much greater than that sorbed by nonhydrating crystalline substances below their critical relative humidities. Typical substances of pharmaceutical interest in this class of solids include celluloses, starches, poly(vinylpyrrolidone), gelatin, and some lyophilized proteins. Although some of these substances exhibit partially crystalline character, they generally contain significant fractions of amorphous material and, thus, fall into this class of substances. A typical isotherm for microcrystalline cellulose is shown in Fig. 4. Note the significant amounts of water that are sorbed over the entire relative humidity range and that both the sorption and desorption isotherms are characterized by the classical sigmoidal shape often observed with the physical adsorption of gases. Also apparent is the hysteresis between the sorption and desorption portions of the isotherm (i.e., the amount of water associated with the solid is greater for the desorption isotherm than the sorption isotherm for a given relative

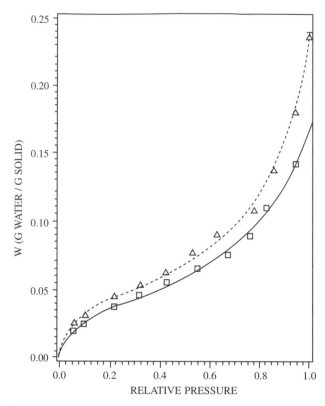

Fig. 4 Water vapor sorption (□) and desorption (△) isotherms for microcrystalline cellulose at 20°C. Solid line: GAB fit to sorption data; Dashed line: GAB fit to desorption data.

Table 3 W_m Values for various starches obtained from BET analysis of moisture uptake isotherms

Starch	W_m (g/g)	Reference
Corn	0.095[a]	(39)
Corn	0.083	(63)
Potato	0.085	(19)
Wheat	0.080	(19)

[a]This value is taken from the desorption isotherm. Others are from sorption isotherms.
(From Ref. 61.)

pressure). This is typical for these types of materials and is generally attributed to either kinetic effects or to a change in the polymer chain conformation caused by plasticization effects of sorbed water (19, 59–62).

Fig. 4 also shows the excellent fit to the GAB equation (Eq. 10) of the sorption and desorption isotherms for microcrystalline cellulose. In this regard, this equation offers considerable practical utility in fitting isotherms for these types of materials over the entire relative humidity range, especially in contrast to the BET equation, which usually only fits uptake data up to about 40% relative humidity. As previously mentioned, however, this does not in itself confirm the validity of the GAB model for describing moisture sorption data on these materials. Rather, independent confirmation of the physical meaning is necessary.

Considerable physical insight has been gained into the primary binding mechanism of water onto starches and celluloses from isotherm analyses that yield values for W_m (Eqs. 5, 7, and 10). This is illustrated in Table 3, which gives W_m values for three types of starches (61). Table 3 shows that the values for W_m are quite constant despite

significant morphological differences between the various starches. One value of W_m, taken from a fit of desorption data, appears to be slightly higher than values obtained from sorption data. This might be expected if the availability of primary sorption sites had been increased by previous exposure to elevated relative humidities, with subsequent increased levels of water sorption. As shown by Van den Berg et al. (19, 59, 60), these values of W_m are all close to the value of 0.11 g of water per g of starch, calculated by assuming that one water molecule sorbs per anhydroglucose unit. Because this calculation assumes that all anhydroglucose units are available for primary binding, and because this is not likely to be precisely the case, it is not surprising that the values measured for W_m are slightly less than 0.11 g/g.

Zografi et al. (61, 64) have extended this analysis to the sorption of water by various celluloses. For celluloses, corrections are necessary because only the amorphous regions of cellulose take up water vapor. Table 4 shows the W_m values obtained from isotherm analyses of several cellulosic materials after accounting for the degree of crystallinity. As expected, celluloses with different degrees of crystallinity exhibit different values of W_m

Table 4 W_m Values for various celluloses obtained from BET analysis of moisture uptake isotherms corrected for degree of crystallinity

Cellulose	Crystallinity %	W_m Corr (g/g)	Reference
Cotton	70	0.093	(65)
Cellophane	40	0.098	(65)
MCC	63	0.095	(66)
MCC[a]	49	0.076	(66)
MCC[a]	38	0.107	(66)
MCC[a]	0	0.086	(66)

[a]MCC Ground in a ball mill.
(From Refs. 61 and 66.)

without correction for crystallinity, and all are considerably less than that for the starches. When corrected, however, for the degree of crystallinity, all of the values are in reasonable agreement with each other and with the W_m values obtained for the starches. Especially interesting are the results in Table 4 for microcrystalline cellulose samples having different degrees of crystallinity due to grinding (66). These results suggest that a similar mechanism of water uptake is occurring in starches and the noncrystalline regions of celluloses.

Similar analyses of moisture uptake data available in the literature for other cellulose and starch derivatives used as pharmaceutical excipients are presented in Table 5. Considering the uncertainties associated with the estimated moisture uptake values from published graphs, the values of W_m are all quite consistent with each other and with a stoichiometry of one water molecule per anhydroglucose unit. It is interesting to note that the two samples derived from cellulose, sodium carboxymethylcellulose and sodium croscarmellose, did not require any correction for degree of crystallinity to conform to close to a 1:1 stoichiometry. It appears quite likely, therefore, that the change in chemical structure and the processing of these materials essentially eliminates the crystallinity of cellulose.

The preceding analysis suggests that water, indeed, penetrates throughout the amorphous regions of these materials and undergoes a specific interaction with available sorption sites, most likely the available hydroxyl groups on the anhydroglucose units. Differential heat of sorption results for various starches (19, 63) and cellulose (10, 68) support this model. Data gathered indicates that there is a specific water–solid interaction out to a moisture content of at least the equivalent of 3 times W_m. The water present in this system appears to

exist in a more structured state (i.e., reduced mobility) than bulk water over this range. Interestingly, the heats of sorption exhibit discrete breaks corresponding to stoichiometries of one and two water molecules per anhydroglucose unit. Some differential heat of sorption results are nearly constant over the W_m range, suggesting that binding is homogeneous over this range (10, 19). This is, however, not always the case. This is borne out by heat of vaporization data reported by Etzler and Conners on cellulose samples (70). As measured using simultaneous DSC/TGA, the heat of desorption of water from the matrix continuously increases once the moisture content is less than approximately 0.5 g water/g cellulose (about 3 times W_m). These results suggest that the sorbed water exists in multiple "states" that are energetically distinct.

Other supportive evidence for a specific water–solid interaction is available from thermal studies showing the amount of nonfreezeable water (71–73), nuclear magnetic resonance (39, 74–80), and diffusion studies (81, 82). The evidence is less clear, however, concerning whether there is distinct binding of water to sorption sites with discrete energy levels or whether there is a continuum of states where water interacts to a lesser extent with increasing amount sorbed (61, 83). In any event, it is clear that sorbed water behaves with a considerable degree of mobility, and hence, questions the use of the term "bound water" (61, 84).

Isotherm Analyses as a Function of Temperature

Generally speaking, the absorption of water into amorphous solids as a function of relative humidity decreases as the temperature increases, reflective of an overall exothermic process, normally expected with vapor adsorption processes. Such behavior has been observed with cellulose (85), starch (19), poly(vinylpyrrolidone) (13), and poly(methyl methacrylate) (86). In such cases it is often assumed that the dominant factor is the negative heat of absorption arising from the change in the extent of water binding. The process, however, is made much more complex than this because of the changing morphology of the solid and, hence, an entropy change as well. The complexity of the effects of temperature on water vapor absorption and the possible links to the plasticizing effects of water may be observed in the work of Oksanen and Zografi (13), who have reported that the W_m values for poly(vinylpyrrolidone) over the temperature range of -40–$60°C$ decrease by a factor of three, suggesting that W_m does not reflect the absolute number of available binding sites on the polymer for directly "bound" water.

Table 5 W_m Values for various pharmaceutical excipients obtained from BET analysis of moisture uptake isotherms

Excipient	W_m (g/g)	Reference
Starch 1500	0.074	(63)
Sodium starch glycolate (Explotab®)	0.081	(67)
Sodium starch glycolate (Primogel®)	0.092	(67)
Crosslinked dextrose (CLD-2)	0.098	(68)
Croscarmellose, sodium (Ac-Di-Sol®)	0.094	(68)
Sodium carboxymethylcellulose	0.103	(69)

(From Ref. 61.)

Rather, W_m appears to be related to $W(T_g = T)$, the amount of water sorbed that will reduce the glass transition temperature, T_g, to the temperature of the sample, as the ratio of $W(T_g = T)/W_m$ remains nearly constant at 3.0 over the entire temperature range.

In summary, it is clear that water absorbs into amorphous polymers to a significant extent. Interaction of water molecules with "available" sorption sites likely occurs via hydrogen bonding such that the mobility of the sorbed water is reduced and the thermodynamic state of water is significantly altered relative to bulk water. Yet accessibility of the water to all potential sorption sites appears to be dependent on the previous history and physicochemical properties of the solid. In this regard, the water–solid interaction in amorphous polymer systems is a dynamic relationship depending quite strongly on water activity and temperature.

The Meaning of Specific Surface Areas Calculated from Water Absorption Studies

Simply calculating specific surface areas from the W_m values in Tables 3–5 leads to "apparent" specific surface areas of approximately 300–500 m²/g (61, 64). Specific surface areas obtained from similar analyses of nonpolar gas (nitrogen or krypton) adsorption studies, however, are typically in the range of 1 m²/g, independent of sample pretreatment.

Interestingly, the ball milling studies of microcrystalline cellulose by Nakai (Table 4) (66) have shown that the W_m values obtained from water sorption studies increase to a much greater extent than the increase in surface area because of comminution of the sample. In fact, as discussed earlier, moisture sorption was shown to be proportional to the amount of amorphous character, suggesting that water is absorbed throughout the amorphous regions of this substance. In this regard, artifactual specific surface areas are obtained if calculated from water absorption data (64) for these types of substances.

The Role of Water as a Plasticizer

Absorption of significant amounts of water into the internal structure of a solid has been shown to influence the properties of the solid. This is apparent, for example, in the hysteresis observed between the sorption and desorption isotherms in Fig. 4. This phenomenon becomes exaggerated to a greater extent for materials that consist of higher proportions of amorphous material. Levine and Slade

(14, 87) have demonstrated that water, with a very low glass transition temperature, can act as a plasticizer, thereby lowering the glass transition temperature, T_g, of amorphous polymers. Similar behavior is observed in amorphous low molecular weight solids. Recognizing that the viscoelastic properties of the solid are altered significantly above T_g (rubbery state) relative to below T_g (glass or vitreous state), it is likely that the solid will undergo changes of its physical properties at distinct moisture contents and defined temperatures as a result of this phenomenon (13, 14). Oksanen and Zografi (13) have shown with poly(vinylpyrrolidone) that the moisture content at which the moisture sorption isotherm begins to increase significantly correlates very well with the moisture content that will reduce T_g to the temperature of the isotherm. This is illustrated in Fig. 5, which shows water absorption isotherms for poly(vinylpyrrolidone) over the temperature range of -40 to $60°C$ (13, 88). Clearly, the inflection point at which the isotherm begins

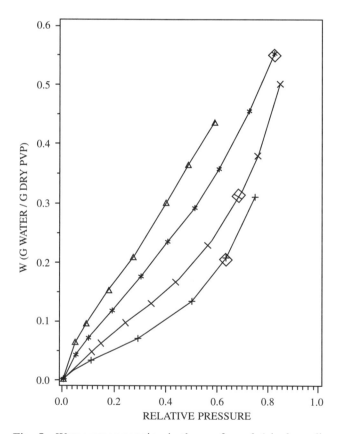

Fig. 5 Water vapor sorption isotherms for poly(vinylpyrrolidone) at 60°C (+); 30°C (×); −20°C (*); −40°C (△). Data were taken from Oksanen and Zografi (76, 78). A ◇ represents the calculated water contents necessary to depress T_g to the temperature of the isotherms.

to turn markedly upward shifts to a higher moisture content as the temperature is reduced. To illustrate this, note that the moisture content (0.674 g/g) necessary to reduce T_g to $-40°C$ has not been attained yet in Fig. 5 and the isotherm appears quite linear over the relative humidity range shown. For further clarity, the moisture contents $[W(T_g = T)]$ corresponding to T_g at $60, 30, -20C$, and $-40°C$ were shown to be about 0.205, 0.313, 0.553, and 0.674 g/g, respectively. Oksanen and Zografi (13) reported that cellulose and elastin (a protein) exhibit similar relationships, where the glass to rubber transitions correspond to the upward inflections in their respective isotherms.

Subsequent studies by Hancock and Zografi (89) demonstrated that the glass transition temperatures for PVP, hydroxypropyl methylcellulose, and poly(methyl methacrylate) were linearly depressed by the weight fraction of sorbed water, according to the simplified Gordon–Taylor/Kelly–Bueche equation (90):

$$\frac{1}{T_g(\text{mix})} = \left(\frac{W_1}{T_{g1}} + \frac{W_2}{T_{g2}}\right) \quad (15)$$

where W_1 and W_2 are the weight fractions of components with T_g values T_{g1} and T_{g2}. The results clearly indicate that the viscoelastic properties of amorphous materials can undergo significant changes as the solid transitions from the glassy to rubbery state. Furthermore, these changes can occur due to elevation of temperature at fixed moisture content or to an increase in moisture content at constant temperature or to a combination of these effects. For dry amorphous substances, molecular mobility of the solid begins to be significantly enhanced relative to the glassy state as low as 50°C below T_g (91). Similar increases in molecular mobility due to the plasticizing effects of absorbed water suggest the need to maintain amorphous systems at least 50°C below the system glass transition temperature to avoid physical, chemical, and/or mechanical property changes over the product shelf life. Some properties that are likely to be affected include tablet compaction (92, 93), gelatin capsule brittleness (14, 94), collapse of lyophilized amorphous powders (88, 95, 96) protein stability (97, 98), and the stability of low molecular weight, moisture sensitive drugs mixed with amorphous polymeric substances (99).

WATER SORPTION BY PHARMACEUTICAL SOLIDS SUBJECTED TO PROCESSING

Understanding the mechanisms of moisture sorption by solids existing in either the crystalline or amorphous states allows a conceptual estimation of critical points where major changes in physical or chemical properties occur (e.g., RH_0, a crystal hydration relative humidity, glass transition temperature). Processing (i.e., milling, spray drying, compaction, lyophilization, etc.) of pharmaceutical solids, however, often induces at least partial conversion of most substances to a high energy form (100–107). Such local disorder has been associated with enhanced chemical reactivity (101–108) and increased solubility (15) relative to the thermodynamically favored crystalline state. These regions have been referred to as "hot" spots of the bulk solid and, when present, leave the solid in an "activated state" (15, 100–107, 109, 110–113).

This nonhomogeneity that exists in processed solids complicates the study of moisture sorption phenomena in these materials, as more than one mechanism of uptake must be considered. This is especially difficult, and often frustrating, for cases in which only a small amount of amorphous material is present, as the experimental techniques required to complete these analyses are labor intensive (114, 115). Yet, relatively low percentages of amorphous material can absorb considerable amounts of water into their structure, with these regions undergoing considerable change and a consequent effect on the overall properties of the bulk substance (100). This is especially important for low molecular weight substances that have the ability to readily recrystallize due to their overall greater mobility relative to higher molecular weight polymeric materials. This has been demonstrated for sodium chloride and sodium salicylate ground for 15 min in a mortar and pestle (48). Whereas recrystallized materials exhibited no change in specific surface areas with increasing relative humidities, the ground samples exhibited significant reductions in specific surface areas as relative humidities were increased. Figure 2 illustrates the differing moisture uptake profiles for the recrystallized and ground sodium chloride samples, normalized for specific surface area (48). Whereas the ground material sorbed significantly more water at lower relative humidities than the recrystallized sample, the recrystallized material sorbed greater amounts at higher relative humidities. This relative reduction in sorption capacity of the ground sample is attributed to a reduction in surface area as relative humidity increased, due to the consequent recrystallization of the disordered surface material (48). Fukuoka et al. (116) have demonstrated that a variety of pharmaceutical substances indeed can be made amorphous and, furthermore, exhibit glass transition temperatures over a range from 243 to 354 K. For example, aspirin, progesterone, phenobarbital, and sulfadimethoxine exhibit T_g values of 243, 279, 321, and 339 K, respectively.

Similar to amorphous polymeric systems, low molecular weight amorphous substances also exhibit a reduction in T_g as moisture content increases (117), thereby leading to favorable conditions for recrystallization to occur. Indeed, low molecular weight amorphous solids possess sufficient molecular mobility well below T_g (118). In some systems with multiple solid states possible, the water activity/moisture content can influence the crystallized form of the solid (119). Unfortunately, recrystallization of nonhydrating, low molecular weight amorphous systems can lead to the liberation of significant amounts of water to the headspace (15, 48, 103, 104, 120). Such "moisture dumping" can have additional impact on the physical, chemical, and mechanical properties of the system (17, 48, 100).

To illustrate this more quantitatively, consider the hypothetical sucrose example discussed by Ahlneck and Zografi (100). Assuming that all the sorbed water is taken up by the amorphous portion of material, 0.1% total moisture would correspond to approximately 20%, 10%, 4%, and 2% moisture content in the amorphous material, respectively, for 0.5%, 1%, 2.5%, and 5% of amorphous solid. The glass transition temperatures for the amorphous portions of these systems range from 9 to 49°C, respectively (87, 100). Hence, significant changes in the solid state properties are expected at room temperature if relatively small amounts of amorphous material (i.e., < 1%) are initially present. This example illustrates that even for low moisture content materials, significant changes can occur in localized amorphous regions of a solid, which may affect properties of the material influenced by molecular mobility (100).

Inhibition of events resulting from increased molecular mobility due to increased moisture absorption and a subsequent reduction in T_g can be accomplished by formulating such materials with amorphous substances of higher T_g. The net effect is to increase molecular interaction and raise the system T_g to a level where molecular mobility is again sufficiently low (high viscosity) such that the undesired property changes do not occur (107, 121, 122).

The recrystallization of amorphous low molecular weight systems can be convoluted by the impact of structural changes on the material. For example, spray drying α-lactose monohydrate typically produces a material that is completely amorphous as determined by powder X-ray diffraction. However, lactose undergoes anomeric rotation in solution, causing a change in the fundamental structure of the molecule. The impact of this structural change on the uptake and equilibration of water to the amorphous lactose is significant. As expected, an increase in moisture content will result in the suppression of the glass transition temperature to the point where instantaneous crystallization occurs. However, the material produced is nonuniform as there are two different forms of lactose present, one of which is anhydrous in the crystalline state. Furthermore, at elevated humidity, the crystalline β-anhydrate can undergo structural change in the solid state and produce the α-monohydrate. Evaluation of data gathered needs to be completed in the context of a careful characterization of the possible solid forms (16, 17, 123–125).

TRANSFER OF WATER BETWEEN SOLID COMPONENTS VIA THE HEADSPACE

Combining solids that have previously been equilibrated at different relative humidities results in a system that is thermodynamically unstable because there will be a tendency for moisture to distribute in the system so that a single relative humidity is attained in the headspace. As shown in Fig. 6, moisture will desorb into the headspace from the component initially equilibrated at a higher relative humidity and sorb to the component initially equilibrated at a lower relative humidity. This process will continue until both solids have equilibrated at the final relative humidity. The final relative humidity can be predicted a priori by the sorption–desorption moisture transfer model (SDMT) model (126) if one has moisture uptake isotherms for each of the solid components, their initial moisture contents and dry weights, headspace volume, and temperature. Final moisture contents for each solid can then easily be estimated from the isotherms for the respective solids.

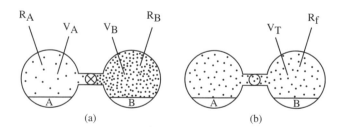

Fig. 6 Schematic representation of moisture transfer between solid components, A and B, respectively. (a) Headspaces isolated from one another; (b) Headspaces allowed to equilibrate. R_A and R_B are initial relative humidities above A and B, respectively; V_A and V_B are headspace volumes above A and B, respectively; R_f and V_T are final relative humidity and headspace volume above A and B, respectively. (From Ref. 126.)

The SDMT model has practical utility in aiding the rational optimization of the initial moisture contents of individual components in a system to attain the final desired relative humidity. Practical applications to date have included adjustment of the initial formulation LODs prior to capsule filling to avoid gelatin capsule brittleness (94, 127), selecting the appropriate formulation moisture content and amount of desiccant to maintain the relative humidity inside a container below a defined value (128), and selection of appropriate dry powder inhaler design and packaging conditions for optimal stability (129).

SUMMARY

Moisture is present in all solid pharmaceutical drugs and dosage forms and in most processing techniques. Understanding where the water resides, its state, and the manner in which it affects the properties of individual materials, their mixtures, and ultimately, final product performance and integrity are essential for the developmental scientist to better understand the role of water in a particular system. Especially important are the kinetics of moisture uptake or loss, "equilibrium" uptake values as a function of relative humidity, whether the water resides externally or is absorbed into the material, its degree of binding with the solid, and the tendency for water to redistribute in a system consisting of more than one solid. Although water–solid interaction(s) can be extremely complex in pharmaceutical systems, application of these fundamental concepts to product development can greatly aid in understanding the role of moisture in affecting the physicochemical properties of solid materials.

ACKNOWLEDGMENTS

The authors thank Professor George Zografi, Dr. Cindy Oksanen, and Dr. Frank Etzler for their technical contributions to this chapter and Ms. Linda Schweikardt for her graphical support.

REFERENCES

1. Carstensen, J.T. *Pharmaceutics of Solids and Solid Dosage Forms*; John Wiley & Sons: New York, 1977; 11–15.
2. Lewis, G.N.; Randall, M.; Pitzer, K.S.; Brewer, L. *Thermodynamics*; McGraw-Hill: New York, 1961.
3. Gal, S. *Vapor Sorption Equilibria and Other Water-Starch Interactions: A Physico-Chemical Approach*; Van den Berg, C., Ed.; Agricultural University: Wageningen, The Netherlands, 1981; 10.
4. Brunauer, S.; Emmett, P.H.; Teller, E. J. Am. Chem. Soc. **1938**, *60*, 309.
5. Langmuir, I. J. Am. Chem. Soc. **1918**, *40*, 1361.
6. Fowler, R.; Guggenheim, E.A. *Statistical Thermodynamics*; Cambridge University Press: Cambridge, UK, 1939.
7a. Hill, T.L. J. Chem. Phys. **1946**, *14*, 263.
7b. J. Am. Chem. Soc. **1946**, *68*, 535.
8a. Cassie, A.B.D. Trans. Faraday Soc. **1945**, *41*, 450.
8b. Trans. Faraday Soc. **1945**, *41*, 458.
9. Lowell, S. *Introduction to Powder Surface Area*; John Wiley & Sons: New York, 1979.
10. Hollenback, R.G.; Peck, G.E.; Kildsig, D.O. J. Pharm. Sci. **1978**, *67*, 1599.
11. Guggenheim, E.A. *Applications of Statistical Mechanics*; Clarendon Press: Oxford, 1966.
12. deBoer, J.H. *The Dynamical Character of Adsorption*, 2nd Ed.; Clarendon Press: Oxford, 1968.
13. Oksanen, C.A.; Zografi, G. Pharm. Res. **1990**, *7*, 654.
14. Levine, H.; Slade, L. *Water Science Reviews*; Franks, F., Ed.; Cambridge University Press: Cambridge, UK, 1987; 3, 79–185.
15. Makower, B.; Dye, W.B. Agr. Fd. Chem. **1956**, *4*, 72.
16. Buckton, G.; Darcy, P. Int. J. Pharm. **1996**, *136*, 141.
17. Buckton, G.; Darcy, P. Int. J. Pharm. **1997**, *158*, 157.
18. Anderson, R.B. J. Am. Chem. Soc. **1946**, *68*, 686.
19. Van den Berg, C. *Vapor Sorption Equilibrium and Other Water-Starch Interactions: A Physico-Chemical Approach*; Agricultural University: Wageningen, The Netherlands, 1981.
20. Flory, P.J. *Principles of Polymer Chemistry*; Cornell University Press: Ithaca, New York, 1953.
21. Hailwood, A.J.; Horrobin, S. Trans. Faraday Soc. **1946**, *42B*, 84.
22. Vrentas, J.S.; Vrentas, C.M. Macromolecules. **1994**, *27*, 4684.
23. Vrentas, J.S.; Vrentas, C.M. Macromolecules. **1994**, *27*, 5570.
24. Hancock, B.C.; Zografi, G. Pharm. Res. **1993**, *10*, 1262.
25. Van den Berg, C.; Bruin, S. *Water Activity: Influences on Food Quality*; Rockland, L.B., Stewart, G.F., Eds.; Academic Press: New York, 1981.
26. Venkateswaren, A. Chem. Rev. **1970**, *70*, 619.
27. Martin, A.; Swarbrick, J.; Cammarata, A. *Physical Pharmacy*; Lea & Febiger: Philadelphia, 1983; 510–512.
28. Fisher, L.R.; Israelachvili, J.N. Chem. Phys. Lett. **1980**, *76*, 325.
29. Zografi, G. Drug Devel. Ind. Pharm. **1988**, *14*, 1905.
30. Etzler, F.M.; Fagundus, D.M. J. Colloid Interface Sci. **1983**, *93*, 585.
31. Greenspan, L. J. Res. N.B.S. **1977**, *81A*, 89.
32. Rockland, L.B.; Nishi, S.K. J. Food Technol. **1980**, *34*, 43.

33. Winston, P.W.; Bates, D.H. Ecology **1960**, *41*, 232.

34. Stokes, R.H.; Robinson, R.A. Ind. Eng. Chem. **1949**, *41*, 2013.

35. Weast, R.C., Ed. *Handbook of Chemistry and Physics*, 6th Ed.; Chemical Rubber Co.: Cleveland, 1986–1987; E-42.

36. Ward, G.H.; Schultz, R.K. Pharm. Res. **1995**, *12*, 773.

37. Bergren, M. *Water–Solid Interactions*; AAPS Short-course: Orlando, FL, 1993.

38. Spancake, C.W.; Hastedt, J.E.; Venero, A.F. Pharm. Res. **1993**, *10*, S-280.

39. Kontny, M.J. *Water Vapor Sorption Studies on Solid Surfaces*; University of Wisconsin-Madison: Madison, WI, 1985.

40. Van Campen, L.; Zografi, G.; Carstensen, J.T. Int. J. Pharm. **1980**, *5*, 1.

41. Van Campen, L.; Amidon, G.L.; Zografi, G. J. Pharm. Sci. **1983**, *72*, 1381, 1388, 1394.

42. *Handbook of Chemistry and Physics*; Weast, R.C., Ed.; Chemical Rubber Co.: Cleveland, 1986–1987, D-189–190.

43. Kontny, M.J.; Zografi, G. J. Pharm. Sci. **1985**, *74*, 124.

44. Bergren, M. Int. J. Pharm. **1994**, *103*, 103.

45. Barraclough, P.B.; Hall, P.G. Surf. Sci. **1974**, *467*, 393.

46. Walter, H.U. Zeitschrift fur Physikalische Chemie Neue Folge Bd. **1971**, *75*, S287.

47. Ladd, R.A. Surf. Sci. **1968**, *12*, 37.

48. Kontny, M.J.; Grandolfi, G.P.; Zografi, G. Pharm. Res. **1987**, *4*, 104.

49. Byrn, S.R. *Solid State Chemistry of Drugs*; Academic Press: New York, 1982; 149.

50. Saleki-Gerhardt, A.; Stowell, J.G.; Byrn, S.R.; Zografi, G. J. Pharm. Sci. **1995**, *84*, 318.

51. Conners, J.J. Unpublished data.

52. Cox, J.S.G.; Woodard, G.D.; McCrone, W.C. J. Pharm. Sci. **1971**, *60*, 1458.

53. Kontny, M.J. Unpublished data.

54. Ross, K.D. Food Technol. **1975**, *29*, 26.

55. Edgar, G.; Swan, W.O. J. Am. Chem. Soc. **1922**, *44*, 570.

56. Adams, J.R.; Merz, A.R. Ind. Eng. Chem. **1929**, *21*, 305.

57. Prideaux, E.B.R. J. Soc. Chem. Ind. **1920**, *39*, 182.

58. Markowitz, M.M.; Boryta, D.A. J. Chem. Eng. Data **1961**, *6*, 16.

59. Van den Berg, C.; Kaper, F.S.; Weldring, J.A.G.; Wolters, I. J. Food Technol. **1975**, *10*, 589.

60. Van den Berg, C. *Water Activity: Influences on Food Quality*; Rockland, L.B., Stewart, G.F., Eds.; Academic Press: New York, 1981; 1–61.

61. Zografi, G.; Kontny, M.J. Pharm. Res. **1986**, *3*, 187.

62. Hancock, B.C.; Zografi, G. Pharm. Res. **1994**, *11*, 471.

63. Wurster, D.E.; Peck, G.E.; Kildsig, D.O. Starch **1984**, *36*, 294.

64. Zografi, G.; Kontny, M.J.; Yang, A.Y.S.; Brenner, G.S. Int. J. Pharm. **1984**, *18*, 99.

65. Stamm, A.J. *Wood and Cellulose Science*; The Ronald Press Co.: New York, 1964.

66. Nakai, Y.; Fukuoka, E.; Nakajima, S.; Hasegawa, J. J. Chem. Pharm. Bull. **1977**, *25*, 96.

67. Mitrevej, A.; Hollenback, R.G. Pharm. Tech. **1982**, *6*, 48.

68. Gordon, R.E.; Peck, G.E.; Kildsig, D.O. Drug Devel. Ind. Pharm. **1984**, *10*, 833.

69. Callahan, J.C.; Cleary, G.W.; Elefant, M.; Kaplan, I.; Kensler, T.; Nash, R.A. Drug Devel. Ind. Pharm. **1982**, *8*, 355.

70. Etzler, F.M.; Conners, J.J. Therm. Acta **1991**, *189*, 185.

71. Rupley, J.A.; Yank, P.-H.; Tollin, G. *Water in Polymers*; Rowland, S.P., Ed.; American Chemical Society: Washington, DC, 1980; 111–132.

72. Nagashima, N.; Suzuki, E.-I. Appl. Spectroscopy Rev. **1984**, *20*, 1.

73. Duckworth, R.B. J. Food Technol. **1971**, *6*, 317.

74. Hennig, H.J.; Lechert, H. J. Colloid Interf. Sci. **1977**, *62*, 199.

75. Mousseri, J.; Steinberg, M.P.; Nelson, A.I.; Wei, L.S. J. Food Sci. **1974**, *39*, 114.

76. Tait, M.J.; Ablett, S.; Wood, F.W. J. Colloid Interf. Sci. **1972**, *41*, 594.

77. Tait, M.J.; Ablett, S.; Franks, F. *Water Structure at the Water–Polymer Interface*; Jellinek, H., Ed.; Plenum Press: New York, 1972; 29–38.

78. Carles, J.E.; Scallan, A.M. J. Appl. Poly. Sci. **1973**, *17*, 1855.

79. Hsi, E.; Voight, G.J.; Bryant, R.G. J. Colloid Interf. Sci. **1979**, *70*, 338.

80. Froix, M.F.; Nelson, R. Macromolecules. **1975**, *8*, 726.

81. Fish, B.P. *Fundamental Aspects of the Dehydration of Foodstuffs*; Soc. Chem. Ind. (S.C.I.): London, 1958; 143–157.

82. Duckworth, R.B.; Smith, G.M. *Recent Advances in Food Science*; Leitch, J.M., Rhodes, D.N., Eds.; Butterworths: London, 1962; 3, 230–238.

83. Etzler, F.M. J. Colloid Interf. Sci. **1983**, *92*, 43.

84. Oksanen, C.A.; Zografi, G. Pharm. Res. **1993**, *10*, 791.

85. Urquart, A.R.; Williams, A.M. J. Textile Inst. **1924**, *15*, 550.

86. Smith, L.S.A.; Schnitz, V. Polymer. **1988**, *29*, 1871.

87. Slade, L.; Levine, H. Pure Appl. Chem. **1988**, *60*, 1841.

88. Mackenzie, A.P.; Rasmussen, D.H. *Water Structure at the Water–Polymer Interface*; Jellineck, H.H.G., Ed.; Plenum: New York, 1972; 146–172.

89. Hancock, B.C.; Zografi, G. Pharm. Res. **1994**, *11*, 471.

90. Gordon, M.; Taylor, J.S. J. Appl. Chem. **1952**, *2*, 493.

91. Hancock, B.C.; Shamblin, S.L.; Zografi, G. Pharm. Res. **1995**, *12*, 799.

92. Shukla, A.J.; Price, J.C. Pharm. Res. **1991**, *8*, 336.

93. Amidon, G.E.; Houghton, M.E. Pharm. Res. **1995**, *12*, 923.

94. Kontny, M.J.; Mulski, C.A. Int. J. Pharm. **1989**, *54*, 79.

95. Mackenzie, A.P. *Freeze Drying and Advanced Food Technology*; Goldblith, S.A., Rey, L., Rothmayr, W., Eds.; Academic Press: New York, 1975; 277–307.

96. Costantino, H.R.; Curley, J.G.; Wu, S.; Hsu, C.C. Int. J. Pharm. **1998**, *166*, 211.

97. Hageman, M.J. Drug Devel. Ind. Pharm. **1988**, *14*, 2047.

98. Hageman, M.J.; Possert, P.L.; Bauer, J.M. J. Agr. Food Chem. **1992**, *40*, 342.

99. Kararli, T.T.; Catalano, T. Pharm. Res. **1995**, *12*, 923.

100. Ahlneck, C.; Zografi, G. Int. J. Pharm. **1990**, *62*, 87.

101. Vadas, E.B.; Toma, P.; Zografi, G. Pharm. Res. **1991**, *8*, 148.

102. Levine, H.; Slade, L. J. Chem. Soc. Faraday Trans. I **1988**, *84*, 2619.

103. Huttenrauch, R. Acta Pharm. Technol. **1988**, *34*, 1.

104. Huttenrauch, R.; Frike, S.; Zeielke, P. Pharm. Res. **1985**, *2*, 302.

105. Otsuka, M.; Kaneniwa, N. Int. J. Pharm. **1990**, *62*, 65.

106. Hersey, J.A.; Krycer, I. Int. J. Pharm. Technol. & Prod. Manuf. **1980**, *1*, 18.

107. Hancock, B.C.; Zografi, G. J. Pharm. Sci. **1996**, *85*, 246.

108. Shalaev, E.Y.; Zografi, G. J. Pharm. Sci. **1996**, *85*, 1137.

109. Carstensen, J.T.; Van Scoik, K. Pharm. Res. **1990**, *7*, 1278.

110. Waltersson, J.-O.; Lundgren, P. Acta Pharm. Suec. **1985**, *22*, 291.

111. Prout, E.G.; Tompkins, F.C. Trans. Faraday Soc. **1944**, *40*, 489.

112. Ng, W.-L. Aust. J. Chem. **1975**, *28*, 1169.

113. Hasegawa, J.; Hanano, M.; Awazu, S. Chem. Pharm. Bull. **1975**, *23*, 86.

114. Saleki-Gerhardt, A. *Estimation of Percent Crystallinity in Milled Samples of Sucrose*; University of Wisconsin-Madison: Madison, WI, 1991.

115. Buckton, G.; Darcy, P. Int. J. Pharm. **1999**, *179*, 141.

116. Fukuoka, E.; Makita, M.; Yamamura, S. Chem. Pharm. Bull. **1989**, *37*, 1047.

117. Saleki-Gerhardt, A.; Zografi, G. Pharm. Res. **1994**, *11*, 1166.

118. Andronis, V.; Zografi, G. Pharm. Res. **1998**, *15*, 835.

119. Andronis, V.; Yoshioka, M.; Zografi, G. J. Pharm. Sci. **1997**, *86*, 346.

120. Lehto, V.-P.; Laine, E. Pharm. Res. **2000**, *17*, 701.

121. Yoshioka, M.; Hancock, B.C.; Zografi, G. J. Pharm. Sci. **1995**, *84*, 983.

122. Shamblin, S.L.; Zografi, G. Pharm. Res. **1999**, *16*, 1119.

123. Angberg, M.; Nystrom, C.; Castensson, S. Int. J. Pharm. **1991**, *73*, 209.

124. Briggner, L.-E.; Buckton, G.; Bystrom, K.; Darcy, P. Int. J. Pharm. **1994**, *105*, 125.

125. Schmitt, E.A.; Law, D.; Zhang, G.G.Z. J. Pharm. Sci. **1999**, *88*, 291.

126. Zografi, G.; Grandolfi, G.P.; Kontny, M.J.; Mendenhall, D.W. Int. J. Pharm. **1988**, *42*, 77.

127. Kontny, M.J. Drug Devel. Ind. Pharm. **1988**, *14*, 1991.

128. Kontny, M.J.; Koppenol, S.; Graham, E.T. Int. J. Pharm. **1992**, *84*, 261.

129. Kontny, M.J.; Conners, J.J.; Graham, E.T. *Proceedings of Respiratory Drug Delivery IV*; Interpharm Press: Engelwood, CO, 1994.

WAXES

Roland A. Bodmeier

Freie Universität Berlin, Berlin, Germany

INTRODUCTION

The term wax generally refers to a substance that is a plastic solid at room temperature and a liquid of low viscosity above its melting point. Strictly speaking, a wax is chemically defined as an ester of a monohydric long chain fatty alcohol and a long chain fatty acid. However, generally the term wax has been applied to a broad group of chemically heterogeneous materials. Waxes usually contain a wide variety of materials including glycerides, fatty alcohols, fatty acids, and their esters. In the pharmaceutical literature, the terms waxes, fats, or lipids have often been used interchangeably and no consistent terminology has been established. They have in common their lipophilic character and their insolubility in water and solubility in nonpolar solvents. Besides natural materials, many semisynthetic products such as fatty acids or alcohols or surfactants are derived from lipids.

Waxes have been used by the pharmaceutical industry for many years. Their applications in semisolid preparations, including ointments, creams, or lotions, and in suppositories are well known and numerous publications exist on this topic. Because of their lipophilic properties, waxes have been used in sustained-release single or multiple unit solid dosage forms. This article reviews the different uses of waxes as sustained-release carrier or coating materials.

WAXES IN PHARMACEUTICAL DOSAGE FORMS

Waxes are obtained from various sources and are generally classified into animal, insect, vegetable, mineral, and synthetic waxes (1–7).

The most familar animal wax is probably lanolin, which is obtained from the wool of the sheep. It consists primarily of esters of C_{18}–C_{26} alcohols and fatty acids, sterols (cholesterol), and terpene alcohols. It is frequently used in topical preparations. Until recently, spermaceti was another commonly used animal wax. Spermaceti is obtained through the precipitation of the head oil from the sperm whale on cooling. It consists primarily of cetyl palmitate. Because of public concerns with animal-derived products, spermaceti has been replaced with other natural or synthetic products.

The most commonly used insect wax is beeswax. It is obtained from the honeycomb of the bee. White and yellow beeswax are GRAS-listed and consist of mixtures of various esters of straight chain monohydric alcohols with even number carbon chains (C_{24}–C_{36}) esterified with straight chain fatty acids. The major ester is myricyl palmitate. Beeswax also contains free acids and carbohydrates. White wax is obtained through bleaching of yellow wax with oxidizing agents or with sunlight. The National Formulary 18 (NF18) (8) specifications list a melting range of 62–65°C, an acid value of 17–24, and an ester value of 72–79. It is practically insoluble in water, sparingly soluble in ethanol, and soluble in chloroform and various oils. Beeswax is used as a stiffening agent in topical preparations, as a stabilizer of w/o-emulsions, and as a polishing agent in sugar coating.

Carnauba wax is plant-derived and is obtained from the carnauba palm tree, indigenous to Brazil. The wax is obtained from the surface of dried leaves. It is widely used in food, cosmetic, and pharmaceutical products. It consists of a complex mixture of high-molecular-weight esters of acids and hydroxyacids. Carnauba wax is very hard and brittle, and has a high melting point. The NF18 specifications list a melting range of 81–86°C, an acid value of 2–7, and a saponification value of 78–95. It is insoluble in water, slightly soluble in boiling ethanol, and soluble in warm chloroform. Besides the sustained-release applications described later, it is used as a polishing agent in sugar coating because of its high gloss, and in topical preparations. Other, less used vegetable-derived waxes include candelilla wax and castor wax.

Hydrogenated vegetable oils are prepared by hydrogenation of refined vegetable oils. Hydrogenated vegetable oil consists of mixtures of triglycerides, with two types being defined in the USP23. Type II includes partially hydrogenated vegetable oils and has a lower melting range and a higher iodine value than Type I. Type I melts in the range of 57–70°C and has iodine value of 0–5, while Type II has a melting range of 20–50°C and an iodine value of 55–80. They are used as lubricants, as sustained-release matrix materials, as viscosity modifiers in semisolid formulations, to enhance

Encyclopedia Pharmaceutical Technology

the solidification of suppositories, and to minimize the sedimentation of dispersed drug.

Two commonly used mineral-derived waxes are petroleum wax, which is microcrystalline, and paraffin wax, which is crystalline. They are both obtained from petroleum: the quality and quantity of the wax depends on the source of the crude oil and the refining process. Microcrystalline wax (petroleum ceresin or wax) consists of straight chain and branched saturated alkanes with a chain length range C_{41}–C_{57}. The NF18 specifications list a melting range of 54–102°C; it comes in plastic and hard grades. It is insoluble in water, slightly soluble in ethanol, and soluble in chloroform. Besides its use as a sustained-release carrier, it is used as a stiffening agent in topical preparations. Because of its high viscosity and melting point, it increases the consistency of creams and ointments. Paraffin wax (hard paraffin) is a mixture of solid straight chain alkanes. It is used in ointments or creams as a base or stiffening agent. It congeals between 47 and 65°C. Various grades with different melting ranges are available. It is insoluble in acetone, ethanol, and water and soluble in chloroform and most warmed fixed oils. Low-molecular-weight polyethylenes (MW < 10,000) have wax-like properties and are used in topical preparations, for example, as gelling agents in Plastibase.

CHARACTERIZATION

Because the harvesting of vegetable or insect waxes is often from wild, noncultivated sources and because of their complex composition, it is important to characterize the chemical and physical properties of the waxes (1–6). The composition of natural materials often varies with location, weather, season of harvesting, and age. A good quality control of the raw materials is of upmost importance in order to obtain pharmaceutical products of high quality.

The chemical methods to characterize waxes include the determination of the acid, saponification, iodine, hydroxyl, and peroxide values. Various tests, often yielding different values, are available to measure the melting point of waxes. Since waxes are nonhomogeneous in chemical composition, a melting range rather than a clear melting point is most observed. The melting point of glycerides generally increases with increasing hydroxyl number, decreasing degree of unsaturation, and increasing molecular weight of the fatty acid. The melting point of many waxes can be determined with capillary tubes. The slip point is defined as the temperature at which a column of the testing material starts raising in an open-ended capillary tube, which is dipped in water filled in a beaker

and heated under specific conditions. The drop-point test can be used; however, it is not reliable for more viscous waxes. The congealing point of a wax is the temperature at which the molten wax stops to flow upon cooling. Thermal methods such as differential scanning calorimetry (DSC) are widely used to characterize the heating and cooling profiles of waxes in a qualitative and quantitative manner. Potential polymorphic transitions and recrystallization during processing can be simulated by running different temperature profiles.

The contraction of suppository bases during cooling within the mold is a well-described phenomenon. The expansion or contraction of waxes is also important during the processing of wax melts, for example, during the preparation of microparticles by spray congealing, hot-melt coating, or hot-melt filling of hard gelatin capsules. The dilatation of waxes or thermal expansion during the transition from the solid to the liquid state can be measured with a dilatometer. The hardness of a wax is measured with a penetration test, whereby the depth of penetration of a needle under a given weight is measured, preferably at different temperatures. The viscosity of the molten wax is an important parameter, especially for processes such as hot-melt coating or spray congealing, where wax melts are processed. In an ASTM monograph (D 88), the time that a certain quantity of molten wax requires to flow through an orifice of specified dimensions is measured.

The color of the wax will affect the color of the finished product. A Lovibond Tintometer is often used for color measurements, whereby the color of the raw material is compared against a series of colored standard glasses, under a standard light source. The color of the solidified wax of the same sample may be different depending on the amount of occluded air, the rate of cooling, or surface finish. Therefore, the color of many waxes is best measured in the molten state. Two ASTM color standards are used to measure dark-brown to off-white color and off-white to pure white. The refractive index and the specific gravity are other parameters often determined.

The structural and physical properties, in particular, the solid and liquid state behavior of lipids, and the optical and spectral characteristics of waxes have been described in detail (4).

PHARMACEUTICAL APPLICATIONS

Waxes in Matrix-Type Drug Delivery Systems

The incorporation of drugs into inert matrices is a popular approach to prolong the drug release. Sustained-release wax matrix drug delivery systems include wax granules or beads prepared by granulation or extrusion/spheroniza-tion, tablets, and wax-filled hard gelatin capsules.

Wax Granules and Beads

Drug-containing wax granules were prepared by melt congealing, by congealing in chloroform, by granulation, and by aqueous dispersion (9–11). In the congealing method, the drug was suspended in the molten wax. This suspension was cooled gradually while stirring until a solid mass formed, which was then comminuted into granules. Granules made by congealing in chloroform were prepared similarily, the drug being suspended in a chloroformic solution of the wax. This mixture was agitated until the solvent evaporated, and was then comminuted into granules. In the granulation method, the powdered wax and drug were granulated with chloroform. In the last method, heated water was given to the molten drug–wax mixture until phase inversion occurred. The emulsion was cooled and the particles were separated from the aqueous phase by filtration. The melt-congealing method gave the largest retardation in drug release, probably because of the denser structure of the granules when compared to granules prepared by the other methods.

Sustained-release nitrofurantoin granules containing stearic acid and glycerol monostearate as matrix materials were prepared by either a fusion, solvent evaporation, or melt granulation technique (12). Various channelling agents including Aerosil, Avicel, dibasic calcium phosphate dihydrate (Emcompress), and sodium chloride were investigated in order to increase the drug release. In the fusion method, the lipid was melted and the drug was added to the melt. After cooling, the congealed mass was granulated through standard sieves. In the solvent evaporation method, the drug and the wax carriers were dissolved in dimethyl formamide. The solution was cast and the solvent was evaporated at 70°C. The resulting mass was granulated as described previously. In the melt granulation method, the drug and carriers were mixed at high speeds; the temperature increased by friction and granulation occurred by sintering of the fatty materials near their melting point. The cooled granules were crushed and sieved. Sustained release could only be obtained with granules prepared by the fusion method. The solvent evaporation method and, surprisingly, melt granulation resulted in granules with a fast drug release.

Drug-containing beads were prepared by extrusion/spheronization of powder blends of 10% drug (chlorpheniramine maleate or acetaminophen), 60% Avicel PH-101, and 30% wax (13). Thermally treating the beads at 80°C for 30 min resulted in the melting and recongealing of the wax within the beads and in a decrease in the drug release, probably because of a densification and redistribution of the wax within the beads. The drug release was dependent on the treatment temperature and the level of the wax, with an increase in both resulting in a decrease in drug release. The beads were subsequently compressed into tablets, which had slower release rates when compared to the release from the corresponding beads. While nontreated compacts mainly disintegrated into the beads, thermal treatment of the compacts resulted in nondisintegrating matrices.

Diclofenac sodium–carnauba wax matrix granules containing various release-controlling agents such as hydroxyporpylcellulose, Eudragit L-100, or NaCl were prepared with a twin-screw extruder and evaluated in vitro and in vivo (14, 15). The drug release depended strongly on the composition of the granules: the mechanical strengths of the wetted granules was high, and a good correlation was obtained between in vitro dissolution parameter and in vivo parameters.

Wax Matrix Tablets

Wax matrix tablets are prepared either by compression of the wax granules or beads described in the previous section, or, with the higher melting waxes available in powder form, by direct compression of powder blends. When compared with polymeric matrix materials, the amount of waxes within the tablet is limited because of fusion and sticking to the punches at higher wax concentrations. This problem could possibly be overcome by compression at lower temperatures.

Matrix tablets containing ephedrine hydrochloride and hydrogenated castor oil were prepared either by compression of a physical mixture or by compression of a congealed melt (16–18). In the second method, the drug was added to the molten hydrogenated castor oil at 100°C, this molten mass was poured onto a glass plate and congealed, comminuted and then compressed into a matrix. A surfactant, 0.1% alkyltrimethylammonium bromide, was added to the dissolution medium to enhance the wetting of the wax matrix. The drug release increased with increasing amounts of drug in the matrix because of an increased porosity, and followed the square root of time relationship (Fig. 1). The release was slower from the matrix prepared by the melt method. This was attributed to a higher tortuosity and lower porosity of the melt matrix when compared to the matrix prepared from the physical mixture. Increasing the pressure decreased the release rate with both preparation processes; however, the effect was much more pronounced for the matrix prepared from

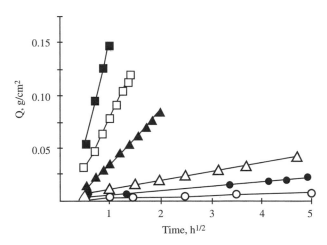

Fig. 1 Effect of concentration of ephedrine hydrochloride on release from matrixes compressed at 7 MPa (48,265 psi). (○) 5%; (●) 10%; (△) 20%; (▲) 30%; (□) 40%; (■) 50%. (From Ref. 17.)

the physical mixture. The processing method also altered the mechanism and rate of release; a matrix diffusion mechanism was dominant with the melt process while a boundary layer diffusion was effective with matrices prepared by the compression of physical mixtures. In the first case, the drug release was independent of stirring speed, while it was dependent in the second case.

Sustained-release nifedipine tablets based on Gelucires were developed (19). A drug-PVP coprecipitate was either added to a solution of Gelucire in chloroform with the subsequent removal of the solvent or it was added to the molten Gelucire with subsequent cooling of the paste. The mixtures were then granulated through a 0.5-mm sieve and tableted. No difference in the release profiles from the two granulates were observed; however, the melting method was preferred because of the absence of organic solvents. Accelerated stability studies on the tablets as a function of temperature and relative humidity revealed no changes in chemical stability; however, the dissolution profiles changed. The changes occurring after storage at high humidities and temperatures were attributed to the formation of nifedipine microcrystals and to structural changes in the wax vehicle.

A combination of ethylcellulose and paraffin wax or hydrogenated castor oil was used as carrier material in sustained-release aminophylline tablets (20). The tablet granulation was prepared by a wet granulation procedure with hot ethanol. The tablets were further coated with Eudragit RL/RS or HPMC/ethyl cellulose. An annealing step at 70°C significantly decreased the drug release due to fusion within the tablet core. Hydrogenated castor oil was superior to paraffin wax. Increasing the wax content and

decreasing the amount of ethyl cellulose or increasing the drug content resulted in faster drug release.

In order to overcome the disadvantage of hydrophilic matrices of uncontrollable erosion of the hydrated polymer gel on the tablet surface, a combined polymer-wax carrier material was evaluated by Huang et al. (21). Carnauba wax was combined with the enteric acrylic polymer, Eudragit L 100, and investigated as a carrier material for diphenhydramine HCl. The drug and Eudragit L100 were mixed, added to the molten wax, followed by compression of the congealed granules. The polymer provided an insoluble structure for the wax. The drug release was significantly retarded with increasing amounts of the anionic polymer. The cationic drug, diphenhydramine HCl, interacted with the anionic Eudragit L within the wax matrix and formed a complex after water penetration. While the drug release from tablets prepared from only the drug and the enteric polymer was highly dependent on the pH of the dissolution media, the drug release was almost independent of pH after the inclusion of carnauba wax in the matrix. Besides the retarding effect of the wax, at low pH, the release was retarded through the enteric polymer and at high pH, the drug formed a less soluble complex with the enteric polymer, thus negating the effect of pH on the drug release.

Matrix minitablets based on starch/microcrystalline wax mixtures were prepared by melt granulation in a hot-stage screw extruder, followed by milling and compression (22). This technique was preferred over the production of pellets.

Surfactants were incorporated into wax matrices in order to increase drug release (23). The drug and surfactant were added to a molten mixture of carnauba wax and stearyl alcohol. Water-insoluble surfactants such as glycerol monostearate had no effect on the dissolution rate, slightly soluble surfactants such as sodium stearate or dioctyl sodium sulfosuccinate moderately increased the drug release, while polyoxyethylene 23 lauryl ether significantly increased the drug release. The drug release occurred via a leaching mechanism; drug diffusion through the matrix did not occur. It was speculated that the surfactant created more channels for the drug to leach into the dissolution medium by increasing the porosity of the matrix.

While the drug release from wax matrix tablets followed the square root of time relationship, approximately zero-order release of ephedrine hydrochloride and procaine hydrochloride could be obtained with multi-layered matrices of hydrogenated castor oil containing different concentrations of the active compound in each layer (24).

A bioadhesive lozenge containing cetylpyridinium chloride was developed based on a multilayered tablet (25). One layer contained the bioadhesive polymer, carbopol, and the other layer contained the drug and a wax (spermaceti or Precirol ATO-5).

Wax Implants

Besides polymers such as polylactides, waxes have the potential as biocompatible/biodegradable carriers in implants. Standard tableting equipment can be used to prepare wax compacts.

Various lipids including triglycerides (e.g., trilaurin, trimyristin, tripalmitin and tristearin) and fatty acids were evaluated as carrier materials in sustained-release insulin implants (26). The drug/wax powder blend was compressed into a disc and implanted subcutaneously into Wistar rats. Monoglycerides tested eroded too fast and were not suitable. The triglycerides only sustained-the insulin release briefly. The best sustained-release properties were obtained with palmitic and stearic acids as the carrier materials.

The drug release of the model protein, bovine serum albumin (BSA), from compressed stearic acid pellets was investigated as function of drug loading, drug and carrier particle size, and compression force (27). At low loadings (5%), the drug release increased with increasing BSA particle size irrespective of the particle size of stearic acid. At high loading (20%), the drug release was higher with larger stearic acid particles. More BSA was released with increasing BSA particle size only when the stearic acid particle size was small. The compression force did not show any effect in the range investigated. In a series of articles, the same research group investigated cholesterol–lecithin implants as a delivery system for antigens (28–31).

Labrafil 1944 CS (derivatized vegetable oil)–Precirol ATO 5 (glyceryl ester of fatty acids) gels were shown to be biocompatible and biodegradable and resulted in controlled release of steroids for prolonged periods of time in vivo (32).

Hard Gelatin Capsules Filled with Waxes

Waxes are difficult to compress at higher levels. The energy imparted during compaction causes melting of the waxes, resulting in sticking and picking of the formulation. This necessitates dilution of the drug-wax granules with inert fillers; high-dose drugs requiring high amounts of wax in order to obtain sustained-release properties are therefore difficult to formulate into tablets. As an alternative to compressed tablets, hard gelatin capsules have been liquid-filled with solutions or dispersions of drugs in molten waxes. On cooling, drug–wax plugs are obtained. Some of the advantages of liquid filling of hard gelatin capsules, when compared to solid-filled capsules, include a better weight uniformity, and the elimination of dust hazards and cross-contamination via airborne particles. The drug–carrier system should not interact with the gelatin shell in the molten as well as in the congealed state, and the physical state of the drug and wax should not change during storage. The melting point of the wax has to be low enough to avoid degradation of the drug and damage to the capsule shell.

A Zanasi hard gelatin powder filling capsule machine (model LZ64) was modified in order to allow the filling of molten or thixotropic formulations into hard gelatin capsules (33, 34). This technique resulted in excellent fill weight uniformity and overcame many of the problems frequently associated with the filling of conventional capsules.

The release of liquid or deliquescent drugs (benzonatate, nicotinic acid, chloral hydrate, and paramethadione) incorporated into Gelucire bases within hard gelatin capsules was related to the behavior of the carriers in simulated gastric fluid (35). Gelucires are semisynthetic glycerides with varying amphiphilic properties and are derived from natural hydrogenated food grade fats and oils. They are characterized by their melting point (range: 33–64°C) and HLB value (range: 1–13). The drugs were released faster from the Gelucires with the higher HLB value and with lower melting points. The Gelucires either dissolved completely or remained intact but softened.

It is well known that wax-based dosage forms can experience physical instabilities. Suppository bases often show an increase in melting point, accompanied by a hardening process. This hardening can result in a reduced release rate, which could also affect the in vivo performance. Melt-filled hard gelatin capsules were evaluated by DSC, dissolution, and hardness properties as expressed by a relative penetration (36). Ketoprofen dissolved in the wax, Gelucire 50/13, and apparently formed a solid solution at room temperature as indicated by the absence of crystalline drug by DSC and microscopy. The melting point of the wax increased during storage and was accompanied by a hardening process. However, the release rate increased, which was attributed to an increased rate of matrix erosion. The observed in vitro changes did not affect the in vivo performance of the wax matrix.

As an alternative to hot-melt filling of capsules, sustained-release wax matrices were formed in a novel way within hard gelatin capsules through fluidization in a heated air stream within a fluidized bed (37). A drug–wax powder blend was filled into hard gelatin capsules, which were then suspended in an upward-moving, heated airstream and circulated within the chamber of a fluidized bed unit. The capsules rotated during fluidization at temperatures above the melting point of the wax and centrifugal forces caused the drug–wax melt to flow into the ends of the capsules. The molten mixture then solidified after ending the heating and two solid wax matrices with dissolved/dispersed drug were obtained in the ends of the capsules. Good control over the drug release was obtained by using blends of waxes with different amphiphilic properties (HLB-values). Gelucire 50/13 (m.p. = 50°C, HLB = 13) and Precirol ATO-5 (m.p. = 53°C, HLB = 2) were selected as the drug carriers. The drug release increased with increasing proportion of the more hydrophilic wax. After cooling of the drug-containing wax melt, the drug could be dispersed, dispersed/dissolved, or dissolved in the wax matrix. DSC studies were used to characterize the physical state of the drugs after formation of the wax matrix. A linear relationship existed between the heat of fusion and the amount of drug in the wax matrix (Fig. 2). The solubility of the drug in the matrix at its melting point corresponds to the intercept of the line. Propranolol HCl was insoluble and dispersed in the Precirol ATO-5 matrix while theophylline was partially dissolved in the wax.

Coating with Waxes

Besides their predominant use in matrix preparations, waxes have also been used as coatings for granules and pellets. Solid dosage forms are often coated to sustain the drug release, to improve the stability, or to mask the taste of poorly tasting drugs. The coating with waxes has various advantages when compared to the coating with polymer solutions or dispersions. The waxes can be applied without organic solvents, and, in the case of hot melts, with a high application rate and therefore shorter processing time. Many food grade natural or semisynthetic waxy materials are available.

Waxes can be applied onto solid dosage forms in the form of hot melts, hot emulsions, aqueous suspensions (colloidal wax particles), or organic solutions. Coating processes include dip coating, pan coating, or fluidized-bed coating. The coating of drug particles by spray congealing is discussed in the section on microencapsulation with waxes.

Coating with Hot Melts

With regard to coating processes, various fluidized-bed techniques and their modifications were evaluated for hot-melt coating (38–40). The fluidized-bed techniques include the top, bottom, and the tangential spray or rotary fluidized-bed modes. The particles to be coated are suspended in a heated high-velocity air stream, and the molten wax is applied in the form of atomized liquid droplets.

The top spray mode, in which the wax melt is sprayed downward on upward moving particles, is the system of choice for hot-melt coating (Fig. 3). The product temperature can be kept closest to the congealing temperature of the wax when compared to the other two spray modes. The wax has to be kept in a molten state in

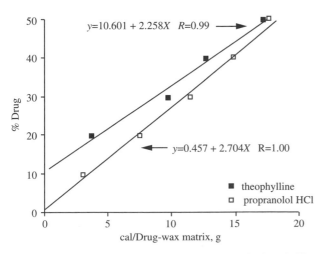

Fig. 2 Relationship of propranolol HCl and theophylline loading and the heat of fusion. (From Ref. 37.)

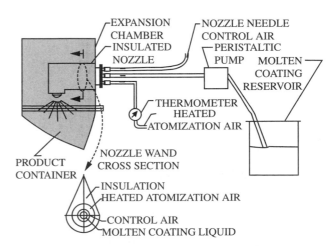

Fig. 3 Insulated nozzle and wand for top-spray hot-melt coating. (From Ref. 38.)

order to be atomized into the fluidized bed. A special nozzle had to be developed. The nozzle wand had a triaxial structure with a center tube for the molten liquid, which is surrounded by a small air space for the delivery of high-pressure, low-volume air to control the valve in the nozzle, which opens when the pump was running. Both of these tubes were surrounded by a larger air space through which the heated atomization air was supplied. The nozzle should be placed as closely as possible to the substrate bed in order to minimize the distance that the molten droplets had to travel prior to contacting the substrate surface.

Substrates with poor fluidization characteristics such as larger particles and/or particles of higher density are difficult to coat with the top spray mode, and the bottom spray mode should be preferred. With the tangential spray process, the product temperatures have to be maintained lower than with the top spray technique in order to avoid adherence of the coated particles to the product container. The tangential spray method is more stressful on the substrates than the other two techniques.

Important process and formulation variables include the product bed temperature, the atomization conditions, the type of substrate, the properties of the coating materials, and the desired release rates (immediate or sustained release). In order to obtain good coatings, the atomization air has to be heated to the same temperature as the molten wax in order to avoid premature congealing. The droplets must remain in a liquid state until they hit the substrate surface. The product bed temperature is very critical to the successful coating of solid dosage forms with molten materials. At low product temperatures, premature congealing of the molten droplets results in poor spreading of the coating on the substrate surface and, in the extreme case, in the failure of the adherence of the coating to the surface. Rough and porous surface structures are obtained, resulting in faster drug release when compared to substrates with smooth coatings. At too high product temperatures, excessive particle agglomeration or clogging of the outlet filter bags is a result of inadequate congealing and hardening of the coating. The product bed temperature can be regulated through the fluidization air temperature. It is recommended to use inlet air temperatures 10–15°C below the melting point of the coating and temperatures for the atomization air and the molten wax of 40–60°C above the melting point.

Droplet size and uniformity are also critical for a successful coating process. The size of the molten droplet is dependent on the viscosity of the melt and the atomization air pressure. Smaller particles require smaller droplet sizes and therefore higher atomization air pressures in order to minimize agglomeration or granulation. In order to obtain small droplets, the viscosity of

the molten material can be decreased by increasing the temperature of the melt. At the same atomization conditions, low feed rates also result in smaller droplets. The spray rate of melts is generally much lower when compared to coating solutions or dispersions. The lower spray rate, however, is offset by the application of pure coating material. The application rate therefore is still higher when compared to polymer solutions or dispersions, with which solvents have to be evaporated.

After the application of the melt, the fluidization is reduced and the product bed is cooled. The cooling circle should be short in order to avoid attrition of the coated product. Rapid cooling, however, may result in cracks in the coating because of contraction of the coating material, and it may also result in unstable polymorphic forms of the wax.

The important variables for the selection of the waxes include the melting point, the melting range, and the viscosity of the melt. The wax should have a melting point of less than 85°C because the melt is usually kept at temperatures of 40–60°C above its melting point. Materials with a broad melting point range can become tacky during spraying because of the broad range of product temperatures and the presence of low melting point fractions. The coating materials include various hydrogenated vegetable oils, beeswax, paraffin wax, carnauba wax, and polyethylene glycol.

Coating with hot emulsions, aqueous suspensions, or organic wax solutions

The coating with hot emulsions has various advantages when compared to the hot-melt process (41, 42). The wax remains in the molten state and premature congealing of the wax could be eliminated because of the presence of hot water. This facilitated the transport of the wax to the spray nozzle and therefore the experimental setup. In addition, the temperatures of the wax emulsion are lower then the comparable wax melts. o/w-Emulsions of various waxes (e.g., glyceryl behenate-Compritol-888 and glyceryl palmitostearate-Precirol-ATO 5) with a solids content of up to 50% were prepared. The emulsions were passed through a microfluidizer to further reduce the particle size of the oil phase. The hot emulsion was then either sprayed directly on the beads or cooled to form a "wax pseudolatex" prior to the coating process. The disadvantages, when compared to hot-melt coating, include the amount of water to be evaporated and therefore longer processing times, and the presence of surfactants in the wax coating. The surfactants, which were needed to stabilize the emulsions, could affect the drug release. The use of liquid surfactants such as various Tween/Span combinations resulted in sticky beads. Solid surfactants such as sodium lauryl sulfate were more suitable. The guaifenesin release from coated pellets decreased with increasing hydrophobicity of the wax and increasing coating level. The coating conditions (e.g., temperature, spray rate, curing) and the particle size of the emulsion/suspension primarily influenced the microstructure of the wax coatings and hence the drug release. When compared to polymer coatings, thicker coatings have to be applied with waxes to obtain the same sustained release profiles.

Bagaria prepared emulsions with waxes including carnauba, paraffin, ceresin, beeswax, and hydrogenated castor, soybean, or cottonseed oil, which were then coated onto drug-containing nonpareil beads (43). The term emulsions was actually misleading because the final products were aqueous suspensions of the waxes with partially submicron particle size (wax pseudolatex). Similar to aqueous polymer dispersions, the wax dispersions were converted into powders by spray drying. The release from beads coated with the redispersed spray dried powder was then compared to beads coated with the original dispersion. With almost all preparations, 100% drug was released within 2–4 h.

Like with organic polymer solutions, the wax can be dissolved in an organic solvent and then be sprayed onto the solid dosage form. In most studies, waxes such as beeswax, hydrogenated castor oil, microcrystalline wax, or glyceryl mono- and distearate were dissolved in chlorinated organic solvents such as chloroform, carbon tetrachloride, or trichlorethane and applied in coating pans at elevated temperatures (44–46). Mixtures of ethyl cellulose with different waxes such as castor, carnauba, or paraffin wax in chloroform were evaluated as sustained-release coatings (47). A lower ratio of ethyl cellulose to wax was used with drugs of high-molecular weight and/or low solubility and a higher ratio for drugs of low-molecular weight and/or high solubility to achieve the desired release properties at a 10% coating level. As the date of the references shows, the coating with organic solutions is obsolete because of the undesirable use of organic solvents.

Microencapsulation with Waxes

Wax microparticles have been prepared primarily by aqueous and nonaqueous melt dispersion techniques or spray congealing/spray drying. These techniques are briefly reviewed below.

Microparticles prepared by melt-dispersion techniques

In the melt dispersion technique, the drug-containing molten wax phase is emulsified into a heated, emulsifier-containing external phase. Depending on the solubility of the drug, the external phase can be either aqueous (for water-insoluble drugs) or nonaqueous (for water-soluble drugs). On cooling the emulsion, the liquid droplets congeal and a suspension of the wax microparticles is formed. The microparticles are then separated, mostly by filtration or centrifugation, sometimes washed to remove free drug crystals and surfactants, dried and sized.

Ibuprofen-wax (carnauba wax, paraffin wax, beeswax, Gelucire 64/02, or Precirol ATO5) microparticles were characterized with respect to drug loading and morphological and release properties (48). Microparticles of the more hydrophilic waxes, Gelucire 64/02 and Precirol ATO5, could be prepared without surfactants, while the other waxes rapidly coalesced and formed big lumps on cooling. With the other waxes, increasing the amount of sodium lauryl sulfate in the external aqueous phase decreased the drug loading because of drug solubilization. This was not the case when poly(vinyl alcohol) was used as stabilizer. During emulsification, the drug will partition into the external aqueous phase until its solubility at the emulsification temperature is reached. During cooling of the emulsion, the drug could precipitate in the aqueous phase because of a decreased drug solubility. The type of wax, the rate of cooling, the stirring time, and the temperature of the aqueous phase had no significant effect on the drug loading because of the low solubility of ibuprofen in the external aqueous phase. Actual drug loadings close to 60% could be achieved. The drug release was controlled by the hydrophobicity of the wax (Gelucire 64/02 > Precirol ATO5 > beeswax > carnauba wax > paraffin wax) (Fig. 4). These wax microparticles could be

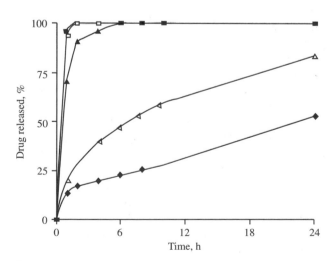

Fig. 4 Ibuprofen release from different wax microparticles (actual drug loading): (■) Precirol ATO5 (35.3%), (□) Gelucire 64/02 (35.4%), (▲) beeswax (37.7%), (△) carnauba wax (37.3%), (◆) paraffin wax (35.0%). (From Ref. 48.)

formulated into aqueous sustained-release oral suspension dosage forms because of the low solubility of the drug.

A modified USP method using mini baskets was used to study the effect of formulation variables, such as type of wax, type of modifier, drug loading, size, on the ibuprofen release from wax microspheres (49). The drug release was in the order of beeswax > ceresine wax > refined paraffin wax > microcrystalline wax. After an initial burst release, the drug release was slow from microparticles prepared with the last two waxes. The dissolution studies were performed in simulated intestinal fluids, because sink conditions could not be maintained in simulated gastric fluids because of the drug solubility. To increase the drug release from the wax microspheres, glycerol monostearate or stearyl alcohol were added prior to the preparation of the microparticles. The addition of these release modifiers also reduced the tendency of the waxes to agglomerate (50). Ibuprofen dissolved in the molten wax and did not crystallize during congealing and microsphere formation, as indicated by DSC studies.

In a modified melt-dispersion method, sulfamethoxazole particles were dispersed in heated water, and powdered beeswax was added. The molten wax droplets collected the drug particles, and spherical agglomerates with sustained-release properties were obtained after cooling. Alternatively, the agglomerates could also be formed at room temperature by using solutions of the wax in a water-immiscible solvent (51).

Water-soluble drugs cannot be encapsulated with the O/W-emulsion technique because the drug would be lost to the external aqueous phase. Two methods have been described for the encapsulation of hydrophilic drugs; one is based on using an external oil phase and the other one on the formation of the microparticles by a w/o/w-melt dispersion technique.

Carnauba-wax microspheres containing 5-fluorouracil for chemoembolization were prepared by a melt dispersion process with an external silicone oil phase (52). The drug was dispersed in the molten carnauba wax and emulsified into silicone oil at temperatures above the melting point of carnauba wax (85°C). The resulting emulsion was cooled through the addition of cold silicone oil and immersion of the beaker in an ice-water bath. After solidification, the microspheres were separated from the oil phase by centrifugation and washed with cyclohexane to remove the silicone oil. 5-Fluorouracil is a hydrophilic drug; an external aqueous phase would have resulted in drug partitioning and therefore low encapsulation efficiencies. However, even with silicone oil, an external phase in which the drug was insoluble, only up to 5% drug could be encapsulated within the carnauba-wax microspheres. This was attributed to the poor wetting of the drug crystals by

the molten wax and therefore the loss of drug crystals to the external silicon oil phase. Various surfactants were added to the wax phase in order to improve the wettability of the drug by the molten wax.

A technique based on the formation of a multiple emulsion with an external aqueous phase was developed for the encapsulation of water-soluble drugs in order to replace the external oil phase (53). Possible unwanted interactions between the oil and the emulsified wax such as swelling or dissolution of the wax, clean-up requirements of the final product, and recovery of the oil phase could be eliminated. In analogy to the encapsulation of water-soluble drugs within polymeric microparticles by a w/o/w-solvent evaporation method, a molten wax phase was used instead of an organic polmer solution. A heated aqueous solution of pseudoephedrine HCl was emulsified into the molten carnauba wax, followed by the emulsification of this w/o-emulsion into a heated external aqueous phase. The temperature of the internal and external aqueous phases had to be kept above the melting temperature of the wax in order to avoid premature congealing and to assure the formation of an emulsion. The microparticles formed after congealing of the wax. A key for high encapsulation efficiencies was the formation of ultrafine internal aqueous phase droplets by sonication. The wax acted as a diffusion barrier between the internal and the external aqueous phases and therefore minimized drug partitioning into the external aqueous phase. Because of the high solubility of the drug in the external aqueous phase, the contact time of the droplets/microparticles with the continuous aqueous phase had to be minimized in order to avoid the drug loss; the microparticles were separated from the aqueous phase within minutes after their formation.

Generally, the wax phase is emulsified into a heated external phase to avoid premature congealing. However, sulfamethazine-japanese synthetic wax particles were prepared by dispersing the drug in the molten wax, followed by slowly pouring the wax phase into a precooled external aqueous phase (54). The microparticles were then separated by filtration after 3 min. Beeswax microparticles were prepared by a phase inversion technique, whereby an aqueous solution of sorbitan monooleate and polysorbate 80 was added to the drug-containing molten wax phase to first form a w/o-emulsion prior to phase inversion. Smaller microparticles were obtained at higher temperatures, with increased amounts of continuous phase, with slower rates of cooling, and with higher speeds of mixing (55).

Suspensions of lipid nanoparticles can be prepared by reducing the size of the molten or dissolved drug containing lipid phase into the colloidal size range by high-pressure homogenization (56, 57). After cooling or solvent evaporation, the nanoparticles are obtained.

The suspensions of the nanoparticles can be converted into powders through freeze or spray drying. The nanoparticles can act as carriers for poorly water-soluble drugs and apparently could result in controlled release over longer periods of time. However, because of the small size and therefore high surface area of the particles, an increase in dissolution rate would be expected unless very low loadings are used.

Microparticles prepared by spray drying and spray congealing

Similar to organic polymer solutions, drug-containing organic wax solutions were spray dried to give sustained-release microparticles (58). The drug could be either dissolved or dispersed in the organic wax solutions. Spray drying is a single step, rapid drying process, which can be scaled up and be used for heat-sensitive drugs. The use of organic solvents, however, is undesirable because of solvent hazards, solvent residuals, and cost. Because of the low melt viscosity, wax microparticles can also be prepared without organic solvents by spray-congealing drug-containing wax melts.

Sulfaethylthiadiazole-hydrogenated castor oil particles were prepared by spray congealing, using a centrifugal wheel atomizer (59). The wax powder was then suspended into water to give an oral sustained-release suspension. In a subsequent article, the effect of various process and formulation variables on the particle size was investigated using a centrifugal wheel atomizer (60). The particle size was directly proportional to the feed rate and inversely proportional to the feed viscosity and the wheel velocity.

In a series of publications, sulfaethylthiadiazole-wax microparticles prepared by spray-congealing were evaluated. The most important factor affecting the drug release was the type of wax used (61). The effect of surfactant on the drug release from spray congealed wax microparticles was investigated by John and Becker (62). White wax-USP, a synthetic wax-like ester, and 1:1 combinations of these two waxes were used as sustained-release matrices. The particle size of the microparticles could be controlled through the nozzle size, with the larger nozzles resulting in larger particles with slower rates of dissolution. Up to 4% sorbitan monooleate apparently softened the particles and promoted wetting, thus resulting in an increase in drug release. However, at a surfactant level of 10%, the slowest release rate was observed. This was partly attributed to the tackiness of the particles, which resulted in agglomeration and a reduction in total surface area available for drug release. The addition of the surfactant allowed the compression of the microparticles into tablets, which was difficult with the surfactant-free microparticles (63). The surfactant-free microparticles adhered or stuck to the punch surface, and resulted in a high friability of the finished tablets. No additives were incorporated into the tablets; nondisintegrating wax matrix tablets were obtained.

A palatable suspension of the bitter-tasting drug, remoxipride, was developed based on microparticles prepared by spray congealing (64). Because of the high water solubility of the drug, the microparticles were formulated into an external oil phase. Unfortunately, neither the nature of the wax nor of the oily vehicle was revealed.

With lipid drug delivery systems, polymorphic transformations may occur during the preparation of the dosage form and during subsequent storage. The polymorphic behavior of lipid micropellets prepared from glycerides and phospholipids by spray drying or spray congealing and their surface structure were evaluated by DSC and scanning electron microscopy (65–67). The rapid solvent evaporation during spray drying can influence the crystallization of the lipid carrier and different polymorphic structures could be obtained. Similarily, during spray congealing and solidification of the melt, the lipid can crystallize in different polymorphic forms, depending on the composition of the lipid and the cooling rate. The major polymorphic forms of the glycerides are the α-, β-, and β′-forms. Rapid cooling rates generally result in the unstable α-form. The transition of the melt first to the α- and β′-forms and then to the β-form represents the transformation of triglycerides into the most stable form.

The spraying process, especially the spray congealing was simulated by cooling the molten samples rapidly at 320°C/min. A DSC thermogram of pure tristearin heated at 10°C/min revealed a single endothermic peak representing the β-form. After rapid cooling of the melt and reheating, an endothermic peak for the α-form and an exothermic peak indicating the recrystallization of the α-form into the β-form, followed by the endothermic peak for the β-form, were detectable. The DSC thermogram of spray-dried tristearin micropellets was similar to the one of the melt-quenched sample. A crystalline modification therefore took place during spray drying because of the rapid solvent removal. The micropellets were then stored at different temperatures to investigate the effect of storage temperature on the polymorphic transitions. Increasing the storage temperature to 37°C resulted in a complete transformation of the unstable polymorphic form into the stable polymorphic form. The melting endotherm of the α-form disappeared. The effect of various emulsifiers such as lecithin or monoglycerides was investigated in order to prevent or delay the transformation of the unstable form into the stable β-form. Adding lecithin to the formulation resulted in a delay of the transformation. The type of glyceride (composition and chain length), solvent, and drugs encapsulated affected the polymorphic transformation, its rate of transformation, and also the surface structure of the microparticles. Spray-congealed lipid micropellets showed a similar thermal behavior as the spray-dried pellets. The smooth surface of the sprayed lipid micropellets was attributed to the unstable polymorphic form. The unstable α-form has various thin and small crystals, resulting in a smooth surface of the crystallized sample. The β- and β′s-forms have larger crystals, therefore causing irregular structures of the micropellets. During ageing at elevated temperatures, the lipid micropellets lost their smooth surface structures because of polymorphic transformations.

Novel oral controlled release microspheres using polyglycerolesters of fatty acids and hydrogenated cottonseed oil (HCSO), stearic acid, stearyl alcohol, or glycerol monostearate as carriers were prepared by spray chilling using a rotating disc (68). The drug release was related to the hydrophobicity of the wax; the release rate decreased in the following order: stearyl alcohol > stearic acid > glycerol monostearate > carnauba wax > hydrogenated cottonseed oil. Adding increasing amounts of lactose to HCSO increased the drug release as a result of the leaching of lactose.

A new atomizer operating with ultrasonic energy was used as an alternative to traditional atomizers to prepare wax microparticles by spray congealing (69).

REFERENCES

1. Bennett, H. *Industrial Waxes, Vol. I–Natural and Synthetic Waxes, Vol. II–Compound Waxes and Technology*; Chemical Publishing Company: New York, 1975.
2. Wade, A.; Weller, P.J. *Handbook of Pharmaceutical Excipients*; American Pharmaceutical Association, The Pharmaceutical Press: London, Washington, 1994.
3. Lechter, C.S. Waxes. *Encyclopedia of Chemical Technology*; Kirk-Othmer, Ed.; John Wiley & Sons: New York, 1984; 24, 466–481.
4. Gunstone, F.D.; Harwood, J.L.; Padley, F.B. *The Lipid Handbook*; Chapman and Hall: London, 1986.
5. Knowlton, J.; Pearce, S. *Handbook of Cosmetic Science and Technology*; Elsevier: Amsterdam, 1993; 21–32.
6. Warth, A.H. *The Chemistry and Technology of Waxes*; Reinhold Publishing Corporation: New York, 1956.
7. Kolattukudy, P.E. *Chemistry and Biochemistry of Natural Waxes*; Elsevier: Amsterdam, 1976.
8. In *United States Pharmacopeia, USP23 NF18*; The United States Pharmacopeial Convention: Rockville, MD, 1995.
9. Asker, A.F.; Motawi, A.M.; Abdel-Khalek, M.M. A Study of Some Factors Affecting the In-Vitro Release of Drug from Prolonged Release Granulations. Part 1. Effect of Method of Preparation. Pharmazie 1971, 26, 170–172.
10. Asker, A.F.; Motawi, A.M.; Abdel-Khalek, M.M. A Study of Some Factors Affecting the In-Vitro Release of Drug from Prolonged Release Granulations. Part 2. Effect of Dissolution Retardant. Pharmazie 1971, 26, 213–214.
11. Asker, A.F.; Motawi, A.M.; Abdel-Khalek, M.M. A Study of Some Factors Affecting the In-Vitro Release of Drug from Prolonged Release Granulations. Part 3. Effects of Particle Size, Enzymatic Contents of Pepsin and Pancreatin, Bile and Ionic Concentration. Pharmazie 1971, 26, 215–217.
12. El-Shanawany, S. Sustained Release of Nitrofurantoin from Inert Wax Matrixes. J. Control. Rel. 1993, 36, 11–19.
13. Ghali, E.S.; Klinger, G.H.; Schwartz, J.B.; Drug Dev. Ind. Pharm. 1989, 15, 1311–1328.
14. Miyagawa, Y.; Okabe, T.; Yamaguchi, Y.; Miyajima, M.; Sato, H.; Sunada, H. Controlled-Release of Diclofenac Sodium from Wax Matrix Granule. Int. J. Pharm. 1996, 138, 215–224.
15. Miyagawa, Y.; Sato, H.; Okabe, T.; Nishiyama, T.; Miyajima, M.; Sunada, H. In Vivo Performance of Wax Matrix Granules Prepared by a Twin-Screw Compounding Extruder. Drug Dev. Ind. Pharm. 1999, 25, 429–435.
16. Foster, T.P.; Parrott, E.L. Effect of Processing on Release from an Inert, Heterogeneous Matrix. Drug Dev. Ind. Pharm. 1990, 16, 1309–1324.
17. Foster, T.P.; Parrott, E.L. Release of Highly Water-Soluble Medicinal Compounds from Inert, Heterogenous Matrixes. I: Physical Mixture. J. Pharm. Sci. 1990, 79, 806–810.
18. Foster, T.P.; Parrott, E.L. Release of Highly Water-Soluble Medicinal Compounds from Inert, Heterogenous Matrixes. II: Melt. J. Pharm. Sci. 1990, 79, 938–942.
19. Remunan, C.; Bretal, M.J.; Nunez, A.; Vila Jato, J.L. Accelerated Stability Study of Sustained-Release Nifedipine Tablets Prepared with Gelucire®. Int. J. Pharm. 1992, 80, 151–159.
20. Boles, M.G.; Deasy, P.B.; Donnellan, M.F. Design and Evaluation of Sustained-Release Aminophylline Tablet. Drug Dev. Ind. Pharm. 1993, 19, 349–370.
21. Huang, H.-P.; Mehta, S.C.; Radebaugh, G.W.; Fawzi, M.B. Mechanism of Drug Release from an Acrylic Polymer-Wax Matrix Tablet. J. Pharm. Sci. 1994, 83, 795–797.
22. De Brabander, C.; Vervaet, C.; Fiermans, L.; Remon, J.P. Matrix Mini-Tablets Based on Starch/Microcrystalline Wax Mixtures. Int. J. Pharm. 2000, 199, 195–203.
23. Dakkuri, A.; Schraeder, H.G.; DeLuca, P.P. Sustained Release from Inert Wax Matrixes. II: Effect of Surfactants on Tripelennamine Hydrochloride Release. J. Pharm. Sci. 1978, 67, 354–357.
24. Foster, T.P.; Parrott, E.L. Constant Release Rate from Inert Heterogeneous Matrixes by Means of Position-Dependent Loading. Drug Dev. Ind. Pharm. 1990, 16, 1633–1648.
25. Collins, A.E.; Deasy, P.B. Bioadhesive Lozenge for the Improved Delivery of Cetylpyridinium Chloride. J. Pharm. Sci. 1990, 79, 116–119.

26. Wang, P.Y. Lipids as Excipient in Sustained Release Insulin Implants. Int. J. Pharm. **1989**, *54*, 223–230.

27. Kaewvichit, S.; Tucker, I.G. The Release of Macromolecules from Fatty Acid Matrices: Complete Factorial Study of Factors Affecting Release. J. Pharm. Pharmacol **1994**, *46*, 708–713.

28. Khan, M.Z.I.; Tucker, I.G.; Opdebeek, J.P. Cholesterol and Lecithin Implants for Sustained Release of Antigen: Release and Erosion In Vitro, and Antibody Response in Mice. Int. J. Pharm. **1991**, *76*, 161–170.

29. Khan, M.Z.I.; Tucker, I.G.; Opdebeek, J.P. Evaluation of Cholesterol-Lecithin Implants for Sustained Delivery of Antigen: Release In Vivo and Single-Step Immunisation of Mice. Int. J. Pharm. **1993**, *90*, 255–262.

30. Opdebeek, J.P.; Tucker, I.G. A Cholesterol Implant Used a Delivery System to Immunize Mice with Bovine Serum Albumin. J. Control. Rel. **1993**, *23*, 271–279.

31. Walduck, A.K.; Opdebeeck, J.P.; Benson, H.E.; Prankerd, R. Biodegradable Implants for the Delivery of Veterinary Vaccines: Design, Manufacture and Antibody Responses in Sheep. J. Control. Rel. **1998**, *51*, 269–280.

32. Gao, Z.; Crowley, W.R.; Shukla, A.J.; Johnson, J.R.; Reger, F. Controlled Release of Contraceptive Steroids from Biodegradable and Injectable Gel Formulations: In Vivo Evaluation. Pharm. Res. **1995**, *12*, 864–868.

33. Walker, S.E.; Ganley, J.A.; Bedford, K.; Eaves, T. The Filling of Molten and Thixotropic Formulations into Hard Gelatin Capsules. J. Pharm. Pharmacol. **1980**, *32*, 389–393.

34. McTaggert, C.; Wood, R.; Bedford, K.; Walker, S.E. The Evaluation of an Automatic System for Filling Liquids into Hard Gelatin Capsules. J. Pharm. Pharmacol. **1984**, *36*, 119–212.

35. Doelker, C.; Doelker, E.; Buri, P.; Waginaire, L. Drug Dev. Ind. Pharm. **1986**, *12*, 1553–1565.

36. Proceedings of the 15th International Symposium on Controlled Release of Bioactive Materials, Basel, Switzerland, Aug 15–19, 1988, The Controlled Release Society, Illinois1998, No. 223, 390–391.

37. Bodmeier, R.; Paeratakul, O.; Chen, H.; Zhang, W. Formation of Sustained Release Wax Matrices Within Hard Gelatin Capsules in a Fluidized Bed. Drug Dev. Ind. Pharm. **1990**, *16*, 1505–1519.

38. Jones, D.M.; Percel, P.J. Coating of Multiparticulates Using Molten Materials. *Multiparticulate Oral Drug Delivery*; Ghebre-Sellassie, I., Ed.; Marcel Dekker, Inc.: New York, 1994; 113–142.

39. Jozwiakowski, M.J.; Jones, D.M.; Franz, R.M. Characterization of a Hot Melt Fluid Bed Coating Process for Fine Granules. Pharm. Res. **1990**, *7*, 1119–1126.

40. Barthelemy, P.; Laforêt, J.P.; Farah, N.; Joachim, J. Compritol® 888 ATO: An Innovative Hot-Melt Coating Agent for Prolonged-Release Drug Formulations. E. J. Pharm. Biopharm **1999**, *47*, 87–90.

41. Bhagwatwar, H.; Bodmeier, R. The Coating of Drug-Loaded Sgura Beads with Various Wax Formulations. Pharm. Res. **1989**, *6*, PT 713–S-73.

42. Bhagwatwar, H. *M.S. Thesis*; The University of Texas at Austin: Austin, 1991.

43. Bagaria, S.C., Ph. D. *Dissertation*; Rutgers University, The State University of New Jersey: New Brunswick, 1986.

44. Blythe, R.H. Sympathomimetic Preparation, US Patent 2,738,303, March 13, 1956.

45. Rosen, E.; Swintosky, J.V. Preparation of A ^{35}S Labelled Trimeprazim Tartrate Sustained Action Product for Its Evaluation in Man. J. Pharm. Pharmacol. **1960**, *12*, 237T–244T.

46. Heimlich, K.R.; MacDonnell, D.R. Method of Preparing Sustained Release Pharmaceutical Pellets and Product Thereof, US Patent 3,119,742, January 28, 1964.

47. Peters, D.; Goodhart, F.W.; Lieberman, H.A. Sustained Release Dosage in the Pellet Form and Process Thereof. US Patent, 3,492,397, January 27, 1970.

48. Bodmeier, R.; Wang, J.; Bhagwatwar, H. J. Process and Formulation Variables in the Preparation of Wax Microparticles by a Melt Dispersion Technique I. Oil-in-Water Technique for Water-Insoluble Drugs. Microencapsulation **1992**, *9*, 89–98.

49. Adeyeye, C.M.; Price, J.C. Development and Evaluation of Sustained-Release Ibuprofen-Wax Microspheres. II. In Vitro Dissolution Studies. Pharm. Res. **1994**, *11*, 575–579.

50. Adeyeye, C.M.; Price, J.C. Development and Evaluation of Sustained-Release Ibuprofen-Wax Microspheres. I. Effect of Formulation Variables on Physical Characteristics. Pharm. Res. **1991**, *8*, 1377–1383.

51. Kawashima, Y.; Ohno, H.; Takenaka, H. Preparation of Spherical Matrixes of Prolonged Release Drugs from Liquid Suspensions. J. Pharm. Sci. **1981**, *70*, 913–916.

52. Benita, S.; Zouai, O.; Benoit, J.-P. 5-Flourouracil: Carnauba Wax Microspheres for Chemoembolization: An in Vitro Evaluation. J. Pharm. Sci. **1986**, *75*, 847–851.

53. Bodmeier, R.; Wang, J.; Bhagwatwar, H.J. Process and Formulation Variables in the Preparation of Wax Microparticles by a Melt Dispersion Technique. II. W/O/W Multiple Emulsion Technique for Water-Soluble Drugs. Microencapsulation **1992**, *9*, 99–107.

54. Kowarski, C.R.; Volberger, B.; Versanno, J.; Kowarski, A. Am. J. Hosp. Pharm. **1964**, *21*, 409–410.

55. Draper, E.B.; Becker, C.H. Some Wax Formulations of Sulfaethylthiadiazole Produced by Aqueous Dispersion for Prolonged-Release Medication. J. Pharm. Sci. **1966**, *55*, 376–380.

56. Lucks, S.; Müller, R. Medication Vehicles Made of Solid Lipid Particles (Solid Lipid Nanospheres) SLN. PCT Application, WO93/05768 April 1,1993.

57. Westesen, K.; Siekmann, B. Process for Producing Detergent Tablets. PCT Application, WO94/20072 March 17, 1994.

58. Asker, A.F.; Becker, C.H. Some Spray-Dried Formulations of Sulfaethylhiadiazole for Prolonged-Release Medication. J. Pharm. Sci. **1966**, *55*, 90–94.

59. Robinson, M.J.; Swintosky, J.V. J. Am. Pharm. Assoc. **1959**, *48*, 473–478.

60. Scott, M.W.; Robinson, M.J.; Pauls, J.F.; Lantz, R.J. Spray Congealing: Particle Size Relationships Using a Centrifugal Wheel Atomizer. J. Pharm. Sci. **1964**, *53*, 670–675.

61. Cusimano, A.G.; Becker, C.H. Spray-Congealed Formulations of Sulfaethyliadiazole (SETD) and Waxes for Prolonged-Release Medication. J. Pharm. Sci. **1968**, *57*, 1104–1112.

62. John, P.M.; Becker, C.H. Surfactant Effects on Spray-Congealed Formulations of Sulfaethylthiadiazole-Wax. J. Pharm. Sci. **1968**, *57*, 584–589.

63. Hamid, I.S.; Becker, C.H. Release Study of Sulfaethylhiadiazole (SETD) from a Tablet Dosage Form Prepared from Spray-Congealed Formulations of SETD and Wax. J. Pharm. Sci. **1970**, *59*, 511–514.

64. Sjoqvist, R.; Graffner, C.; Ekman, I.; Sinclair, W.; Woods, J.P. In Vivo Validation of the Release Rate and Palatability of Remoxipride-Modified Release Suspension. Pharm. Res. **1993**, *10*, 1020–1026.

65. Eldem, T.; Speiser, P.; Hincal, A. Optimization of Spray-Dried and -Congealed Lipid Micropellets and Characterization of the Surface Morphology by Scanning Electron Microscopy. Pharm. Res. **1991**, *8*, 47–54.

66. Eldem, T.; Speiser, P.; Altorfer, H. Polymorphic Behavior of Sprayed Lipid Micropellets and Its Evaluation by Differential Scanning Calorimetry and Scanning Electron Microscopy. Pharm. Res. **1991**, *8*, 178–184.

67. Eldem, T.; Speiser, P.; Hincal, A. Proceedings of the 15th International Symposium on Controlled Release of Bioactive Materials Basel Switzerland, Aug 15–19, 1988, The Controlled Release Society, Illinois No. 247, 1988, 436–437.

68. Akiyama, Y.; Yoshioka, M.; Horibe, H.; Hirai, S.; Kitamori, N.; Toguchi, H.J. Novel Oral Controlled-Release Microspheres Using Polyglycerol Esters of Fatty Acids. Control. Rel. **1993**, *26*, 1–10.

69. Rodriguez, L.; Passerini, N.; Cavallari, C.; Cini, M.; Sancin, P.; Fini, A. Description and Preliminary Evaluation of a New Ultrasonic Atomizer for Spray Congealing Process. Int. J. Pharm. **1999**, *183*, 133–143.

WORLD HEALTH ORGANIZATION (WHO) CONTINUES GLOBAL HARMONIZATION OF REQUIREMENTS FOR MEDICINAL PRODUCTS

Juhana E. Idänpään-Heikkilä

Council for International Organizations of Medical Sciences, WHO, Geneva, Switzerland

INTRODUCTION

The World Health Organization (WHO) is an intergovernmental specialized agency of the United Nations with 193 member states. Regarding pharmaceutical and biological products, WHO has the global mandate to develop, establish, and promote quality, safety, and efficacy standards and codes of good practices for all medicinal products. Vigorous harmonization of quality, safety, efficacy, and nomenclature requirements on a worldwide basis has continued in 1998–2000 as the explicit responsibility of WHO. The content of the constitutional mandate, expertise involved, working practices and rules, consultative processes, and role of the governing bodies regarding WHO's normative work was described in detail in the Encyclopedia of Pharmaceutical Technology, Vol. 18 (1). This review gives an update on ongoing harmonization activities since 1998 and outlines the new harmonization initiatives.

International Nonproprietary Names (INNs)

The International Nonproprietary Names (INNs) identifies pharmaceutical substances by unique, globally recognized names. A single internationally recognized name for an active drug substance is a starting point for its pharmacopeial monograph, safe prescribing and dispensing, and easy communication among scientists and health professionals worldwide. The INN is for common use without restrictions (except as a trademark); it is distinctive in sound and spelling and not too long. In 1998–1999, WHO published more than 270 new INNs in its quarterly publication, WHO Drug Information (2) and issued a revised Guidelines on the Use of International Nonproprietary Names (INN) for Pharmaceutical Substances (3). The revision of the procedure included the introduction of a service fee, improvements in Procedures to raise objections to proposed INNs, and the replacement of a recommended INN.

Naming the biotechnology-derived substances and products received increasing attention. Prevention of INNs from using trademarks has now been strengthened in collaboration with the World Intellectual Property Organization (WIPO). A new point of collaboration was the protection of INNs against misuse of Internet domain names (4).

International Pharmacopoeia—50 Years Old

Publication of the International Pharmacopoeia has continued now for 50 years. Its role has been to fulfill a need in developing countries where use of less technically advanced tests using simple instrumentation is common practice for specific substances and preparations. Publishing monographs for finished products has also been useful. In 1999, the Expert Committee recommended that less-advanced methods should be developed in parallel with modern analytical techniques because in some developing countries, more sophisticated methods could be useful (4). Volume 5 of the International Pharmacopoeia is in print. WHO has completed monographs for several antimalarials including artemisin derivatives. Basic tests for pharmaceutical substances, medicinal plant materials, and dosage forms (including 345 tests for substances, 208 for dosage forms, and four for plant materials) were published in 1998 (5). The 69 International Infrared Reference Spectra (IIRS) have been made available from the WHO Collaborating Centre for Chemical Reference Substances (Kungens Kurva, Sweden). The list of reference substances and infrared reference spectra is updated regularly and is now available on the World Wide Web (http://www.who.int/dmp/irintro.htm).

A revised guideline on Good Practices for National Pharmaceutical Control Laboratories (GPCL) was published in 1999. It takes into account guidances from ISO 17025, EN 45001, and OECD–GLP and recommendations published by the Pharmaceutical Inspection Convention (PIC) (4).

WHO GMP and Quality Assurance

In 1998, WHO began a special project to assist in implementing of GMP in member states with limited resources. Countries interested in upgrading their manufacturing have been identified, and training material on basic GMP principles has been prepared together with training modules for advanced GMP topics and inspections. Several regional training workshops for trainers in GMP have been organized, together with missions to concerned countries (4).

The following guidelines have been completed: GMP for Sterile Pharmaceutical Products, Guideline on Pre-Approval Inspection (before granting marketing authorization), Quality System for National GMP Inspectorate, and General Aspects of Packaging Pharmaceuticals (4).

In 1999, WHO published a report on the control and safe trade of starting materials for pharmaceutical products in English, French, Spanish, Russian, Chinese, and Arabic, based on recommendations from a meeting of experts in Geneva in May 1998 (6). The meeting was inspired by several recent incidents of contamination with highly toxic solvent diethylene glycol.

Because of their increasing use worldwide, plant materials used in over-the-counter preparations, home remedies, or as raw materials for pharmaceutical preparations are receiving more and more attention. In 1998, WHO published a book, Quality Control Methods for Medicinal Plant Materials to fulfill the needs of quality control laboratories and to provide a basis for the development of national standards (7).

A compendium of WHO guidelines and related materials entitled Quality Assurance of Pharmaceuticals, Volume 1, was published (8) and the next volume is in print.

Counterfeit drugs

In 1999, WHO published guidelines on the detection and prevention of counterfeit and substandard products (9). Vigilance and reporting of counterfeit products to WHO were enhanced by setting up a liaison officer network among drug regulatory authorities and WHO.

The WHO Certification Scheme

The WHO Certification Scheme on the Quality of Pharmaceutical Products Moving in International Commerce (1) was used in increasing the number of countries as a model instrument to exchange information among authorities in importing and exporting countries. In 1999,

WHO completed a model certificate of analysis to be used for trade of starting materials intended for drug manufacturing, and manufacturers of pharmaceutical substances, excipients, and medicinal products (4).

Comparator product system for equivalence testing

The use of generic pharmaceutical products has increased in many countries. Consequently, drug regulatory authorities are increasingly involved in the assessment of the scientific documentation submitted for marketing approval of generic medicinal products. WHO has stated that the quality, safety, and efficacy of a generic product must comply with the same requirements applied to the innovator (10). Consequently, the therapeutic equivalency and interchangeability with the innovator must be proven with valid comparative in vivo bioequivalence studies. To assist both manufacturers and drug regulators in this, WHO has developed a list of international comparator products. The information on comparator products was collected first from drug regulatory agencies, and a provisional list of candidate products was consulted with the innovator companies concerned. The companies were requested to designate the market and trademark that best represented the quality, manufacturing, and labeling of the product. The current list thus far contains 147 products from the WHO Model List of Essential Drugs, complemented with detailed instructions for use and a decision tree for special situations (11). The list will be updated periodically by WHO.

The WHO Model List of Essential Drugs

The Model List of Essential Drugs was created in 1975, and the most recent assessment and updating of the list took place in 1997 and 1999 (12, 13). The following additions to the list were made including aciclovir for use in herpes infections; amoxicillin + clavulanic acid for the treatment of infections resistant to the production of β-lactamase; dextrometorphan for the treatment of cough; ephedrine for treatment of hypotension in spinal anesthesia during delivery; imipenem + cilastatin for the treatment of Pseudomonas; ipratropium bromide for the treatment of asthma; metformin for the treatment of noninsulin-dependent diabetes; triclabendazole for the treatment of liver and lung flukes; and nevirapine and zidovudine to reduce or prevent mother-to-child transmission of HIV infection. The value of lipid-lowering agents was discussed; however, because of their high costs, they were not included in the list, with a recommendation that each country make its own decisions for use in high-risk patient populations (12).

Sale and promotion of medical products on the internet

The Internet is a rapidly expanding medium that has many uses and great potential for disseminating and obtaining information regarding a variety of subjects such as new treatments, institutions offering care, and medical products available. Individuals can get this information more quickly and conveniently than in traditional ways, such as in medical journals and textbooks. Organizations, pharmaceutical companies, and individuals post and exchange information about their aims, activities, or products and sometimes offer to sell their products, including medical products. However, have the products been approved for marketing? Are they safe, effective, properly labeled, and of good quality? Reported cases show that dangerous, harmful, unreliable, low-quality, substandard, fake, counterfeit, and mislabeled products have been available on the Internet (14).

The World Health Assembly (the annual summit of Ministries of Health of 193 member states of WHO) recognized in May 1997 the increasing use of electronic communication by the general public to shop and gather information on health education, diseases, treatments, and medical products (15). The Assembly was concerned about reported cases of inappropriate use of the Internet, which had caused a potential hazard for public health, and decided to convene a WHO ad hoc working group to formulate recommendations for action. The working group met in September 1997 in Geneva and consisted of representatives of health and drug regulatory authorities, consumer groups, professional associations, the pharmaceutical industry, experts in legal and ethical matters, marketing, and other interested parties. The group reviewed the situation and made several recommendations regarding cross-border advertising, promotion, and sale of medical products. Based on these recommendations, in May 1998 (16) the World Health Assembly urged all member states to review existing legislation, regulations, and guidelines to ensure that they are applicable and adequate to cover the promotion and sale of medical products over the Internet. Member states were asked to set up monitoring and surveillance systems for the Internet. Collaboration was recommended among countries to identify difficult cases and disseminate information through WHO. The availability of scientific, validated information to consumers by competent health authorities was determined to be necessary.

The Assembly appealed to the pharmaceutical industry, health professional and consumer organizations, and other interested parties to promote the formulation and use of good information practices consistent with the principles of the WHO Ethical Criteria for Medicinal Drug Promotion; monitor and report problem cases and aspects of cross-border advertising, promotion, and sale of medical products using the Internet; and maintain legal and ethical standards in these activities.

WHO was requested to encourage the international community to formulate self-regulatory guidelines for good information practices and to develop a model guide for member states. The guide should educate and instruct people using the Internet on how to best obtain reliable, independent, and compatible information on medical products through this medium. The WHO model guide, *Medical Products and the Internet*, was published in 1999 (17).

Biologicals

WHO's normative work for biological substances used in medicinal products, including vaccines, blood products, and diagnostic procedures, has resulted in a number of globally applicable specifications, guidelines, and guiding principles. In 1999, WHO published guidelines for the production and quality control of synthetic peptide vaccines for human use to ensure their consistent safety and efficacy (18). The guidelines address control of starting materials including background data on the synthesis of the peptide of interest and control of the manufacturing process and the final product. WHO requirements for tick-borne encephalitis vaccine (inactivated) were formulated to take into account current manufacturing practices and control procedures in place and to give guidance on how these practices and procedures could be updated (18). Requirements for hepatitis B vaccines made by recombinant DNA techniques have been amended to reflect recent developments in assay methodology, as well as for specifications for Hemophilus type b conjugate vaccines. Under development were guidelines for standardization and calibration of cytokine immunoassays, and requirements for tetravalent dengue vaccine (live) and oral poliomyelitis vaccine (18).

In 1999, WHO published requirements for production and control of *Haemophilus influenzae* type b (Hib) conjugate vaccine and the acellular perussis component of monovalent or combined vaccines. The requirements for oral polio vaccine (OPV) were also revised in 1999, with several additions. WHO published new and replacement International Standards and Reference Materials covering a wide range of products (19).

WHO, ICH, and Regional Harmonization

The role of WHO as an observer of the ICH and its contribution as a global, intergovernmental organization to tripartite ICH activities involving 17 WHO member states have been described in detail (1).

With strong support from WHO, the ICH Steering Committee decided in 1997 to accept the participation of experts from the International Generic Pharmaceutical Alliance (IGPA) and the World Self-Medication Industry (WSMI) in the designated expert working groups (20). This was a first step toward a more comprehensive harmonization procedure. Since 1998, WHO participated as an observer in drafting a guideline for good manufacturing practices for active pharmaceutical ingredients based on preliminary work by the Pharmaceutical Inspection Co-operation Scheme (PIC/S). Australia, China, and India, known for their extensive production of pharmaceutical substances and excipients, were invited to participate in this exercise. The draft guideline is still in development and was an ICH step 2 document in February 2000.

Because Common Technical Document (CTD) (content and format of a new drug application) was accepted as a new ICH topic in 1998, WHO asked a WHO regional adviser for pharmaceuticals from each of the six WHO regions to coodinate among ICH CTD working groups and drug regulatory authorities WHO regions (20). This is an important development because the CTD will undoubtedly have an impact on new drug applications in non-ICH countries and industries. The CTD expert working groups succeeded in 1999 to sign -off as step 2 document tables of contents for all three sections of the CTD, namely quality, safety, and efficacy. Significant work remains to be done, and the progress has been slowest in the quality section.

In 1999, the ICH began a major revision of its existing stability testing guideline. To make this guideline practical and useful for all countries, WHO suggested that it should address not only new molecular entities and associated drug products but also stability testing of generic pharmaceutical products in its new revised form Furthermore, WHO proposed that it should address, in addition to its current coverage of only climatic zones I and II, the remaining critical climatic zones, namely zone III (hot/dry) and zone IV (hot/humid). The WHO guidelines on stability testing of pharmaceutical products containing well-established (generic) drug substances in conventional dosage forms cover all four climatic zones (21).

REFERENCES

1. Idänpään-Heikkilä, J.E. WHO and the Harmonization of Regulatory Requirements for Medicinal Products. *Encyclopedia of Pharmaceutical Technology*, 1st Ed.; Swarbrick, J., Boylan, J.C., Eds.; suppl. 1. Marcel Dekker, Inc.: New York, 1999; 18, 353–360.
2. WHO. International Nonproprietary Names for Pharmaceutical Substances (INN). *WHO Drug Information*; 13, 1999; 1–4, WHO: Geneva, 1998; 12.
3. WHO. *Guidelines on the Use of International Nonproprietary Names (INN) for Pharmaceutical Substances*; WHO/PHARM S/NOM 1570, WHO: Geneva, 1997.
4. WHO. Technical Report Series. *Report of the WHO Expert Committee on Specifications for Pharmaceutical Preparations*; WHO: Geneva, 2000.
5. WHO. *Basic Tests for Drugs, Pharmaceutical Substances, Medicinal Plant Materials and Dosage Forms*; WHO: Geneva, 1998.
6. WHO. *Starting Materials for Pharmaceutical Products: Control and Safe Trade*; WHO/PHARM/98.605, WHO: Geneva, 1998.
7. WHO. *Quality Control Methods for Medicinal Plant Materials*; WHO: Geneva, 1997.
8. WHO. *Quality Assurance of Pharmaceuticals*; WHO: Geneva, 1997; 1.
9. WHO. *Guidelines for the Development of Measures to Combat Counterfeit Drugs*; WHO/EDM/QSM/99.1, WHO: Geneva, 1999.
10. WHO . Drug Information **1999**, *13*, 158–162.
11. WHO. International Comparator Products for Bioequivalence Testing. Drug Information **1999**, *13*, 158–162.
12. WHO. Model List (revised in December 1997). Drug Information **1998**, *12*, 22–35.
13. WHO. Model List (revised in November 1999). Drug Information **1999**, *13*.
14. Idänpään-Heikkilä, J.E. Marketing Pharmaceuticals on the Internet. *Medicines on the Internet. Communication from the Industry to the Patients, Nordic Council on Medicines*, 52, NLN: Stockholm, 2000, 63–67.
15. WHO. *Cross-Border Advertising, Promotion and Sale of Medical Products Through the Internet*; WHO/WHA 50.4, WHO: Geneva, 1997.
16. WHO. *Cross-Border Advertising, Promotion and Sale of Medical Products Using the Internet*; WHO/WHA 51.9, WHO: Geneva, 1998.
17. WHO. *Medical Products and the Internet, A Guide to Finding Reliable Information*; WHO/EDM/QSM/99.4, WHO: Geneva, 1999.
18. WHO. Technical Report Series, No. 889. *Expert Committee on Biological Standardization*; WHO: Geneva, 1999.
19. WHO. Progress in Biological Standardization. Drug Information **1999**, *13*, 86–90.
20. Idänpään-Heikkilä, J.E. ICH and the Common Technical Document (CTD). WHO Drug Information **1999**, *13*, 78–81.
21. WHO. Technical Report Series No. 863, Expert Committee on Specifications for Pharmaceutical Preparations. WHO: Geneva, 1996.
22. Idänpään-Heikkilä, J.E. Pharmaceutical Products: The International Harmonization and Collaboration Perspective. *Focus on Pharmaceutical Research, Policy and Law*; Valverde, J.L., Fracchia, G.N., Eds.; IOS Press, 1999, 25–34.

X-RAY POWDER DIFFRACTOMETRY[a]

Raj Suryanarayanan

University of Minnesota, Minneapolis, Minnesota

Suneel Rastogi

Forest Laboratories, Inc., Inwood, New York

INTRODUCTION

X-rays are electromagnetic radiation lying between ultraviolet and gamma rays in the electromagnetic spectrum. The wavelength of the X-ray region is considered to be between 0.01 and 100 Å (1).

There are two broad applications of X-rays in the characterization of materials: (i) X-ray spectrometry and (ii) X-ray diffractometry. The former technique is used for chemical analysis and has found only limited use in the characterization of pharmaceuticals. On the other hand, X-ray diffractometry, by providing a means for the study of the structure of crystalline materials, is extensively used to characterize pharmaceutical solids. There are two principal applications of X-ray diffractometry. X-ray crystallography is concerned with the structure determination of crystalline phases. Single crystals are usually used for this purpose. On the other hand, in X-ray powder diffractometry, the sample is usually in the form of a powder. X-ray powder diffractometry is recognized as a powerful technique for the identification of crystalline phases. The technique can also be used for the quantitative analyses of solids. This article will be restricted to the principles and applications of X-ray powder diffractometry (XRD) in the characterization of pharmaceutical solids.

Diffraction is a scattering phenomenon. When X-rays are incident on crystalline solids, they are scattered in all directions. In some of these directions, the scattered beams are completely in phase and reinforce one another to form the diffracted beams (1, 2). The Bragg law describes the conditions under which this would occur. It is assumed that a perfectly parallel and monochromatic X-ray beam, of wavelength λ, is incident on a crystalline sample at an angle θ. Diffraction will occur if:

$$n\lambda = 2, d \sin \theta \qquad (1)$$

where d = distance between the successive planes in the crystal lattice, expressed in Å, and n = order of reflection (an integer).

X-ray patterns can be obtained using either a powder diffractometer or a camera. Currently, diffractometers find widespread use in the analysis of pharmaceutical solids. The technique is usually nondestructive in nature. The theory and operation of powder diffractometers is outside the scope of this discussion, but these topics have received excellent coverage elsewhere (1–4). Instead, the discussion will be restricted to the applications of X-ray powder diffractometry (XRD) in the analysis of pharmaceutical solids. The United States Pharmacopeia provides a brief but comprehensive introduction to X-ray diffractometry (5). The use of XRD in the physical characterization of pharmaceutical solids (6) and in the characterization of controlled release delivery systems have been discussed earlier (7).

QUALITATIVE ANALYSIS

Since the X-ray diffraction pattern of every crystalline form of a compound is unique, the technique is widely used for the identification and characterization of solid phases. XRD is the technique of choice to identify different polymorphic forms of a compound (Fig. 1) (8). It can also be used to identify the solvated and unsolvated (anhydrous) forms of a compound, provided their lattice structures are different. The technique can also reveal differences in the crystallinity of compounds. The XRD pattern of an amorphous (noncrystalline) compound will consist of one or more broad diffuse halos (see Fig. 2; upper panel) (9).

The United States Pharmacopeia contains the XRD patterns of two anhydrous forms (Form 1 and Form 2) of

[a]Some parts of this article have been reproduced from the chapter, "X-ray Powder Diffractometry," written by R. Suryanarayanan in "Physical Characterization of Pharmaceutical Solids," edited by H. Brittain. This was Vol. 70 of *Drugs and Pharmaceutical Sciences*, Editor: J. Swarbrick, Marcel Dekker, Inc., New York, 1995.

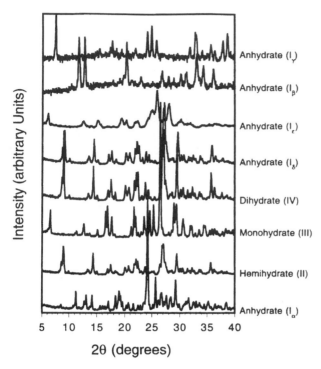

Fig. 1 X-ray powder diffraction (XRD) patterns of the different solid forms of AG337. (From Ref. 8.)

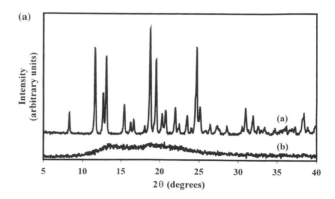

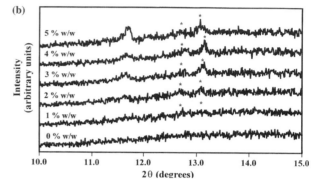

Fig. 2 Upper panel: XRD patterns of (a) crystalline and (b) amorphous sucrose. Lower panel: XRD patterns of the physical mixtures of crystalline and amorphous sucrose. The sucrose content ranged between 0 and 5 wt%. The 12.7 and 13.1°2θ peaks were used for the quantitative analyses. (Bottom panel reproduced from Ref. 9.)

ampicillin, ampicillin trihydrate and amorphous anhydrous ampicillin (5). The powder patterns of these four solid phases reveal pronounced differences, which can form the basis of their identification.

XRD was a powerful tool for the characterization of the different solid phases of AG337 (a 5-substituted quinazolinone; dihydrochloride salt). In addition to several polymorphic forms of the anhydrate ($C_{14}H_{12}N_4OS \cdot 2HCl$), the compound existed as a hemihydrate ($C_{14}H_{12}N_4OS \cdot 2HCl \cdot 0.5H_2O$), a monohydrate ($C_{14}H_{12}N_4OS \cdot 2HCl \cdot H_2O$), and a dihydrate ($C_{14}H_{12}N_4OS \cdot 2HCl \cdot 2H_2O$) (8). The hemihydrate, the dihydrate, and one of the polymorphic forms of the anhydrate (I_δ) had identical lattice structures (Fig. 1).

While the amorphous and crystalline solid forms of sucrose can be readily distinguished by XRD (Fig. 2, upper panel), the technique is also capable of revealing the presence of small amounts of crystalline sucrose in the presence of amorphous sucrose (9). This is evident from the XRD patterns of physical mixtures of amorphous and crystalline sucrose wherein the crystalline sucrose content ranged between 1 and 5 wt% (Fig. 2, lower panel).

Six crystalline solid phases of fluprednisolone and an amorphous phase were characterized using XRD, IR spectroscopy, and differential scanning calorimetry (10). Three of these six crystalline phases were anhydrous, two were monohydrates, and one was a tert-butylamine

disolvate. The differences in the powder patterns of the phases were readily evident. This study demonstrated the unique ability of XRD for the identification of (a) an anhydrous compound existing in both crystalline and amorphous states, (b) different polymorphic forms of the anhydrate, (c) the existence of solvates, where the solvent of crystallization is water (hydrate) or an organic solvent (in this case, tert-butylamine), and (d) polymorphism in the hydrate.

Reference Diffraction Patterns

The International Centre for Diffraction Data (ICDD, Newtown Square, PA) maintains a collection of single-phase X-ray powder patterns (11). There are separate listings of inorganic and organic compounds. The X-ray diffraction data of ibuprofen, as a representative example is given here (Table 1).

The card pattern contains the Powder Diffraction File (PDF) number (Region 1); quality mark of the data (Region 2); the chemical formula and the specimen name

(Region 3); the experimental conditions under which the powder pattern was obtained and the source of the data (Region 4); physical data that include crystallographic system, space group, lattice parameters, and interaxial angles (Region 5); general comments, Crystal Data cell (if different from that reported in Region 5); Pearson Symbol Code (PSC), Merck Index number, etc. (Region 6); and a table of interplanar spacings, relative intensities, and the Miller indices (Region 7).

There are also several indicators of the quality of the data. The highest quality data are given*. To qualify for this mark, the chemistry of the compound must be well characterized. The intensities of the X-ray lines must be measured objectively and instrumentally and there must be no unindexed, space group extinct or impurity lines. Lines with d-spacings of ≤2.50 Å must retain at least three significant digits after the decimal point. To qualify for the "i" mark, there can be a maximum of two unindexed, space group extinct or impurity lines provided none of these belong to the strongest eight. Again there must be no serious systematic errors and lines with d-spacings ≤2.00 Å must retain at least three significant digits after the decimal point. If the data are of low precision or if the data are due to a poorly characterized or multiphase system, an "O" mark is assigned. Patterns that do not meet the criteria for "*," "i," or "O" are left blank. When the powder pattern is calculated from structural parameters, the pattern is marked "C." Extensive details about the quality mark guidelines can be found in ICDD publications (12).

Another important database for pharmaceuticals is the Cambridge Structural Database (CSD). Maintained by the Cambridge Crystallographic Data Centre, CSD is a compilation of single-phase data containing structural information including unit cell parameters, crystal system, and space group. The structural information can be used to

Table 1 The card pattern of ibuprofen

1 ← 32 - 1723 * → 2

	$C_{13}H_{18}O_2$	d Å	Int	h k t	d Å	Int	h k t
		14.41	85	100	2.886	4	$\bar{3}13$
3 ←	Ibuprofen	7.24	15	200	2.792	2	213
		6.93	9	$\bar{1}10$	2.665	2	$\bar{4}21$
	Rad. CuKα₁ λ 1.5406 Filter Ni d-sp	6.33	15	011	2.664	3	004
	Cut off Int. Diffractometer I/I_cor.	6.02	10	$\bar{1}11$	2.533	6	$\bar{1}31$
4 ←	Ref. Cong. P. Polytechnic Insititute of New York.	5.34	100	210	2.504	4	$\bar{4}22$
	Brooklyn. New York. USA. *JCPDS Grant-in-Aid*	5.01	45	$\bar{2}11$	2.437	3	$\bar{3}23$
	Report. (1981)	4.73	10	102	2.409	2	113
	Sys. Monoclinic S.G. P2₁/c (14)	4.65	15	$\bar{2}02$	2.379	4	502
	a 14.667 b 7.899 c 10.731 A 1.8568 C 1.3585	4.55	30	211	2.280	2	512
5 ←	α β 99.46 γ Z 4 mp	4.40	75	012	2.193	2	232	→ 7
	Ref. Ibrd	4.12	2	$\bar{3}10$			
	D_x 1.117 D_m SS/FOM F30=33.0 (.0114.80)	4.06	4	112			
	Color White	3.973	40	202			
	Reported by McConnell. *Cryst. Struct. Commun..* **3**	3.897	4	$\bar{3}02$			
6 ←	73 (1974) as: a = 14.667. b = 7.886, c = 10.730, β = 99.36,	3.811	2	120			
	Space Group = P2₁/c, Z=4. Sillicon used as internal	3.664	4	311			
	standard. PSC: mP132. Merck Index. 9th Ed., 4796.	3.617	4	400			
	To replace 30.1757.	3.546	9	212			
		3.466	4	$\bar{2}20$			
		3.373	1	$\bar{2}21$			
		3.290	4	410			
		3.219	15	221			
		3.053	3	320			
		3.015	3	411			

(From Ref. 11.)

calculate powder diffraction patterns. The ICDD and the Cambridge Crystallographic Data Centre have a cooperative program. This allows the ICDD to calculate powder patterns for inclusion in the Powder Diffraction File, from the data recorded in the CSD.

Phase Identification in Solid Dosage Forms

In addition to the active ingredient, solid dosage forms usually contain one or more excipients. In such powder mixtures, each crystalline phase produces its pattern independently of the other constituents in the mixture. Thus, the unique advantage of XRD is that it combines absolute specificity with a high degree of accuracy. Shell pioneered the use of XRD in the characterization of pharmaceutical dosage forms (13). The recent advances in instrumentation and software have substantially enhanced the utility of the technique. XRD was used to simultaneously identify the three active ingredients, acetaminophen, aspirin, and caffeine, in a commercially available tablet formulation (Excedrin®). The three active ingredients together constituted 83 wt% of the formulation (14). The XRD pattern contained numerous peaks in the angular range of 7–37° 2θ (Fig. 3d). In an effort to identify the components in the dosage form, the XRD patterns of acetaminophen, aspirin, and caffeine were obtained (Fig. 3a–c). Acetaminophen could be readily identified by two unique lines with d-spacings of 6.48 and 4.92 Å (2θ values of 13.65 and 18.00°, respectively). At these 2θ values, the XRD patterns of aspirin and caffeine contained no peaks. Similarly, aspirin could be readily identified by two unique lines with d-spacings of 11.54 and

3.95Å (2θ values of 7.65 and 22.45°, respectively). Caffeine had an intense line with a d-spacing of 7.55 Å (2θ value of 11.70°) and two intense lines with d-spacings of 3.39 and 3.31Å (2θ values of 26.25 and 26.85°, respectively). Since at these 2θ values, peaks due to aspirin and acetaminophen occurred, unambiguous identification of caffeine was not possible. An added complication was that caffeine constituted only 8.9 wt% of the formulation.

In order to identify caffeine, the XRD patterns of acetaminophen and aspirin were selectively subtracted from the XRD pattern of the formulation. The details of the pattern subtraction procedure are described in the literature (14). When the subtracted profile (Fig. 4a) was compared with that of caffeine (Fig. 4b), the high intensity peaks of caffeine at 11.70, 26.25, and 26.85° 2θ were readily discernible. However, an amorphous halo was observed over the angular range of 18–23° 2θ. The formulation contained numerous excipients including microcrystalline cellulose, hydroxypropyl methylcellulose, and hydroxypropyl cellulose. The XRD pattern of microcrystalline cellulose exhibited a broad halo over the angular range of 18–25° 2θ (Fig. 5c). While amorphous halos were also observed in the XRD patterns of hydroxypropyl methylcellulose (Fig. 5b) and hydroxypropyl cellulose (Fig. 5a), their angular range did not match that of the formulation (Fig. 5d). Therefore, microcrystalline cellulose is likely to be the major contributor to the observed halo. Thus, XRD not only permitted simultaneous identification of all the active ingredients in the dosage form, but it also provided information about the excipients in the formulation.

The authors also evaluated the sensitivity of the method, using chlordiazepoxide HCl (hereafter referred to

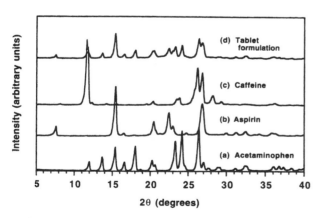

Fig. 3 (a) The XRD pattern of acetaminophen powder. (b) The XRD pattern of aspirin powder. (c) The XRD pattern of caffeine powder. (d) The XRD pattern of a powdered tablet formulation containing acetaminophen, aspirin, and caffeine (Excedrin®). (From Ref. 14.)

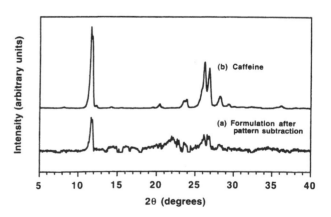

Fig. 4 (a) The residual XRD pattern after proportional subtraction of acetaminophen and aspirin XRD patterns from that of the powdered tablet formulation. (b) The XRD pattern of caffeine powder. (From Ref. 14.)

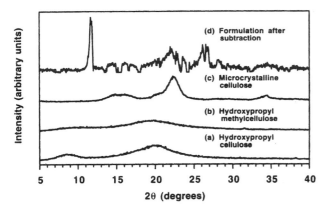

Fig. 5 (a) The XRD patterns of hydroxypropyl cellulose powder. (b) The XRD pattern of hydroxypropyl methylcellulose powder. (c) The XRD pattern of microcrystalline cellulose powder. (d) The residual XRD pattern after proportional subtraction of acetaminophen and aspirin XRD patterns from that of the powdered tablet formulation. (From Ref. 14.)

as chlordiazepoxide) as the model compound (14). While chlordiazepoxide was crystalline (Fig. 6a), microcrystalline cellulose exhibited a broad amorphous halo (Fig. 6c). Identifying chlordiazepoxide was no problem so long as its weight fraction was ≥0.10. When the drug weight fraction was decreased to 0.05, its presence was not readily discernible (Fig. 6b). Using the pattern subtraction technique, the XRD pattern of microcrystalline

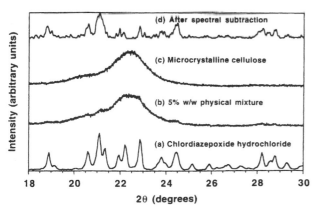

Fig. 6 (a) The XRD pattern of chlordiazepoxide hydrochloride powder. (b) The XRD pattern of a powder mixture of chlordiazepoxide hydrochloride (5 wt%) and microcrystalline cellulose (95 wt%). (c) The XRD pattern of microcrystalline cellulose powder. (d) The residual XRD pattern after proportional subtraction of the microcrystalline cellulose XRD pattern from that of the physical mixture (b). The full scale in this case is different from that of the other three XRD patterns. (From Ref. 14.)

cellulose was subtracted from the XRD pattern of the drug-microcrystalline cellulose mixture (Fig. 6d). This permitted ready identification of chlordiazepoxide (compare Fig. 6d with Fig. 6a).

Phase Transitions Induced During Processing

The components of a dosage form, both active ingredients and excipients, can undergo a variety of physical transformations during pharmaceutical processing and storage. These include polymorphic transformations, alterations in crystallinity, and changes in the state and degree of hydration. XRD is well-suited for analyses of such transformations, provided the analytes are crystalline. In most cases, the dosage forms can be analyzed directly with minimal or no sample pretreatment. There is no need to extract the active ingredient from the dosage form, since it can be usually characterized in presence of the excipient(s). The technique will permit simultaneous identification and quantification of more than one active ingredient in formulations. Finally, XRD can provide quantitative information about the degree of crystallinity.

When theophylline monohydrate was dehydrated, it formed a metastable anhydrous phase, which then transformed to the stable anhydrate (15). The XRD patterns of the two anhydrate phases and the monohydrate were sufficiently different so that all three of them could be simultaneously identified in a sample (Fig. 7; upper panel). Anhydrous theophylline was granulated with an aqueous solution of PVP. During the wet-massing stage, the anhydrate transformed to the monohydrate. When the granules were dried, there was dehydration resulting in the formation of the metastable anhydrate, which then transformed to the stable anhydrate. All three phases were simultaneously monitored by XRD (Fig. 7; lower panel).

DEGREE OF CRYSTALLINITY

Solids may be either crystalline or noncrystalline. The crystalline state is characterized by a perfectly ordered lattice and the noncrystalline (amorphous) state is characterized by a disordered lattice. These represent two extremes of lattice order and intermediate states are possible. The term degree of crystallinity is useful in attempts to quantify these intermediate states of lattice order.

XRD is widely used to determine the degree of crystallinity of pharmaceuticals. The procedure developed by Hermans and Weidinger (16) is based on three assumptions. First, it must be possible to demarcate and

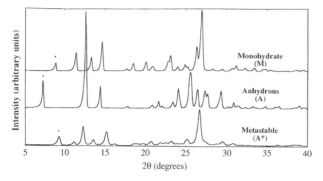

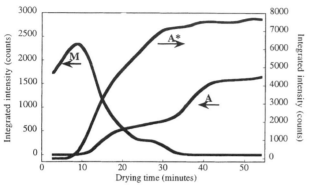

Fig. 7 Upper panel: XRD patterns of theophylline phases. M, A, and A* refer to theophylline monohydrate, stable anhydrous theophylline, and metastable anhydrous theophylline respectively. Lower panel: Phase transitions during the drying of theophylline granules. PVP was the granulating agent. The integrated intensities of the 8.9, 9.4, and 7.0° 2θ peaks unique to M, A*, and A respectively were simultaneously monitored as a function of the drying time. (From Ref. 15.)

measure the crystalline intensity (I_c) and amorphous intensity (I_a) from the powder pattern. Usually, the integrated line intensity (area under the curve), rather than the peak intensity (peak height), is measured. Second, there is a proportionality between the experimentally measured crystalline intensity and the crystalline fraction (x_c) in the sample. Finally, a proportionality exists between the experimentally measured amorphous intensity and the amorphous fraction (x_a) in the sample. The degree of crystallinity (or percent crystallinity), x_{cr}, is given by the expression,

$$x_{cr} = \frac{I_c 100}{1_c + \frac{qI_a}{p}} \qquad (2)$$

where p and q are proportionality constants. The values of I_a and I_c can be determined for samples of varying degrees of crystallinity. A plot of the measured values of I_a against those of I_c will result in a straight line, and

the intercepts on the y- and x-axes will provide the intensity values of the 100% amorphous and 100% crystalline materials, respectively. This method was used by Nakai et al. (17) to estimate the degree of crystallinity of lactose that had been milled for various time periods (Fig. 8). If the value of (q/p) is known, the degree of crystallinity of an unknown sample can be calculated from the experimentally determined values of I_c and I_a. The degree of crystallinity of microcrystalline cellulose and digoxin milled for various time periods were also determined (18, 19). The problems and limitations of this method have been discussed in the literature (6).

A number of drugs and excipients exist in the amorphous state. However, the physical instability of amorphous compounds can lead to their crystallization resulting in partially crystalline materials. In recent years, several techniques have been developed to quantify low levels of an amorphous compound in presence of its crystalline counterpart. Using sucrose as a model compound, an XRD method was developed to detect and to quantify crystalline sucrose when it occurred as a mixture with amorphous sucrose (9). The XRD patterns of amorphous and crystalline sucrose were presented earlier (Fig. 2). Standards consisting of amorphous and crystalline sucrose were prepared wherein the crystalline sucrose content ranged between 1 and 5 wt%. The sum of the background subtracted integrated intensities of the 12.7° 2θ (6.94 Å) and 13.1° 2θ (6.73 Å) peaks of sucrose

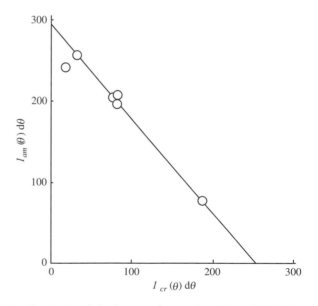

Fig. 8 A plot of the integrated amorphous intensity (I_{am}) as a function of the integrated crystalline intensity (I_c) for lactose samples milled for various time periods. (From Ref.17.)

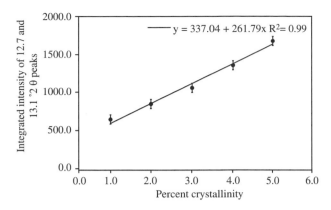

Fig. 9 Plot of the sum of the intensities of the 12.7 and 13.1° 2θ peaks as a function of the weight percent of crystalline sucrose in mixtures of amorphous and crystalline sucrose. (From Ref. 9.)

(these peaks have been marked with an asterisk in Fig. 2) were linearly related to the weight percent of sucrose (Fig. 9).

The limits of detection and quantitation of crystalline sucrose were determined to be 0.9 and 1.8 wt% respectively. Water sorption and FT–Raman spectroscopy also appear to be very sensitive with detection possible down to levels of 1 wt% (20, 21).

PHASE QUANTIFICATION (QUANTITATIVE ANALYSIS)

The Direct Method (No Internal Standard)

Alexander and Klug developed the theoretical basis of the quantitative analyses of powder mixtures (3). Although a powder mixture may be composed of several components, it can be regarded as being composed of just two components: Component 1 (which is the unknown) and the sum of the other components (which is designated as the matrix). The relationship between the intensity of peak i of the unknown component (I_{i1}) and its weight fraction (x_1) in the mixture is given by the equation:

$$I_{i1} = \frac{Kx_1}{\rho_1[x_1(\mu_1^* - \mu_M^*) + \mu_M^*]} \tag{3}$$

where K is a constant, ρ_1 is the density of Component 1, and μ_1^* and μ_M^* are the mass attenuation coefficients of Components 1 and the matrix respectively. The mass attenuation coefficient of a substance is the weighted average of the mass attenuation coefficients of its constituent elements.

Let us first consider a two-component mixture, where $\mu_1^* \neq \mu_M^*$. One example is a mixture of the anhydrous

and hydrated forms of a compound. It is first necessary to determine the intensity of peak i of a sample consisting of only the analyte [$(I_{i1})_0$]. Next, Equation (3) is modified so that the relative intensity of the XRD peak of Component 1 [expressed as $[(I_{i1})/(I_{i1})_0]$ is expressed as:

$$\frac{I_{i1}}{(I_{i1})_0} = \frac{x_1 \mu_1^*}{x_1(\mu_1^* - \mu_M^*) + \mu_M^*} \tag{4}$$

It is possible to calculate the mass attenuation coefficients of the analyte and the matrix based on their chemical compositions (2). This enables the calculation of the relative intensity [$I_{i1}/(I_{i1})_0$] as a function of the weight fraction of the analyte in the mixture and thus generate a theoretical curve. This eliminates the need for the preparation of experimental standard curves. An added advantage of this approach is that there is no requirement of an internal standard.

This approach was used to determine the weight fractions of anhydrous carbamazepine and carbamazepine dihydrate when they occurred as mixtures (22). Based on the mass attenuation coefficients of the anhydrate and the dihydrate, the intensity ratios [$I_{i1}/(I_{i1})_0$] were calculated as a function of the anhydrate content in the mixture (the line in Fig. 10). These were in good agreement with the experimentally obtained values of [$I_{i1}/(I_{i1})_0$].

A simpler system is a two component mixture, where $\mu_1^* = \mu_M^*$. This occurs when the analyte and the matrix have the same molecular formula, as in polymorphic mixtures. In such cases, Equation (4) reduces to:

$$\frac{I_{i1}}{(I_{i1})_0} = x_1 \tag{5}$$

Therefore a plot of the relative intensity as a function of the analyte weight fraction would be linear. This approach was used to determine the weight fractions of anhydrous α-carbamazepine and β-carbamazepine when they occurred as mixtures (23). While studying the polymorphism of 1,2-dihydro-6-neopentyl-2-oxonicotinic acid, Chao and Vail (24) used XRD to quantify Form I in mixtures of Forms I and II. They estimated that Form I levels as low as 0.5 wt% can be determined by this technique. Similarly the α-inosine content in a mixture consisting of α-and β-inosine was achieved with a detection limit of 0.4 wt% for α-inosine (25).

Internal Standard Method

In this method, an internal standard is added, and its weight fraction is maintained constant in all the mixtures. This method was used to simultaneously quantify the S(+)-enantiomer and the racemic compound of ibuprofen (26).

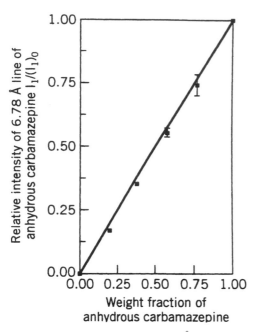

Fig. 10 The relative intensity of the 6.78 Å line of anhydrous carbamazepine (β-form) as a function of its weight fraction in binary mixtures of anhydrous carbamazepine (β-form) and carbamazepine dihydrate. The line is based on theoretical values, while the data points are experimental measurements. (From Ref. 22.)

Selection of Internal Standard

Success in quantitative XRD may hinge on the selection of an appropriate Internal Standard. The following properties are desired in an internal standard (13). (i) The compound must have high crystal symmetry so that strong, but few, diffraction peaks are produced. (ii) The high-intensity lines in the analyte and the internal standard that are to be used for quantitative purposes should not overlap with one another, but they should be close to each other. (iii) The density of the internal standard should be close to that of the system ingredients so that homogeneous mixtures can be prepared for analysis. (iv) The internal standard must be chemically stable in the experimental system. When dealing with organic pharmaceutical systems, an organic internal standard is preferred. Since the XRD patterns of organic compounds usually contain numerous lines, it might not be possible to identify lines unique to the analyte and the internal standard that are completely separated from one another. Therefore, inorganic compounds such as corundum (α-Al_2O_3), silicon, lithium fluoride, and zinc oxide are often used as internal standards. Methenamine, an organic compound, has several of the properties desired in an internal standard (13). However, it has not found widespread use in the analyses of pharmaceuticals.

Whole Powder Pattern Analyses

In the pharmaceutical community, quantitative analyses has conventionally been based on the intensity of a characteristic peak of the analyte. It is now recognized that phase quantification will be more accurate if it is based on the *entire* powder pattern (27, 28). This forms the basis for the whole-powder-pattern analyses method developed in the last few decades. Of the available methods, the Rietveld method is deemed the most powerful since it is based on structural parameters. This is a whole-pattern fitting least-squares refinement technique that has also been extensively used for crystal structure refinement and to determine the size and strain of crystallites.

Simultaneous quantitative analyses, of complex pharmaceutical mixtures, has been accomplished by the Rietveld method (29). Using lithium fluoride as an internal standard, mixtures consisting of anhydrous β-carbamazepine, anhydrous α-carbamazepine, and carbamazepine dihydrate were subjected to quantitative analyses (Table 2). When the analyte concentration was high ($\geq$ 20%), the method was accurate, with a relative error $< \pm 5\%$. However, when the analyte concentration was low ($<5\%$), the method lacked accuracy.

NONAMBIENT XRD

Conventionally, XRD patterns are obtained at room temperature under ambient conditions. Variable temperature XRD is a technique where XRD patterns are obtained while the sample is subjected to a controlled temperature program. It is also possible to control the environment and maintain the sample under the desired relative humidity. Recent advances in commercially available instrumentation have greatly facilitated the study of pharmaceutical systems under nonambient conditions. Experiments can be carried out both at elevated temperatures and under subambient conditions.

High Temperature XRD

In the characterization of pharmaceutical systems, high temperature XRD has been used extensively. The phase transitions of theophylline monohydrate were discussed earlier in the section dealing with Phase Transitions Induced During Processing (Fig. 7). High temperature XRD was used to investigate the dehydration of theophylline monohydrate (Fig. 11). This technique revealed that dehydration resulted in a metastable

Table 2 Measured composition of carbamazepine mixtures and the residuals obtained by the Rietveld analysis

Actual composition of carbamazepine (wt %):				Measured composition of carbamazepine (wt %):				
α	β	Dihydrate	Lithium fluoride	α	β	Dihydrate	Lithium fluoride	R^awp (%)
	80		20		79		21	20.0
	80		20		79		21	22.7
	80		20		80		20	20.7
	79.6	0.4	20		78	1	21	21.5
	79.2	0.8	20		80	1	19	21.4
	79.2	0.8	20		78	2	21	20.9
	79.2	0.8	20		78	2	21	21.4
0.4	79.6		20	<1	79		20	20.7
0.4	79.6		20	<1	79		21	21.3
0.4	79.6		20	<1	78		22	20.9
0.8	79.2		20	1	78		21	20.9
0.4	78.8	0.8	20	<1	77	1	21	21.3
0.8	78.8	0.4	20	<1	78	1	21	20.1
4	72	4	20	3	73	5	19	15.5
4	72	4	20	2	71	7	19	26.9
4	72	4	20	2	71	7	19	26.9
4	40	36	20	2	41	36	20	22.3

[a] Weighted profile residual.
(From Ref. 29.)

anhydrous phase, which then transformed to the stable anhydrate (30). Theophylline has been in widespread use for many years and its solid-state properties have been the subject of numerous investigations. Without high temperature XRD, it is unlikely that this metastable phase would have been identified.

Kinetics of Solid-State Reactions

Solid-state reactions in pharmaceuticals can be broadly classified into chemical decompositions and physical transformations. The chemical decomposition of drugs has received adequate attention in the pharmaceutical literature. The active ingredient in a solid dosage form can also undergo a variety of physical transformations including polymorphic transitions, alterations in degree of crystallinity, and alterations in degree of solvation. These transformations can affect pharmaceutically important properties such as solubility, stability, powder flow, and tabletting behavior, which ultimately can cause variations in the performance of the product. There are strict pharmacopeial standards, which govern not only the chemical purity of drugs and excipients, but also the drug content in dosage forms. On the other hand, very few compounds have pharmacopeial standards that govern their physical form. However, it is increasingly recognized that the physical form of a compound and physical transformations in a dosage form can profoundly affect product performance. An added complication is that

conventional analytical techniques such as HPLC, which are used for monitoring chemical decomposition reactions are unsuitable to monitor solid-state physical transformations. This is because of their inability to distinguish between the different solid forms of a compound. Both chemical decomposition as well as physical transitions can occur simultaneously during the processing or storage of solid formulations. Therefore, it would be ideal if an analytical technique can simultaneously monitor both types of transformations. XRD is one such technique.

Conventionally, thermoanalytical techniques, specifically differential scanning calorimetry and thermogravimetric analysis, have been used to investigate the kinetics of solid-state reactions. These techniques have several limitations. They do not unambiguously identify crystalline phases and are incapable of providing quantitative information about the degree of crystallinity. Intermediate phases, if formed, may not be readily identified. The techniques may therefore be unsuitable for discerning the reaction mechanism. When two or more gaseous products are simultaneously evolved, thermal analysis alone is not very helpful in the study of reaction kinetics. In such cases, thermal analysis should be used in conjunction with other techniques for evolved gas analysis (e.g. infrared spectroscopy, mass spectroscopy, or gas chromatography). It is often realized that solid-state reactions take place through complex mechanisms involving intermediates and the same end product is obtained through multiple pathways. In such cases, thermoanalytical

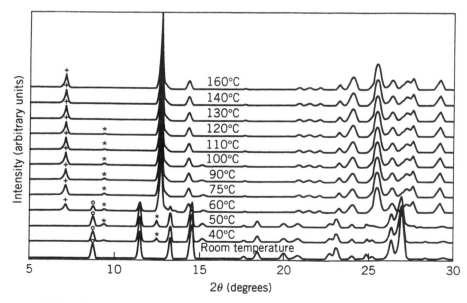

Fig. 11 High temperature XRD of theophylline monohydrate. XRD patterns were obtained at the temperatures indicated in the figure. The "*", "+," and "○" marks indicate peaks unique to metastable anhydrous theophylline (referred to as A* in Fig. 7), stable anhydrous theophylline (A in Fig. 7), and theophylline monohydrate (M in Fig. 7) respectively. (Adapted from Ref. 30.)

techniques yield complex profiles because of overlapping thermal events. Often, it is difficult to separate the reaction steps and study the kinetics of the individual steps. XRD does not suffer from these limitations and can therefore serve as an excellent complement to thermoanalytical techniques. Recent advances in instrumentation have enabled simultaneous and independent control of the temperature and the water vapor pressure in the sample chamber.

The dehydration kinetics of theophylline monohydrate ($C_7H_8N_4O_2 \cdot H_2O$) and ampicillin trihydrate ($C_{16}H_{19}N_3O_4S \cdot 3H_2O$) were studied by XRD (31). Dehydration of theophylline monohydrate resulted in a crystalline anhydrous phase, while the ampicillin trihydrate formed an amorphous anhydrate. In the case of theophylline, simultaneous quantification of both the monohydrate and the anhydrate was possible. By carrying out the reaction at several temperatures, the activation energy for the dehydration reaction was determined.

The enantiomers of pseudoephedrine were observed to react in the solid state to form the racemic compound (32). While the powder patterns of the enantiomers were identical, the racemic compound exhibited a different powder pattern. XRD permitted the simultaneous quantification of the disappearance of the enantiomers and the subsequent appearance of the racemic compound. The rate of disappearance of the enantiomers followed a diffusion-controlled reaction model. During the kinetic experiment, the sum of the weight fractions of the enantiomers and the racemic compound progressively decreased from an initial value of unity, suggesting the formation of an intermediate noncrystalline phase. This was confirmed by a steady increase in the background counts in the powder pattern.

The sweetener aspartame exists as a hemihydrate ($C_{14}H_{18}N_2O_5 \cdot 0.5H_2O$; ASH), under ambient conditions. When heated, ASH converted to aspartame anhydrate (ASA), which on further heating decomposed to form a diketopiperazine (DKP) derivative (33). The XRD patterns of ASH, ASA, and DKP showed pronounced differences (Fig. 12). XRD was used to simultaneously quantify the (i) disappearance of ASH and appearance of ASA in the first reaction and (ii) disappearance of ASA and appearance of DKP in the second reaction. For studying the kinetics of the first reaction, the peaks unique to ASH at 15.9 and 16.4°2 θ and the 17.1° 2θ peak of ASA were used. For the second reaction, the sum of the integrated intensities of the peaks at 10.2, 11.0, and 11.8° 2θ of ASA and the 13.0° 2θ peak of DKP were used. While the dehydration of ASH appeared to follow first-order kinetics, the cyclization of ASA was a nucleation-controlled process. Figs. 13 and 14 contain the dehydration and cyclization data at 118 and 180°C respectively. Since the concentrations of the

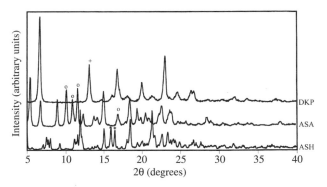

Fig. 12 XRD patterns of aspartame hemihydrate (ASH), aspartame anhydrate (ASA) and diketopiperazine derivative (DKP). "*," "○" and "+" denote the peaks unique to aspartame hemihydrate, aspartame anhydrate, and diketopiperazine derivative respectively. (From Ref. 33.)

crystalline reactant as well as the product were simultaneously monitored, mass balance calculations of the crystalline phases were possible at each time point. The reaction rate constants were obtained at several temperatures, which permitted the calculation of the activation energies of dehydration and cyclization from the Arrhenius plots.

Drug–Excipient Interactions

XRD is an excellent technique to study drug–excipient interactions, provided the drug and the excipients are crystalline. In a solid mixture, the powder pattern of each crystalline phase is produced independently of the other constituents. Thus the diffraction pattern of a powder mixture will be the summation of the diffraction patterns of the individual constituents. If the drug–excipient interaction results in a crystalline product, this will be characterized by the appearance of new peaks in the powder pattern. However, if the interaction results in an amorphous product, this will become evident from the broad halos in the pattern. Thus, irrespective of the nature of the product phase, XRD is capable of revealing such interactions.

Low Temperature XRD

The use of a cooling accessory permits XRD patterns to be obtained under subambient conditions. In pharmaceutical systems, the greatest utility of the technique is to monitor the crystallization of solutes in frozen solutions. Conventionally, differential scanning calorimetry has been the most popular technique for the characterization of frozen systems. However, as mentioned earlier, this

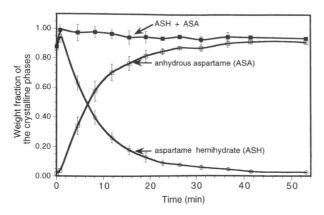

Fig. 13 Weight fractions of ASH and ASA as a function of time following storage of ASH at 118°C. The curves are drawn only to assist in visualizing the trends. (From Ref. 33.)

technique has some drawbacks: (i) It does not enable direct identification of crystalline solid phase(s). Moreover, it is difficult to draw any definitive conclusions about the degree of crystallinity. (ii) The interpretation of DSC curves is very difficult if there are overlapping thermal events. Low temperature XRD was found to be an excellent complement to differential thermal analysis in the characterization of water–glycine–sucrose ternary systems (34).

When sodium nafcillin solutions were frozen, the solute did not crystallize (35). However, annealing caused solute crystallization. It was also possible to monitor the amount of sodium nafcillin crystallizing as a function of annealing time. XRD was also useful to characterize the behavior of buffer solutions. While disodium hydrogen phosphate crystallized when an aqueous solution was frozen, the presence of monosodium hydrogen phosphate inhibited the crystallization of the former.

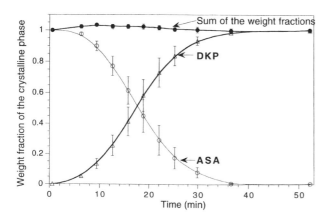

Fig. 14 Weight fractions of ASA and DKP as a function of time, following storage of ASA at 180°C. (From Ref. 33.)

In situ freeze-drying

The low temperature stage of the X-ray powder diffractometer was modified so that the sample chamber could be evacuated. As a result, the entire freeze-drying process was carried out *in situ* in the sample chamber of the XRD. The advantage of such a set-up is that the alterations in the solid state *during* the various stages of the freeze-drying process (cooling, primary, and secondary drying) were monitored (36). As mentioned earlier, annealing of frozen aqueous solutions of sodium nafcillin resulted in the crystallization of sodium nafcillin hydrate (the hydrate stoichiometry was not known). During the primary drying, there was partial dehydration resulting in the formation of partially crystalline sodium nafcillin hemihydrate (Fig. 15). It was possible to simultaneously monitor the disappearance of sodium nafcillin hydrate as well as the appearance of sodium nafcillin hemihydrate (Fig. 16). XRD revealed that this reaction was complete in about 40 min. The technique was also used to monitor the phase transitions during the freeze-drying of mannitol.

Implications in the Design of Freeze-Dried Formulations

Most solid-state characterization studies investigate the starting material and the freeze-dried end product. It will be useful and relevant to study alterations in the solid state *during* the different stages of the freeze-drying process, and this is enabled by low temperature XRD. The physical characterization of the phases at different stages of freeze-drying will not only aid in the optimization of the freeze-drying cycle, but will also facilitate the production of formulations that are physically and chemically stable.

ISSUES AND CHALLENGES IN XRD

Most materials of pharmaceutical interest are organic compounds. Jenkins has comprehensively discussed the problems associated with the X-ray diffractometric analysis of organic materials (37): 1) The unit cells of organic compounds are often large, resulting in low angle lines (large d-spacings). The accuracy of d-spacing data tends to decrease as the d-spacing increases, particularly when the d-spacing value is higher than 8 Å. 2) The unit cells are often of low symmetry resulting in complex powder patterns. 3) Since organic compounds usually have low mass attenuation coefficients, the X-rays can penetrate

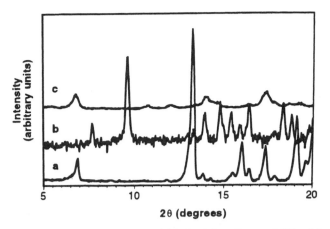

Fig. 15 The XRD patterns of (a) "as is" sodium nafcillin, (b) frozen solution of sodium nafcillin (40 wt%) annealed at $-4°C$ for 1 h, and (c) after freeze-drying the annealed system. The "as is" sodium nafcillin was a monohydrate. Annealing is believed to result in the crystallization of a higher hydrate of sodium nafcillin (unknown stoichiometry). The freeze-dried material was partially crystalline sodium nafcillin hemihydrate. (From Ref. 35.)

deep into the specimen leading to large beam transparency errors. 4) Finally, organic compounds are especially prone to preferred orientation (preferred orientation is discussed in the next section).

Sample Preparation

There are many different methods of sample preparation. Most of the sample holders contain a cavity into which the

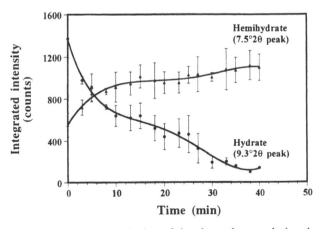

Fig. 16 Real time monitoring of the phase changes during the freeze-drying of sodium nafcillin by in situ XRD. The disappearance of sodium nafcillin hydrate ("Hydrate") and the appearance of sodium nafcillin hemihydrate ("Hemihydrate") were simultaneously quantified. The curves were drawn to assist in visualizing the trends. (From Ref. 36.)

powder sample is filled, usually from the top. However, the side-loading (also referred to as side-drift) method is considered the best packing method (1, 38). Unfortunately, many commercial sample holders do not permit sample filling by this method. As a result, holders have been specially fabricated for this purpose (23). Since organic compounds predominantly consist of atoms with low atomic numbers, there will be significant penetration of X-rays. This can result in peak displacement as well as broadening. Detailed information on sample preparation is available in the literature (4).

When only a very small amount of powder sample is available, the use of a low-background (also referred to as zero background) support is advisable. The support is a quartz or silicon plate cut along a nondiffracting crystallographic direction, which is then polished (1). This results in a very low background and improves the signal-to-noise ratio and enables XRD patterns to be obtained with extremely small amounts of sample.

Sources of Error

There are numerous sources of error in XRD. Two of these are discussed hereafter.

Preferred orientation

Reliable and reproducible results can only be obtained if the sample is prepared carefully. When a sample is packed in an X-ray holder, the distribution of crystal orientations can be nonrandom, and this condition is referred to as preferred orientation. Jenkins and Snyder (1) have elegantly illustrated this point in Fig. 17. Atoms bond together, in a unique manner, to form unit cells. If the unit cells are grouped so as to have long-range order, a crystalline material is obtained. In the absence of long-range order, the material is amorphous (noncrystalline). A powder sample is composed of crystallites. When the crystallites in a sample are oriented in some particular (nonrandom) manner, they are said to exhibit preferred orientation (1). Ideally, random orientation of individual crystallites is desired. It is recognized that preferred orientation is a commonly encountered condition in powdered samples (2).

Grinding the sample and thereby reducing the particle size can decrease preferred orientation. However, grinding can cause lattice disorder (decrease in crystallinity) and also induce other undesirable transitions, such as polymorphic transformations. Moreover, when the particle size is very small, particle size induced peak broadening can be observed. This effect, observed when the particle size is <10,000 Å (1 μm), is simply a consequence of the

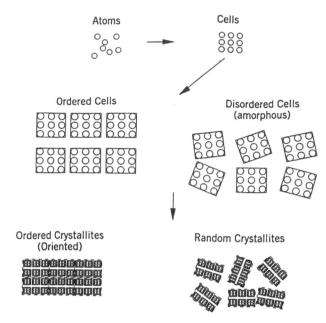

Fig. 17 The structural makeup of solids. (From Ref. 1.)

Measurement of line intensity

When measuring intensity, the integrated line intensity (peak area) and not the maximum intensity (peak height) must be measured. Variations in lattice strain and particle size can significantly influence the line shape, but their effect on the integrated intensity will generally be minimal (2).

Other sources of error

There are numerous other sources of error that are particularly relevant while conducting quantitative XRD studies. These are discussed in detail in the literature (Refs. 1–3, 6).

ACKNOWLEDGMENT

We thank Mr. Rahul Surana for his assistance in the preparation of the manuscript.

limited number of planes that are diffracting X-rays (Fig. 18). The particle (crystallite) size is related to the X-ray line width according to the Scherrer equation (1). It is important to recognize the fact that line broadening can be brought about by a loss in crystallinity as well as a decrease in particle size. In the pharmaceutical literature, there is a tendency to automatically attribute line broadening to loss in crystallinity. Such a conclusion, while usually correct, can be occasionally erroneous.

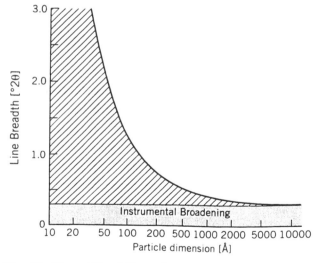

Fig. 18 The width of X-ray lines as a function of particle dimension. (From Ref. 1.)

REFERENCES

1. Jenkins, R.; Snyder, R.L. *Introduction to X-Ray Powder Diffractometry*; Wiley: New York, NY, 1996.
2. Cullity, B.D. *Elements of X-Ray Diffraction*, 2nd Ed.; Addison-Wesley: Reading, MA, 1978.
3. Klug, H.P.; Alexander, L.E. *X-Ray Diffraction Procedures for Polycrystalline and Amorphous Materials*, 2nd Ed.; Wiley: New York, NY, 1974.
4. Buhrke, V.E.; Jenkins, R.; Smith, D.K. *A Practical Guide for the Preparation of Specimens for X-Ray Fluorescence and X-Ray Diffraction Analysis*; Wiley-VCH: New York, NY, 1998.
5. *The United States Pharmacopeia;* 24th Rev. U.S. Pharmacopeial Convention: Rockville, MD, 1999.
6. Suryanarayanan, R. X-Ray Powder Diffractometry. *Physical Characterization of Pharmaceutical Solids*; Brittain, H.G., Ed.; Marcel Dekker, Inc.: New York, NY, 1995.
7. Rastogi, S.; Suryanarayanan, R. Characterization of Delivery Systems—X-Ray Powder Diffractometry. *The Encyclopedia of Controlled Drug Delivery*; Mathiowitz, E., Ed.; Wiley: New York, NY, 1999.
8. Rastogi, S.; Zamansky, I.; Roy, S.; Tyle, P.; Suryanarayanan, R. Solid-State Phase Transitions of AG337, an Antitumor Agent. Pharm. Dev. Technol. **1999**, *4* (4), 623–632.
9. Surana, R.; Suryanarayanan, R. Quantitation of Crystallinity in Substantially Amorphous Pharmaceuticals and Study of Crystallization Kinetics by X-Ray Powder Diffractometry. Powder Diffr. **2000**, *15* (1), 2–6.
10. Haleblian, J.K.; Koda, R.T.; Biles, J.A. Isolation and Characterization of Some Solid Phases of Fluprednisolone. J. Pharm. Sci. **1971**, *60* (10), 1485–1488.
11. McClune, W.F., Ed. *Powder Diffraction File, Inorganic Phases, Organic and Organometallic Phases Search*

Manual; International Centre for Diffraction Data: Newtown Square, PA, 1993.

12. Powder Diffraction File: Set 43. *Inorganic and Organic Databook*; McClune, W.F., Ed.; International Centre for Diffraction Data: Newtown Square, PA, 1993.

13. Shell, J.W. X-Ray and Crystallographic Applications in Pharmaceutical Research, II. J. Pharm. Sci. **1963**, *52*, 24–39.

14. Phadnis, N.V.; Cavatur, R.K.; Suryanarayanan, R. Identification of Drugs in Pharmaceutical Dosage Forms by X-Ray Powder Diffractometry. J. Pharm. Biomed. Anal. **1997**, *15* (7), 929–943.

15. Tank, J. *Changes in the Solid-State of Theophylline Upon Aqueous Wet Granulation*; M.S. Thesis Department of Pharmaceutics, University of Minnesota: Minneapolis, MN, 1997.

16. Hermans, P.H.; Weidinger, A. Quantitative X-Ray Investigation on the Crystallinity of Cellulose Fibres. A Background Analysis. J. Appl. Phys. **1948**, *19*, 491–506.

17. Nakai, Y.; Fukuoka, E.; Nakajima, S.; Morita, M. Physicochemical Properties of Crystalline Lactose. I. Estimation of the Degree of Crystallinity and the Disorder Parameter by an X-Ray Diffraction Method. Chem. Pharm. Bull. **1982**, *30* (5), 1811–1818.

18. Nakai, Y.; Fukuoka, E.; Nakajima, S.; Hasegawa, J. Crystallinity and Physical Characteristics of Microcrystalline Cellulose. Chem. Pharm. Bull. **1977**, *25* (1), 96–101.

19. Black, D.B.; Lovering, E.G. Estimation of the Degree of Crystallinity in Digoxin by X-Ray and Infrared Methods. J. Pharm. Pharmacol. **1977**, *29* (11), 684–687.

20. Saleki-Gerhardt, A.; Ahlneck, C.; Zografi, G. Assessment of Disorder in Crystalline Solids. Int. J. Pharm. **1994**, *101*, 237–247.

21. Taylor, L.S.; Zografi, G. Quantitative Analysis of Crystallinity using FT-Raman Spectroscopy. Pharm. Res. **1998**, *15*, 755–761.

22. Suryanarayanan, R. Determination of the Relative Amounts of Anhydrous Carbamazepine and Carbamazepine Dihydrate in a Mixture by Powder X-Ray Diffractometry. Pharm. Res. **1989**, *6* (12), 1017–1024.

23. Suryanarayanan, R. Determination of the Relative Amounts of α-Carbamazepine and β-Carbamazepine in a Mixture by Powder X-Ray Diffractometry. Powder Diffr. **1990**, *5* (3), 155–159.

24. Chao, R.S.; Vail, K.C. Polymorphism of 1,2-Dihydro-6-Neopentyl-2-Oxonicotinic Acid: Characterization, Interconversion, and Quantitation. Pharm. Res. **1987**, *4* (5), 429–432.

25. Doff, D.H.; Brownen, F.L.; Corrigan, O.I. Determination of α-Impurities in the β-Polymorph of Inosine using Infrared Spectroscopy and X-Ray Powder Diffraction. Analyst (London) **1986**, *111* (2), 179–182.

26. Phadnis, N.V.; Suryanarayanan, R. Simultaneous Quantification of an Enantiomer and the Racemic Compound of Ibuprofen by X-Ray Powder Diffractometry. Pharm. Res. **1997**, *14* (9), 1176–1180.

27. Anwar, J. Analysis of Time-Resolved Powder Diffraction Data using a Pattern-Decomposition Method with Restraints. J. Appl. Crystallogr. **1993**, *26* (3), 413–421.

28. Rietveld, H.M. Profile Refinement Method for Nuclear and Magnetic Structures. J. Appl. Crystallogr. **1969**, *2*, 65–71.

29. Iyengar, S.S.; Phadnis, N.V.; Suryanarayanan, R. Quantitative Analyses of Complex Pharmaceutical Mixtures by the Rietveld Method. Powder Diffr. *in press*.

30. Phadnis, N.V.; Suryanarayanan, R. Polymorphism in Anhydrous Theophylline-Implications for the Dissolution Rate of Theophylline Tablets. J. Pharm. Sci. **1997**, *86* (11), 1256–1263.

31. Shefter, E.; Fung, H.-L.; Mok, O. Dehydration of Crystalline Theophylline Monohydrate and Ampicillin Trihydrate. J. Pharm. Sci. **1973**, *62* (5), 791–794.

32. Duddu, S.P.; Khin-Khin, A.; Grant, D.J.W.; Suryanarayanan, R. A Novel X-Ray Powder Diffractometric Method for Studying the Reaction between Pseudoephedrine Enantiomers. J. Pharm. Sci. **1997**, *86* (3), 340–345.

33. Rastogi, S.; Zakrzewski, M.; Suryanarayanan, R. Investigation of Solid-State Reactions using Variable Temperature X-Ray Powder Diffractometry. I. Aspartame Hemihydrate. Pharm. Res. **(2001)**, *18* (3), 267–273.

34. Shalaev, E.Y.; Malakhov, D.V.; Kanev, A.N.; Kosyakov, V.I.; Tuzikov, F.V.; Varaksin, N.A.; Vavilin, V.I. Study of the Phase Diagram Water Fraction of the System Water–Glycine–Sucrose by DTA and X-Ray Diffraction Methods. Thermochim. Acta **1992**, *196* (1), 213–220.

35. Cavatur, R.K.; Suryanarayanan, R. Characterization of Frozen Aqueous Solutions by Low Temperature X-Ray Powder Diffractometry. Pharm. Res. **1998**, *15* (2), 194–199.

36. Cavatur, R.K.; Suryanarayanan, R. Characterization of Phase Transitions during Freeze-Drying by in Situ X-Ray Powder Diffractometry. Pharm. Dev. Technol. **1998**, *3* (4), 579–586.

37. Jenkins, R. New Directions in the X-Ray Diffraction Analysis of Organic Materials. Adv. X-Ray Anal. **1992**, *35*, 653–660.

38. McMurdie, H.F.; Morris, M.C.; Evans, E.H.; Paretzkin, B.; Wong-Ng, W.; Hubbard, C.R. Methods of Producing Standard X-Ray Diffraction Powder Patterns. Powder Diffr. **1986**, *1* (1), 40–43.

ZETA POTENTIAL

Luk Chiu Li

Abbott Laboratories, Abbott Park, Illinois

Youqin Tian

Alcon Research, Ltd., Fort Worth, Texas

INTRODUCTION

Dispersion systems represent an important class of pharmaceutical dosage forms such as emulsions, suspensions, microspheres, liposomes, and nanoparticles. The medium of these systems is mainly aqueous in nature and the dispersed phase can be either solid particles or immiscible liquid droplets. Electrical charges are developed by several mechanisms at the interface between the dispersed phase and the aqueous medium (1). The two most common mechanisms are the ionization of surface functional groups and the specific adsorption of ions. These electrical charges play an important role in determining the interaction between particles of the dispersed phase and the resultant physical stability of the systems, particularly for those in the colloidal size range. For dispersed systems which are used as drug carriers, i.e., liposomes and microparticles, their in vivo fate and therapeutic efficacy are both affected by these surface charges. Therefore, the understanding of this electrical phenomenon becomes essential in developing these systems.

The presence of these surface charges influences an uneven distribution of charges (ions) surrounding the particle and the development of an electrical potential (or an electrical field) between the surface and the electrically neutral bulk-solution phase of the system. The surface charge and the counterions in its vicinity give rise to an electric double layer as shown in Fig. 1. The double layer is divided into two parts separated by a plane called the Stern layer which is located at about a hydrated-ion radius from the surface. Usually, the number of ions in the Stern layer is smaller than that needed to achieve neutralization of the surface charge and the balance of the neutralization occurs in a Gouy–Chapman layer outside the Stern layer. The surface potential (ψ_0) and the Stern potential (ψ_d) are not readily measured experimentally; instead, the potential between a stationary fluid layer enveloping the particle and the bulk-solution phase can be determined by measuring the mobility of the particle in an applied electrical field.

The potential between the tightly bound surface liquid layer (shear plane) of the particle and the bulk phase of the solution is called zeta potential (ζ). It can provide a measure of the net surface charge on the particle and potential distribution at the interface. Zeta potential serves as an important parameter in characterizing the electrostatic interaction between particles in dispersed systems and the properties of the dispersion as affected by this electrical phenomenon.

METHOD AND INSTRUMENTATION

Microelectrophoresis

The most common method for determining the zeta-potential is the microelectrophoretic procedure in which the movements of individual particles under the influence of a known electric field are followed microscopically. The zeta potential can be calculated from the electrophoretic velocity of the particles using the Helmholtz–Smoluchowski equation,

$$U_{rmp} = V_{rmp}E = zeta \epsilon \eta \tag{1}$$

where U_p is the electrophoretic mobility, V_p is the electrophoretic velocity, E is the electric-field strength, ζ is the zeta potential, ε is the permittivity, and η is the viscosity of the medium.

It is important to realize that the observed electrophoretic migration is the sum of two contributions, one of which is the electro-osmotic flow of the medium through the cell. The glass of the sample cell generally bears negative charges, so that a diffuse layer of cations exists adjacent to them. This sets up an electro-osmotic flow through the cell (with or without particles). This flow has its maximum value at the center, since the layer of fluid adjacent to the walls is stationary. The particles tracked at the center of the cell therefore possess the maximum increment in velocity because of the electro-osmotic flow. Since there is no net liquid flow through the closed cell,

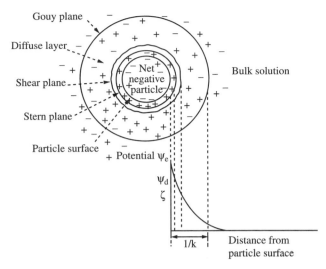

Fig. 1 A schematic representation of the electric double layer around a particle with negative surface charges and electrical potentials surrounding the particle.

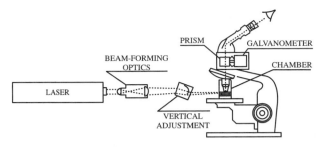

Fig. 3 A diagram of light paths in the rotating prism method of microelectrophoretic measurement.

a back-pressure builds up which causes fluid flow in the reverse direction in the core of the cell. In the steady state, these flows balance, giving rise to a velocity profile as shown in Fig. 2. Therefore, the tracking of particles at a location where the medium experiences no net flow becomes important in yielding an accurate electrophoretic mobility measurement. A velocity profile has been derived for the liquid contained in a cylindrical electrophoretic cell. The location with zero liquid flow is shown to be 14.6% of the cell diameter inside the surface of the capillary. The location of the surface of zero liquid flow in cells of rectangular cross section has also been determined. For a cell in which the direction of migration is relatively long compared to the width of the cell, the surface with zero liquid flow lies 21.1% of the cell depth above the bottom and below the top of the working compartment. Experimentally, particles tracked at these positions of the sample cell will display their mobility uncomplicated by the electro-osmotic effect.

The rate of particle migration can be determined by measuring with a stopwatch the time required for a particle

to travel between the marks of a calibrated graticule in the microscope eyepiece. Since many particles are usually measured in order to get good statistical results, the measurement of a sample may take 30 min or even longer. As the time of measurement increases, however, the susceptibility to errors also increases. For example, a long measurement time will cause convection currents generated by heating of the sample, air-bubble formation, settling of particles, and electrode reactions. These potential errors can be avoided if the measurement is taken much more quickly without loss of accuracy. A rotating prism method employed by the Lazer Zee Meter (Model 50,1 Pen Kem, Inc.), allows the operator to measure more than 10 particles simultaneously. Data are thereby attained more rapidly and, consequently, with fewer time-dependent errors. Fig. 3 shows a diagram of light paths in the rotating prism method (2). The microscope is focused on the stationary layer of the cell (with no fluid flow). Special cylindrical optics compress the laser beam into an illumination sheet of laser light. A vertical adjustment is provided to vary the height so that it coincides with the focal plane of the microscope. A cube prism inside the microscope causes the viewed image to translate at a rate proportional to the prism's speed of rotation. The applied electric field causes the particle to move at an electrophoretic velocity proportional to the mobility and the applied voltage. Adjustment of the potentiometer causes the prism to rotate at a rate proportional to potentiometer voltage times applied voltage. When the image velocity caused by prism rotation is equal and opposite to the mean electrophoretic velocity, the cloud of particles appears stationary. The applied voltage is therefore proportional to the mean particle electrophoric mobility. The mobility value is scaled by an appropriate constant in the digital meter and the computed zeta potential is displayed on the 3-digit readout.

In spite of a major improvement gained from the rotating prism method, there are still serious limitations in the use of microelectrophoresis in determining zeta potential. First, this technique cannot be applied to dense dispersions, i.e., the number density of the particles must

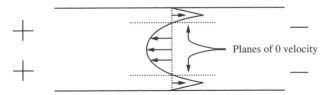

Fig. 2 The velocity profile of fluid flow in an electrophorectic cell.

be very low. This can sometimes, but not always, be remedied by filtering the sample and diluting a small amount of the original dispersion with a large volume of filtrate. Second, it cannot be applied to particles less than about 0.2 μm in diameter because they are not easily visible in the ultramicroscope, though the particle-size range may be extended by adsorbing the colloidal particles (i.e., protein molecules) on suitable carrier particles. An additional and unresolvable problem with very small particles is the blurring effect imparted by Brownian motion. Furthermore, the microelectrophoretic technique cannot be used to determine mobility distributions or to separate mutlimodal mobility distributions.

Electrophoretic Light-Scattering (3–5)

Electrophoretic light-scattering is a technique which determines the electrophoretic velocities by measuring the Doppler shifts of scattered laser light. The electrophoretic mobility can be expressed by

$$U_p = \Delta \nu \lambda_0 / 2\, n\, E \sin(\theta/2) \qquad (2)$$

where U_p is electrophoretic mobility, $\Delta \nu$ is the Doppler frequency shift, λ_0 is the wavelength of the laser in a vacuum, n is the index of refraction of the medium, E is the electric field applied, and θ is the scattering angle. Since a He–Ne laser light has a frequency of about 6.0×10^{14}, a direct measurement of frequency shifts ranging from zero to several hundred Hz may be problematic because of the difficulty in measuring a small difference between large quantities. However, this can be overcome by using the principle of heterodyning, which measures the difference in frequency resulting from a reference beam and the Doppler-shifted beam.

When the Brownian motion of the particles is negligible, the power spectrum which is generated by the autocorrelation function of the scattered light has a very narrow peak. However, the actual spectral peak has considerable line width attributable to the Brownian motion of the particles and a distribution of electrophoretic mobilities. The separation of these two sources of spectral-peak broadening is critical because, without such a separation, a measurement of electrophoretic mobility at a single angle provides information only about the peak position (Doppler shift). The shape of the peak (Doppler broadening), being attributable to either of the two effects, cannot be interpreted with a single-angle measurement. Simultaneous multiple-angle measurements allow peak shapes to be analyzed to give accurate measurement of the electrophoretic mobility and the subsequent determination

of zeta potential according to the Helmholtz–Smoluchowski equation (Eq. 1).

The DELSA 440 (Coulter Scientific Instruments) is a laser-scattering particle electrophoretic analyzer that measures the electrophoretic mobility distribution and zeta-potential distribution (6). This instrument provides simultaneous measurements of line widths at four different angles so that the motion of the particle can be decomposed with high resolution into components caused by electrophoretic and diffusional motions. Therefore, particle sizing can also be carried out by the same instrument simultaneously with electrophoretic mobility determinations. Fig. 4 presents a schematic diagram of the DELSA 440 system. Other commercially available electrophoretic analyzers using the laser light-scattering principles are the Zetasizer 3 (Malvern Instruments), ZetaPlus (Brookhaven Instruments), System 3000 (PenKem, Inc.), and NICOMP 380/ZLS (Particle Sizing Systems).

Electrokinetic Sonic Analysis (3, 6, 7)

When a colloidal dispersion is subject to ultrasonic waves, a density difference between the dispersed phase and the continuous phase will cause relative motion between the particles and the surrounding fluid. This relative motion means that there will be a periodic interchange of the charged particle surface and the oppositely charged counter-ions in the electric double layer. This interchange results in the development of an alternating dipole at the frequency of the applied ultrasound wave. This effect is termed the ultrasound vibration potential (UVP). The UVP effect in colloids is also referred to as the colloid vibration potential or CVP. An effect opposite that of CVP is generated, when an alternating electric field is applied to a colloidal dispersion, creating an acoustic wave which, by means of a piezoelectric device, may be transduced into an alternating potential of a certain amplitude, depending on the dispersion and the electric double-layer properties. This is called the electrokinetic sonic amplitude (ESA). These two phenomena are both known as electro-acoustic effects.

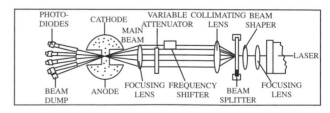

Fig. 4 A schematic diagram of the DELSA 440 system.

The magnitude of these effects is directly proportional to the electrophoretic mobility of the particles. The mobility determined by either electro-acoustic effect is the dynamic or AC mobility of the particle.

The dynamic mobility which is determined by the electro-acoustic effects differs from the low-frequency or DC mobility that is determined by electrophoresis because of the effects of particle inertia which cause particle velocities in an alternate field to become out of phase with the applied field. The higher the frequency, the greater is the phase lag between the particle and the applied field. Dynamic mobility (U_d) is a function of frequency, particle size, particle density, and particle zeta potential. These inertial effects arise in both ESA and CVP measurements. In the case of spherical particles with thin double layers and low zeta potential, the equation below can be applied:

$$U_d = (\epsilon\zeta/\eta)G(\alpha) \tag{3}$$

where $G(\alpha)$ is the inertial term. The formula for dynamic mobility is identical to the well-known Helmholtz–Smoluchowski equation (Eq. 1) for DC electrophoretic mobility except for the $G(\alpha)$ term.

A linear relationship exists between the ESA or CVP amplitude and the volume fraction of the suspended particles. At relatively high-volume fractions, hydrodynamic and electric double-layer interactions lead to a non-linear dependence of these two effects on volume fraction. Generally, non linear behavior can be expected when the electric double-layer thickness is comparable to the interparticle spacing. In most aqueous systems, where the electric double layer is thin relative to the particle radius, the electro-acoustic signal will remain linear with respect to volume fraction up to 10% by volume. At volume-fractions that are even higher, particle-particle interactions lead to a reduction in the dynamic mobility.

The commercial systems for zeta-potential determination using these electro-acoustic effects are typified by the AcoustoSizer 8000 (Matek Applied Sciences) consisting of five main components (Fig. 5). The synthesizer

produces a continuous sinusoidal voltage which feeds into the gated amplifier. This creates a sinusoidal voltage pulse across the cell which contains the dispersion. The resulting ESA sound waves are converted by a pressure transducer in the cell to an electrical signal, which then passes to the signal processing electronics. The electronics extract the amplitude and the phase of the ESA signal, storing them in the computer housed in the AcoustoSizer.

A schematic diagram of the cell is shown in Fig. 6. The dispersion is located in the region between the pair of electrodes. The pulse from the gated amplifier is applied across these electrodes, generating the ESA sound waves. Voltage pulses rather than continuous sinusoids are applied to avoid interference by the sound wave emanating from the electrodes. The use of pulsed signals also avoids electrical heating of the suspension and the complications of multiple reflections of the waves at the electrodes and at the ends of the rods. The voltage pulse produced by the sound wave in the transducer on the right passes into the signal-processing electronics, which measures the amplitude and phase of the sinusoidal component of the pulse. These data are passed to the computer where it is stored for subsequent processing.

Since the ESA signal depends on particle motion and also on the acoustic property of the dispersion, the determination of particle motion from the ESA signal requires knowledge of the acoustic impedance of the dispersion. This parameter is measured using sensors associated with the rod on the left immediately after each ESA measurement. The signals from these two rods are stored in the computer and are subsequently converted to a particle-velocity spectrum, and from that the zeta potential and size information is determined. The AcoustoPhor 8000 (PenKem, Inc.) is another example of a commercial system which determines zeta potential and the particle size of dispersions using these electro-acoustic effects.

APPLICATIONS

The practical significance of zeta-potential measurement lies in the fact that strong empirical correlation exists between the measured zeta potential of the system and the properties of the system which are the manifestation of the electrostatic interfacial phenomenon. Since the measurement of zeta potential can be conveniently performed, it becomes an ideal parameter for use in routine testing. Zeta-potential control has been successfully applied to various technical fields involving colloidal and non-colloidal systems.

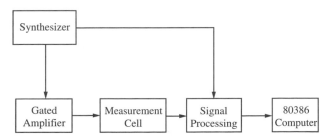

Fig. 5 An AcoustoSizer signal processing block diagram.

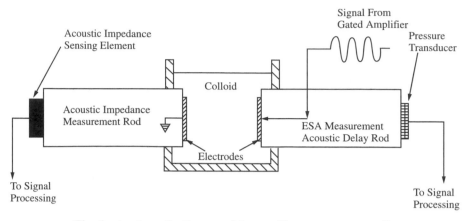

Fig. 6   A schematic diagram of AcoustoSizer measurement cell.

Colloid Stability (3, 8, 9)

The physical stability of a colloidal system is determined by the balance between the repulsive and attractive forces which is described quantitatively by the Deryaguin–Landau–Verwey–Overbeek (DLVO) theory. The electrostatic repulsive force is dependent on the degree of double-layer overlap and the attractive force is provided by the van der Waals interaction; the magnitude of both are a function of the separation between the particles. It has long been realized that the zeta potential is a good indicator of the magnitude of the repulsive interaction between colloidal particles. Measurement of zeta potential has therefore been commonly used to assess the stability of colloidal systems.

Electrostatic repulsive energy, V_R, at a given inter-particle distance is the work which must be performed to bring the particles to a specific point. Using the Debye–Huckel low-potential approximation and assuming equal spheres, V_R can be described by

$$V_R = 2\pi\epsilon a\psi_d{}^2 \ln(1 + \exp[-\kappa H]) \tag{4}$$

where a is the particle radius, H is the distance of separation between the two particles, and κ is the Debye parameter. The magnitude of V_R decreases in an approximately exponential fashion with increasing H and that its range decreases by increasing κ (i.e., by increasing electrolyte concentration and/or counter-ion charge number). V_R can be also influenced by other specific factors. Counter-ion adsorption in the Stern layer may cause a reversal of charge, so that V_R will be zero at the reversal-of-charge concentration and will be positive (repulsion) at both below and above this concentration.

The attractive-force component between particles in a colloidal system is developed by summation of the London dispersion forces between all atom pairs in the particles. Neglecting retardation effects, the expression for the attractive energy V_A between two particles of radius a at a distance of separation H_0, for $a \gg H_0$, is

$$V_{rmA} = A, a12H_0 \tag{5}$$

where A is the effective Hamaker constant describing the attraction between the particles and the dispersion medium. It is apparent that V_A decreases as an inverse power of the distance between the particles.

According to DLVO theory, the total energy of interaction between colloidal particles is given by the sum of the attraction (V_A) and repulsion (V_R) energies:

$$V_T = V_R + V_A \tag{6}$$

Fig. 7a shows the total interaction energy curve for a colloidal system. At very close distances between the particles, the Born repulsion between adjoining electron clouds predominates, and the net interaction is repulsion. However, at slightly greater distances, the van der Waals attraction predominates over the electrostatic repulsion, and the net interaction is strong attraction as shown by the deep potential energy minimum V_P. At even greater distances, the net interaction is moderate attraction (a shallow secondary minimum V_S) because with increasing distance between two particles, electrostatic repulsion weakens more rapidly than the van der Waals attraction energy. At intermediate distances, the electrostatic repulsion predominates and the net interaction becomes repulsion, with an energy barrier, V_m.

The attraction energy arising from van der Waals forces does not vary significantly with changes in the surface potential and electric double-layer properties of the colloidal particles. By contrast, changes in these two parameters have significant impact on the repulsion energy

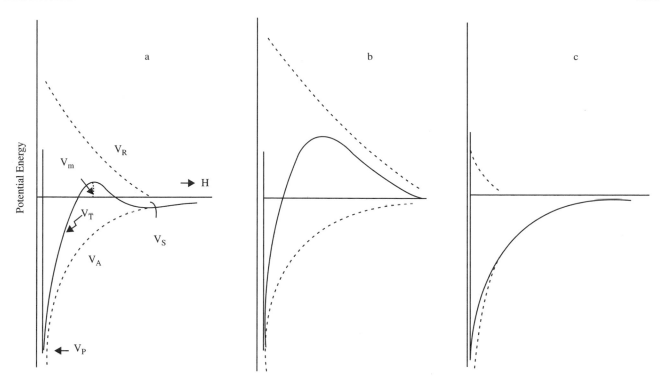

Fig. 7 Variation of the attraction and repulsion energies and the total energy of interaction between two colloidal particles with interparticle distance.

component of the total interaction energy. Therefore, at greater distances, a further increase in electrostatic repulsion will result in a total repulsive net interaction curve without the secondary minimum (Fig. 7b). However, as the repulsive component of the interaction energy diminishes (i.e., the electrolyte concentration increases), the interaction curve becomes totally attractive and rapid coagulation (controlled by particle-diffusion rate) of the colloidal particles takes place (Fig. 7c).

An empirical relationship was developed between the zeta potential and the coagulation behavior of a variety of systems. Deryaguin shows that a rapid decrease in stability can be expected when the following conditions are met (3).

$$4\pi\varepsilon\xi^2/\kappa[A \qquad (7)$$

For a given system, A and ε are fixed; therefore, varying the electrolyte (in type and concentration) should produce instability at a particular value of ξ^2/κ. The validity of using zeta potential in describing the coagulation process should come as no surprise because it characterizes the potential of the diffuse part of the electric double layer which is involved in double-layer overlap and which plays an important role in the coagulation process. When the zeta potential is sufficiently high to produce a potential

barrier opposing coagulation, the rate of coagulation is slowed by a factor W, called the stability ratio, defined as the ratio of the total number of particle collisions to the number of collisions forming permanent doublets. Wiese and Healy reported an excellent correlation between the theoretical values for W (calculated from the zeta potential) and the experimental values for TiO_2 and Al_2O_3 sols as a function of pH (Fig. 8) and electrolyte (KNO_3) concentration (10). Rapid coagulation, whether induced by pH or KNO_3 concentration changes, occurs at a value of $|\zeta| \leq 14 \pm 4$ mV, corresponding to $\zeta^2/\kappa = 6 \times 10^{-4}$ (mV)^2 cm.

Pharmaceutical Systems

Most of the pharmaceutical dispersions can be classified as colloidal systems, although this depends upon the size of their dispersed phase. Therefore, in general, the theoretical and empirical relationships between zeta potential and colloid stability are applicable to the physical stability of these pharmaceutical systems. However, the practical aspects of applying zeta potential to these systems may vary because of differences in the chemical composition and physical state of their dispersed and continuous phases. In addition, the practical significance of zeta-potential

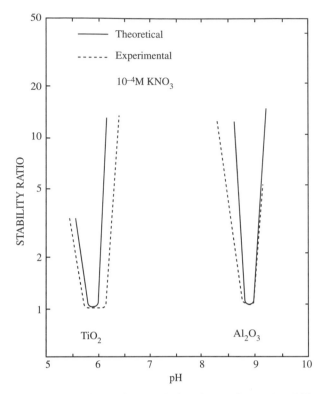

Fig. 8 Comparison of theoretical and experimental stability ratios for TiO^2 (0.05 g/L) and Al$_2$O$_3$ (0.15 g/L) colloids in 10^{-4} M KNO$_3$.

measurement may be different for products which differ in their clinical requirements such as route of administration and consequent in vivo disposition.

Emulsions

Emulsions have been widely used as vehicles for oral, topical, and parenteral delivery of medications. Although the product attributes of an emulsion dosage form are dependent on the route of administration, a common concern is the physical stability of the system, in particular the coalescence of its dispersed phase and the consequent alteration in its particle-size distribution and phase separation. The stabilization mechanism(s) for an emulsion is mainly dependent on the chemical composition of the surfactant used. Electrostatic stabilization as described by DLVO theory plays an important role in emulsions (O/W) containing ionic surfactants (11). For O/W emulsions with low electrolyte content in the aqueous phase, a zeta potential of 30 mV is found to be sufficient to establish an energy maximum (energy barrier) to ensure emulsion stability (11). For emulsions containing nonionic surfactants (polymers), the principal stabilization mechanism is the repulsion between the adsorbed polymer chains on the surface of the oil globules called steric stabilization (11). In such a case, zeta-potential measurement may have limited values with respect to emulsion stability.

In the past, injectable emulsions were administered intravenously to provide patients with vegetable oils as a major energy source in nutrition therapy (12). In recent years, injectable emulsions have been found to be very effective vehicles for the parenteral delivery of water-insoluble drugs (13). Because of toxicological considerations, surfactants which are used in the formulation of injectable emulsions have been largely limited to mixtures of phospholipids which are either derived from egg (egg yolk lecithin) or soybean (soybean lecithin). The majority of the phospholipids (80–90%) are phosphatidylcholine (PC) and phosphatidylethanolamine (PE), which are uncharged at physiological pH. But the presence of small quantities (2–5%) of acidic components, largely phosphatidylserin (PS) and phosphatidylglycerol (PG), which are ionized at pH 7, confers a surface charge of approximately -40 to -50 mV on the emulsion particles (14). Therefore, the stability of these emulsions is mainly attributable to electrostatic stabilization. Any factors which alter the surface potential are likely to have an impact on overall emulsion stability. The physical instability of an injectable emulsion as manifested by an increase in particle size (>5 μm) will result in serious clinical consequences such as formation of pulmonary emboli (15). Therefore, the extent of electrostatic stabilization of an injectable emulsion as measured by its zeta potential has been an important parameter in the characterizing and monitoring of its physical stability.

A relative wealth of information relating to the application of zeta potential to injectable emulsions has been documented with respect to the use of total nutrient admixtures (TNA) (16). Total nutrient admixtures are prepared by mixing the lipid emulsion with other components (i.e., dextrose, amino acids, and electrolytes) in a single container prior to administration. Depending on composition, the mixtures vary widely in their stability and may show clinically unacceptable coalescence after different periods of storage time.

When the electrostatic stabilization of the emulsion is considered, the electrolytes (monovalent and divalent) added to the mixture are the major destabilizing species. The zeta potential of the emulsion particles is a function of the concentration and type of electrolytes present. Two types of emulsion particle-electrolyte (ions) interaction are proposed: nonspecific and specific adsorption (16). In nonspecific adsorption the ions are bound to the emulsion particle only by electrical double-layer interactions with the charged surface. As the electrolyte concentration is increased, the zeta potential asymptotes to zero. As

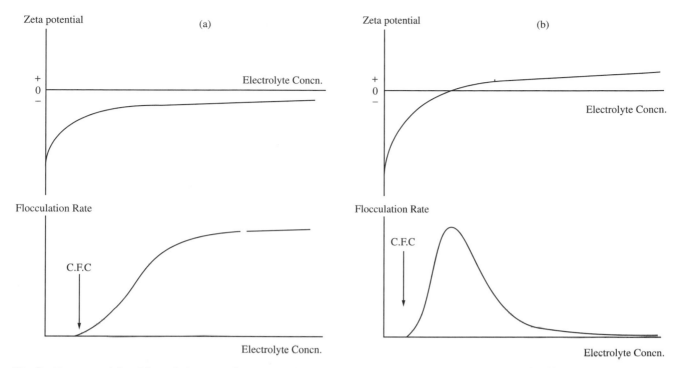

Fig. 9 Zeta potential and flocculation rate of a parenteral emulsion in the presence of a nonspecifically adsorbing electrolyte (a) and a specifically adsorbing electrolyte (b).

the electrostatic repulsion decreases, a point can be found where the attractive van der Waals force is equal to the repulsive electrostatic force and flocculation of the emulsion occurs (Fig. 9a). This point is called the critical flocculation concentration (CFC).

DLVO theory predicts that the CFC should vary inversely with the sixth power of the ion charge. The application of CFC alone fails to correlate the TNA stability with electrolytes in the mixtures. This is because divalent ions (calcium and magnesium) adsorbed specifically on the emulsion particles through their complexation with the negatively charged acidic phospholipids. Fig. 9b demonstrates the relationship between the concentration of a specifically adsorbed ion and the zeta potential and flocculation rate of an injectable emulsion. The increase in electrolyte concentration causes the particle charge to pass through zero; this is referred to as the point of zero charge (PZC). At this point the flocculation rate is at maximum; a further increase in electrolyte concentration causes a surface-charge reversal of the particles and increases in zeta potential (opposite sign) as well as a decrease of the flocculation rate from its maximum value.

The effect of pH on the stability of an injectable emulsion was also followed by measuring its zeta potential (Fig. 10). At pH 7 the ionization of PS and PG imparts a surface negative charge (-30 to -50 mV) to the emulsion

particles. As the pH is reduced, this ionization is suppressed until the charge is zero at a pH of 3.2. Further decreases in pH cause the protonation of the phospholipid and a positive surface charge (positive zeta potential). Significant progress has been made in relating the electrokinetic properties of phospholipid-stabilized emulsions to their instability when influenced by other TNA ingredients (17, 18). Washington and his coworkers have attempted to develop a model to predict emulsion stability in TNAs using DLVO-based methods in the measurement of the zeta potential of the system (19).

Suspensions

Pharmaceutical suspensions are dispersions of solid particles in a suspending medium or vehicle (usually aqueous in nature). When the suspended solids are less than 1 μm, the system is referred to as a colloidal suspension. When the particle sizes are greater than about 1 μm, the system is called a coarse suspension. The practical upper limit for particles in a coarse suspension is approximately 50–75 μm. Depending on the affinity or interaction between the dispersed phase and the dispersion medium, a colloidal dispersion can be classified as lyophilic (hydrophilic) or lyophobic (hydrophobic) (20).

The dispersion of hydrophilic particulate solids in water occurs spontaneously and gives rise to a thermodynamically

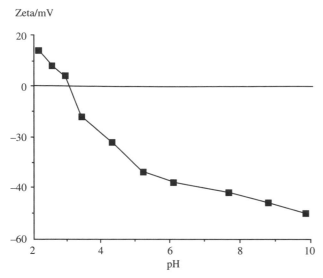

Fig. 10 Zeta potential of a parenteral emulsion as a function of pH.

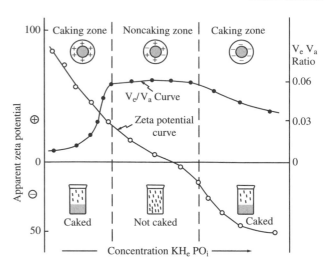

Fig. 11 A caking diagram showing the flocculation of a bismuth subnitrate suspension by means of the flocculating agent, potassium monobasic phosphate.

stable system such as colloidal silicone dioxide or microcrystalline cellulose. Hydrophobic solids are not easily wetted and are not dispersed spontaneously in water as sulfur, clays, and most nonpolar organic compounds. The van der Waals attractive forces between particles cause them to aggregate, since the solvation forces which promote dispersal in water are weak. Therefore, aqueous dispersions of hydrophobic solids can only be stabilized kinetically to resist flocculation and coagulation, which can be defined by referring to the total interaction energy curve (Fig. 7). Flocculation indicates the association of particles in the secondary minimum and coagulation is the aggregation of particles in the primary minimum. Since the attractive forces between particles in a flocculated system are relatively week, they can be redispersed and the process is reversible. In contrast, coagulation is irreversible as attractive forces operating between particles in the primary minimum are difficult to overcome.

When electrostatic repulsion is predominant between particles in a suspension, it is called a deflocculated system. For particles with a diameter of 2–5 μm, Brownian movement counteracts sedimentation to a measurable extent at room temperature by keeping the dispersed particles in random motion. This results in a system which is physically stable with respect to sedimentation and flocculation (20). However, in a deflocculated suspension consisting of larger particles (coarse), gravitational force counteracts Brownian movement and sedimentation occurs (21). At the bottom of the container, a compact sediment with strong attractive forces between the particles is formed and it cannot be easily

redispersed. This phenomenon is referred to as caking. The prevention of caking has been one of the main objectives in preparing stable coarse suspensions (21, 22). Although flocculation is referred to as a physical instability of colloids, flocculated suspensions are pharmaceutically acceptable since they are noncaking. In a flocculated suspension, particles attract each other (at the secondary minimum) loosely to form flocs which tend to settle together, creating a distinct boundary between the sediment and the supernatant. Particles in flocs are thereby easily redispersed after settling.

Controlled flocculation is a process by which flocculation of particles in a suspension is purposely produced by adding flocculating agents. One of the most effective methods of achieving controlled flocculation is to reduce the electrostatic repulsive forces between particles (21, 22). Electrolytes have been shown to be effective flocculating agents. Zeta-potential measurement has been a valuable tool in monitoring and evaluating the influence of various electrolytes on the flocculation phenomena in coarse suspensions (23). Sedimentation volume F, which is the ratio of the volume of sediment to the original volume of the suspension, is a useful parameter in measuring the extent of flocculation of the suspension. An excellent correlation between the zeta potential, sedimentation volume, and caking was found for a series of bismuth subnitrate suspensions containing various concentrations of potassium phosphate monobasic (Fig. 11) (24). The addition of potassium phosphate monobasic causes a decrease in the zeta potential of the suspension because of partial neutralization of the positive surface charge on the bismuth subnitrate particles. With the decrease in the zeta potential (positive), the suspension becomes flocculated and noncaking, accompanied by an increase in the sedimentation volume. The continued addition of electrolyte causes the zeta potential to fall to zero and then increases in a negative direction. The suspension remains flocculated until the zeta potential becomes sufficiently negative to effect deflocculation of the system, which is shown by a decrease in the sedimentation volume and an increase in caking tendency.

Zeta potential has also found an application in relating the surface-charge characteristics of a suspension to properties other than physical stability. Heyd and Dhabhar improved the fluidity of concentrated antacid suspensions by adding a colloidal polyelectrolyte (carrageenan sodium) which is called a fluidizing agent (25). As the concentration of the fluidizing agent increases, the zeta potential of the suspension changes from positive to negative, accompanied by a reduction in viscosity of the suspension. The mechanism for this viscosity-thinning phenomenon is believed to be the selective adsorption of the negatively charged fluidizing agent onto the positively charged antacid particles. This imparts an electronegative charge (as measured by the zeta potential) onto the antacid particles, decreasing the demand for water.

In the literature, the reported use of zeta potential measurement for nonaqueous suspensions is relatively infrequent because nonaqueous suspensions only represent a small percentage of all medicated suspensions. Su and others evaluated the flocculation–deflocculation behavior of cefazolin sodium in nonaqueous media and the effect of surfactants as measured by zeta potential along with sedimentation and porosity measurements (26). A significant difference in zeta potential was observed when the particles were dispersed in peanut oil and ethyl oleate. The addition of lecithin reduced the zeta potential of cefazolin sodium, resulting in a deflocculated state accompanied by a decrease in sedimentation volume. The effect of surfactant excipient on the zeta potential of salbutamol in trichlorofluoroethane (P113) for metered-dose inhalation was determined (27). Although the zeta potential of the particles is decreased (more negative) by the addition of oleic acid, the overall zeta potential is too low to be effective in providing the system with adequate electrostatic stabilization, particularly in media with a low dielectric constant (organic solvents).

Microparticulate drug-delivery systems, including microspheres and nanoparticles, are suspensions when they are administrated in a liquid medium. Microspheres are solid particles containing dispersed drug in either solution or microcrystalline form and range in size from 1 to 1000 μm. Although most microspheres are outside the conventional colloidal size range, in pharmaceutical literature microspheres with sizes up to approximately 15 μm are still considered as colloidal delivery systems (28). Nanoparticles are similar to microspheres but have particle sizes in the range of 0.01–1 μm; therefore, they form colloidal suspensions when dispersed in a liquid medium (29). Zeta-potential measurement is an important surface-characterization technique which provides information regarding the surface charge of these microparticulate systems. The effect of surface charge (zeta potential) on the physical stability of these systems (i.e., aggregation) can be predicted using the DLVO theory, although steric stabilization plays an important role in systems with surface-adsorbed macromolecules.

When the microparticles are administered intravenously, surface change is an important parameter affecting the interaction between the microparticles and other biological components of the body and their subsequent in vivo distribution and disposition (30). Tabata and Ikada reported that phagocytosis of polymer microspeheres by macrophages is enhanced as the absolute value of zeta potential increases for both the negatively charged and the positively charged surfaces, while the lowest phagocytosis is shown for the surface with a zeta potential of zero (31). The uptake of charged serum components by nanoparticles (opsonization) in blood is considered to be the first step leading to phagocytosis by liver and spleen macrophages. Muller and his coworkers determined the increase in zeta potential of nonparticles in serum as a measure of the extent of opsonization and used this as selection criteria for i.v. drug carriers avoiding liver/spleen uptake (32).

Liposomes

Liposomes are phospholipid-based vesicles which have been studied as delivery systems to target drugs to specific sites in the body (33–35). The surface of a liposome can be neutral or negatively or positively charged, depending on the composition of lipids used. For charged liposomes, their surface potential is a critical factor affecting their physical stability and in vivo performance. Instead of their surface potential, zeta-potential measurement is frequently used in the investigation of the behavior of liposomes as influenced by their surface charge. Liposomes in aqueous dispersions have a tendency to aggregate and subsequently fuse on storage. This physical instability potentially limits their application as dosage forms.

Crommelin incorporated charge-inducing components in liposome bilayers to produce electrostatic repulsion between liposomes, thus increasing the shelf life of the dispersion (36). He investigated the effect of including stearylamine or phosphatidylserin on the zeta potential of phosphatidylcholine-cholesterol–containing liposomes. A correlation between the aggregation stability of negatively charged liposomes and the increments in the surface-charge density at both low and high ionic strength was established, whereas the positive liposome dispersions were found to be unstable.

Carrion and his coworkers investigated the effect of incorporating phosphatidic acid on the zeta potential and aggregation of large unilamellar vesicle liposomes of phosphatidylcholine in the presence of neutral electrolytes (37). Their results show that increasing concentrations of phosphatidic acid in lipid bilayers resulted in high zeta potential and enhanced physical stability of the liposomes. The destabilizing effect of divalent cations (i.e., calcium ions) on charged liposomes has been well documented and is attributable to the reduced surface potential of the liposomes as the result of cation binding (38–40).

The effect of calcium ions on the aggregation behaviors of neutral liposomes composed of egg phosphatidyl-choline and dipalmitoylphosphatidylcholine was investigated by Mosharraf and coworkers (41). Both systems displayed a high negative zeta potential in deionized water, probably the result of adsorption of hydroxyl ions. A reasonable correlation was found in both cases between particle-size increase and zeta potential decrease of the system, suggesting that the mechanism by which the aggregation takes place is related to the surface-charge characteristics. Although it has long been established that liposomes composed of neutral phospho-lipids acquire negative surface charge via anion adsorption, Makino and his group in Japan found that neutral liposomes exhibit negative zeta potential in buffer solution containing no chloride ion (42). They also reported that changes in the ionic strength and temperature causes the zeta potential of neutral liposomes to reverse sign. They proposed that the reversal of zeta potential is triggered by changes in the direction of the dipole connecting the negative charge of the phosphatidyl group and the positive charge of the choline group consisting the head group of a lipid molecule.

The study of the effect of drug-loading on the zeta potential of liposomes provides information regarding the drug-liposome interaction. Lawrence and others reported that the loading of polymyxin B, a polycationic antibiotic in negatively charged liposomes, results in the decrease of zeta potential, indicating electrostatic attraction between the positive drug and the negative lipid bilayer (43). That the highest drug-loading is found in negatively charged liposomes in comparison to positively charged and neutral liposomes further supports this electrostatic drug-liposome interaction. Beschiaschvili and Seelig investigated the binding of a cyclic somatostatin analogue, a positively charged peptide, to negatively charged mutilamellar liposomes (44). From the binding isotherm and the zeta-potential measurement, they were able to describe a partition equilibrium between the peptide and the negatively charged membrane with a surface-partition constant. They concluded that most of the peptide molecules are embedded in the headgroup region with little penetration into the lipid core.

The measurement of the zeta potential of liposomes provides valuable information relating to their in vivo performance because, in addition to size, the surface charge of liposomes is an important determinant of their clearance from the general circulation and their tissue disposition after parenteral administration. Large multi-lamellar liposomes are cleared from the circulation much more rapidly than small unilamellar liposomes. Among small unilamellar liposomes, however, those with a negative surface charge are cleared rapidly, but positively charged or uncharged liposomes remain in the circulation for longer periods (45). Rahman and his coworkers compared the pharmacological and therapeutic effects of adriamycin entrapped in positively charged and negatively charged liposomes in rats (46). They found that less cardiotoxicity was associated with the drug entrapped in the positively charged liposomes which exhibited lower in vivo uptake by cardiac tissue. When liposomes are employed to target drugs to lymph nodes, their surface charge has been shown to affect their lymphatic uptake from subcutaneous and intraperitonial injection sites (47). Patel showed that negatively charged liposomes yield the highest localization in the lymph nodes, followed by positively charged and neutral ones. The drainage of negatively charged liposomes has also shown to be faster than that of positive liposomes after intraperitoneal administration (48).

SUMMARY

Zeta-potential measurement has long been recognized as an excellent tool for characterizing colloidal systems. Its practical significance stems from the fact that it allows the quantitation of the electrostatic repulsion between particles, which is one of the most important forces governing the behavior and physical stability of colloidal systems. In recent years, the concept of zeta potential has been applied to areas beyond classical colloidal sciences and industrial processes. Pharmaceutical sciences are the new fields to which the application of zeta potential has been extended. The expanding role of zeta potential in

Z

these fields is attributable to the advance in modern instrumentation of zeta potential measurement, the rapid development of colloidal drug-delivery systems, and the emphasis on interdisciplinary basic research. While good correlation has been demonstrated for zeta potential and in vitro properties of colloidal drug-carrier systems, the understanding of the impact of zeta potential in organ distribution and in vivo clearance of these systems has been the focus of additional research efforts.

REFERENCES

1. Shaw, D.J. *Introduction to Colloid and Surface Chemistry*, 4th Ed.; Butterworth Heinemann Ltd.: Oxford, 1992.
2. Goetz, P.J.; Penniman, J.G. A New Technique for Microelectrophoretic Measurements. Jr. Am. Lab. **Oct. 1976**.
3. Hunter, R.J. *Zeta Potential in Colloid Science, Principles and Applications*, Academic Press: London, 1981.
4. Uzgiris, E.E. *Progress in Surface Science*, Pergamon Press: New York, 1981; X.
5. Oja, T.; Bott, S.; Sugrue, S. Doppler Electrophoretic Light Scattering Analysis Using the Coulter DELSA 440. Coulter Electronics: Luton, 1989.
6. O'Brien, R.W. J. Fluid Mech. **1988**, *190*, 71–86.
7. Babchin, A.J.; Chow, R.S.; Sawatzky, R.P. Electrokinetic Measurements by Electroacoustical Methods. Adv. Colloid Interface Sci. **1989**, *111–151*, 30.
8. Hiemenz, P.C. *Principles of Colloid and Surface Chemistry*, 2nd Ed.; Marcel Dekker, Inc.: New York, 1986.
9. Hirtzel, C.S.; Rajagopalan, R. *Colloidal Phenomena, Advanced Topics*, Noyes Publications: New Jersey, 1985.
10. Wiese, G.R.; Healy, T.W. Coagulation and Electrokinetic Behavior of TiO_2 And Al_2O_3 Colloidal Dispersions. J. Colloid Interface Sci. **1975**, *51*, 427–433.
11. Friberg, S.E.; Goldsmith, L.B.; Hilton, M.L. *Theory of Emulsion in Pharmaceutical Dosage Forms: Dispersion Systems*, Lieberman, H.A., Reiger, M.M., Banker, G.S., Eds.; Marcel Dekker, Inc.: New York, 1988; I.
12. Wretlind, A.J. Development of Fat Emulsions. Parenter. Enteral. Nutr. **1981**, *5*, 230–235.
13. Davis, S.S.; Washington, C.; West, P.; Illum, L.; Liversidge, G.; Sternson, L.; Kirsh, R. Ann. N.Y. Acad. Sci. **1987**, *507*, 75–88.
14. Washington, C.; Chawla, A.; Christy, N.; Davis, S.S. The Electrokinetic Properties of Phospholipid-Stabilized Fat Emulsions. Int. J. Pharm. **1989**, *54*, 191–197.
15. Burnham, W.R.; Hansrani, P.K.; Knott, C.E.; Cook, J.A.; Davis, S.S. Stability of a Fat Emulsion Based Intravenous Feeding Mixture. Int. J. Pharm. **1983**, *13*, 9–22.
16. Washington, C. The Stability of Intravenous Fat Emulsions in Total Parenteral Nutrition Mixtures. Int. J. Pharm. **1990**, *66*, 1–21.
17. Washington, C.; Athersuch, A.; Kynoch, D.J. The Electrokinetic Properties of Phospholipid Stabilized Fat Emulsions. IV. The Effect of Glucose and of pH. Int. J. Pharm. **1990**, *64*, 217–222.
18. Washington, C.; Connolly, M.A.; Manning, R.; Skerratt, M.C.L. The Electrokinetic Properties of Phospholipid Stabilized Fat Emulsions. V. The Effect of Amino Acids on Emulsion Stability. Int. J. Pharm. **1991**, *77*, 57–63.
19. Washington, C.; Ferguson, J.A.; Irwin, S.E. Computational Prediction of the Stability of Lipid Emulsions in Total Nutrient Admixtures. J. Pharm. Sci. **1993**, *82*, 808–812.
20. Zograft, G.; Schott, H.; Swarbrick, J. Dispersion Systems. *Remington's Pharmaceutical Sciences*, 18th Ed.; Mack Publishing Company: Pennsylvania, 1990.
21. Hiestand, E.N. Theory of Coarse Suspension Formulation. J. Pharm. Sci. **1964**, *53*, 1–18.
22. Falkiewicz, M.J. Theory of Suspensions in Theory of Emulsion. *Pharmaceutical Dosage Forms: Dispersion System*, Lieberman, H.A., Reiger, M.M., Banker, G.S., Eds.; Marcel Dekker, Inc.: New York, 1988; I.
23. Nash, R.A.; Haeger, B.E. Zeta Potential in the Development of Pharmaceutical Suspension. J. Pharm. Sci. **1966**, *55*, 829–837.
24. Martin, A.; Swarbrick, J. *American Pharmacy*, 6th Ed.; Lippincott: Philadelphia, 1966.
25. Heyd, A.; Dhabhar, D.J. Enhancing Fluidity of Concentrated Antacid Suspensions. J. Pharm. Sci. **1975**, *64*, 1697–1699.
26. Su, K.S.E.; Quay, F.; Campanale, K.M.; Stucky, J.F. Nonaqueous Cephalosporin Suspension for Parenteral Administration: Cefazolin Sodium. J. Pharm. Sci. **1984**, *73*, 1601–1602.
27. Clarke, J.G.; Wicks, S.R.; Farr, S.J. Surfactant Mediated Effects in Pressurized Metered Dose Inhalers Formulated as Suspensions. I. Drug/Surfactant Interactions in a Model Propellant Systems. Int. J. Pharm. **1993**, *93*, 221–231.
28. Burgess, D.J.; Hickey, A.J. Microsphere Technology and Applications. *Encyclopedia of Pharmaceutical Technology*, 1st Ed.; Swarbrick, J., Boylan, J.C., Eds.; Marcel Dekker, Inc. New York, 1994; 10.
29. Kreuter, J. Nanoparticles. *Encyclopedia of Pharmaceutical Technology*, 1st Ed.; Swarbrick, J., Boylan, J.C., Eds.; Marcel Dekker, Inc.: New York, 1994; 10.
30. Wilkins, D.J.; Meyers, P.A. Studies on the Relationship Between the Electrophoretic Properties of Colloids and their Blood Clearance and Organ Distribution in the Rat. Br. J. Exp. Pathol. **1966**, *47*, 568–576.
31. Tabata, Y.; Ikada, Y. Effect of the Size and Surface Charge of Polymer Microspheres on their Phagocytosis by Macrophage. Biomaterials **1988**, *9*, 356–362.
32. Müller, R.H.; Wallis, K.H.; Tröster, S.D.; Kreuter, J. In Vitro Characterization of Poly(Methyl-Methacrylate) Nanoparticles and Correlation to their In Vivo Fate. J. Contr. Rel. **1992**, *20*, 237–246.
33. Riaz, M.; Weiner, N.; Martin, F. Liposomes in Theory of Emulsion. *Pharmaceutical Dosage Forms: Dispersion Systems*, Lieberman, H.A., Reiger, M.M., Banker, G.S. Eds.; Marcel Dekker, Inc.: New York, 1989; 2.
34. Gregoriadis, G.; Florence, A.T. Liposomes in Drug Delivery. Drugs **1993**, *45*, 15–28.
35. Barenholz, Y.; Crommelin, D.J.A. Liposomes as Pharmaceutical Dosage Forms. *Encyclopedia of Pharmaceutical Technology*, 1st Ed.; Swarbrick, J., Boylan, J.C., Eds.; Marcel Dekker, Inc.: New York, 1994; 9.

36. Crommelin, A.J.A. Influence of Lipid Composition and Ionic Strength on the Physical Stability of Liposomes. J. Pharm. Sci. **1984**, *73*, 1559–1563.

37. Carrion, F.J.; De La Maza, A.; Parra, J.L. The Influence of Ionic Strength and Lipid Bilayer Charge on the Stability of Liposomes. J. Colloid Interface Sci. **1994**, *164*, 78–87.

38. Düzgünes, N.; Sur, S.; Wilschut, J.; Bentz, J.; Newton, C.; Portis, A.; Papahadjopoulos, D. Calcium-and Magnesium-Induced Fusion of Mixed Phosphatidylserine/Phosphatidylcholine Vesicles: Effect of Ion Binding. J. Membr. Biol. **1981**, *59*, 115–125.

39. Hope, M.J.; Walker, D.C.; Cullis, P.R. Ca^{2+} and pH Induced Fusion of Small Unilamellar Vesicles Consisting of Phosphatidylethanolamine and Negatively Charged Phospholipids: A Freeze Fracture Study. Biochim. Biophys. Res. Commun. **1983**, *110*, 15–22.

40. Minami, H.; Inque, T.; Shimozawa, R. Aggregation Kinetics of Dimyristoylphosphatidylglycerol Vesicles Induced by Divalent Cations. J. Colloid Interface Sci. **1993**, *158*, 460–465.

41. Mosharraf, M.; Taylor, K.M.G.; Craig, D.Q.M. Effect of Calcium Ions on the Surface Charge and Aggregation of Phosphadylcholine Liposomes. J. Drug Target. **1995**, *2*, 541–545.

42. Makino, K.; Yamada, T.; Kimura, M.; Oka, T.; Ohshima, H. Temperature and Ionic Strength-Induced Conformational Changes in the Lipid Head Group Region of Liposomes as Suggested by Zeta-Potential Data. Biophy. Chem. **1991**, *41*, 175–183.

43. Lawrence, S.M.; Alpar, H.O.; McAllister, S.M.; Brown, M.R.W. Liposomal (MLV) Polymyxin B: Physicochemical Characterization and Effect of Surface Charge on Drug Association. J. Drug Target. **1993**, *1*, 303–310.

44. Beschiaschvilli, G.; Seelig, J. Peptide Binding to Lipid Bilayers. Binding Isotherms and ζ-Potential of a Cyclic Somatostatin Analogue. Biochemistry **1990**, *29*, 10995–11000.

45. Juliano, R.L.; Stamp, D.; McCullough, N. Pharmacokinetics of Liposome-Encapsulated Antitumor Drugs and Implications for Therapy. Ann. N.Y. Acad. Sci. **1978**, *308*, 411–425.

46. Rahman, A.; Kessler, A.; More, N.; Sikic, B.; Rowden, G.; Woolley, P.; Schein, P.S. Liposomal Protection of Adriamycin-Induced Cardiotoxicity in Mice. Cancer Research **1980**, *40*, 1532–1537.

47. Hawley, A.E.; Davis, S.S.; Illum, L. Targeting of Colloids to Lymph Nodes: Influence of Lymphatic Physiology and Colloidal Characteristics. Adv. Drug Delivery Rev. **1995**, *17*, 129–148.

48. Patel, H.M.; Boodle, K.M.; Vaughan-Jones, R. Assessment of the Potential Uses of Liposomes for Lymphoscintigraphy and Lymphatic Drug Delivery. Biochim. Biophys. Acta **1984**, *801*, 76–86.

Index

jacket, 2602
  poststerilization phases, 2603
    ampoule tightness tests, 2603
    cooling, 2603
    drying-cooling final vacuum, 2603
  process, 2602-2604
    controllers, 2603-2604
  sterilization, air entering chamber, 2603
Saw palmetto, 42
Scalar coupling, nuclear magnetic resonance
    spectroscopy, 1903-1904
Scale-up, postapproval
  changes, 175, 954-955, 2396-2400
  chemical tests, 2398
  controls tests, 2398
  documentation, 2397
  efficacy, surrogate measures of, 2399
  levels of change, 2397-2398
  manufacturing tests, 2398
  stability, 2398-2399
Scaling, tumbling blenders, 1802-1803
Scanning electron microscopy, sample
    preparation, 2406-2409
Scheduling
  in project management, 2316-2318
  technology transfer, 2763
Scientists, clinical evaluation, drugs, 451
Scintillation detectors, in radiation detec-
    tion, 2357
  efficiency, 2358
Scopolamine hydrobromide, 381
  isotonicity, 2821
Screening, 2882
  adverse drug reaction and, 41
Sealing, liquid oral preparations, 1684
Seal integrity, container-closure, 1064
  rubber compounds, 1064
Secobarbital, 408
  elixir, 381
  sodium, 381, 408
Secondary drying, freeze drying, 1309-1312
  factors impacting drying rate, 1310-1311
  moisture content during storage, 1311-1312
  optimum residual moisture, 1309-1310
  product temperature control, glass tran-
    sitions, 1309
Secondary electron microscopy, 2401-2435
  application, 2409-2430
  coatings, 2421-2423
  dry syrup preparations, 2416-2417
  electrons in, types of, 2401-2402
    absorbed electrons, 2401
    backscattered electrons, 2401
    cathodoluminescence, 2401-2402
    secondary electrons, 2401
    transmitted electrons, 2401
    X-ray photons, 2401
  freeze-dried products, 2426-2427
  implants, 2427-2429
  injection, microparticles for, 2427
  pellets, 2417-2418
  powder mixtures, 2415-2416
  sample preparation, scanning electron
    microscopy, 2406-2409
  specimen preparation, 2406-2409
  spray-dried products, 2423-2426
  starting materials, 2410-2415
    disintegrants, 2413-2415
    filler/binders, 2410-2413
    lubricants, 2415
  tablets, 2418-2421
Second generation emulsions, blood
    substitutes, 269-270
Second-order models, optimization methods and,
    statistical experimental designs
    for, 1928-1930
Secretions, 13-14

Security, electronic documents, 1987
  corporate network security, 1987
  database security, 1987
  file security, 1987
  folder security, 1987
  version security, 1987
Sedative-hypnotic, 71
Sedatives, 26-28
  adverse effects, 27
  alcohol, 27
  barbiturates, 26
  benzodiazepines, 26-27
  chronic abuse, 27
  cross-tolerance, dependence, 28
  history, 26
  mechanism of, 28
  synergy, 28
  tranquilizers, 27
Sedimentation, 2882
Sedimentation techniques, particle-size
    characterization, 2000-2003
Segregation, intensity of, tumbling blenders, 1804
Selectivity coefficients,
    potentiometry, 2256-2257
Selenious acid, 408
Self-regulating delivery systems, 831
Semiconductor silicon diodes, in ultraviolet spec-
    trophotometry, 2562
Semisolids, 2436-2457
  compounding, 581-582
  dissolution, 726-727
  dosage forms, 757
  gels, 2443-2444
  manufacturing methods, 2444-2452
    emulsion products, 2446-2450
    fusion process, 2445-2446
    industrial scale, 2445
    laboratory scale, 2444-2445
    ointments, 2444-2445
  ointments, creams, 2436-2443
    absorption bases, 2439
    anionic emulsifiers, 2440
    cationic emulsifiers, 2440
    gelled petrolatum base, 2438
    hydrocarbon bases, 2436-2438
    hydrophilic ointment, 2440
    light mineral oil, 2438
    microemulsions, 2441-2442
    mineral oil, 2438
    nonionic emulsifiers, 2440-2441
    ophthalmic ointments, 2438
    soft petrolatum base, 2438
    vanishing cream, 2440
    water-removable bases, 2439-2441
    water-soluble bases, 2442-2443
    white ointment, 2438
    white petrolatum, 2437
    yellow petrolatum, 2437
  packaging, 2453-2454
  pastes, 2443
  preservatives, 2452-2453
    parabens, 2452-2453
  quality control, 2454
  stability, 2454-2456
  sustained drug release, 850
  vesicular systems, topical route, 952-953
Semisynthetic polymers, 1338
  gels, 1338-1339
    hydroxypropyl methylcellulose, 1338-1339
    methylcellulose, 1339
Senior management, 2320-2321
Senna concentrate, 2215
Sensitive teeth, 701-702
Sensitivity, changes in, in geriatrics, 1353
Separation techniques, analysis-gas
    chromatography, 373-375
  special techniques, 373-374

temperature programming, 373
Seprafilm, 219
Sepsis, hypoalbuminemia with, 37
Sequencing, human genome, 2392-2394
Sequential simplex optimization, 1934-1935
Seragen, biotechnology company, 220
Serine, 408
Serono, biotechnology company, 220
Serostim, 216
Serum drug concentrations, pediatric
    administration, 2052-2053
Sesame oil, 408
Sex. *See* Gender
Shaft, dissolution, 721-722
Shake-flask method
  extraction, partition coefficients, 2018
  Hansch-Fujita constant, partition coeffi-
    cients, 2015
  partition coefficients, 2013-2014
  Leo-Hansch f constant, 2015-2017
  peptides, partition coefficients of, 2018-2019
Shear, three-dimensional tumblers, 1800
Shear cells, flow properties, 1276-1280
Sheep, ectoparasiticide dosage, 2962
Shelf life
  cosmetics, 655
  statistical determination of, long-term storage
    data, 214-1215
Shields, collagen, delivery of drugs from, 865-866
Shikimate pathway, biosynthesis, 181-185
Siberian ginseng, 42
Sickle cell anemia, oxygen delivery, blood sub-
    stitutes, 249
Side effects, reduction of, complexation, 541
Sieve fractionation, particle-size characteriz-
    ation, 2000
Sieving, 2882
Signal processing, in fluorescence
    spectroscopy, 2514-2515
Signatures, electronic, 1990-1992
Silicon dioxide colloidal silicon dioxide, 408
Silicone, 867
  properties of, 2528
Silver
  consumable anode, 1577
  as preservative, 2279
Silver anodes, chloride ion management
    with, 1577-1578
Silver bromide, properties of, 2528
Silver chloride
  consumable cathode, 1578
  properties of, 2528
Silver nitrate, isotonicity, 2821
Simethicone, 408
Simplex
  experimental domain, optimization methods
    and, 1931
  mathematical models, 1713-1714
Simulation of data, 1709-1711
  integration methods, 1709-1711
    laplace transforms, 1710
    methods for still equations, 1711
    multistep methods, 1711
    numerical integration, 1710-1711
    point-slope methods, 1710-1711
    Runge-Kutta methods, 1711
Simulect, 218
Single-dose studies, *versus* multiple-dose studies,
    bioavailability, 132-133
Single particle optical sizers, metered dose inha-
    ler, 1750
Single photon emission computed tomography,
    misconceptions of, 2370-2371
SIPAC. *See* Scale-up, postapproval changes
Site-targeting delivery systems, 831-832
Size characterization, 1998-2009
  fine-powder fractionation, 2006-2008

Brief Contents